HEMATOLOGY
of INFANCY *and* CHILDHOOD

edited by

DAVID G. NATHAN, M.D.

Chief, Division of Hematology and Oncology,
Children's Hospital Medical Center;
Pediatrician-in-Chief,
Children's Cancer Research Foundation;
Professor of Pediatrics,
Harvard Medical School, Boston

FRANK A. OSKI, M.D.

Professor and Chairman of the Department
of Pediatrics, State University of New York,
Upstate Medical Center College of Medicine, Syracuse

W. B. SAUNDERS COMPANY   1974
Philadelphia, London, Toronto

W. B. Saunders Company: West Washington Square
Philadelphia, PA 19105

12 Dyott Street
London, WC1A 1DB

833 Oxford Street
Toronto, Ontario M8Z 5T9, Canada

Library of Congress Cataloging in Publication Data

Nathan, David G

Hematology of infancy and childhood.

1. Pediatric hematology.   I. Oski, Frank A., joint author.
   II. Title.   [DNLM: 1. Hematologic diseases — In infancy
   and childhood.   WS300 N274h 1974]

RJ411.N37   618.9'21'5   73–89190

ISBN 0–7216–6660–4

Hematology of Infancy and Childhood   ISBN 0-7216-6660-4

Last digit is the print number: 9   8   7   6   5   4   3   2   1

CONTRIBUTORS

NEIL ABRAMSON, M.D.
Associate Professor of Medicine, University of Florida. Chief, Jacksonville Hospitals Educational Program (JHEP), Division of Hematology and Medical Oncology, Gainesville, Florida.

FRED H. ALLEN, JR., M.D.
Senior Investigator, The New York Blood Center. Clinical Associate Professor of Pediatrics, Cornell University Medical College; Genetics Faculty, Cornell University Graduate School of Medical Sciences, New York, New York.

CHESTER A. ALPER, M.D.
Associate Professor of Pediatrics, Harvard Medical School. Scientific Director, Center for Blood Research; Associate in Medicine, Children's Hospital Medical Center, Boston, Massachusetts.

ROBERT L. BAEHNER, M.D.
Professor of Pediatrics, Indiana University School of Medicine. Director, Pediatric Hematology-Oncology Division, The James Whitcomb Riley Hospital for Children, Indianapolis, Indiana.

MICHAEL C. BRAIN, M.D.
Professor of Medicine, McMaster University. Coordinator for Hematology, McMaster University Medical Center, Hamilton, Ontario, Canada.

LARS-ERIC BRATTEBY, M.D., Ph.D.
Associate Professor of Pediatric Clinical Physiology, University of Uppsala. Chief of Perinatal Research Unit of Pediatric Department, University Hospital, Uppsala, Sweden.

JAN L. BRESLOW, M.D.
Assistant Professor of Pediatrics, Harvard Medical School. Associate in Medicine, Children's Hospital Medical Center, Boston, Massachusetts.

H. FRANKLIN BUNN, M.D.
Associate Professor of Medicine, Harvard Medical School. Senior Associate in Medicine, Peter Bent Brigham Hospital, Boston, Massachusetts.

PETER R. DALLMAN, M.D.

Associate Professor of Pediatrics, University of California School of Medicine, San Francisco, California.

VIRGINIA H. DONALDSON, M.D.

Professor of Pediatrics and Medicine, University of Cincinnati College of Medicine and Children's Hospital Research Foundation. Staff Physician at Children's Hospital and Cincinnati General Hospital, Cincinnati, Ohio.

STEPHEN A. FEIG, M.D.

Assistant Professor of Pediatrics, University of California at Los Angeles, Center for Health Sciences, Los Angeles, California.

BERNARD G. FORGET, M.D.

Assistant Professor of Pediatrics, Harvard Medical School. Associate in Medicine (Hematology), Children's Hospital Medical Center, Boston, Massachusetts.

FRANK H. GARDNER, M.D.

Professor of Medicine, University of Pennsylvania School of Medicine. Director of Hematology Research Laboratory, and Director of Department of Medicine, Presbyterian–University of Pennsylvania Medical Center; Consultant in Hematology, Philadelphia Veterans Administration Hospital, Philadelphia, Pennsylvania.

LARS GARBY, M.D., Ph.D.

Professor of Physiology, University of Odense, Odense, Denmark.

PARK S. GERALD, M.D.

Professor of Pediatrics, Harvard Medical School. Chief, Clinical Genetics Division, Children's Hospital Medical Center, Boston, Massachusetts.

JEFFREY A. GOTTLIEB, M.D.

Assistant Professor, University of Texas System Cancer Center, M.D. Anderson Hospital and Tumor Institute. Head, Section of Chemotherapy, M.D. Anderson Hospital, Houston, Texas.

ROBERT I. HANDIN, M.D.

Assistant Professor of Medicine, Harvard Medical School. Associate in Medicine, Peter Bent Brigham Hospital, Boston, Massachusetts.

CHARLES A. JANEWAY, M.D.

Thomas Morgan Rotch Professor of Pediatrics, Harvard Medical School. Physician-in-Chief and Chief of Medicine, Children's Hospital Medical Center, Boston, Massachusetts.

YUET WAI KAN, M.D.

Associate Professor of Medicine, University of California School of Medicine. Chief, Hematology Service, San Francisco General Hospital, San Francisco, California.

ALAN S. KEITT, M.D.
Associate Professor of Medicine, University of Florida College of Medicine. Consultant, Gainesville Veterans Administration Hospital, Gainesville, Florida.

SHERWIN V. KEVY, M.D.
Associate Professor of Pediatrics, Harvard Medical School. Director of Transfusion Service, Children's Hospital Medical Center, Boston, Massachusetts.

C. THOMAS KISKER, M.D.
Associate Professor of Pediatrics, University of Iowa. Director of Pediatric Hematology, University of Iowa Hospitals, Iowa City, Iowa.

BEATRICE C. LAMPKIN, M.D.
Associate Professor of Pediatrics, University of Cincinnati College of Medicine. Director, Hematology-Oncology Division, The Children's Hospital Research Foundation, Cincinnati, Ohio.

SAMUEL E. LUX, M.D.
Assistant Professor of Pediatrics, Harvard Medical School. Associate in Medicine, Children's Hospital Medical Center, Boston, Massachusetts.

ALVIN M. MAUER, M.D.
Professor of Pediatrics, University of Tennessee School of Medicine. Medical Director, St. Jude Children's Research Hospital, Memphis, Tennessee.

NANCY B. McWILLIAMS, M.D.
Assistant Professor of Pediatrics, Medical College of Virginia, Richmond, Virginia.

WILLIAM C. MENTZER, JR., M.D.
Assistant Professor of Pediatrics, University of California School of Medicine. Pediatric Hematologist, San Francisco General Hospital, San Francisco, California.

SCOTT MURPHY, M.D.
Assistant Professor of Medicine, University of Pennsylvania School of Medicine. Associate Director of Hematology Research Laboratory, Presbyterian–University of Pennsylvania Medical Center, Philadelphia, Pennsylvania.

DAVID G. NATHAN, M.D.
Professor of Pediatrics, Harvard Medical School. Chief, Division of Hematology and Oncology, Children's Hospital Medical Center and Pediatrician-in-Chief, Children's Cancer Research Foundation, Boston, Massachusetts.

FRANK A. OSKI, M.D.
Professor and Chairman, Department of Pediatrics, State University of New York. Chief of Pediatrics, Upstate Medical Center, Syracuse, New York.

ROBERTSON PARKMAN, M.D.
Assistant Professor of Pediatrics, Harvard Medical School. Associate in Medicine, Children's Hospital Medical Center, Boston, Massachusetts.

HOWARD A. PEARSON, M.D.

Professor and Chairman, Department of Pediatrics, Yale University Medical School. Chief, Department of Pediatrics, Yale–New Haven Hospital, New Haven, Connecticut.

SERGIO PIOMELLI, M.D.

Professor of Pediatrics, New York University School of Medicine. Attending Physician and Director of Pediatric Hematology, Bellevue Hospital and New York University Hospital, New York, New York

JOEL M. RAPPEPORT, M.D.

Instructor in Medicine, Harvard Medical School. Junior Associate in Medicine, Peter Bent Brigham Hospital and Children's Hospital Medical Center, Boston, Massachusetts.

STEPHEN H. ROBINSON, M.D.

Associate Professor of Medicine, Harvard Medical School. Chief, Hematology Unit, Beth Israel Hospital, Boston, Massachusetts.

FRED S. ROSEN, M.D.

James L. Gamble Professor of Pediatrics, Harvard Medical School. Chief of Immunology Division, Children's Hospital Medical Center, Boston, Massachusetts.

ELIAS SCHWARTZ, M.D.

Professor of Pediatrics, University of Pennsylvania School of Medicine. Director, Division of Hematology, and Senior Attending Pediatrician, Children's Hospital of Philadelphia; Consulting Hematologist, Philadelphia General Hospital and Children's Seashore House, Philadelphia, Pennsylvania.

STEPHEN BYRON SHOHET, M.D.

Associate Professor, University of California. Chief of Hematology, and Director of Hematology Laboratories, Moffitt Hospital, San Francisco, California.

IRVING SCHULMAN, M.D.

Professor and Chairman of Pediatrics, Stanford University Medical Center, Palo Alto, California.

HOWARD R. SLOAN, M.D.

Head, Section on Genetics and Lipid Biochemistry, Molecular Disease Branch, National Lung & Heart Institute, National Institutes of Health, Bethesda, Maryland.

ALVIN ZIPURSKY, M.D.

Professor, Department of Pediatrics, McMaster University. Active Staff, McMaster University Medical Center, Hamilton, Ontario, Canada.

WOLF W. ZUELZER, M.D.

Professor of Pediatric Research, Wayne State University School of Medicine. Pathologist, Hematologist, and Director of Laboratories, Children's Hospital of Michigan; Consultant in Pediatrics, Sinai Hospital; Director, Child Research Center of Michigan; Medical Director, Michigan Community Blood Center, Detroit, Michigan.

INTRODUCTION
AND
ACKNOWLEDGMENTS

This book is the result of the prodding of research fellows, medical students, and our colleagues in pediatric hematology who have insisted that there is a need to collate the massive amount of hematologic pathophysiology that has accumulated in many laboratories, particularly during the past decade. The flow of new information in molecular and membrane biology, genetics, and enzymology has revolutionized pediatric hematology and has changed it from a descriptive clinical specialty, dependent almost entirely upon morphology, to a vibrant biomedical discipline interdigitated with basic information from multiple scientific disciplines.

The editors have shared the excitement of the past decade. Working together in Boston under the guidance and encouragement of Dr. Louis K. Diamond and Dr. Frank H. Gardner, two men who saw the wisdom of the alliance of medicine and pediatrics in hematology, we particularly benefited from the new thrust of biomedical science in our field. The range of potentially soluble problems seemed to us unlimited, and that sense of excitement remains.

Though we are now separated by 300 miles of solid (and usually frozen) New England and Middle Atlantic soil, the telephone, the jet aircraft, and our friends who have labored to write the chapters have enabled us to submit this compilation to Mr. John Dusseau of W. B. Saunders Company, our remarkably helpful publisher.

The decisions that have been made during the development of this book have led to a different approach than is usually found in most of the textbooks of hematology that are currently available. Most of the chapters are primarily intended to provide the reader with a broad base of biomedical knowledge. The clinical disorders serve to illustrate these basic principles. It is hoped that this approach will provide the reader with a rational basis for both differential diagnosis and treatment. The references, though numerous, are selective rather than exhaustive. Other general textbooks of hematology should be consulted by the reader who seeks a complete literature survey. The book is not a clinical laboratory manual, nor is it a morphology text. There are other smaller books available which serve those specific purposes admirably.

Although most chapters are quite independent of the others, understanding of some is aided by examination of others. For example, the chapter by Dr. William C. Mentzer, Jr. on red cell enzymes could be difficult for the average reader unless he first consults the chapters by Dr. Alan S. Keitt and by Dr. Stephen B. Shohet and Dr. Samuel E. Lux. The chapters on the abnormal hemoglobins should be read as a unit after review of the genetics of hemoglobin described by Dr. Park S. Gerald and also emphasized by Dr. Bernard G. Forget and Dr. Yuet Wai Kan.

As we concluded the editing of this book, we realized that we had largely ignored the beginnings of pediatric hematology in our efforts to present an up-to-date review of present information. For that task we turned to Dr. Wolf W. Zuelzer, whose accomplishments and personal contact with the leaders of the field make him an ideal historian of this short but exciting period in medicine. The editors are particularly grateful to him for his incisive account of the development of the field.

That we are grateful to our chapter writers goes without saying. They tolerated our ceaseless urging and caviling with minimal murmurs of discontent. Several members of the staff of the Division of Hematology of The Children's Hospital Medical Center, particularly Dr. Arthur W. Nienhuis, and some of our colleagues in hematology in Boston gave freely of their time as reviewers, as did Dr. Marie Stuart in Syracuse. We hope they are now finally satisfied with the revisions. We thank them for their waspish words and unstinting efforts.

As the complexity of the book increased, Dr. Blanche P. Alter assumed increasingly important editorial responsibility. Many of the chapter writers have already thanked her for her efforts. The editors are also very grateful.

To Ann Buckley we offer our heartfelt thanks. Patiently and efficiently she waded through the myriads of revisions and countless details that are the frustrating concomitants of this sort of effort. Without her the birth of this volume would have ended in dystocia totalis.

Certainly we must thank our research fellows, medical students, and colleagues whose questions stimulated us to make the effort. We hope we have helped to organize this complex but fascinating field for their benefit and that physicians caring for patients will find themselves more aware of new developments and therapeutic possibilities as a result of their perusal of the book.

Both of us wish to extend to Dr. Louis K. Diamond, Dr. Charles A. Janeway, and Dr. William B. Castle our gratitude and profound respect. They showed us the way and shared a deep commitment to research and patient care with us. We were fortunate indeed to have served with them.

DAVID G. NATHAN
FRANK A. OSKI

CONTENTS

Section II
RED CELL PRODUCTION

Section III
RED CELL DESTRUCTION: DISORDERS OF MEMBRANE AND METABOLISM

Chapter 6

THE RED BLOOD CELL MEMBRANE AND MECHANISMS OF HEMOLYSIS

by Stephen B. Shohet and Samuel E. Lux

Chapter 7

DESTRUCTION OF RED CELLS BY THE VASCULATURE AND THE RETICULOENDOTHELIAL SYSTEM

by Michael C. Brain

Chapter 8

IMMUNOHEMOLYTIC ANEMIA

By Neil Abramson

Section IV

RED CELL DESTRUCTION: DISORDERS OF HEMOGLOBIN

II   THE WHITE CELL

Chapter 16

DISORDERS OF LEUKOCYTE FUNCTION AND DEVELOPMENT 493
by Robert L. Baehner

III   COAGULATION

IV   INVASIVE AND STORAGE DISORDERS

IV BLOOD TRANSFUSION THERAPY

Chapter 30

PLATELET TRANSFUSION 867
by Robert I. Handin

Chapter 31

GRANULOCYTE TRANSFUSION 875
by Joel M. Rappeport

Pediatric Hematology
in Historical Perspective

by Wolf W. Zuelzer

As a subspecialty of pediatrics and a *sine qua non* of the modern teaching institution, pediatric hematology is a latecomer, naturally enough, for diseases of the blood were a minor problem—one is tempted to say a mere hobby of a few inquisitive and far-seeing minds—compared with the great challenges of infectious and nutritional disorders that faced the pioneers of pediatrics. As a serious concern of investigators, however, it is as old as scientific pediatrics as a whole, though its early history is too closely interwoven with that of general hematology to be traced separately. Its tools as well as its basic concepts came largely from internal medicine and from the experimental sciences, and one needs only to mention names like Ehrlich, Metchnikoff, Landsteiner, Chauffard, Downey, Minot, Castle, Whipple, and Wintrobe to appreciate the magnitude of this debt.

The discoveries of these and many other men were applied to the special problems of infancy and childhood by investigators who, with few exceptions, were pediatricians with diverse interests rather than hematologists with a specialized background. This is true even of those whose names are familiar through eponymic usage, for example, von Jaksch, Lederer, Cooley, Blackfan, and Fanconi. Those who labored patiently in the vineyards without stumbling on a buried syndrome are mostly forgotten, though it is among them that one finds the first true pediatric hematologists. A case in point is that of Heinrich Lehndorff, who grew up in the Vienna of von Pirquet and Escherich and devoted his

life to the study of both normal and abnormal hematologic conditions in childhood, publishing his first paper at the age of 29 in 1906 and his last at the age of 86 in 1963. His interest was in the blood of the newborn, in the anemias of infancy, and in leukemia. Like that of most of his contemporaries, his work was almost entirely descriptive, but he was a good morphologist and clinical observer. Lehndorff left Vienna in 1939 at the age of 63, found temporary shelter with Leonard Parsons—then the leading figure of pediatric hematology in England—at Birmingham, came to the United States during World War II, and ended his career as an octogenarian with an honorary appointment at the New York Medical College. *Sic transit gloria mundi.*

From the very beginning, the unique blood picture of the newborn received special attention. In one of the oldest hematologic texts, *Du Sang et de ses Altérations Anatomiques,* published in Paris in 1889, Hayem—known to this day as the inventor of Hayem's solution but deserving to be remembered for more important contributions—discussed the blood at birth in great detail, giving the number of red and white corpuscles and platelets on the basis of his own counts, describing macrocytosis, anisocytosis, and a tendency toward spherocytosis, and attributing the high hemoglobin level to hyperactivity of the bone marrow. The title of a paper by E. Schiff in the *Jahrbuch für Kinderheilkunde* of 1892, "Newer contributions to the hematology of the neonate, with special reference to the time of ligation of the umbilical cord," implies the existence of earlier

1

studies and anticipates those of Windle and his associates some 50 years later.

The hematology of the neonate remained a cardinal concern of investigators for many decades. Progress was slow, perhaps in part because of the tediousness of the methods used, in part because of variables in obstetric and pediatric practice and differences in the timing of observations. Schiff himself, working successively in Prague and Budapest, found hemoglobin levels on the first day to average 104 per cent in one city and 144 per cent in the other. Much controversy arose over normal values because the early workers did not come to grips with the problems of individual variation and frequency distribution. A German author, H. Flesch (1), wrote despairingly in 1909, "The differences in the hemoglobin values of different observers according to the ages of the children are so considerable that one is really in no position to give definite normal figures." It was difficult, moreover, to draw a line between normal and abnormal conditions. ABO hemolytic disease, for example, was unknown until 1944, when Halbrecht (2) in Hadera recognized the relationship between "icterus praecox" and incompatibility of the major blood groups of mother and child. Prior to the studies of Lippman (3) in 1924, on the other hand, the transient normoblastemia of normal full-term infants was considered pathologic, although Neumann (4) had observed it in 1871 and König (5) had written about it in 1910. Supravital staining, introduced by Ehrlich in 1880, was not utilized until 1925, when Friedländer and Wiedemer (6), writing in the *American Journal of Diseases of Children*—then the only major pediatric journal in the United States—reported reticulocytosis as a regular feature of neonatal blood. Although it was known by then that reticulocytes were young forms, the belief still prevailed that the high hemoglobin at birth was due solely to hemoconcentration rather than to active erythropoiesis, as postulated by Hayem.

Conversely, the postnatal drop in hemoglobin was taken as evidence of accelerated hemolysis, which in turn was held by some to be the cause of physiologic jaundice. That puzzling phenomenon was long thought to signify the entry of bile into the blood, as a result of temporary mechanical obstruction by a mucous plug in the common bile duct or a "desquamative catarrh" of the small radicals, or liver damage from bacterial toxins from the recently colonized intestine of the newborn. The noted Finnish neonatologist, Ylppö (7), however, had demonstrated increased bilirubin levels in the cord blood as early as 1913 and had concluded that icterus neonatorum was due to a "functional inferiority" of the liver. All theories involving the regurgitation of bile became untenable in 1922, when Erwin Schiff and Färber (8), pupils of the renowned Adalbert Czerny, showed that "during the period of bilirubinemia only the indirect van den Bergh reaction is positive." The alternative that the jaundice was due to increased blood destruction, however, could not be proved. Summarizing the argument in 1928, the Viennese pediatric hematologist, Eugen Stransky (9), wrote, "Although the morphologic stigmata of a hemolytic icterus [i.e., spherocytosis] are lacking and the red blood counts do not permit a firm explanation, a hematogenous origin of icterus neonatorum nevertheless seems likely. Why destruction of red corpuscles takes place is still an unsolved question."

One must sympathize with these early investigators who formulated the alternatives clearly enough but could not solve the riddle of neonatal jaundice with the means at their disposal. To them, icterus meant either regurgitation of bile or increased destruction of blood. Hemolysis seemed indeed a plausible explanation for the combination of bilirubinemia of the indirect variety with a falling hemoglobin and a regenerative blood picture, all the more because mild forms of hemolytic disease were undoubtedly included in studies of infants presumed to be normal. The life span of fetal—or for that matter adult—red cells remained an unknown quantity, even after Winifred Ashby had measured it in adults with the differential agglutination technique in 1919, for the range of 30 to 100 days reported by her was too great to be of practical value. This was also true of the blood volume of the newborn, which William Palmer Lucas and B. F. Dearing (10) of San Francisco had actually attempted to measure in the same year, using the brilliant vital red dilution method. They obtained a range of values from 107 to 195 ml. per kg. of body weight, almost twice that found in 1950 by Mollison (11) and his associates with a method combining isotope and dye dilution. The mere fact that they concerned themselves with such questions in 1919 puts them ahead of their pediatric contemporaries. Neither of the first two books devoted specifically to pediatric hematology, that of Ferruccio Zibordi of Modena, *Ematologia Infantile Normale e Patologica* (12), which appeared in 1925, and that of Baar and Stransky of Vienna, *Die Klinische Hämatologie des Kindesalters* (1), published in 1928, mentioned blood volume or red cell survival. The name of Lucas deserves recognition in any survey of pediatric hematology, for, apart from looking after patients with blood diseases in the Children's Department of the University of California Hospital before such specialization had become accepted elsewhere, he was an enterprising and thoughtful investigator. His chapters on blood in Abt's *Pediatrics* of 1924, written with E. C. Fleischner (13), are outstanding in their emphasis on physiologic processes, clarity of thought, and absence of semantic claptrap, and in these respects superior to the two works just cited.

As for the solution of the puzzle of neonatal jaundice, the functional inferiority of the liver postulated so long ago by Ylppö could not be defined, of course, until Hijmans van den Bergh's two pigments had been identified as free and glucuronide-conjugated bilirubin through the independent studies of Billing and Lathe (14), Schmid (15), and Talafant (16) in 1956; the results of the preceding demonstration of the role of UDPGA as a glucuronide donor by Dutton (17) and others could be applied to bilirubin, and the enzymatic reactions involved in the conjugation process could be investigated as a function of hepatic maturation (18).

Traditionally, the history of pediatric hematology begins in 1889 with von Jaksch's report (19) on the condition that bears his name, which he designated *anemia pseudoleucaemica infantum*. By a strange irony not only the term but the very syndrome has long since vanished from the horizon, though in its day it had an enormous vogue and was considered by some to be the characteristic anemia of infancy *par excellence*. Within the same year, 1891, it was described independently by Hayem (20) and his compatriot Luzet (21), so that their names were also attached to it. The clinical picture was overshadowed by severe nutritional disturbances, wasting, diarrhea, rickets, and, as a rule, chronic infections of the respiratory tract, otitis media, pyoderma, and the like. The findings suggestive of leukemia were marked splenomegaly, anemia, and what later hematologists would call a leukemoid reaction, leukocytosis, and immature granulocytes. It was Luzet who noted the normoblastemia that led to the use of the term "erythroblastic anemia," until that term was temporarily preempted by Cooley for the anemia that *he* described. At that time, the combination of splenomegaly and leukocytosis meant leukemia, and von Jaksch's paper was therefore a distinct step forward, though its essence was the simple observation that some of the patients survived, a remarkable fact in itself, given their general condition and the paucity of therapeutic means then available.

Von Jaksch was not a hematologist, and, except for a follow-up report in 1890, he made no further contributions to the understanding of the disease that made him famous. He practiced pediatrics in Prague, then the capital of the Austrian province of Bohemia, and held an appointment at the Charles University, where, as a legendary octogenarian, he was pointed out to this writer in 1934, a tall aristocratic figure with a massive white head who bore his fame with a casual elegance reminiscent of the old Hapsburg Empire. The riddle of von Jaksch's anemia was never properly solved. It was at one time common in central Europe and in France, less so in England, and still less in the United States. Its disappearance paralleled the gradual improvement in child health and care. As Lehndorff (22) wrote many years afterward in an almost nostalgic epitaph on the extinct entity, it was a "poor people's disease." In truth, it was not an entity at all but a convenient diagnostic wastebasket, though an interesting one. The contemporaries finally agreed that it was a nonspecific response of the infantile organism to the horrendous combinations of infectious and nutritional insults that were so common at the time and so difficult to sort out.

Far more lasting and important, of course, was the contribution made to pediatric hematology—and indeed to medical science as a whole—by Thomas B. Cooley of Detroit in 1925 (23), when he salvaged from this wastebasket the distinct entity now known as thalassemia. He soon abandoned his original designation of "erythroblastic anemia," for he realized that the conspicuous normoblastemia which had first attracted his attention was neither a specific nor a central feature of the disorder, and in his later publications he emphasized the fragmentation and shape anomalies of the red cells and the paucity and uneven distribution of the hemoglobin. He did not know, of course, that the ultimate disturbance was one of hemoglobin, let alone beta chain, synthesis, but he came to conceive of the disease as a fundamental disorder of hemopoiesis and was fully aware of its genetic nature from the beginning. He himself had originally proposed a recessive mode of inheritance, anticipating the classical study of Valentine and Neel of 1944 (24). Strangely enough, he did not investigate the seemingly normal parents of the propositi, and later was led to defer judgment by reports of transmission by a single affected parent, which he doubted but could neither verify nor disprove.

Cooley was, in any case, profoundly interested in the genetic aspects of the anemias and was, in this respect, far ahead of most contemporary hematologists. He corresponded with geneticists, used such terms as "heterozygote" for humans at a time when their use was still largely restricted to plants and Drosophila, and for years pondered the then wholly puzzling relationship between "sicklemia" and sickle cell anemia. He reported the first instance of sickle cell disease, which this writer later had occasion to identify as a case of sickle-thalassemia, in a Greek family (25), and he proposed a sex-linked mode of inheritance, backed by pedigree studies over five generations, for familial hypochromic anemia in a kindred first described by him (26) and later restudied and published by Rundles and Falls (27) at Ann Arbor. In accepting the term "Mediterranean anemia," which Whipple had suggested at a time when the known cases were restricted to Italian and Greek families, Cooley (28) made an interesting and prophetic reservation: "We are not inclined," he wrote in 1932, "to lay great stress on the limitation of this or any similar disease to a particular race. We have found that sickle cell anemia, formerly supposed to be peculiar to Negroes, occurs in Greeks, and it seems likely to us that any disease in which there is a hereditary element, as presumably there is in this disease, is limited more by locality and association than by race."

The style is as characteristic of the man as the thought. Cooley was articulate, well educated—he spoke or at least read four languages and maintained a global correspondence—and highly intelligent. He came from a family of distinguished jurists, the only one to eschew the law and enter the medical profession. Born in Ann Arbor, the son of a future justice of the Michigan Supreme Court, he obtained his degree in medicine at the University of Michigan, worked for three years in "clinical chemistry," interned at Boston City Hospital, spent a year visiting clinics in Germany, returned to Boston for prolonged training in contagious diseases, then was appointed Assistant Professor of Hygiene at his alma mater. Except for a stint with the Children's Bureau of the American Red Cross in France during the first World War, he remained in Michigan for the rest of his life, first as a practicing pediatrician and, after the death of Raymond Hoobler in 1936, as a professor of pediatrics in Detroit. Throughout these years he was closely associated with The Children's Hospital, whose pediatrician-in-chief he ultimately became.

As mentioned, Cooley had no formal training in hematology and very little technical help. He and his faithful associate of many years, Pearl Lee, examined blood smears, roentgenograms, and, of course, the patients themselves, making sketchy notes on index cards and keeping the bulk of their observations in their heads. His equipment consisted of a monocular microscope of ancient vintage, a staining rack, a rather small card file, and—in an otherwise vacant upstairs room intended for the affairs of the Child Research Council of the American Academy of Pediatrics—a couch on which he took siestas and did much of his thinking. His daughter Emily, a gifted and artistic young woman, made the beautiful camera lucida and freehand drawings with which he illustrated his papers. She also chauffeured him about town, went to the library for him, and accompanied him to meetings. His home in Detroit's "Indian Village" and his garden, professionally landscaped by Emily, were oases of good taste. He owned a cottage on the coast of Maine where he spent his summers. He liked music, knew his wines, enjoyed good food, and was an excellent conversationalist. He knew how to live.

Cooley's influence extended well beyond the field of hematology. His was the conception behind the series of studies on the chemical composition of the red cell stroma carried out in the 1930's by Erickson and her associates in the laboratories of Icie Macy Hoobler, which earned high praise from Eric Ponder. He was one of the founders of the Academy of Pediatrics, and, long before the time was ripe, saw the role of pediatrics in terms of preventive medicine. Politically he was a liberal, scientifically a radical, personally a patrician. Combined with a rather haughty expression, an irrepressible wit, and an utter lack of reverence for established authority, these traits were bound to earn him enmities on the part of town and gown alike, but his enemies respected and his friends admired him. He was well ahead of his time, a lucid thinker and a giant in the history of pediatric hematology.

An entirely different personality was George Guest, for many years one of the mainstays of the Children's Hospital Research Foundation in Cincinnati, whose contributions were equally important, if less spectacular. Guest was as much a physiologist as a hematologist, interested in the basic aspects of blood during growth, a stickler for precise measurements, a patient investigator who set himself long-term goals and took a systematic approach to reach them. The meticulous studies he conducted between 1932 and 1942 on the hemoglobin levels, red blood counts, and packed cell volumes of a large group of infants and young children of widely different social and economic backgrounds are a model of intelligent and purposeful data-gathering, the purpose being both physiologic and clinical. In the face of the rather arbitrary definitions and therapeutic practices then prevailing, Guest set out to ascertain the range of normal variation and to delineate optimal values

against hypoferric states. Such data were badly needed then and have remained valid to this day. In serial studies (29) involving among other things intra-family and twin comparisons, he showed convincingly that a fall of the MCV and MCH in the presence of seemingly adequate hemoglobin levels could be reversed or altogether prevented by the administration of iron and is therefore a sensitive indicator of an incipient deficiency state rather than a physiologic phenomenon. He concluded that iron deficiency anemia was far commoner among infants than had been previously thought and advocated the general use of prophylactic treatment. His earlier observations on glycolysis and the rise of inorganic phosphorus in stored blood (30) and his joint investigations with Sam Rapoport (31) on the role of the pH in the breakdown of diphosphoglycerate were milestones in the understanding of red cell metabolism. He also made significant contributions to the knowledge of the osmometric properties of erythrocytes (32), both normal and abnormal, devising a method that was, typically, both practical and precise and permitted simultaneous determinations of hemolysis and red cell volume at each stage of the procedure.

Apart from these accomplishments, George Guest was a delightful friend and, with the help of his wife, a perfect host, so perfect that the house on Dana Avenue became a kind of unofficial headquarters for the entertainment of the many visitors to the Children's Hospital. Here they were offered the *vin d'honneur* from a well stocked wine cellar decorated with frescoes by an artist friend—the owners' pride and the first and last stop for the visitor—and here they would find good conversation, interesting people, and an exquisite cuisine. The Guests were passionate Francophiles, and the cooking was French, unless a keg of oysters had just arrived from the East to be prepared in endless variations, or unless Jesse, the houseman, more friend than butler, just happened to have shot—illegally, of course—a fat squirrel from one of the magnificent old trees in the garden. George, a short, stocky, quiet man, understood the art of good fellowship, but the soul of the house and its social genius was "M.L.," a handsome woman with red hair, a passion for poetry, and a gift for conversation. They had met in Europe after the First World War as young and idealistic members of the Hoover Relief team, were drawn together by their love for all things French, and remained deeply devoted to one another. A large part of each summer was spent in France visiting friends, traveling through the countryside, and sampling wines. George Guest was the only American member of the French Pediatric Society, a fact in which he took greater pride than in his other achievements, and though his French accent left much to be desired, he liked to attend meetings and even present papers in such delightful places as Bordeaux, Lyon, and Paris. When M.L. died about 1964, the house was sold and an era passed.

It would be instructive to trace in detail the thinking of earlier observers concerning the iron deficiency of infancy, to whose definition Guest made such a solid contribution, but which remained an object of controversy, confusion, and neglect for generations of pediatricians. Although Bunge had proposed an essentially correct explanation as early as 1889, the nature of the commonest anemia of infancy eluded investigators for many years. The reasons for this paradox are enlightening. One was the belief that not only mild anemia but also hypochromasia was a physiologic condition. "That the hemoglobin content suffers more than the red blood count," Heinrich Baar wrote in 1927 (33), "is surely a purposeful mechanism, for the same quantity of hemoglobin can serve its function better when it is distributed over a larger number of red corpuscles." More important, no doubt, is the fact that among the clinic patients on whom most studies were conducted, pure iron deficiency was rare. In the face of the multiple ailments to which such patients were prone, failure to respond to iron alone was common, and it was easy to draw erroneous conclusions from therapeutic trials. Conversely, of course, a rise of the hemoglobin following the administration of iron was just as uncritically taken as proof of its efficacy on the principle of *post hoc propter hoc,* though it was believed that iron was a bone marrow "stimulant" rather than a specific substance effective only when correcting or preventing a deficiency.

Much of the problem was semantic in nature. While French pediatricians described iron-responsive hypochromic anemias in infants as *"chlorose du jeune âge,"* or *"chlorose alimentaire,"* most German and Austrian authors rejected this concept, if only because "chlorosis occurs only during puberty and only in females." The highly influential Czerny, in particular, set the clock back by stating categorically that a whole group of alimentary anemias existed which could be influenced by diet but in which iron was utterly ineffective. Baar wrote: "If it appears *a priori* unjustified to group together, and attribute to direct or indirect lack of iron, anemias of the most diverse origin solely because they are all hypochromic, fail to show nucleated red cells in the peripheral blood and lack splenomegaly, the notion of a chlorosis of alimentary origin was definitely refuted by Czerny's findings." If this was to pour out the child with the bathwater, to use the German expression, Baar retreated from his aprioristic position to the extent of recognizing a "pseudochlorosis infantum" or infantile iron deficiency anemia as an "etiologically uniform type to be separated from the rest of the alimentary anemias of infancy." This was rare, however, he said, in comparison with "the overwhelming majority [which] remains uninfluenced by iron administration, though nevertheless improved or cured by appropriate changes in diet." In reading such statements, one must remember that even fresh air and sunshine were still considered essential adjuncts to the treatment of anemia. Moreover, no less an authority than Haldane (34) had asserted earlier that "recovery affords no ground for assuming that iron is built up into hemoglobin," and that "in typical cases [of chlorosis] the curative factor of iron salts must be exercised otherwise than simply in building up the hemoglobin. The essential process in the cure of chlorosis is the reduction in the volume of the plasma [*sic*]." In addition, the notion of toxic hemolysis due to the fatty acids in cow's milk and especially in goat's milk had a prolonged vogue on the Continent, where "cow's milk anemia" and "goat's milk anemia" were accepted entities.

Related to the semantic difficulties was the problem of classification. Ever since Hayem had introduced the color index in 1877, hypochromasia had been used to characterize certain anemias, and it was soon apparent that most anemias of older infants were of this type, but the difficulty of relating morphologic criteria to pathogenetic mechanisms and of recognizing in turn that different etiologic factors could operate through identical pathways proved too much. Not until the work of Minot and Castle established the characteristic response of hemoglobin and reticulocytes to specific hematinics, and Wintrobe put the morphologic classification on the firm basis of red cell measurements, did pediatric hematologists gradually abandon such terms as "alimentary-infectious" anemia. In 1936 Hugh Josephs (35) still used it as a common denominator which, to him, included deficient hemoglobin formation, deficient erythropoiesis and deficient stimulation of erythropoiesis, deficient maturation (the "erythroblastoses"), and blood destruction. Such usage, apart from the vagueness of the etiologic concept, was bound to delay both the understanding of the pathogenesis and the development of a workable classification of the anemias. It was an internist who said that "the infant bleeds into his own increasing blood volume," and the importance of the hemoglobin mass at birth was not appreciated until later. When Blackfan and Diamond's *Atlas of the Blood in Children* finally appeared in 1944 (36), it used Wintrobe's classification and described the principal anemia of infancy under the title "iron deficiency anemia."

One cannot leave the subject of iron deficiency without mentioning Hugh Josephs, a strange figure and in his day an authority in the field of American pediatric hematology. It is remarkable that this should have been the case, for he published little and confined his work largely to the relationship between iron metabolism and anemia in infancy. His chapters on diseases of the blood in Holt and McIntosh's textbook were excellent, but on the whole his mind had a somewhat pedantic cast and a tendency to look for profound meanings underneath simple facts. His forte was a thorough knowledge of the literature, which he analyzed in erudite but unconscionably lengthy reviews, complete with foreword, statement of scope and purpose, introduction, presentation of fundamental concepts, summary, table of contents, and a bibliography which in one instance exceeded 750 titles. He was Associate Professor of Pediatrics in Dr. Park's department and published mostly in the Johns Hopkins Bulletin. His manner and appearance were those of a college professor or a don—mild, pleasant, serious, single-minded, a slight, grayhaired man who smoked a pipe, wore soft collars and a velvet jacket with elbow patches, and received his visitors in a drab office in the old Harriet Lane Home, cluttered with books, magazines, and reprints.

Curiously enough, Josephs came to the unshakable conclusion that the hypochromic iron deficiency anemia of infants was not due to depletion of iron but to its diversion to unknown sites by unknown mechanisms (37). He based this on theoretical calculations which proved that an anemic baby of 18 months should have an excess of 200 mg. of unused iron—other than the necessary tissue iron—somewhere in his body; *ergo* the baby suffered from "iron deficiency without depletion." This hypothetical baby, he said, "is starving in the midst of plenty. Give this baby a small amount of iron by mouth and he will utilize it avidly for hemoglobin formation, and may as a result use even more than he was given." In the absence of infection, the unavailability of iron might be due, he thought, to hormonal, histotrophic, or even emotional factors. In 1956, three years after these speculations, Philip Sturgeon (38) calculated on the basis of the same data that had been available to Josephs that a seemingly normal newborn could easily have a hemoglobin mass low enough to account for severe anemia in later infancy. Earlier, Bruce Chown (39) of Winnipeg had documented the occurrence of massive transplacental hemorrhage. Soon afterward, Kleihauer and Betke (40) devised their ingenious method for demonstrating fetal cells in maternal blood by the acid elution technique. Subsequent studies by Cohen and Zuelzer (41) and others showed that moderate and repeated fetal bleeds were not at all rare. A mechanism for depriving the fetus of hemoglobin iron without necessarily causing overt anemia at birth but capable of explaining the later development of iron deficiency in the absence of further blood loss seemed to offer a simpler solution than the tortuous hypothesis of "iron deficiency without depletion." The modern age had arrived.

Their semantic difficulties did not keep the earlier pediatricians from devising eminently practical methods of treatment, as exemplified by the story of pediatric transfusion therapy. The technical problems of transfusing infants were overcome in various ways. In 1915, Helmholz of the Mayo Clinic advocated the use of the superior sagittal sinus, and in 1925 Hart of the Sick Children's Hospital of Toronto used this route for the first exchange transfusion ever given for "icterus gravis" (42). Though his patient recovered, exchange transfusion was not again used for this indication until Wallerstein revived it in 1946 on the grounds that "the removal of most of the Rh-positive cells and of the circulating antibody shortly after birth prevents the incidence of the more severe pathological and physiological changes." Wallerstein (43), then Director of the Erythroblastosis Fetalis Clinic of the Jewish Memorial Hospital in New York, had used the sagittal sinus for most of his cases, but stated that "the umbilical vessels should be an excellent route for both the withdrawal and replacement procedures," with the strange proviso that they could be used "only if the decision to perform the substitution is made before birth . . ." J. B. Sidbury (44), a pediatrician at the Babies' Hospital in Wrightsville, North Carolina, in a little-noticed report had described a simple transfusion via the umbilical vein in the case of a bleeding newborn in 1923. It was Diamond (45) who later established the umbilical route as the safest and simplest for exchange transfusion in hemolytic disease and who, with Allen and Vaughan (46), was the first to recognize that the prevention of kernicterus was the main rationale of the procedure. It is interesting to recall that exsanguination transfusion through the fontanelle or the femoral vein was used on a large scale at the Sick Children's Hospital in Toronto for the treatment of burns, erysipelas, and other conditions since 1921. It was introduced by Bruce Robertson, who in 1916 during the campaign in France had observed two soldiers recover from severe carbon monoxide poisoning after venesections followed by transfusions. By March of 1924, when Robertson was already dead, 501 exsanguination trans-

fusions had been performed at Sick Children's (47).

In the late 1950's there was a small flurry of papers reporting successful transfusions by the intraperitoneal route. This subject had been thoroughly explored in two studies, one experimental (48), the other clinical (49), in 1923 by a young pediatric resident in Minneapolis, David Siperstein, whose concise and accurate summary read as follows: "1. The intraperitoneal transfusion of citrated blood is a therapeutic procedure of possible merit. 2. It can apparently be utilized in cases in which transfusion is indicated, when other routes are unavailable." The author documented the effective reabsorption of the transfused cells not only with serial red counts and hemoglobin determinations but also with photomicrographs showing the dual populations of hypochromic recipient and normochromic donor cells. In his review of the literature he found that intraperitoneal transfusion was first used by Ponfick of Berlin in 1875, and that Hayem in 1884 had performed ingenious experiments involving cross transfusions of dog and rabbit blood in order to prove absorption from the peritoneal cavity. Although technical progress has since made the procedure obsolete, Siperstein's work deserves to be rescued from oblivion, if only to show that there is nothing new under the sun. Passing mention should also be made of the use of bone marrow transfusions as a means of sidestepping technical difficulties, especially for the general pediatrician with little practice in "needlework," in transfusing infants. The method had its day in England and particularly in Denmark, where Heinild (50) in 1947 described the experience of 4 years, during which 686 blood transfusions were given without a single mishap. He stated that the risk of osteomyelitis was limited to continuous infusions. One hesitates to argue with success and realizes that, in places and under conditions in which the required skills or supplies are lacking, it is better to apply unorthodox means than to let a baby die for lack of blood.

A less desirable development that took place in the late 1920's and continued until the early 1940's was the practice of giving newborn infants intramuscular injections of adult blood as a prophylactic measure against hemorrhagic disease of the new-born. During those years, according to recollections provided by James L. Wilson, who for many years was Dr. Blackfan's right arm at The Children's Hospital in Boston, hemorrhagic disease of the newborn was becoming so large a problem that prophylactic measures seemed indicated. The blood was given without typing or cross-matching, and the procedure undoubtedly was responsible for a significant number of sensitizations against the Rh factor that did not come to light until these infants had grown up. The decline in hemorrhagic disease of the newborn coincided with both the introduction of vitamin K and a significant improvement in obstetric practices, and since the condition has now become rare and its definition was always vague and without clear distinction between traumatic hemorrhages and those primarily attributable to a coagulation difficulty, the mystery of its upsurge and the reasons for its decline have never become quite clear.

If pediatricians proved resourceful in the matter of blood transfusions, it must be said that they showed little innovative spirit in certain other respects. It is a curious fact that the study of bone marrow in children was neglected, especially in the United States, long after its usefulness had been amply demonstrated in adults. Thus Cooley, for example, never looked at anything but the peripheral blood, Blackfan and Diamond's otherwise very complete *Atlas* has not a single illustration of bone marrow, and this writer remembers visiting a prominent Eastern pediatric center about 1946 and finding half a dozen patients on the wards suspected of having leukemia and awaiting surgical biopsies—to be performed if and when they stopped bleeding. His own interest in the cytology of the bone marrow, which led to the recognition of megaloblastic anemia of infancy and its reversal by folic acid (51), had been stimulated by many "curbstone" discussions with Lawrence Berman, a student of Downey and himself an outstanding morphologist. It should be noted that Amato of Naples (52) gave an excellent description of infantile megaloblastic anemia independently in the same year as Zuelzer and Ogden, though he did not have folic acid at his disposal and concluded from the response to potent liver extract that he was dealing with

true pernicious anemia or at least with a temporary deficiency of intrinsic factor. An even earlier report by Veeneklaas (53) of Holland had the misfortune of being prevented from reaching readers abroad because of World War II.

This is the place to pay tribute to the memory of Katsuji Kato, pupil and associate of Downey, a superb morphologist and illustrator, who was the first student of the infantile bone marrow in the United States. In 1937, Kato (54) published a definitive study based on bone marrow aspirations in 51 normal infants and children. He commented on the lymphocytosis in the younger subjects and gave the myeloid-erythroid ratios for the various ages. He also illustrated the diagnostic value of the procedure with a case of leukemia and one of Niemann-Pick disease. Kato was on the staff of Bobs Roberts Memorial Hospital in Chicago and often made the long trek to the North Side to participate in Dr. Brennemann's grand rounds. One remembers him, a jolly, round-faced, smiling figure reminiscent of the *Hotei-Sama* statuettes of his native Japan, a rapid speaker with an atrocious accent but interesting ideas, showing off his delicate colored drawings with as much aesthetic pleasure as scientific pride and at the same time implying by his self-deprecating manner that it was all quite simple and hardly worth the honorable listeners' attention. The War put an end to his career. He returned to Japan and was lost from sight.

Perhaps it was Kato's unfortunate choice of the sternum, making the procedure unnecessarily difficult and unpleasant in pediatric practice, that kept others from emulating him. Except for the enterprising Peter Vogel at Mount Sinai Hospital in New York, whose study with Frank Bassen (55) in 1939 covered 113 examples of diverse conditions, including leukemia, Gaucher's disease, and metastatic neuroblastoma, illustrated by excellent photomicrographs, American authors virtually ignored Kato's work. In Europe, and especially in Switzerland under the influence of Rohr and Moeschlin, pediatric hematologists were more curious. Zürich, where Naegeli had created a strong tradition, had already become a Mecca of continental hematology. "The painstaking exploration of every case [of unexplained anemia] with old and new methods, which include bone marrow puncture, handled at the Zürich [Children's] Clinic with consummate skill by my *Oberarzt, Dozent* Willi, promises to uncover new, sharply defined entities," Guido Fanconi (56) declared in 1937. In the short span between 1935 and 1938, H. Willi (57) published four excellent studies on the bone marrow in thrombocytopenic purpura, leukemia, and various anemias of childhood. Fanconi had the satisfaction of seeing his prophecy fulfilled, in part by his next *Oberarzt*, Conrad Gasser. In addition to megaloblastic anemia of infancy, a whole series of conditions came to light or were clarified through bone marrow studies, among them the acute erythroblastopenia described in 1949 by Gasser (58), chronic neutropenia, also studied by Gasser (59) and later by Zuelzer and Bajoghli (60), Kostmann's infantile genetic agranulocytosis (61), "myelokathexis" (62) or "ineffective granulopoiesis" (63), and the aplastic and hypoplastic anemias.

Hematology occupied a special place among Fanconi's far-flung interests, and in giving encouragement and support to his associates—in this respect not unlike Blackfan—he contributed as much to progress in this field as he had done earlier with the recognition of the anemia that bears his name (64). A tall, handsome man, every inch the professor yet gracious and outgoing, capable of charming an audience in six languages, a lively and eclectic spirit, Fanconi was—and is—a superb clinician and an excellent organizer to whom pediatric hematology owes much. With Fanconi one must rank his colleague in Bern, Glanzmann (65), whose report in 1918 on "hereditary hemorrhagic thrombasthenia" as a condition characterized by prolonged bleeding time and poor clot retraction in the presence of a normal platelet count opened the era of platelet function studies. Glanzmann postulated the existence of a platelet factor specifically involved in clot retraction. He contributed greatly to the knowledge of the various purpuras. The term "anaphylactoid purpura" stems from him (66) and was based partly on clinical observations and similarities with human serum sickness, partly on his interpretation of Hayem's findings in dogs injected intravenously with bovine serum.

Conrad Gasser as one of the ablest and most productive pediatric hematologists in Europe deserves more than passing mention in this narrative. Apart from his discovery of acute erythroblastopenia—known until then only from the report of Owren (67) as a complication of congenital spherocytosis—and his study of chronic neutropenia, he added greatly to our knowledge of hemolytic anemias in childhood. His monograph, *Die Hämolytischen Syndrome des Kindesalters* (68), which appeared in 1951, ranks in quality if not in scope with Dacie's well-known book. In 1948 in a paper with Grumbach (69), Gasser described spherocytosis as a feature of ABO hemolytic disease. In the same year, he gave a detailed report of anemia with spontaneous Heinz body formation in a premature infant (70), a condition then unknown except for a brief note by Willi. In his book and in subsequent publications, he added a large case material, described the detailed morphologic picture of the abnormal red cells—which were identical with the "pyknocytes" later observed by Tuffy, Brown, and Zuelzer (71) in full-term infants as well, but which he called more graphically "ruptured eggshells"—and determined their incidence in the blood of normal prematures. He coined the term "hemolytic-uremic syndrome," being among the first to recognize that condition.

One reports with regret that so fruitful a career was disrupted by the exigencies of an academic system that, at the time at least, provided insufficient "room at the top" and effectively eliminated key people upon the retirement of their chief unless they happened to be chosen to succeed him. Gasser, a modest man with a quiet sense of humor and a *gemütlich* Alemannic temperament, today practices pediatric hematology in a small private office in Zürich. Similar reasons prematurely ended the academic career of Sansone in Genoa, author of a book on favism and one of the most promising pediatric hematologists in Italy.

It is manifestly impossible in the allotted space to do justice to, or even name, all those who contributed to the evolution of pediatric hematology. Among European workers one would like to dwell on Sir Leonard Parsons as a central figure in England, an original thinker who refused to accept the confused semantics of childhood anemias and created his own system along pathophysiologic lines, the first to recognize, in 1933, the hemolytic nature of erythroblastosis fetalis and to defend that concept (72) even against the authority of Castle and Minot, who, along with Diamond, Blackfan and Baty, Josephs, and others, regarded it as a defect of hemopoiesis in a class with Cooley's anemia and other "erythroblastoses." One would like to describe the achievements of his associates, Hawksley and Lightwood, of Cathie, Gairdner, Walker, Hardisty, and so many other British colleagues; of Lichtenstein in Sweden, an early student of the anemia of prematurity, which he was the first to call physiologic and to separate from the later phase of iron deficiency; of his compatriots Wallgren and Vahlquist; of Plum of Copenhagen, the discoverer of vitamin K and originator of the thesis of its temporary deficiency as the cause of hemorrhagic disease of the newborn; of van Creveld of Amsterdam, a pioneer in the study of coagulation factors in the newborn; of Betke, then in Tübingen, who with Kleihauer developed the acid elution technique for the demonstration of fetal hemoglobin in individual cells and who later, in Munich, developed his department as a base for a strong program in pediatric hematology; of Jonxis in Leyden, an imaginative investigator, who among other things organized a comparative study of the incidence of sickling in Curaçao and Dutch Guiana to test Allison's hypothesis of the selective effect of malaria in two genetically similar populations exposed for centuries to different risks of infection.

To return closer to home, credit must be given to James M. Baty as a member, with Blackfan and Diamond, of the triumvirate at The Boston Children's Hospital which set the pattern for the development of pediatric hematology in the United States. Their collaborative effort resulted, among other things, in the recognition of hydrops, icterus gravis, and anemia as related conditions (73), a crucial step toward the understanding of hemolytic disease. After Baty moved to the Floating Hospital and Blackfan died an untimely death, Diamond emerged as the American pediatric hematologist *par excellence,* a man whose role cannot be described solely in terms of his publications—too numerous to be listed

here—but who become the mentor of a whole generation of pediatric hematologists now holding key positions in teaching institutions throughout the country. Directly or indirectly we all owe him a debt of gratitude, even those who from time to time disagreed with him on specific points. This writer remembers his first meeting with him when, as an intern in 1935, he consulted him in connection with a case of Cooley's anemia, then an unheard-of rarity in the small New England hospital where he served. He made the pilgrimage to The Children's Hospital—under Blackfan, forbidden territory to those who had not graduated from Harvard, Yale, Columbia, or Johns Hopkins—with apprehensions that were not allayed when he laid eyes on Dr. Diamond, rather fierce-looking in a dark, Assyrian sort of way. They *were* allayed when Diamond proved to be a most amiable consultant, willing to discuss the case with an insignificant intern without condescension or conceit, and, what is more, to confirm his diagnosis. Of Diamond's specific contributions one need mention here only the "Diamond-Blackfan" syndrome of hypoplastic anemia (74), the numerous studies on the nature, diagnostics, and treatment of hemolytic disease, and the *Atlas,* an outstanding work for its day, which was his work rather than Blackfan's.

The memory of the late Carl Smith is too recent to need restoring. His book, *Blood Diseases of Infancy and Childhood* (75), was the first of its kind in the United States, an excellent reference work that is still current. His most important contribution was the description of infectious lymphocytosis. He took a great interest in thalassemia and established a model outpatient transfusion service at New York Hospital. Carl Smith was a modest and generous man, always willing to praise and to give credit even when credit was not due. Through his untiring efforts, Cornell became one of the important centers of pediatric hematology.

The prime mover in the field on the West Coast was Philip Sturgeon, who was then creating the hematology department at the Children's Hospital of Los Angeles. He first emerged about 1950 as a student of the infantile bone marrow, providing quantitative measurements that were badly needed at that time (76) and promoting the diagnostic use of marrow aspiration at an early stage. A great traveler and sportsman in private life, Sturgeon combined in his work the elements of common sense and scientific curiosity, establishing the outstanding hematology clinic which today is carried on by his successor, Hammond. Wiser than most of us, he recently announced his early retirement to Zermatt in Switzerland.

The state of the art cannot be measured solely in terms of publications. An equally important indicator is the standard of practice and research in the field. The fact that a major pediatric teaching institution in the United States today is almost unthinkable without its pediatric hematologist reflects the influence of a few model institutions. The establishment of a Diamond "school" of pediatric hematology has been referred to above. The only center of comparable importance in producing research-oriented and practically competent men and women in this field has been the Hematology Service at the Children's Hospital of Michigan, which this writer has been privileged to direct and which has turned out well over a hundred fellows in the last quarter of a century, many of them today directing services of their own here and abroad. The impending creation of a subspecialty board in pediatric hematology may or may not be desirable as a means of stimulating further progress, but it is a sure indication that, between Boston, Detroit, and a number of smaller centers, a sufficiency of manpower has been developed to provide service, teaching, and research at a high level of excellence for the future.

One cannot end this fragmentary account without emphasizing some of the contributions made to pediatric hematology by scientists in other fields. The most striking example by far is the history of hemolytic disease of the newborn. In 1938, Ruth Darrow, a pathologist who had a deep personal interest in the subject, having experienced a series of stillbirths, sat down and reflected on the pathogenesis of what was then called erythroblastosis fetalis (77). Assembling all the then known facts, notably the sparing of the first child, the involvement of subsequent pregnancies after the birth of an afflicted baby, and the range of clinical and hematologic manifestations, she discarded all the current theories and concluded that the disease could only be explained as the result of maternal sensitiza-

tion to an as yet unknown fetal antigen—a splendid example of the value of intelligent speculation.

Within three years Darrow's hypothesis was confirmed, and the Rh factor, described in a brief communication by Landsteiner and Wiener (78) in 1940, was identified as the offending antigen. Wiener (79), and independently Levine (80), observed transfusion reactions after administration of ABO-compatible blood that could be attributed to Rh antibodies. It was Levine, observing such a reaction in a woman who had received no prior transfusions (81) but had received blood from her husband after delivering a stillborn fetus, who recognized the relationship between Rh and hemolytic disease of the newborn (82). He showed that mothers of affected infants possessed antibodies which reacted with the majority of random bloods and those of their husbands and children but not with each other's. A gentle, unassertive, scholarly man, he characteristically sought the opinion of those experienced in neonatal pathology before publishing his epochal discovery. This writer remembers Levine's visit to Detroit in this connection some time in 1941. Bubbling with excitement yet reluctant to attack established dogma, he was visibly reassured when his attention was called to Darrow's paper. Though a former associate of Landsteiner and a man whose contributions entitled him to a prestigious position, he had withdrawn from the Rockefeller Institute and fallen back on a mundane bread-and-butter job in an unlikely Newark hospital, surely the most unambitious and modest genius in his field. Content to pursue his research, a devoted *paterfamilias*, amateur pianist, and bridge player, he has continued to reside in New Jersey, off the beaten track, to produce scientific gems, and to make national and international meetings more tolerable by his benign, avuncular presence.

The names of Levine and Wiener were antithetically linked for the generation that witnessed their ascent, largely because both had worked with Landsteiner and both contributed enormously to immunohematology and genetics, though they went their separate ways. This is not the place to assess the totality of their achievements. Wiener's role in the technical and conceptual development of hemolytic disease, both Rh and ABO, cannot be exaggerated, but his obsession with nomenclature, his tendency to pile hypothesis upon hypothesis without bothering to inform the reader that he was discarding—as in a game of jacks—pieces from the bottom without toppling the edifice, and his imperviousness to conflicting opinions and to the needs of those less sophisticated than he isolated him from the mainstream of clinical investigation. Of Wiener's enormous output— [by 1954 when the theory of Rh isoimmunization was essentially complete, he had published over 333 papers, and a typical Wiener bibliography might contain 60 references by A. S. Wiener (with or without *et al.*) out of 80 titles]—the contributions relevant to pediatrics were above all those dealing with the "blocking" Rh antibodies (83), which he discovered and named "univalent," recognizing that they alone could pass the placental barrier and cause disease in the fetus (84). He was one of the pioneers of exchange transfusion (85) and personally performed the procedure countless times at the Brooklyn Jewish Hospital, but his technique involving transection of the radial artery and the use of heparinized blood did not gain general acceptance. Less reticent to invade the domain of the clinician and the pathologist than Levine, he proposed ingenious but purely speculative theories of the pathophysiology of hemolytic disease that did not stand the test of time and tended to detract from his brilliant achievements in his proper field of blood group immunology. Personally a likeable, friendly, unpretentious man, he was always in the thick of a battle in which he was his own worst enemy.

The modern era of leukemia therapy begins with the work of the late Sidney Farber (86), formerly pathologist at The Children's Hospital of Boston and the leading pediatric pathologist in the country and indeed the world, who in 1948 developed the conception of cancer chemotherapy. He had the good fortune of finding in Subarov a chemist able to give him the antifol compounds he needed, but the idea of antimetabolites was his, and he pursued and promoted it with single-minded energy. It led him to the creation of the Children's Cancer Research Foundation and to the organization of a vast program of clinical and fundamental research. Although mar-

ried to a charming woman of great artistic talent, and father of gifted and lively children, Farber was a man of almost monastic dedication to his work, a magnificent hermit who spent day and night in his rather resplendent cell in the Jimmy Fund building planning new approaches, an indefatigable optimist who was convinced that a cure for leukemia would come forth and who did much to bring it nearer.

In 1949, by coincidence, two papers bearing on the same subject from different angles appeared within a few months of each other; they were to have a decisive influence on the direction of pediatric hematology. One was Pauling's demonstration (87) of the nature of sickle hemoglobin as a discrete protein, separable in the sickle trait from normal hemoglobin. The other was the study of Neel (88), solving at last the genetics of sickle cell anemia and the sickle trait. Their findings meshed and became the starting point of a veritable flood of investigations in the new field of the hemoglobinopathies and in human genetics at large. The subsequent work of Ingram identified the point mutation in the structure of the sickle hemoglobin molecule and added another dimension to genetic research. Though the riddle of thalassemia is still unsolved, Ingram's conception of alpha and beta chain thalassemias proved extraordinarily fruitful.

Another point of departure was the report of Carson and his associates (89) in 1956 on the enzymatic defect in primaquine-sensitive erythrocytes, which soon afterwards Zinkham (90) showed to be the basis of the then common hemolytic anemia associated with naphthalene poisoning, described earlier by Zuelzer and Apt (91). The exploration of enzymopathies proceeded rapidly thereafter. In 1962 Tanaka and Valentine (92) established the association of still another enzymatic defect, pyruvate kinase deficiency, with nonspherocytic hemolytic anemia, and other defects in the Embden-Meyerhof pathway and its collaterals began to be looked for and found. Largely through the work of Kirkman (93), the polymorphism at the G6PD locus became apparent. Today the well-equipped pediatric hematology laboratory must be able to perform enzyme studies as a matter of course.

Still another area of investigation was opened by the discovery of the nature of the defect in the leukocytes of patients with chronic granulomatous disease, in which area contributors to this volume played a role. The importance of such phenomena as phagocytosis, chemotaxis, and other functions studied long ago by Metchnikoff and his contemporaries has been rediscovered. Cellular immunity and its disturbances have become of importance to the hematologist. And finally, the role of oncogenic viruses, so amply documented in animals, has become relevant to human leukemia and perhaps to immunodeficiency states with hematologic components.

In summary, it is apparent that pediatric hematology has come into its own. After a prolonged infancy beset by morphologic and semantic woes, it has moved out of its descriptive phase into an era of functional and physiologic concepts well beyond the fondest dreams of the pioneers. It seems fitting that a volume that brings together these modern concepts should begin with a tribute to those who did the best they could with the tools available to them and on whose work the new generation is building.

References

1. Flesch, H., quoted by Baar, H., and Stransky, E.: *Die Klinische Hämatologie des Kindesalters*. Leipzig, Franz Dueticke, 1928.
2. Halbrecht, I.: Role of hemo-agglutinins anti-A and anti-B in pathogenesis of the newborn (icterus neonatorum praecox). Am. J. Dis. Child. 45:1, 1964.
3. Lippman, H. S.: A morphologic and quantitative study of the blood corpuscles in the new-born period. Am. J. Dis. Child. 27:473, 1924.
4. Neumann, N. A., quoted by Baar, H., and Stransky, E.: *Die Klinische Hämatologie des Kindesalters*. Leipzig, Franz Dueticke, 1928.
5. König, H.: Die Blutbefunde bei Neugeborenen. Folia Haematol. (Leipz.). 9:278, 1910.
6. Friedländer, A., and Wiedemer, C., quoted by Baar, H., and Stransky, E.: *Die Klinische Hämatologie des Kindesalters*. Leipzig, Franz Dueticke, 1928.
7. Ylppö, A.: Icterus Neonatorum. Z. Kinderheilk. 9:208, 1913.
8. Schiff, E., and Färber, E.: Beitrag zur Lehre des Icterus Neonatorum. Jb. Kinderheilk. 97:245, 1922.
9. Stransky, E., in Baar, H., and Stransky, E.: *Die Klinische Hämatologie des Kindesalters*. Leipzig, Franz Dueticke, 1928.
10. Lucas, W. P., and Dearing, B. F.: Blood volume in infants estimated by the vital dye method. Am. J. Dis. Child. 21:96, 1921.
11. Mollison, P. O., Veall, W., et al.: Red cell volume and plasma volume in newborn infants. Arch. Dis. Child. 24:242, 1950.
12. Zibordi, F.: *Ematologia Infantile*. Milano, Instituto Editoriale Scientifico, 1925.
13. Lucas, W. P., and Fleischner, E. C., In Abt, I. A.: *Pediatrics*. Philadelphia, W. B. Saunders Company, 1924, pp. 406–623.
14. Billing, B. H., and Lathe, G. H.: The excretion of bilirubin as an ester glucuronide, giving the direct van den Bergh reaction. Biochem. J. 63:6P, 1956.
15. Schmid, R.: Direct-reacting bilirubin, bilirubin glucuronide in serum, bile and urine. Science 124:76, 1956.
16. Talafant, E.: On the nature of direct and indirect bilirubin. V. The presence of glucuronic acid in the direct bile pigment. Chem. Listg. 50:1329, 1956.
17. Dutton, G. J.: Uridine-diphosphate-glucuronic acid and ester glucuronide synthesis. Biochem. J. 60:XIX, 1955.
18. Brown, A. K., Zuelzer, W. W., et al.: Studies on the neonatal development of the glucuronide conjugating system. J. Clin. Invest. 37:332, 1958.
19. von Jaksch, R., quoted by Baar, H., and Stransky, E.: *Die Klinische Hämatologie des Kindesalters*. Leipzig, Franz Dueticke, 1928.
20. Hayem, G., quoted by Baar, H., and Stransky, E.: *Die Klinische Hämatologie des Kindesalters*. Leipzig, Franz Dueticke, 1928.
21. Luzet, C.: Etude sur L'Anémie de la Première Enfance et sur l'Anémie Enfantile Pseudoleucémique. Thèse de Paris, 1891.
22. Lehndorff, H.: Jaksch-Hayem anaemia pseudoleucaemica infantum. Helv. Paediatr. Acta 18:1, 1963.
23. Cooley, T. B., and Lee, P.: Series of cases of splenomegaly in children with anemia and peculiar bone changes. Trans. Am. Pediatr. Soc. 37:29, 1925.
24. Valentine, W. N., and Neel, J. V.: Hematologic and genetic study of the transmission of thalassemia (Cooley's anemia: Mediterranean anemia). Arch. Intern. Med. 74:185, 1944.
25. Cooley, T. B., and Lee, P.: Sickle cell anemia in a Greek family. Am. J. Dis. Child. 38:103, 1929.
26. Cooley, T. B.: A severe type of hereditary anemia with elliptocytosis. Am. J. Med. Sci. 209:561, 1945.
27. Rundles, L. W., and Falls, H. F.: Hereditary (?sex-linked) anemia. Am. J. Med. Sci. 211:641, 1946.
28. Cooley, T. B., and Lee, P.: Erythroblastic anemia, additional comments. Am. J. Dis. Child. 43:705, 1932.
29. Guest, G. M.: *Hypoferric Anemia in Infancy*. Symposium on Nutrition, Robert Gould Research Foundation, Inc., Cincinnati, Ohio, 1947.
30. Guest, G. M.: Studies of blood glycolysis: sugar and phosphorus in relationships during glycolysis in normal blood. J. Clin. Invest. 11:555, 1932.
31. Guest, G. M., and Rapoport, S.: Organic acid-soluble phosphorus compounds of the blood. Physiol. Rev. 21:410, 1941.

32. Guest, G. M.: Osmometric behavior of normal and abnormal human erythrocytes. Blood 3: 541, 1948.

33. Baar, H.: Die Anämien, in Baar, H., and Stransky, E.: Die Klinische Hämatologie des Kindesalters. Leipzig, Franz Dueticke, 1928.

34. Haldane and Smith, quoted by Lucas, W. P., and Fleischner, E. C., In Abt, I. A.: Pediatrics. Philadelphia, W. B. Saunders Company, 1924, pp. 406–623.

35. Josephs, H. W.: Anaemia of infancy and early childhood. Medicine 15:307, 1936.

36. Blackfan, K. D., and Diamond, L. K.: Atlas of the Blood in Children. New York, The Commonwealth Fund, 1944.

37. Josephs, H. W.: Iron metabolism and the hypochromic anemia of infancy. Medicine 22:125, 1953.

38. Sturgeon, P.: Iron metabolism: A review. Pediatrics 18:267, 1956.

39. Chown, B.: Anaemia in a newborn due to the fetus bleeding into the mother's circulation: Proof of the bleeding. Lancet 1:1213, 1954.

40. Kleihauer, E., and Betke, K.: Praktische Anwendung des Nachweises von Hb F-haltigen Zellen in fixierten Blutausstrichen. Internist 6:292, 1960.

41. Cohen, F., Zuelzer, W. W., et al.: Mechanisms of isoimmunization. I. The transplacental passage of fetal erythrocytes in homospecific pregnancies. Blood 23:621, 1964.

42. Hart, A. P.: Familial icterus gravis of the newborn and its treatment. Can. Med. Assoc. J. 15:1008, 1925.

43. Wallerstein, H.: Erythroblastosis foetalis and its treatment. Lancet 2:922, 1946.

44. Sidbury, J. B.: Transfusion through the umbilical vein in hemorrhage of the newborn. Am. J. Dis. Child. 25:290, 1923.

45. Diamond, L. K., Allen, F. H., Jr., et al.: Erythroblastosis fetalis. VII. Treatment with exchange transfusion. New Engl. J. Med. 244:39, 1951.

46. Allen, F. H., Jr., Diamond, L. K., et al.: Erythroblastosis fetalis. VI. Prevention of kernicterus. Am. J. Dis. Child. 80:779, 1950.

47. Robertson, B.: Exsanguination—transfusion: A new therapeutic measure in the treatment of severe toxemias. Arch. Surg. 9:1, 1924.

48. Siperstein, D. M., and Sansby, T. M.: Intraperitoneal transfusion with citrated blood: An experimental study. Am. J. Dis. Child. 25:107, 1923.

49. Siperstein, D. M.: Intraperitoneal transfusion with citrated blood: A clinical study. Am. J. Dis. Child. 25:203, 1923.

50. Heinild, S., Søndergaard, T., et al.: Bone marrow infusion in childhood. J. Pediatr. 30:400, 1947.

51. Zuelzer, W. W., and Ogden, F.: Megaloblastic anemia in infancy. Am. J. Dis. Child. 71:211, 1946.

52. Amato, M.: Rilievi anamnesto-clinici . . . su 25 casi di anemie ipercromiche megaloblastiche osserrate in bambini della prima infanzia. Pediatria 54:71, 1946.

53. Veeneklaas, G. M. H.: Über Megalozytäre Mangelanämien bei Kleinkindern. Folia Haematol. (Leipz.) 65:203, 1940.

54. Kato, K.: Sternal marrow puncture in infants. Am. J. Dis. Child. 54:209, 1937.

55. Vogel, P., and Bassen, F. A.: Sternal marrow of children in normal and in pathologic states. Am. J. Dis. Child. 57:246, 1939.

56. Fanconi, G.: Die primären Anämien und Erythroblastosen im Kindesalter. Monatsschr. Kinderheilkd. 68:129, 1937.

57. Willi, H.: quoted to Rohr, K., Das Menschliche Knochenmark. Stuttgart, Georg Thieme Verlag, 1949.

58. Gasser, C.: Akute erythroblastopenie. Helv. Paediatr. Acta 4:107, 1949.

59. Gasser, C.: Die Pathogenese der essenthiellen chronischen Granulocytopenie. Helv. Paediatr. Acta 7:426, 1952.

60. Zuelzer, W. W., and Bajoghli, M.: Chronic granulocytopenia in childhood. Blood 23:359, 1964.

61. Kostmann, R.: Infantile genetic agranulocytosis (agranulocytosis infantilis hereditaria). A new recessive lethal disease in man. Acta Paediatr. 45(Suppl. 105):1, 1956.

62. Zuelzer, W. W.: "Myelokathexis"—A new form of chronic granulocytopenia. Report of a case. New Engl. J. Med. 270:699, 1964.

63. Krill, C. E., Jr., Smith, H. D., et al.: Chronic idiopathic granulocytopenia. New Engl. J. Med. 270:973, 1964.

64. Fanconi, F.: Familiäre infantile Pernizosaartige Anämie (Perniziöses Blutbild und Konstitution). Jb. Kinderheilk. 117:257, 1927.

65. Glanzmann, E.: Hereditäre hämorrhagische Thrombasthenie. Jb. Kinderheilk. 88:113, 1918.

66. Glanzmann, E.: Die Konzeption der Anaphylaktoiden Purpura. Jb. Kinderheilk. 91:371, 1920.

67. Owren, P. A.: Congenital hemolytic jaundice. The pathogenesis of the "hemolytic crisis." Blood 3:231, 1948.

68. Gasser, C.: Die Hämolytischen Syndrome des Kindesalters. Stuttgart, Georg Thieme Verlag, 1951.

69. Grumbach, A., and Gasser, C.: ABO-Inkonpatibilitäten und Morbus Haemolyticus Neonatorum. Helv. Paediatr. Acta 3:447, 1948.

70. Gasser, C., and Karrer, J.: Deletäre Hämolytische Anämie mit "Spontan-Innenköper" Bildung bei Frühgeburten. Helv. Paediatr. Acta 3:387, 1948.

71. Tuffy, P., Brown, A. K., et al.: Infantile pyknocytosis, a common erythrocyte abnormality of the first trimester. Am. J. Dis. Child. 98:227, 1959.

72. Parsons, L. G.: The haemolytic anaemias of childhood. Lancet 2:1395, 1938.

73. Diamond, L. K., Blackfan, K. D., et al.: Erythroblastosis foetalis and its association with universal edema of the fetus, icterus gravis neonatorum and anemia of the newborn. J. Pediatr. 1:269, 1932.

74. Diamond, L. K., and Blackfan, K. D.: Hypoplastic anemia. Am. J. Dis. Child. 54:464, 1938.

75. Smith, C. H.: Blood diseases of Infancy and Childhood. 2nd ed. St. Louis, Mo., C. V. Mosby Co., 1966.

76. Sturgeon, P.: Volumetric and microscopic pattern of bone marrow in normal infants and children. II. Cytologic pattern. Pediatrics 7:642, 1951.

77. Darrow, R. R.: Icterus gravis neonatorum. An

examination of etiologic considerations. Arch. Pathol. 25:378, 1938.

78. Landsteiner, K., and Wiener, A. S.: An agglutinable factor in human blood recognized by human sera for rhesus blood. Proc. Soc. Exp. Biol. Med. 43:223, 1940.

79. Wiener, A. S., and Peters, H. R.: Hemolytic reactions following transfusions of blood of the homologous group with 3 cases in which the same agglutinogen was responsible. Ann. Intern. Med. 13:2306, 1946.

80. Levine, P., Katzin, E. M., et al.: Atypical warm isoagglutinins. Proc. Soc. Exp. Biol. Med. 45:346, 1940.

81. Levine, P., Katzin, E. M., et al.: Isoimmunization in pregnancy, its possible bearing on the etiology of erythroblastosis fetalis. J.A.M.A. 116:825, 1941.

82. Levine, P., Burnham, L., et al.: The role of isoimmunization in the pathogenesis of erythroblastosis fetalis. Am. J. Obstet. Gynecol. 42:825, 1941.

83. Wiener, A. S.: A new test (blocking test) for Rh sensitization. Proc. Soc. Exp. Biol. Med. 56:173, 1944.

84. Wiener, A. S.: Pathogenesis of congenital hemolytic disease (erythroblastosis fetalis) I. Theoretic considerations. Am. J. Dis. Child. 71:14, 1946.

85. Wiener, A. S., and Wexler, I. B.: The use of heparin in performing exchange transfusions in newborn infants. J. Lab Clin. Med. 31:1016, 1946.

86. Farber, S., Diamond, L. K., et al.: Temporary remissions in acute leukemia in children produced by folic acid antagonist, 4-aminopteroylglutamic acid (aminopterin). New Engl. J. Med. 238:787, 1948.

87. Pauling, L., Itano, A. H., et al.: Sickle cell anemia, a molecular disease. Science 110:543, 1949.

88. Neel, J. V.: The inheritance of sickle cell anemia. Science 110:64, 1949.

89. Carson, P. E., Flanagan, C. L., et al.: Enzymatic deficiency in primaquine-sensitive erythrocytes. Science 124:484, 1956.

90. Zinkham, W. H., and Childs, B.: A defect of glutathione metabolism in erythrocytes from patients with a naphthalene-induced hemolytic anemia. Pediatrics 22:461, 1958.

91. Zuelzer, W. W., and Apt, L.: Acute hemolytic anemia due to naphthalene poisoning, a clinical and experimental study. J.A.M.A. 141:185, 1949.

92. Tanaka, K. R., Valentine, W. N., et al.: Pyruvate kinase (PK) deficiency hereditary nonspherocytic hemolytic anaemia. Blood 19:267, 1962.

93. Kirkman, H. W., Riley, H. D., Jr., et al.: Different enzymic expressions of mutants of human glucose-phosphate dehydrogenase. Proc. Natl. Acad. Sci. USA 46:938, 1960.

I

THE
RED
CELL

Red Cell Morphology

The following collection of 18 photomicrographs by Dr. Arthur W. Nienhuis is designed to acquaint the reader with the salient features of red cell morphology as they are described in this section of the book. In certain chapters other photomicrographs are presented, but most of the important examples of morphologic principles are presented in this collection. Reference is made to this group of photomicrographs in the following chapters devoted to disorders of the red cell.

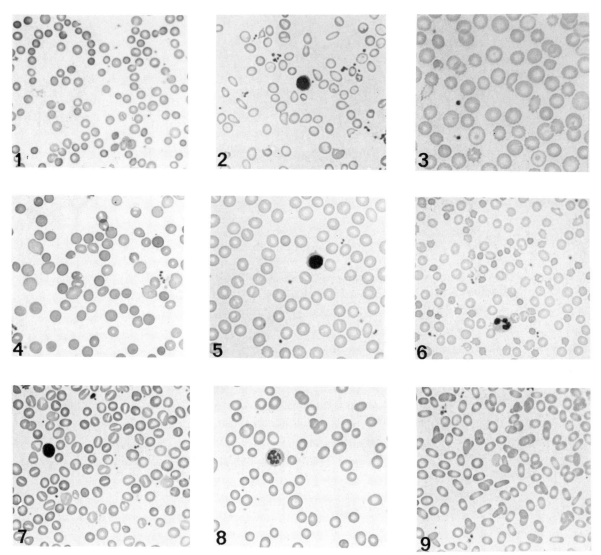

Figure 1. 1, *Hereditary spherocytosis before splenectomy.* Note the variability of cell size and shape. The larger cells are reticulocytes, and the small, dense microspherocytes have been "conditioned" by the spleen. 2, *Iron deficiency anemia.* Note hypochromia and microcytosis (compare red cell diameter with that of the mature lymphocyte). Increased numbers of platelets are also noted. 3, *Biliary atresia.* Note spur cells and target cells. 4, *Acquired immunohemolytic anemia.* Note large numbers of spherocytes. 5, *Normal blood smear.* Compare red cell size with that of mature lymphocyte. 6, *Abetalipoproteinemia.* Note acanthocytosis. 7, *Stomatocytosis.* Note slit shape instead of biconcavity. From a case of hemolytic anemia with high sodium red cells. 8, *Megaloblastic anemia.* In this case of juvenile pernicious anemia, ovoid macrocytosis (red cells with nearly the diameter of a granulocyte) and a polylobulated neutrophil are evident. Thrombocytopenia, so often a complication, is not evident on this smear. 9, *Hereditary elliptocytosis.* Note the variability of the expression of the morphologic change.

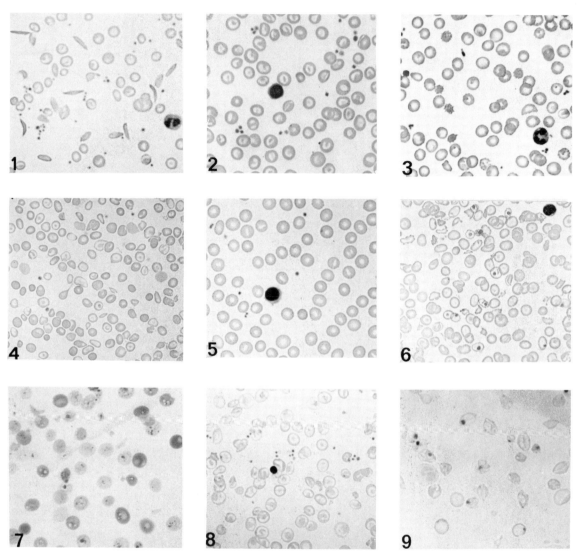

Figure 2. 1, *Sickle cell anemia.* Irreversibly sickled cells, hypochromia, and target cells are present. There is little evidence of fragmentation in this particular smear. A better example may be found in Chapter 14, Figure 14–1. 2, *Hemoglobin C disease.* Note target cells. 3, *Pyruvate kinase deficiency after splenectomy.* Note irregularly contracted cells. 4, *Homozygous beta thalassemia before splenectomy.* Note marked anisocytosis and anisochromia together with "tear drop" cells. The well-hemoglobinized cells probably contain large amounts of fetal hemoglobin which is heterogeneously distributed. 5, *Normal smear.* 6, *Hemoglobin H disease after splenectomy.* Note hypochromia and the presence of large, single inclusions of hemoglobin H in many of the most hypochromic cells. 7, *Homozygous beta thalassemia after splenectomy (Betke:Kleihauer stain for fetal hemoglobin).* Note heterogeneous distribution of fetal hemoglobin. The largest inclusions representing precipitated alpha chains are in the cells with the least amount of fetal hemoglobin. 8, *Homozygous beta thalassemia after splenectomy.* Hypochromia and target cells are prominent. Tear drop forms are less evident. 9, *Homozygous beta thalassemia after splenectomy (methyl violet stain).* Note large inclusions of precipitated alpha chains.

Red Cell Renewal

Chapter 1

Red Cell Maturation and Survival:

Factors Governing Red Cell Life Span

by Alan S. Keitt

INTRODUCTION

The erythron, which has been defined as the total mass of erythroid cells in all stages of development within the body (1), is a large, diffuse, complex organ system which lacks a discrete anatomic framework. It is my hope in this chapter to provide a conceptual framework depicting the ecology of the erythron by identifying the important interactions among its parts (Fig. 1–1). The organization of the red cell into three interdependent systems—hemoglobin, membrane, and metabolism—and the interactions of these systems with each other and with certain environmental factors, specifically the plasma, the bone marrow, and the spleen, will be described. Whenever possible, the mediators by which one system affects another have been selected for special emphasis. Detailed descriptions of many of the individual components of the erythron are presented in other chapters and in many current reviews, which will be cited below. It is hoped that

an understanding of some of the interactions among the components of the erythron will help the reader predict the consequences of a malfunction in any one part.

I shall take liberties with my chapter title by dwelling on many pathologic mechanisms, since it is largely by analogy with disordered processes that the factors underlying normal red cell maturation and survival are currently understood. The reader should be cautioned that development and senescence of the normal red cell are subtle processes as yet incompletely understood, and our concepts of them are subject to change as further information accrues. Before discussing some explicit points of intersection in the ecosystem portrayed in Figure 1–1, a narrative biography of the normal red cell from its conception to its final dissolution will be drawn in order to dramatize where and when things can go wrong. Certain definitions and methodologies upon which our concepts of the life and death of the red cell are based will also be described.

23

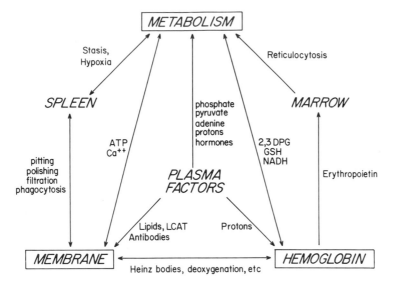

Figure 1–1. A schematic erythron. Some mediators of the interactions between the components are identified.

A Biographical Sketch of the Normal Red Cell

Admirers of the red cell often endow it with human properties, perhaps because of the seeming ingenuity evident in the intricacies of its structure and function. Such anthropomorphic descriptions not only are fun but also can be conceptually useful, particularly in a text designed for pediatricians firmly grounded in human growth and development.* While intrinsic wisdom has not yet been isolated from the red cell, it is not an exaggeration to state that considerable biologic wisdom can be gleaned through studying its life cycle and biologic functions. A thorough understanding of the many facets of the red cell requires and provides a firm grounding in modern biology.

Conception

Conception for the red cell involves an as yet poorly understood encounter between a nondescript, sometimes migratory,

*In order to avoid substituting levity for clarity, it must be emphasized that the following discussion concerns the life cycle of the red cell within a *mature* individual. Thus subsequent references to "fetal" or "neonatal" red cells should not be confused with developing red cells in the human fetus or neonate. Special considerations of fetal erythropoiesis and erythrocytes are covered in Chapter 2.

pluripotential stem or precursor cell and a trophic hormone, erythropoietin. The significance of this liason lies in the irreversible pregnancy of the stem cell, which is thereafter firmly committed to erythroid development. Erythropoietin appears to enhance the proliferation of cells committed to erythroid development. As we shall see, erythropoietin will continue to affect developing red cells at various stages during their sojourn in the bone marrow (2). As with many other hormones, recent evidence indicates that cyclic AMP may be involved in some actions of erythropoietin upon developing red cells (3). It appears that, in addition to erythropoietin, other factors in the "microenvironment" of the bone marrow stimulate the development of the pluripotential stem cell along the pathway of erythropoiesis (4).

In Utero

The earliest recognizable product of this episode, the proerythroblast, resides deep within the bone marrow cords with other embryonic cells of the granulocytic and megakaryocytic series. This prenatal dwelling allows the young red cells a chance to develop outside the rigorous challenges of the peripheral circulation. The bone marrow is a large, teeming Okefenokee-like structure, full of "fugitive vessels" (5), which has been called the most unstable organ in the body because of the irregularity and apparent motility of both its internal and external boundaries (6). The cordal compartments are considered extravascular, filling the marrow spaces between a series of radially oriented sinuses which drain into a central longitudinal vein and thence into the general circulation. The structure in cross section of rat femurs has been likened to a wheel, with an outer bony rim fed by arterioles and an endosteal sinusoidal bed, and spokes, represented by penetrating sinuses, around an axle, the central vein (5). The lining surfaces separating cord from sinus, which will serve as the birth canal when the developing red cell emerges into the sinus and thence into the circulation, are composed of sinusoidal lining cells, a discrete but highly rarified basement membrane, and adventitial reticular cells in intimate association with the developing marrow cells. Adventitial cells, which project from the lining surface into the cordal space like so many placental villi, are often surrounded with developing red cells and may participate in the transfer of iron into the cells for hemoglobin synthesis. Similar clones of developing red cells also surround free reticular cells within the cords, which serve a role which Bessis and Breton-Gorius have likened to that of a "nurse" cell (7). The completeness of the sinusoidal/cordal partition varies markedly in different areas and with differing hemo poietic requirements. Normally, however, the fetal cells are scrupulously retained within the cords and out of the general circulation.

Life in utero for a developing red cell usually represents an orderly process of three or four cell divisions in the span of three to four days. Thus each proerythroblast normally gives rise to 8 to 16 mature red cells. Most hemoglobin synthesis occurs early in fetal development by a process, stimulated by erythropoietin, which involves a ribosomal protein synthetic apparatus dependent on mitochondrial energy production in the form of ATP produced by oxidative phosphorylation. This complex metabolic system, dependent on oxygen and versatile in its metabolic substrate requirements, contrasts markedly with the specialized, anaerobic, glucose-dependent adult red cell. The process of erythroblast maturation is characterized morphologically by a progressive decline in cytoplasmic basophilia as the ribosomes and mitochondria are dismantled for extrusion or are catabolized, perhaps by lysosomal organelles which have been found in young red cells (8). The cell nucleus also progressively self-destructs, forming a dense homogeneous detritus, which normally will be extruded just before or during delivery of the cell into the sinus as a reticulocyte. It is apparent that this attenuation of the cell's capacity to synthesize proteins and to divide severely limits its ability for self-repair and obliterates its ability to regenerate. Only by entrance of new stem cells into the sequence can erythropoiesis continue.

Quickening

Fetal movements have been observed in marrow reticulocytes by time-lapse cinematography (9). These studies suggest that these near-term babies are capable of approaching and penetrating the sinusoidal wall by an active process. At about the same time that motility is observable in fetal red cells, their cell membrane undergoes a dramatic physical alteration that greatly enhances its intrinsic flexibility, presumably setting the stage for its impending squeeze into the intravascular sinusoids (10). While easy deformability remains an essential characteristic of the mature red cell, motility is lost. However, there is some evidence that it retains the elements of a primitive system that allows contraction and propulsive movement in other cells in the form of certain microfibrillar proteins which are precipitable with agents such as vinblastine, colchicine, and strychnine (11). These may have evolved into the structural elements which confer a unique discoid shape upon the mature red cell.

Birth and the Neonatal Period

Birth for a red cell, as for a fetus, may be a traumatic event. It represents the first of many subsequent encounters with the elaborate trabeculations of the vascular system. It has been suggested that extrusion of the nucleus may frequently occur as the red cell passes through narrow fenestrations in the sinusoidal wall (12). The possible role of the sinusoidal lining or adventitial cell as midwife here has clear analogies with the similar role of the sinusoidal lining cells of the spleen in removing other kinds of particulate material from circulating cells, a process known as "pitting" (see below). While delivery of the red cell into the sinus and retention of its nucleus in the adventitial cell may occur as a single event, it is apparent from the many anucleate reticulocytes lining the cordal surface of the sinusoidal wall that many red cells extrude their nuclei before traversing this barrier (13). Whether adventitial cells or free reticular cells also play a role in the extrusion of nuclei from these marrow reticulocytes is unclear, but they rapidly phagocytize and destroy bare nuclei which are only rarely found in the marrow.

The normal neonatal red cell is called a reticulocyte because it contains residual precipitable material or reticulum, largely ribosomal RNA, in its cytoplasm. It is capable of a small amount of hemoglobin synthesis, albeit at a minute rate when compared with its marrow precursors. It retains both major metabolic options, i.e., oxidative phosphorylation and anaerobic glycolysis, for meeting its rapidly dwindling energetic needs. Thus it can withstand the metabolic inhibition of either, but not both, of its energy-producing pathways (14).

As with its human counterpart, the maximal rate of red cell postnatal development occurs during the initial 1 to 2 per cent of its life span. However, for the reticulocyte, maturation signifies loss or attenuation rather than acquisition or enhancement of many of its vital processes. Thus certain metabolic pathways, such as oxidative phosphorylation and protein synthesis, disappear completely, while the activities of many glycolytic and other enzymes decrease drastically during the first 24 hours of postnatal life.

Term reticulocytes contain more membrane lipid and cell water than the average mature red cell and as a result are larger and less dense. Most studies of the properties of reticulocytes have exploited these differences to achieve a partial separation of these young cells by centrifugal sedimentation. Considerable remodeling of these cells occurs during the first several days after their release from the marrow with loss of membrane and water (15), a process which concludes a similar but more drastic remodeling of prenatal reticulocytes within the bone marrow (16).

When the marrow is stimulated by erythropoietin, either in response to a severe peripheral deficit of red cells or by injection of large amounts of the partially purified hormone, large "stress" or macroreticulocytes emerge which, in contrast to the "term reticulocyte," can be readily discerned on a conventional blood smear by their large size and the stainable basophilia of their cytoplasm (17). When superimposed on the cytoplasmic hemoglobin, a characteristic grayish-pink or "polychromatophilic" hue appears. The presence of polychromatophilic macroreticulocytes indicates the premature delivery of reticulocytes that are normally present in the marrow (18), as well as of even younger reticulocytes which have skipped one cell division (6). It is not clear whether this premature release of red cells, a third action of erythropoietin (in addition to its effects on proliferation and differentiation), is directed at the developing red cell or at the sinusoidal/cordal partition of the marrow.

Previous studies of the properties of macroreticulocytes suggested that they had a shortened life span, but more recent data indicate that they lose significant quantities of hemoglobin and membrane without any apparent morbidity (19). It has been shown that the spleen may substitute in part for the marrow in this remodeling process (15).* It seems likely that the premature macroreticulocyte is released before its membrane is sufficiently flexible for immediate and prolonged general circulation. As will be developed later, the spleen is a remarkably efficient detector of relatively rigid and sticky red cells and may serve as an incubator for some macroreticulocytes for a period until they are sufficiently agile to escape and remain in the general circulation.

Extreme red cell prematurity occurs in a number of situations which reflect the importance of maternal factors in the de-

---

*Dr. John Parker has suggested that "circumcision" would be a suitable name for this process.

livery of red cells to the circulation. The dynamic alterations in marrow architecture in response to the stress of hemolytic anemia have been beautifully characterized by Weiss (5). By either migration or breakdown of the sinusoidal/cordal partitions, whole clones of premature red and white cells may be rather suddenly "intravascularized," proliferating within the sinuses, thereby allowing ready access of macroreticulocytes and even nucleated red blood cells to the peripheral circulation. Intrusion of fibrous tissue, granuloma, or tumor cells may also upset the intimate microvascular anatomy of the marrow so as to allow the escape of nucleated red cells.

Adulthood and Senescence

While reticulocyte maturation is a distinct and easily quantifiable phenomenon, the gradual transition from robust maturity to senescence is subtle and remains incompletely understood. Adult life for the red cell is a repetitious encounter with the tortuous ramifications of various capillary beds throughout the body. Survival of the normal red cell can be drawn in broad terms as the balance between the "wear and tear" of some 175 miles of constant travel (6) within the circulation against its rather limited, though finite, capacity for self-repair. The red cell is probably unique amongst tissue cells in fulfilling its prime function of gas transport without any directly linked expenditure of energy. Rather, it diverts its main energetic equivalent, ATP, into processes which either reduce the wear and tear by maintaining its shape and ready deformability or, which repair, as best they can, insults to its membrane.

As will be shown subsequently, ultimate removal of the "normal" red cell from a "normal" vascular bed is largely an age-dependent rather than a random process. At present, it is a moot point whether the travail of the red cell's travels finally exceeds its reparative capacities or whether metabolic failure alters its physical properties sufficiently to preclude continued circulation. A large body of literature exists in which many metabolic and membrane alterations have been associated with aging [see Bunn (20) for references]. In general, such studies have exploited minor differences in cell density to physically separate cells by centrifugation. It should be noted that the aforementioned changes during the first day or two in the circulation are vastly greater than subsequent changes in surface constituents and metabolic capabilities, which have been reported as concomitants and putative determinants of cell death.

Nevertheless, studies in rats in which an aged cohort of cells was attained by a method which does not rely on differential cell density (16) indicate that loss of hemoglobin and volume resumes in older cells prior to their removal from the circulation. The mechanism of this senile fragmentation of aged red cells is not certain, but it is presumably analogous to the pathologic fragmentation of red cells which will be described below.

The search for THE lesion of aging will doubtless continue, but its elusiveness should not unduly upset us. Clearly, the number of terminal cells within the circulation will depend on the rate at which they acquire the critical lesion and on the threshold of the body for recognizing and clearing these cells. It is probable that both normal and pathologic cells do not remain in the circulation long once they reach a certain degree of malfunction unless removal mechanisms become saturated. The intimate relationships between the physical features of the cell, which determine its "circulatability," and its metabolic functions, which will be developed subsequently, set the stage for a vicious cycle that will lead to a very brief agonal period in the circulation.

Necrology

It is perhaps more disconcerting that there is no solid consensus as to the exact site of destruction for the more than 1 million normal human red cells which leave the circulation each second. It is clear that the graveyard lies within the general confines of the reticuloendothelial system, and an educated guess as well as a certain body of evidence strongly implicates the spleen. However, removal of a normal spleen does not increase red cell longevity. As we shall see, the spleen is the organ par excellence for detecting a subtle increase in the rigidity of altered red cells, which is among the most important risk factors in the red cell mortality tables. Within the spleen, the moribund red cell encounters an environment not at all unlike that in which it was born, i.e., a sinusoidal/cordal system richly endowed with phagocytes.

The ultimate dissolution of the red cell begins within a phagocytic reticuloendothelial cell and yields a number of distinct products which will be put to widely differing uses. The particulate stromal components associated with the cell membrane are most likely degraded by lysosomes within the scavenger's cytoplasm. Hemoglobin, the red cell's essence, is split into heme and globin, and the amino acid constituents of globin are hydrolyzed for return to the general revenue (an inheritance tax, as it were). Heme is attacked by a recently characterized microsomal enzyme, heme oxygenase, which splits the porphyrin ring at the so-called α-methene bridge, with stoichiometric formation of carbon monoxide, iron, and the tetrapyrrol biliverdin (21). Surviving red cells then serve as pallbearers for transport of the carbon monoxide to the lung for excretion, a process which has been exploited for quantitative studies of heme turnover (22). The iron is efficiently transported by the carrier globulin transferrin to the marrow where it provides an important legacy to the next generation of developing red cells. The remainder of the estate, biliverdin, is converted within the reticuloendothelial cell to bilirubin by an NADPH-dependent biliverdin reductase (21). Bilirubin enters the circulation and becomes bound to albumin for transport to the liver, where it undergoes conjugation with two glucuronyl groups which render it soluble for excretion in the bile. The tightly bound, unconjugated ("indirect") bilirubin does not pass the glomerulus of the kidney and thus accumulates in the plasma whenever the red cell death rate exceeds the liver's capacity to conjugate and excrete bilirubin. The subsequent reductive conversion of bilirubin diglucuronide to urobilinogen in the gut by its bacterial flora is described in detail in a recent review (23) and in Chapter 3. A certain amount of the fecal urobilinogen is reabsorbed from the gut and recirculated, allowing a small and variable excretion in the urine. However, measurement of urine urobilinogen has proved a rather unreliable correlate of increased red cell destruction, as it depends on many other factors, including the excretory capacity of the liver, the bacterial flora of the small bowel, and the urine pH (23).

Methodologic Bases for Current Concepts of Hemolysis and Survival

Red cells suffer from a variety of afflictions — stone (Fig. 1–2), pocks (24), dropsy (25), bile (26), sunburn (27), worms (28, 29), opisthotonos (Fig. 1–3), asphyxiation (30), poison (31), trauma (32), snake bite (33), and corpulence (Fig. 1–4), as well as iatrogenocide (34). These maladies arise either from inborn errors of the cell or from accidents encountered by normal cells in the circulation. Some are rapidly fatal, others are subacute or chronic, while others are merely cosmetic.

Hemolysis in its broadest definition means red cell death, while survival is its reciprocal function. Hemolysis may occur in a variety of sites and at any temporal stage in the life cycle which has just been drawn. Our concepts of hemolysis and survival have largely been derived from certain methodologies which have allowed rough quantitation of the production of cells within the marrow, the survival of those cells which reach the peripheral circulation, and the turnover of hemoglobin pigments derived from deceased or remodeled red cells. It is useful, therefore, to consider these various methods for determining survival of red cells in relation to the cell's life cycle.

The most primitive condition which qualifies as "hemolytic" is the rather rare occurrence of certain types of acquired pure red cell aplasia. Until recently, this disorder was considered to represent failure of conception; however, antibodies have been detected in some individuals which seem to attack the earliest proerythroblasts (35). The specificity of the antibody, as indicated by the normal white cell and platelet proliferation, indicates that it is probably acting immediately after the pluripotential stem cell has undergone erythroid differentiation

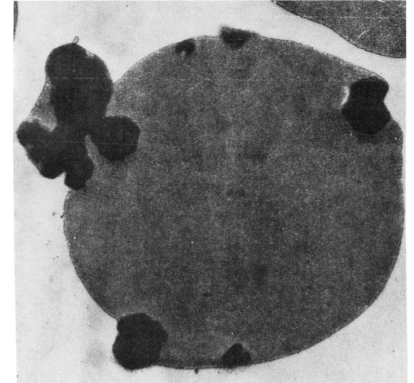

Figure 1–2. End-stage Heinz bodies lying under and distorting the plasma membrane of a mature erythrocyte (× 26,000). (From Rifkind, R. A., and Danon, D.: Heinz body anemia —An ultrastructural study. I. Heinz body formation. Blood 25:885–896, 1965, by permission of Grune & Stratton.)

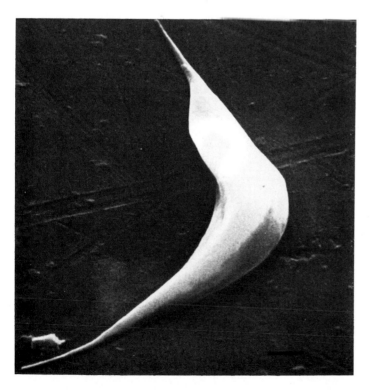

Figure 1–3. Sickled cell (scanning electron micrograph, × 7500). (Courtesy of Dr. Lawrence S. Lessin.)

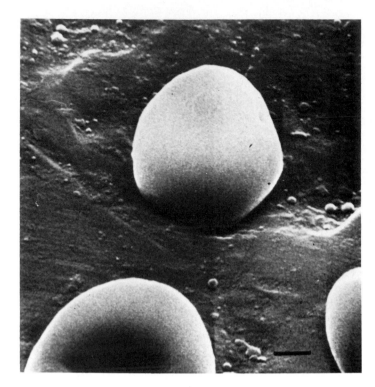

Figure 1–4. Spherocyte. A normal discoid cell is in the foreground (× 10,500). (Courtesy of Dr. Lawrence S. Lessin.)

to inhibit erythroid proliferation and hemoglobin synthesis, since there is no indication of increased turnover of hemoglobin in such patients.

Intramedullary Hemolysis and Ineffective Erythropoiesis

Death in utero of red cells is a prominent feature in a number of more common conditions, including thalassemia and the anemias of vitamin B_{12} or folic acid deficiency. Here cell destruction primarily occurs after maturation and hemoglobin synthesis have begun, so that the bone marrow is filled with erythroid precursors. While the descriptive terms "intramedullary hemolysis" and "ineffective erythropoiesis" are both used to describe this phenomenon, they are not synonymous, as we shall see. Those methods which quantitate the turnover of hemoglobin, namely, the production of bilirubin (36), its degradation to fecal urobilinogen and stercobilin, and the formation of endogenous carbon monoxide (22), are markedly enhanced, while procedures measuring the survival of red cells that reach the circulation, such as tagging the cells with ^{51}chromium, do

not reveal sufficient shortening to account for the increased marrow activity. The number of premature cells which do escape into the circulation as reticulocytes is often much smaller than would be expected in the face of severe hyperplasia of the bone marrow. The nearly normal survival of some of these cells doubtless reflects the marked heterogeneity of the developing cells whereby only the most fit escape into the circulation.

The existence of ineffective erythropoiesis had been suspected well before the pathophysiologic basis for the destruction of "fetal" erythrocytes in the bone marrow was elucidated in such disorders as the thalassemias (37). The basis for this concept was derived from studies of the incorporation in vivo of radioactive glycine into circulating hemoglobin and the timing of its appearance in bilirubin or in fecal stercobilin, the ultimate reductive product of bilirubin in the feces (38).

In vivo labels, such as ^{15}N-glycine and ^{14}C-leucine,* are called cohort labels since they are actively incorporated only into

---

*As a precursor for heme synthesis, ^{14}C-glycine is incorporated into both heme and globin, while ^{14}C-leucine is incorporated only into the globin fraction.

those cells which are synthesizing hemoglobin at the time when the material is injected. Thus the cells which become labeled are all of a similar age, which is an important distinction between them and labels such as ^{51}chromium, which are bound to the entire spectrum of circulating red cells. The classic studies of London, West, Shemin, and Rittenberg established that 10 to 20 per cent of the radioactivity from ^{15}N-glycine that had been injected into humans appeared as fecal stercobilin before any radioactivity emerged in circulating hemoglobin (39). This so-called "early labeled peak" has subsequently been shown with reasonable certainty to reflect at least two separate processes. The earliest label appears to represent the rapid turnover of heme proteins other than hemoglobin which derive primarily from the liver, while the 3- to 5-day stercobilin represents the catabolism of hemoglobin derived from red cells within the bone marrow (19). Part of this latter component may reflect loss of hemoglobin during the remodeling of reticulocytes or from the thin "corona" of hemoglobin surrounding the nucleus after its extrusion, and thus it is a part of the normal life cycle of the red cell rather than an indicator of fetal wastage (40). As such it could be termed ineffective erythropoiesis but not intramedullary hemolysis. However, in disorders such as pernicious anemia, thalassemia, and certain refractory sideroblastic anemias, the inordinate increase in this early fraction undoubtedly represents the death of many developing red cells within the marrow.

Probably the commonest cohort label in clinical usage is ^{59}iron. The timing of the disappearance of radioiron from plasma and its subsequent reappearance in circulating red blood cells has allowed many insights into the functional state of the bone marrow in various disorders of the erythron. However, ^{59}iron is a rather poor label for estimation of red cell life span, since it is very efficiently reutilized many times by new red cells and thus suffers as a true cohort label. It is most useful in detecting the presence of ineffective erythropoiesis when there is rapid uptake of ^{59}Fe by the marrow but reduced incorporation into circulating red cells.

A curious form of ineffective erythropoiesis, in which selective hemolysis of immature cells occurs after they have been released from the marrow, has been described in several cases of red cell pyruvate kinase (PK) deficiency (30). This phenomenon depends on the presence of an intact spleen, which appears to participate in the removal of premature reticulocytes from the circulation. Before splenectomy, radiochromium studies of peripheral red cell survival may be nearly normal despite evidence of severe hemolysis, as judged by anemia, hyperplasia of the bone marrow, and the accumulation of unconjugated bilirubin in the serum (41). Removal of the spleen is associated in some of these patients with extraordinary sustained reticulocytosis and significant improvement in the level of circulating hemoglobin (14). Reinfusion of the peripheral blood from a patient after splenectomy into a normal recipient with a spleen demonstrates a marked shortening of red cell survival with selective loss of the many of the youngest cells (42). A possible metabolic basis for the vulnerability of the PK reticulocyte in the spleen will be discussed subsequently. As in thalassemia, it appears that there is marked heterogeneity in the genetic endowment of cells with inborn enzyme defects. When the lesion is so severe as to destroy the developing red cell prior to its escape from the marrow or the spleen, there will be a marked error in estimation of hemolysis by any techniques involving just the determination of the rate of disappearance of peripheral cells from the circulation.

Estimates of Survival of Circulating Red Cells

Most hemolytic disorders involve a more orderly cycle in which the terminal lesion occurs in circulating red cells, because of either exhaustion of limited resources in a congenitally defective cell or accidents encountered in the circulation. When this is the case, the previously mentioned measurements of hemoglobin catabolism agree reasonably well with survival measurements made on circulating red cells. Under ordinary circumstances, about 75 per cent of heme turnover as measured by carbon monoxide or bilirubin techniques is derived from hemoglobin (43); the remainder represents the turnover of other heme proteins, which comprise part of the "early labeled peak" of bile pigment. Generally, increases in carbon monoxide production and bilirubin turnover represent increased red cell destruction, but it is noteworthy that increases in nonhemoglobin heme turnover, such as occur in certain porphyrias (44) or after induction of the microsomal heme oxygenase system with drugs such as Dilantin and phenobarbital (45), can confuse the interpretation.

In theory, when the death of the cell occurs after a reasonably constant period of time in the circulation (e.g., 120 ± 5 days for a normal cell), the line relating the proportion of randomly labeled cells remaining in the circulation with time is a straight one. On the contrary, when damage is random and affects cells of any age, the disappearance curve is exponential, reflecting the destruction of a reasonably constant percentage of all the remaining cells each day.

The original and still most precise method for determining cell survival, the so-called Ashby technique, led to the first real understanding of the difference between intracorpuscular and extracorpuscular red cell defects. The method exploits antigenic differences in red cells, so that red cells infused from one individual into another can be recovered and quantitated using specific antisera. By this cross-transfusion technique, abnormalities can be localized to the donor cells or to the recipient's circulation. Careful Ashby survival curves first established the linear disappearance of normal red cells in a normal recipient and established red cell longevity as 120 days (46).

The most widely used technique for measuring red cell survival in clinical practice is the radiochromium method. Chromium in trace amounts binds to hemoglobin tightly but not irreversibly. A complicating factor, therefore, in the interpretation of ^{51}chromium survival curves is the finite rate of elution of bound ^{51}chromium from the labeled red cells, which amounts to approximately 1 per cent each day but may exceed 3 per cent per day in certain patients with abnormal hemoglobins (47). As a result, the disappearance of ^{51}chromium from normal blood after labeling and reinjection of a small sample of cells is not a linear process, and corrections must be applied to achieve a semiquantitiative measure of red cell survival. In practice, however, this correction is rarely made, and the survival is generally reported as the half-life of ^{51}chromium in the blood (corrected for radioactive decay but not elution), which is normally between 28 and 38 days.

The use of ^{51}chromium as a red cell label has three valuable adjuncts that may actually have more frequent clinical utility than measuring red cell survival. These are (1) the detection of small amounts of blood in the stool by the presence of ^{51}chromium when there is occult blood loss in the GI tract; (2) the determination of the primary sites of red cell destruction by body surface scanning; and (3) the easy estimation of red cell mass by determining the dilution of the labeled cells after complete mixing. The problems of elution of ^{51}chromium from the cell can be overcome with the use of $DF^{32}P$, an irreversible red cell label, most of which binds to the membrane acetylcholinesterase. However, the technique is sufficiently more demanding than the ^{51}chromium label that it is much less commonly employed. It is important to realize that none of the labeling methods which only follow the disappearance of cells from the circulation can distinguish between accelerated cell destruction and chronic blood loss.

Extravascular Versus Intravascular Hemolysis

The concepts of intravascular and extravascular hemolysis were also largely defined methodologically before the actual sites and mechanisms of hemolysis were appreciated. These entities, which are rarely perfectly separable clinically, have been distinguished by contrasting routes of hemoglobin catabolism. The extravascular pattern, mediated by the reticuloendothelial system, has already been described as a feature of normal cell death.

When a circulatory accident is sufficiently severe that death ensues before the cell can make it back to the reticuloendothelial system or the system is saturated, hemoglobin is liberated into the plasma, initiating a series of events which have recently been explicitly reviewed by Bunn (20) and by Pimstone (48). Free plasma hemoglobin is rather rapidly oxidized within the circulation to methemoglobin, a process which facilitates both its dissociation into dimers (half-molecules) and the dissociation of heme groups from globin. Hemoglobin dimers bind to a circulating glycoprotein called haptoglobin. The resulting complex is cleared from the circulation by cells of the reticuloendothelial system. When the rate of liberation of hemoglobin into plasma exceeds the synthetic capacity of the liver for haptoglobin, depletion of haptoglobin occurs, which is a common finding in many acute and chronic hemolytic states. Depletion of haptoglobin allows the passage of unbound hemoglobin dimers (molecular weight, 32,000) across the renal glomeruli. Renal tubular cells actively reabsorb filtered hemoglobin up to a maximal rate that is reached when the unbound plasma hemoglobin exceeds 90 to 100 mg./100 ml. This reabsorbed hemoglobin is not returned to the circulation but is catabolized by the renal tubular cell in a manner which is very similar to the reticulocndothelial cell with one important exception. Hemoglobin iron is not readily reclaimed from the kidney, and significant quantities appear in the urine in the form of hemosiderin within the tubular cells as they are sloughed. Thus hemosiderinuria is a sensitive indicator of acute intravascular hemolysis, and iron deficiency may be a sequel of a chronic process. It should be apparent that free hemoglobin will appear in the urine only after the combined thresholds of haptoglobin binding and tubular reabsorption are exceeded.

When heme becomes dissociated from free circulating hemoglobin dimers, it may bind to one of two plasma proteins, albumin or hemopexin. The presence of methemalbumin is sometimes sought to detect intravascular hemolysis, but it is measurable only transiently in severe hemolytic processes. Hemopexin apparently transports ferriheme to the liver for excretion. Depletion of plasma hemopexin also occurs only with rather severe intravascular hemolysis.

Methodologic Bases for Current Concepts of Hemolytic Mechanisms

Colloid Osmotic Hemolysis

Historically our concepts of hemolytic mechanisms in various disorders of the erythron have also been based on certain in vitro techniques. Thus, prior to about 1965, definitive discussions of hemolysis (49) revolved around the concept of colloid osmotic hemolysis as originally defined by Wilbrandt (50). The currently fashionable importance of alterations in red cell deformability has largely superseded osmotic theories of hemolysis in vivo. Nevertheless, an understanding of colloid osmotic hemolysis and of its quantitiative expression, the osmotic fragility test, is still vitally important for grasping the red cell's functional organization.

It has been known for many years that the red cell behaves as though it were a nearly perfect osmometer; that is, its volume, within certain limits of cell size, maintains an inverse linear relationship with the external osmolarity of the suspending medium. This relationship reflects the rapid movement of water across the cell membrane in such a direction as to maintain osmotic equilibrium. The red cell concentrates K^+ ion as its main osmotically active solute and regulates its own volume by varying its K^+ content. The very high concentration gradient for K^+ between cells and plasma results in a slow but finite leakage of K^+ out of the cell, which normally is just matched by the active transport of K^+ into the cell by a membrane-bound cation pump. Na^+ ion is normally transported out of the cell by a similar linked mechanism. When the pump fails or is overwhelmed by an increase in leakage of cations into the cell, equalization of osmotic pressure can only occur by passage of water into the cell, with a consequent increase in cell volume. The increase in cell volume is limited by the surface area of the cell, since the membrane, while normally quite flexible, cannot stretch. When the cell has reached its maximal volume, it assumes the shape of a sphere, the geometric figure which has the highest possible volume to surface ratio. Any further osmotic gradient induces drastic changes in membrane permeability, allowing rapid and sequential equilibration of cations, phosphate esters, enzymes, and hemoglobin across the membrane, a process known as colloid osmotic hemolysis.

Osmotic Fragility

Colloid osmotic hemolysis also occurs when cells with a normal cation content

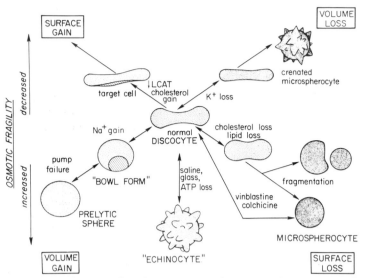

Figure 1–5. Acquired alterations in surface and volume of normal red cells. All of these changes can be induced in vitro under isotonic conditions, and many have in vivo counterparts. With the exception of fragmentation, all of these changes are reversible.

This is a potentially confusing figure which deserves considerable study. The relationship between the "echinocyte" and the "crenated microspherocyte" is not well established. The latter cell may represent a later stage of the former, i.e., a contracted cell which is depleted of ATP and has lost most of its intracellular potassium. Depending on the conditions, the terminal stage of this sequence probably results in a smooth, contracted spherocyte which has lost surface as well as volume (this relationship is not shown). The older term "disc-sphere transformation" and the newer "discocyte-echinocyte transformation" therefore probably describe different stages of the same basic phenomenon. It is essential to consult the recent, concise review by Brecher and Bessis (63) for the current status and nomenclature of this process.

are suspended in solutions of sufficiently low osmolarity. This is the basis of the osmotic fragility test, in which red cells are suspended in a series of buffered solutions of decreasing osmolarity and the per cent hemolysis is determined for each tube by comparing the supernatant hemoglobin with a totally hemolyzed sample. The osmotic fragility of a cell is an indirect measure of how much it can swell before reaching its spherical or critical hemolytic volume. Some factors influencing red cell osmotic fragility have been shown diagrammatically in Figure 1–5; two independent axes represent changes in cell surface area and changes in cell volume. While red cells may have inborn tendencies for altered surface to volume relationships, e.g., the hereditary spherocyte or the thalassemic target cell, the alterations shown in Figure 1–5 represent *acquired changes* which can be induced in normal red cells in vitro and in vivo by appropriate manipulations. The message from Figure 1–5 is twofold: first, the surface to volume ratio of normal red cells within the circulation is maintained by numerous dynamic processes, and second, both the surface area and volume of red cells may expand or contract independently of each other. An excess of surface area relative to the volume of its intracellular contents is associated with decreased osmotic fragility

regardless of the absolute value of either parameter. The processes which mediate these changes in cell volume and surface, many of which are vital determinants of cell survival, are the subject of the subsequent sections of this chapter.

Red Cell Deformability

The beautifully quantitative studies of colloid osmotic hemolysis in vitro provided no adequate insight into the effects on the red cell of its repetitious encounters with the various capillary beds of the body organs. Studies of the filtrability of red cell suspensions by Jandl et al. (51) indicated that abnormal flow properties of individual red cells might underlie the premature death of sickle cells and hereditary spherocytes. However, it was the ingenious technique of Rand and Burton (52), measuring the intrinsic flexibility of individual red cells, and its subsequent application by Weed and LaCelle which dramatized and firmly established alterations in red cell deformability as a unifying factor in many hemolytic disorders (53). This advance came by applying simple, quantitative, physical techniques to individual red cells rather than to red cell suspensions. Micropipets with precisely calibrated cylindrical tips are applied to the surface of a free floating red cell, and the negative pressure required to induce a hemispheric convexity of the cell surface within the pipet and that pressure required to completely aspirate the cell into the pipet are determined. Red cell deformability, measured by Rand and Burton's method, has been shown to depend on three discrete factors: cell shape (spheroidicity), the internal viscosity of the cell (e.g., of hemoglobin), and the intrinsic deformability of the cell membrane (54).

The hypothesis that impaired deformability of individual red cells is a primary cause of red cell death is an attractive one for several reasons. First, it has unified our pathophysiologic concepts of hemolytic mechanisms, since virtually every hemolytic disorder, whether due to abnormal metabolism, hemoglobin, membrane, or trauma, can be shown to affect one or more of the three factors, e.g., shape, internal viscosity, or intrinsic membrane deformability, which determine cellular deformability. Second, it incorporates the capillary beds and phagocytic cells of various body organs into the destructive mechanism in a way which simple colloid osmotic hemolysis could not.

SELECTED EXAMPLES OF THE INTERDEPENDENCE OF THE VARIOUS COMPONENTS OF THE ERYTHRON

Metabolic Support of Membrane Function — ATP-Mediated Functions

ATP occupies an essential role in the economy of the red cell and can be considered the key mediator by which its metabolism, specifically the Embden-Meyerhof pathway, affects the function of the cell membrane. It has additional pervasive influences in the other metabolic pathways of the red cell as an essential cofactor for the initial reactions of anaerobic glycolysis, for the synthesis of glutathione, and for the incorporation and maintenance of red cell adenine nucleotides. The position of ATP in the Embden-Meyerhof pathway is shown in Figure 1–6. The numerous enzymatic defects in this sequence that jeopardize ATP synthesis in affected red cells are explicitly reviewed in Chapter 10.

ATP and Active Cation Transport

A voluminous body of literature, recently reviewed (55), has firmly linked the active transport of sodium and potassium ions with a membrane-bound enzyme system, which is usually designated the Na^+- and K^+-activated adenosine triphosphatase or the membrane cation pump. We have seen previously that the red cell depends on the active transport of these cations against a concentration gradient to maintain its osmotic equilibrium. It has been proposed that the ATPase reaction is a two-step affair by which Na^+ facilitates the transfer of the terminal or γ phosphate group of ATP to an as yet undefined intermediate, while K^+ promotes the cleavage of the intermediate, forming inorganic phosphate and regenerating the reactive "carrier" compound. Ouabain and other cardiac glycosides have been shown to specifically inhibit the terminal step of this sequence. Under "normal" circumstances in vitro, about 2 mEq. of K^+ are transported per hour across the membranes of a liter of red cells, while 3 mEq. of Na^+ are removed from the cell. The process accounts for only a minor portion of the potential ATP formed in the Embden-Meyerhof pathway.

Accumulating information suggests that the linkage between red cell glycolysis and the membrane cation pump may have a precise anatomic orientation. The studies of Parker and Hoffman (56) originally indicated that the locus of this interaction was at the site where the glycolytic enzyme, phosphoglycerate kinase (PGK), was attached to the inner membrane surface. A significant fraction of the activity of this enzyme had been previously shown by Schrier (57) to come down with the stromal or membrane-bound fraction of hemolysates. Parker and Hoffman were able to show, as had Whittam and Ager (58), that ouabain inhibited glycolytic formation of lactate, presumably by blocking ATP consumption and ADP generation by the cation pump. When the control point for this effect was sought, it was noted that glycolytic inter-

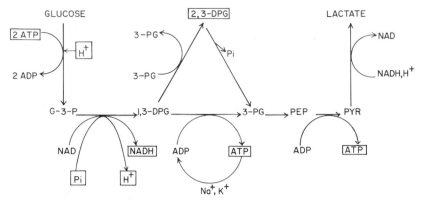

Figure 1–6. The Embden-Meyerhof pathway of red cells. Some important mediators with their sites of production or action are indicated by boxes.

mediates proximal to PGK accumulated in the presence of ouabain, with the exception of ADP which did not change. Parker accordingly surmised that control of the rate of the PGK reaction was mediated by a local or compartmentalized pool of ADP that was not in equilibrium with the main cytoplasmic nucleotide pool and that was specifically generated by the activity of the cation pump. This finding strongly implied an anatomic relationship between the two enzymes and represents the most explicit description of the linkage between glycolysis and the active transport of cations.

Cation flux studies in red cells from a patient with phosphoglycerate kinase deficiency have not revealed a marked deficit in Na^+ or K^+ transport (59). This may be due to the small but significant amount of substrate flow passing through the residual enzyme.

ATP and "Leak"

The passive movement of cations across the red cell membrane, i.e. "leak," is also affected by metabolic processes, and again ATP may be considered the mediator. This mechanism is closely linked to calcium homeostasis within the red cell and is apparently independent of the Na^+- and K^+-activated ATPase. The metabolic dependence of the passive component of red cell membrane flux was first appreciated when red cells were exposed to certain metabolic inhibitors, such as fluoride and iodoacetate, which under certain conditions induce a

drastic increment in K^+ leakage out of the red cell. This phenomenon, which is often termed the "Gardos effect" (60) by workers in the area, is remarkably selective for K^+, since Na^+ leak is not increased. A common requirement for this selective K^+ loss is exhaustion of intracellular ATP and the availability of external Ca^{2+} in the medium, since chelation of external Ca^{2+} by EDTA abolishes the effect.

Certain membrane-active agents, such as lead, triose reductone, and valinomycin, may also induce selective K^+ loss but probably act by different mechanisms than those of the "Gardos effect." Numerous other agents which interact with the cell membrane (e.g., detergents and sulfhydryl oxidants) induce simultaneous leakage of both Na^+ and K^+ ions. Such agents act independently of the metabolic apparatus of the red cell, although they may induce compensatory activation of cation pumping with a secondary depletion of ATP.

The profoundly differing effect of selective K^+ loss on the red cell, as compared with loss of permeability barriers to both Na^+ and K^+, is apparent by studying the "volume axis" in Figure 1–5. As the major internal cation, K^+ contributes importantly to intracellular osmotic pressure. Thus rapid equilibration of K^+ across the membrane is necessarily accompanied by a drastic decrease in intracellular water, with consequent shrinkage of the cell, a process which has been termed "dessicytosis" (61). In contrast, when gradients for both Na^+ and K^+ are abolished, cation exchange occurs with a somewhat slower influx of water, causing the cell to swell. The osmotic fragility of the cells will reflect their change in total internal solute and water. It is probable that the marked decrease in osmotic fragility, which occurs during sterile incubation of red cells from patients with glycolytic enzyme deficiencies, lead poisoning, and thalassemia, represents a transient, selective K^+ leak. The result is a skewing of the incubated osmotic fragility curve with the coexistence of both fragile and resistant populations.

Most models which have been put forward to explain the relative impermeability of the red cell membrane to cations embrace the "charged pore" hypothesis by which positively charged pores electrostatically repel cations, thus preventing their penetration of the cell membrane. However, no adequate anatomic model has been proposed which incorporates the remarkable ability of the red cell to discriminate between such similar ions as Na^+ and K^+ under conditions of ATP depletion. Recent work by Blum and Hoffman (62) has shown that this rapid movement of K^+ may be carrier-mediated, which would seem to offer a more satisfactory explanation for its specificity than would the "charged pore" hypothesis alone.

The genesis of these acquired alterations in red cell volume has been described in some detail, because they appear to have pathologic significance in certain hemolytic processes. The probable in vivo counterpart of the sodium-leaking cell is the swollen "bowl form" depicted in Figure 1–5, which occurs in the peripheral blood of patients with "high-sodium red cells" (25) (see Chapter 6). The converse situation at the other end of the volume axis is the crenated microspherocyte, which may be found in varying numbers in blood smears of patients with red cell glycolytic enzyme deficiencies. The exact relationship between these in vitro models and their occurrence in vivo, while highly suggestive (61), is still in some dispute (63).

ATP and Phospholipid Exchange

The concept of "membrane repair" in red cells has only recently emerged, and its pathologic importance has still to be defined. However, it is now very apparent that the red cell membrane is a dynamic system and that its lipid constituents are constantly turning over by both active and passive processes, which can profoundly influence its physical properties. The energetics of membrane lipid renewal have recently been reviewed by Shohet (64) and are covered in Chapter 6.

The original convincing observation that intact fatty acids bound to albumin in the plasma could be incorporated into phospholipids within the red cell membrane was made by Oliviera and Vaughan, who demonstrated that this exchange depended on both coenzyme A and red cell ATP (65). The reaction involves "acylation" of a preformed membrane lysophosphatide (i.e., a glycerophospholipid containing only one fatty acid in the first position of the glycerol moiety) by an activated fatty acid derived from plasma. The source of the lysophosphatide is presumably a membrane phospholipid moiety that is deprived of its fatty acid in the second position by the action of a phospholipase. This series of reactions has been calculated to represent a turnover of 2 per cent of red cell phospholipids per hour and to expend approximately 5 per cent of the potential energy derived as ATP from glycolysis (66). Although the concentration requirements for ATP are not well established, it is clear that, below a critical ATP level, the inability of the red cell to renew its lipid surface could have disastrous consequences to its integrity.

ATP and Red Cell Deformability

Studies in vivo of capillary blood flow have clearly demonstrated the extreme deformation of individual red cells within capillaries where they characteristically travel single file in a streamlined, parachute-shaped configuration rather than as bioconcave discs. Frequently cells must fold over double to squeeze past promontories or to negotiate sharp turns. This ability to fold its membrane is now widely held to be one of the most important requisites for continuing circulation of the red cell. The studies of LaCelle and Weed have demonstrated that ATP is also an important mediator of this parameter (67).

The physical alterations in the red cell membrane induced when ATP is exhausted are complex and multiple. These may be

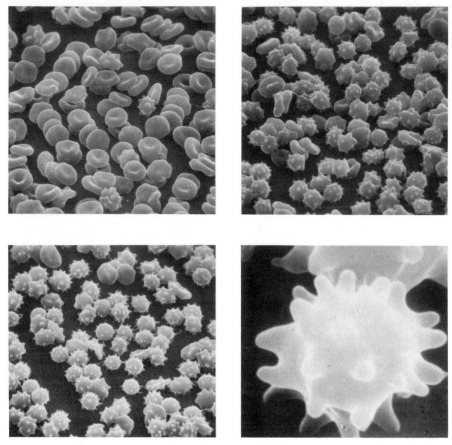

Figure 1-7. Scanning electron micrographs of the in vitro production of echinocytes by prolonged incubation. (From Hochmuth, R. M., and Mohandas, N.: Microvasc. Res. 4:295, 1972.)

grouped under the general term "disc-sphere transformation" (Fig. 1–7), which is in itself a composite of at least three identifiable processes, as pointed out by Szasz (68): loss of biconcavity (sphering), loss of smooth contour (echinocyte formation), and decrease in cell diameter (contraction). These alterations and the resulting increase in membrane rigidity all require the presence of internal Ca^{2+}. The product of these transformations has been called an "echinocyte" by Lessin and Bessis (69) (Fig. 1–5).

In contrast to the active transport of cations and phospholipid exchange, the maintenance of cell shape and deformability does not seem to depend entirely on the expenditure of ATP; rather, ATP seems to act in part by its ability to chelate Ca^{2+}. Thus EDTA, when introduced intracellularly into red cells by the technique of reversible hemolysis, completely prevents the changes in shape and plasticity in ATP-depleted ghosts. It appears that, consequent to the depletion of intracellular ATP, there is an internal redistribution of Ca^{2+} ions. LaCelle and Weed have proposed that Ca^{2+} and ATP are acting reciprocally to influence conversion from a pliable sol to a more rigid gel at the inner surface of the red cell membrane (70). An additional process associated with the "disc-sphere transformation," the contraction of the red cell membrane, may involve ATP expenditure by a separate contractile protein with Ca^{2+}-dependent ATPase activity (71). Reports of the semi-isolation of a contractile protein from red cell membranes support this interpretation. However, as noted by Shohet (64), free Ca^{2+} has important interactions with lipids in experimental membranes, and similar interactions may contribute to the effects of ATP depletion on the physical properties of the red cell membrane.

An additional facet of the relationship between ATP and Ca^{2+} emanated from the discovery of Schatzmann that Ca^{2+} is actively transported out of red cells by an ATPase which is not inhibitable by ouabain (72). The Ca^{2+} requirement for activation of this Ca^{2+} pump is very low (73, 74), and the process is efficient enough to keep the intracellular concentration of free Ca^{2+} within the cell at extremely low levels. It is probably through failure of this pump that net inward movement of Ca^{2+} occurs in ATP-depleted states, with resulting increases in membrane K^+ permeability. The exact relationship between this Ca^{2+} transport system and the previously mentioned contractile proteins with Ca-dependent ATPase activity has not yet been determined.

The intimate interactions between the red cell membrane, ATP, and Ca^{2+} ion are summarized in Table 1–1. It is very apparent that research in this area is gaining speed and will doubtless provide greatly increased insight into the fundamental molecular bases of red cell membrane function in the near future.

Metabolic Support of Hemoglobin Function — 2,3-DPG, NADH, and Glutathione

The question has often been raised as to why hemoglobin needs to be enclosed within an external membrane at all rather than circulate as a free solution. Although mechanical and rheologic explanations are often invoked, it is becoming increasingly apparent that the internal milieu of the red cell is carefully controlled for the optimal function and protection of hemoglobin in a way which is much more efficient than changes involving the entire intravascular space. The roles of NADH in methemoglobin reduction and of 2, 3-DPG in regulating hemoglobin-oxygen affinity are discussed in other chapters and will not be recapitulated here, since they have to do more with cell function than survival.

The Role of Glutathione

Jandl first noted the paradoxical situation whereby the red cell, whose prime function is to transport large quantities of a potent oxidant, molecular oxygen, must maintain a relatively reduced environment in order to survive and function (75). In addition to the heme iron, which can only bind oxygen when in the ferrous state, several reactive sulfhydryl groups on red cell macromolecules, such as hemoglobin, the membrane, and certain glycolytic enzymes, must be scrupulously maintained in the reduced state for proper function. An important mediator for this critical role is the tripeptide glutathione (GSH), the functional end of which is the sulfhydryl group of cysteine. Glutathione is perhaps best considered as a "redox buffer," which preferentially reacts with intracellular oxidants so as to spare the key SH groups of functional proteins. Perhaps the most important oxidant with which the red cell must deal is hydrogen peroxide, a potent oxidant which is slowly generated in normal red cells and may accumulate rapidly in the presence of

TABLE 1–1. MEMBRANE PHENOMENA INVOLVING ATP AND Ca^{2+}

	Ca^{2+} DEPENDENCE	REFERENCE
Processes Requiring ATP		
1. Active cation transport (Na^+- and K^+-activated ATPase)	Ca^{2+} inhibits, $K_i 10^{-4}$ M	73
2. Active Ca^{2+} transport (Ca^{2+}-activated ATPase)	K_M for Ca^{2+} 6×10^{-6} M	73
Processes Requiring Absence of ATP		
1. Loss of biconcave shape	Requires presence of internal free Ca^{2+}	74
2. Loss of smooth contour	Unknown	
3. Contraction	Requires internal free Ca^{2+}	68
4. Decrease in deformability	Requires internal free Ca^{2+}	67
	Accelerated by external Ca^{2+}	73
5. Selective K^+ leak	Requires external free Ca^{2+}	60

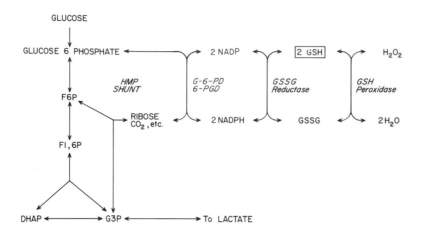

Figure 1–8. Glutathione metabolism in red cells.

numerous exogenous compounds, such as primaquine (76). The presence and importance of the red cell enzyme, glutathione peroxidase, which provides an enzymatic basis for the preferential oxidation of GSH to its disulfide form, GSSG, is now generally accepted (77).

The linkage between glycolysis and GSSG reduction is outlined in Figure 1–8. The system is shown to require the generation of NADPH, which in the red cell is exclusively limited to the first two dehydrogenase reactions of the hexose monophosphate shunt. This pathway then serves a critical reducing function against various oxidant stresses, and a breakdown, such as by an enzyme deficiency, anywhere between G6PD and GSH peroxidase, or an overwhelming oxidant stress initiates a series of cell lesions which can involve both hemoglobin and the cell membrane. The extent to which hemoglobin or membrane is damaged depends on the particular oxidant involved, on its concentration, and on the reactivity of intracellular hemoglobin (78).

Another important reaction of GSH in the red cell is the formation of a mixed disulfide with the exposed β93 cysteine (SH) groups of hemoglobin in the presence of hydrogen peroxide. The glutathione reductase of red cells in the presence of NADPH may cleave the mixed disulfide bonds, regenerating functionally normal hemoglobin (79). If this defense perimeter is overwhelmed, i.e., the β93 cysteine residues remain oxidized, the dissociation equilibrium between heme and globin is markedly shifted, with a resulting decrease

in heme-globin affinity (80). Loss of heme has dire consequences for the structural integrity of hemoglobin because of the extensive bonding between heme and globin. When these stabilizing forces are ruptured, the globin chains begin to unwind, and many previously buried nonpolar amino acid groups are exposed, drastically reducing the solubility of the molecule. The resulting amorphous, electron-dense precipitates or Heinz bodies eventually become attached to the red cell membrane (Fig. 1–2), with important consequences which will be described subsequently.

Metabolic Consequences of Hemoglobin Oxidation

Certain metabolic correlates have been described in cells containing Heinz bodies, most of which follow logically from the above sequence. Increased activity of the hexose monophosphate shunt has been reported to occur in association with hemoglobin Köln, which forms mixed disulfides with GSH (81). This presumably stems from the increased regeneration of NADPH consequent to its oxidation by glutathione reductase. Heinz body–forming cells containing mutant hemoglobins which are unduly sensitive to oxidation may have reduced levels of free GSH as well, although the total glutathione is elevated because of the large amount bound to hemoglobin as the disulfide (82). The Embden-Meyerhof pathway is also very active in these cells, reflecting the high proportion of reticulocytes consequent to the increased turnover of the cells, and the increased rate of cation pumping, possibly due to alteration in membrane sulfhydryl content (83).

Some Interactions Between Red Cell Metabolism and the Plasma Environment

Perhaps because of the ease with which red cells can be washed and studied ex vivo, the importance of variations in certain plasma factors on their metabolism has only been recognized rather recently. Some reasonably well-defined interactions have been selected for discussion here, but it should be noted that hormonal and drug influences on red cell metabolites are being found with increasing frequency. It is through the mediation of these plasma factors that the red cell reflects many of the diverse metabolic states of the body.

Protons

Because protons diffuse rapidly across the cell membrane, the internal pH of red cells is dependent on the extracellular pH and the H^+ gradient across the red cell membrane. Because of the Donnan equilibrium, the normal internal pH of the red cell is about 0.2 pH units below the external pH. Protons affect many red cell functions but are crucial in three areas: control of red cell glycolysis, the oxygen affinity of hemoglobin via the Bohr effect, and the flexibility of the red cell membrane. All three parameters are decreased in the presence of increased protons (i.e., decreased pH).

The primary locus of interaction between glycolysis and hydrogen ions is the cytoplasmic enzyme, phosphofructokinase, which is strongly inhibited by protons and may be virtually inactive at the low pH levels attainable under certain conditions in vivo, such as in the spleen (84). A secondary effect of low pH occurs as a result of the increase in G6P level accumulating behind the inhibited PFK. G6P strongly inhibits hexokinase, so that ordinarily hexokinase and PFK act in concert to regulate glycolytic rate within red cells. The hexose monophosphate shunt reactions are much less pH-dependent, as judged by the resto-

ration in large part of glucose consumption at low pH by diverting G6P through the shunt with methylene blue (85).

Phosphate

The normal concentration of inorganic phosphate within the cells is in the order of 0.4 mM, which is much lower than the prevailing extracellular phosphate concentration of about 1.2 mM. This gradient seems not to depend on the active transport of phosphate ion out of the cell, as is the case for Na^+ ion. Rather, the slow rate of diffusion of phosphate across the cell membrane relative to its incorporation into phosphorylated intermediates accounts for this imbalance (86). It is now generally believed that the major point of incorporation of inorganic phosphate into the glycolytic sequence is at G3PD, with the phosphate diffusing across the membrane into a general intracellular pool of inorganic phosphate.

Under conditions of increased incorporation of inorganic phosphate into organic phosphate esters, such as during the consumption of inosine by nucleoside phosphorylase, inorganic phosphate drops to very low levels and may become the limiting factor in the glycolytic rate (87). Similarly, when extracellular phosphate levels fall, as by ingestion of excess antacids for renal failure (88), or during intravenous hyperalimentation (89), the gradient for diffusion of phosphate into the cell is diminished, with marked consequences for cell function and survival. Two important glycolytic mediators, ATP and 2,3-DPG, as well as the entire glycolytic reaction rate fall drastically under these conditions. A marked increase in the affinity of hemoglobin for oxygen occurs, which may have consequences in total body oxygen transport. Also, not unexpectedly, spherocytic hemolytic anemia has been reported in a patient with very low red cell ATP secondary to hypophosphatemia (90).

Travis and her co-workers (91) have proposed that the locus of the effect of very low levels of serum phosphate on red cell glycolysis is at the G3PD reaction, where inorganic phosphate is incorporated into the glycolytic sequence. Accordingly, an accumulation of red cell glycolytic intermediates proximal to G3PD in the Embden-Meyerhof pathway could be demonstrated in a patient with severe hypophosphatemia.

In contrast, when the plasma phosphate concentration is continuously elevated, the concentrations of ATP (and usually 2,3-DPG) are increased. Thus a highly significant correlation has been found between red cell ATP and serum inorganic phosphate in growing children up to 12 years of age whose plasma phosphate and red cell ATP levels exceed those of normal adults (92). Similarly in chronic uremia ATP levels are commonly elevated up to twice normal (93).

The Adenine Nucleotide Precursor

It is now well established that the adenine nucleotides (ATP, ADP, and AMP) of circulating red cells undergo continuous turnover (94) and that their maintenance depends on an external supply of a preformed adenine moiety, since mature red cells lack the enzymatic capability for de novo purine synthesis (95). The size of the adenine nucleotide pool of red cells is clearly sensitive to changes in plasma inorganic phosphate. It is not clear, however, whether the locus of this action of phosphate lies in the glycolytic sequence (i.e., at G3PD) or in the reactions by which the adenine nucleotide precursor is incorporated into AMP. Both adenine and adenosine can be incorporated into red cell adenine nucleotides by the reactions shown in Figure 1–9. The requisite cofactor for adenine incorporation is phosphoribosyl pyrophosphate (PRPP), a product of ribose-5-phosphate derived from the hexose monophosphate shunt and ATP. PRPP synthetase, which is a logical point of control for the incorporation of adenine nucleotides into red cells, is inhibited by several red cell metabolites acting at their physiologic concentrations (96). This inhibition, which has allosteric properties, is strikingly alleviated by inorganic phosphate, thus offering an attractive explanation for at least part of the observed dependence of red cell adenine nucleotides on external plasma phosphate concentration. A weakness in this formulation is the paucity of convincing evidence that adenine occurs in normal plasma, although it is conceivable that a rapid transfer from liver cell to red cell could occur.

By contrast, adenosine has been found in normal plasma draining the myocardium (97). This compound can also enter the red cell adenine nucleotide pool via the enzyme adenosine kinase (98). It is noteworthy that both of these possible precursors for ATP require the expenditure of ATP (reactions 3, 4, and 5 in Fig. 1–9) and thus a functioning glycolytic pathway. Thus part of the observed phosphate dependence of adenine nucleotide incorporation could result from the effects of phosphate on glycolytic rate at the level of G3PD.

At least one other regulator than phosphate must be operative in the regulation of red cell adenine nucleotide levels since they have been shown to be elevated in severe anemia. This elevation occurs in normal cells transfused into an anemic recipient and does not therefore represent the presence of young red cells or a developmental abnormality in the marrow. It has been postulated that fluctuations in plasma adenine account for this increment (99), but the presence of adenine in anemic plasma needs confirmation.

Lactate and Pyruvate

Considerable confusion has arisen from ex vivo experiments in which red cells are incubated with various glycolytic stimulants or inhibitors which for various reasons alter the availability of NAD. In an Erlenmeyer flask with glucose or nucleosides as substrate, the G3PD reaction and the LDH reaction of red cells are usually strictly coupled, because the substrate for the latter reaction, pyruvate, is generated exclusively by glycolytic reactions which pass through the former reaction, G3PD. Since the total pool of NAD-NADH is very small in red cells, any combination of circumstances leading to the accumulation of 2,3-DPG, such as incubation with phosphate or in alkaline pH, soon exhausts the available NAD and severely limits the rate of G3PD. The result may be an extraordinary accumulation of triose phosphates proximal to G3PD. Extrapolation of this phenomenon to the in vivo situation, however, is not possible, since red cells in the circulation are

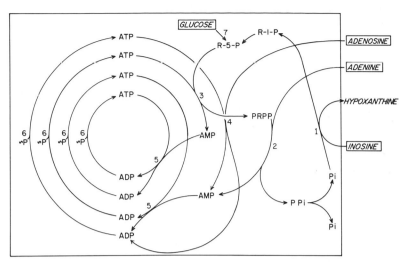

Figure 1–9.   Adenine nucleotide metabolism in red cells. Important substrates are in boxes. Numerals represent the following enzymes: (1) purine nucleoside phosphorylase (EC 2.4.2.1.); (2) adenine phosphoribosyl transferase (EC 2.4.2.7.); (3) ribose phosphate pyrophosphokinase or PRPP synthetase (EC 2.7.6.1.); (4) adenosine kinase (EC 2.7.1.20); (5) adenylate kinase (EC 2.7.4.3); (6) ATP generating reactions of anaerobic glycolysis: phosphoglycerate kinase (EC 2.7.2.3) and pyruvate kinase (EC 2.7.1.40); (7) dehydrogenase reactions of the hexose monophosphate shunt: glucose-6-phosphate dehydrogenase (EC 1.1.1.49) and phosphogluconate dehydrogenase (EC 1.1.1.44). (This figure has been modified by adding the adenosine loop to the figure of Minakami, S., and Yoshikawa, H.: *Proceedings 11th Congress of the International Society of Blood Transfusion.* Basel: S. Karger, 1968, pp. 168–177.)

continuously exposed to exogenous pyruvate, which freely permeates the red cell membrane and does not depend on the glycolytic production through red cell G3PD. Thus triose accumulation, which is a rather constant accompaniment of incubations in vitro with glycolytic stimulants, does not occur under similar circumstances in vivo. The NAD/NADH ratio of red cells is dependent on the *plasma* lactate/pyruvate ratio and is apparently independent of red cell glycolytic reactions. It is unlikely that physiologic or pathologic alterations in lactate and pyruvate are ever of sufficient magnitude to significantly affect red cell glycolysis, in constrast to protons and phosphate.

Effect of the Spleen on Red Cell Metabolism

Several observations point to the potential importance of the spleen in inducing metabolic alterations in red cells. It has been reported that the level of 2,3-DPG in red cells from patients with hereditary spherocytosis prior to splenectomy is low or barely normal despite anemia and reticu-

locytosis, both of which characteristically are associated with increased 2,3-DPG levels (100). As will be described subsequently, the spleen serves as a giant, hostile detention center for spherocytic cells of various types. The particular environmental properties of the spleen which may affect red cell metabolism are (1) possible glucose deprivation, (2) acidotic pH, and (3) hypoxia. The level of 2,3-DPG has been shown to be very sensitive to the intracellular pH of the red cell, tending to fall with acidosis and rise in alkalosis (101). It seems likely, therefore, that prolonged repetitious exposure of red cells to the acidotic environment of the spleen may cause sufficient lowering of the level of 2,3-DPG to be detected in those cells which are "out on bail" in the general circulation.

Another example of how the spleen may affect the metabolism of certain red cells is the peculiar case of the PK-deficient reticulocyte, to which allusion has already been made. The critical factor in the premature destruction of these cells seems to be hypoxia, since the young PK cell has been shown to be inordinately sensitive to interruption of its oxidative energy-producing pathways (14, 102). ATP production in these cells ceases at oxygen tensions well above those which might prevail within splenic cords jammed with rapidly respiring reticulocytes (102). Since PK-deficient reticulocytes seem to do quite well without glucose (14), it is very likely that hypoxia is their main splenic detriment.

Interactions Between Membrane and Hemoglobin

Normal Hemoglobin

The normal relationships between hemoglobin and membrane remain to be clarified. It is clear that they are in extremely close contiguity and that numerous interactions which might affect the function of either hemoglobin or the membrane are possible. One example is the observation of Sirs (103), which has been confirmed by LaCelle and Weed (104), that deoxygenation of red cells is associated with increased rigidity of the cell membrane. LaCelle has attributed this effect to increased binding of intracellular ATP by deoxyhemoglobin. This, in turn, is postulated to upset the delicate equilibrium between membrane, ATP, and Ca^{2+}, inducing a conformational change in the "structural protein" underlying the red cell membrane. An alternative possibility, that deoxyhemoglobin itself binds to red cell membranes in such a way as to alter its deformability, has not been excluded.

Numerous examples of pathologic interactions between abnormal hemoglobins and their surrounding membranes have been described which have clarified the hemolytic mechanisms operating in these disorders. In general, these interactions reflect alterations in the physical properties of the mutant hemoglobins. Three general processes have been recognized: gelation (hemoglobin S), crystallization (hemoglobin C), and denaturation (hemoglobin Köln and other unstable hemoglobins and alpha chains in beta thalassemia which form Heinz bodies).

Hemoglobin S

The polymerization of hemoglobin S into long, linear aggregates with a helical structure has been well demonstrated by electron microscopy (6). It is not surprising that these relatively ordered structures should drastically alter the rheologic properties of individual sickled cells by changing their internal viscosity. It has not been appreciated until recently, however, that the repeated sickling and unsickling of affected red cells eventually damages the cell membrane in a manner which no longer depends on the presence of sickled hemoglobin (105). An early consequence of sickling is a rapid increase in the leakage of intracellular potassium out of the cell (106). As the process is repeated, the cells can be shown to lose portions of membrane containing varying amounts of hemoglobin during reoxygenation and the restoration of discoid form (107). Since continuous loss of fragments of the cell inevitably alters the surface to volume ratio, a progressively more spherocytic and undeformable cell results. Eventually these cells become unable to regain their discoid form during reoxygenation and remain "irreversibly sickled cells," even though the hemoglobin loses its parallel fiberlike orientation. Furthermore, if these cells are osmotically hemolyzed and then restored to normal tonicity, they return to their distorted elongated form despite losing most of their hemoglobin. It has been suggested that linear aggregations of helical hemoglobin S are directly attached to the membrane, leaving an imprint on its internal surface when viewed by freeze-etching techniques (108).

Hemoglobin C

The fundamental physical alteration induced by the abnormal cationic lysine group in hemoglobin C is a decrease in its solubility, with a resulting propensity to form crystals. Increased molecular organization approaching a precrystalline state can be viewed with freeze-etching techniques, and actual rhomboid crystals may be seen in the most aged hemoglobin C–containing red cells (109). The surface site of the substitution of the hemoglobin molecule and its strong positive charge probably allows increased electrostatic bonding between adjacent tetramers. The curious morphologic result of this altered physical state is the formation of target cells which demonstrate extensive membranous folds in the center of the discoid C hemoglobin cell. These cells do not seem to have an expanded surface area as is the case in jaundiced patients (see below). Paradoxically, the hemolytic mechanism seems to involve loss of membrane, perhaps in the spleen, so that target cells and spherocytes coexist in the same smear (109). The exact relationship between the mutant hemoglobin and the central protuberance, i.e. targeting, is unknown, but it does not seem analogous to the target cells which occur in hypochromic, asplenic, or jaundiced individuals.

Unstable Hemoglobins

The molecular basis for the denaturation and precipitation of normal hemoglobin during exposure to oxidant compounds has been outlined, and it is now appropriate to resume the sequence of events leading to the ultimate demise of Heinz body–containing cells. The hemoglobin molecule, like many others which must function in aqueous medium, hides many of its reactive and nonpolar groups internally so as to enhance its solubility. Unwinding of the polypeptide chains, therefore, by exposing nonpolar amino acid residues drastically lowers the solubility of the protein and at the same time exposes formerly buried sulfhydryl groups. Electron microscopic studies of oxidant hemolysis in rabbits have shown that these amorphous aggregates form near the center of the cell, but with further denaturation they coalesce and migrate to the periphery (110). The studies of Jacob have clearly shown the avidity of Heinz bodies for the cell membrane and provide convincing evidence that the linkage is a covalent one between reactive sulfhydryl groups on the membrane and on hemoglobin (83). These mixed disulfide bonds persist even after the soluble hemoglobin has been dispersed by osmotic hemolysis, and Heinz body–laden ghosts are strikingly apparent within the spleen of animals following administration of phenylhydrazine (111). A similar sequence of events almost certainly occurs with mutant hemoglobins which are intrinsically unstable and in the various forms of thalas-

semia where excess alpha or beta chains also precipitate and bind to red cell membranes. Jacob has suggested that heme-depleted hemoglobin Köln may blockade membrane SH groups before visible Heinz bodies appear (83).

The functional correlates of these newly recognized interactions can be predicted from studies of cells in which reactive sulfhydryl groups have been blocked by parachloromercuribenzoate (PCMB). It has been shown by such studies that sulfhydryl groups are of critical importance in the maintenance of the normally low cation permeability of the red cell membrane (112). Not surprisingly, therefore, increased cation flux has been noted in Heinz body–containing cells. As previously noted, this probably contributes to the low levels of ATP and rapid glycolysis in these cells because of compensatory stimulation of the membrane cation pump. Heinz bodies have also been shown to render the cell membranes rigid (113) and to provoke rapid selective K^+ leakage out of the cell (114).

Interactions Between Membrane and Spleen

Filtration

The spleen has been integrated into the schematic erythron of Fig. 1–1 in order to dramatize its extensive involvement in the life cycle of the red cell. For detailed yet concise elaboration of the intimate details of this crucial organ, the reader is referred to one of the several articles by Weiss (115) as well as the classic review of Crosby (116). Using Figure 1–10 (from Weiss), the essential structure of this elaborate obstacle course for red cells can be readily ascertained. A simplistic concept which emerges is that a critical juncture for the red cell is its escape from the cordal compartment of the red pulp into the splenic sinuses which, just as with bone marrow, drain into the general circulation. The adventitial endothelial cells lining the sinusoids are arranged longitudinally, with circumferential bands of reticulin forming a rather flimsy basement membrane. The whole structure is aptly described by Weiss as "barrel-like," with elongated sinusoidal lin-

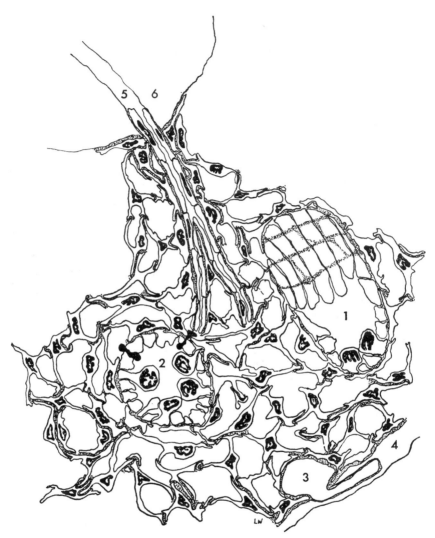

Figure 1–10. A schematic depiction of the reticular connective tissue in a lobule of the spleen. The reticular cells and fibers of the red pulp are drawn in some detail as is a bifurcating arterial vessel (5). The white pulp (6), a pulp vein (3), and trabecula (4) are barely outlined.

The arterial vessel posseses a rather high endothelium. It passes from white pulp, through the marginal zone, and into red pulp. It bifurcates, one branch coming up close to a sinus (2), the other ending rather centrally in the cordal tissue between sinuses 1 and 2. Sinus 2 is cut in cross section; the lining cells are roughly cuboidal in cross section, their nuclear portion protruding deeply into the lumen. The basement membrane is defective, and two erythrocytes may be seen in passage across the sinus wall. Sinus 1 is exposed in longitudinal section above, the cut grazing its basal portion and thereby providing a surface view of the basement membrane and the base of the lining cells. Note the major transverse element in the defective basement membrane. Below, the sinus is seen in cross section. The reticular meshwork tends to be circumferential about the sinus but elsewhere branches in a rather regular way. The reticular cells branch and their cytoplasmic processes overlap those of contiguous cells. As exposed in section, the reticular fibers lie between the overlapping portions of reticular cells. The reticulum is seen to be continuous with the outer or adventitial layer of both sinuses, arterial vessels, and pulp vein as well as with the surface layer of the trabecula.

This scheme shows the fixed elements in a lobule of the spleen with the exception of the two erythrocytes of sinus 2. The meshes of the reticulum are commonly filled with free cells, so solidly, indeed, that the reticular meshwork in most preparations is scarcely discernible. Perhaps it may be best demonstrated with silver or staining methods which selectively reveal the extracellular reticulum. The reticular cells, particularly of the cords and adventitial to the sinus, may be phagocytic, but no effort is made to show this here. (From Wennberg, E., and Weiss, L.: Annu. Rev. Med. *20:*29, 1969.)

ing cells representing staves and the discontinuous reticulin fibers representing hoops. It is between the barrel staves that those red cells which have entered the cordal compartment must squeeze in order to return to the circulation and at which point they are in most jeopardy. The adventitial cells are phagocytic and have an excellent chance for tactile scrutiny of the cells which pass between and among them. In order to filter through these interstices, the red cell must be freely deformable, since the apparent fenestrations are considerably smaller than the diameter of the discoid cell. The spleen, then, represents the body's fine mesh filter, which can recognize and detain cells with very subtle physical defects. The fact that hereditary spherocytes, which have been shown to have definite though subtle defects in deformability, can circulate with impunity only in splenectomized individuals clearly establishes that this "ultrafiltration" is a unique function of the spleen which cannot be assumed by other reticuloendothelial organs.

Pitting

Another unique role of the spleen is its ability to remove particulate inclusions from normal red cells without damaging them, a function which can best be appreciated by studies of red blood cells from splenectomized individuals. Such cells contain various kinds of debris, some of which are left over from early life, e.g., nuclear remnants (Howell-Jolly bodies) or siderotic granules (Pappenheimer bodies), and some of which seem to form continuously during the cell's life. The latter inclusions, which have been called autophagic vacuoles (117), may arise from internalization of the cell membrane (endocytosis). They are particularly prominent in red cells of newborn and premature infants, probably reflecting the functional immaturity of the neonatal spleen (118).

When cells containing these particles are transfused into recipients with normally functioning spleens, the inclusions disappear at a rate which is much faster than that of the transfused red cells which survive normally. The exact dumping site for this rubbish is not known with certainty, but studies of red cells containing Heinz bodies offer suggestive evidence that it lies at the critical sinusoidal/cordal boundary (115).

Resuming the narrative of the Heinz body, which is by now firmly attached to the red cell membrane, there is convincing evidence from electron microscopic studies (Fig. 1–11) that the Heinz bodies are retained in the splenic cords as the red cell squeezes through into the sinusoids. This process causes a considerable wastage of the red cell membrane, which is retained with the rigid concretion and phagocytized by the sinusoidal lining cells. It is not difficult to conceive how repetitious encounters of this sort will result in sphering of cells due to progressive loss of their surface area. Since sphered red cells also lack the requisite deformability to squeeze through the barrel staves, they undergo increasingly long stasis and eventually hemolyze within the spleen.

It is of interest that splenectomy in the Heinz body hemolytic anemias due to unstable hemoglobins does not necessarily result in improved red cell longevity. After splenectomy, Heinz bodies are readily visible in virtually all circulating red cells, while they are absent before splenectomy. Apparently the noxious effect of these retained concretions is about an even trade-off for the morbidity of the recurrent splenic Heinzectomies.

Polishing

Another distinctive morphologic feature of the asplenic state is thinning and "targeting" of red cells due to a redundancy of their membrane. The excess surface area is reflected in a significant increase in both phospholipid and cholesterol and a decrease in osmotic fragility compared with normal red cells, as can be predicted from Figure 1–5 (119). It seems likely, then, that another splenic function is the removal of surface membrane from normal red cells, a process which might be likened to "polishing." The exact timing of this process is not clear at present. It could represent only the remodeling of reticulocytes ("circumcision") or the loss of membrane during the

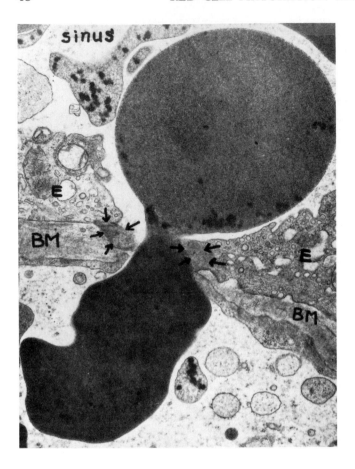

Figure 1–11. An interendothelial slit of the splenic sinus occupied by an erythrocyte is shown transversely. A portion of the erythrocyte with normal density has passed from cord to sinus, leaving a dark portion containing Heinz bodies in the cord. The width of the slit was restricted by the microfilamentous bands (arrows) of the endothelial cells (E). Heinz bodies are induced by a single intraperitoneal injection of phenylhydrazine (0.1 mg. per gm.) into the rat. BM indicates the basement membrane (× 25,000). (From Chen, L. T., and Weiss, L.: Role of the sinus wall in the passage of erythrocytes through the spleen. Blood *41*:529–537, 1973, by permission of Grune & Stratton.)

pitting of autophagic vacuoles, which apparently continues throughout the cell's life span, or both.

Phagocytosis

As a filter, the spleen recognizes and sorts out red cells primarily on the basis of their deformability characteristics. However, a variety of other surface properties can be recognized by macrophages as red cells percolate through the splenic cords. Thus another prime requisite for survival of red cells is their ability to resist the potentially damaging embraces of these voracious scavengers. Such cell-cell interactions have been studied advantageously in vitro with macrophages from various sources. One rather poorly characterized feature of immature reticulocytes is their "stickiness," which may contribute to their predilection to remain in the spleen to undergo further maturation (120). A more discrete surface feature, the presence of

IgG on the red cell membrane, allows intimate contact between macrophages and red cells (see below). Depletion of coating substances by washing red cells in saline also greatly enhances subsequent phagocytosis by macrophages (121). Similarly, metabolic depletion induced by incubating red cells in vitro (122), by aging them in preservatives, or by preparing ATP poor ghosts (123) renders the red cell more palatable to macrophages.

Interactions Between Membrane and Plasma Factors

Cholesterol Exchange

In previous sections we have examined the dynamics of membrane maintenance and repair by active, energy-dependent processes intrinsic to the cell. In addition to the ATP-dependent turnover of fatty acids, there are other significant dynamic exchanges between membrane and plasma cholesterol which appear to be completely passive; these are depicted on the "surface" axis in Figure 1–5. One such process can critically affect the physical properties of the cell membrane by controlling the amount of free cholesterol on the cell surface. The studies of Cooper and Jandl (124) have demonstrated the direct correlation between membrane cholesterol and membrane surface area as judged by the critical hemolytic volume of the red cell. Virtually the entire complement of cholesterol on the cell membrane is unesterified "free cholesterol" and is in dynamic equilibrium with the free cholesterol of plasma.

In some manner which is as yet incompletely understood, an important mediator of this exchange is a plasma enzyme, lecithin-cholesterol acyl transferase (LCAT) (125). In conditions where this enzyme is inhibited or deficient, such as in obstructive liver disease or the inherited LCAT deficiency, cholesterol accumulates in red cell membranes, giving them the characteristic "target cell" morphology on a dried slide. This cell has a relative excess of surface area to volume, and accordingly its osmotic fragility is markedly reduced. However, in most instances its survival within the circulation is unaffected by this acquired ectomorphism.

In a small subgroup of patients with rather severe parenchymal liver disease, extreme membrane cholesterol accumulation occurs, and red cells acquire spiny membrane projections, which has led to their designation as "spur cells" (126). At this point, the expanded cell surface begins to diminish, probably by avulsion of these spiny processes by shearing forces within the circulation. Now the cell begins to lose its agility, and the decreased osmotic fragility returns to normal. As membrane loss progresses further, the cells are destroyed, primarily by the spleen.

It will be appreciated from Figure 1–5 that a microspherocyte and a target cell are essentially opposite cells on the same axis. An interesting clinical correlate of this relationship has been noted by Cooper, who was able to restore cholesterol to the membrane of hereditary spherocytic cells by injecting them into patients with obstructive jaundice, whose own cells were markedly targeted (119). Survival of the membrane-poor spherocytes in the jaundiced recipient was significantly greater than expected, and their osmotic fragility returned toward normal, indicating expansion of their surface area during circulation. The occasional observation of a sudden decrease in hemolysis in patients with hereditary spherocytosis who become jaundiced by an impacted gallstone seems to have its basis in this relationship also.

Incomplete Antibodies

This voluminous topic is beyond the scope of this chapter, but it is discussed in Chapters 8 and 9. However, an important new understanding of the hemolytic mechanism in certain antibody-induced disorders fits nicely within our proposed conceptual framework, since it clarifies a three-way interaction between the cell membrane, antibody, and phagocytes of the spleen and reticuloendothelial system. LoBuglio and co-workers (127), drawing upon the earlier morphologic observations of Policard and Bessis (128) and Archer (129) have demonstrated the binding of red cells coated with IgG antibodies to macrophages in a circumferential ring called a rosette. A striking feature of the in vitro association of the macrophages with coated red cells is the partial sphering of the red cells, which become dense and depleted of membrane. Further studies by Abramson described elsewhere in this volume demonstrate with electron micrographs that fragments of cell membrane are actually engulfed by the macrophage during this period of contact. The phenomenon is relatively specific for certain IgG subtypes (1 and 3) and implies that macrophages have receptor sites on their surfaces which can detect and bind red cells with minute amounts of surface IgG.

These important observations have resolved some confusing aspects of certain types of immune hemolysis by clarifying the importance of the reticuloendothelial cell in the hemolytic mechanism. Spherocytosis is the morphologic hallmark of disorders such as erythroblastosis fetalis and autoimmune hemolytic anemias which are associated with incomplete IgG antibodies on the surface of red cells. Yet when cells are coated with such antibodies in vitro, no exceptional loss of membrane occurs during prolonged incubations. Small aliquots of cells coated with amounts of antibody which are almost undetectable by conventional Coombs' testing are quantitatively removed during a single passage through the spleen (130). However, only when anti–red cell antibodies are injected directly into the circulation in quantities sufficient to coat all circulating red cells does marked peripheral spherocytosis occur (131). The circulating spherocytes in this animal model show marked loss of cell membrane, including both phospholipid and cholesterol. Thus the immune production of circulating spherocytes requires both the coating of red cells with incomplete antibodies and a reticuloendothelial system which is saturated with coated red cells. Only when the ratio of unoccupied phagocytes to coated red cells is relatively low can the partially phagocytized, membrane-depleted red cells escape temporarily into the circulation. Repetitious nibbling of this sort eventually renders the cells so rigid that they will be unable to evade complete phagocytosis.

Complement

Electron microscopy has afforded an extraordinarily graphic portrayal of the devastating effects upon the red cell of activation and completion of the complement sequence. The clinical observation that antibodies which fix complement may be hemolytic in vitro and that intravascular hemolysis may occur without mediation of the host's reticuloendothelial system suggests that a fundamentally different hemolytic mechanism occurs in the presence of such antibodies. Electron micrographs in a number of complement-mediated systems have shown regular, discrete, circular areas of lucency in cell membranes with a uniform diameter of approximately 100 Å (132). In contrast to the apparent ease with which the membrane seals over defects due to pitting or fragmentation of small buds or spines, the complement-induced defects appear to be irreparable. While a single defect does not apparently allow direct leakage of hemoglobin into the medium, it profoundly alters cation permeability and rapidly induces colloid osmotic hemolysis (133).

Most human cells are relatively resistant to the completion of the complement system as compared with those of other species. Thus it is not unusual to detect the presence of C3 on red cells without any evidence of intravascular hemolysis. Although a macrophage receptor site for C3 on red cells has been reported, this has been disputed, and the normal survival of cells heavily coated with C3 makes the significance of such an interaction unlikely (see Chapter 8). Thus the role of complement in extravascular hemolytic processes remains to be clarified.

Fragmentation

The last important concept to be discussed, red cell fragmentation, has only recently come into vogue; in contrast to previously described hemolytic mechanisms, it received its major impetus from a clinical observation rather than an in vitro technique. While the fact that red cells could undergo traumatic fragmentation in vitro had received periodic isolated attention, it was not until the clinical description of microangiopathic hemolytic anemia by Brain et al. (134) that widespread recognition of the importance of this phenomenon in the body was recognized. The observation was a morphologic one, i.e., the presence of helmet cells or schistocytes in the blood of patients with various forms of microvascular disease, such as malignant hypertension and disseminated carcinomatosis. The important deduction which was made by Brain et al. was that the abnormal morphology represented an acquired traumatic injury rather than a manifestation of disordered erythropoiesis. Subsequently, the precise process by which red cells may be transected has been photographed in vitro by forcing cells through a loose fibrin meshwork, a situation closely paralleling the circumstances in diffuse intravascular coagulation (32).

Weed has greatly extended the concept of red cell fragmentation and traced its history (53). Fragmentation occurs by a great many different mechanisms, ranging from the pinching off of buds during unsickling to the partial dissolution of pieces of cell membrane in metabolically depleted red cells. In some instances, membrane may be lost without any loss of hemoglobin, while in others, as demonstrated by the partial phagocytosis of red cells by macrophages, both hemoglobin and membrane are lost. However, whether or not hemoglobin is lost within the fragment, the inevitable result for the cell is a relative loss of membrane, since more surface will be required to enclose the residual hemoglobin. Red cells accomplish this self-sealing job by rounding up and becoming more spherocytic. An inevitable consequence of "sphering," as previously noted, is a decrease in the ability of the red cell to become deformed, since it has less membrane to accommodate its bulk. Repetitious fragmentation then, regardless of cause, renders the red cell at risk in the circulation.

Summary

In attempting to provide connective tissue both for the erythron and for the other chapters of this volume, I have rather arbitrarily extracted what is currently highly ordered collagen from amorphous ground substance. This has been done with the full awareness that future advances in understanding the red cell will probably derive from the latter fraction, and that even collagen undergoes continuous turnover. If this chapter has merit, it lies in its organization rather than its details. Most of what needs to be conveyed can be found in the Table of Contents and by a careful study of the illustrations. Hopefully it will provide the reader with a slightly new way of looking at the red cell in its environment and pull together in one place many concepts which have taken me 10 years to learn.

References

1. Castle, W. B., and Minot, G. R.: *Pathologic Physiology and Clinical Description of the Anemias.* London, Oxford University Press, 1936.
2. Finch, C. A.: *Red Cell Manual.* Seattle, University of Washington, 1969.
3. Fisher, J. W.: Erythropoietin: Pharmacology, biogenesis and control of production. Pharmacol. Rev. 24:459, 1972.
4. Metcalf, D., and Moore, M. A.: *Haemopoietic Cells: Their Origin, Migration and Differ-*
entiation. (Frontiers of Biology Ser., No. 24). Amsterdam, North-Holland, 1971.
5. Weiss, L.: The structure of bone marrow. Functional interrelationships of vascular and hematopoietic compartments in experimental hemolytic anemia: An electron microscopic study. J. Morphol. 117:467, 1965.
6. Harris, J. W., and Kellermeyer, R. W.: *The Red Cell. Production, Metabolism, Destruction: Normal and Abnormal.* Cambridge, Harvard University Press, 1970.
7. Bessis, M., and Breton-Gorius, J.: Nouvelles observations sur l'ilot érythroblastique et la rhophéocytose de la ferritine. Rev. Hémat. 14:165, 1959.
8. Kornfeld, S., and Gregory, W.: The identification and partial purification of lysosomes in human reticulocytes. Biochim. Biophys. Acta 177:615, 1969.
9. Bessis, M., and Bricka, M.: Aspect dynamique des cellules du sang. Son étude par la microcinématographie en contraste de phase. Rev. Hémat. 7:407, 1952.
10. Leblond, P. F., Lacelle, P. L., et al.: Cellular deformability. A possible determinant of the normal release of maturing erythrocytes from the bone marrow. Blood 37:40, 1971.
11. Jacob, H., Amsden, T., et al.: Membrane microfilaments of erythrocytes: Alterations in intact cells reproduces the hereditary spherocytosis syndrome. Proc. Natl. Acad. Sci. USA 69:471, 1972.
12. Skutelsky, E., and Danon, D.: An electron microscopic study of nucleus elimination from the late erythroblast. J. Cell. Biol. 33:625, 1967.
13. Isaacs, R.: Physiologic histology of the bone marrow: The mechanism of the development of blood cells and their liberation into the peripheral circulation. Folia Haematol. (Leipz.) 40:395, 1930.
14. Keitt, A. S.: Pyruvate kinase deficiency and related disorders of red cell glycolysis. Am. J. Med. 41:762, 1966.
15. Shattil, S. J., and Cooper, R. A.: Maturation of macroreticulocyte membranes in vivo. J. Lab. Clin. Med. 79:215, 1972.
16. Ganzoni, A. M., Oakes, R., et al.: Red cell aging in vivo. J. Clin. Invest. 50:1373, 1971.
17. Brecher, G., and Stohlman, F.: Reticulocyte size and erythropoietic stimulation. Proc. Soc. Exp. Biol. Med. 107:887, 1961.
18. Reiff, R. H., Nutter, J. Y., et al.: Relative number of marrow reticulocytes. Am. J. Clin. Pathol. 30:199, 1958.
19. Robinson, S. H.: Formation of bilirubin from erythroid and nonerythroid sources. Semin. Hematol. 9:43, 1972.
20. Bunn, H. F.: Erythrocyte destruction and hemoglobin catabolism. Semin. Hematol. 9:3, 1972.
21. Tenhunen, R.: The enzymatic degradation of heme. Semin. Hematol. 9:19, 1972.
22. Sjöstrand, T.: Endogenous formation of carbon monoxide in man under normal and pathologic conditions. Scand. J. Clin. Lab. Invest. 1:201, 1949.
23. Elder, G., Gray, C. H., et al.: Bile pigment fate in gastrointestinal tract. Semin. Hematol. 9:71, 1972.

24. Holroyde, C. P., Oski, F. A., et al.: The "pocked" erythrocyte. New Engl. J. Med. *281*:516, 1969.

25. Zarkowsky, H. S., Oski, F. A., et al.: Congenital hemolytic anemia with high sodium, low potassium red cells. I. Studies of membrane permeability. New Engl. J. Med. 278:593, 1968.

26. Cooper, R. A., and Jandl, J. H.: Bile salts and cholesterol in the pathogenesis of target cells in obstructive jaundice. J. Clin. Invest. 47:809, 1968.

27. Goldstein, B. D., and Harber, L. C.: Erythropoietic protoporphyria: lipid peroxidation and red cell membrane damage associated with photohemolysis. J. Clin. Invest. *51*: 892, 1972.

28. Kalderon, A. E., Kikkawa, Y., et al.: Chronic toxoplasmosis associated with severe hemolytic anemia. Arch. Intern. Med. *114*:95, 1964.

29. Ricketts, W. E.: Bartonella bacilliformis anemia (Oroya fever). Blood *3*:1025, 1948.

30. Mentzer, W. C., Jr., Baehner, R. L., et al.: Selective reticulocyte destruction in erythrocyte pyruvate kinase deficiency. J. Clin. Invest. *50*:688, 1971.

31. Griggs, R. C.: Lead poisoning: hematological aspects. Progr. Hematol. *4*:117, 1964.

32. Bull, B. S., and Kuhn, I. N.: The production of schistocytes by fibrin strands (a scanning electron microscope study). Blood *35*:104, 1970.

33. Perkash, A., and Sarup, B. M.: Red cell abnormalities after snake bite. J. Trop. Med. Hyg. *75*:85, 1972.

34. Beutler, E.: Drug-induced hemolytic anemia. Pharmacol. Rev. *21*:73, 1969.

35. Krantz, S. B., and Kao, V.: Studies on red cell aplasia. I. Demonstration of a plasma inhibitor to heme synthesis and an antibody to erythroblast nuclei. Proc. Nat. Acad. Sci. USA *58*:493, 1967.

36. Berk, P. D., Howe, R. B., et al.: Studies of bilirubin metabolism in normal adults. J. Clin. Invest. *48*:2176, 1969.

37. Nathan, D. G., and Gunn, R. B.: Thalassemia: the consequences of unbalanced hemoglobin synthesis. Am. J. Med. *41*:815, 1966.

38. London, I. M., and West, R.: Formation of bile pigment in pernicious anemia. J. Biol. Chem. *184*:359, 1950.

39. London, I. M., West, R., et al.: On the origin of bile pigment in normal man. J. Biol. Chem. *184*:351, 1950.

40. Bessis, M., Breton-Gorius, J., et al.: Rôle possible de l'hémoglobine accompagnant le noyau des érythroblastes dans l'origine de la stercobiline éliminée précocement. C. R. Acad. Sci. (Paris) *252*:2300, 1961.

41. Valentine, W. N., and Tanaka, K. R.: Pyruvate kinase deficiency and other enzyme-deficiency hereditary hemolytic anemias, In *The Metabolic Basis of Inherited Disease.* 3rd ed. Stanbury, J. B., Wyngaarden, J. B., et al. (eds.), New York, McGraw-Hill, 1972.

42. Nathan, D. G., Oski, F. A., et al.: Life span and organ sequestration of red cells in pyruvate kinase deficiency. New Engl. J. Med. *278*: 73, 1968.

43. Landaw, S. A., Callahan, E. W., Jr., et al.: Catabolism of heme in vivo: Comparison of the simultaneous production of bilirubin and carbon monoxide. J. Clin. Invest. *49*:914, 1970.

44. Haining, R. G., Cowger, M. L., et al.: Congenital erythropoietic porphyria. I. Case report, special studies and therapy. Am. J. Med. *45*:625, 1968.

45. Coburn, R. F.: Enhancement by phenobarbital and diphenylhydantoin of carbon monoxide production in normal man. New Engl. J. Med. *283*:512, 1970.

46. Ashby, W.: The determination of the length of life of transfused blood corpuscles in man. J. Exp. Med. *34*:127, 1919.

47. Pearson, H. A.: The binding of Cr^{51} to hemoglobin. II. In vivo elution rates of Cr^{51} from Hb CC Hb CS and placental red cells. Blood *28*:563, 1966.

48. Pimstone, N. R.: Renal degradation of hemoglobin. Semin. Hematol. *9*:31, 1972.

49. Jandl, J. H.: Leaky red cells. Blood *26*:367, 1965.

50. Wilbrandt, W.: Osmotische Natur Sogennanter nicht-osmotischer Hämolysen (Kolloidosmotische Hämolyse). Pfluegers Arch. *245*: 22, 1941.

51. Jandl, J. H., Simmons, R. L., et al.: Red cell filtration in the pathogenesis of certain hemolytic anemias. Blood *28*:133, 1961.

52. Rand, R. P., and Burton, A. C.: Mechanical properties of the red cell membrane. I. Membrane stiffness and intracellular pressure. Biophys. J. *4*:115, 1964.

53. Weed, R. I.: Disorders of the red cell membrane: history and perspectives. Semin. Hematol. *7*:249, 1970.

54. LaCelle, P.: Alterations of membrane deformability in hemolytic anemias. Semin. Hematol. *7*:355, 1970.

55. Dunham, P. B., and Gunn, R. B.: Adenosine triphosphate and active cation transport in red blood cell membranes. Arch. Intern. Med. *129*:241, 1972.

56. Parker, J. C., and Hoffman, J. F.: The role of membrane phosphoglycerate kinase in the control of glycolytic rate by active transport in human red blood cells. J. Gen. Physiol. *50*:893, 1967.

57. Schrier, S. L.: Studies of the metabolism of human erythrocyte membranes. J. Clin. Invest. *42*:756, 1963.

58. Whittam, R., and Ager, M. E.: The connection between active cation transport and metabolism in human erythrocytes. Biochem. J. *97*:214, 1965.

59. Segel, G. B., Feig, S. A., et al.: An essential role for phosphoglycerate kinase dependent red cell cation transport (abstract). Accepted for presentation to the American Society of Hematology, Chicago, Illinois. Dec. 1–4, 1973.

60. Gardos, G., and Straub, F. B.: Uber die Rolle der Adenosintriphosphorsäure (ATP) in der K-Permeabilität der menschlichen roten Blutkörperchen. Acta Physiol. Acad. Sci. Hung. *12*:1, 1957.

61. Nathan, D. G., and Shohet, S. B.: Erythrocyte ion transport defects and hemolytic anemia:

"Hydrocytosis" and "dessicytosis." Semin. Hematol. 7:381, 1970.

62. Blum, R. M., and Hoffman, J. F.: Carrier mediation of Ca-induced K transport and its inhibition in red blood cells (abstract). Fed. Proc. 29:663, 1970.

63. Brecher, G., and Bessis, M.: Present status of spiculed red cells and their relationship to the discocyte-echinocyte transformation: A critical review. Blood 40:333, 1972.

64. Shohet, S. B.: Hemolysis and changes in erythrocyte membrane lipids. New Engl. J. Med. 286:577, 1972.

65. Oliviera, M. M., and Vaughan, M.: Incorporation of fatty acids into phospholipids of erythrocyte membranes. J. Lipid Res. 5:156, 1964.

66. Shohet, S. B., Nathan, D. G., et al.: Stages in the incorporation of fatty acids into red blood cells. J. Clin. Invest. 47:1096, 1968.

67. Weed, R. I., LaCelle, P. L., et al.: Metabolic dependence of red cell deformability. J. Clin. Invest. 48:795, 1969.

68. Szasz, I.: Structure and function of erythrocytes. IV. The role of nucleotides and bivalent cations in determining the shape of normal and tryspin treated erythrocytes. Acta Biochim. Biophys. Acad. Sci. Hung. 5:399, 1970.

69. Lessin, L. S., and Bessis, M.: The discocyte-echinocyte equilibrium of the normal and pathological red cell. Blood 36:399, 1970.

70. LaCelle, P. L., and Weed, R. I.: The contribution of normal and pathologic erythrocytes to blood rheology, In Progress in Hematology. Vol VII. Brown, E. B., and Moore, C. V. (eds.), New York, Grune & Stratton, 1971.

71. Rosenthal, A. S., Kregenow, E. M., et al.: Some characteristics of a Ca²⁺-dependent ATPase activity associated with a group of erythrocyte membrane proteins which form fibrils. Biochim. Biophys. Acta. 196:254, 1970.

72. Schatzmann, H. J.: ATP-dependent Ca²⁺ extrusion from human red cells. Experientia 22:364, 1966.

73. Davis, P. W., and Vincenzi, F. F.: Ca-ATPase activation and NaK-ATPase inhibition as a function of calcium concentration in human red cell membranes. Life Sci. 10:401, 1971.

74. Szasz, I., Teitel, P., et al.: Structure and function of erythrocytes. V. Differences in the Ca²⁺ dependence of the ATP requiring functions of erythrocytes. Acta Biochim. Biophys. Acad. Sci. Hung. 5:409, 1970.

75. Jandl, J. H.: The Heinz body hemolytic anemias. Ann. Intern. Med. 58:702, 1963.

76. Cohen, G., and Hochstein, P.: Generation of hydrogen peroxide in erythrocytes by hemolytic agents. Biochemistry 3:895, 1964.

77. Mills, G. C.: Hemoglobin catabolism. I. Glutathione peroxidase, an erythrocyte enzyme which protects hemoglobin from oxidative breakdown. J. Biol. Chem. 222:189, 1957.

78. Kosower, N. S., Marikovsky, Y., et al.: Glutathione oxidation and biophysical aspects of injury to human erythrocytes. J. Lab. Clin. Med. 78:533, 1971.

79. Srivastava, S. K., and Beutler, E.: Glutathione metabolism of the erythrocyte. The enzymic cleavage of glutathione-haemoglobin preparations by glutathione reductase. Biochem. J. 119:353, 1970.

80. Bunn, H. F., and Jandl, J. H.: Exchange of heme among hemoglobin molecules. Proc. Nat. Acad. Sci. USA 56:974, 1966.

81. Grimes, A. J., Meisler, H., et al.: Congenital Heinz body anaemia. Brit. J. Haematol. 10:281, 1964.

82. Jacob, H. S., Brain, M. C., et al.: Altered sulfhydryl reactivity of hemoglobin and red cell membranes in congenital Heinz body hemolytic anemia. J. Clin. Invest. 47:2664, 1968.

83. Jacob, H. S.: Mechanism of Heinz body formation and attachment to red cell membrane. Semin. Hematol. 7:341, 1970.

84. Rose, I. A., and Warms, J. V. B.: Control of glycolysis in the human red blood cell. J. Biol. Chem. 241:4848, 1966.

85. Roigas, H., Zoellner, E., et al.: Regulierende Faktoren der Methylenblaukatalyse in Erythrocyten. Eur. J. Biochem. 12:24, 1970.

86. Vestergaard-Bogind, B.: The transport of phosphate ions across the human red cell membrane. II. The influence of the concentration of inorganic phosphate on the kinetics of the uptake of (³²P) phosphate ions. Biochem. Biophys. Acta 66:93, 1963.

87. Gerlach, E., Deuticke, B., et al.: Phosphat permeabiltät und Phosphat-Stoffwechsel menschlicher Erythrocyten und Möglichkeiten ihrer experimentellen Beeinflussung. Pfluegers Arch. 280:243, 1964.

88. Lichtman, M. A., Miller, D. R., et al.: Erythrocyte adenosine triphosphate depletion during hypophosphatemia in a uremic subject. N. Engl. J. Med. 280:240, 1969.

89. Travis, S. F., Sugarman, H. J., et al.: Alterations of red-cell glycolytic intermediates and oxygen transport as a consequence of hypophosphatemia in patients receiving intravenous hyperalimentation. N. Engl. J. Med. 285:763, 1971.

90. Jacob, H. S., and Amsden, T.: Acute hemolytic anemia with rigid red cells in hypophosphatemia. New Engl. J. Med. 285:1446, 1971.

91. Travis, S. F., Sugerman, H. J., et al.: Alterations of red cell glycolytic intermediates and oxygen transport as a consequence of hypophosphatemia in patients receiving intravenous alimentation. New Engl. J. Med. 285:763, 1971.

92. Card, R. T., and Brain, M. C.: The "anemia" of childhood: Evidence for physiologic response to hyperphosphatemia. New Engl. J. Med. 288:388, 1973.

93. Lichtman, M. A., and Miller, D. R.: Erythrocyte glycolysis, 2,3-diphosphoglycerate and adenosine triphosphate concentration in uremic subjects: Relationship to extracellular phosphate concentration. J. Lab. Clin. Med. 76:267, 1970.

94. Lowy, B. A., Ramot, B., et al.: The biosynthesis of adenosine triphosphate and guanosine triphosphate in rabbit erythrocytes in vivo and in vitro. J. Biol. Chem. 235:2920, 1960.

95. Lowy, B. A., Williams, M. K., et al.: Enzymatic deficiencies of purine nucleotide synthesis in the human erythrocyte. J. Biol. Chem. 237:1622, 1962.

96. Hershko, A., Razin, A., et al.: Regulation of the

synthesis of 5-phosphoribosyl-1-pyrophosphate in intact red blood cells and in cell-free preparations. Biochim. Biophys. Acta. *184*:64, 1969.

97. Rubio, R., and Berne, R. M.: Release of adenosine by the normal myocardium in dogs and its relationship to the regulation of coronary resistance. Circ. Res. *25*:407, 1969.

98. Lerner, M. H., and Rubinstein, D.: The role of adenine and adenosine as precursors for adenine nucleotide synthesis by fresh and preserved human erythrocytes. Biochim. Biophys. Acta *224*:301, 1970.

99. Syllm-Rapoport, I., Jacobasch, G., et al.: On a regulatory system of the adenine level in the plasma connected with red cell maturation and its effect on the adenine nucleotides of the circulating erythrocyte. Lack of relation between ATP-level and life span of the erythrocyte. Blood *33*:617, 1969.

100. Palek, J., Mirčevová, L., et al.: 2,3-Diphosphoglycerate metabolism in hereditary spherocytosis. Brit. J. Haematol. *17*:59, 1969.

101. Rapoport, S., and Guest, J. M.: The decomposition of diphosphoglycerate in acidified blood: Its relationship to the reactions of the glycolytic cycle. J. Biol. Chem. *129*:781, 1939.

102. Mentzer, W. C., Jr., Baehner, R. L., et al.: Selective reticulocyte destruction in erythrocyte pyruvate kinase deficiency. J. Clin. Invest. *50*:688, 1971.

103. Sirs, J. A.: The measurement of the haematocrit and flexibility of erythrocytes with a centrifuge. Biorheology *5*:1, 1968.

104. LaCelle, P. L., and Weed, R. I.: Low oxygen pressure: A cause of erythrocyte membrane rigidity. J. Clin. Invest. *49*:54a, 1970.

105. Bertles, J. F., and Döbler, J.: Reversible and irreversible sickling: A distinction by electron microscopy. Blood *33*:884, 1969.

106. Tosteson, D. C.: Potassium exchange in sickle cell anemia red cells. J. Clin. Invest. *32*:608, 1951.

107. Jensen, W. N.: Fragmentation and the "freakish poikilocyte." Am. J. Med. Sci. *257*:355, 1969.

108. Lessin, L. S., Jensen, W. N., et al.: Ultrastructure of the normal and hemoglobinopathic red blood cell membrane. Arch. Intern. Med. *129*:306, 1972.

109. Lessin, L. S., Jensen, W. N., et al.: Molecular mechanism of hemolytic anemia in homozygous hemoglobin C disease. J. Exp. Med. *130*:443, 1969.

110. Rifkind, R. A., and Danon, D.: Heinz body anemia—An ultrastructural study. I. Heinz body formation. Blood *25*:885, 1965.

111. Rifkind, R. A.: Heinz body anemia: An ultrastructural study. II. Red cell sequestration and destruction. Blood *26*:433, 1965.

112. Jacob, H. S., and Jandl, J. H.: Effect of sulfhydryl inhibition on red blood cells. I. Mechanism of hemolysis. J. Clin. Invest. *41*:779, 1962.

113. Lubin, A., and Desforges, J. F.: Effect of Heinz bodies on red cell deformability. Blood *39*:658, 1972.

114. Orringer, E., and Parker, J.: Increased potassium permeability in red blood cells containing Heinz bodies (abstract). Clin. Res. *21*:94, 1973.

115. Weiss, L., and Tavassoli, M.: Anatomical hazards to the passage of erythrocytes through the spleen. Semin. Hematol. *7*:372, 1970.

116. Crosby, W. H.: Normal function of the spleen relative to red blood cells: A review. Blood *14*:399, 1959.

117. Kent, G., Minick, O. T., et al.: Autophagic vacuoles in human red cells. Am. J. Pathol. *48*:831, 1966.

118. Holroyde, C. P., and Gardner, F. H.: Acquisition of autophagic vacuoles by human erythrocytes. Physiologic role of the spleen. Blood *36*:566, 1970.

119. Cooper, R. A., and Jandl, J. H.: The role of membrane lipids in the survival of red cells in hereditary spherocytosis. J. Clin. Invest. *48*:736, 1969.

120. Jandl, J. H.: Agglutination and sequestration of immature red cell. J. Lab. Clin. Med. *55*:663, 1960.

121. Habeshaw, J., and Stuart, A. E.: Susceptibility of erythrocytes to phagocytosis after exposure to physiological saline. J. Reticuloendothel. Soc. *9*:528, 1971.

122. Stuart, A. E., and Cumming, R. A.: A biologic test for injury to the human red cell. Vox. Sang. *13*:270, 1967.

123. Maruta, H., and Mizuno, D.: Selective recognition of various erythrocytes in endocytosis by mouse periotoneal macrophages. Nature [New Biol.] *234*:246, 1971.

124. Cooper, R. A., and Jandl, J. H.: Bile salts and cholesterol in the pathogenesis of target cells in obstructive jaundice. J. Clin. Invest. *47*:809, 1968.

125. Cooper, R. A.: Lipids of human red cell membrane: Normal composition and variability in disease. Semin. Hematol. *7*:296, 1970.

126. Cooper, R. A.: Anemia with spur cells: A red cell defect acquired in serum and modified in the circulation. J. Clin. Invest. *48*:1820, 1969.

127. LoBuglio, A. F., Cotran, R. S., et al.: Red cells coated with immunoglobulin G.: Binding and sphering by mononuclear cells in man. Science *158*:1582, 1967.

128. Policard, A., and Bessis, M.: Fractionnement d'hématies par les leucocytes au cours de leur phagocytose. C. R. Soc. Biol. (Paris) *147*:982, 1953.

129. Archer, G. T.: Phagocytosis by human monocytes of red cells coated with Rh antibodies. Vox. Sang. *10*:590, 1965.

130. Jandl, J. H., Jones, A. R., et al.: Destruction of red cells by antibodies in man. I. Observations on the sequestration and lysis of red cells altered by immune mechanisms. J. Clin. Invest. *36*:1428, 1957.

131. Cooper, R. A.: Loss of membrane components in the pathogenesis of antibody-induced spherocytosis. J. Clin. Invest. *51*:16, 1972.

132. Humphrey, J. H., and Dourmashkin, R. R.: The lesions in cell membranes caused by complement, In *Advances in Immunology.* Vol. II. Dixon, F. J., Jr., and Kunkel, H. G. (eds.), New York, Academic Press, 1969.

133. Rosse, W. F., and Lauf, P. K.: Effects of immune reactions on the red cell membrane. Semin. Hematol. 7:323, 1970.

134. Brain, M. C., Dacie, J. V., et al.: Microangiopathic hemolytic anemia.: The possible role of vascular lesions in pathogenesis. Brit. J. Haematol. 8:358, 1962.

ACKNOWLEDGMENTS

The author wishes to acknowledge the important contributions of the following individuals in the preparation of this work: Dr. John Parker for his critical review of the manuscript; Dr. Frank Oski for his editorial encouragement and indulgence; Mrs. Jane Heidingsfield and Mrs. Sharon Preston for essential clerical assistance; and all the donors of the figures for their cooperation. One cannot but acknowledge, however indirectly, Dr. John Harris and Dr. Robert Kellermeyer, whose book, *The Red Cell*, looms Everest-like on the horizon for anyone tackling this topic. Hopefully this chapter has been completely purged of any unconscious paraphrasing of their monumental book, which has been a key reference source.

Chapter 2

Development of Erythropoiesis:

Infant Erythrokinetics

by Lars-Eric Bratteby
and Lars Garby

INTRODUCTION

During the last few decades considerable knowledge has been obtained in several fields related to the physiology of the erythron during fetal life and during the first months after birth. The development and structure of different embryonic and fetal hemoglobins have been described, and several of the genetic and biosynthetic mechanisms of cell differentiation and hemoglobin formation have been revealed. The functional properties of hemoglobin F and their relationship to the molecular structure, especially with respect to the interaction with one intracellular ligand, 2,3-diphosphoglycerate, have been partly elucidated. Quantitative studies have yielded information on the rate of red cell (hemoglobin) production and destruction and on how these rates change during the period around the birth. There is also new information concerning the amount of circulating red cells during various times of the development and on the manner in which this amount is related to the production and destruction of the red cells.

This chapter is an attempt to give an account of the physiology of the erythron during prenatal life and during the first months of postnatal life. No attempts have been made to cover the subjects in a com-

prehensive way. Instead, the terms in which the subject is treated are directed towards a deeper understanding of the pathologic changes that are likely to be of importance in clinical practice.

Additional valuable information on various topics in this field of study can be found in the chapters by Kleihauer (1) and by Riegel (2), in the monograph edited by Stave (3), and in the recent second edition of the monograph by Oski and Naiman (4).

THE PRODUCTION OF RED BLOOD CELLS

Prenatal Life

Embryonic red cell formation can be observed 14 days after conception and takes place mainly in the area vasculosa in the yolk sac. Isolated foci of erythropoiesis may be observed throughout the extraembryonic mesoblastic tissue. During the embryonic development, two separate generations, the primitive and the definitive erythroid cell generations, are seen. The yolk sac erythropoiesis appears to embrace both series (5). The cells of the first generation of erythrocytes are very large and hypochromic, and they are delivered to the circulation with

56

intact nuclei. These cells probably retain their nuclei throughout their life span. Thus, at the end of the second gestational month, more than 90 per cent of the circulating red cells are nucleated. Later, the formation of these cells also takes place within intravascular sites of the mesenchyme of the embryo itself; the cells can be found here up to the third month of gestation. The general physiology of these cells remains to be studied; their life span is not known but it must be less than 8 weeks (6). Most of the hemoglobin in the cells is ϵ_4, $\alpha_2 \epsilon_2$ (hemoglobin Gower 1 and 2), or $\gamma_2 \zeta_2$ (hemoglobin Portland). There is an unequal distribution of embryonic and fetal hemoglobin among red cells from embryos and fetuses (1). The ligand binding properties of the ϵ chains and the ζ chains are not known.

During the second and third gestational months, the liver gradually becomes the main source of circulating red cells. During the third and fourth months of fetal life there is also some red cell formation in the spleen. In mice the cell line in the liver, the so-called normoblastic cell generation, is quite different from the primitive cell generation of the mesenchyme (7). In man, the second generation of red blood cells contains much smaller cells which lose their nuclei before or soon after they are delivered to the circulation. Thus, at the end of the third month, only about 2 per cent of the

circulating red cells are nucleated. These cells contain hemoglobin F ($\alpha_2\gamma_2$) and hemoglobin A ($\alpha_2\beta_2$) in varying proportions, but the average content of Hb A is quite low, 5 to 10 per cent. The presence of ϵ or ζ chains after this time is evidence for disturbed synthesis of α chains or for chromosomal aberrations.

The myeloid period of erythropoiesis starts at the end of the fourth month. At the time of birth, most of the red cells are formed in the bone marrow, but there are still numerous hemopoietic foci in the liver; they disappear during the first week of extrauterine life (8). There is no evidence to suggest that the type of cells formed by the liver differs in any principal way from that formed by the bone marrow, although the relative rate of synthesis of hemoglobin F may be larger in the former cells (9).

The development of the different hemoglobin chains and its relation to the change in hemopoietic sites are schematically shown in Figure 2–1 (10).

The mechanisms of erythroid precursor differentiation and proliferation and the associated changes in rate of formation of the different globin chains are still a matter of continued research and are covered in greater detail in Chapters 15 and 25. However, recent studies give strong evidence for the existence of two classes of erythroid precursors: the multipotential stem cells, and the erythropoietin-sensitive stem cells, to

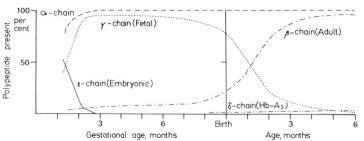
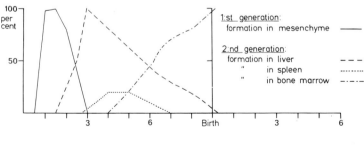

Figure 2–1. Hemopoietic sites and development of different globin chains during fetal life and early infancy. [After Knoll, W., and Pingel, E.: Acta Haematol. (Basel) 2:369, 1949, and Huehns, E. R., Dance, N., et al.: Science 175:134, 1972.]

which the former are occasionally converted by as yet unknown mechanisms. Erythropoietin acts selectively on the latter cells to induce differentiation, cell replication, and hemoglobin formation. The primary effect of the hormone(s) is to stimulate the formation of a variety of species of RNA, which in turn leads to cell replication and, only secondarily, to increased hemoglobin formation (7). An interesting hypothesis, on the molecular-genetic level, to account for the changes in the synthesis of the β-like chains that occur during fetal life has recently been proposed (11). This "looping-out excision" theory assumes intrachromosomal cross-over events, in which the genes for specific globin chains are successively excised from the chromosomes. In this model, as well as in most other models, erythropoietin acts only upon cells already containing the final genetic information.

The differences in the rate of formation of non–α chains, i.e., β, γ, ϵ, and δ chains, during fetal life is presumably also under the influence of the concentration of free heme in the cells. A model for the control of globin formation on the basis of differences in chain affinity for heme and of differences in chain-chain affinity has recently been proposed (12).

The absolute rate of synthesis of hemoglobin or formation of red cells during fetal life is difficult to estimate, since neither the absolute increase in circulating hemoglobin or red cells nor the absolute destruction rate is known. The absolute rate of production of red cells at birth, however, can be estimated fairly well. A value

of 2.5 to 3.0 per cent per day of the circulating red cell mass, or about 4.5 ml. per day in a 3.5 kg. infant, can be calculated on the basis of determinations of the relative number of circulating reticulocytes and determinations of the in vitro mean life span of reticulocytes obtained from cord blood (13). A very similar figure was obtained (14) on the basis of an analysis of the distribution kinetics of radioiron in the plasma and in the red cells (Fig. 2–2). Measurements of the circulating red cell volume (RCV) in newborn infants at various gestational ages (15), shown in Figure 2–3, demonstrated an increase of about 1.5 per cent per day of the RCV. Assuming a mean life span of these cells of 45 to 70 days (see below), these data show a production rate of 3.6 to 4.2 per cent per day of the RCV two months before term, and 2.5 to 3.5 per cent per day of the RCV at term. The combined data, therefore, indicate very strongly that the rate of red cell production during the latter part of fetal life is quite high, about three to five times that of a normal adult subject. This finding is in agreement with the well established fact that, at the same time, all the bones are filled with red marrow and that the concentration of red cell precursors per unit volume of marrow is quite high (16, 17, 18).

Erythropoiesis stimulating factor(s) (ESF) is found in the plasma during fetal life, and the activity is higher than that found in infants (19, 20) after one week of life when the rate of production of red cells is quite low (see below). Newborn infants with anemia due to erythroblastosis have

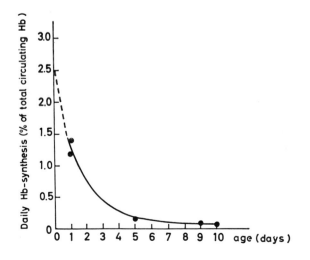

Figure 2–2. The relative rate of hemoglobin synthesis at birth and during the first ten days of life. [From Garby, L., Sjölin, S., et al.: Acta Paediatr. (Stockholm) 52:537, 1963.]

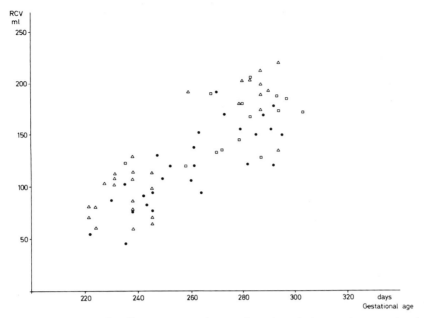

Figure 2-3. The circulating red cell mass in newborn infants in relation to the gestational age. Symbols: ● = by ^{51}Cr-dilution method; △, □ = from plasma volume measurements. [From Bratteby, L.-E.: Acta Paediatr. (Stockholm) 57:132, 1968.]

a higher plasma ESF (21, 22), and fetal lambs have been shown to respond to acute anemia with an increased production of ESF. These data show that the ESF level is mediated by the red cell mass, at least during the latter part of fetal life.

Postnatal Life

The rate of hemoglobin synthesis and production of red cells decreases dramatically during the first few days after delivery. The evidences for this statement have been discussed (14) and include the following: (1) data on the concentration of reticulocytes in peripheral blood (13,16), shown in Figure 2-4; (2) data on the relative amount of red cell precursors in the bone marrow (16), shown in Figure 2-5; and (3) data based on studies of the distribution kinetics of radioiron in plasma and red cells, shown in Figure 2-2 (14). If the data of Seip (13) are reinterpreted and corrected for the finite life span in the marrow of the red cell precursors, all these estimates are in accordance with the view that the production of red cells (or hemoglobin) decreases by a factor of two to three during the first few days after birth and by a factor of about

ten during the first week of life. The mechanism(s) behind this sudden and marked decrease in the red cell production is not known. It may well be initiated by the equally sudden increase in the tissue oxygen tension that takes place at birth. This stimulus may be transmitted to the bone marrow through the virtual disappearance of ESF in the plasma (20), but there are also indications of formation of inhibitors of erythropoiesis in the plasma (23).

At the time of birth, between 55 and 65 per cent of the total hemoglobin synthesis consists of hemoglobin F (24). Thereafter, the synthesis of Hb F decreases much more rapidly than that of Hb A; the time course is seen in Figure 2-6.

The rate of production of red cells (and of hemoglobin), which reaches a minimum during the second week of life, increases during the following months and reaches a maximum, at about 3 months of age, of approximately 2 ml. of packed red cells per day or about 2 per cent per day of the circulating red cell mass. These statements are based on ferrokinetic measurements (14) and on reticulocyte counts (16) (see also Table 2-3), and they are also in accordance with calculations of the change in erythrocyte production during the first five months of life, based on estimations of RCV and

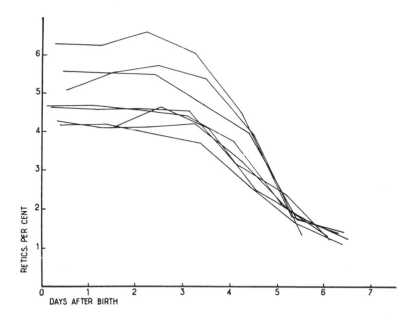

Figure 2–4.   The time course of blood reticulocyte counts in normal infants during the first week of life. [From Seip, M.: Acta Paediatr. (Stockholm) *44*: 355, 1955.]

erythrocyte destruction (see below), as shown in Figure 2–13. The increase in red cell production is associated with an increase in erythropoietin activity in the plasma (19, 20).

Most of the red cells produced during this time, i.e., from about 3 months of age, are presumably identical in character to those produced during adult life with respect to shape, volume, hemoglobin content, hemoglobin type and life span (see below).

THE CIRCULATING RED BLOOD CELLS

Considerations concerning the volume, shape, physical behavior, chemical composition, and metabolic behavior of circu-

lating red blood cells during fetal life and the neonatal period must take into account the mean age of the sampled cells. In particular, differences in any of these characteristics between cells during this period of life and cells from normal adult subjects must be interpreted in the light of differences in mean cell age, as must also the changes that occur during the period in question. The mean age of circulating cells in a normal adult is about 55 days, and the age frequency function is nearly rectangular. The mean cell age during the different phases of fetal life is not known, but it is almost certainly considerably lower. The mean cell age at birth has been estimated to be 20 to 30 days (25). Normalization of the mean cell age and the age frequency distribution towards adult values takes

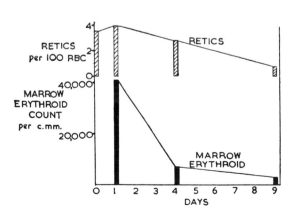

Figure 2–5.   The time course of the reticulocyte and marrow erythroid count in normal infants during the first week of life. (After Gairdner, D., Marks, J., et al.: Arch. Dis. Child. 27:214, 1952.)

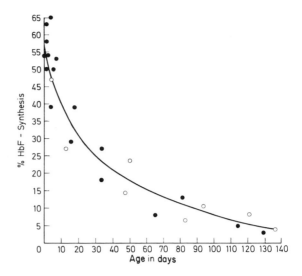

Figure 2–6. The time course of the relative synthesis of Hb F in normal infants during the first 140 days of life. Symbols: ● = Radioiron method; ○ = reticulocyte method. [From Garby, L., Sjölin, S., et al.: Acta Paediatr. (Stockholm) 51:245, 1962.]

place gradually during the first months of life and is probably reached at the age of 6 to 9 months.

The difficulties, due to different age distribution, of interpreting comparisons between red cells from fetuses, infants, and adult subjects could, in principle, be overcome by analysis of cells which have been separated according to age. A critical review of the literature (26) has shown, however, that present methods for cell separation according to age are far from sufficient to reveal other than very marked differences.

Prenatal Life

Characteristics of the red blood cell picture of the human embryo and fetus have been described by several authors (4). Some main features are summarized in Table 2–1. In early fetal life, the red cells are large and have a high corpuscular hemoglobin content. Before the tenth week of gestation most of the cells are nucleated. The concentration of circulating cells, the hemoglobin concentration, and the hematocrit are low compared to the values seen in normal adults. During development, the diameter and volume of the erythrocytes, the corpuscular hemoglobin content (MCH), and the number of nucleated cells decrease. The red cell count, the hemoglobin concentration, and the hematocrit increase fairly rapidly during the first half of the gestation and thereafter more slowly. The mean corpuscular hemoglobin concentra-

tion (MCHC) remains relatively constant during fetal development.

No measurements of the circulating red cell volume (RCV) of human fetuses have been published. Results of measurements of the RCV in newborn infants of different gestational age (15) are shown in Figure 2–3. Part of the fairly large variation seen in this illustration must be due to errors in the determination of the gestational age, and it is likely that the true variation is smaller. In fact, a stronger correlation was found (15) between RCV and birth weight in these same infants. In this study, the amount of red cells remaining in the placental circulation after birth was not estimated.

Postnatal Life

HEMOGLOBIN CONCENTRATION, HEMATOCRIT, AND RETICULOCYTE COUNT. At the time of birth the hemoglobin concentration is 5 to 10 per cent lower in venous blood than in blood sampled by skin prick (27) (Fig. 2–7). The site of venous or skin prick sampling is not critical for this difference, which is present for a few weeks after birth. The reason for the difference is not known, but rheological factors seem to be involved, and hyperemia of the region chosen for skin prick sampling reduces, but does not abolish, the difference (28). The important consequence of the phenomenon is that, whenever possible, venous blood should be used when high precision

TABLE 2–1.   MEAN RED CELL VALUES DURING GESTATION*

Age (in Weeks)	Hb (G./ 100 ml.)	Hemato- crit (%)	RBC (10⁶/ mm.³)	Mean Corpusc. Vol. (μ³)	Mean Corpusc. Hb (γγ)	Mean Corpusc. Hb Conc. (%)	Nuc. RBC (% of RBC's)	Retic. (%)	Diam. (μ)
12	8.0–10.0	33	1.5	180	60	34	5.0–8.0	40	10.5
16	10.0	35	2.0	140	45	33	2.0–4.0	10–25	9.5
20	11.0	37	2.5	135	44	33	1.0	10–20	9.0
24	14.0	40	3.5	123	38	31	1.0	5–10	8.8
28	14.5	45	4.0	120	40	31	0.5	5–10	8.7
34	15.0	47	4.4	118	38	32	0.2	3–10	8.5

*From Oski, F. A., and Naiman, J. L.: *Hematologic Problems in the Newborn.* 2nd ed. Philadelphia, W. B. Saunders Company, 1972, p. 5.

is needed for determinations of hemoglobin, packed cell volume, or red cell count in the newborn or very young infant.

Values for cord blood in normal infants show a considerable variation: 13.7 to 20.5 g. per 100 ml. (29) and 13.9 to 18.0 g. per 100 ml. (30). The source of this variation is not known, but most probably it is due to a combination of a number of factors. One of them is the variation in gestational age. As mentioned previously, there is an increase in hemoglobin concentration during fetal life. Towards term, however, the values show much greater variation than earlier in gestation. The same is true also for the hematocrit and the red cell count (31, 32). It has been claimed (31) that vary-

ing degrees of hypoxia of the fetus towards term contribute to this variation, and higher hemoglobin concentrations were found in postmature infants than in infants born at term; however, this could not be verified (33, 34).

During the first 24 hours of life, even larger variations of the peripheral blood values are found among normal infants. These variations are mainly due to the consequences of differences in the timing of cord clamping, with its effect on the so-called placental transfusion and the subsequent readjustment of the total blood volume. Thirty minutes after birth, the venous hematocrit of nine full-term infants with immediate cord clamping was 47 ± 2 per

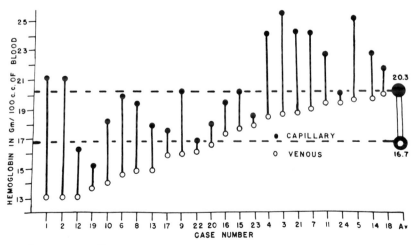

Figure 2–7. Simultaneous capillary and venous hemoglobin determinations in 24 newborn infants. (From Oettinger, L., and Mills, W. B.: J. Pediatr. 35:362, 1949.)

Figure 2–8. Hemoglobin concentration and red cell count in cord blood and in venous blood in normal infants during the first week of life. NS-Blood = cord blood; Kp-Blood = capillary blood; ml = million. [After Künzer, W., In *Blutbildung und Blutumsatz beim Feten und Neugeborenen*. Kepp, R., and Oehlert, G. (eds.), Stuttgart, Ferdinand Enke, 1962, p. 4.]

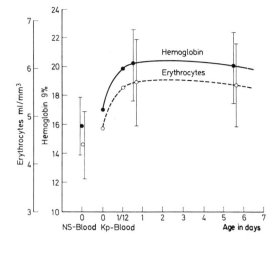

cent (SEM), and that of ten infants with delayed cord clamping 59 ± 1.5 per cent (SEM) (35). During the first hours after delivery, the concentration of red cells increases by some 15 to 25 per cent (Fig. 2–8). This increase is due to readjustment of the blood volume by loss of plasma (35, 36). If the cord is tied early, the change is much less pronounced (35, 37).

After the first 24 hours of life, the concentration of red blood cells is relatively constant for about 5 to 7 days (Fig. 2–8), after which time the well-known decrease takes place. Values for hemoglobin and hematocrit of full-term infants are shown in Table 2–2 (29). This table clearly shows that, also after the first 24 hours of life, the variation in hemoglobin and hematocrit values among normal full-term infants is markedly larger than that found in normal adults. The coefficient of variation in

normal adult populations is usually between 5 and 10 per cent (38), whereas the same figure is 25 per cent for infants at 45 days of age and 15 per cent at 120 days of age. The source of this large variation has not been systematically studied, but several factors can be suspected: variations in placental transfusion of red cells, variations in physical activity, variations in maturation rate of the regulatory systems involved in tissue oxygenation, and, finally, dietary factors. The influence of early clamping has been well established (4) and is also illustrated by a comparison of the values in Table 2–2 with a recent study on apparently healthy full-term infants with early clamping (39), shown in Table 2–3. The values for hemoglobin between the second and twelfth week of age are about 0.5 g. per 100 ml. lower in this study than in that documented in Table 2–2.

The concentration of hemoglobin in peripheral blood and its time course is related to the birth weight (gestational age). Figure 2–9 shows mean values from three different studies (40). The difference between the values of the full-term infants and the prematurely born infants can, at least to some extent, be overcome by iron supplementation to the premature infants. Since an increase with respect to a control value in hemoglobin concentration upon supplementation with iron should be looked upon as due to iron deficiency, this fact shows that some of the hemoglobin values obtained in apparently healthy premature infants are pathologic and due to iron deficiency. The argument also applies to the mean values in a group. When apparently

TABLE 2–2. HEMOGLOBIN AND HEMATOCRIT VALUES (MEAN ± 2 SD) IN NORMAL FULL-TERM INFANTS DURING THE FIRST FOUR MONTHS OF LIFE*

AGE IN DAYS	HEMOGLOBIN (G/100 ML.)	HEMATOCRIT (%)
Cord	17.1 (13.7–20.5)	52.3 (41.7–62.9)
7	18.8 (14.6–23.0)	54.9 (42.5–67.3)
20	15.9 (11.3–20.5)	46.2 (31.8–60.6)
45	12.7 (9.5–15.9)	36.5 (26.9–46.1)
75	11.4 (9.6–13.2)	33.1 (27.9–38.3)
120	11.9 (9.9–13.9)	35.3 (29.1–41.5)

*After Guest, G., and Brown, E. W.: Am. J. Dis. Child. 93:486, 1957. Copyright 1957, American Medical Association.

TABLE 2–3.   NORMAL HEMATOLOGIC VALUES DURING THE FIRST TWELVE
WEEKS OF LIFE IN THE TERM INFANT*

AGE	NO. OF CASES	HB G./100 ML. ± 1 SD	RBC × 10⁶ MM³ ± 1 SD	HCT % ± 1 SD	MCV μ³ ± 1 SD	MCHC % ± 1 SD	RETIC % ± 1 SD
Days							
1	19	19.0 ± 2.2	5.14 ± 0.7	61 ± 7.4	119 ± 9.4	31.6 ± 1.9	3.2 ± 1.4
2	19	19.0 ± 1.9	5.15 ± 0.8	60 ± 6.4	115 ± 7.0	31.6 ± 1.4	3.2 ± 1.3
3	19	18.7 ± 3.4	5.11 ± 0.7	62 ± 9.3	116 ± 5.3	31.1 ± 2.8	2.8 ± 1.7
4	10	18.6 ± 2.1	5.00 ± 0.6	57 ± 8.1	114 ± 7.5	32.6 ± 1.5	1.8 ± 1.1
5	12	17.6 ± 1.1	4.97 ± 0.4	57 ± 7.3	114 ± 8.9	30.9 ± 2.2	1.2 ± 0.2
6	15	17.4 ± 2.2	5.00 ± 0.7	54 ± 7.2	113 ± 10.0	32.2 ± 1.6	0.6 ± 0.2
7	12	17.9 ± 2.5	4.86 ± 0.6	56 ± 9.4	118 ± 11.2	32.0 ± 1.6	0.5 ± 0.4
Weeks							
1–2	32	17.3 ± 2.3	4.80 ± 0.8	54 ± 8.3	112 ± 19.0	32.1 ± 2.9	0.5 ± 0.3
2–3	11	15.6 ± 2.6	4.20 ± 0.6	46 ± 7.3	111 ± 8.2	33.9 ± 1.9	0.8 ± 0.6
3–4	17	14.2 ± 2.1	4.00 ± 0.6	43 ± 5.7	105 ± 7.5	33.5 ± 1.6	0.6 ± 0.3
4–5	15	12.7 ± 1.6	3.60 ± 0.4	36 ± 4.8	101 ± 8.1	34.9 ± 1.6	0.9 ± 0.8
5–6	10	11.9 ± 1.5	3.55 ± 0.2	36 ± 6.2	102 ± 10.2	34.1 ± 2.9	1.0 ± 0.7
6–7	10	12.0 ± 1.5	3.40 ± 0.4	36 ± 4.8	105 ± 12.0	33.8 ± 2.3	1.2 ± 0.7
7–8	17	11.1 ± 1.1	3.40 ± 0.4	33 ± 3.7	100 ± 13.0	33.7 ± 2.6	1.5 ± 0.7
8–9	13	10.7 ± 0.9	3.40 ± 0.5	31 ± 2.5	93 ± 12.0	34.1 ± 2.2	1.8 ± 1.0
9–10	12	11.2 ± 0.9	3.60 ± 0.3	32 ± 2.7	91 ± 9.3	34.3 ± 2.9	1.2 ± 0.6
10–11	11	11.4 ± 0.9	3.70 ± 0.4	34 ± 2.1	91 ± 7.7	33.2 ± 2.4	1.2 ± 0.7
11–12	13	11.3 ± 0.9	3.70 ± 0.3	33 ± 3.3	88 ± 7.9	34.8 ± 2.2	0.7 ± 0.3

MCV   = mean corpuscular volume.
MCH   = mean corpuscular hemoglobin.
MCHC = mean corpuscular hemoglobin concentration.
*From Matoth, Y., Zaizov, R., et al.: Acta Paediatr. (Stockholm) 60:317, 1971.

healthy full-term infants are given supplementary iron, at least some of them will attain a higher value of hemoglobin concentration than that obtained in control infants (41). This fact, together with the convention stated above, shows that part of the so-called physiologic anemia of infancy is due to iron deficiency. Interpretations of the response to supplementary iron in a group of infants will, however, be highly dependent on the dietary intake of iron of the control group, so that it appears impossible at the present time to define the degree and prevalence of iron deficiency anemia during this period of life. In any case, the time course of the hemoglobin values in full-term infants, as depicted in Figure 2–9, would only be slightly influenced by iron supplementation. Since there is no evidence that other dietary factors would influence the time course of the hemoglobin concentration indicated in Figure 2–9, it follows that the great majority of infants showing this time course are not anemic.

Reticulocyte values in apparently healthy full-term infants are shown in Table 2–3. The data included here are in reasonably good agreement with earlier work (4). The high values during the first 3 to 4 days of life reflect, as discussed on p. 58, the intense erythropoiesis during fetal life and the delay in the delivery to the circulation because of the finite life span of the marrow precursors. The time course of the reticulocyte counts during the following months corresponds to the changes in red cell production, as depicted in Figure 2–13.

RED CELL INDICES. The erythrocyte volume, hemoglobin content, and hemoglobin concentration are fairly well known during the neonatal period (29,42). The mean corpuscular volume (MCV) is large in the cord blood and decreases continuously during the first months of life, the values (29) being 113 μ³ in cord blood, 106 μ³ at 7 days and 100 μ³ at 20 days after birth. The decrease is most marked during the first 24 hours. The variability among subjects is quite large and much larger than among normal adults. There is evidence (43,44) that the mean diameter increases immediately after birth, so that the cells become more flat. The mean corpuscular hemoglobin content (MCH) follows the MCV rather closely and is as follows (29):

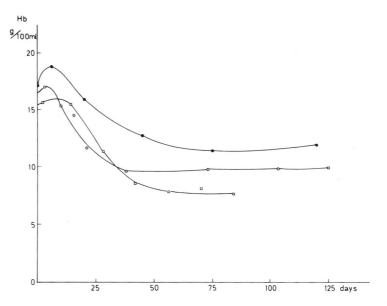

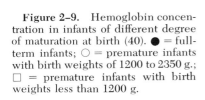

Figure 2–9. Hemoglobin concentration in infants of different degree of maturation at birth (40). ● = full-term infants; ○ = premature infants with birth weights of 1200 to 2350 g.; □ = premature infants with birth weights less than 1200 g.

36.9 $\mu\mu$g. per cell at birth, 36.2 $\mu\mu$g. at 7 days, and 34.4 $\mu\mu$g. per cell at 20 days of age. The mean corpuscular hemoglobin concentration is, accordingly, fairly constant throughout the neonatal period: 32.7, 34.2, and 34.4 g. per 100 ml. of packed cells at birth, 7, and 20 days of age, respectively (29).

The data on MCV reported above (29) are in agreement with earlier works (31,33) but considerably lower than recently reported values (39). In the latter study, the values for the red cell count are lower than obtained in earlier works (4), so that a difference in methods for determining the red cell count may explain the differences in the MCV as calculated from the hematocrit and the red cell count. Values for MCV calculated in this way from the actual data given in (39) do not, however, agree with the values given in the paper (Table 2–3), so that it appears that the latter values derive directly from the electronic size counter used.

The hemoglobin content of individual cord blood red cells was determined by measuring the light absorption of single cells in the Soret band (45). A considerable variation was found among cells from the same sample, and the variation was much larger than that found among cells from normal adults. The hemoglobin content correlated well with red cell volume.

The large variation among subjects in mean erythrocyte volume and hemoglobin content may be explained by interindividual variation in production and destruction of two different cell populations, i.e., the large cells produced during fetal life, and the smaller cells produced after birth. Since it must be assumed that part of the mechanism of cell destruction involves fragmentation (46), variations in the degree of this process must also produce a variation in mean erythrocyte characteristics among subjects. The large variation within subjects of the erythrocyte characteristics should also be viewed in the light of different populations of red cells and of cell fragmentation.

THE BLOOD VOLUME AND THE CIRCULATING RED CELL MASS. The circulating red cell volume of full-term infants during the first 24 hours of life was determined using ^{32}P-labeled red cells (47). In 32 normal infants the mean value was 42 ml. per kg. body weight, with a range of 23 to 58 ml. per kg. body weight. In 28 of these infants, the total blood volume was estimated to be 85 ml. per kg. body weight, with a range of 68 to 100 ml. per kg. The variability of the blood volume was thus considerably smaller than that of the red cell mass, showing that the plasma volume is used to regulate the blood volume. The large variation in red cell volume is most probably a result of differences in the placental transfusion (p. 63). The average venous hematocrit in these infants was 56.8 per cent, with a range of 39.9 to 66.2

per cent. In 9 of these infants, whose hematocrit values were within the normal adult range, i.e., 37.0 to 47.8 per cent, the red cell volume, the plasma volume, and the total blood volume were very close to the values usually present in normal adults, i.e., 29.2, 47.9, and 77.1 ml. per kg. body weight. This fact indicates very strongly that infants at the time of birth have regulation mechanisms for the circulating blood and red cell volumes that are quite similar to those of normal adult subjects. This similarity is also evident from the data (48) showing the relation between circulating red cell mass and venous hematocrit (Fig. 2–10). This relation, which is well described by the simple equation,

red cell mass (ml./kg.) =
$$\text{venous hematocrit (\%)} - 12.0$$

is quite similar to that found in normal adults (48). The standard error of estimate of the predicted red cell mass is not more than 10 per cent and only slightly larger than that found in adults.

The time course of the circulating red cell mass per kg. body weight during the first months of life is shown in Figure 2–11 (49). There is a striking decrease in this quantity during the first 50 days of life, after which time the value remains constant, around 20 ml. per kg. body weight, and with relatively little interindividual variation up to at least 150 days of age. The value of 20 ml. per kg. body weight is considerably lower than that found in normal adult life (29 and 26 ml. per kg. body weight in men and women, respectively). The cause of this difference is not known. The constant low level and the small interindividual variation indicate that powerful regulation mechanisms operate, possibly related to the low, uniform physical activity of the infants during this period of life.

HEMOGLOBIN F AND WHOLE BLOOD OXYGEN AFFINITY. The red cells of the newborn infants contain between 60 and 90 per cent of fetal hemoglobin (Hb F); the remaining hemoglobin is Hb A. The two hemoglobins exist together in all cells

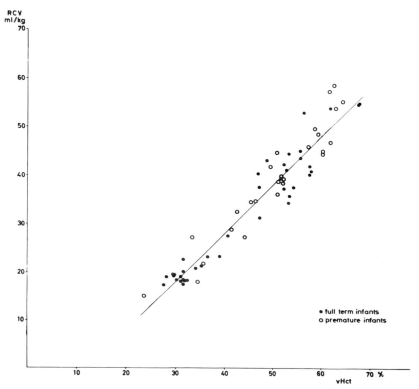

Figure 2–10. The relation between the circulating red cell mass per kg. of body weight and the venous hematocrit. The regression line is given in the text. [From Bratteby, L.-E.: Acta Paediatr. (Stockholm) 57:125, 1968.]

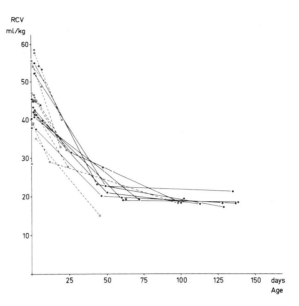

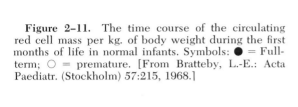

Figure 2–11. The time course of the circulating red cell mass per kg. of body weight during the first months of life in normal infants. Symbols: ● = Full-term; ○ = premature. [From Bratteby, L.-E.: Acta Paediatr. (Stockholm) 57:215, 1968.]

in all proportions (50). The fraction of Hb F in circulating blood decreases slowly during the neonatal period (Fig. 2–12), partly because the synthesis of Hb F decreases proportionately more than that of Hb A (24), but probably also because the red cells dying during this period of life contain more Hb F than Hb A (25, 51).

Hemoglobin F differs from hemoglobin A in several respects (Chapter 13). The molecule consists of four polypeptide chains, of which two, the γ chains, differ from the corresponding β chains in Hb A with respect to the primary structure, i.e., the amino acid composition and sequence. This difference in primary structure implies that there are also differences in the secondary, the tertiary, and the quaternary structures, and that the affinity of the Hb F molecule for the normally occurring ligands, i.e., oxygen, carbon dioxide, protons, and 2,3-diphosphoglycerate (2,3-DPG), should be different from that of the Hb A molecule. The affinity of any one of these ligands depends, through the allosteric effects on the hemoglobin molecule, not only on its intrinsic affinity but also on the medium activity and intrinsic affinity of each of the other ligands. The interaction between these ligands and Hb A has been studied in detail during recent years [see Chapter 13 and (52)], but corresponding studies on Hb F are still lacking. In particular, separate determinations of the effect of protons and of carbon dioxide on the oxygen affinity

of whole blood from newborn infants are lacking. However, studies on the classic Bohr effect, reflecting the combined effect of protons and of carbon dioxide at constant base excess on the oxygen affinity at half oxygen saturation, have given divergent results with respect to blood containing Hb F and blood containing Hb A (2), but most studies show that the effect is at least roughly similar.

On the other hand, the oxygen-linked binding of 2,3 DPG to Hb F is smaller than that to Hb A (53), a fact that accounts for the finding that the effect of 2,3-DPG on the oxygen affinity of Hb F is smaller than that on Hb A (54, 55). The difference in oxygen-linked binding can be explained by the substitution in Hb F by a serine residue instead of a histidine residue at position 123 near the C-terminal ends of the γ chains.

The experimental results (2) that the oxygen affinity of whole blood, at identical plasma activities of protons (pH = 7.40) and of carbon dioxide (pCO₂ = 40 mm. Hg), is higher in blood containing Hb F than in blood containing Hb A can most readily be explained by the differences in oxygen-linked 2,3-DPG–binding between the two hemoglobins. Other factors, such as differences in proton distribution between red cells and plasma and differences in proton binding, may also contribute to the results. In any case, the physiologic significance of this difference in oxygen affinity

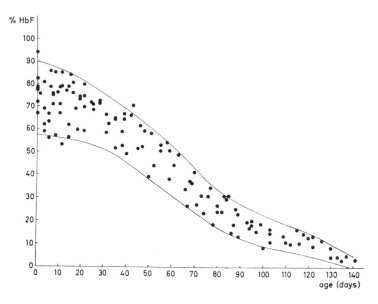

Figure 2–12. The time course of the relative Hb F concentration in blood from normal infants. [After Garby, L., and Sjölin, S.: Acta Paediatr. (Stockholm) *51*:245, 1962.]

between fetal and adult blood remains to be elucidated. The transfer of oxygen from the maternal to the fetal blood takes place under conditions where the pH, pCO_2, pO_2, and oxygen saturation are not well known and where measurements of the ligand interactions have not yet been performed. It is therefore difficult to predict quantitatively the influence of the differences in ligand interaction, because of the differences in oxygenlinked binding of 2,3-DPG, on the actual transfer of oxygen, protons, and carbon dioxide. It is of interest, however, that, if the biochemical regulation mechanisms for the 2,3-DPG level were the same in fetal and adult red cells, an oxygen-linked binding of 2,3-DPG to Hb F of the same magnitude as that to Hb A, together with the fact that circulating fetal blood is much more deoxygenated than maternal blood in vivo, would lead to extremely high values of 2,3-DPG in the fetal cells and thus render this blood unsuitable for oxygen uptake in the placenta (56).

The erythrocyte content of 2,3-DPG at the time of birth is quite similar to that found in normal adult subjects, i.e., between 5.0 and 5.5 mmoles per liter of packed red cells (57). Thus the level remains relatively constant during the first 6 months of life (57). During the second half-year, the level increases up to about 7.5 mmoles. In premature infants, the red cell 2,3-DPG level is lower at birth, and there is an increase to

supernormal levels during the first weeks of life (57).

Values of the oxygen affinity of whole blood in vivo in newborn infants and during the neonatal life have not yet been published. Values for the oxygen tension at half saturation in vitro at specified plasma pH and pCO_2 are somewhat difficult to interpret at the present time, since values for the proton- and carbamino-linked oxygen affinity for blood containing a high proportion of Hb F have not yet been established. However, the value of 30.3 mm. Hg at half saturation at a plasma pH of 7.40 for full-term infants at the age of 8 to 11 months (57) indicates strongly that the oxygen affinity of whole blood in vivo is considerably lower at that age than during adult life. This decrease in oxygen affinity is most probably associated with the reported increase in the red cell 2,3-DPG at that age (57), and may be taken as evidence for the regulation of the relative oxygen release capacity in response to a high physical activity in relation to a relatively low hemoglobin level. Anemias respond, in general, with an increased 2,3-DPG level and a decreased oxygen affinity, and it may be asked if the changes found during the second half-year of life can be taken as evidence for an uncomfortably low hemoglobin level. As discussed on p. 000, a certain proportion of infants in this age period respond to iron supplementation with an increased hemoglobin level. The relation between this response and the actual oxygen affinity in vivo is, however, not known.

Destruction of Red Cells

The rate of destruction of red cells during the early part of fetal life is not known. During the third trimester, a rough estimation, based on an analysis of data on circulating red cell mass and estimates of the production rate (25), gives a figure of about 1 to 2 ml. of packed red cells per day.

In newborn infants, the rate of red cell destruction has been estimated by two independent methods. The rate of excretion of carbon monoxide was shown (58,59) to be about 14 μl. per day and per kg. body weight. If all the excreted carbon monoxide derives from the breakdown of circulating red cells, this estimate corresponds to a red cell destruction rate of 230 mg. of hemoglobin per day and per kg. or 2.5 ml. per day in a 3.5-kg. infant. The initial slope of the disappearance of randomly labeled cells from the circulation, which is a direct estimate of the fractional red cell destruction in both the stationary and the nonstationary state, was shown (60) to be about 2 per cent per day or about 3.0 ml. per day in a 3.5-kg. infant. Both these estimates are likely to be somewhat too high, the first one because some of the excreted carbon monoxide must have originated from breakdown of heme not associated with circulating red cells, and the second one because of some early elution of label or destruction of damaged red cells.

The rate of red cell destruction decreases rather markedly during the following weeks, as estimated from measurements of the excretion of carbon monoxide (58), and attains a minimum of less than 0.5 per cent per day of the circulating red cell mass at the end of the fourth month. This low destruction rate, i.e., less than 0.5 ml. of packed cells per day, is due to the fact that most of the red cells produced during fetal life have already died and that very few cells produced after birth have reached the end of their life span at that time (Fig. 2–13).

RED CELL LIFE SPAN. The life span and manner of destruction of red cells formed during the early part of fetal life is not known. There is good evidence to show, however, that the cells formed during the latter part of fetal life and present in the circulation during the first weeks after birth have a mean cell life span considerably shorter than that of cells formed in adult life. The evidence comes from several sources of experimental data, the most important being the combined data on the survival of labeled cells from newborn subjects in the circulation of normal adults or infants and on the increase in the red cell mass during the latter part of fetal life. The data and their use for calculation of the

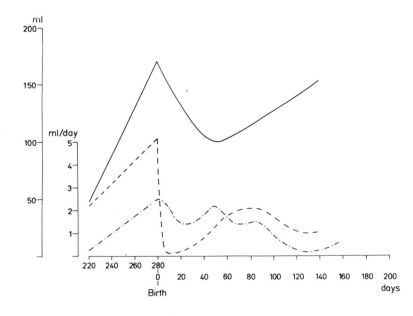

Figure 2–13. The time course of the circulating red cell mass (—), the rate of red cell production (----), and the rate of red cell destruction (—·—·—·) in normal fetuses and infants. The data represent results of measurements and calculations described in several papers (14,15,25,48, 49,51,60).

mean cell life span as well as the life span distribution have been discussed in detail (25). The results show that the mean life span of these cells is between 45 and 70 days, and that the distribution of life spans around the mean value is skewed with the majority of cells dying before the end of the mean life span.

Several findings make it unlikely that the short life span of these cells is due to extrinsic factors (25). Rather, the data favor the hypothesis that intrinsic factors are more important. If this hypothesis is accepted, it follows that the intrinsic factors, or cell deficiencies, are distributed very differently among the cells formed during the period in question, i.e., the latter part of fetal life. The biochemical and biophysical counterparts of these intrinsic factors are not known. However, it is of considerable interest to note that the macrocytic erythrocytes produced in rats and rabbits in response to large doses of erythropoietin (61) and to low barometric pressure (62) also seem to survive for only short periods. Furthermore, macrocytic cells produced by administration of phenylhydrazine in rabbits not only have a very short mean life span but also show a wide distribution of life spans around the mean value (63). The similarity between the red cells produced under these experimental conditions of stress and those produced by the human fetus during the last weeks before birth is striking with respect to production rate, mean size, size distribution, and survival behavior. Little is known about the mechanisms by which these cells are removed from the circulation. Erythrocyte fragmentation with rapid removal of fragments from the circulation would explain the size distribution and to some extent also the rapid disappearance of tracer in survival studies. Trapping of the cells in the reticuloendothelial system due to increased cell rigidity (46) presents an interesting possibility but has not yet been explored experimentally. There is good evidence that the mean cell content of adenosine triphosphate is normal or even increased (64), but this observation does not exclude the presence of a large proportion of cells with a low content of ATP.

The red cells formed after birth have a normal or near-normal life span, as determined by cohort-labeling with ^{15}N-glycine or ^{59}Fe (51, 65, 66). These cells are produced at a much lower rate than those produced before birth and are presumably identical in character with cells produced during normal adult life.

Biochemical Characteristics of the Fetal Erythrocyte

The erythrocytes produced during the period of intrauterine life differ in both their metabolism and membrane structure and function from the red cells produced in later infancy, childhood, or adulthood. Many of the salient features of these cells are listed in Table 2–4.

Studies of the red cells of both the term infant and the premature infant are hampered by the heterogeneity of the red cell population. Interpretation of results is frequently confounded by the fact that the investigator is dealing with a population of very young erythrocytes; and thus it is necessary to distinguish those features which are characteristic of young red cells in general from those that are peculiar to cells produced in utero. The blood at birth is a mixture of cells, some produced late in gestation and some produced one to three months earlier. Despite these difficulties of investigation, many differences remain apparent.

The red cells of the newborn infant possess greater activities of the glycolytic enzymes—glucose phosphate isomerase, glyceraldehyde-3-phosphate dehydrogenase, phosphoglycerate kinase, and enolase—than can be explained by their young red cell age (67–70). Red cell phosphofructokinase activity is significantly reduced (67,68,71,72).

Despite the fact that these young red cells of the newborn consume more glucose than the mature erythrocytes of normal adults, they consume less glucose than would be anticipated in cells of a similar young red cell age (73). When these cells are incubated in the presence of increased quantities of inorganic phosphate (74) at a pH of 7.8 to 8.0 (75) or after depletion of red cell 2,3-diphosphoglycerate (76), their glycolytic rate increases substantially and resembles those of other young erythrocytes. These metabolic features of the cell appear to be primarily of developmental

TABLE 2-4. METABOLIC CHARACTERISTICS OF THE ERYTHROCYTES OF THE
NEWBORN

Carbohydrate Metabolism
Glucose consumption increased.
Galactose more completely utilized as substrate both under normal circumstances and for methemoglobin reduction.[*]
Decreased activity of sorbitol pathway.[*]

Glycolytic Enzymes
Increased activity of hexokinase, phosphoglucose isomerase,[*] aldolase, glyceraldehyde-3-phosphate dehydrogenase,[*] phosphoglycerate kinase,[*] phosphoglycerate mutase, enolase,[*] pyruvate kinase, lactic dehydrogenase, glucose-6-phosphate dehydrogenase, 6-phosphogluconic dehydrogenase, galactokinase, and galactose-1-phosphate uridyltransferase.
Decreased activity of phosphofructokinase.[*]
Distribution of hexokinase isoenzymes differs from that of adults.[*]

Nonglycolytic Enzymes
Increased activity of glutamic-oxaloacetic transaminase and glutathione reductase.
Decreased activity of NADP-dependent methemoglobin reductase,[*] catalase,[*] glutathione peroxidase,[*] carbonic anhydrase,[*] and adenylate kinase.[*]

ATP and Phosphate Metabolism
Decreased phosphate uptake,[*] slower incorporation into ATP and 2,3-diphosphoglycerate.[*]
Accelerated decline of 2,3-diphosphoglycerate upon red cell incubation.[*]
Increased ATP levels.
Accelerated decline of ATP during brief incubation.

Storage Characteristics
Increased potassium efflux and greater degrees of hemolysis during short periods of storage.[*]
More rapid assumption of altered morphologic forms upon storage or incubation.[*]

Membrane
Decreased ouabain-sensitive ATPase.[*]
Decreased potassium influx.[*]
Decreased permeability to glycerol and thiourea.[*]
Decreased membrane deformability.[*]
Increased sphingomyelin, decreased lecithin content of stromal phospholipids.
Decreased content of linoleic acid.[*]
Increase in lipid phosphorus and cholesterol per cell.
Greater affinity for glucose.[*]

Other
Increased methemoglobin content.[*]
Increased affinity of hemoglobin for oxygen.[*]
Glutathione instability.[*]
Increased tendency for Heinz body formation in presence of oxidant compounds.[*]

[*]Appears to be a unique characteristic of the newborn's erythrocytes and not merely a function of the presence of young red cells.

interest and are probably not responsible for the shortened life span of the fetal erythrocyte.

Another characteristic feature of these cells is their extreme sensitivity to compounds which are direct- or indirect-acting oxidants. This sensitivity is reflected by the methemoglobinemia, Heinz body formation, and hemolysis they induce. Many of the enzymatic reactions involved in the detoxification of oxidants are less active in the cells of the newborn. These include the relative deficiencies of NADH-dependent methemoglobin diaphorase (77), glutathione peroxidase (78), and catalase (79). Although the reduced activity of the NADH-dependent methemoglobin diaphorase may be responsible for the increased methemoglobin levels observed in newborns, current evidence suggests that neither the catalase nor glutathione deficiencies, which are only 15 to 25 per cent less than those of normal adults, are responsible for the Heinz body formation and hemolysis induced by compounds such as menadione (80, 81).

The membrane of the neonate's erythrocyte is both structurally and functionally different from that of cells produced later in life. The membrane contains less ouabain-inhibitable ATPase activity (82) and has reduced cholinesterase activity (83). These cells have reduced binding sites for the absorbed system of Lewis antigens, have less exposed A and B antigenic sites, and have less I antigen on their membrane (84). The cells leak more potassium during storage than do the cells from adults and have a decreased rate of active potassium influx (85).

The membrane is less permeable to the nonelectrolytes, glycerol and thiourea (86) and demonstrates differences in its kinetics of glucose transport (87). In addition, either the number or stability of membrane thiol groups appears to be reduced (80). It has been proposed that the latter feature may be the primary basis for the cells' vulnerability to oxidant compounds (80).

Another feature of these red cells is their decreased deformability (88). Like the cells of the adult, these cells become even less deformable at reduced pH and oxygen tension.

It remains to be determined if any one of these factors is primarily responsible for the reduced life span of these cells, or if many of these metabolic handicaps work in concert to shorten the cells' survival.

References

1. Kleihauer, E.: The hemoglobins, In *Physiology of the Perinatal Period.* Vol. I. Stave, U. (ed.), New York, Appleton-Century-Crofts, 1970.
2. Riegel, K. P.: Respiratory gas transport characteristics of blood and hemoglobin, In *Physiology of the Perinatal Period.* Vol. I. Stave, U. (ed.), New York, Appleton-Century-Crofts, 1970.
3. Stave, U.: *Physiology of the Perinatal Period.* New York, Appleton-Century-Crofts, 1970.
4. Oski, F. A., and Naiman, J. L.: *Hematologic Problems in the Newborn.* (2nd ed.). Philadelphia, W. B. Saunders Company, 1972.
5. Metcalf, D., and Moore, M. A. S.: *Hemopoietic Cells.* Amsterdam, North-Holland Publishing Co., 1971.
6. Knoll, W.: Der Gang der Erythropoese beim menschlichen Embryo. Acta Haematol. (Basel) 2:369, 1949.
7. Marks, P. A., and Rifkind, R. A.: Protein synthesis: Its control in erythropoiesis. Science *175*: 955, 1972.
8. Langley, F.: Haemopoiesis and siderosis in the fetus and newborn. Arch. Dis. Child. 26:64, 1951.
9. Thomas, E. D., Lochte, H. L., Jr., et al.: In vitro synthesis of foetal and adult haemoglobin by foetal haematopoietic tissues. Nature (London) *185*:396, 1960.
10. Huehns, E. R., Dance, N., et al.: Human embryonic hemoglobins. Cold Spring Harbor Symp. Quant. Biol. *24*:327, 1964.
11. Kabat, D.: Gene selection in hemoglobin and in antibody-synthesizing cells. Science *175*: 134, 1972.
12. Winterhalter, K. H.: Structure and synthesis of heme and references to globin synthesis, In *Synthesis, Structure and Function of Hemoglobin.* Martin, H., and Nowicki, L. (eds.), München, J. F. Lehmann, 1972.
13. Seip, M.: The reticulocyte level and the erythrocyte production judged from reticulocyte studies in newborn infants during the first week of life. Acta Paediatr. (Stockholm) 44: 355, 1955.
14. Garby, L., Sjölin, S., et al.: Studies on erythrokinetics in infancy. III. Plasma disappearance and red cell uptake of intravenously injected radioiron. Acta Paediatr. (Stockholm) 52:537, 1963.
15. Bratteby, L.-E.: Studies on erythrokinetics in infancy. X. Red cell volume of newborn infants in relation to gestational age. Acta Paediatr. (Stockholm) 57:132, 1968.
16. Gairdner, D., Marks, J., et al.: Blood formation in infancy. II. Normal erythropoiesis. Arch. Dis. Child. 27:214, 1952.
17. Sturgeon, P.: Volumetric and microscopic pattern of bone marrow in normal infants and children. I. Volumetric pattern. Pediatrics 7:577, 1951.

18. Sturgeon, P.: Volumetric and microscopic pattern of bone marrow in normal infants and children. II. Cytologic pattern. Pediatrics 7:642, 1951.

19. Halvorsen, S.: Plasma erythropoietin levels in cord blood and in blood during the first weeks of life. Acta Paediatr. (Stockholm) 52:425, 1963.

20. Mann, D. L., Sites, M. D., et al.: Erythropoietic stimulating activity during the first ninety days of life. Proc. Soc. Exp. Biol. Med. 118:212, 1965.

21. Finne, P. H.: Erythropoietin levels in cord blood as an indicator of intrauterine hypoxia. Acta Paediatr. (Stockholm) 55:478, 1966.

22. Finne, P. H.: Erythropoietin production in fetal hypoxia and in anemic uremic patients. Ann. N. Y. Acad. Sci. 149:497, 1968.

23. Skjaelaaen, P., and Halvorsen, S.: Inhibition of erythropoiesis by plasma from newborn infants. Acta Paediatr. (Stockholm) 60:301, 1971.

24. Garby, L., and Sjölin, S.: Studies on erythrokinetics in infancy. II. The relative rate of synthesis of hemoglobin F and A during the first months of life. Acta Paediatr. (Stockholm) 51:245, 1962.

25. Bratteby, L.-E., Garby, L., et al.: Studies on erythrokinetics in infancy. XIII. The mean life span and the life span frequency function of red blood cells formed during fetal life. Acta Paediatr. (Stockholm) 57:311, 1968.

26. Hjelm, M.: Aging of erythrocytes. Methodological aspects on current procedures to separate erythrocytes into age groups, In Cellular and Molecular Biology of Erythrocytes. Nakao, M., and Rapoport, S. M. (eds.), (in press).

27. Oettinger, L., and Mills, W. B.: Simultaneous capillary and venous hemoglobin determinations in the newborn infant. J. Pediatr. 35:362, 1949.

28. Oh, W., and Lind, J.: Venous and capillary hematocrit in newborn infants and placental transfusion. Acta Paediatr. (Stockholm) 55:38, 1966.

29. Guest, G., and Brown, W.: Erythrocytes and hemoglobin of the blood in infancy and childhood. Am. J. Dis. Child. 93:486, 1957.

30. Künzer, W.: Rotes Blutzellsystem bei Feten und Neugeborenen, In Blutbildung und Blutumsatz beim Feten und Neugeborenen. Kepp, R., and Oehlert, G. (eds.), Stuttgart, Ferdinand Enke, 1962.

31. Walker, J. L., and Turnbull, E. P. N.: Haemoglobin and red cells in the human fetus and their relation to the oxygen content of the blood in the vessels of the umbilical cord. Lancet 2:312, 1953.

32. Thomas, D. B., and Yoffey, J. M.: Human foetal haematopoiesis. I. The cellular composition of foetal blood. Br. J. Haematol. 8:290, 1962.

33. Marks, J., Gairdner, D., et al.: Blood formation in infancy. III. Cord blood. Arch. Dis. Child. 30:117, 1955.

34. Rooth, G., and Sjöstedt, S.: Haemoglobin in cord blood in normal and prolonged pregnancy. Arch. Dis. Child. 32:91, 1957.

35. Usher, R., Shephard, M., and Lind, J.: The blood volume of the newborn infant and placental transfusion. Acta Paediatr. (Stockholm) 52:497, 1963.

36. Steele, M. W.: Plasma volume changes in the neonate. Am. J. Dis. Child. 103:10, 1962.

37. Mollison, P. L., and Cutbush, M.: Haemolytic disease of the newborn: criteria of severity. Br. Med. J. 1:123, 1949.

38. Garby, L.: The normal haemoglobin level. Br. J. Haematol. 19:429, 1970.

39. Matoth, Y., Zaizov, R., et al.: Postnatal changes in some red cell parameters. Acta Paediatr. (Stockholm) 60:317, 1971.

40. O'Brien, R. T., and Pearson, H.: Physiologic anemia of the newborn infant. J. Pediatr. 79:132, 1971.

41. Sjölin, S., and Wranne, L.: Iron requirements during infancy and childhood, In Occurrence, Causes and Prevention of Nutritional Anaemias. Blix, G. (ed.), Uppsala, Almqvist & Wiksells, 1968.

42. Vahlquist, B.: Das Serumeisen. Eine pädiatrisch-klinische und experimentelle Studie. Acta Paediatr. (Stockholm) 28(Suppl. 5):1, 1941.

43. Weicker, H., Wagner, J., et al.: Der Erythrozytendurchmesser der Kinder. Acta Haematol. (Basel) 10:50, 1953.

44. Hanssler, H., and Rieger, K.: Studien zur Blutmorphologie des Neugeborenen. Klin. Wochenschr. 32:741, 1954.

45. Ambs, E.: Durchmesser und Hämoglobingehalt der Erythrozyten. Acta Haematol. (Basel) 15:302, 1956.

46. Weed, R.: Disorders of the red cell membrane. History and perspectives. Semin. Hematol. 7:249, 1970.

47. Mollison, P. L., Veall, N., et al.: Red cell volume and plasma volume in infants. Arch. Dis. Child. 25:212, 1950.

48. Bratteby, L.-E.: Studies on erythrokinetics in infancy. IX. Prediction of red cell volume from venous hematocrit in early infancy. Acta Paediatr. (Stockholm) 57:125, 1968.

49. Bratteby, L.-E.: Studies on erythrokinetics in infancy. XI. The change in circulating red cell volume during the first five months of life. Acta Paediatr. (Stockholm) 57:215, 1968.

50. Betke, K., Kleihauer, E., et al.: Zytologische Untersuchungen zur perinatalen Ablösung von HbF durch HbA und ihre beziehungen zur Makrozytose des Neugeborenen. Pädiatr. u. Pädol. 1/1:17, 1965.

51. Garby, L., Sjölin, S., et al.: Studies on erythrokinetics in infancy. V. Estimation of the life span of red cells in the newborn. Acta Paediatr. (Stockholm) 53:165, 1964.

52. Rörth, M., and Astrup, P.: Oxygen Affinity of Hemoglobin and Red Cell Acid-Base Status. Copenhagen, Munksgaard, and New York, Academic Press, 1972.

53. de Verdier, C.-H., and Garby, L.: Low binding of 2,3-diphosphoglycerate to hemoglobin F. A contribution to the knowledge of the binding site and an explanation for the high oxygen affinity of foetal blood. Scand. J. Clin. Lab. Invest. 23:149, 1969.

54. Bauer, C., Ludwig, I., et al.: Different effects of 2,3-diphosphoglycerate and adenosine tri-

phosphate on the oxygen affinity of adult and foetal human haemoglobin. Life Sci. 7:1339, 1968.

55. Tyuma, I., and Shimizu, K.: Different response to organic phosphates of human fetal and adult hemoglobins. Arch. Biochem. 129:404, 1969.

56. de Verdier, C.-H., and Garby, L.: Binding of DPG to haemoglobin F and its physiological significance. Försvarsmedicin 5:192, 1969.

57. Delivoria-Papadopoulos, M., Roncevic, N. P., et al.: Postnatal changes in oxygen transport of term, premature and sick infants: The role of red cell 2,3-diphosphoglycerate and adult hemoglobin. Pediatr. Res. 5:235, 1971.

58. Wranne, L.: Studies on erythrokinetics in infancy. VII. Quantitative estimation of the haemoglobin catabolism by carbon monoxide technique in young infants. Acta Paediatr. (Stockholm) 56:381, 1967.

59. Maisels, M. J., Pathak, A., et al.: Endogenous production of carbon monoxide in normal and erythroblastotic newborn infants. J. Clin. Invest. 50:1, 1971.

60. Bratteby, L.-E., Garby, L., et al.: Studies on erythrokinetics in infancy. XII. Survival in adult recipients of cord blood red cells labelled in vitro with di-isopropyl fluorophosphonate (DF³²P). Acta Paediatr. (Stockholm) 57:305, 1968.

61. Stohlman, F., Jr.: Humoral regulation of erythropoiesis. VII. Shortened survival of erythrocytes produced by erythropoietin or severe anemia. Proc. Soc. Exp. Biol. Med. 107:884, 1961.

62. Fryers, G. R., and Berlin, N. I.: Mean red cell life of rats exposed to reduced barometric pressure. Am. J. Physiol. 17:465, 1952.

63. Card, R. T., and Valberg, L. S.: Characteristics of shortened survival of stress erythrocytes in the rabbit. Am. J. Physiol. 213:566, 1967.

64. Stave, U., and Clara, J.: Adenosinphosphat in Blut Frühgeborener. Biol. Neonate 3:160, 1961.

65. Dancis, J., Danoff, S., et al.: Hemoglobin metabolism in the premature infant. J. Pediatr. 54:748, 1959.

66. Vest, M., Stebel, L., et al.: The extent of "shunt" bilirubin and erythrocyte survival in the newborn infant measured by the administration of ¹⁵N-glycine. Biochem. J. 95:11C, 1965.

67. Konrad, P. N., Valentine, W. N., et al.: Enzymatic activities and glutathione content of erythrocytes of the newborn: Comparison with red cells of older normal subjects and those with comparable reticulocytosis. Acta Haematol. (Basel) 48:193, 1972.

68. Oski, F. A.: Red cell metabolism in the newborn infant. V. Glycolytic intermediates and glycolytic enzymes. Pediatrics 44:84, 1969.

69. Witt, I., Muller, H., et al.: Vergleichende biochemische Untersuchungen an Erythrocyten aus Neugeborenen- und Erwachsenen-Blut. Klin. Wochenschr. 45:262, 1967.

70. Cotte, J., Nivelon, J. L., et al.: Les enzymes de la glycolyse intraerythrocytaire chez le prémature. Ann. Pediatr. (Paris) 73:3158, 1967.

71. Gross, R. T., Schroeder, E. A. R., et al.: Energy metabolism in the erythrocytes of premature infants compared to full-term newborn infants and adults. Blood 21:755, 1963.

72. Caruso, P., Conti, F., et al.: Diagramma della attivita enzimatiche endoeritrocitarie nel neonato, nel lattante, nel bambino. Minerva Pediatr. 15:1136, 1963.

73. Oski, F. A., Smith, C., et al.: Red cell metabolism in the premature infant. III. Apparent inappropriate glucose consumption for cell age. Pediatrics 41:473, 1968.

74. Bentley, H. P., Jr., Alford, C. A., Jr., et al.: Erythrocyte glucose consumption in the neonate. J. Lab. Clin. Med. 76:311, 1970.

75. Oski, F. A., and Travis, S. F.: Effect of pH on glycolysis in the erythrocytes of the newborn infant. Soc. Pediatr. Res. (abstract), 1972, p. 106.

76. Oski, F. A., Urmson, J., et al.: 2,3-Diphosphoglycerate (DPG) and the control of red cell glycolysis. Soc. Pediatr. Res. (abstract), 1973, p. 122.

77. Ross, J. D.: Deficient activity of DPNH-dependent methemoglobin diaphorase in cord blood erythrocytes. Blood 21:51, 1963.

78. Gross, R. T., Bracci, R., et al.: Hydrogen peroxide toxicity and detoxification in erythrocytes of newborn infants. Blood 29:481, 1967.

79. Jones, P. E. H., and McCance, R. A.: Enzyme activities in the blood of infants and adults. Biochem. J. 45:464, 1949.

80. Schroter, W.: Drug susceptibility and the development of erythrocyte enzyme systems, In Nutricia Symposium. Metabolic processes in the fetus and newborn infant. Jonxis, J. H. P., Visser, H. K. A., et al. (eds.), Leiden, Stenfert-Kroese N. V., 1971, p. 73.

81. Glader, B., Winn, L., et al.: Glutathione instability of cyanate-treated red blood cells in vitro. Pediatr. Res. (abstract) 6:365, 1972.

82. Whaun, J., and Oski, F. A.: Red cell stromal adenosine triphosphatase (ATPase) of newborn infants. Pediatr. Res. 3:105, 1969.

83. Burman, D.: Red cell cholinesterase in infancy and childhood. Arch. Dis. Child. 36:363, 1961.

84. Mollison, P. L.: Blood Transfusion in Clinical Medicine. 4th ed. Oxford, Blackwell, 1967, p. 275.

85. Blum, S. F., and Oski, F. A.: Red cell metabolism in the newborn infant. IV. Transmembrane potassium flux. Pediatrics 43:396, 1969.

86. Hollan, S. R., Szeleny, J. G., et al.: Structural and functional differences between human foetal and adult erythrocytes. Haematology 4:409, 1967.

87. Moore, T. J., and Hall, N.: Kinetics of glucose transfer in adult and fetal human erythrocytes. Pediatr. Res. 5:356, 1971.

88. Gross, G. P., and Hathaway, W. E.: Fetal erythrocyte deformability. Pediatr. Res. 6:593, 1972.

Chapter 3

Disorders of Heme Metabolism:

Porphyria and Hyperbilirubinemia

by Stephen H. Robinson

The porphyrins are products related to the biosynthesis of heme. Defects in heme synthesis are implicated in several types of hypochromic anemia and in a group of rather rare and interesting diseases, the porphyrias, about which much has been learned in the past several years. The bile pigments, of which bilirubin is the most important in human biology, are excretory products that result from heme degradation. Jaundice, the retention of increased amounts of bilirubin in the blood with staining of tissues, is primarily a sign of underlying hematologic or hepatic disease. However, in the newborn period, jaundice takes on particular importance since increased levels of unconjugated bilirubin may be the cause of infant mortality or severe deficits in neurologic function. Detailed reviews of the pathophysiology of porphyrin and bile pigment metabolism have been published elsewhere (1–6). It is the aim of the present chapter to review the normal pathways of heme metabolism in rather general terms, then to relate them to defects encountered in the hypochromic anemias, porphyrias, and hyperbilirubinemic states.

HEME BIOSYNTHESIS (PORPHYRINS)

Normal Pathways

The general structures of the porphyrinogens, porphyrins, bile pigments, and their basic substituent, the pyrrole ring, are shown in Figure 3–1, and a schematic outline of heme biosynthesis is presented in Figure 3–2 (82). A major advance in our knowledge of the pathways of heme synthesis was made in the late 1940's (7) when Shemin and his co-workers found that glycine is a precursor of heme, in a reaction in which glycine and succinyl CoA are condensed to form an unstable intermediate, which is quickly converted to δ-aminolevulinic acid (ALA). Several facts about this initial reaction bear emphasis. ALA synthetase, which mediates this condensation, is a mitochondrial enzyme. Pyridoxal phosphate, derived from vitamin B_6, is a cofactor. Most important, ALA synthetase is the critical rate-limiting enzyme in the pathway of heme synthesis. It is a rather common mechanism in biochemistry that the end product of a reaction sequence (heme in this instance) regulates the rate of its own formation by modulating the activity of a very early step.

Heme appears to act on ALA synthetase in two ways. First, by so-called end-product repression an excess of heme causes a decrease in the formation of new enzyme protein, and since ALA synthetase has a very rapid rate of turnover, enzyme levels fall quickly. As a result, less ALA is formed and there is decreased substrate available for continued heme synthesis. Secondly, by a process known as end-product inhibition, heme interacts directly with ALA synthetase, rendering it inactive; this mechanism is operative in certain microorganisms, and

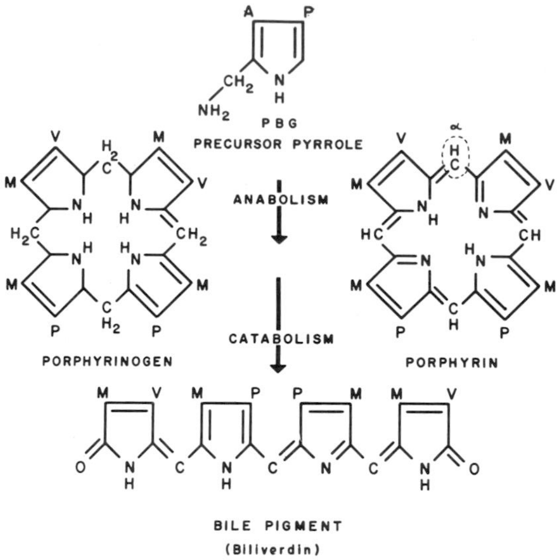

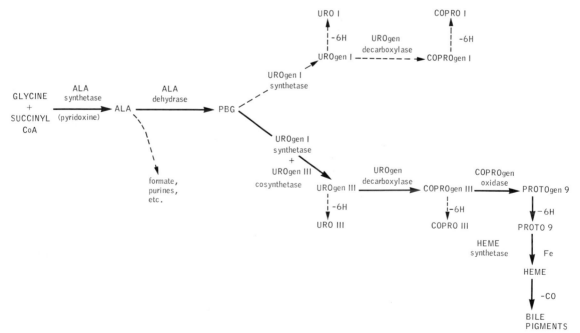

Figure 3–1. Structures of porphobilinogen, protoporphyrinogen 9, protoporphyrin 9, and biliverdin. Bile pigment is formed by cleavage of α-methene bridge in Fe-protoporphyrin 9 (heme). [From Robinson, S. H., In *Harvard Pathophysiology Series, Vol. I. Hematology.* Beck, W. S. (ed.), Cambridge, M.I.T. Press, 1973, p. 51.]

there is growing evidence that it plays some role in the regulation of heme synthesis in mammalian cells as well.

It is of interest that the last two enzymes in the heme biosynthetic sequence, COPROgen oxidase and heme synthetase (or ferrochelatase), are, like ALA synthetase, located in the mitochondria, whereas all of the intervening steps take place in the cytoplasm. Hence, heme synthesis both begins and ends in the mitochondria, an arrangement eminently suited to the process of end-product inhibition. It is possible of course that this anatomic arrangement may be only the vestige of a mechanism that is important primarily in more primitive species.

Two moles of ALA are condensed to form

Figure 3–2. Biosynthesis of heme. Bold arrows show main pathway. Dashed arrows show by-pathways. Abbreviations: ALA, δ-aminolevulinic acid; PBG, porphobilinogen; UROgen, COPROgen, and PROTOgen, the porphyrinogens; URO, COPRO, and PROTO, the porphyrins.

the basic pyrrole substructure of the porphyrins and heme, porphobilinogen (PBG), by a cytoplasmic enzyme, ALA dehydrase. Four PBG's are then joined to form a cyclic or ring tetrapyrrole structure in the presence of the enzyme UROgen I synthetase, otherwise called PBG deaminase. This brings us to the critical branch point in Figure 3–2, at which porphyrinogens of either the type I or III isomeric series are formed. There are theoretically four isomers of UROgen or COPROgen, although only types I and III are found in nature. During normal heme synthesis virtually all of the porphyrinogen formed is type III. COPROgen I cannot undergo progressive oxidation to protoporphyrin and hence to heme (Fig. 3–2); consequently, the little type I material formed must be excreted as a by-product. The difference between the I and III isomers is in the arrangement of the side groups of the D ring (Fig. 3–3); there is a regular alternation of acetic and propionic acid side groups in each of the four rings in UROgen I, but this sequence is reversed in the D ring of UROgen III, a rearrangement mediated by a second enzyme, UROgen III cosynthetase, otherwise called the isomerase enzyme. If this enzyme is deficient, as occurs in congenital erythropoietic porphyria, porphyrinogen synthesis is diverted into the type I pathway. If the activity of the synthetase is impaired but that of the cosynthetase is intact, as now appears to be true in acute intermittent porphyria, type III isomer is produced but at a potentially diminished rate.

It should be noted that we are referring to porphyrinogens, not porphyrins, in this discussion of normal heme biosynthesis. Porphyrins, which are formed from porphyrinogens by the loss of six hydrogen atoms, are by-products of heme biosynthesis. Once formed, they are lost from this pathway as obligatory excretory products. The one exception is protoporphyrin. The distinction between porphyrinogens and porphyrins has considerable significance for the pathophysiology of the porphyrias. The cardinal differences are noted in Table 3–1. Porphyrinogens are unstable and colorless and are true intermediates in heme biosynthesis. Porphyrins, by contrast, are stable, are highly colored and fluorescent (both their color and fluorescence are red), and are by-products of heme biosynthesis. The basis of these properties is that the loss of six hydrogens leads to the formation of a resonating ring structure comprised of a regular alternation of single and double bonds (Fig. 3–1). Resonating molecules are favored thermodynamically, and the oxidation reaction by which porphyrinogens may be converted to porphyrins is therefore downhill and irreversible. Thus any porphyrin formed cannot gain reentry to the main biosynthetic pathway. The cells in which heme synthesis is taking place must therefore maintain defenses against such oxidation. They do so quite successfully under normal circumstances by maintaining a high reducing environment and by excluding light, since the oxidation process is in part photocatalytic. In the porphyrias there is an excess of porphyrins in the excreta and in various tissues, in part because these reducing mechanisms are overwhelmed by overproduction of porphyrinogens and in part because porphyrinogens are oxidized after leaving their sites of origin. Alternatively, it is possible that defects in the reducing mechanisms themselves might be the cause of the increased porphyrin production in some of the porphyrias.

The colored and fluorescent properties of the porphyrin molecules are also a result of their resonating structure, which permits them to absorb and reemit quanta of light energy. These properties have direct clinical significance. In those forms of porphyria

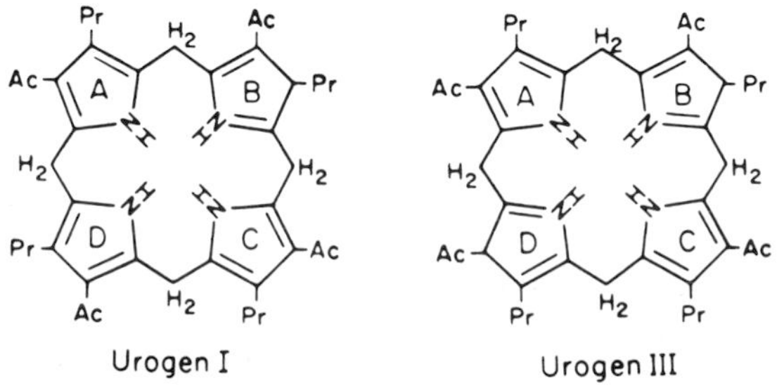

Figure 3–3. Structures of UROgen I and III. The difference lies in the orientation of the D-ring side groups.

Urogen I   Urogen III

TABLE 3–1.

PORPHYRINOGENS	$\xrightarrow{-6H}$	PORPHYRINS
Reduced forms		Irreversibly oxidized forms
On biosynthetic pathway		By-products of heme biosynthesis*
Nonresonating molecules		Resonating molecules
Unstable		Stable
Colorless		Colored (red)
Nonfluorescent		Fluorescent (red)

*Exception: protoporphyrin.

in which there is an increased excretion of uroporphyrin, the urine has a characteristic red color and manifests dramatic red fluorescence when examined under ultraviolet light. Moreover, the sensitivity to sunlight and, often, severe dermatitis that characterize many of the porphyrias are directly attributable to these properties of the porphyrin molecules. Using monochromatic light sources, Magnus et al. have shown that the specific wavelengths of light in which the porphyrins absorb cause excitation of excess porphyrin in the skin of porphyric patients and thereby elicit the characteristic skin manifestations of these diseases (8).

We now return to the heme biosynthetic pathway. The conversion of UROgen to COPROgen and then to PROTOgen is the result of a series of decarboxylation and oxidation steps. UROgen has acetic and propionic acid side groups (Fig. 3–3). With the conversion of UROgen to COPROgen, all of the acetic acid residues are decarboxylated to methyl groups. With formation of PROTOgen, the two topmost propionic acid groups are oxidized to vinyls (Fig. 3–1). There are now three kinds of side groups —methyls, propionic acids, and vinyls— and there are now 15 rather than four possible isomers of PROTOgen. Only the ninth is found in nature, and this is derived solely from COPROgen III. Thus all the PROTOgen, heme, and bile pigment found in man is of the type 9 series.

There is an exception to the rule that porphyrins are not on the main biosynthetic pathway. Under physiologic conditions PROTOgen 9 is oxidized to PROTO 9, and it is this porphyrin which is chelated with iron to form heme, the end product of the reaction sequence.

Before proceeding to a discussion of disorders of heme synthesis, three aspects of the normal metabolic pathway merit reemphasis: (1) the role of ALA synthetase in regulating the rate of heme synthesis; (2) the balance normally present between the UROgen synthetase and cosynthetase enzymes that leads to the preferential formation of porphyrinogens of the physiologic type III series; and (3) the distinctions between the porphyrinogens and their oxidized counterparts, the porphyrins, with respect both to their roles in the biosynthetic sequence and to their physicochemical properties and potential biological effects.

Disorders of Heme Biosynthesis

Defects in heme biosynthesis may be considered to be of two general types: those interfering with net heme production in erythroid cells, resulting in hypochromic anemia, and the porphyrias, in which a normal or even increased rate of heme synthesis is maintained but at the expense of increased production of intermediates in the pathway, often with disastrous consequences to the patient.

Hypochromic Anemia

The hypochromic anemias are discussed in detail in Chapter 4 and will be mentioned here only briefly. In iron deficiency anemia the final substrate iron is lacking, leading to impairment of the synthesis of hemoglobin heme. In the hypochromic anemia sometimes encountered with chronic illness (infection, inflammatory disease, malignancy), iron is again in short supply, but now because of a defect in iron release from the reticuloendothelial cells in which senescent red cells are destroyed.

In both of these forms of iron deficient erythropoiesis, red cell free protoporphyrin is increased. In the thalassemic syndromes the impairment of hemoglobin production is due primarily to defective globin synthesis, although there is also a decrease in ALA synthetase activity (9), perhaps secondary to transient excesses of heme as compared to globin in immature erythroid cells. Finally, there is a group of disorders, the sideroblastic anemias, characterized by hypochromic red cells in the peripheral blood and ringed sideroblasts in the bone marrow (10). By electron microscopy the latter are normoblasts with iron-laden mitochondria, which have a perinuclear distribution in early erythroid cells. It is to be remembered that these organelles are the sites of both initiation and completion of heme synthesis. Retention of iron in the mitochondria and the associated hypochromic anemia suggest a defect in the heme biosynthetic pathway. However, the precise mechanisms underlying this relationship are far from clear in all but a few specific types of sideroblastic anemia. The exceptions are pyridoxine-responsive anemia, the sideroblastic anemia of the alcoholic, and the anemia of chronic lead intoxication. In most other causes of sideroblastic anemia, no defect in heme biosynthesis can yet be demonstrated.

Pyridoxine-responsive anemia is itself probably not a single disorder, since many patients with sideroblastic anemia respond to large doses of pyridoxine to a greater or lesser extent. A defect in ALA synthesis, which can be partially reversed by supraphysiologic doses of pyridoxine, has been demonstrated in several patients who respond to this agent (11, 12). The response is usually incomplete, and both hypochromia and ringed sideroblasts frequently persist. Moreover, these patients often relapse soon after pyridoxine is withdrawn. Hence, this is not simple pyridoxine deficiency. Decreased ALA synthetase activity appears to explain both the diminution in hemoglobin heme synthesis and the iron-loading of mitochondria, where the final assembly of iron and protoporphyrin takes place. A minor defect in heme synthetase has also been described in one such patient (13). The latter defect disappeared after excess iron had been removed by extensive phlebotomy and appears to have been an acquired abnormality due to iron engorgement of the mitochondria. One might therefore question whether the greater defect in ALA synthetase activity is indeed primary or whether it, too, is not the result of some more general mitochondrial abnormality.

The reversible sideroblastic change seen in acute alcoholism also appears to be due to impaired ALA synthetase activity. It has recently been reported that these patients may be unable to convert pyridoxine to its active coenzyme form, pyridoxal phosphate (14).

The anemia of lead intoxication is also associated with hypochromia and ringed sideroblasts, findings which are explicable on the basis of known defects produced by lead. This heavy metal chelates sulfhydryl groups and presumably in this manner inhibits several enzymes in the heme biosynthetic sequence—primarily ALA dehydrase and heme synthetase, but also COPROgen oxidase and possibly ALA synthetase (15). A decrease in net heme synthesis would result in both hypochromia and clogging of mitochondrial cristae with unused iron. [It should be pointed out, however, that in some experimental studies mitochondria were found to be swollen and empty, presumably because of impaired intracellular transfer of iron (16, 17).] Red cell stippling in chronic lead intoxication represents aggregated ribosomes often associated with iron deposits. Evidence differs as to whether the abnormal mitochondria are also involved. The characteristic increase in urinary ALA and COPRO III excretion in these patients can be explained by appropriate blocks at early and late steps in the heme synthetic pathway. It is of interest in this regard that many of the symptoms of chronic lead intoxication, including the encephalopathy, neuropathy, and abdominal colic, resemble those of acute intermittent porphyria. Whether these resemblances are coincidental or point to some underlying similarity in the pathophysiology of these disorders is yet to be determined.

The Porphyrias

In this group of disorders there is no hypochromia and often no anemia. Heme synthesis is normal or sometimes increased. One may look upon the porphyrias as disorders of unbalanced heme synthesis, in which different intermediates are produced and excreted in excess. Recent observations have demonstrated that at least some of these disorders are due to circumscribed enzyme defects; compensatory mechanisms maintain a normal rate of heme synthesis at the expense of increased elaboration of intermediates proximal to the lesion. The pathophysiology of the different forms of porphyria is determined by two factors: the biochemical location of the defect and hence the nature of the intermediates produced in excess, and the anatomic tissue in which the defect occurs.

It must be emphasized that, although most heme is synthesized in erythroid precursors in the bone marrow, heme synthesis also takes place in other tissues. Heme is a prosthetic group of a variety of proteins, which include most of the cytochromes, catalase, peroxidase, tryptophan pyrrolase, and myoglobin, in addition to hemoglobin. All of these heme proteins undergo turnover, i.e., they are regularly degraded and newly synthesized at more or less regular and unique rates. Virtually all cells are therefore sites of some porphyrin and heme production. Second to the bone marrow, the liver is the richest source of heme synthesis.

The porphyrias are disorders of heme synthesis in either the bone marrow or the liver, or in some instances both organs, and anatomic location provides a convenient basis for classifying these diseases. The hepatic porphyrias are more common than the erythropoietic types. In addition, these disorders may be classified as inherited or acquired; most are inherited. Finally, the porphyrias may be divided into two general types with regard to pathophysiology, depending on whether porphyrin precursors or true porphyrins are produced in excess. In many of these diseases there is overproduction of true porphyrins. If these are excreted in the urine (e.g., URO and to a lesser extent COPRO), the urine is red and fluoresces red under ultraviolet light. The physicochemical properties of the porphyrins also lead to photosensitivity and dermatitis and, in some instances in which red cell porphyrin content is high, to hemolytic anemia as well. In a second group

of so-called porphyrias there is no true porphyrin excess, but instead there is overproduction of the porphyrin precursors, ALA and PBG. In these disorders the freshly passed urine is not discolored, although it may change color with time, and there is no photosensitivity, dermatitis, or hemolytic anemia. Instead, there is a sometimes bizarre constellation of symptoms, the basis of which is not understood, but which appears to be related to neurologic and endocrine dysfunction; this will be described in more detail in the discussion of acute intermittent porphyria. In a few diseases, such as variegate porphyria and coproporphyria, both pathophysiologic types of porphyria may coexist.

A simplified classification of the porphyrias according to these three criteria is presented in Table 3–2. This is elaborated briefly in the following discussion. The reader is referred to specialized texts (1, 2, 18) for a more complete description of these diseases.

CONGENITAL ERYTHROPOIETIC PORPHYRIA. This is a rare disease, inherited as an autosomal recessive, and characterized chiefly by severe, sometimes mutilating dermatitis and photosensitivity, porphyrin staining of the teeth (erythrodontia), hemolytic anemia with splenomegaly, and the passage of red urine. The evolution of the skin lesions characterizes the pathophysiology of this disorder. Blisters develop on exposed parts of the skin; these contain porphyrin, as demonstrated by pink fluorescence under ultraviolet light. The blisters tend to break down, frequently become superinfected, and often go on to scarification and contracture – all the result of increased concentrations of resonating porphyrin molecules in the skin. Similarly, the hemolysis may be due to photo-oxidative effects mediated by porphyrins in and around red cells as they traverse superficial blood vessels.

An excess of URO and, to a lesser extent, COPRO I is found in the marrow, red cells, and urine. Fluorescence microscopy reveals porphyrin fluorescence in the nuclei of approximately half of the normoblasts present in the marrow. Clearly, this disorder is due to a defect at the branch point in Figure 3–2, with too much type I isomer formed in erythroid precursors. Recent investigations indicate that this is due to de-

TABLE 3–2. CLASSIFICATION OF PORPHYRIAS

	ERYTHROPOIETIC	HEPATIC
Inherited	Congenital erythropoietic porphyria[p]	Acute intermittent porphyria[a] Variegate (mixed) porphyria[p,a] Coproporphyria[p,a] Congenital erythrohepatic porphyria[p]
Acquired	Lead intoxication[*]	Symptomatic porphyria (porphyria cutanea tarda symptomatica)[p]† Hexachlorobenzene intoxication[p]

[p]True porphyrias with cutaneous disease and light sensitivity. Red urine and hemolytic anemia in some of these disorders (see text).

[a]Disorders of precursor (ALA, PBG) excess, with acute neuropsychiatric symptomatology.

[*]Relation to true porphyrias unclear.

†May be genetic predisposition in some instances.

creased UROgen III cosynthetase (isomerase) activity (19). This defect causes a shift from the type III to the type I series, which would tend to impair the synthesis of heme. Heme synthesis is in fact increased in this disorder in response to the hemolytic anemia, and this is presumably mediated by enhancement of ALA synthetase activity. However, much of the ALA and PBG formed as the result of this enzyme induction is siphoned off into URO and COPRO I, the price paid by the patient to maintain adequate production of the physiologic type III isomers and hence of heme. Splenectomy ameliorates the hemolytic anemia and thus decreases the need for accelerated heme synthesis; not surprisingly, therefore, splenectomy often leads to decreased URO and COPRO I excretion and to improvement in the dermatologic as well as the hematologic manifestations of this disorder.

CONGENITAL ERYTHROHEPATIC PROTOPORPHYRIA. As implied in this recently revised name, the increased production of PROTO 9 and to a lesser extent COPRO III appears to arise in both the marrow and the liver (20), not just in the marrow as originally thought. This disorder is inherited as an autosomal dominant and is probably not uncommon. However, it was only recently described, and patients with protoporphyria are often considered to have a primary dermatologic disease called solar urticaria or solar eczema. This is partly because PROTO and COPRO are excreted preferentially via the bile into the feces, and the urine is therefore not discolored. Hence, analysis of fecal and erythrocyte

porphyrins is necessary to establish the diagnosis.

Clinical manifestations consist primarily of relatively mild skin changes in those portions of the body most exposed to sunlight. Only a rare patient has hemolytic anemia, although red cells from these patients can be readily hemolyzed in vitro on exposure to ultraviolet irradiation. The basic biochemical defect is unknown. A defect in heme synthetase would appear to explain the chemical changes, but the relatively crude assays now available fail to support this supposition.

ACUTE INTERMITTENT PORPHYRIA (AIP). This disorder is not a true porphyria and is thus misnamed. There is little if any excess production of porphyrins, and hence there is no photosensitivity or dermatitis, and the freshly passed urine is normal in color. Instead, these patients overproduce and excrete in their urine large quantities of the porphyrin precursors, ALA and PBG. The diagnosis is made presumptively by the Watson-Schwartz test, in which a red color develops when urine containing an excess of PBG is mixed with Ehrlich's reagent. The color is not extractable into chloroform (that formed with urobilinogen is), and false-positive results are further eliminated by failure to extract the pigment into butanol. An excess of PBG in the urine may also cause a dark color to develop when the urine is allowed to stand in the light. This is the result of the formation of porphobilin, an oxidation product of PBG, and probably also of some nonenzymatic conversion of PBG to uroporphyrin.

Clinically, patients with AIP suffer from

a constellation of symptoms and signs, including abdominal colic, constipation, hypertension, peripheral neuropathies, neuroses, and psychoses. Death may ensue from respiratory paralysis and attendant complications. In addition, these patients may evince a variety of changes apparently ascribable to hypothalamic or endocrine dysfunction, including inappropriate ADH secretion, high levels of protein-bound iodine due to increases in thyroid-binding globulin, and imbalances in the secretion of growth hormone and ACTH.

The clinical disorder is more common in women, virtually never commences before the menarche, and often regresses at the time of menopause. In addition, some patients experience exacerbations in relation to the menstrual cycle, and administration of estrogens may cause the disease to flare. It is not yet clear what relationship these findings have to the basic disturbance in heme biosynthesis. Indeed, the pathophysiology of the entire clinical complex of AIP is obscure, since neither ALA nor PBG when given in excess will induce the symptoms and signs of acute intermittent porphyria.

AIP is inherited as an autosomal dominant, but the biochemical disorder is more common than the clinical disease, i.e., many patients have "latent" disease. Latent cases may be made overt or overt cases made worse with the administration of a wide variety of drugs or with carbohydrate deprivation. The latter may occur with the anorexia that accompanies intercurrent illnesses. The inciting drugs include, among many others, barbiturates, meprobamate, sulfonamides, estrogens, and griseofulvin. All these agents are inducers of hepatic ALA synthetase activity in a variety of experimental systems. Fasting, too, facilitates induction of this enzyme.

It seemed possible, therefore, that the biochemical defect in AIP involved an abnormality at the level of ALA synthetase. Indeed, Tschudy et al. observed a marked increase in enzyme activity in the liver of a woman who had just expired from this disorder (21), and this finding has now been reconfirmed in several other studies. Recent evidence suggests that the increase in ALA-synthetase activity is not primary, but is the result of a more distal block at the level of UROgen I synthetase (PBG deaminase) (22, 23). A partial defect here would interfere with heme production and thus would lead to a secondary rise in ALA synthetase activity. ALA and PBG would be overproduced, but porphyrinogens occurring beyond the block would not be formed in excess. This formulation requires further confirmation. Moreover, although it accounts for the biochemical findings, it leaves unexplained the interesting and often devastating neurologic dysfunction that besets patients with this disorder.

VARIEGATE (MIXED) PORPHYRIA. This disorder, very common in the Afrikaner population of South Africa but present throughout the world, is inherited as an autosomal dominant, has a high incidence of latency as in AIP, and is characterized clinically by chronic cutaneous true porphyria sometimes accompanied by acute intermittent attacks identical to those seen in AIP. The dermatologic condition is associated with increased excretion of COPRO III and PROTO 9, primarily in the feces, although the urine contains increased amounts of COPRO as well. Exposed portions of the skin are highly susceptible to trauma, and there is often hypertrichosis, hyperpigmentation, and hirsutism in addition to chronic scarring. Acute attacks are usually precipitated by the same drugs that provoke attacks of AIP, and the clinical and chemical findings are then identical to those of AIP except that they are engrafted upon a true cutaneous porphyria. The basic defect (or defects), which is unknown, will have to explain both the differences from, and the similarities to, AIP.

COPROPORPHYRIA. This recently described disorder is similar in virtually all respects to variegate porphyria, except for a much more selective increase in COPRO III excretion.

ACQUIRED (SYMPTOMATIC) CUTANEOUS PORPHYRIA. These porphyrias of diverse origin are discussed together because they share many features. Most commonly, acquired hepatic porphyria is due to alcoholic liver disease. In fact, patients with liver disease not uncommonly exhibit porphyrinuria (asymptomatic, excessive porphyrin excretion in the urine), although only few have porphyric dermatitis. The same is true for a variety of neoplastic diseases. This has led to the concept that some, or possibly all, cases of "porphyria cutanea tarda symptomatica" (symptomatic cutaneous porphyria of late onset) have a hereditary predisposition that is brought to light by an acquired insult, usually to the liver.

There is a particularly high incidence of acquired hepatic porphyria in the Bantus of South Africa. Urinary excretion of URO III is elevated, in contrast to the findings in variegate porphyria in which COPRO and PROTO are increased. The urine is therefore frequently red. Typically, there are ulcerative lesions, scars, hyperpigmentation, and hypertrichosis of exposed portions of the skin. Liver biopsy characteristically shows cirrhosis with increased iron deposits. Removal of excess iron by phlebotomy often leads to amelioration of both the increased URO excretion and the skin disorder, suggesting that there may be a causal relationship between the iron-loading state and porphyrin overproduction. In contrast to several of the other forms of hepatic porphyria, symptomatic cutaneous porphyria may not be associated with enhanced ALA synthetase activity. However, evidence differs regarding this point. The underlying metabolic defect is unknown, although it has been conjectured that there may be excessive oxidation of porphyrinogens to porphyrins.

There is at least one clear-cut example of truly acquired porphyria—the "epidemic" of severe cutaneous porphyria that occurred in Turkey in the 1950's. This outbreak was traced to hexachlorobenzene, a fungicide that had recently been introduced into the grain in portions of that country. Hexachlorobenzene has subsequently been found to be a potent stimulator of ALA synthetase activity and, when given to rats, to cause marked porphyrin overproduction (24).

HEME DEGRADATION (BILE PIGMENTS)

Normal Pathways

Bilirubin Formation

Recent observations have led to an understanding of the enzymatic mechanisms that mediate the conversion of heme to bile pigment (25). The critical enzyme, microsomal heme oxygenase, is linked to a so-called mixed-function oxidase system and is found in the microsomal fraction of a variety of tissues. The specific activity of this enzyme is highest in the spleen, whereas total organ enzyme content is greatest in the liver. Both hepatic parenchymal and sinusoidal cells contain the enzyme, and it has also been found in kidney, bone marrow, and isolated macrophages. The enzyme is inducible by heme and by a variety of other agents. Its action is to mediate schism of the topmost or α-methene bridge in the heme molecule, with formation of carbon monoxide and the linear tetrapyrrole, biliverdin (Fig. 3-1). The biliverdin is then rapidly reduced to bilirubin by a second enzyme, biliverdin reductase, which is present in the soluble fraction of the same cells. Thus it is the yellow bilirubin molecule that enters the plasma, an obligatory excretory product destined for excretion by the liver.

Heme is the only known source of bile pigment, i.e., there is probably no synthesis of these linear tetrapyrroles directly from pyrrolic or porphyrinic precursors. As described earlier, there are many heme proteins, and these are present in virtually all tissues. Each of these hemes is potentially a source of bile pigment production, the magnitude of which is a function of the size of the specific heme pool and its rate of turnover. Hemoglobin heme in erythroid cells is, of course, the major contributor to bile pigment production. Next in importance are the nonhemoglobin hemes in hepatic cells.

With the use of isotopically labeled glycine and ALA, three general sources of bilirubin production have now been identified (26). These may be referred to as erythrocytic, hepatic, and erythropoietic. Glycine is a cohort label that is incorporated into newly synthesized heme (Fig. 3-2), including the hemoglobin heme of developing erythroid cells. The latter enter the circulation as labeled reticulocytes and then survive for an average of 120 days (Fig. 3-4). When they reach the end of their physiologic life span, the labeled cells are removed from the peripheral blood, and simultaneously a large, late peak of labeled bile pigment is produced (Fig. 3-4) (27-29). This late peak, representing degradation

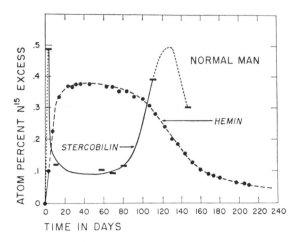

Figure 3–4. Labeling of peripheral blood hemoglobin hemin and fecal stercobilin in a human subject given ^{15}N-glycine at time 0. (From London, I. M., West, R., et al.: J. Biol. Chem. *184*:351, 1950.)

of hemoglobin from senescent red blood cells, accounts for the major fraction of the total labeled pigment. In addition there is a small early-labeled peak, comprising 10 to 20 per cent of the total labeled pigment, that is formed before there is significant label in circulating erythrocytes (Fig. 3–4) (27–29). Recent studies have demonstrated that this early-labeled fraction is heterogeneous in origin and consists of at least two general components (Fig. 3–5) (26, 29–31, 83). There is a very rapidly formed peak which originates almost entirely from the turnover of nonhemoglobin hemes in extraerythroid tissues, primarily the liver (29–32). A slower "plateau" phase follows this initial sharp component. In rats this later fraction also appears to be derived largely from nonerythroid sources, presumably from heme proteins with a slower rate of turnover. In addition, the plateau phase contains an erythropoietic component which is related to the process of hemoglobin synthesis and red cell production in the bone marrow. The magnitude of the erythropoietic component has been a matter of some controversy. It appears to be quite small in rats under normal conditions (29), but may comprise a larger proportion of the early-labeled fraction in species such as man and the dog (30, 31). In all species studied, however, the erythropoietic component may assume major proportions with alterations in red cell production (26, 29–31, 33). It should be pointed out that some labeled pigment continues to be formed at a slow rate between the early and late labeling periods (27–29). The origin of this intermediate fraction is not known with certainty, although in all likelihood it is derived both from nonhemoglobin hemes, such as myoglobin, with a slow rate of turnover, and from some random destruction of circulating erythrocytes.

Bilirubin Excretion

The three main pathways of bilirubin production, feeding into the plasma bili-

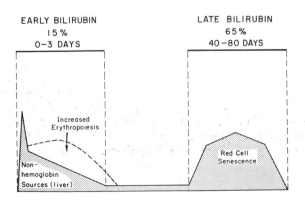

Figure 3–5. Detailed analysis of the sources of bile pigment production in the rat, based on studies with glycine-2-^{14}C. A similar scheme applies to humans, although the early-labeled fraction extends to 4 to 5 days, and the late fraction is formed between 90 to 150 days in man. [From Robinson, S. H., In *Hemopoietic Cellular Proliferation.* Stohlman, F., Jr. (ed.), New York, Grune & Stratton, 1970, p. 180, by permission.]

rubin pool, are indicated schematically in Figure 3–6. Bilirubin in plasma is bound to albumin (34, 35). There is an equilibrium between free and albumin-bound bilirubin which markedly favors the bound state. The plasma bilirubin is transported to the liver, where the excretory process is conveniently viewed as occurring in three phases: hepatic uptake, conjugation, and secretion of the conjugate into the bile. There is growing evidence that these three steps are closely interrelated.

During hepatic uptake bilirubin is dissociated from albumin and enters the hepatic parenchymal cell. There the pigment is bound to two cytoplasmic proteins, known as Y and Z (36, 37). These same globulins also bind a variety of other materials that undergo hepatic excretion, including cortisol, BSP, cholecystographic agents, and flavaspidic acid. Although the Y and Z proteins are clearly implicated in bilirubin binding within the liver cell, they probably do not account for the initial uptake process (37). Southdown sheep are jaundiced because of a defect in hepatic

uptake but apparently have normal concentrations of Y and Z. It is likely that another mechanism, perhaps involving carrier transport, mediates the passage of bilirubin across the plasma membrane of the hepatocyte.

The unconjugated bilirubin taken up by the liver cell is now esterified with two glucuronic acid molecules (38–40). (There is growing evidence that some monoglucuronide is also formed, and that some bilirubin is conjugated with a variety of other sugars.) Conjugation is mediated by the enzyme, bilirubin uridine diphosphate (UDP)-glucuronyl transferase, which is located in the smooth endoplasmic reticulum of the liver cell. A variety of materials undergo similar glucuronidation, and it is not yet clear whether different substrates are handled by different specific glucuronyl transferases or by a small number of enzymes with varying specificities.

The major differences between conjugated and unconjugated bilirubin are shown in Table 3–3. The unconjugated pigment is nonpolar, relatively water insoluble,

FORMATION AND DEGRADATION OF HEME

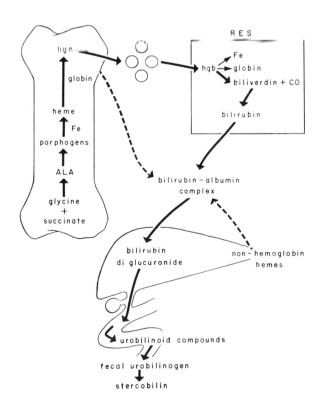

Figure 3–6. [From Robinson, S. H., In *Harvard Pathophysiology Series, Vol. I. Hematology.* Beck, W. S. (ed.), Cambridge, M.I.T. Press, 1973, p. 51.]

TABLE 3–3.   UNCONJUGATED VERSUS CONJUGATED BILIRUBIN

UNCONJUGATED	CONJUGATED
Nonpolar	Polar
Limited solubility in water	Water-soluble
Lipid-soluble	Lipid-insoluble
Passes lipid membranes	Does not pass lipid membranes
No urinary excretion	Urinary excretion
Indirect diazo reaction	Direct diazo reaction

and lipid soluble. It therefore does not gain access to the urine but readily crosses biological membranes. However, its binding to albumin normally prevents bilirubin from escaping from the plasma and extracellular fluid. Unconjugated bilirubin requires both methanol and time for the development of full purple color on diazotization with sulfanilic acid, i.e., it gives an "indirect" diazo reaction. Conjugated bilirubin, on the other hand, is a polar molecule that is water soluble but lipid insoluble. It therefore will not penetrate lipid membranes but may gain access to the urine; like unconjugated bilirubin, the conjugated pigment in the plasma is primarily bound to albumin, but there is a small dialyzable fraction that can be excreted by the kidney (41). Conjugated bilirubin gives a "direct" diazo reaction; color develops immediately without addition of methanol. Thus, in the van den Bergh test used for measurement of serum bilirubin concentration, the conjugate is estimated by the direct color reaction, and total bilirubin (both conjugated and unconjugated) by the color recorded 30 minutes after the addition of methanol. Subtraction of the direct from the total value yields the indirect-reacting fraction, an estimate of the concentration of unconjugated pigment.

In the third phase of hepatic bilirubin excretion, the conjugated pigment is secreted from the liver cell into the bile canaliculus. The precise mechanism by which this occurs is not yet understood, but several facts are known. Secretion appears to be an active, energy-requiring process. It also ap-

pears to be the rate-limiting step in the entire excretory pathway. Finally, the secretory process is highly vulnerable to injury. Thus a defect in the excretion of conjugated bilirubin into the bile is observed very commonly in acquired liver disease due to viral disease, alcohol, or a variety of drugs and is manifested by "regurgitation" of conjugated pigment into the plasma and thence into the urine.

After the conjugated pigment is excreted into the bile, it is transported through the biliary system to the duodenum. Reabsorption from bile or intestinal fluid does not occur because of the solubility properties of the conjugated material. On reaching the lower intestinal tract, bilirubin undergoes a series of reduction reactions, mediated by the intestinal bacteria, which lead to the formation of a group of colorless compounds collectively known as urobilinogen or stercobilinogen. The link with glucuronic acid is largely hydrolyzed during this process. On excretion into the feces, the urobilinogens are oxidized to orange substances, called urobilin or stercobilin. Measurement of daily "fecal urobilinogen" excretion provides a crude but useful estimate of the total biliary excretion of bilirubin; however, a substantial fraction of the total bilirubin cannot be recovered in this form, presumably because some is converted to other compounds. The test involves reduction of urobilin to urobilinogen and measurement of the latter with the same Ehrlich's aldehyde reaction used to assay for porphobilinogen; however, urobilinogen, unlike porphobilinogen, is extracted into chloroform.

Some of the urobilinogen produced in the intestinal tract undergoes an "enterohepatic circulation," i.e., it is absorbed into the portal venous system, extracted by the liver, and then excreted back into the intestine via the bile (Fig. 3–7). A small fraction normally escapes hepatic extraction, enters the systemic circulation via the hepatic vein, and is then excreted by the kidney. Two mechanisms may lead to increased urinary urobilinogen excretion: increased bilirubin production and hence increased formation and recirculation of urobilinogen from the gut, and hepatic cell dysfunction causing decreased extraction of urobilinogen as it passes through the liver. The latter mechanism is commonly

ENTEROHEPATIC CIRCULATION OF UROBILINOGEN

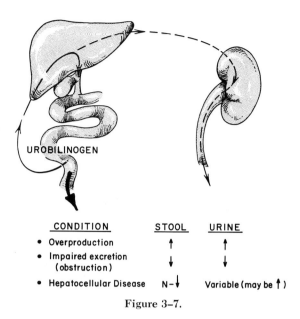

CONDITION	STOOL	URINE
• Overproduction	↑	↑
• Impaired excretion (obstruction)	↓	↓
• Hepatocellular Disease	N–↓	Variable (may be ↑)

Figure 3–7.

observed with hepatocellular disease (e.g., hepatitis) and may sometimes lead to an increase in urine urobilinogen despite a decrease in urobilinogen excretion into the stools. Unfortunately, the clinical value of the urine urobilinogen test is impaired because a variety of factors, such as urinary pH, also influences the clearance of this product.

Developmental Aspects of Bilirubin Metabolism

Bile pigment metabolism changes dramatically during the transition from fetus to infant. Evidence primarily from animal investigations indicates that most or all phases of the hepatic excretory process are in abeyance during fetal life. Although most emphasis has been placed on the immaturity of the conjugating system, it now seems clear that there is also a diminution in the Y protein (42) involved in hepatic uptake or storage of bilirubin, as well as a decreased capacity to secrete conjugated bilirubin into the bile (43). The bilirubin produced by the fetus is excreted by the mother. The unconjugated product is able to pass through the placental barrier, after which it is excreted by the maternal liver

into the maternal bile (43). With birth the infant must quickly develop the normal mechanisms for hepatic bilirubin excretion, and these usually become mature by the tenth to fourteenth day of life. There is evidence that development of the capacity to conjugate bilirubin is at least partly due to substrate induction, as the level of serum unconjugated bilirubin rises after severance of the placenta (44, 45).

In addition to the "immaturity" of the excretory pathway, there is an apparent increase in the early-labeled fraction of bile pigment production during the first few days of extrauterine life (46). Some bilirubin may also be reabsorbed from the intestinal tract after hydrolysis of the glucuronide link, since there are initially no bacteria to mediate conversion to urobilinogen (47). For all of these reasons, the newborn child normally manifests mild unconjugated hyperbilirubinemia. Serum bilirubin concentrations are usually maximal by the fifth day of life, rarely exceed 10 to 12 mg. per 100 ml., and fall to normal levels during the second week. Both the degree of the hyperbilirubinemia and the time required for the jaundice to clear are increased with prematurity.

Disorders of Bilirubin Metabolism (Hyperbilirubinemia)

Each of the sources of bilirubin production and each of the steps in the excretory pathway represent a potential avenue for hyperbilirubinemia. There are several inherited forms of hyperbilirubinemia which are generally rather rare. In these there is often a single, circumscribed defect. Indeed, study of such patients has led to the delineation of many of the mechanisms involved in normal bile pigment metabolism. Acquired causes of jaundice are much more common, and their pathophysiology is more complex since multiple defects are frequently involved. In addition to classifying hyperbilirubinemia as inherited or acquired, it is useful to ask two rather broad questions: is the increased level of bilirubin due to overproduction or to underexcretion, and is the retained bilirubin primarily unconjugated or conjugated in type? The first question can usually be answered by standard tests of hematologic and hepatic function. Measurement of fecal urobilinogen may also be helpful. The second question is answered by measurement of total and direct bilirubin or use of other fractionation procedures, or, more simply, by testing the urine for bilirubin; only conjugated bilirubin is excreted by the kidneys. Unconjugated hyperbilirubinemia is not associated with bilirubinuria, is relatively uncommon, and implicates an abnormality in bilirubin production or in hepatic bilirubin uptake or conjugation, i.e., a defect at or proximal to the conjugation step. Conjugated hyperbilirubinemia is typically associated with bilirubinuria, is quite common, and implicates a problem at the level of the secretory process or more distally in the biliary tree. Frequently, elevated levels of conjugated bilirubin are associated with increases in the unconjugated fraction as well. Some of the major causes of hyperbilirubinemia are listed in Table 3–4 and are described briefly below.

UNCONJUGATED HYPERBILIRUBINEMIA

Bilirubin Overproduction

ERYTHROCYTIC SOURCES. An increased rate of hemoglobin degradation in hemolytic disorders is the most common cause of overproduction jaundice and probably the most common cause of unconjugated hyperbilirubinemia. Serum bilirubin concentrations rarely exceed 6 to 7 mg. per 100 ml., and there is no significant excretion of bilirubin into the urine.

HEPATIC SOURCES. An increase in the hepatic fraction of early-labeled bilirubin

TABLE 3–4. DEFECTS IN BILIRUBIN METABOLISM

UNCONJUGATED HYPERBILIRUBINEMIA WITHOUT BILIRUBINURIA

A. Overproduction
    1. Hemolysis
    2. Increase in early-labeled bilirubin
        a. Hepatic sources
        b. Ineffective erythropoiesis

B. Impaired Excretion
    1. Defects in hepatic uptake
        a. Drugs (flavaspidic acid, etc.)
        b. Congenital unconjugated hyperbilirubinemia, mild type (Gilbert-Lereboullet syndrome)[*]
        c. Post-hepatitis hyperbilirubinemia[*]
    2. Defects in conjugation
        a. Physiologic jaundice of newborn (see text)
        b. Drugs and hormonal agents (maternal serum factor, breast milk factor)
        c. Congenital unconjugated hyperbilirubinemia, severe type (Crigler-Najjar syndrome, Gunn rat)
        d. Congenital unconjugated hyperbilirubinemia, moderate type (Arias)
        e. Congenital unconjugated hyperbilirubinemia, mild type (Gilbert-Lereboullet syndrome)[*]

PREDOMINANTLY CONJUGATED HYPERBILIRUBINEMIA WITH BILIRUBINURIA

    3. Defects in secretion and/or canalicular function
        a. Dubin-Johnson and Rotor syndromes
        b. Recurrent jaundice of pregnancy
        c. Benign recurrent cholestasis
        d. Drugs (chlorpromazine, androgenic and estrogenic hormones, etc.)
        e. Cholestatic form of viral hepatitis
    4. Extrahepatic obstruction
        a. Stone, stricture, or carcinoma affecting common duct
        b. Congenital atresia of bile ducts

C. Multiple Defects
    1. Most forms of acquired hepatocellular disease (hepatitis, cirrhosis)

[*]Nature of defect(s) still uncertain (see text).

(Figs. 3–5 and 3–6) has been observed in rats under a variety of conditions affecting liver function (48). A similar explanation has been proposed for the enlarged early-labeled peak found in a patient with protoporphyria (49). It seems possible that increased bilirubin production from non-hemoglobin sources may be a sensitive index of liver dysfunction. Whether such changes occur commonly in human subjects and whether they may be of sufficient magnitude to cause or contribute to clinical hyperbilirubinemia are questions that still await resolution.

ERYTHROPOIETIC SOURCES. Enlargement of the erythropoietic bilirubin fraction occurs in two settings: with physiologically regulated erythroid hyperplasia and with hematologic diseases associated with "ineffective erythropoiesis" (destruction of immature erythroid cells in or soon after leaving the marrow, with impairment of net red cell production). The unconjugated hyperbilirubinemia found in patients with pernicious anemia (50), thalassemia (51, 52), sideroblastic anemia (33), and isolated instances of more unusual hematologic disorders (53, 54) is due largely to the destruction of abnormal erythroid precursors, with conversion of their newly synthesized hemoglobin to early-labeled bile pigment (Fig. 3–8). Pathologic ineffective erythropoiesis may be recognized by erythroid hyperplasia of the bone marrow out of proportion to the degree of reticulocytosis and by evidence of increased bile pigment production (unconjugated hyper-

bilirubinemia, increased fecal urobilinogen excretion), although there is usually little or no hemolysis (55). Ferrokinetic studies characteristically reveal rapid disappearance of ^{59}Fe from the plasma, an increased rate of iron turnover, but decreased incorporation of ^{59}Fe into circulating red cells (55). Studies with glycine-2-^{14}C are laborious and are therefore performed only rarely, but they reveal an increase in the early-labeled bilirubin fraction (26, 33, 50–54).

It has been suggested that a physiologic degree of ineffective erythropoiesis also explains the erythropoietic bilirubin fraction in normal subjects and the increase in this component found with the normal marrow response to blood loss, hemolysis, or hypoxia. However, there has been little direct evidence to substantiate this concept. Indeed, recent observations have suggested that the increased production of erythropoietic bilirubin found with erythroid hyperplasia is due to surface remodeling of reticulocytes and perhaps also earlier erythroid cells, a process by which these large cells lose significant portions of their plasma membrane, accompanied by small fragments of hemoglobinized cytoplasm (56, 57).

Bilirubin Underexcretion

DEFECTS IN HEPATIC UPTAKE. Perhaps the most clear-cut example is the unconjugated hyperbilirubinemia produced by

Figure 3–8. Production of labeled bile pigment (fecal stercobilin) and red cell hemoglobin heme from glycine-2-^{14}C in a girl with thalassemia minor, unconjugated hyperbilirubinemia, and severe ineffective erythropoiesis. The early-labeled peak accounts for over 80 per cent of the total labeled pigment, as compared to only 10 to 20 per cent with normal subjects. (From Robinson, S. H., Vanier, T., et al.: New Engl. J. Med. 267:523, 1962.)

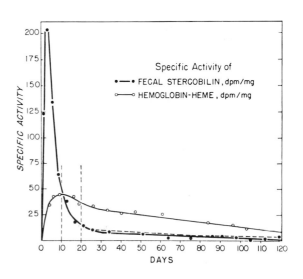

certain drugs, such as the oral cholecystographic dyes and flavaspidic acid, an antihelminthic agent. These apparently act by competing with bilirubin for receptor sites on the Z protein (36). A decreased concentration of the Y protein has been described in neonatal animals and probably contributes to physiologic jaundice of the newborn (42). It may be argued that these do not represent true uptake defects, since the Y and Z proteins probably function just distal to the uptake step. It has been suggested that benign constitutional unconjugated hyperbilirubinemia (Gilbert-Lereboullet syndrome) and the apparently similar disorder, post-hepatitis hyperbilirubinemia, are due to impaired bilirubin uptake. However, these have also been attributed to a mild conjugating defect and are discussed under that heading.

DEFECTS IN BILIRUBIN CONJUGATION. Several entities may be classified here. Certain drugs, such as novobiocin, interfere with the conjugation process and may lead to mild, reversible, unconjugated hyperbilirubinemia. In addition, hormonal factors are implicated in two forms of neonatal jaundice. In a rare disorder, severe jaundice sometimes leading to kernicterus is caused by a factor transmitted to the child from the maternal plasma (58). This factor inhibits conjugation in vitro and appears to be a progestational steroid (58). In breast milk hyperbilirubinemia, a milk-born factor, probably a congener of pregnanediol, leads to unconjugated hyperbilirubinemia which disappears rapidly with cessation of breast-feeding (59). Jaundice is mild to moderate, does not lead to kernicterus, and disappears spontaneously after 1 to 2 months despite continued breast-feeding.

The three forms of *congenital unconjugated hyperbilirubinemia* comprise an interesting and instructive spectrum. They are compared in Table 3–5, which is derived largely from the observations of Arias and co-workers (60). The mild disorder, *Gilbert-Lereboullet syndrome,* or, more simply, Gilbert's syndrome, was thought perhaps to be an abnormality of bilirubin uptake, but recent assays of liver biopsy specimens showed low levels of bilirubin UDP-glucuronyl transferase, implicating a defect in conjugation (61). Studies of labeled bilirubin disappearance from the plasma have suggested that there may, in fact, be problems of both uptake and conjugation (62); indeed, it seems possible that the entire excretory pathway is underdeveloped in these patients. In addition, there is some bilirubin overproduction as the result of mild hemolysis in some of these patients. It is probable that Gilbert's syndrome is not a single disease entity, and that otherwise unexplained, sometimes familial, unconjugated hyperbilirubinemia may be due to different causes in different groups of patients. Indeed, great care must be taken to exclude other disorders associated with mild unconjugated hyperbilirubinemia (see preceding sections) before making such a diagnosis.

In familial cases, Gilbert's syndrome is inherited as an autosomal dominant trait.

TABLE 3–5. CONGENITAL UNCONJUGATED HYPERBILIRUBINEMIA

	MILD (GILBERT-LEREBOULLET)	MODERATE (ARIAS)	SEVERE (CRIGLER-NAJJAR)
Inheritance	Dominant°	Dominant°°	Recessive
Serum bilirubin (mg./100 ml.)	1–6	6–20	13–48 (usually >20)
Kernicterus	No	Rare	Yes
Conjugated bilirubin in bile	Yes†	Yes	No
Response to phenobarbital	Yes	Yes	No
Bilirubin conjugation	Reduced‡	Very reduced	Absent

°Many cases without familial incidence.
°°"Variable expressivity."
†Assumed to be present.
‡Other defects may coexist (see text).

However, a familial incidence cannot be documented in many instances. It is a benign, asymptomatic disorder characterized by unconjugated hyperbilirubinemia without bilirubinuria (63). Some patients complain of fatigue or vague abdominal discomfort, but these symptoms often disappear with reassurance. Serum bilirubin levels can reach approximately 6 mg. per 100 ml., are usually less than 3 mg. per 100 ml., frequently fluctuate with time, and may intermittently fall within the range of normal. Liver function tests and liver biopsy are normal, although there may sometimes be mild abnormalities on testing with BSP. Hyperbilirubinemia is exacerbated by intercurrent illnesses, certain drugs, including alcohol, and fasting. Indeed, restriction of caloric intake to 400 calories per day for 1 to 2 days has been proposed as a presumptive test for Gilbert's syndrome, since this will elevate the concentration of serum unconjugated bilirubin to levels above normal in all patients with this disorder. However, fasting will also raise serum bilirubin concentrations in normal subjects, and this test is probably not of diagnostic value. The mechanism of this effect may be inhibition of hepatic bilirubin uptake (64), although an increase in hepatic bilirubin production might also play a role.

The *intermediate syndrome,* referred to as type II by Arias (60), clearly seems to be due to a partial defect in bilirubin conjugation (60, 65). Pedigrees of such patients sometimes contain individuals who resemble those with Gilbert's syndrome but never include patients with the most severe disorder, the *Crigler-Najjar syndrome* (type I in the Arias classification). Kernicterus is largely a function of the level of unconjugated hyperbilirubinemia and therefore is uncommon in the moderate disorder in which serum bilirubin levels are usually less than 20 mg. per 100 ml. Patients with type I disease, the Crigler-Najjar syndrome, characteristically have serum levels of unconjugated bilirubin exceeding 20 mg. per 100 ml. starting soon after birth. Kernicterus is therefore the rule in this disorder.

Patients with the Crigler-Najjar syndrome fail to respond to phenobarbital with a fall in serum bilirubin levels (60). This observation, together with the total absence of conjugated bilirubin from the bile, has been taken as evidence that these patients are completely deficient in bilirubin UDP-glucuronyl transferase activity. This conclusion is further substantiated by direct measurements of enzyme activity in Gunn rats, mutant Wistar rats with a disorder virtually identical to that of patients with the Crigler-Najjar syndrome. Patients with the intermediate type II syndrome do respond to phenobarbital, often with quite striking reductions in the level of jaundice (66, 67), and do have some conjugated bilirubin in the bile (60). These findings suggest an only partial diminution in conjugating activity which can then be augmented by pharmacologic stimulation (60). Although these conclusions appear valid, it is now clear that phenobarbital has multiple effects on liver function. In addition to inducing increased activity of bilirubin UDP-glucuronyl transferase, it has stimulatory effects on the concentration of the Y protein (68) and on the secretory process (69, 70) and augments production of the hepatic component of early-labeled bilirubin as well (26, 71).

Physiologic jaundice of the newborn is classically categorized as a conjugation defect, although it now appears that the entire excretory pathway is immature, as discussed in the preceding section, Developmental Aspects of Bilirubin Metabolism. The transient, moderate, unconjugated hyperbilirubinemia typically observed during the first week after birth is innocuous. However, the underlying causes may lead to severe complications if there is a superimposed alteration in bilirubin metabolism. This is most commonly due to Rh incompatibility and attendant hemolysis but may also be related to deficiency of glucose-6-phosphate dehydrogenase or other congenital hemolytic anemias. The level of unconjugated bilirubin climbs precipitously in the absence of an effective excretory pathway. Since the unconjugated pigment readily traverses the blood-brain barrier, bilirubin encephalopathy (kernicterus) becomes a grave danger. Pediatricians agree that serum bilirubin levels in excess of 20 mg. per 100 ml. must be avoided, and there is some evidence that neonates who have more moderate levels of hyperbilirubinemia—even in the range of 10 to 15 mg. per 100 ml.—may be at risk with regard to future neurologic and intellectual development, particularly if the infant is ill or premature.

Some discussion of the treatment of severe neonatal jaundice, as encountered with erythroblastosis fetalis or congenital defects in pigment conjugation, is in order before we leave the subject of unconjugated hyperbilirubinemia. Several complications are to be avoided if possible. Hypoxia predisposes patients to bilirubin encephalopathy. Decreased caloric intake may increase the level of hyperbilirubinemia, as described earlier. Certain drugs, including salicylates and sulfonamides, displace unconjugated bilirubin from its bond with albumin and make more free pigment available for diffusion across the blood-brain barrier (72). Similarly, a decrease in pH or hypoalbuminemia may cause an increase in the unbound pigment fraction. Conversely, infusions of albumin have been advocated to retain more bilirubin within the vascular compartment, particularly when serum albumin is depressed, as with prematurity. Phenobarbital treatment of mothers during the last few weeks of pregnancy, or of infants soon after birth, has been shown in some studies to accelerate the development of the normal excretory mechanisms and to decrease the level of neonatal jaundice (73, 74). However, the small magnitude of the effect and the latent period of several days to several weeks before the drug is maximally effective probably make this an impractical means of dealing with severe degrees of hyperbilirubinemia. Oral agar has also been shown to reduce the level of neonatal hyperbilirubinemia (47) by retaining bilirubin in the intestinal tract; this observation would appear to be of more theoretical than practical importance.

The mainstays of therapy are phototherapy and exchange transfusion. The blue lights now used so frequently in the nursery act by causing photodegradation of the unstable bilirubin molecule in the skin to products that do not require conjugation for excretion (75, 76). They may also cause an increase in the diffusion of small amounts of unconjugated bilirubin into bile by mechanisms that are not well understood (76). Despite the fact that phototherapy is now quite commonly used, it has not been proved with certainty that the breakdown products formed are entirely innocuous to the infant. On the other hand, exchange transfusion serves to remove three different products: unconjugated bilirubin, antibody to the infant's red cells, and, probably most important, sensitized red cells, hemolysis of which is the source of the excess bilirubin production.

PRIMARILY CONJUGATED HYPERBILIRUBINEMIA

Bilirubin Underexcretion

DEFECTS IN SECRETION AND/OR CANALICULAR FUNCTION. At this stage of our knowledge, it is difficult to discriminate defects in excretion of conjugated pigment intrinsic to the liver cell from those just distal to the cell membrane at the level of the bile canaliculus. The precise anatomic location of the abnormalities that account for the disorders discussed in this section are therefore still somewhat hypothetical.

The *Dubin-Johnson syndrome* is an autosomal dominant disorder in which there is inhibition of the hepatic excretion of a variety of materials, including conjugated bilirubin, conjugated BSP, and oral cholecystographic dyes (77, 78). The secretory defect is apparently within the hepatocyte. There is a characteristic brown-black discoloration of the liver due to melanin or a melanin-like substance, which similarly cannot be secreted normally into the bile. The level of jaundice may vary considerably in a single patient with this disease. There is a characteristic abnormality on testing with BSP: the concentration of dye in the plasma is normal or, more often, moderately elevated at 45 minutes, but values rise again at 1.5 to 2 hours, and BSP may then be excreted in the urine. The late-appearing dye is BSP that has been conjugated in the liver but then regurgitated back into the plasma because of the defect in secretory function.

The Dubin-Johnson syndrome is benign but may mimic gallbladder disease, particularly since these patients may have some abdominal discomfort and frequently have nonvisualization of the gallbladder with oral cholecystographic agents. In addition, the liver may sometimes be enlarged and tender. Although there is some dispute about this point, the Rotor syndrome is probably identical to the Dubin-Johnson syndrome except for the absence of liver pigmentation.

Recurrent jaundice of pregnancy is an interesting disorder in which conjugated hyperbilirubinemia and bilirubinuria recur during the third trimester of each pregnancy and disappear soon after parturition (79). Unlike the Dubin-Johnson and Rotor syndromes, the defect apparently resides at the level of the bile canaliculus rather than within the parenchymal cell. This is an example of true intrahepatic cholestasis, i.e., all of the symptoms and signs of extrahepatic biliary obstruction are present. There is evidence of bile stasis on liver biopsy, the serum alkaline phosphatase is elevated, and the patients characteristically have pruritus as the result of bile salt retention—findings that are absent in the Dubin-Johnson syndrome. Many patients with pruritus gravidarum have recurrent jaundice of pregnancy in anicteric form. Administration of estrogens to patients with this disorder when they are not pregnant leads to recurrence of the syndrome. Estrogens are known to inhibit hepatic excretory function, and recurrent jaundice of pregnancy appears to represent a particular sensitivity to the effect of these agents.

Perhaps not surprisingly, it has recently been reported that many women who develop jaundice during pregnancy or during use of oral contraceptives have the Dubin-Johnson syndrome, frequently unnoticed until the superimposed effects of estrogen make the disorder manifest (80). The clinical aspects of this syndrome run true to form during pregnancy and thus differentiate it from the true cholestatic lesion found with recurrent jaundice of pregnancy.

Benign recurrent cholestasis (81) resembles recurrent jaundice of pregnancy in almost all respects except for the absence of a regular relationship to pregnancy. A variety of drugs also may cause impairment of hepatic secretory function, usually with the clinical picture of intrahepatic cholestasis. Offending agents include the phenothiazines and androgenic and estrogenic hormones, to name but a few. The defect is almost always reversible on withdrawal of the drug. In addition, some patients with viral hepatitis have an obstructive picture with only little hepatic necrosis; these subjects are said to have cholestatic infectious hepatitis.

EXTRAHEPATIC BILIARY OBSTRUCTION. Biliary obstruction is most commonly due to stone, stricture, or carcinoma occluding the common bile duct and is in general uncommon in the pediatric age group. Children with gallstones should be investigated for hemolytic anemia. In infants evidence of biliary obstruction should lead to consideration of atresia of the bile ducts. The clinical and chemical picture of extrahepatic biliary obstruction resembles that described above for intrahepatic cholestasis in virtually all respects.

MIXED DEFECTS: ACQUIRED LIVER DISEASE. In acute hepatitis and chronic liver disease, defects at several points contribute to hyperbilirubinemia. There is frequently some hemolysis, and thus the erythrocytic and, to a lesser extent, the erythropoietic fractions of bile pigment formation are often increased. In addition, the hepatic bilirubin component may be enlarged, if recent observations in laboratory animals prove applicable to man. Presumably, the uptake and conjugation phases of the hepatic excretory pathway are also deranged to some extent. Despite these multiple causes of unconjugated hyperbilirubinemia, a substantial portion of the serum bilirubin is typically conjugated in patients with acquired insults to the liver. This appears to be due to the particular vulnerability of the secretory pathway to injury and also to physical obstruction of small bile radicles by architectural distortion and edema.

References

1. Marver, H. S., and Schmid, R.: The porphyrias, In *Metabolic Basis of Inherited Disease.* 3rd ed. Stanbury, J. B., Wyngaarden, J. B., et al. (eds.), New York, McGraw-Hill, 1972, p. 1087.
2. Porphyria and disorders of porphyrin metabolism. Semin. Hematol. 4: no. 4, 1968.
3. Schmid, R.: Hyperbilirubinemia, In *Metabolic Basis of Inherited Disease.* 3rd ed. Stanbury, J. B., Wyngaarden, J. B., et al. (eds.), New York, McGraw-Hill, 1972, p. 1141.
4. Physiology and disorders of hemoglobin degradation. Semin. Hematol. 9: nos. 1 and 2, 1972.
5. Lester, R., and Troxler, R. F.: Recent advances in bile pigment metabolism. Gastroenterology 56:143, 1969.

6. Fleischner, G., and Arias, I. M.: Recent advances in bilirubin formation, transport, metabolism and excretion. Am. J. Med. 49:576, 1970.

7. Shemin, D., and Rittenberg, D.: The biological utilization of glycine for the synthesis of the protoporphyrin of hemoglobin. J. Biol. Chem. 166:621, 1946.

8. Magnus, I. A., Porter, A. D., et al.: Action spectrum for skin lesions in porphyria cutanea tarda. Lancet 1:912, 1959.

9. Vavra, J. D., Mayer, V. K., et al.: In vitro heme synthesis by human blood: abnormal heme synthesis in thalassemia minor. J. Lab. Clin. Med. 63:736, 1964.

10. MacGibbon, B. H., and Mollin, D. L.: Sideroblastic anaemia in man: Observations on seventy cases. Br. J. Haematol. 11:59, 1965.

11. Harris, J. W., and Horrigan, D. L.: Pyridoxine-responsive anemia—prototype and variations on the theme, In Vitamins and Hormones. Vol. 22. Harris, R. S., Wool, I. G., et al. (eds.), New York, Academic Press, 1964, p. 721.

12. Vogler, W. R., and Mingioli, E. S.: Heme synthesis in pyridoxine-responsive anemia. New Engl. J. Med. 273:347, 1965.

13. Vogler, W. R., and Mingioli, E. S.: Porphyrin synthesis and heme synthetase activity in pyridoxine-responsive anemia. Blood 32:979, 1968.

14. Hines, J. D., and Cowan, D. H.: Studies on the pathogenesis of alcohol-induced sideroblastic bone-marrow abnormalities. New Engl. J. Med. 283:441, 1970.

15. Goldberg, A.: Lead poisoning as a disorder of heme synthesis. Semin. Hematol. 4:424, 1968.

16. Bessis, M. C., and Breton-Gorius, J.: Iron metabolism in the bone marrow as seen by electron microscopy: A critical review. Blood 19:635, 1962.

17. Griggs, R. C.: Lead poisoning: hematologic aspects, In Progress in Hematology. Vol. IV. Moore, C. V., and Brown, E. B. (eds.), New York, Grune and Stratton, 1964, p. 117.

18. Dean, G.: The Porphyrias. 2nd ed. Philadelphia, J. B. Lippincott, 1971.

19. Romeo, G., and Levin, E. Y.: Uroporphyrinogen III cosynthetase in human congenital erythropoietic porphyria. Proc. Natl. Acad. Sci. USA. 63:856, 1969.

20. Scholnick, P., Marver, H. S., et al.: Erythropoietic protoporphyria: Evidence for multiple sites of excess protoporphyrin formation. J. Clin. Invest. 50:203, 1971.

21. Tschudy, D. P., Perlroth, M. G., et al.: Acute intermittent porphyria: The first "overproduction disease" localized to a specific enzyme. Proc. Natl. Acad. Sci. USA. 53:841, 1965.

22. Stroud, L. J., Felsher, B. F., et al.: Heme biosynthesis in intermittent acute porphyria: Decreased hepatic conversion of porphobilinogen to porphyrias and increased δ-aminolevulinic acid synthetase activity. Proc. Natl. Acad. Sci. USA. 67:1315, 1970.

23. Miyagi, K., Cardinal, R., et al.: The serum porphobilinogen and the hepatic porphobilinogen deaminase in normal and porphyric individuals. J. Lab. Clin. Med. 78:683, 1971.

24. Ockner, R. K., and Schmid, R.: Acquired porphyria in man and rat due to hexachlorobenzene intoxication. Nature (Lond.) 189:449, 1961.

25. Tenhunen, R., Marver, H. S.: The enzymatic conversion of heme to bilirubin by microsomal heme oxygenase. Proc. Natl. Acad. Sci. USA 61:748, 1968.

26. Robinson, S. H.: Formation of bilirubin from erythroid and nonerythroid sources. Semin. Hematol. 9:43, 1972.

27. London, I. M., West, R., et al.: On the origin of bile pigment in normal man. J. Biol. Chem. 184:351, 1950.

28. Gray, C. H., Neuberger, A., et al.: Studies in congenital porphyria. 2. Incorporation of ^{15}N in the stercobilin in the normal and in the porphyric. Biochem. J. 47:87, 1950.

29. Robinson, S. H., Tsong, M., et al.: The sources of bile pigment in the rat: Studies of the "early-labeled" fraction. J. Clin. Invest. 45:1569, 1966.

30. Israels, L. G., Yamamoto, T., et al.: Shunt bilirubin: Evidence for two components. Science 139:1054, 1963.

31. Schwartz, S.: Quantitation of erythropoietic and non-erythropoietic contribution to early labeling of bile pigments, In Bilirubin Metabolism. Bouchier, I. A. D., and Billing, B. H. (eds.), Oxford, Blackwell, 1967, p. 15.

32. Robinson, S. H., Owen, C. A., Jr., et al.: Bilirubin formation in the liver from non-hemoglobin sources. Blood 26:823, 1965.

33. Barrett, P. V. D., Cline, M. J., et al.: The association of the urobilin "early peak" and erythropoiesis in man. J. Clin. Invest. 45:1657, 1966.

34. Ostrow, J. D., and Schmid, R.: The protein-binding of C^{14}-bilirubin in human and murine serum. J. Clin. Invest. 42:1286, 1963.

35. Schmid, R., Diamond, I., et al.: Interaction of bilirubin with albumin. Nature (Lond.) 206:1041, 1965.

36. Levi, A. J., Gatmaitan, Z., et al.: Two hepatic cytoplasmic protein fractions, Y and Z, and their possible role in the hepatic uptake of bilirubin, sulfobromophthalein, and other anions. J. Clin. Invest. 48:2156, 1969.

37. Reyes, H., Levi, A. J., et al.: Studies of Y and Z, two hepatic cytoplasmic organic anion-binding proteins: Effect of drugs, chemicals, hormones, and cholestasis. J. Clin. Invest. 50:2242, 1971.

38. Schmid, R.: Direct-reacting bilirubin, bilirubin glucuronide, in serum bile and urine. Science 124:76, 1956.

39. Billing, B. H., Cole, P. G., et al.: The excretion of bilirubin as a diglucuronide giving the direct van den Bergh reaction. Biochem. J. 65:774, 1957.

40. Talafant, E.: Properties and composition of bile pigment, giving direct diazo reaction. Nature (Lond.) 178:312, 1956.

41. Fulop, M., Sandson, J., et al.: Dialyzability, protein binding, and renal excretion of plasma conjugated bilirubin. J. Clin. Invest. 44:666, 1965.

42. Levi, A. J., Gatmaitan, Z., et al.: Deficiency of hepatic organic anion-binding protein, im-

paired organic anion uptake by liver and "physiologic" jaundice in newborn monkeys. New Engl. J. Med. 283:1136, 1970.

43. Schenker, S., Dawber, N. H., et al.: Bilirubin metabolism in the fetus. J. Clin. Invest. 43: 32, 1964.

44. Bakken, A. F.: Effects of unconjugated bilirubin on bilirubin-UDP-glucuronyl transferase activity in liver of newborn rats. Pediatr. Res. 3:205, 1969.

45. Thaler, M. M.: Substrate-induced conjugation of bilirubin in genetically deficient newborn rats. Science 170:555, 1970.

46. Vest, M., Strebel, L., et al.: The extent of "shunt" bilirubin and erythrocyte survival in the newborn infant measured by the administration of ¹⁵N-glycine. Biochem. J. 95:11c, 1965.

47. Poland, R. L., and Odell, G. B.: Physiologic jaundice: The enterohepatic circulation of bilirubin. New Engl. J. Med. 284:1, 1971.

48. Robinson, S. H.: Increased bilirubin formation from nonhemoglobin sources in rats with disorders of the liver. J. Lab. Clin. Med. 73: 668, 1969.

49. Gray, C. H., Kulczycka, A., et al.: Isotope studies on a case of erythropoietic protoporphyria. Clin. Sci. 26:7, 1964.

50. London, I. M., and West, R.: The formation of bile pigment in pernicious anemia. J. Biol. Chem. 184:359, 1950.

51. Grinstein, M., Bannerman, R. M., et al.: Hemoglobin metabolism in thalassemia. In vivo studies. Am. J. Med. 29:18, 1960.

52. Robinson, S. H., Vanier, T., et al.: Jaundice in thalassemia minor: A consequence of "ineffective erythropoiesis." New Engl. J. Med. 267:523, 1962.

53. Israels, L. G., and Zipursky, A.: Primary shunt hyperbilirubinaemia. Nature (Lond.) 193:73, 1962.

54. Berendsohn, S., Lowman, J., et al.: Idiopathic dyserythropoietic jaundice. Blood 24:1, 1964.

55. Giblett, E. R., et al.: Erythrokinetics: Quantitative measurement of red cell production and destruction in normal subjects and patients with anemia. Blood 11:291, 1956.

56. Ganzoni, A., Hillman, R. S., et al.: Maturation of the macroreticulocyte. Br. J. Haematol. 16: 119, 1969.

57. Come, S. E., Shohet, S. B., et al.: Surface remodelling of reticulocytes produced in response to erythroid stress. Nature [New Biol.] 236:157, 1972.

58. Arias, I. M., Wolfson, S., et al.: Transient familial neonatal hyperbilirubinemia. J. Clin. Invest. 44:1442, 1965.

59. Arias, I. M., Gartner, L. M., et al.: Prolonged neonatal unconjugated hyperbilirubinemia associated with breast feeding and a steroid, pregnane-3(alpha), 20 (beta)-diol, in maternal milk that inhibits glucuronide formation in vitro. J. Clin. Invest. 43:2037, 1964.

60. Arias, I. M., Gartner, L. M., et al.: Chronic nonhemolytic unconjugated hyperbilirubinemia with glucuronyl transferase deficiency: Clinical, biochemical, pharmacologic, and genetic evidence for heterogeneity. Am. J. Med. 47: 395, 1969.

61. Black, M., and Billing, B. H.: Hepatic bilirubin UDP glucuronyl transferase activity in liver disease and Gilbert's syndrome. New Engl. J. Med. 280:1266, 1969.

62. Berk, P. D., Bloomer, J. R., et al.: Constitutional hepatic dysfunction (Gilbert's syndrome). Am. J. Med. 49:296, 1970.

63. Foulk, W. T., Butt, H. R., et al.: Constitutional hepatic dysfunction (Gilbert's disease): Its natural history and related syndromes. Medicine 38:25, 1959.

64. Felsher, B. F., Rickard, D., et al.: The reciprocal relation between caloric intake and the degree of hyperbilirubinemia in Gilbert's syndrome. New Engl. J. Med. 283:170, 1970.

65. Arias, I. M.: Chronic unconjugated hyperbilirubinemia without overt signs of hemolysis in adolescents and adults. J. Clin. Invest. 41: 2233, 1962.

66. Yaffe, S. J., Levy, G., et al.: Enhancement of glucuronide-conjugating capacity in a hyperbilirubinemic infant due to apparent enzyme induction by phenobarbital. New Engl. J. Med. 275:1461, 1966.

67. Crigler, J. F., Jr., and Gold, N. I.: Effect of sodium phenobarbital on bilirubin metabolism in an infant with congenital nonhemolytic unconjugated hyperbilirubinemia, and kernicterus. J. Clin. Invest. 48:42, 1969.

68. Reyes, H., Levi, A. J., et al.: Organic anion-binding protein in rat liver: Drug induction and its physiologic consequence. Proc. Natl. Acad. Sci. USA. 64:168, 1969.

69. Roberts, R. J., and Plaa, G. L.: Effect of phenobarbital on the excretion of an exogenous bilirubin load. Biochem. Pharmacol. 16:827, 1967.

70. Robinson, S. H., Yannoni, C., et al.: Bilirubin excretion in rats with normal and impaired bilirubin conjugation. Effect of phenobarbital. J. Clin. Invest. 50:2606, 1971.

71. Schmid, R., Murver, H. S., et al.: Enhanced formation of rapidly labeled bilirubin by phenobarbital: Hepatic microsomal cytochromes as a possible source. Biochem. Biophys. Res. Commun. 24:319, 1966.

72. Diamond, I., and Schmid, R.: Experimental bilirubin encephalopathy: The mode of entry of bilirubin-¹⁴C into the central nervous system. J. Clin. Invest. 45:678, 1966.

73. Maurer, H. M., Woff, J. A., et al.: Reduction in concentration of total serum-bilirubin in offspring of women treated with phenobarbitone during pregnancy. Lancet 2:122, 1968.

74. Trolle, D.: Decrease of total serum-bilirubin concentration in newborn infants after phenobarbitone treatment. Lancet 2:705, 1968.

75. Callahan, E. W., Thaler, M. M., et al.: Phototherapy of severe unconjugated hyperbilirubinemia: Formation and removal of labeled bilirubin derivatives. Pediatrics 46:841, 1970.

76. Ostrow, J. D.: Photocatabolism of labeled bilirubin in the congenitally jaundiced (Gunn) rat. J. Clin. Invest. 50:707, 1971.

77. Dubin, I. N.: Chronic idiopathic jaundice. Am. J. Med. 24:268, 1958.

78. Sprinz, H., and Nelson, R. S.: Persistent nonhemolytic hyperbilirubinemia associated with lipochrome-like pigment in liver cells: Report of four cases. Ann. Intern. Med. 41:952, 1954.

79. Adlercreutz, H., Svanborg, A., et al.: Recurrent jaundice in pregnancy. I. A clinical and ultrastructural study. Am. J. Med. *42*:335, 1967.

80. Cohen, L., Lewis, C., et al.: Pregnancy, oral contraceptives, and chronic familial jaundice with predominantly conjugated hyperbilirubinemia (Dubin-Johnson syndrome). Gastroenterology *62*:1182, 1972.

81. Summerskill, W. H. J., and Walshe, J. M.: Benign recurrent intrahepatic "obstructive" jaundice. Lancet *2*:686, 1959.

82. Robinson, S. H.: Heme metabolism: The porphyrias, bilirubin production, In *Harvard Pathophysiology Series, Vol. I. Hematology.* Beck, W. S. (ed.), Cambridge, Mass., Massachusetts Institute of Technology Press, 1973, p. 51.

83. Robinson, S. H.: Ineffective erythropoiesis and the erythropoietic component of early-labeled bilirubin, In *Hemopoietic Cellular Proliferation.* Stohlman, F., Jr. (ed.), New York, Grune and Stratton, 1970, p. 180.

Red Cell Production

Chapter 4

The Nutritional Anemias

by Peter R. Dallman

INTRODUCTION

Malnutrition has always affected a large segment of the world's population. Yet only in the last few decades has there been a widespread awareness that dietary insufficiency can interfere, often permanently, with normal growth and development. The manifestations of malnutrition are usually most severe in the growing child, whose nutritional needs are greatest but whose capacity to adapt to deficiency states is in many ways most restricted. The pathophysiology of the nutritional anemias is therefore a topic of importance, not only for the management of individual young patients but also for planning necessary public health measures to improve the diet.

This chapter deals first with those general topics that apply to the pathophysiology and management of all forms of nutritional anemia. Then follow sections on three deficiency states that are recognized primarily through their association with anemia. Of these, iron deficiency is by far the most common cause of anemia in children and will be discussed in most detail. Folate lack is next in prevalence, and vitamin B_{12} deficiency is rare. Then there are brief discussions of copper and vitamin E

deficiency. Though the clinical importance of these conditions remains uncertain, the pathogenesis of both deficiency states is interesting and is becoming better understood. Protein-calorie deficiency is considered at some length because it is the most prevalent of all nutritional deficiency states. Lastly, excessive lead absorption as a cause of anemia is included since lead is a common dietary contaminant, even though it cannot be considered a nutrient. Since none of these topics is comprehensively covered, references for each section are carefully selected to fill gaps and amplify important points. In addition, general references and reviews that deal with the subject of nutritional anemias are cited (1–8).

INTERPRETATION OF ANEMIA

Definition of Anemia and Derivation of Normal Values

Anemia is a lower than normal concentration of hemoglobin, per cent packed red cell volume, or number of red cells per cubic mm. The limit is generally set two standard deviations below the mean for the normal population. By this definition, 2.5 per cent of normal individuals will be mistakenly considered anemic. Conversely, the values of deficient individuals will have a distribution that will bring some within the normal range. These persons will be recognized only if their production of hemoglobin is increased in response to treatment with a dietary essentiality such as iron.

The designation of normal values for hemoglobin and hematocrit at various ages has a profound influence on estimates of the prevalence of nutritional anemias. Until recently normal values were compiled from a superficially healthy population but one that was not systematically screened to exclude individuals with mild deficiencies of iron, folate, and other nutrients. This type of sampling has usually led to a nongaussian distribution, with a skew toward low values (9, 10), since individuals with subclinical deficiencies outnumber those with polycythemia due to hypoxia and other causes. This helps to explain why, until recently, a hemoglobin concentration of 10 g. per 100 ml. was the accepted lower limit of normal in children.

If individuals making up the lower portion of a frequency distribution curve respond to treatment with iron (9, 11) (Fig. 4–1) or iron plus folate with a significant

TABLE 4–1. HEMOGLOBIN AND HEMATOCRIT: LOWER LIMITS OF NORMAL AT SEA LEVEL

	HB, G./100 ML.	HCT, %
6 months to 4 years*	11	33
4 years to puberty	11.5	34.5
Postpubertal males	14	42
Postpubertal females	12	36
Late-pregnancy females	11	33

*Earlier age groups are covered in Chapter 2 and are rarely subject to nutritional anemia.

From Iron deficiency in the United States. Council on Foods and Nutrition. J.A.M.A. 203:407, 1968.

increase in hemoglobin production, as shown in some studies, then the original values cannot legitimately be included in establishing a normal range. Recent surveys in which those individuals with other laboratory evidence of malnutrition (low transferrin saturation, serum folate, or serum vitamin B_{12}) have been systematically excluded, yield higher values with a normal, symmetrical distribution (12) (Fig. 4–2). As a result, there is increasing agreement concerning childhood and adult values for normal hemoglobin and hematocrit. Table 4–1 shows the values below which anemia may be considered to exist at sea level.

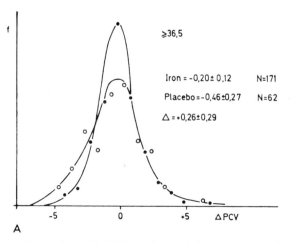

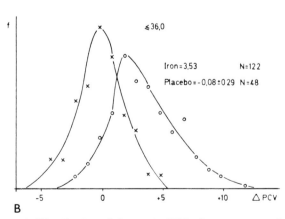

A   B

Figure 4–1. Definition of anemia by response to therapy: *A*, Distribution of change in PCV after treatment of women with initial values of 36.5 or more (●, iron; ○, placebo). *B*, Distribution of change in PCV after treatment of women with initial values of 36.0 or less (○, iron; x, placebo). There is a significant increase in PCV in the iron-treated group. [From Garby, L., and Killander, A., In *Symposia of the Swedish Nutrition Foundation. VI. Occurrence, Causes, and Prevention of Nutritional Anaemias.* Blix, G. (ed.), Stockholm, Almqvist & Wiksell, 1968, p. 13.]

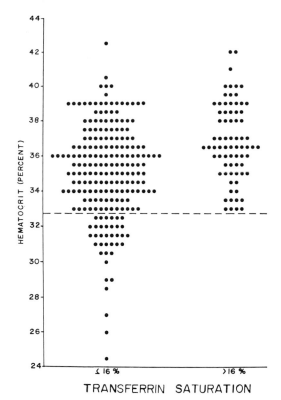

TRANSFERRIN SATURATION

Figure 4–2. Definition of anemia based on exclusion of individuals with low transferrin saturation. Distribution of hematocrits in infants 6 to 18 months of age in association with transferrin saturation ≤ 16 per cent (left) and > 16 per cent (right). (From Hunter, R. E., and Smith, N. J.: J. Pediatr. *81*:710, 1972.)

It should be noted that the period of puberty is one of transitional values, since the increase to adult values coincides with the variable onset of sexual maturity.

Classification of Nutritional Anemias

Anemias can be classified either on the basis of the responsible mechanism or by red cell morphology (8). By the former classification, anemia can be due either to decreased production of red cells or to increased loss of cells through hemorrhage or hemolysis. Most nutritional anemias, including those of iron, folate, and vitamin B_{12} deficiency, are associated with a decrease in the release of red blood cells from the bone marrow, characteristically manifested by a decrease in the number of reticulocytes. Lack of the essential nutrient restricts cell proliferation or differentiation. However, each of these three deficiencies

is also complicated by an important component of red cell destruction, both in the bone marrow and in the peripheral blood. In the bone marrow, the acceleration of both production and destruction of red cells, with a diminished release of cells to the circulation, is termed ineffective erythropoiesis (see Chapter 3). In the peripheral blood, the survival time of red cells is also moderately shortened, sometimes to 50 per cent or less of the normal 120 days. These abnormalities manifest themselves in an increased cellularity of the bone marrow, with an abundance of red cell precursors. Occasionally mild jaundice is a consequence of increased red cell destruction, even though the overall mechanism of these anemias is best classified as a failure of production. Protein-calorie malnutrition, copper deficiency, and lead poisoning also result in decreased production of red cells. In protein-calorie malnutrition, the decreased rate of proliferation of red cells is part of a systemic process in which the growth or division or both of many cell populations is restricted by lack of essential amino acid substrates. The only nutritional anemia characterized primarily by red cell destruction is vitamin E deficiency, in which oxidative damage to the red cell membrane results in hemolysis (see individual subject sections for references).

The morphologic classification of the nutritional anemias is particularly useful in *differential diagnosis.* Hypochromic, microcytic cells are found when the synthesis of hemoglobin is impaired, most commonly as a result of iron deficiency, less frequently with lead poisoning, and very rarely due to copper deficiency. Macrocytosis results from a decreased number of cell divisions during the development of erythroid precursors. This is seen in folate and vitamin B_{12} deficiency, presumably as a result of a diminished rate of DNA synthesis. Normochromic, normocytic nutritional anemias include protein-calorie malnutrition and vitamin E deficiency.

Mixed and Masked Deficiencies

Most research and teaching in nutrition deals with deficiencies of single nutrients, a natural consequence of the relatively recent beginnings of this field. The concept of vitamins was not proposed until the first years of this century, and essential vitamins and minerals have only been catalogued in recent decades. The classic method of studying the physiologic role of a dietary component has been to determine the consequences of omitting only that substance from the diet. In man, however, a diet lacking in one component is almost invariably deficient in other respects as well. This is most evident in the severe forms of malnutrition prevalent in underdeveloped countries but is also characteristic of the mild deficiencies that are common, particularly among the poor, in the United States. It is a disappointment to find clinical circumstances more tangled and complex than textbook classifications had led one to anticipate. In the field of nutrition, this is frequently the case.

When a mineral or vitamin deficiency involves only a single component, it usually has not resulted from a deficient diet. Thus, the iron deficiency of chronic blood loss is likely to be relatively uncomplicated by a lack of other nutrients. Pernicious anemia may be a specific deficiency of vitamin B_{12}, since it results from a failure in the absorption of only that vitamin rather than from an unbalanced diet.

Marked variations in the manifestations of protein-calorie malnutrition throughout the world are largely attributable to different coexisting mineral and vitamin deficiencies. For example, iron deficiency anemia is a common and severe problem concurrent with protein deficiency in low-altitude tropical areas, such as Ceylon, because of the prevalence of chronic blood loss from heavy hookworm infestation. In contrast, anemia is less common in patients with protein-calorie malnutrition in regions of Ethiopia where the intake of iron is high and hookworm is not a major factor.

The manifestations of the most severe and limiting dietary lack usually dominate the clinical picture and often obscure the clinical and laboratory characteristics of the milder ones. The interaction between iron and folic acid, for instance, is such that the more severe and limiting deficiency presumably masks the milder one by depressing red cell production. This reduces the requirement for the less deficient component and allows it to accumulate in the serum. Thus, in infants who develop overt

iron deficiency after prolonged and almost exclusive milk intake, a coexisting deficiency of folic acid may not become apparent until treatment with iron is underway. Although hypersegmented neutrophils can be recognized initially, the serum folate may become decreased only after initiation of iron therapy. Under such circumstances, both iron and folate treatments are required to achieve a complete hematologic response. In infants fed goat's milk, folate deficiency is apt to be more severe. The extremely low content of both folic acid and iron in goat's milk favors the development of an anemia, the megaloblastic features of which may not at first be noticed. When iron alone is administered, the anemia becomes obviously megaloblastic.

An analogous phenomenon is observed in patients with pernicious anemia who have a concurrent masked iron deficiency. When erythropoiesis is depressed by a lack of vitamin B_{12}, the utilization of iron for hemoglobin synthesis is diminished, and iron accumulates in the serum. Thus a normal or elevated serum iron may delay the diagnosis of concurrent iron deficiency until treatment with vitamin B_{12} restores hematopoiesis. The resulting demand for iron then causes its serum concentration to fall into the subnormal range characteristic of iron deficiency.

The recognition of masked deficiencies is of great importance in the design of nutritional supplements for use in prevention and treatment of malnutrition. With the relatively mild forms of malnutrition that are most common in the United States, harmful consequences of omitting minor components from a rehabilitation regimen are rarely recognized. The possibility of doing harm with an incomplete, unbalanced regimen is greater in severe protein-calorie malnutrition, particularly during periods normally characterized by rapid growth. The retardation of growth that is an early response to protein-calorie deficiency is an adaptation that reduces the requirement for other nutrients. However, the smaller than normal quantities of vitamins and minerals that suffice during restricted growth are inadequate to support the accelerated growth that accompanies nutritional rehabilitation with protein and calories. Thus aggravation of keratomalacia with a risk of blindness can occur during protein realimentation of severely vitamin A–deficient patients if the concurrent deficiency of vitamin A is not also treated. Similar harm can result through mistaken treatment with a component that was not the primary cause of malnutrition. Thus the neurologic manifestations of pernicious anemia can be aggravated by treatment with large doses of folic acid.

Better laboratory methods are needed to evaluate mixed deficiencies and unmask minor ones. Progress in this area may come from studies of bacteria and mammalian cells in tissue culture. In such single-cell systems, a uniform sequence of metabolic events can be discerned in response to a large variety of inadequacies in nutrient medium the ultimate result of which is failure of growth. Thus the development of tests to screen for general nutritional adequacy is within the realm of possibility.

At our present state of knowledge, a careful nutritional history and an awareness of local nutritional patterns are particularly important. Laboratory methods cannot yet provide an accurate or complete nutritional assessment. A broad vitamin and mineral supplement is indicated in the treatment of severe malnutrition, particularly if an increased rate of body or tissue growth is anticipated and the history or clinical findings or both suggest a combination of dietary deficiencies (see Protein-Calorie Malnutrition).

Individual Variations in Dietary Requirements (13–18)

Marked cultural differences in diet indicate that the individual is able to vary the intake of essential nutrients within wide limits without apparently jeopardizing his health. Nevertheless, people differ markedly in their dietary requirements (13) according to age, sex, level of energy expenditure, and a variety of environmental factors. Furthermore, individual genetic differences may play a role in more subtle individual differences in dietary requirements. An analogy may be drawn to the better known variations in response to drugs. A specific dose may be ineffective in one individual but toxic in another. A genetic basis for such individual differences has been inferred from familial drug idiosyncrasies and from the observation that identical twins tend to have similar drug responses.

Present methods for establishing optimum requirements for essential nutrients are still crude. As more precise methods develop, there is increasing evidence that nutritional intake in the "normal" range influences normal metabolic reactions. As a result, the traditional impression of a broad range of normality within which the level of intake has no metabolic consequences is gradually being modified. Thus physiologic variations in dietary riboflavin can alter glutathione reductase activity in the red blood cell (14). Similarly, in the experimental animal, variations in protein intake that do not influence rate of growth nevertheless alter the activity of the urea cycle enzymes and affect the extent to which amino acids are either used for protein synthesis or burned for energy. Thus small variations in dietary pattern may have definite metabolic consequences, even though their effect upon growth, development, and physiologic function may be undetectable. The composite of many interrelationships such as these plays a role in what is termed "biochemical individuality" and lends support to the dictum, "you are what you eat."

Factors known to influence specific dietary requirements include (1) rate of body growth, (2) rate of energy expenditure, (3) rate of proliferation of certain cell populations, as in the hemolytic anemias, (4) the quantity of other nutrients in the diet, and (5) inherited biochemical abnormalities (vitamin dependency states) that can be partially corrected by administration of large doses of a vitamin.

ROLE OF BODY GROWTH. On the basis of body weight, the estimated nutrient requirements of the growing infant for many vitamins and minerals are 5 to 15 times greater than those in the adult and are often close to adult requirements in absolute amounts (6). Consequently, dietary inadequacy often has its most obvious manifestations in the rapidly growing infant. Other periods of fast growth, as in the preschool child, the adolescent, and the pregnant female, are also frequently characterized by nutritional deficiency.

RATE OF ENERGY EXPENDITURE. The difference in energy expenditure between a sedentary life and one of active exercise is large and has a profound influence on caloric requirement as well as on the direction and magnitude of substrate flow through various metabolic pathways. In addition to raising the need for calories, exercise can also increase the requirements for other dietary components. Anemia and hypoproteinemia are reported to develop in Japanese athletes during muscle training (15). Presumably the protein required for muscle hypertrophy contributes to a temporary protein deficiency, since both anemia and hypoproteinemia can be prevented by increasing the protein content of the diet to 2 g. per kg. per day.

RATE OF CELL PROLIFERATION. With chronic hemolysis, as in sickle cell anemia or thalassemia, increased DNA synthesis and cell division in the erythroid series of the bone marrow require additional folic acid and vitamin B_{12}, vitamins that are associated with nucleic acid synthesis. Serum folic acid, in particular, is often decreased in hemolytic anemias. Since these circumstances are analogous to those of rapid, overall body growth, it is likely that individuals with hemolytic anemia will have increased requirements for other dietary factors as well. Iron is an obvious exception, since its absorption from the intestine is increased in association with accelerated hematopoiesis.

INFLUENCE OF ONE NUTRIENT ON REQUIREMENT FOR ANOTHER. All essential nutrients interact to some extent in the metabolism of the body, although few interrelationships among dietary components are understood in detail. One example of interest to the hematologist is the interaction of vitamin E and dietary lipid. Vitamin E functions as an antioxidant and suppresses lipid peroxidation, particularly in the lipid-rich membranous portions of the cell. When dietary polyunsaturated fatty acids are increased, there follows a concomitant change in the fatty acid composition of lipids within the cell membranes. Increased vitamin E is then required to provide effective in vivo inhibition of membrane peroxidation. The vitamin E content of natural fats and oils tends to be proportional to the degree of unsaturation. When such important foods as infant formulas become increasingly modified, this relationship can deviate markedly from normal and may have to be corrected artificially by vitamin E supplementation (see Vitamin E Deficiency).

Essential nutrients can also interact with abnormal dietary constituents. The common association of iron deficiency and lead poisoning is of interest in this regard. Animal studies indicate that similar quantities of ingested lead may be more toxic in the presence of iron deficiency (see Lead Poisoning).

Dietary components may also interact in the intestinal lumen before they are absorbed (16). Thus the absorption of iron is profoundly influenced by the compound in which it is supplied and by other factors in the foods with which it is eaten (see Iron Deficiency).

VITAMIN-DEPENDENCY STATES. A group of rare inherited abnormalities can be partially corrected by administration of unusually large doses of vitamin (ten or more times the normal). In the evaluation of nutritional anemia it is important to be aware of the existence of a microcytic, hypochromic anemia that is pyridoxine-responsive, of a thiamine-responsive megaloblastic anemia, and of a methylmalonic aciduria which is partially corrected by vitamin B_{12}. These interesting abnormalities are reviewed elsewhere (17).

Anemia: Only One Manifestation of a Systemic Disease

The ease with which blood can be sampled and the consequent widespread use of hematologic studies make it easy to forget that anemia is only one manifestation of a systemic disease. Malnutrition may have equally important consequences in other tissues, but these are more difficult to ascertain because biopsies are rarely essential for diagnosis or for evaluation of therapy. Consequently, many of the systemic effects of iron and protein deficiency, for example, are best delineated in animal models that invariably differ from the human condition in some aspects. However, certain useful generalizations emerge when the limited data in man are pieced together with more easily controlled and extensive studies in the experimental animal. Thus we are beginning to understand how the turnover of cells, subcellular organelles, and individual proteins may determine the rates of both production and repair of deficiency states.

In man, the systemic manifestations of the megaloblastic anemias were recognized many years ago, particularly with respect to long-term neurologic sequelae. Therefore, we are well prepared for the evidence that megaloblastic changes affect not only the red blood cell but also the cells of the intestinal lining and probably cells of other tissues in a similar manner. Our understanding of these and other systemic manifestations of nutritional deficiency states remains rudimentary. Fortunately, this does not prevent the successful nutritional rehabilitation of patients with anemia. However, intelligent planning of future public health measures and of preventive programs in nutrition requires more detailed information, particularly to identify the most susceptible periods of tissue growth and development and to determine the correctibility of damage due to malnutrition.

Permanent Sequelae (19–24)

The reversibility of nutritional anemia following treatment may lead to a false sense of security because all of the easily measured clinical laboratory studies have been corrected. In recent years, however, the possibility of long-term sequelae is deservedly receiving more attention. It is generally agreed that severe protein calorie malnutrition in early life may result in a permanent deficit in growth and intellectual function. This conclusion is based on studies involving a large number of patients, but it is difficult to exclude the influence of social and environmental factors. Indeed, a strong potential for recovery from a finite period of severe malnutrition alone is indicated by a careful survey showing that prenatal exposure to the Dutch famine of 1944–45 had no discernable relationship to mental performance at age 19 (24).

In the individual patient, it is even more difficult than in large groups to determine deficits in growth and intellectual performance since there is no measure of what his full potential might have been if he had always been well nourished. Only very large deviations from normal with a corroborating history make it convincing that nutritional rather than other environmental or genetic factors are responsible. Specific sequelae may be easier to detect. Thus, in severe vitamin B_{12} deficiency, the neurologic changes are sufficiently distinctive to identify in the individual patient. In iron deficiency, long-term residua, if present, are likely to be subtle. None has been definitely documented. However, of pertinence to this problem is the description of poor scholastic performance among mildly anemic students presumed to have iron deficiency (24a). If these findings are confirmed, it will be important also to determine the reversibility of the defect with improved nutrition.

The association of long-term sequelae following dietary deficiency in early development has made nutrition a matter of particular importance in pregnant women and children. The mechanisms responsible for permanent defects are poorly understood, and most of our information is descriptive. Abnormal morphogenesis in the fetus which results in congenital malformations can be inferred to be a consequence of maternal malnutrition in animal experiments using vitamin antagonists or antimetabolites, such as methotrexate. Tissue damage is also known to follow even brief periods of hypoglycemia or hypocalcemia. Another type of permanent deficit is that of body growth and cell number following protein-calorie malnutrition. In none of these examples is the persistence of biochemical abnormalities a readily apparent feature. It seems, rather, that many permanent defects result from some manner of irreversible tissue damage, presumably initiated by a temporary biochemical event. When the diet improves, the biochemical abnormalities tend to correct themselves gradually as a result of the dynamic state of most body constituents.

IRON DEFICIENCY (25–35)

Iron deficiency remains the most common cause of anemia in the world today. There is no evidence that its high incidence and widespread distribution have changed substantially during the several decades that iron-lack has been recognized as a public health problem. In recent years the goal of preventing iron deficiency has been pursued more actively, especially with increasing evidence of the efficacy of iron fortification of staple foods in reducing the incidence of iron deficiency. Intelligent planning of such broad public health programs, as well as proper management of individual patients with iron deficiency, is dependent on a familiarity with iron metabolism and with the changes in iron status during development.

Metabolism and Pathogenesis

IRON COMPOUNDS IN THE BODY: DISTRIBUTION AND METABOLIC FUNCTION. The iron-containing compounds in the body are conveniently grouped into two categories: (1) those known to serve a metabolic or enzymatic function, and (2) those associated with iron storage and transport. The approximate quantities of iron present in these compounds are shown in Figure 4–3. The first category of iron compounds consists almost entirely of heme proteins, i.e., proteins with an iron-porphyrin prosthetic group. The function of all heme proteins is related to oxidative metabolism.

Hemoglobin is the most abundant of this group and accounts for more than 65 per cent of body iron. Its function is to transport oxygen via the bloodstream, and it is most readily available for sampling. Hemoglobin is a tetramer made up of four globin chains, each of which is associated with a heme group that contains one iron atom. The total molecular weight is 64,450. Hemoglobin accounts for over 99 per cent of the protein of the red cell.

Myoglobin, the red pigment of muscle, stores oxygen for utilization during muscle contraction. This protein accounts for less than 5 per cent of the total body iron. Myoglobin has a molecular weight of 17,000. Its structure is closely related to the monomeric units of hemoglobin, e.g., it is made up of one globin chain attached to a heme group with a single iron atom. The myoglobin concentration in human muscle is of the order of 1 to 3 mg. per g. of tissue.

Cytochromes, the electron transport enzymes, are located in the mitochondria as well as in other cellular membranes. Cytochromes *a, b,* and *c* are present in all aerobic cells within the cristae of mitochondria and are essential for the oxidative production of cellular energy in the form of ATP. Cytochrome *c,* the best characterized of the cytochromes, is a pink protein with a molecular weight of 13,000. Like myoglobin, it is made up of one globin chain and one heme group containing an atom of iron. Its concentration in man ranges between 5 and 100 μg. per g. of tissue. The highest concentrations are in tissues such as heart muscle, that have a high rate of oxygen utilization. Cytochrome P-450 is located primarily within microsomal membranes of the liver and is involved in oxidative degradation of drugs and endogenous substrates. Cytochrome b_5 is a component of many membranes and is also present in the matrix of the red blood cell. In the latter, it is believed to function in the reduction of methemoglobin, whereas in the endoplasmic reticulum it probably provides energy for protein synthesis. This large group of essential, iron-containing enzymes ac-

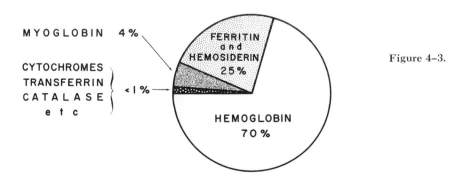

DISTRIBUTION OF IRON IN MAN

(Adult male: ~3.5 grams)

MYOGLOBIN 4%

CYTOCHROMES
TRANSFERRIN
CATALASE
e t c

<1%

FERRITIN and HEMOSIDERIN 25%

HEMOGLOBIN 70%

Figure 4–3.

counts for a fraction of 1 per cent of the total body iron.

A similarly small percentage is made up of *catalase* and *peroxidase,* which are widely distributed in the body and function in the reduction of endogenously generated hydrogen peroxide. Catalase is a large molecule, having a molecular weight of about 240,000, which contains 4 heme groups, each with one iron atom. Catalase is particularly abundant in the red cell and in the liver. An absence of catalase or a markedly decreased concentration is found in the inherited condition called *acatalasia* (see Chapter 1). Surprisingly, most individuals with this disorder are asymptomatic; in others, septic and necrotic lesions of the mouth are the only overt manifestations. The composition of various peroxidases is not well-defined. The myeloperoxidase of the granulocyte is known to contain iron, but the presence of iron in the glutathione peroxidase of the red cell has not been established.

Also in the first category of the metabolically active compounds is a less well-characterized group of iron proteins which have an enzymatic function but in which the iron is not in the form of heme. In mitochondria, nonheme compounds account for far more iron than the cytochromes. A portion of this iron is in a group of compounds designated as metalloflavoproteins. These compounds, which include NADH dehydrogenase and succinate dehydrogenase, are all involved in oxidative metabolism and contain iron and flavin prosthetic groups. Other enzymes of this group which are not attached to cellular structures are xanthine oxidase and aldehyde dehydrogenase.

The second category of iron compounds includes the storage compounds, *ferritin* and *hemosiderin* (36, 37), which are present primarily in the liver and reticuloendothelial cells, and the erythroid precursors of the bone marrow. About one-third of storage iron is in the liver, one-third in bone marrow, and the remaining third in the spleen and other tissues. The total amount of storage iron in the body is subject to marked variations. It may be reduced to near zero before iron deficiency anemia develops and increased more than fortyfold in iron overload. Storage iron exists primarily in ferric salt–protein complexes. The protein portion of ferritin, apoferritin, is homogeneous in any given organ. It is believed to consist of 24 identical subunits, with a total molecular weight of 450,000. The subunits form a spherical cluster around variable amounts of hydrated ferric phosphate in a central colloidal core to make up ferritin. Ferritin contains up to 25 per cent iron and has a molecular weight as high as 900,000, depending on its iron content. Ultrastructurally, ferritin has a characteristic appearance, consisting of electron-dense particles about 5 nm. in diameter, often appearing in clusters of four. In hematologically normal adults, ferritin accounts for about half of the storage iron present in the liver.

Hemosiderin, which makes up the other half, is a rather ill-defined, chemically heterogeneous group of large iron-salt-protein aggregates. Often the term is applied to water-insoluble iron remaining in the residue after ferritin has been extracted. As iron stores become abnormally large, hemosiderin makes up an increasingly greater proportion of the total. The contribution of both compounds to total body iron can vary widely, less than 5 per cent or more than 30 per cent. Unless the stores are exhausted, their size has no discernible influence on any physiologic or biochemical function other than iron absorption.

Transferrin also belongs in this category of components but only accounts for a small fraction of 1 per cent of the total body iron. Transferrin is a β_1 globulin with a molecular weight of 74,000, capable of binding two atoms of ferric iron. Its major role is to transport iron released from hemoglobin catabolism in the spleen or elsewhere or absorbed from the intestinal lumen to the bone marrow for synthesis of hemoglobin in developing red blood cells.

Assessment of iron status is generally restricted to hemoglobin, transferrin-bound iron, and bone marrow storage iron. These categories account for, or are representative of, well over 90 per cent of body iron. While they do not necessarily reflect the status of the remaining iron-containing compounds, one can conclude that the iron supply does not limit the production of any "metabolic or enzymatic" iron protein when storage iron is present and the hemoglobin concentration is normal.

SYNTHESIS AND TURNOVER OF IRON COMPOUNDS (38). All aerobic cells have the complete enzymatic apparatus for heme synthesis and synthesize their own complement of heme proteins. The longevity of a heme protein is limited by and, in general, is similar to the lifespan of the cell or subcellular structure of which it is a component. For example, hemoglobin and red cell catalase have a finite lifespan, similar to the 120 days of the red cell. The release of iron from the breakdown of almost 1 per cent of the total number of red cells per day is about 20 to 25 mg. per day. The iron from hemoglobin breakdown, as well as amino acids, can be almost completely reutilized. Heme, on the other hand, is degraded to bilirubin and largely lost via the bile.

In contrast to hemoglobin and catalase in the red cell, heme proteins in long-lived cells do not appear to have a finite life span. Rather, they seem to be subject to random degradation at an exponential rate that is in accord with the rate of turnover of the subcellular structure in which they are contained. Thus the turnover of myoglobin approximates that of other myofibrillar components. The mitochondrial cytochromes are degraded at a rate similar to mitochondrial DNA or total mitochondrial protein, with a half-life of six to eight days in heart and liver, but probably longer in the muscle and brain of the rat. The half-life of liver catalase corresponds closely to the seven-day half-life of the peroxisome, of which it is a major component.

The microsomal cytochromes of the liver have a shorter half-life, less than two days, corresponding to the more rapid rate of replacement of the endoplasmic reticulum. Although the microsomal cytochromes of the liver probably account for no more than 0.05 per cent of total body iron, they may contribute significantly to bilirubin production by virtue of this very rapid turnover, roughly a hundred times greater than that of hemoglobin (see discussion of "early-labeled peak" of bilirubin in Chapter 3).

The implication of the dynamic state of heme protein constituents is that tissue deficits are ultimately reparable through the production of new subcellular structures. However, the rates of repair in individual tissues may differ markedly from those of hemoglobin.

The rate at which deficits of heme protein can be replaced depends on the rate of synthesis and turnover of heme proteins.

In hemoglobin, the rate can be modified within a wide range, particularly in disease states. During recovery from iron-, folate-, or vitamin B_{12}-deficiency, with acclimation to high altitude, and in response to blood loss or hemolytic states, hemoglobin synthesis increases severalfold. Conversely, a decrease in net hemoglobin production occurs in the dietary deficiency states, in infection, and in descent from altitude. Modulations in rates of synthesis and degradation are also characteristic of other heme proteins but are not yet as well delineated.

Storage iron can be depleted or replenished apparently without an analogous restriction by synthetic rates of the cell structures with which it is associated. However, some anatomic compartmentalization is suggested by kinetic studies showing that recently established stores are most available for meeting the requirements of heme protein synthesis.

IRON COMPOUNDS DURING DEVELOPMENT (38). The normal developmental changes in concentration of hemoglobin and of other heme proteins are not a function of variations in iron supply. However, with insufficiency of iron, the production of several heme proteins can be depressed, particularly at ages when these compounds are normally increasing in absolute amount as well as in concentration. Except for hemoglobin, all heme proteins are present in low concentrations during intrauterine development, reach peak concentrations in the young adult, and generally decrease somewhat with old age. However, the timing of these developmental changes is very distinct, not only from one heme protein to another, but also according to the organ or cell type in which they are located. Rates of synthesis are influenced by the timing of cell differentiation, by systemic metabolic changes such as those which occur at birth, and by oxygen availability. Most of the information concerning tissue heme protein is derived from experimental animals. Fortunately, the developmental sequences tend to be similar in man, when comparative data are available.

Hemoglobin and Storage Iron. The developmental changes in production of hemoglobin are best considered in conjunction with iron stores, since the two make up 92 to 95 per cent of body iron.

In the fetus, the accumulation of hemoglobin and storage iron is remarkably independent of the mother's iron status. Transferrin is more saturated with iron in the fetus than in the mother. The maintenance of this gradient probably ensures that, regardless of maternal iron nutrition, the fetal iron saturation rarely drops below about 15 per cent, the range in which iron lack is likely to be limiting upon hemoglobin production. The accumulation of fetal iron stores is also thought to be favored by the lack of xanthine oxidase activity in the fetal liver. This iron-containing enzyme is thought to be essential for mobilization of liver iron stores. Its lack would presumably make iron deposition in the liver irreversible until the enzyme increases in activity shortly after birth. Severe maternal iron deficiency may be reflected in decreased liver iron stores at birth, but this remains controversial and cannot be of great quantitative consequence because of the small size of this iron compartment compared to hemoglobin.

At birth, the term infant has a total body iron content of about 75 mg. per kg. (Fig. 4–4). Liver iron stores, though variable, are always present and contribute approximately 25 per cent of this amount. The delivery of blood from the placenta to the newborn, particularly after the infant's first breath, is an additional but variable source of iron for the newborn. The time at which the umbilical cord is clamped has a profound influence on the infant's red cell mass. For example, very prompt clamping

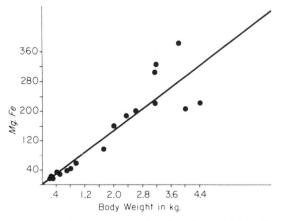

Figure 4–4. Iron content and body weight in the fetus and newborn child. There is a linear relationship between the two. (From Widdowson, E. M., and Spray, C. M.: Arch. Dis. Child. 26:205, 1951.)

yields an average value of 31 ml. per kg. at three days of age, in contrast to 49 ml. per kg. with late clamping. However, after three months of age there is no evidence that cord clamping influences hemoglobin concentration. Presumably, since iron losses are minimal, any difference in total body iron would manifest itself in the size of iron stores.

The newborn is relatively polycythemic (mean hemoglobin, 16.8 g. per 100 ml.; hematocrit, 53 per cent). This is believed to reflect fetal erythropoietin production in response to a relatively hypoxic intrauterine environment. Erythropoiesis is active in a maximally expanded marrow compartment that occupies almost all tubular and membranous bones as well as extramedullary tissues, particularly the liver and spleen.

After birth, arterial oxygen saturation increases, as there is improved access to oxygen via the lungs. During the first few days of life, erythropoietin activity and the rate of erythropoiesis decrease. The percentage of erythroid precursor cells in the bone marrow declines from about 30 per cent at birth to less than 10 per cent, and extramedullary hematopoiesis comes to a halt by one week of age. In the peripheral blood, these changes are reflected in the disappearance of nucleated red blood cells and a precipitous fall in the reticulocyte count. The virtual cessation of erythropoiesis continues for six to eight weeks following birth (39), and the concentration of hemoglobin drops concurrently at a rate that largely reflects the survival of fetal red blood cells. Iron from this red cell breakdown is salvaged by the reticuloendothelial system and augments the neonatal iron stores.

After six to eight weeks, an abrupt increase in the reticulocyte count heralds the resumption of active erythropoiesis at a rate sufficient to maintain relatively constant mean values of 12.5 g. per 100 ml. hemoglobin and 37 per cent hematocrit during the tripling of weight that marks the first year of life. The low iron content of the milk-rich diet customarily provided during this year contributes to a depletion of iron stores, initiating the marginal period of iron nutrition (Figs. 4–5 and 4–6).

In the premature infant, the total body iron is less than in the full-term new-

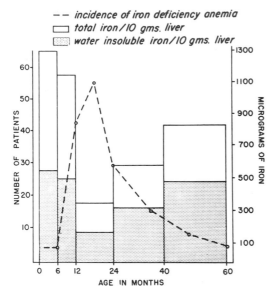

Figure 4-5. Relationship of iron stores to the incidence of iron deficiency anemia during infancy and early childhood. Iron deficiency is most common at the age when iron stores are lowest. (From Smith, N. J., Rosello, S., et al.: Pediatrics 16:166, 1955.)

born, though the proportion of iron to body weight remains relatively constant. Infants of low birth weight generally have a more rapid than normal rate of postnatal growth. Unless the diet is iron-supplemented, the proportionately smaller neonatal iron stores become more rapidly depleted than in a full-term infant, and iron deficiency develops after two to three months.

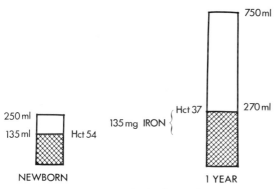

Figure 4-6. Iron needs for hemoglobin synthesis during the first year of life schematically represented. The height of the bar indicates blood volume, and the cross-hatched portion the red cell mass. About 1 mg. of iron is required to make 1 ml. of packed red blood cells. The doubling of red cell mass and the maintenance of a normal hematocrit for the age require about 135 mg. of iron.

In the preschool and preadolescent child, the iron status is, on the average, improved since there is an increased opportunity to obtain iron from a mixed diet. Erythropoiesis keeps pace with growth, and the hemoglobin concentration remains stable at a mean of 12.5 g. per 100 ml. Total body iron averages about 35 mg. per kg. If the diet is adequate, storage iron accumulates during this period.

Adolescence is another period of marginal iron nutrition. From the high incidence of mild iron deficiency anemia in adolescents, one can infer that average iron stores are low in this group as a whole. Not only must hemoglobin production in the male keep pace with the accelerated growth that accompanies sexual maturation, but its concentration increases disproportionately to reach substantially higher adult values. The incidence of deficiency is similar in young men and women. This is because the iron requirement for the male's greater hemoglobin increment in adolescence is balanced against the female's increased requirement for the replacement of iron lost in menses. Iron lack continues to be prevalent until the early twenties, as shown in surveys of Armed Services personnel.

With cessation of somatic growth, there is an opportunity for the accumulation of storage iron over the course of many years. The iron content of the average 70-kg. adult male is about 3.5 g., or 50 mg. per kg. The corresponding figures for the 60-kg. female average a total of 2.1 g., or 35 mg. per kg. The difference is due to both a lower hemoglobin concentration and the smaller size of the stores, which average about 1000 mg., or 30 per cent of total iron in the male, compared to approximately 300 mg., or 15 per cent in the female.

Other Heme Proteins. The developmental patterns of other heme proteins follow a simpler curve than that of hemoglobin. Tissue concentration of myoglobin, the cytochromes, and catalase are generally low during fetal life, then increase to adult values at various periods of development and, in some cases, decrease slightly in old age. Of particular relevance to iron nutrition is the fact that concentrations of the mitochondrial cytochromes and skeletal muscle myoglobin increase at more rapid rates than that of body growth during childhood. This is one explanation for the susceptibility of these heme proteins to iron lack, particularly during early development.

IRON BALANCE. Body iron is normally maintained within narrow limits at each stage of growth and development, largely through regulation of intake, first in the fetus at the placental interface, and after birth by the intestinal mucosa. The quantity of iron absorbed from the diet is a function of (a) the quantity and form of iron present in the food, and the interaction of food iron with other dietary components and with the intestinal secretions, and (b) the regulation of iron transport by the intestinal mucosa.

Food Iron. The iron content of a mixed American or European diet is very close to 6 mg. per 1000 calories. In physically active individuals, a high caloric intake generally assures an adequate supply of iron. However, in recent decades an increasingly sedentary way of life in children and adults has resulted in a diminution of caloric intake. This is an appropriate adaptation to decreased energy needs, but the concurrent reduction in dietary iron often leads to a marginal supply since iron requirements are almost independent of physical activity.

In the infant, predominance of milk in the diet is another factor favoring a borderline intake of iron. Breast milk and cow's milk contain less than 1.5 mg. iron per 1000 calories (0.5 to 1.0 mg. per L.). Even the early introduction of solid foods, including iron-fortified cereals, rarely compensates for the almost uniquely low iron content of milk. The commercial availability of cow's milk in the last century has favored an abnormally prolonged period of feeding an iron-poor diet.

Iron in food is primarily in the form of ferric complexes. A smaller amount is in the heme proteins, hemoglobin and myoglobin, which are present in meat. In the process of digestion, the ferric iron complexes are partly broken down, and the iron is reduced to the more readily absorbed ferrous form. This is facilitated in the stomach by the hydrochloric acid–containing gastric juice, and continues in the small intestine. Assimilation of ionic iron is enhanced by the formation of readily absorbed complexes with other components of the diet, such as fructose, ascorbic acid, and, probably most important, the amino acids, histidine and lysine. On the other hand,

absorption is decreased by the formation of insoluble phosphates and oxalates, which is favored by the alkaline environment of the small intestine. More than half the phosphorus in cereals and legumes is in the form of phytic acid (inositol hexaphosphoric acid). Phytic acid forms salts with food or medicinal iron and can reduce iron absorption by 50 per cent or more (16). The gradual formation of insoluble salts as food is moved down the small bowel may help explain why iron is absorbed largely in the duodenum, with diminishing amounts being assimilated toward the ileum.

Dietary iron in the form of heme protein is handled in a different manner. Heme is split from the globin portion of the molecule in the intestinal lumen. The heme is then assimilated intact, and a heme-splitting enzyme within the mucosal cell releases ionic iron.

The form of iron in the diet influences the percentage of iron that is assimilated. The range of iron absorption from biosynthetically labeled food is 1 per cent to 22 per cent (Fig. 4–7). Food of vegetable origin is at the lower end of this range, whereas meat and animal products are at the upper end. About 10 per cent of the small amount of iron normally present in milk is absorbed.

The combination of foods in a meal also influences the utilization of iron. Iron absorption from beans may be enhanced by the presence of animal products. However, assimilation of iron from meat is not more than modestly depressed by a concurrent ingestion of beans (Table 4–2).

The absorption of an iron salt, such as ferrous sulfate, added to a food product in order to prevent iron deficiency is equivalent to but may be greater than the utilization of the naturally occurring iron in that food. Supplemented milk products are an important source, from which about 10 per cent of ferrous sulfate is absorbed.

In response to iron deficiency, the absorption of iron is increased to from 15 to 30 percent of the dose. The magnitude of the response depends on the type of food. Utilization of iron from wheat and other vegetable products increases only slightly, whereas the absorption from animal sources may double (Fig. 4–8). The utilization of iron salts, provided in small doses, may exceed 40 per cent.

Medicinal iron is best absorbed if given

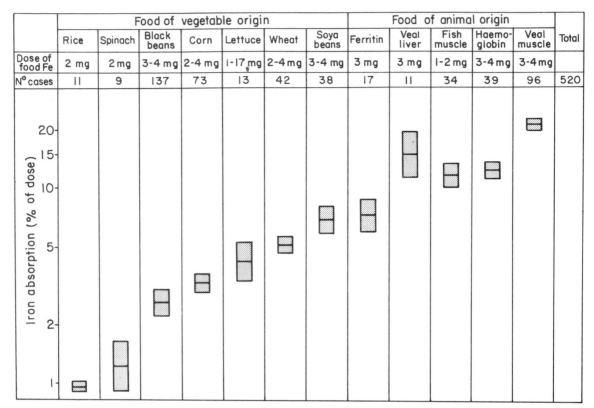

	Food of vegetable origin							Food of animal origin					
	Rice	Spinach	Black beans	Corn	Lettuce	Wheat	Soya beans	Ferritin	Veal liver	Fish muscle	Haemo-globin	Veal muscle	Total
Dose of food Fe	2 mg	2mg	3-4 mg	2-4 mg	1-17 mg	2-4mg	3-4 mg	3 mg	3 mg	1-2 mg	3-4mg	3-4mg	
N° cases	11	9	137	73	13	42	38	17	11	34	39	96	520

Figure 4-7. Iron absorption from biosynthetically labeled food. Collaborative study of the Departments of Botany and Medicine, University of Washington at Seattle, U.S.A., and the Department of Pathophysiology, Instituto Venezolano de Investigaciones Científicas, Caracas, Venezuela. The thick horizontal line represents the geometrical mean, and the cross-hatched area shows the limits of one standard error. (From WHO Tech. Rep. Ser., #503, 1972.)

alone between meals. However, the benefit of more efficient utilization is often justifiably overridden by considerations of convenience and the fact that intestinal intolerance is less likely when iron is given with food. Ascorbic acid has often been administered with iron, either in a hematinic or in the form of orange juice. Although this may result in some increase in iron absorption, it needlessly complicates therapy.

Intestinal Absorption (40–42). From an

TABLE 4-2.   EFFECT OF FOOD COMBINATIONS ON IRON ABSORPTION[*]

FOOD OR FOOD COMBINATION	NORMALS		FE-DEFICIENT	
	NO.	ABSORPTION, %	NO.	ABSORPTION, %
Black beans (Fe[59]) 4 mg. Fe	4	3.2 (1.7–8.2)	7	9.2 (1.7–24.3)
Black beans (Fe[59]) 1 mg. Fe + beef 3 mg. Fe	4	15.4 (9.3–22.8)	3	11.3 (4.9–17.4)
Beef (Fe[59]) 4 mg. Fe	4	19.5 (12.7–23.9)	7	23.7 (15.2–31.4)
Beef (Fe[59]) 3 mg. Fe + black beans 1 mg. Fe	4	20.5 (14.4–25.0)	3	15.6 (9.8–20.7)

[*]Beef enhances iron absorption from black beans. Conversely, iron absorption from beef is either unaffected or modestly decreased by the concurrent ingestion of black beans.

Data of Roche and Layrisse, adapted from Moore, C. V., In *Symposia of the Swedish Nutrition Foundation. VI. Occurrence, Causes and Prevention of Nutritional Anaemias.* Blix, G. (ed.), Stockholm, Almqvist & Wiksell, 1968, p. 98.

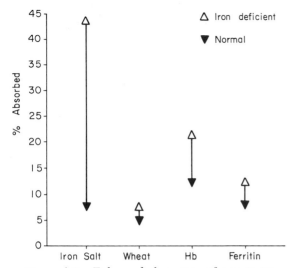

Figure 4-8. Enhanced absorption of iron in iron-deficient patients. The iron salt used was ferrous ascorbate; individual test doses contained 2 to 6 mg. iron. The average absorption of each form of iron in normal subjects is indicated by the solid arrowhead, and in iron-deficient subjects by the open arrowhead. (Data from Walker, Layrisse, Clark, and Finch in Moore, C. V., In *Symposia of the Swedish Nutrition Foundation. VI. In Occurrence, Causes, and Prevention of Nutritional Anaemias.* Blix, G. (ed.), Stockholm, Almqvist & Wiksell, 1968, p. 96.)

evolutionary perspective, iron excess has probably been more of a hazard than iron lack; the earth's crust contains about 4.5 per cent iron, whereas the human body contains less than 0.005 per cent. The exclusion of excess iron from the body is accomplished primarily within the mucosal cell (Fig. 4–9). The mucosal cell, by virtue of its two- to three-day life span, constitutes a temporary holding zone for iron between the intestinal lumen and the blood. In the iron-loaded individual, iron is taken up and largely retained by the mucosal cell, to be returned to the luminal contents by desquamation. In contrast, in iron deficiency, iron crosses through the mucosa into the circulation, and very little is retained within the cell to be lost by desquamation. Normally the diet contains 5 to 20 times the amount absorbed. Most of the iron is absorbed 1 to 30 hours after it is ingested.

The homeostatic characteristics of mucosal regulation are most effective within the physiologic ranges of iron intake and iron stores. Thus about 7 per cent of a 5-mg.

dose of ferrous salt is absorbed by an adult male with iron stores approximating 1000 mg., while an average of 18 per cent is absorbed by women of childbearing age with stores averaging 300 mg. Developmental increments in iron absorption mark those periods which are usually characterized by a rapid rate of growth and consequently diminishing iron stores, e.g., infancy and adolescence. At any time, the more iron that is ingested, the more is absorbed, although the percentage absorbed decreases (Fig. 4–10).

Iron absorption is also enhanced in response to increased hematopoiesis. This normally has the beneficial effect of facilitating the recovery from blood loss. However, in chronic hemolytic states, such as thalassemia and sickle cell anemia, it may lead to iron overload, even with ingestion of a normal diet.

With a normal rate of erythropoiesis, body iron is maintained at a relatively constant level over a wide range of iron intake, but it is not known how much unwanted iron can be excluded. The intestinal mucosa offers little protection against acute iron poisoning and cannot completely exclude large doses of medicinal iron. However, a severalfold excess over the average iron intake can apparently be well tolerated for many years unless another disease coexists, such as protein malnutrition, alcoholism, or severe hemolytic anemia.

Iron transport across the intestinal mucosa is dependent upon active metabolic processes. It remains unclear by what mechanism the mucosal regulation of iron absorption is accomplished. Ferritin in the intestinal mucosa, presumably in equilibrium with the larger body iron stores, has been thought to play a controlling role. Recent studies indicate that this is not so but do not provide a satisfactory alternate hypothesis.

Iron Losses. Iron losses from the body are small and relatively fixed, in contrast to wide variations in iron intake and lesser fluctuations in absorption. Careful measurements in the adult male after administration of isotopically labeled iron indicate that total losses average less than 1 mg. per day, or 13 μg. per kg. per day. About two-thirds of this is from extruded cells of the intestinal mucosa, the remainder from desquamated cells of the skin and urinary tract. Iron losses are greater in the infant

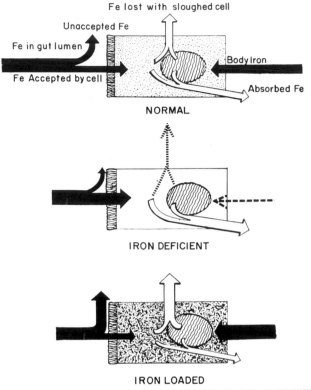

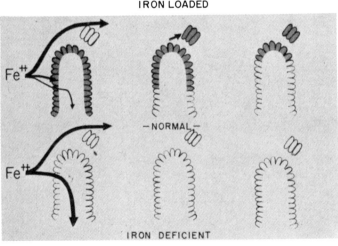

Figure 4–9.   Regulation of iron absorption at the intestinal mucosa. In normal individuals, iron from a systemic source is deposited in the mucosal cell. This iron is believed to regulate—within the physiologic range—the amount of iron that can enter from the intestinal lumen. A portion of the iron enters the body, whereas the remainder is lost when the cell is sloughed into the intestinal lumen at the end of its two- to three-day lifespan. In the iron-deficient patient, more iron, primarily from the lumen, enters the cells to be transferred to the body, and little iron is retained in the cell to be lost by desquamation. In iron-loaded individuals, increased iron from systemic sources is incorporated into the developing mucosal cell, and absorption of dietary iron is decreased (except in hemolytic anemia). The iron in the cell is then lost with cell death. (From Conrad, M. E., Jr., and Crosby, W. H.: Intestinal mucosal mechanisms controlling iron absorption. Blood 22:406–415, 1963, by permission of Grune & Stratton.)

and the postpubertal female. In the normal infant, the loss of iron is at least 20 μg. per kg. per day (43); in addition, as many as 8 per cent of "normal" infants reportedly have occult intestinal blood loss detectable by the guaiac test (44), a finding that in some cases is related to ingestion of large volumes of cow's milk (45, 46).

In the mature female, menses account for an average of 43 ml. blood loss per month, raising the total iron losses to an average of 1.5 mg. per day. Pregnancy requires a mean of about 700 mg. iron for the fetus, placenta, and perinatal blood loss; averaged over the last two trimesters of pregnancy, this represents a loss of 3.5 mg. per day. An additional 450 mg. of iron is required during pregnancy for an expanded maternal red cell mass, but this iron is available for later reutilization and does not represent a net loss. After delivery, lactation removes 0.5 to 1.0 mg. per day, somewhat more than is saved by the temporary cessation of menses. All of these losses are relatively

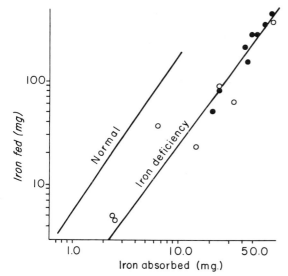

Figure 4-10. Absorption of iron salts. As the dose of iron is raised, a decreasing percentage is absorbed, but the absolute amount absorbed increases. (From Bothwell, T. H., and Finch, C. A.: *Iron Metabolism.* Boston, Little, Brown & Company, 1962, p. 338.

Iron Requirements. Estimates of iron requirement have been based on two types of procedures or calculations. One involves the determination of the lowest dietary iron intake which results in maximal hemoglobin concentrations (Fig. 4-11) (47); this amount is considered to be the minimum requirement. The second method is based on the normal amount of body iron which accumulates during a period of development; the net increase in body iron indicates how much must be ingested over that period if iron absorption is assumed to average 10 per cent. Both methods yield similar results for the first year of life, and have led to the recommendation of 1.0 mg. per kg. per day to a maximum of 15 mg. in full term infants and 2 mg. per kg. per day to a maximum of 15 mg. for low birth weight infants (33). As is generally true of nutritional guidelines, these amounts are generous enough to encompass individual variations within two standard deviations from the mean. An unusually rapid rate of growth or much greater than average intestinal iron loss results in a larger need for dietary iron.

Between one year of age and full adulthood there is less experimental information on which to base precise recommendations. A total of 10 mg. per day in children and of 15 to 20 mg. per day in adolescents is generally accepted as adequate. In the mature adult male, 15 mg. per day is considered a normal intake, and 10 mg. per day a minimum, on the basis of long-term iron balance and food iron absorption data.

fixed and are influenced only slightly by the iron status of the mother. Thus the fetus and nursing infant are remarkably independent of the iron status of the mother. Iron deficiency during pregnancy interferes with hemoglobin production in the mother, but placental transport of iron remains near normal as judged by concentrations of hemoglobin in the newborn. Similarly, iron in breast milk is depressed by no more than about 10 per cent, even in severe maternal iron deficiency.

Figure 4-11. Estimation of iron requirements. Distribution of hemoglobin concentration in infants 12 months old who had received different amounts of iron in the food. The daily iron intakes were as follows: group A, 20 mg.; group B, 8 to 13 mg.; group C, 5 to 8 mg.; group D, uncontrolled iron supply. [From Moe, P. J.: Acta Paediatr. (Stockholm) (Suppl. 150):1, 1963.]

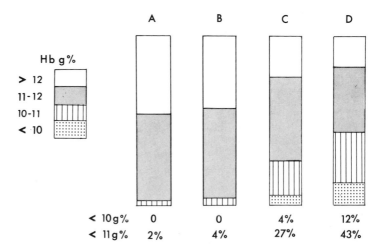

A comparable minimum intake for a non-pregnant female is 18 mg. per day, about double this amount during the latter two trimesters of pregnancy, and an intermediate amount during lactation. More important than the amount of iron ingested is the amount that is absorbed. This depends on many factors, including the amount of animal-derived food in the diet. The World Health Organization recommendations commensurately vary according to the quantity of animal protein ingested.

CAUSES OF IRON DEFICIENCY. The most common factors that contribute to the development of iron deficiency in children are rapid growth, insufficient dietary intake of iron, and blood loss; many cases result from a combination of all three. Growth and diet are usually of primary importance, since hemoglobin iron normally remains roughly proportional to body weight, and the periods of most rapid weight gain are often characterized by an iron-poor diet. Though intestinal blood loss is frequently a contributing factor, it is rarely associated with a gross anatomic lesion, such as an ulcer or a carcinoma, as is commonly true in an adult population.

In the full-term infant, iron deficiency is uncommon for the first six months of life, since storage iron is rarely exhausted during this interval. Iron lack usually develops later, between six months and two years of age, when neonatal iron stores have been utilized but have not been replenished by dietary iron. The need for new iron is large since body weight and blood volume more than double during this period, even though the rate of growth is decelerating. In infants of low birth weight (premature infants and twins), iron deficiency is more common and develops earlier than in the full-term infant. The relationship of diet and rate of growth to the prevalence of iron deficiency at various ages is discussed under Iron Compounds During Development.

Iron loss as a cause of deficiency in children is less important than in the adult. In the adult male, iron exchange with the environment is so slow (of the order of 12 per cent per year) that the discovery of iron deficiency suggests blood loss secondary to another disease. In children, blood loss is a common cause of iron deficiency, primarily in areas where hookworm infes-

tation is prevalent. In low altitude tropical regions, such as Ceylon, blood loss due to hookworm infestation may be almost universal and is the major factor responsible for an average hemoglobin concentration well below 10 g. per 100 ml. in a primary school age population. However, blood loss of lesser severity is also common in dietary iron deficiency uncomplicated by parasitic infestation. Over 50 per cent of iron-deficient infants in the United States have guaiac-positive stools (44). It is uncertain to what extent this is cause or effect. In some patients, there is good evidence that blood loss represents an intestinal intolerance to large amounts of cow's milk (Fig. 4–12) (45, 46). Alternatively, it has been postulated that intestinal blood loss is secondary to the effects of iron deficiency on the mucosal lining (48), as, for example, through a deficiency of iron-containing enzymes in this tissue. What distinguishes this bleeding from that associated with gross anatomic lesions is that it ceases shortly after initiation of treatment with iron if the milk provided concurrently is heat-processed (46).

Blood loss due to anatomic lesions is easy to overlook in children because of its rarity. It should be suspected when intestinal blood loss or anemia persists or recurs after iron treatment or when severe anemia is detected after the period of peak incidence in infancy. Causes of bleeding in the perinatal period include fetal-maternal hemorrhage, placental injury around the time of delivery, and twin-to-twin transfusion through placental communications. Beyond infancy, recurrent iron deficiency, particularly in the absence of symptomatology, should suggest a Meckel's diverticulum, often a cause of intermittent bleeding and the most common lesion associated with painless intestinal blood loss in children. Other congenital anomalies, such as intestinal duplications and hemorrhagic telangiectasia, are less common but may also result in iron deficiency anemia. Bleeding ulcers, as in the adult, are usually symptomatic, but they are relatively rare in children.

Primary pulmonary hemosiderosis, another unusual condition involving iron loss, should be considered when chronic pulmonary disease and hypochromic anemia coexist. In this case, though the chronic loss of blood is into the lung parenchyma

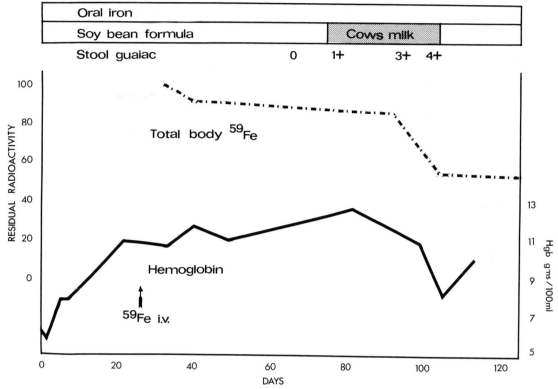

Figure 4-12. Enteric blood loss in a 3-month-old infant with severe hypochromic anemia on cow's milk. The use of a whole body counter to quantitate iron loss allows precise measurement of blood loss after labeling of red cells with a small dose of ^{59}Fe, without the inaccuracies of methods relying on stool collection. The daily blood loss, calculated from total body counts and counts in the peripheral blood, averaged 0.66 ml. per day when the infant was fed a soybean formula, and 21.2 ml. per day after challenge with pasteurized milk. (From unpublished data of Mentzer, W. L., 1972.)

rather than lost from the body, the iron is unavailable for reutilization. This is also the case in Goodpasture's syndrome (progressive glomerulonephritis with intrapulmonary hemorrhage).

Rare disorders of iron metabolism may result in a hypochromic microcytic anemia, even though there is no blood loss or lack of dietary iron. Such defects include abnormalities of iron mobilization from storage sites (49) and a congenital lack of transferrin. Failure to absorb iron is rare except as part of a generalized malabsorption syndrome.

Mild iron deficiency of any cause tends to be self-correcting since iron absorption from food is increased as iron stores in the body diminish. In severe iron deficiency, however, certain factors have a self-perpetuating or accelerating effect on the proc-

ess. Occult intestinal blood loss related to iron deficiency per se has been mentioned. An additional observation of particular interest is that severely iron-deficient children and chronically deficient animals may lose the normal adaptation of absorbing increased amounts of iron. There seems to be a point of diminishing return beyond which iron absorption, at least from heme, no longer increases but decreases below the normal for that age (48). However, this abnormality is promptly corrected after treatment with iron and is unlikely to interfere significantly with the clinical effectiveness of orally administered iron.

Diagnosis

The development of iron deficiency proceeds in a well-defined sequence that facilitates its diagnosis and staging (Fig. 4–13) (8). An initial depletion of iron stores is followed by a fall in the iron saturation of serum transferrin and ultimately results in a decreased net production of heme protein that is recognized as anemia (50).

STORAGE IRON (36, 37, 51). Storage iron is most commonly evaluated by *Prussian blue staining* of iron in a bone marrow aspirate or biopsy, quantitated on a 0 to 4+ scale, or by the percentage of sideroblasts, i.e., erythroblasts containing stainable iron, or both. This represents the reserve that is available for the synthesis of hemoglobin, and its abundance parallels the reserve of iron stores in the reticuloendothelial system as a whole. Non-heme iron in the erythroblast is shown by electron microscopy to be partly in the form of ferritin, which is located mainly in vesicles as large as 1μ in diameter. This localization is also in accord with the pattern of iron staining seen by light microscopy, which is present as readily visible particles rather than diffusely distributed. Under normal circumstances storage iron is not visible in mitochondria, where it is utilized for heme synthesis. In the normal adult male there are 30 per cent to 60 per cent sideroblasts; less than 8 per cent sideroblasts are seen when transferrin saturation drops below 15 per cent. The counts are difficult to reproduce in a clinical laboratory and are primarily of research use. Iron is also present in the reticuloendothelial cells of the bone marrow. Some of this iron is not readily mobilized and may remain, even in the face of iron deficiency anemia.

A biopsy specimen of the liver can also be stained for iron in a similar manner or used for the chemical determination of non-heme iron. This provides a good indication of body iron stores, but the procedure is rarely warranted for diagnostic use.

Diminished iron stores generally result in increased intestinal absorption of iron, an observation that has been experimentally utilized for early detection of iron defi-

THE SEQUENCE OF EVENTS IN IRON DEPLETION

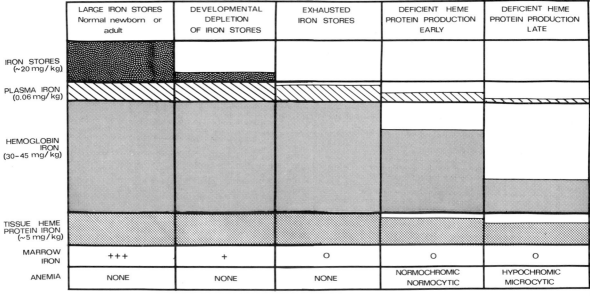

	LARGE IRON STORES Normal newborn or adult	DEVELOPMENTAL DEPLETION OF IRON STORES	EXHAUSTED IRON STORES	DEFICIENT HEME PROTEIN PRODUCTION EARLY	DEFICIENT HEME PROTEIN PRODUCTION LATE
IRON STORES (~20 mg/kg)					
PLASMA IRON (0.06 mg/kg)					
HEMOGLOBIN IRON (30–45 mg/kg)					
TISSUE HEME PROTEIN IRON (~5 mg/kg)					
MARROW IRON	+++	+	o	o	o
ANEMIA	NONE	NONE	NONE	NORMOCHROMIC NORMOCYTIC	HYPOCHROMIC MICROCYTIC

Figure 4–13. The sequence of events in iron depletion. Iron stores are normally reduced during periods of rapid growth, especially infancy and adolescence (second column). Only after iron stores are essentially exhausted can iron deficiency be detected by a depression in plasma iron concentration (third column). When plasma iron saturation remains below 16 per cent, production of hemoglobin and probably of other heme proteins is reduced; this is first manifested as a mild anemia that may still be normochromic, normocytic (fourth column). Marked hypochromic, microcytic anemia and changes in epithelial tissues result from prolonged and severe iron deficiency (fifth column). (Adapted from Harris, J. W., and Kellermeyer, R. W.: *The Red Cell.* Cambridge, Harvard University Press, 1970, p. 117.)

ciency in the adult. A dose of ^{59}Fe is given orally under strictly standardized conditions, and its absorption is followed in a whole body counter. The complexity and expense of the procedure, as well as the need for radioactive isotopes, are likely to restrict it to research use.

Of great promise as a simple measurement of iron status is the assay of *serum ferritin* (52, 53). Ferritin is normally present in serum but in such small quantities (5 to 100 ng. per ml.) that it remained undetected until recently (52). The size of iron stores and the serum ferritin concentration are correlated in several conditions (52, 53) (Table 4–3). Normal males have higher average values than females, in accord with known differences in iron stores. Furthermore, the developmental curve of serum ferritin concentration from birth to adult life also parallels changes in iron stores (53, 53a). A low concentration is associated with iron deficiency. High values are found in patients with iron overload due to thalassemia and sickle cell anemia. In certain disease states, ferritin concentration may be elevated without evidence of concomitant change in iron status. These conditions include respiratory infection and malignancy (53).

After blood loss, serum ferritin falls before there is a change in the saturation of iron in serum, suggesting that it is an early indicator of depletion in iron stores (52). The apparent correspondence with iron stores throughout a wide range should therefore make this assay, when it becomes more generally available, useful for the early diagnosis of iron deficiency.

TRANSFERRIN SATURATION (PER CENT SATURATION OF TOTAL IRON-BINDING CAPACITY). Iron-binding capacity normally ranges between 200 and 450 μg. per 100 ml. plasma [except in the newborn (4)]. Since 1 g. of transferrin can bind 1250 μg. of iron, serum iron-binding capacity of 300 μg. per 100 ml. is equivalent to about 0.24 g. per 100 ml. of transferrin. Transferrin saturation falls only after iron stores of ferritin and hemosiderin are essentially exhausted. The per cent of transferrin saturation is a more sensitive index of iron status than serum iron alone, since total transferrin usually increases in iron deficiency, whereas serum iron decreases. Furthermore, the per cent saturation most accurately reflects

the availability of iron for hematopoiesis. When transferrin saturation drops below 15 or 16 per cent, iron lack becomes limiting to hemoglobin production.

Major developmental variations in serum iron and iron-binding capacity are restricted to the first week of life, when they are unlikely to cause confusion because of the extreme rarity of iron deficiency during this period (25, 39). At birth, serum iron falls precipitously from 160 μg. per 100 ml. in cord blood with an iron-binding capacity of 250 μg. per 100 ml. to a value of about 50 μg. per 100 ml. at one day of age. Between three days and two months of age, serum iron and iron-binding capacity again approach adult values. This is followed by a period of lower serum iron (down to 75 μg. per 100 ml.) that coincides with the period of depleted iron stores (between three to six months and two years).

Transferrin saturation is a particularly useful diagnostic tool in the pediatric age group. Determination of the bone marrow iron stores is less useful in infants and adolescents than in adults, since storage iron is normally marginal during rapid growth and there is insufficient distinction between the normal and deficient individual. Furthermore, a low transferrin saturation is relatively specific for iron deficiency. Infection and protein-calorie malnutrition pose a problem in that they result in a prompt diminution of serum transferrin due to a decrease in its rate of production. In protein-calorie malnutrition, the per cent of transferrin saturation usually remains high, even though there may be a coexisting iron deficiency. Consequently, the diagnosis of iron deficiency is more likely to be missed rather than mistakenly diagnosed when the two conditions coexist. Infection is likely to depress serum iron as well as transferrin and is, therefore, a greater potential source of confusion.

Infection appears to impair the reutilization of iron for the synthesis of hemoglobin. Although iron from degraded hemoglobin is readily deposited in the reticuloendothelial system, the subsequent release of iron to circulating transferrin is decreased. Thus an anemia resembling that of iron deficiency may develop, even though storage iron is not depleted. Serum iron is also decreased within one day of surgical procedures, possibly on a similar basis, but

TABLE 4–3.   SERUM FERRITIN CONCENTRATION IN CHILDREN AGED
6 MONTHS TO 15 YEARS

| | | SERUM FERRITIN | |
	NUMBER OF CHILDREN	Median (ng./ml.)	Range (ng./ml.)
Normal°	486	30	7–142‡
Iron deficiency anemia	13	3.4	1.5–9
Latent iron deficiency†	6	11	4.5–41
Respiratory infection (mild, acute)	19	128	18–510
Sickle cell anemia	14	163	49–180
Thalassemia major	7	850	590–1830

°No anemia.
†No anemia, but serum iron saturation < 16 per cent.
‡95 per cent confidence limits.
From Siimes, M. A., Addiego, J. E., et al.: Ferritin in serum: Diagnosis of iron deficiency and iron overload in infants and children. Blood, 1974 (in press).

this is of insufficient duration to cause anemia.

An important consideration in interpreting transferrin saturation is the marked diurnal variation in serum iron, whereas total transferrin remains stable. Thus, at 8:00 A.M., serum iron normally averages 140 μg. per 100 ml., yielding a saturation of about 47 per cent. This falls throughout the course of the day to a low of 40 μg. per 100 ml. by 10:00 P.M., or a saturation of 13 per cent. In iron depletion or overload, diurnal variations are less striking. Nevertheless, it is apparent that transferrin saturation should be studied at standardized times, particularly in public health surveys.

There are several practical disadvantages of determining serum transferrin saturation that detract slightly from its usefulness. The colorimetric determination of iron requires about 5 ml. of blood, a quantity that is often difficult to obtain in infants. Determination of iron by atomic spectroscopy is more sensitive and thus requires less blood, but this method is not yet generally available. An additional problem with any serum iron assay is the necessity of applying scrupulous precautions against iron contamination. A further difficulty in clinical management is that in most laboratories iron determinations are not done in sufficient volume to warrant daily assays. Consequently, it is often expedient to initiate

therapy before the confirmatory laboratory test is completed, in effect constituting a therapeutic trial.

ANEMIA.   Anemia is a delayed manifestation of iron deficiency, clinically evident only after months of suboptimal hemoglobin production, since red cells that are produced under conditions of iron adequacy live out their normal 120-day lifespan. Furthermore, as long as the transferrin saturation is only slightly depressed, the production of new red cells may be normochromic and normocytic, and it proceeds at a rate that remains close to normal. As anemia becomes pronounced, the newly produced red blood cells gradually become smaller and less well-filled with hemoglobin (see Table 4–1 for lower limits of normal hemoglobin and hematocrit).

The anemia of iron deficiency results primarily from a decrease in the number of red cells released by the bone marrow, but there is also an associated component of ineffective erythropoiesis and hemolysis (54). Within the bone marrow, the rate of red cell production and destruction are both accelerated, as indicated by isotopic studies. The increased cellularity of the bone marrow, usually with a predominance of erythroid precursors, is in accord with these results and does not merely reflect a maturation arrest, as was previously postulated. There is an increased number of immature erythroid forms. Mature normoblasts have scant and irregular cytoplasm and basophilic staining, indicative of deficient production of hemoglobin. Nuclear abnormalities can be striking and include multinuclearity, budding, and fragmentation.

The *laboratory diagnosis* of iron deficiency is based primarily on the detection of anemia. The microhematocrit, the spectrophotometric assay of hemoglobin as cyanmethemoglobin, and electronic red cell sizing and counting are accurate and suitable for rapid handling of many samples. Of the red cell indices, the mean corpuscular hemoglobin (MCH) and mean corpuscular hemoglobin concentration (MCHC) have been the most useful since the per cent deviation from normal is greater than that of the mean corpuscular volume (MCV) as the hemoglobin decreases. However, electronic counting has made the MCHC an unreliable figure in most clinical laboratories. The other indices remain of value in distinguishing the hypochromic microcytic anemias from other types (Table 4–4). The blood smear, by revealing a hypochromic microcytic picture, is of great diagnostic value (see Red Cell Morphology, Fig. 1, 2). If anemia is characterized by either or both methods as hypochromic and microcytic, a low transferrin saturation helps to establish the diagnosis of iron deficiency, particularly in the absence of infection. Most other causes of hypochromic microcytic anemia, such as thalassemia and lead poisoning, are associated with an elevated transferrin saturation.

The three principal causes of microcytosis in the United States are iron deficiency, alpha or beta thalassemia minor, and lead poisoning. The development of a simple, micromethod for the measurement

of free erythrocyte porphyrin has proved useful in distinguishing between these disturbances. In both iron deficiency anemia and lead poisoning, the level of free erythrocyte porphyrin is elevated, while it remains normal in patients with thalassemia minor. The level of free erythrocyte porphyrin tends to be higher in lead poisoning than in iron deficiency and is elevated at blood lead levels in excess of 40 μg. per 100 ml. (55). Patients with MCV's of less than 75 μ^3 can be rapidly separated into those with and those without thalassemia minor on this basis.

OTHER RED CELL CHANGES (38). Decreased survival of red cells released to the circulation is detectable when anemia becomes severe (56). This may result in part from an abnormal stiffening of the usually pliable red cell membrane, associated with a low concentration of ATP (57). In iron-deficient rabbits, for example, erythrocytes, despite their smaller volume, have a decreased ability to squeeze through a millipore filter with a 5-μ pore diameter. This lack of pliability may favor trapping of the cells within the narrow vascular channels of the spleen. In accord with this concept is the normal survival of red cells from iron-deficient patients that are injected into asplenic recipients. There is no known enzymatic basis for decreased red cell ATP and loss of pliability. The enzymes of glycolysis and of the pentose shunt are either normal or increased in activity in iron deficiency.

Other than hemoglobin, catalase is the heme protein present in largest amounts in the red cell. According to most reports, red cell catalase activity is decreased in iron deficiency when expressed on the basis of whole blood or red cell number. The results are more variable when expressed on the basis of hemoglobin. This may at first suggest that iron deficiency has little effect on this heme protein. However, when it is realized that hemoglobin, the standard of reference, is decreased, it becomes clear that catalase production must also be diminished to a comparable extent just to maintain the normal proportionality between the two. Glutathione peroxidase in red cells appears to be more markedly decreased.

Free *protoporphyrin* accumulates in the

TABLE 4–4. RED CELL INDICES

TYPE OF ANEMIA	MCV (μ^3)	MCH ($\mu\mu$g.)	MCHC (%)
Macrocytic	97–160	35–40	32–36
Normocytic	80–96	26–34	32–36
Microcytic, hypochromic	50–79	12–29	24–31

Reproduced by permission from Cartwright, E. D.: *Diagnostic Laboratory Hematology.* 4th ed. New York, Grune & Stratton, 1968, p. 119.

Editor's Note: The color of the serum may also be valuable. The serum is of normal straw color in thalassemia trait and lead poisoning and is clear and colorless in iron deficiency.

erythrocyte when iron deficiency limits hemoglobin synthesis. This determination has recently been proposed for clinical use. Improvements in methodology over the previously time-consuming assay may make it a potentially useful diagnostic tool. The advantage of the free protoporphyrin determination is that it does not fluctuate as much as serum iron and transferrin saturation in response to recent dietary intake. Unfortunately, the test lacks specificity since levels also become elevated with infection and lead poisoning. In the absence of infection, free protoporphyrin can be used to screen for both iron deficiency and lead poisoning (55).

TISSUE HEME PROTEINS (38, 58, 59). Tissue heme protein production is depressed along with that of hemoglobin during the progression of iron deficiency. Though these changes are clinically difficult to assess, they undoubtedly contribute to the manifestations of the disorder. However, in view of the obscurity of symptomatology in iron deficiency, it is hardly surprising that attribution of specific physical findings to tissue heme protein deficiency is purely speculative.

In man, *cytochrome oxidase* activity is decreased in the mucosal lining of the mouth and the intestine. The sampling of most other solid tissues is hard to justify in the management of iron deficiency. Thus much of our information on the systemic effects of iron deficiency is derived from animal models that invariably differ from the human situation in some respects but often provide useful insights. In the rat, for example, it is clear that the effect of iron deficiency on the concentration of a heme protein varies from tissue to tissue. Thus *cytochrome c*, which is present in all aerobic cells in the body, falls to less than half of normal concentrations within two weeks in skeletal muscle and intestinal mucosa in the growing rat. At the same time there is no detectable effect in tissues such as brain and heart muscle. Similarly, *myoglobin* concentration is more depressed in skeletal muscle than in diaphragmatic or heart muscle. Factors that seem to favor the development of deficiency in a tissue include rapid growth or rapid cell turnover or both. Tissues that are most resistant are those that are already fully grown and those subjected to a continuing obligatory work load, especially of a nature that is essential to survival.

Even in the same tissue, some heme proteins become deficient while others are extraordinarily resistant. Thus the microsomal heme proteins of the liver, cytochromes b_5 and P-450, in spite of their extremely rapid turnover (a half-life of about two days), remain normal in concentration while the mitochondrial cytochromes are decreased. Indeed, the deficient rat responds to phenobarbital administration with the same fourfold increase in cytochrome P-450 concentration that is observed in the normal animal. Why these rapidly synthesized cytochromes have such an unusually high priority for iron is unexplained. It is conceivable that, by virtue of their location in the endoplasmic reticulum, they have preferential access to iron released in the liver by red cell degradation.

Ultrastructural changes in iron deficiency are most apparent in the mitochondria of erythroid precursors in man, and in liver and heart muscle in the rat. The mitochondria are enlarged, rounded, and electron-lucent. The mitochondrial enlargement in heart muscle of severely anemic animals is so marked that it accounts, in large part, for the heart hypertrophy present.

Gross morphologic changes in epithelial and endothelial structures are included in the next section.

CLINICAL MANIFESTATIONS. The symptomatology of iron deficiency is nonspecific. Mild iron deficiency is usually diagnosed on the basis of laboratory studies alone, and the findings in severe iron deficiency anemia are likely to be similar to those of other anemias. Fatigue, irritability, loss of appetite, and pallor may be noted. The gradual onset of the findings characteristic of nutritional iron-lack may escape the notice of even the observant physician and parent. Tachycardia and cardiomegaly may be found on physical examination but are rarely the initial clues to the diagnosis.

Manifestations not readily attributable to anemia (38, 58, 59) are most likely to be evident in epithelial or endothelial tissues, but these are not consistently observed, even with severe anemia. The fingernails may be thin and brittle and assume a concave shape (koilonychia or spoon nail). The papillae of the tongue are sometimes atrophied. Inflammation of the mucous membranes of the mouth, vagina, and anus is even more unusual than in the adult population, where the frequency of these findings is reported to be decreasing. Abnormalities of intestinal function, however, are not unusual. Decreased absorption of fat, vitamin A, and xylose is well documented and may be associated with an atrophic appearance of the villi in the small intestine (60). In some cases, there is a depletion of serum protein and of serum copper, probably on the basis of exudative loss through the intestinal mucosa (61).

Treatment (62)

The treatment of choice for most cases of iron deficiency is oral administration of ferrous sulfate. This iron salt remains the standard against which the efficacy of a multitude of other compounds is measured. It is low in cost and is as well tolerated as comparable amounts of iron in other therapeutically effective preparations. Intolerance to oral iron salts is very rare in children. If it occurs, a reduction of the dose or administration of the medication with meals will generally solve the problem. Iron-staining of the teeth may occur, but it is not permanent; it can be minimized by administering the medication on the back of the tongue.

The *dosage of oral iron* is based on the amount which will be adequate for a maximal hematologic response. A generous estimate is 6 mg. per kg. per day of elemental iron, divided into three doses to reduce the likelihood of gastrointestinal intolerance. Assuming a value of 20 per cent for absorption in the iron-deficient patient, this provides over 1 mg. per kg. per day, an amount which is ample for the production of 0.4 g. per 100 ml. per day of hemoglobin. The calculation assumes a blood volume of about 70 ml. per kg. and the presence of 3.4 mg. of iron in 1 g. hemoglobin.

In infancy, dietary iron deficiency accounts for most anemias in individuals who are otherwise healthy. This discourages an elaborate diagnostic evaluation in the typical case; a trial of iron medication is often justified on the basis of a hemoglobin or hematocrit determination alone. If the child seems otherwise well, this is an economical, practical, and safe course, with the stipulation that the results of the therapeutic trial are monitored after two weeks to one month. In order to avoid iron overloading, the *duration of therapy* should not extend beyond one or two months after anemia is reversed; this is sufficient time to allow for the restitution of depleted iron stores, particularly if the cause of the deficiency has been corrected.

Use of *intramuscular iron* in the form of iron-dextran (Imferon) is rarely warranted except when administration of oral iron medications cannot be relied upon. The injections are often painful, skin discoloration is common if special care is not taken to avoid backflow into subcutaneous tissue, and the therapeutic response is not significantly more rapid than with oral medication. Furthermore, severe anaphylactic reactions have been reported, rarely resulting in death. Therefore, this preparation should only be used when there is a good reason to substitute it for oral medication, as for example after there has been an apparent lack of response to oral therapy. Malabsorption is rare, but failure to administer medication is relatively common.

The total dose of Imferon (50 mg. per ml. of elemental iron) is distributed over at least two to three daily injections and can be calculated by estimating the iron deficit as follows: (1) it requires about 2.5 mg. of elemental iron per kg. to raise the hemoglobin concentration 1 g. per 100 ml., and (2) an additional 10 mg. per kg. should be added to allow for iron stores to be replenished and for incomplete absorption from the site of injection.

In infants with concurrent vitamin E deficiency, iron-dextran administration may result in hemolysis (63). The biochemical basis for this is probably the role of ionic iron as a cofactor in peroxidation of lipid in the red cell membrane. On the basis of studies in vitro, such an effect might be anticipated if the capacity of transferrin to bind iron is temporarily exceeded, leaving free ionic iron in the medium.

Very rarely, *blood transfusion* is indicated as an adjunct in the treatment of iron deficiency to correct an anemia more rapidly than is possible with iron medication alone. The severely anemic infant with a hemoglobin below 4 to 5 g. per 100 ml. has very little margin for safety between cardiovascular compensation and heart failure.

If the risk of blood transfusion is warranted to improve the clinical status rapidly, it can be given as packed red cells, either at a slow rate or, alternatively, at the same rate at which the patient's anemic blood is withdrawn. This method of partial exchange transfusion avoids a sudden change in blood volume and can be accomplished within one to two hours. Vital signs should be carefully monitored and no more than 10 to 20 ml. per kg. exchanged in this manner.

Nutritional counseling to prevent recurrence of a dietary deficiency is often of value, but it is important to realize that culturally based eating patterns are not modified easily ("It may be easier to change a person's religion than his dietary habits"). However, in infants who have been milk-fed, an improved appetite and weaning from the bottle as the child gets older will provide a more iron-rich diet.

A *response to iron therapy* can be detected in the bone marrow in less than 24 hours. Erythroid precursors change from the pretreatment predominance of immature basophilic forms to include many normoblasts, with generous amounts of hemoglobin evident in the cytoplasm. Reticulocytes increase in the peripheral blood after a lag of as little as two to three days in children, perhaps a somewhat shorter period than in the adult. The rate of reversal of anemia is limited by the rate at which new red cells can be produced (Fig. 4–14). New hemoglobin-replete cells gradually replace old hypochromic ones which have lost their protein-synthetic apparatus and therefore are unable to replenish their hemoglobin. After one to two weeks of treatment of a severe deficiency, a double population of red cells can be seen on the blood smear: hypochromic microcytic cells

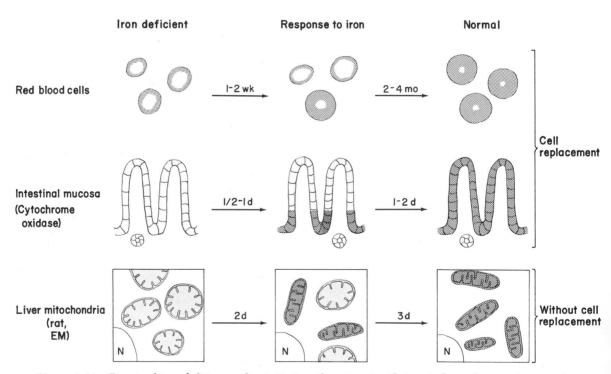

Figure 4–14. Repair of iron deficiency after initiation of treatment with iron is dependent on the rate of turnover of cells and subcellular structures. Newly produced, hemoglobin-replete red cells gradually replace the senescent, hypochromic, microcytic cells which are unable to replenish their hemoglobin. There is a double population of cells until replacement of the hypochromic, microcytic cells is complete.

Cells of the intestinal mucosa that are deficient in cytochrome oxidase are similarly replaced by new cells that have normal cytochrome oxidase activity. The life span of mucosal cells is about two days. (From data of Dallman, P. R., and Schwartz, H. C.: J. Clin. Invest. *44*:1631, 1965.)

Liver cells have a long life span and are not replaced to a significant degree. However, mitochondria within the cell are replaced at a rapid rate. In the rat, ultrastructural abnormalities of the mitochondria are reversed without the production of new cells. (From data of Dallman, P. R., and Goodman, J. R.: J. Cell. Biol. *48*:79, 1971.)

that were produced during the deficient period and larger, well-filled normal cells that have matured during the recent period of iron adequacy.

The *rate of recovery* may be 0.25 to 0.4 g. per 100 ml. per day of hemoglobin or a 1 per cent per day rise in hematocrit, also more rapid than is anticipated in the adult (Fig. 4–15) (64). If iron deficiency is discovered as an incidental finding in a patient with an infection, the response to iron is often delayed until the infection is resolved. Protein deficiency may similarly interfere with iron utilization. The enzyme xanthine oxidase is believed to be required for the mobilization of iron from storage compounds. This enzyme is profoundly depressed by protein deficiency. Consequently, a defect in the capacity to mobilize iron may partially explain the frequent finding of adequate marrow iron, even when iron-lack complicates protein deficiency. Under these circumstances, iron deficiency may become unmasked only after two to three weeks of treatment with an adequate protein intake.

Since iron deficiency is a systemic dis-

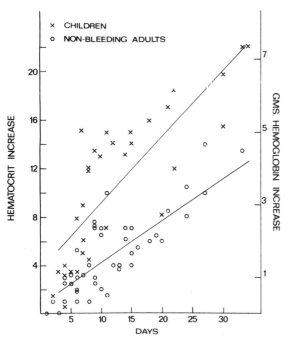

Figure 4–15. Rate of hemoglobin and hematocrit response to iron therapy. Children appear to recover more rapidly than adults. [Adapted from Stevens, A. R., In *Iron in Clinical Medicine.* Wallerstein, R. O., and Mettier, S. R., (eds.), Berkeley, University of California Press, 1958, p. 150.]

ease, it follows that correction of the disorder is a function of other factors in addition to the response in hemoglobin production. The reversal of deficiencies in other heme proteins proceeds at rates that are generally related to the rate of replacement of the cellular or subcellular structure in which the deficient substance is located (Fig. 4–14). Thus, in man, deficient cytochrome oxidase activity in the basal layer of the buccal mucosa and in the intestinal mucosa is back to normal within one to three days of iron treatment, before there is an appreciable change in hemoglobin concentration. In the intestinal mucosa, histochemical stains for cytochrome oxidase show that recovery begins in the newly differentiating cells at the base of the villi and progresses as these cells migrate toward the tip of the villus, gradually replacing the deficient cells (65). The prompt recovery is consistent with the rate of replacement of these cells, which is much more rapid than that of the red cell.

Reports on the recovery of red cell catalase with iron treatment are conflicting, but the weight of evidence seems to indicate that it occurs at the same rate as the reversal of anemia. Presumably, the newly produced red cells that are normal in respect to hemoglobin are also the first to have a normal complement of catalase.

The relationship of the rate of reversal of other deficiencies in tissue heme proteins to the turnover of cells or subcellular structures can be inferred from biochemical and ultrastructural studies in the rat (38). In skeletal muscle, a tissue with a negligible rate of cell turnover, the return to normal myoglobin and cytochrome *c* concentrations takes about five times as long as the reversal of anemia (Fig. 4–16). In the liver there is a more rapid recovery of cytochrome *c* concentration, which is not surprising since liver mitochondria are known to have a rapid rate of turnover. The cytochrome *c* response to iron treatment is consistent with this rate, and suggests that repair proceeds as new mitochondria or mitochondrial enzyme complexes are synthesized.

Ultrastructural studies of the rat liver similarly show that production of new cells is not a prerequisite to recovery as it is with hemoglobin (Fig. 4–14). Two days after the start of iron treatment, the mitochondria

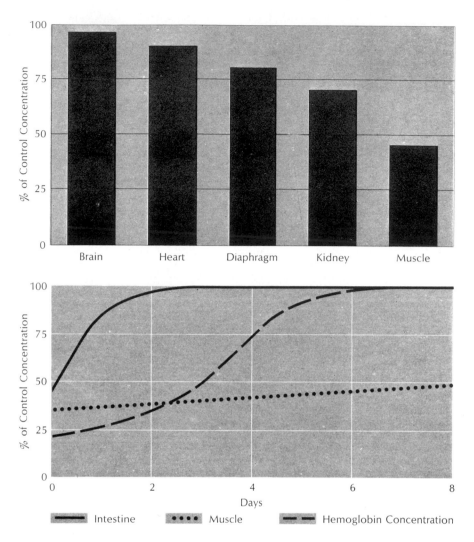

Figure 4–16. Iron deficiency has been shown to depress tissue concentrations of heme proteins, such as the cytochromes, that are essential to cellular metabolism. Graph at top indicates levels of cytochrome *c* found in rats fed an iron-deficient diet, as compared with control values in normally fed rats. As lower graph shows, adding iron to the diet converts cytochrome *c* concentrations to normal rather promptly in the intestine (hemoglobin concentration also returns to normal), but recovery in muscle is slow. (Data from Dallman, P. R., and Schwartz, H. C.: J. Clin. Invest. *44*:1631, 1965.)

have a heterogeneity of appearance in any given cell. Some mitochondria retain the electron-lucent, swollen, and rounded appearance characteristic of iron deficiency, some have reverted to the normal configuration, whereas others are intermediate. The implication of these findings is that repair may be a gradual process, even within long-lived cells.

Prevention

Iron lack is unique among the classic deficiency syndromes first recognized 40 to 50 years ago in that its overall prevalence is stable or may actually be increasing, while scurvy, rickets, and pellagra have become rarities. The focus of interest is therefore shifting from treatment to prevention. Table 4–5 lists the recommended daily dietary allowances for iron according to age and sex (6). Among two groups, the growing child and the female between adolescence and menopause, iron intakes far below these amounts are common.

In the United States the incidence of iron deficiency, according to large surveys, ranges between 5 per cent and 45 per cent

TABLE 4–5. RECOMMENDED DAILY
DIETARY ALLOWANCES (RDA)
FOR IRON (1968)

GROUP	AGE RANGE (YR.)	RDA FOR IRON (MG.)
Infants	0–1/6	6
	1/6–1/2	10
	1/2–1	15
Children	1–3	15
	3–10	10
Males	10–12	10
	12–18	18
	18–75+	10
Females	10–55	18
	55–75+	10
Pregnancy		18
Lactation		18

among various age groups in childhood and adolescence, with the peak incidence between six months and two years of age (33, 66–68). No socioeconomic group is spared. Children of low-income families are generally reported to have the highest incidence, but the relationship of prevalence to income is still a matter of some dispute. The high incidence of iron deficiency during early adolescence, another period of rapid growth, has been appreciated only recently. Iron deficiency is present in well over 10 per cent of high school students in areas where low-income families predominate. Among young male and female military recruits there is also a similar, surprisingly high prevalence of anemia.

In this country, cow's milk often dominates the infant's diet during the first two years of life and results in an iron intake that may be less than 5 per cent of the recommended amount. The impact of nutritional counseling on altering this dietary pattern has been disappointing. Bottle feeding is accepted readily by infants and can be carried out largely unattended. Thus, even when an increasingly mixed diet is recommended after three to six months of age, excessive reliance on bottle feeding is the path of least resistance.

There is no doubt that absorbable forms of iron added to foods will improve iron balance and prevent iron deficiency. In the United States, *food supplementation with iron* (69–74) is in use in infant cereals, commercial milk formulas, and in "enriched" flour and other cereal products. For about 30 years, infant cereals have been fortified with reduced iron of relatively large particle size or with sodium ferric pyrophosphate. Recent studies indicate that negligible amounts of this iron are absorbed. In contrast, milk-based infant formulas are supplemented with 12 mg. of iron as ferrous sulfate per reconstituted quart, which is effectively utilized. At present, these commercial formulas are used primarily during the first four months of life, prior to the peak incidence of iron deficiency. Recently, iron-supplemented milk products, intended for use after early infancy, have been marketed. Some physicians oppose the iron supplementation of milk on the grounds that it lends sanction to the excessive use of milk in the diet and that it is a poor substitute for improving the diet through nutritional counseling. In any case, none of the above measures to increase iron intake has had a major effect on the high prevalence of iron deficiency in infants. The failure is partly attributed to the fact that these foods do not adequately reach the lower socioeconomic groups, and their use among other segments of the population is generally restricted to a brief period. Consequently, the Committee on Nutrition of the Academy of Pediatrics has recommended that iron-fortified formulas be used routinely, at least until one year of age (33). In addition, it is urged that iron-fortified whole milk or evaporated milk be marketed for infant feeding. Marketing trials of iron-supplemented pasteurized milk have been successful and have helped to dispel the concern that the product would be unacceptably discolored. It may prove important to treat such a milk product at a higher temperature than used during pasteurization since this appears to prevent intestinal blood loss that is often associated with the ingestion of large volumes of pasteurized milk. Folic acid would then have to be added to compensate for losses by heating.

Some reservations have been expressed in regard to the use of any form of milk as a vehicle for iron supplementation. First, there is evidence that the bacteriostatic properties of milk are abolished when its iron-binding proteins, lactoferrin and transferrin, are saturated with iron (75). It is postulated that this bacteriostatic effect may play an important role in preventing enteric infections during early development. Theoretically, saturation of the two iron-binding proteins could occur in the intestinal tract if iron is fed with milk. Second, it may be unwise to rely on a uniquely lactose-rich food as a vehicle for iron since a large percentage of Blacks and Spanish-Americans have a relative lactose intolerance. In spite of these reservations, one is reassured by the extensive experience of the last ten years with iron supplementation of infant formulas, which has shown only beneficial effects. The recommendations of the Academy of Pediatrics are therefore reasonable for the present and are justifiably gaining increased support.

Prevention of iron deficiency in infancy has been successfully accomplished in much of Scandinavia by programs of medicinal iron supplementation, monitored largely in neighborhood health centers. In the United States it is difficult to reach the most susceptible segments of the population in this manner. Other disadvantages of a program based on medicinal iron are an already high incidence of accidental acute iron poisoning in children and the uncertainty that any medication will be taken as prescribed over a long period of time.

The greatest impact on iron nutrition during the next decade is likely to result from proposals by the Food and Nutrition Board of the National Academy of Sciences to increase iron supplementation in a broad range of flour products from the present level of 13.0 to 16.5 mg. per lb. to between 40 and 60 mg. per lb. (70, 71). These recommendations are based on the 1965 food consumption survey of the U. S. Department of Agriculture. Daily consumption of grain products averages one-fifth pound in young adult females and one-third pound in males. This should assure an adequate iron supply for preschool children and postpubertal females (Table 4–6). The mature male, however, may receive more than twice his minimum requirement, but it is doubtful that this constitutes a significant hazard. However, some fear exists that the increment in iron intake may harm those with problems of iron overload, i.e., alcoholics

TABLE 4–6. PROJECTION OF IRON INTAKE WITH IRON SUPPLEMENTATION OF 12 MG./L. OF MILK AND 40 MG./LB. OF FLOUR

	PRESENT (MG./DAY)	PROJECTED (MG./DAY)
Infants (age 1)	5	12–15
Females (aged 10–55)	11	17
Males	15	25–30

with cirrhosis, those with hemolytic anemia or hemochromatosis, and perhaps even the normal individual whose capacity to exclude unwanted dietary iron may be exceeded. Current plans for a continuous system of nutritional surveillance of the general population under the auspices of governmental agencies should help in the evaluation of the efficacy of this program.

Prevention of iron deficiency is a more complex and urgent problem in the underdeveloped countries. The prevalence of hookworm and the predominance of cereals and starches in the diet are responsible for a high incidence of iron deficiency. Vehicles for supplementation are limited, since most food products do not go through commercial processing. Cereal staples, such as rice and wheat, and such products as sugar have been utilized as vehicles where they form a relatively constant and predictable fraction of the diet. The form of iron that is ideal for the supplementation of these foods remains to be experimentally determined.

MEGALOBLASTIC ANEMIA: FOLATE DEFICIENCY (76–83)

Folate deficiency is the most common cause of megaloblastic anemia in childhood. Predisposing factors include marginal intake during infancy, limited storage capacity (compared to iron and vitamin B_{12}), and increased requirements during rapid growth. Folate is also deficient in several forms of intestinal malabsorption.

Metabolism and Pathogenesis

STRUCTURE AND METABOLIC ROLE. Folate in plant and animal food exists primarily as pteroic acid derivatives, conjugated with peptides composed of one to ten glutamic acid residues (Fig. 4–17). This is probably also a storage form of folate in man. The active form of the vitamin is a free or monoglutamic conjugate of folate, in which the double bonds at positions 5, 6 and 7, 8 are both reduced to tetrahydro compounds.

The conversion of the inactive dietary form of folate begins with digestion of the polyglutamate peptide, which requires the action of so-called conjugase enzymes. This takes place either within the lumen or in the mucosa of the proximal small intestine. The resulting monoglutamate is then largely converted to a tetrahydrofolate form (primarily 5-methyltetrahydrofolate) before release into the circulation. Total folate stores in the adult normally range between 5 to 10 mg., about half of this being in the liver.

Folates serve as cofactors in reactions that involve the transfer of single carbon units. N5-N10 methylene tetrahydrofolic acid, for example, is the methyl donor in the conversion of deoxyuridylate to thymidylate, the nucleotide that is unique to DNA. This key role of folate in DNA synthesis is probably responsible for the megaloblastic cell morphology so characteristic of folate deficiency. Not only hematopoietic cells but also other rapidly replicating cell populations, such as intestinal mucosa, show an increase in cell size and a disordered maturation. These cells accumulate RNA but require extra time to synthesize sufficient DNA to enter mitosis. Rapidly dividing cells are a small proportion of the total in the adult, where most cells are either incapable of further division (neurons), or divide primarily in response to injury or partial resection (liver, muscle, kidney). During early development, however, almost all cell populations go through periods of rapid division. The essential role of folate in cell replication may account for the high requirement for this vitamin in infants. It also suggests that the cellular consequences of folate lack may prove to be more widespread in the infant than in the adult. The teratogenic effects of folate antagonists on the fetus warn us that growing and irreplaceable cell populations can be subject to permanent damage, in contrast to the more familiar, reversible damage in blood and epithelial tissues.

REQUIREMENTS AND DIETARY SOURCES. The adult requirement for folate is a minimum of 50 to 100 μg. per day; a mixed adult diet contains about 1 mg. per day, a com-

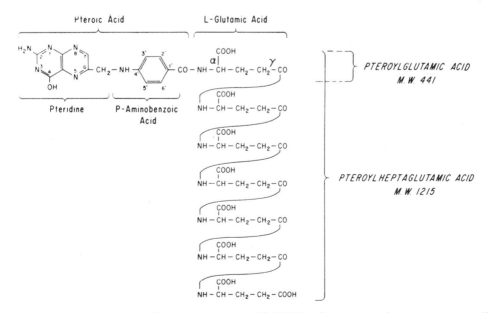

Figure 4–17. Folic acid. Structure of pteroylglutamic acid (PGA) and its principal conjugate, pteroylheptaglutamic acid. The number of glutamic acid residues varies in naturally occurring folates.

fortable margin over the minimum requirement. About ten times as much folate on a body weight basis is required by the infant as by the adult, e. g., 20 to 50 μg. per day. Folate is widely distributed in foods. Liver is a particularly rich source and contains about 300 μg. per 100 g.; other meat products, fresh vegetables, whole grain cereals, and dried beans are also adequate sources, with 10 to 100 μg. per 100 g.

Milk is a poor source of folate. Breast milk or pasteurized cow's milk contains approximately 35 μg. per L. (3.5 μg. per 100 g.) below the amount present in most foods and near the minimum required to sustain rapid growth in infancy. Heat treatment lowers the folate content of milk further. Thus sterilization of formula by boiling halves the folate, and evaporated milk has less than 20 μg. per reconstituted liter.

Bacteria are a rich, potential source of folate. Experimental folate deficiency in the rat is produced by preventing coprophagia and by reducing the number of intestinal bacteria with broad-spectrum antibiotics. There is also a bacterial contribution to human folate intake, but its magnitude is not known. Folate-containing bacteria reside mainly in the colon, a site from which the vitamin is poorly absorbed. Nevertheless, the partial elimination of intestinal bacteria by prolonged use of broad-spectrum antibiotics is also associated with folate deficiency.

Mild folate deficiency is common in the pregnant woman. However, as in the case of iron, there is a placental gradient favorable to the fetus. Folate in the cord blood is normally over twice as high as that in the mother. After birth there is an exponential drop in both blood and serum folate and a period of marginal folate nutrition follows (84–89). By two weeks of age, the stores established during fetal life become depleted, as reflected by mean values for blood and serum folate which are slightly below those of the normal adult. These remain somewhat depressed throughout the first year of life and then return toward adult values. In the premature infant, the depression of blood and serum folate below adult values is even more marked, especially between one and three months of age, when 68 per cent of infants below a birth weight of 1700 g. are reported to have low serum folate levels. These values suggest that the folate intake of the infant is marginal and is likely to be deficient if heat-treated or evaporated milk forms the bulk of the diet.

CAUSES AND CLASSIFICATION OF FOLATE DEFICIENCY. These fall into the categories of deficient dietary intake, malabsorption, and drug interactions.

A *dietary lack* of folate generally results from a loss of the vitamin during cooking rather than from its deficiency in food. Folate lack is most common under circumstances that increase the requirement, e.g., rapid body or cell growth. This is most dramatic in the premature infant, during pregnancy, and in severe chronic hemolytic states (90, 91).

Folate deficiency due to *malabsorption* is common in such chronic diarrheal states as tropical sprue, gluten intolerance, and idiopathic steatorrhea, particularly in infancy. A combination of factors is likely to be responsible. First, there is apparently a loss of intestinal conjugase activity in these conditions, since a small dose of monoglutamic folate will produce a prompt therapeutic response, whereas large doses of the polyglutamic folates that are present in food are poorly absorbed. Second, loss of intestinal flora through use of broad-spectrum antibiotics or through diarrhea may reduce the contribution of bacteria as a supplementary source of folate. Finally, diarrhea may interfere with the absorption and normal enterohepatic circulation of folate through an excessively rapid intestinal passage. Self-filling bowel loops can also be associated with a related form of folate deficiency. Since broad-spectrum antibiotics may improve folate status in these cases, it is inferred that the deficiency results from accumulation of dietary folate by the abundant bacterial growth in the stagnant bowel contents.

DRUG INTERACTIONS (92). Folate analogs, such as methotrexate, react with dihydrofolate reductase and interfere with the conversion of the normal dihydrofolate substrates to the active tetrahydro forms. Consequently, hypersegmentation of neutrophils and megaloblastic changes in the bone marrow and peripheral blood are common concomitants of this form of antimetabolite therapy.

A different mechanism is responsible for

the folate deficiency associated with the use of oral contraceptives or diphenylhydantoins and other anticonvulsants. These drugs interact with polyglutamates in the intestinal lumen and interfere with their digestion to the absorbable monoglutamate form. Administration of pteroylglutamic acid (PGA) reverses the folate deficiency, whereas an increase in dietary polyglutamic folates is ineffective unless the drug is also stopped.

Diagnosis

A folate-deficient diet (less than 5 μg. per day) in an adult (93) will first result in a fall in serum folate (assayed with *Lactobacillus casei*). Hypersegmentation of neutrophils then develops in the bone marrow after five weeks of the diet but is not detected in the peripheral blood until seven weeks. By this time the bone marrow begins to show megaloblastic changes which progress over the next 11 weeks. Red cell folate does not fall until the seventeenth week of the regimen. At this time macrocytosis also becomes evident on the peripheral smear. Not until after the eighteenth week is there a significant anemia and the appearance of symptoms of sleeplessness, forgetfulness, and irritability. Significantly detectable anemia and symptomatology are delayed over three months beyond the first evidence of disordered cell maturation, e.g., hypersegmentation. Thus cell pathology is present long before a skilled clinician may suspect the abnormality. No comparable data are available in children, but one anticipates a more rapid progression of deficiency because of the additional demand for folate imposed by growth. The prompt development of folate deficiency in the premature infant indicates that this is the case.

The anemia of folate deficiency is largely due to a deficient net release of red blood cells from the bone marrow. But there is also a component of ineffective erythropoiesis. The mild jaundice that may be one of the manifestations of severe folate deficiency is attributed to a markedly increased release of heme degradation products, primarily from the bone marrow.

Hypersegmentation of the neutrophils in peripheral blood is the single most useful laboratory aid to early diagnosis. It is often evident, even in mixed deficiency states with an iron and protein lack, whereas red cell indices and the serum folate are less reliable. An average of more than 3.42 lobes per cell in 100 neutrophils is considered abnormal. More frequently, hypersegmentation is a subjective impression which prompts confirmation of the diagnosis by serum studies, bone marrow aspiration, or a therapeutic trial (see Red Cell Morphology, Fig. 1, 8).

Although *serum folate* reflects recent dietary changes, it may be too sensitive to normal dietary fluctuations to be an ideal test of chronic folate status. Nevertheless, it remains the best way of confirming the existence of an early folate deficiency when hypersegmentation is observed. *Red cell folate* levels do not respond rapidly enough to be of value in early diagnosis. The folate content of newly produced red cells appears to reflect current body folate stores. As in the case of hemoglobin, the folate complement of the red cell is established during its early development. Therefore, a deficiency does not become evident until new folate-deficient cells replace most older cells that live out their normal lifespan. For this reason, red cell folate is a better index of chronic folate status independent of short-term improvement in diet.

The commonly used microbiologic assay of folate with *Lactobacillus casei* responds to essentially all forms of the vitamin in the blood. However, the assay of folate in foods requires prior enzymatic digestion, since polyglutamic conjugates with a chain length of more than three will not be detected. A serum folate below 3 ng. per ml. is subnormal. The corresponding lower limit for whole blood folate is 50 ng. per ml. Marrow morphology is megaloblastic in more than half the infants, with a value below 20 ng. per ml. whole blood.

Measurement of serum or red cell folate or both and serum vitamin B_{12} will usually distinguish between the two major causes of megaloblastic anemia. A concurrently low vitamin B_{12} activity may be misleading, since it can occasionally be corrected by folate treatment alone. This is one of several interactions between the two vitamins that are incompletely understood and are extensively reviewed elsewhere.

The development of macrocytic indices (MCV over 100 μ^3) occurs later, usually concurrently with anemia and with other noticeable abnormalities in red cell morphology. Variations in cell size are marked in megaloblastic anemia (Fig. 4–18). Most cells are larger than normal, but many are small and distorted in shape.

Megaloblastic changes in the bone marrow are similar in folate and vitamin B_{12} deficiency. All cell lines are affected, with changes the most marked in the erythroid series. Many large erythroid precursors contain nuclei with a finely granular chromatin pattern and prominent nucleoli. The cytoplasm usually appears too mature for the nucleus and has the eosinophilic staining characteristic of abundant hemoglobin. Cells of the myelocytic series, myelocytes and metamyelocytes particularly, are also enlarged and have immature appearing nuclei.

The measurement of formiminoglutamic acid (FIGLU), an intermediate in the conversion of histidine to glutamic acid, is less useful than previously thought in the diagnosis of folate deficiency. The FIGLU reacts with tetrahydrofolate in the last step of this pathway. In folate deficiency urinary FIGLU is elevated, particularly after a loading dose of histidine. However, its diagnostic applicability is limited, since abnormal values can also be seen in vitamin B_{12} and iron deficiency. The test is also poorly reproducible, especially during pregnancy.

Treatment

A therapeutic dose of folate, 0.5 to 1.0 mg. per day of pteroylglutamic acid (PGA) (1 to 20 times the daily requirement), is ample when the deficiency is primarily one of folic acid. Folic acid is now available in 1-mg. tablets; liquid preparations for infants will soon be available containing 0.2 mg. per ml. (1 mg. per ml. available at present is unnecessarily concentrated). As in iron deficiency, marrow morphology shows a return toward normal within one or two days. The timing of the reticulocytosis and the rate of rise in hemoglobin and hematocrit are also comparable to the response to treatment of iron deficiency.

Iron and folate deficiencies are commonly combined, and one or the other can be masked. The transferrin saturation and the blood smear may then reveal iron deficiency several weeks after initiation of treatment with folate alone.

When a *therapeutic trial* is being used to distinguish between folate and vitamin B_{12} deficiency, either 50 to 100 μg. of folate per day orally or parenterally or 1 to 5 μg. per day of vitamin B_{12} parenterally is adequate to produce a prompt reticulocyte response

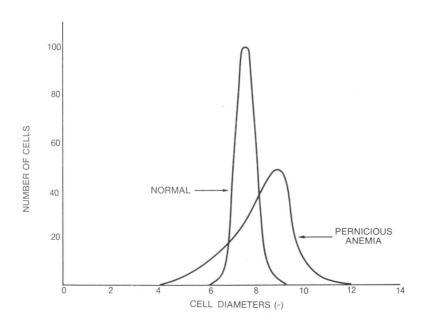

Figure 4–18. Idealized Price-Jones curves comparing a normal population of erythrocytes with those found in pernicious anemia. (From Lewis, A. E.: *Principles of Hematology.* New York, Appleton-Century-Crofts, 1970, p. 122.)

that is specific to each of the corresponding deficiencies.

A deficiency of folate beyond infancy often calls attention to a diet inadequate in many other aspects (94). A multiple vitamin and mineral supplement, including no more than 0.1 mg. folate per day, may be appropriate, particularly if vitamin B$_{12}$ lack can be excluded. A larger dose of folate can correct anemia due to vitamin B$_{12}$ deficiency but may aggravate neurologic manifestations. Nutritional counseling should include a warning against overheating milk and overcooking other foods.

Prevention

The prevalence of folate deficiency is a by-product of two important developments in pediatric care: (1) the extensive use of a folate-poor food, such as cow's milk, for infant feeding and its further reduction in folate content by heat treatment; and (2) an improved survival of small prematures, who have a high requirement for folate to support their unusually rapid extrauterine growth.

Several of the multivitamin preparations available in dropper form for premature and full-term infants contain vitamin B$_{12}$, but none now contain folate, for which there is a greater need. At present, folic acid must be supplied as a separate preparation. An appropriate maintenance dose to prevent folate deficiency in a premature is 0.05 to 0.1 mg. per day. This dose is adequate for prevention of the folate deficiency that commonly accompanies hemolytic anemias.

Folate loss after terminal sterilization of cow's milk formulas can be avoided by the use of commercially prepared, ready-to-feed infant formulas to which extra folate is added to compensate for losses due to heat treatment in processing. This type of formula can be poured into presterilized bottles and simply warmed as needed.

In many underdeveloped countries and among certain ethnic groups, prolonged cooking of dried beans, rice, and other starch staples converts them into poor sources of folate. Processing of these foods can eliminate the need for lengthy cooking and save scarce fuel as well. One such product being developed in Central America is an inexpensive "instant" bean meal that can be prepared rapidly and that should therefore retain a large percentage of its ample folate content.

MEGALOBLASTIC ANEMIA: VITAMIN B$_{12}$ DEFICIENCY (95–97)

Metabolism and Pathogenesis

Vitamin B$_{12}$ deficiency is a very rare cause of megaloblastic anemia in children. Nevertheless, it assumes importance because of the danger of irreversible neurologic damage unless it is diagnosed and treated early, and because most causes of the deficiency require continuing therapy throughout life. Most cases of vitamin B$_{12}$ deficiency involve a defect in absorption. Deficient dietary intake of the vitamin is very unusual.

STRUCTURE AND METABOLIC ROLE. Vitamin B$_{12}$ is one of a group of biologically active cobalamins or compounds which contain cobalt at the center of a tetrapyrrole ring structure similar to that of heme. Attached to the cobalt atom is a nucleotide group. The cobalamins differ according to the other chemical group attached to the cobalt atom, a cyanide group in the case of cyanocobalamin. Although animal protein is the source of vitamin B$_{12}$ for man, the vitamin is not synthesized by mammalian cells. It is unique among vitamins in that it enters the food chain entirely through bacterial synthesis, particularly in the intestines of ruminants. This process requires cobalt in the diet of the animal as an essential building block for the vitamin.

Many of the metabolic functions of vitamin B$_{12}$ are closely linked to those of folate. Indeed, the delayed synthesis of DNA associated with megaloblastic changes in blood and endothelial cells (98) is attributed to the effect of B$_{12}$ deficiency on tetrahydrofolate regeneration. Impairment in the tetrahydrofolate-dependent conversion of ribonucleotides to deoxyribonucleotides consequently limits DNA synthesis.

REQUIREMENTS AND DIETARY SOURCES. The normal human diet contains a severalfold excess of vitamin B$_{12}$ over the daily minimum of less than 1 μg. in the adult and 0.1 μg. in the infant that is necessary for normal erythropoiesis. Even among populations suffering from protein malnutrition, vitamin B_{12} deficiency is rare except among strict vegetarians (vegans) who avoid all animal products, including milk and eggs. Among such groups, megaloblastic anemia with neurologic changes has been observed even in breast-fed babies because of a subnormal concentration of vitamin B_{12} in the maternal milk.

The absorption of physiologic amounts of vitamin B_{12} is dependent upon the vitamin forming a complex with a specific mucoprotein (intrinsic factor) produced by the parietal cells of the stomach. The complex is taken up specifically by the distal ileum. Vitamin B_{12} freed from the complex is then released into the circulation. In the plasma, vitamin B_{12} is bound to a β-globulin transport protein (transcobalamin II). The vitamin is stored primarily in the liver. In the newborn liver these stores are large, averaging about 25 μg., and are rarely depleted before one year of age.

CAUSES OF VITAMIN B_{12} DEFICIENCY. With the exception of the rare dietary deficiency, most cases of vitamin B_{12} deficiency result from an absence or abnormality of intrinsic factor from the gastric mucosa, or from interference with absorption of the vitamin–intrinsic factor complex

(Table 4–7) (99). The term "pernicious anemia" is generally reserved for those cases in which there is a deficiency of intrinsic factor. Two types of pernicious anemia are distinguished in children (96). In both types, absorption of vitamin B_{12} becomes adequate if intrinsic factor is supplied.

The so-called *juvenile pernicious anemia* occurs in older children and is the same in most respects as pernicious anemia in the adult. Gastric atrophy and decreased secretion of acid and pepsin are commonly associated with demonstrable antibodies to intrinsic factor or to parietal cells. Concurrent endocrinopathies may also be present. Often there are associated manifestations of immune deficiency, such as selective IgA deficiency, chronic candidiasis, or abnormal cellular immunity as manifested by a lack of responsiveness of lymphocytes in vitro to phytohemagglutinin. It has been postulated that the immune deficiency may be the primary defect leading to parietal cell or endocrine and tissue damage or both. Although there is no clear inheritance pattern, endocrinopathies or immune deficiencies may be present in siblings.

In contrast, there is a group of patients designated as having *congenital pernicious anemia,* in whom pernicious anemia is

TABLE 4–7. VITAMIN B_{12} DEFICIENCY IN CHILDREN

	EARLIEST AGE AT ONSET	FAMILIAL INCIDENCE	ABNORMAL SCHILLING TEST
I. *Diet*			
A. Related to maternal deficiency	Less than 4 months		
B. Related to child's diet	Over 6 months		
II. *Inadequate Absorption*			
A. Lack of intrinsic factor			
1. Congenital	Over 6 months	X	X
2. Addisonian type (juvenile)	Over 10 years	*	X
B. Competition for vitamin B_{12} in intestinal lumen—fish tapeworm or bacteria in blind loops	Over 6 months		
C. Abnormality of absorptive site—ileal resection or regional ileitis	Over 6 months		X
D. Abnormality of transcobalamin II, the serum vitamin B_{12} transport protein	Less than 1 month	X	X
E. Unknown mechanism			
1. Syndrome of vitamin B_{12} malabsorption and proteinuria	Over 6 months	X	X
2. Associated with pancreatic insufficiency, celiac disease, and other forms of less specific malabsorption	Over 6 months	X	X

*Endocrinopathy in siblings.

usually evident before three years of age. Though secretion of normally active intrinsic factor is lacking, the gastric mucosa is normal with respect to morphology and secretory function. There are no demonstrable antibodies or associated endocrinopathies, and long-term follow-up does not show progression to the typical adult form of pernicious anemia. An autosomal recessive inheritance pattern is suggested by a high incidence of consanguinity and the occurrence in siblings.

Other causes of deficiency are not properly called pernicious anemia since there is no lack of intrinsic factor. These include removal of the vitamin from the contents of the intestinal lumen by parasites or bacteria. This is a well-documented cause of megaloblastic anemia in individuals with a heavy infestation with fish tapeworm (*Diphyllobothrium latum*). It is restricted to areas where raw or smoked fresh water fish form an important part of the diet, as in parts of Scandinavia. Bacterial consumption of vitamin B$_{12}$ in intestinal diverticuli or blind loops also can result in removal of the vitamin before it is absorbed.

Vitamin B$_{12}$ is unusual among nutritional constituents in having an absorptive site restricted to a small segment of the intestine, the distal half of the ileum. Surgical removal of this area of bowel for treatment of intussusception, regional enteritis, or congenital malformation results in a severe and lifelong deficiency. Chronic disease of this tissue, most commonly due to regional enteritis, can also produce a deficiency of vitamin B$_{12}$, but usually one that is mild and manifested primarily by a low serum concentration of vitamin B$_{12}$.

Vitamin B$_{12}$ absorption and transport are also decreased in a rare inherited deficiency or abnormality of transcobalamin II (100). Presumably the transport protein is necessary as an acceptor in order to assure normal transport of the vitamin across the ileal mucosa.

An additional cause of vitamin B$_{12}$ deficiency in children is an apparently specific absorptive defect for the vitamin, with normal small bowel morphology usually associated with proteinuria (101). It is postulated that these may be only two manifestations of a more widespread defect in membrane transport. Consanguinity is associated,

and an autosomal recessive pattern of inheritance is suspected.

Progression of vitamin B$_{12}$ deficiency is very slow since neonatal liver stores are normally ample. Exceptions are the development of megaloblastic anemia in the infant of a mother with pernicious anemia (102) and the inherited deficiency of transcobalamin II (100). If intrinsic factor is present, as in dietary vitamin B$_{12}$ deficiency, the onset of deficiency is even more delayed because of intestinal reabsorption of the vitamin lost in bile and pancreatic juice. Depression of serum vitamin B$_{12}$ and the appearance of hypersegmented neutrophils are the earliest clinical manifestations. Late findings of vitamin B$_{12}$ deficiency include megaloblastic anemia, leukopenia, thrombocytopenia, and jaundice and are similar to those of folate deficiency. However, the neurologic manifestations are generally quite distinct from those of folate lack. They include posterior and lateral column demyelinization in the spinal cord and associated paresthesias, sensory deficits, loss of deep tendon reflexes, slowing of mental processes, confusion, and memory defects. Neurologic changes may antecede anemia. The biochemical basis for the neuropathy is uncertain. Inappropriate administration of moderate or large doses of folate (well in excess of 0.1 mg. per day in an adult) to vitamin B$_{12}$–deficient individuals can aggravate neurologic disease (103).

Diagnosis

Diagnosis of vitamin B$_{12}$ deficiency can be suspected when serum B$_{12}$ is less than 100 pg. per ml. The serum folate is usually normal or elevated. As in folate deficiency, hypersegmentation of neutrophils is an early finding, whereas megaloblastic changes in the peripheral blood or bone marrow are characteristic of chronic or severe disease. If the dietary history indicates a normal vitamin B$_{12}$ intake, then absorption of ^{57}Co-labeled B$_{12}$ may be determined by the Schilling test. A standard dose (0.5 μg.) of the labeled vitamin is given orally after an overnight fast; two hours later a "flushing dose" of 1000 μg. of vitamin B$_{12}$ is given parenterally. This allows the excretion of labeled vitamin B$_{12}$ into the urine in readily detectible amounts. Less than 7 per cent of the administered label is recovered in the urine in 24 hours if there is a lack of intrinsic factor or a defective absorption of vitamin B_{12} for other reasons. If absorption is impaired, the Schilling test is repeated with oral intrinsic factor. Enhancement of urinary excretion of the label confirms the diagnosis of pernicious anemia or intrinsic factor deficiency. The availability of assays for intrinsic factor in gastric juice provides an additional diagnostic tool. Absence of acid in gastric secretions after histamine stimulation may be helpful in distinguishing between the two forms of pernicious anemia in children, although a gastric biopsy provides a more definitive answer. The excretion of methylmalonic acid is increased in vitamin B_{12} deficiency and is a useful means of detecting the deficiency state.

Megaloblastic anemias produced by deficiencies of folic acid or vitamin B_{12} must be distinguished from the rare disorder of pyrimidine biosynthesis, hereditary orotic aciduria. This defect may manifest itself with megaloblastic anemia, leukopenia, retarded growth and development, and the excessive urinary excretion of orotic acid. Eight cases have been reported to date and are the subject of a recent extensive review (104). In seven of eight patients, the activities of both orotate phosphoribosyltransferase and orotidine 5'-phosphate decarboxylase were markedly diminished in red cells (type I). Both enzyme deficiencies were also demonstrable in leukocytes, liver, and cultured fibroblasts. In the eighth patient, initial studies revealed only a deficiency of the decarboxylase enzyme (type II). The disturbance appears to be inherited as an autosomal recessive trait. The heterozygotes are detectable by enzyme assays but are hematologically normal and without symptoms.

Patients with this disorder are unresponsive to therapy with folic acid or vitamin B_{12} but may improve when fed yeast extracts containing uridylic and cytidylic acid.

Treatment

Most cases of vitamin B_{12} deficiency require treatment throughout life. Optimal doses for children are not as well-defined as those for adults. For a therapeutic trial as little as 0.1 to 0.5 μg. of vitamin B_{12} (cyanocobalamin or hydroxycobalamin) per day may be employed. If the diagnosis is firmly established, several daily doses of 25 to 100 μg. may be used to initiate therapy. Alternatively, in view of the ability of the body to store vitamin B_{12} for long periods, maintenance therapy can be started with the first of a series of monthly intramuscular injections. Doses ranging between 50 μg. and 1000 μg. have been successfully employed. The hematologic response to treatment is described under Folate Deficiency.

COPPER DEFICIENCY

Copper deficiency is a common cause of hypochromic anemia among farm animals in several parts of the world where there is copper-poor soil. In man, the deficiency has been recognized primarily under unusual or iatrogenic dietary circumstances, e.g., when copper is inadvertently omitted from a chronic, intravenous, alimentation regimen (105) or when powdered milk, a poor source of copper, is used to treat cases of severe combined nutritional deficiency states (106). Hypocupremia has also been reported in association with exudative enteropathy.

Metabolism and Pathogenesis

Copper balance, in contrast to iron balance, is regulated by excretion as well as by absorption (107, 108). About 30 per cent is absorbed from a 1-mg. dose of a copper salt, an amount that corresponds to what is present in the normal daily diet. Much of the absorbed copper is promptly excreted in the bile, with a lesser amount lost through the intestinal mucosa.

One hundred to 150 mg. of copper is present in the adult. The highest concentration is in the liver which, together with muscle and bone marrow, accounts for 50 to 75 per cent of the total. Plasma copper remains much more constant than plasma iron and exists in two forms. A small amount is loosely bound to albumin and is probably involved in transport, while a larger fraction is tightly bound to an α_2-globulin, designated as ceruloplasmin or ferroxidase.

As with iron, the fetus accumulates large stores of copper towards term, particularly in the liver, where concentrations are five to ten times greater at birth than in the adult. Normally these stores do not drop to adult levels until 5 to 15 years of age. Copper is an essential component of cytochrome oxidase, the terminal oxidase of the electron transport chain that converts oxygen to water. It is, therefore, essential for the oxidative production of ATP. The enzyme tyrosinase is also a copper-containing protein and is required for melanin synthesis. Thus, in animals, the activity of cytochrome oxidase in most tissues is markedly decreased, and loss of hair pigment is a readily apparent consequence of copper deficiency.

Copper deficiency mimics certain of the findings of iron deficiency, such as low serum iron and hypochromic anemia (109). The role of copper in iron transport now provides a reasonable explanation for the development of these manifestations of copper deficiency in spite of abundant iron stores. Ceruloplasmin, the blue-green copper-containing serum protein, is an enzyme that catalyzes the oxidation of ferrous iron (110, 111). This step is required for the conversion of ferrous storage iron from the liver and the intestinal mucosa to the ferric transport form (transferrin) in the plasma. Copper also plays a role in the intracellular transport of iron in erythroblasts (112). It is required to mobilize iron from ferritin storage sites in membrane-bound cytoplasmic vesicles to the mitochondria, where it is utilized for heme synthesis.

The normal copper intake is 2 to 5 mg. per day in an adult, and 0.04 to 0.15 mg. per kg. per day in the growing child. The low copper content of milk (0.1 to 0.15 mg. per L.) makes it a particularly copper-poor food. A high intake of milk to the exclusion of other foods provides a setting for marginal copper nutrition or deficiency during late infancy, particularly in premature infants with low copper stores. Chronic diarrhea also aggravates copper deficiency by interfering with its enterohepatic circulation.

Copper deficiency can also be the consequence of an inherited defect in copper absorption as in the condition, "Menkes's syndrome" or "kinky hair syndrome" (113). This potentially treatable disorder is characterized by a low serum copper, slow growth, kinky hair, cerebral degeneration, and an X-linked pattern of inheritance. Death before age three is usual. There is a striking similarity between the clinical features of this syndrome and severe nutritional copper deficiency in experimental animals.

Diagnosis and Treatment

Copper deficiency in man is often obscured by other dietary abnormalities, particularly iron deficiency. A low concentration of serum copper is the earliest manifestation. The normal ranges are 68 to 161 μg. per 100 ml. in the adult and 45 to 110 μg. per 100 ml. in the newborn. Anemia is not consistently found, but when present it is generally mild and hypochromic. Leukopenia with very marked neutropenia is particularly characteristic of copper deficiency and should suggest the diagnosis.

Treatment of the deficiency with 0.2 mg. per kg. per day (two or three times the estimated daily requirement) in the form of 0.5 per cent copper sulfate (about 2 mg. of copper per ml.) given orally results in prompt reticulocytosis and correction of the anemia and neutropenia. Menkes's syndrome will require intramuscular treatment; optimal regimens have not been established. Generally, the dietary circumstances which lead to the deficiency can be corrected when copper lack is recognized.

VITAMIN E DEFICIENCY

Vitamin E deficiency is implicated as a cause of hemolytic anemia, particularly in the premature infant and in individuals exposed to high oxygen concentrations under hyperbaric conditions. The extent to which vitamin E deficiency is of broader clinical importance remains controversial (114, 115).

Metabolism and Pathogenesis

The vitamin E compounds are antioxidants, one of whose metabolic roles is to protect the lipids in biological membranes against oxidative damage. The most biologically active of this group is *α-tocopherol*, which is also the most abundant of these compounds in foods.

As in the case of other fat-soluble vitamins, absorption from the intestinal tract requires fat in the diet and the presence of bile. The latter is the basis for vitamin E deficiency in biliary atresia and for the proposal of the red cell hemolysis test as an aid to its diagnosis (116).

The requirement for vitamin E depends on the degree of saturation of fats in the diet. Diets particularly high in unsaturated fats produce a corresponding change in the composition of the fatty acids in cellular and intracellular membranes. The membranes are then more susceptible to damage resulting from lipid peroxidation, and the requirement for the antioxidant effect of vitamin E is increased. Thus 5 mg. per day of α-tocopherol is the recommended intake for an adult if the diet contains little unsaturated fatty acid, but 30 mg. per day is suggested if the diet is rich in unsaturated fats. During infancy, 5 mg. per day is currently recommended. The content of vitamin E in naturally occurring fats is often appropriately highest in those fats which are most unsaturated.

Manifestations of vitamin E deficiency are more conclusively demonstrated in the experimental animal than in man. Oxidative damage to membranes is most clearly manifest as hemolytic anemia, with a modest decrease in red cell survival (117). The anemia also may have a component of depressed hemoglobin synthesis. The basis for this may be the reported vitamin E dependence of δ-aminolevulinic acid synthetase, a rate-limiting enzyme of the heme synthetic pathway. Furthermore, treatment of the deficiency with vitamin E results in an increased reticulocyte count within a week (118), suggesting recovery from a maturation arrest. However, interpretation of this response is complicated by the fact that vitamin E administration results in a prolonged survival of the reticular structure within the red cell, presumably as a result of membrane stabilization (119). Thus an increased reticulocyte count might represent a prolonged persistence of reticulum or increased red blood cell production or both.

In the experimental animal, sterility and muscular dystrophy are among many systemic effects of the deficiency. The former appears to be related to abnormal production of the centriole, a microtubular cell structure required for mitosis. Whether these manifestations of the deficiency are also attributable to membrane peroxidation is still uncertain.

Diagnosis

Diagnostic criteria for vitamin E deficiency in man are not well established (118–124). Hematologic manifestations include a normochromic, normocytic anemia and an elevation of the reticulocyte count, though usually not above 10 per cent. Thrombocytosis may also be present (124). Red cell morphology is characterized by the presence of acanthocytes. These are defined as cells with up to eight irregular, pointed, thorny projections from an irregular central mass. Acanthocytes are also a relatively common and reversible finding in infants with an adequate supply of vitamin E and are therefore of limited help in establishing a diagnosis during this period of borderline vitamin E nutrition. Acanthocytes or "spur" cells are to be distinguished from echinocytes or "burr" cells. The latter are covered by about 30 regularly spaced, short, rounded spicules and are most commonly artifacts of preparing a dried blood smear.

One of the physical manifestations of the deficiency reported in infants is edema of the legs, labia, and eyelids (124). A serum concentration of α-tocopherol below 0.5 mg. per 100 ml. has arbitrarily been considered as evidence of a vitamin E lack. However, the lipid composition of cellular membranes is an equally important factor in individual resistance to oxidative damage. The red cell *peroxide hemolysis test* provides a crude estimate of this by measuring the resistance of the red cell membrane to incubation in hydrogen peroxide. The results of these two assays are often closely correlated. However, the peroxide hemolysis test may also be abnormal in conditions other than vitamin E lack, such as spherocytosis, thalassemia, sickle cell anemia, and other hemolytic states. Such red cell disorders must therefore be excluded on the basis of clinical findings, blood smear, or additional laboratory studies.

The importance of vitamin E deficiency as a cause of anemia in man is controversial largely because of the difficulty in establishing diagnostic criteria and therapeutic response. Experimental deficiency in man has produced few of the abnormalities observed in animals. Once α-tocopherol stores are established, they are extremely hard to deplete. It may be a year before a vitamin E-deficient regimen in an adult produces a fall in the serum α-tocopherol and an abnormal red cell peroxide hemolysis test. On the other hand, an increased exposure of membranes to oxidative damage can rapidly produce a relative deficiency of vitamin E. Thus hemolysis of red cells under conditions of hyperbaric oxygen in subjects given a normal diet can be prevented by additional vitamin E.

Treatment and Prevention

Deficiency of vitamin E is most likely to occur in the infant, particularly in the premature infant, in whom body stores of α-tocopherol at birth are disproportionately low: 3 mg. in a 1000-g. premature infant, compared with 20 mg. in a 3500-g. term infant. The premature infant, therefore, embarks upon a period of rapid growth with a small store of α-tocopherol and is dependent on a single source of nourishment. Thus it is important to scrutinize the relationship of vitamin E to fatty acid composition in prepared infant formulas. Breast milk, the ideal model for infant formulas, contains a low proportion of polyunsaturated fats, including only 8 per cent linoleate. In contrast, in many artificial formulas in which milk fat is replaced by vegetable oil, linoleate accounts for over 50 per cent of the fatty acids. The dietary proportions of fatty acid are reflected in corresponding changes in the fatty acid composition of cell membranes and adipose tissue over the course of a few weeks to several months. It is likely that an enrichment of the infant's tissues with polyunsaturated fats increases the requirement for vitamin E beyond that provided in the artificial formula. The vitamin E content of breast milk and unsupplemented prepared formulas may be quite similar, 1 to 2 mg. of α-tocoph-

erol per 100 ml. However, after one month of formula feedings rich in unsaturated fatty acids, serum α-tocopherol concentrations are significantly lower than in the breast-fed infant. There is a corresponding increase in sensitivity of erythrocytes to peroxide hemolysis, even though other evidence of vitamin E deficiency is lacking. These considerations have led to more careful monitoring of vitamin E content in proprietary formulas. Many products have been routinely supplemented with vitamin E within the last few years. This seems to be a prudent course of action, since the lipid composition of most formulas otherwise makes them less adequate in respect to vitamin E content than breast milk.

The daily requirement for α-tocopherol during the first year of life has been tentatively set at about 0.4 mg. per day if butterfat is the major source of dietary lipid, and 1.5 mg. per day if polyunsaturated fats predominate, as in most artificial formulas.

Oxygen therapy is commonly used in infants with respiratory distress. Whether pulmonary damage associated with prolonged use of high oxygen concentrations can be modified by vitamin E has not been determined. Nevertheless, since lung "stiffening" may represent oxidative damage to pulmonary tissues, the use of a formula or vitamin supplement that contains an adequate and possibly protective quantity of vitamin E (5 mg. per day) seems to be an easy form of insurance.

The role that vitamin E deficiency might play in aggravating the anemia of prematurity is hard to assess. Anemia is particularly difficult to evaluate at one to two months of age when the deficiency is also likely to be most pronounced. During this period, the postnatal low point in hemoglobin concentration and hematocrit is reached. Then increased erythrocyte production commences, and there is a corresponding rise in the reticulocyte count that varies in its magnitude and timing. Against the background of these rapid changes in normal hematopoiesis, the therapeutic effect of vitamin E is not easy to evaluate. If vitamin E deficiency is suspected, an oral therapeutic dose of 10 to 20 mg. of α-tocopherol acetate or the same number of I.U. of vitamin E, in a water emulsion, is generous in relation to the recommended daily allowance. However, in the individual premature infant the absorption of this form of vitamin E is unreliable until after three months of age (125). Other oral preparations as well as intramuscular regimens are being tested in order to circumvent this finite period of malabsorption of α-tocopherol acetate, the form of vitamin E that is currently being used in vitamin preparations and infant formulas. A single intramuscular dose should not exceed 50 I.U., and that dose should not be repeated more than twice a week. There is new evidence in animals that vitamin E excess can interfere with wound healing, presumably through an inappropriate stabilization of the lysosomal membrane (125a). It therefore seems prudent not to administer more than ten times the recommended daily allowance of 5 I.U. per day. Correction of the peroxide hemolysis test merely demonstrates that the vitamin has been assimilated. Correction of anemia, thrombocytosis, and edema constitutes more convincing evidence of a therapeutic response.

PROTEIN
DEFICIENCY (126–132)

Definition

Protein deficiency is the most common form of malnutrition in the world. It is almost invariably accompanied by some degree of caloric insufficiency, not only because of cultural and economic factors but also because loss of appetite is one of the early consequences of a lack of protein. Protein-calorie malnutrition is, therefore, a convenient term, even though the characteristics of the disorder vary markedly according to which of the two deficiencies, protein or caloric, predominates. Two types of such malnutrition are distinguished: (1) *kwashiorkor,* which refers to a severe lack of protein in a diet with a relatively unrestricted supply of calories, largely derived from carbohydrates; and (2) *marasmus,* which refers to varying degrees of starvation from a more uniform lack of all major dietary components. Most cases are intermediate. Many classifications have been proposed, but none has gained widespread acceptance. Many investigators feel that

discord over terminology is distracting attention from more important matters. Edema is the sine qua non for the diagnosis of kwashiorkor. Hypoalbuminemia is also given some weight, whereas hepatomegaly and skin and hair changes are given different emphases in different parts of the world. Marasmus is defined by some as a weight less than 50 per cent of normal for age without evidence of edema or depigmentation.

There are marked regional and seasonal differences, particularly in the hematologic manifestations of protein-calorie malnutrition, which can often be attributed to associated deficiencies of vitamins and minerals. In tropical regions where hookworm infestation is common, iron deficiency due to blood loss is superimposed on the protein-calorie deficiency. Consequently, hypochromic, microcytic anemia is common. In other areas, megaloblastic anemia commonly indicates an associated folate deficiency. Less frequent is the megaloblastic anemia of the strict vegetarians (vegans) who avoid all animal protein and thus lack a dietary source of vitamin B_{12}. Seasonal changes may correspond with altered availability of foods in relation to harvest time and rainy season. This is especially evident where a market economy is underdeveloped or where food preservation is ineffective. In parts of Gambia, for example, food supplies are inadequate during the rainy season due to difficulties in transport. As a result, there are dramatic seasonal variations in weight gain among children. After six months of age (when breast-feeding diminishes) there is often a weight loss or no gain during the rainy season, followed by a greater than normal "catch-up" growth during the dry months.

Metabolism and Pathogenesis

There is no known tissue store of protein as there is for carbohydrate, fat, and many vitamins and minerals. Thus lack of dietary protein requires immediate metabolic adaptations to provide the amino acid raw materials for the large number of protein-synthetic processes that continue unabated. The manner in which certain of these adaptive changes take place must be examined at several levels of organization: (1) in the body as a whole; (2) in individual organs;

(3) in specific types of cells, including the red blood cell; (4) in subcellular fractions; and (5) in individual proteins.

BODY GROWTH. Growth retardation is an early consequence of protein-calorie malnutrition, though it may become obvious only with time. In the experimental animal during periods of rapid growth it is detectable within a day. In man a similarly early depression of the rate of body growth is noted only in the rapidly growing newborn. With normal slowing of growth after one year of age, it may be difficult to document growth retardation, even with careful serial measurements over a period of several months. Since children with malnutrition generally come from a population that receives little medical attention, changes in the rate of body growth are rarely evident. However, the cumulative effect of malnutrition on stature becomes statistically apparent in studies of large groups, particularly in underdeveloped countries. An indication that small stature is not primarily genetic comes from the repeated demonstration of its higher incidence among the poor, who are more subject to protein-calorie lack, than among an economically favored, well-fed group of the same ethnic background.

Growth retardation due to malnutrition is most apparent in children between one and five years of age when carbohydrate-rich diets generally replace breast milk. The abnormality in weight is almost invariably greater than the deficit in height, even when edema is present. For this reason and because serial measurements are rarely available, the relationship of weight to height is used widely to estimate the severity of malnutrition.

It is essential to bear in mind that retardation of growth is not necessarily nutritional, but that other environmental factors may be responsible or contributory. Thus parental neglect may be associated with slow growth, apparently more on an emotional than on a nutritional basis. Intrauterine infection is also a cause of long-term depression of growth and is most prevalent among the same populations that suffer from malnutrition.

GROWTH OF ORGANS AND TISSUES. Within the body as a whole, protein-calorie malnutrition results in a gradual redistribution of protein among organs and tissues.

In the rat, the liver loses 30 per cent of its protein during the first three days of a protein-free diet. After this, the liver remains relatively stable in weight, while skeletal muscle, the major protein depot of the body, gradually loses weight in supplying amino acids to meet systemic energy needs and the large demands imposed by essential protein-synthetic processes. Muscular activity decreases concurrently. Other tissues whose continued function is more essential to survival, such as heart or diaphragmatic muscle and red cell mass, tend to retain their normal proportionality to total body weight or lean body weight.

In the experimental animal as well as in man, the brain preserves its normal size longer than other tissues. Thus, in a marasmic patient, the brain accounts for a much larger than normal percentage of the body weight. An important factor in the brain's resistance to undernutrition may be the fact that its cells usually approach the adult number and size during the relatively protected period of transplacental nutrition and nursing. Tissues retain a surprisingly good capacity to respond to an increased work load or to the need for repairing tissue damage in spite of malnutrition. Muscles in the protein-deficient animal undergo hypertrophy with the imposition of obligatory work, evidently by commanding a high priority for scarce amino acids needed for protein synthesis. Similarly, after blood loss and after resection of one kidney or of a large segment of the liver, there is compensatory proliferation of the remaining tissue, though it is somewhat slower or less complete or both than in animals eating a normal diet.

CELL GROWTH AND PROLIFERATION. During early development, cell growth and proliferation proceed throughout the body. Both processes are depressed in response to protein lack within as short a time as one day. A deficit in cell number and in overall growth may be permanent, even with the reinstitution of a normal diet (133). A different situation prevails with advancing age, as cell proliferation gradually becomes restricted to a few tissues, such as blood cells, epithelial tissues, and the intestinal lining. The bulk of tissues, as exemplified by liver and skeletal muscle, contain very few proliferating cells except in response to injury. Malnutrition in the adult tends to decrease the size of cells in nonproliferating tissues and the rate of proliferation in cells that normally continue to divide. The decrease in body weight, cell size, and rate of cell proliferation in the adult can all be corrected with institution of an adequate diet. Malnutrition in children lies in an intermediate category; hence, there is concern about the permanence of systemic sequelae, particularly in respect to nonreplaceable tissues in the younger age groups.

RED CELL PRODUCTION AND THE SYNTHESIS OF HEMOGLOBIN. These two factors retain a relatively high priority during the progression of protein deficiency (134). Patients with relatively uncomplicated protein-calorie malnutrition have only a moderate degree of anemia, with hemoglobin concentrations from 8 to 12 g. per 100 ml. (135, 136). The plasma volume per kilogram body weight is disproportionately increased; consequently the actual deficit in hemoglobin is slight. Nevertheless, when expressed on the basis of weight, height, or surface area, the total circulating hemoglobin, total red cell mass, and total blood volume are all reduced to some extent in the malnourished child (136). If, on the other hand, total circulating hemoglobin or red cell mass is expressed on the basis of lean body tissue (estimated on the basis of creatinine excretion), there is little or no change. A similar proportional relationship between the above two parameters and basal oxygen consumption is retained. The production of hemoglobin and red cells therefore seems appropriate to the reduced oxygen needs of the body, which has lost a large fraction of its tissue.

The morphology of red blood cells is generally normochromic and normocytic, often with some degree of aniso- and poikilocytosis. Bone marrow morphology is· characterized by a decreased erythroid-to-myeloid ratio. In severe malnutrition, the volume of active red marrow is decreased centripetally, being replaced peripherally by fat. Red blood cell survival is normal.

Erythropoietin levels and reticulocyte counts are variable. It has been postulated that this is a function of the duration of protein deficiency. Whereas lean body mass decreases rapidly in response to deficiency, the red cell mass or total hemoglobin decreases slowly. Even if the rate of erythropoiesis is reduced promptly, anemia can only develop gradually because hemoglobin is synthesized only in young, differentiating red cells. The mature cells survive normally and retain their original complement of hemoglobin for their entire life span. Thus, during early deficiency, the concentration of hemoglobin can be inappropriately high for lean body mass; as a result, erythropoietin and the reticulocyte count may be low. During later stages of deficiency the effect of decreased erythropoiesis finally results in a decreased hemoglobin concentration.

REPLACEMENT OF SUBCELLULAR ORGANELLES. Most cells in the body other than red blood cells synthesize and degrade their subcellular organelles and most other protein constituents throughout their life span. This process of protein turnover or replacement remains normal or may actually be accelerated in protein-calorie deficiency, even though growth and proliferation of the cells is severely curtailed. One infers that continued renewal of such structures as mitochondria, ribosomes, and endoplasmic reticulum is a prerequisite for maintenance of cell function and for the production of cellular energy. These structures tend to retain their normal proportions to tissue mass. The capacity of the cell for oxidative phosphorylation, RNA synthesis, and synthesis of cellular structures also tends to remain normal.

The continued synthesis of protein components of cell organelles in almost all tissues, even in the central nervous system, indicates that there must be a generous supply of substrates from other than dietary sources to meet this demand. This supply is maintained through a markedly increased reutilization of amino acids that are released by protein degradation in tissues such as liver and skeletal muscle. Thus, in the rat, after one to two days of fasting, as much as 90 per cent of the free amino acid pool available for synthesis of protein in the liver is derived from protein degradation instead of the normal 50 per cent.

Amino acid metabolism is modified in a manner that promotes this conservation of substrate. Depressed activity of degradative enzymes, such as the urea cycle enzymes and xanthine oxidase, manifests itself as a decreased loss of amino acid from the body through degradation to urea.

The differences among organs in their responses to malnutrition are reflected in correspondingly distinctive metabolic changes. Thus the activity of the degradative enzyme amino acid oxidase is increased in muscle when there is a decrease in the liver. This contributes to a continuing loss of muscle protein at a time when the liver weight has stabilized. It also helps to provide a large amount of substrate for hepatic protein synthesis, both for endogenous purposes and for export to the plasma.

PROTEIN SYNTHESIS. Even though many of the metabolic adaptations to protein deficiency favor the maintenance of a constant internal milieu, the synthesis of individual protein, such as albumin and transferrin, is decreased disproportionately to body weight. While these changes are not specific, they are among the earliest clinically detectable biochemical abnormalities and are thus diagnostically useful.

Diagnosis

CLINICAL MANIFESTATIONS. Retardation of growth is estimated by comparing the height and weight of the individual to standards obtained in a normally nourished population, preferably of the same ethnic background. Since such standards are unavailable in many parts of the world, the growth curves developed by the Harvard School of Public Health from white children of primarily Northern European origin are generally used. In those areas where both types of standards are available for comparison, the two correspond very closely.

Severity of protein-calorie malnutrition is often graded according to the deficit in body weight. Thus first-, second-, and third-degree protein-calorie malnutrition are classified as corresponding to body weights of 90-75, 75-60, and less than 60 per cent of the Boston fiftieth percentile, respectively. Another approach is the expression of weight, height, and head circumference as "developmental age," the age at which an average normal child would have the same measurements. The developmental age divided by the chronological age then yields a "developmental quotient" indicative of the degree of retardation in respect to various parameters of growth.

The creatinine height index (137) is another means of quantitating growth retardation. This is designed to overcome misinterpretation of body weight due to edema. Creatinine excretion over a period of one to three days is used to estimate lean body mass; the index is the ratio of this value to that of normal children of the same height. The usefulness of the index as a physiologically relevant parameter is suggested by its tendency to remain essentially proportional to basal oxygen consumption and to total hemoglobin or red cell mass.

Among the most striking *physical findings* of protein-calorie malnutrition are abnormalities of epithelial tissues. Hair is discolored, often developing red hypopigmented bands when it is normally black. The distance of these bands from the hair root can pinpoint the timing of greatest nutritional inadequacy. The diameter of hairs may be less than half of normal, and they are easily pulled out and broken. Tensile strength and hair diameter have been proposed as diagnostic measures suitable for field studies. The skin may also be hypopigmented, shiny, and atrophic. Angular stomatitis and cheilosis are common. The abdomen is often protuberant, with an enlarged liver.

Signs of infection, diarrhea, dehydration, or all three are also often present. Although the incidence of these conditions may be not much greater than that in a well-fed, similarly exposed population, they are associated with a markedly prolonged period of negative nitrogen balance, much greater morbidity, and a higher risk of mortality that is particularly striking with measles or shigellosis.

LABORATORY DIAGNOSIS. Because protein-calorie malnutrition is a disease primarily of poor people and poor nations, laboratory studies are most useful if they are low in cost and easy to perform in large volume. Ideally, the samples should be easy to obtain and transport to a central laboratory, even from remote areas. In addition, the assay should be sensitive enough to be helpful in milder forms of malnutrition, yet not so sensitive that it responds to variations in the most recent meal or in the diet of the preceding few days.

Blood is most commonly used for diagnostic purposes. Serum *albumin* and *transferrin* are among the most useful laboratory studies. Concentrations of each decrease to less than half of the normal range (albumin, 3.5 to 4.5 g. per 100 ml., and transferrin, 200 to 350 mg. per 100 ml.) when the weight-to-height index declines below 80 per cent of normal. These changes, though not specific, occur earlier than those in hemoglobin and are of greater magnitude than can be attributed to the increase in plasma volume that is usually present. The decreased concentration of transferrin often results in a relatively high iron saturation in spite of a low serum iron and may, therefore, help to mask iron deficiency. Serum globulins are less depressed than albumin and transferrin.

Hemoglobin and *hematocrit* are only moderately depressed by protein-calorie deficiency per se, and a large part of this depression is attributable to an increased plasma volume. However, their measurement is very useful because they indicate a commonly concurrent deficiency of iron or folate or both if the anemia is marked.

The *ratio of essential to nonessential amino acids* in the serum is another diagnostic tool (138, 139). This ratio increases promptly in response to protein-calorie malnutrition, largely because of a fall in concentration of the branched-chain amino acids (valine, leucine, and isoleucine) and an increase in the concentration of serine. A paper chromatographic method to detect a change in the ratio has been proposed for use in screening for protein deficiency. The disadvantages are its relative complexity, its apparent failure to include those patients who suffer primarily from calorie deprivation, and its fluctuation with the diet immediately preceding the test.

Within the red blood cell, most amino acids are reported to be higher than normal in concentration, whereas the converse is true of the plasma. This seems to indicate an alteration in membrane transport favoring delivery of amino acid to the cell.

There are no red cell enzyme changes that are specific for protein-calorie deficiency. In the white cell there is a depression of enzyme activity in the pentose shunt, particularly of glucose-6-phosphate dehydrogenase and 6-phosphogluconate dehydrogenase. This may be of potential diagnostic value if the assays can be adapted to routine use.

Other serum abnormalities include decreased activities of amylase and lipase, reflecting a marked decrease in the production of pancreatic enzymes. In severe deficiency, this manifestation of pancreatic damage may be permanently affected. Depression of blood urea may also prove a useful early indicator of protein malnutrition, as suggested by animal studies.

Urinary manifestations include a marked decrease in nitrogen excretion—a reflection of low nitrogen intake as well as more effective conservation. The decrease is observed within 2 to 3 days of a protein-deficient diet in the infant and in about one week in the adult.

Treatment and Prevention

Most children with severe protein malnutrition go untreated for lack of access to adequate medical care. Even in well-staffed and well-equipped wards, the mortality rate is rarely below 10 to 20 per cent. The high mortality is undoubtedly related to the decreased adaptability of the body to normal and abnormal challenges from the environment. Since the progression of severe protein-calorie malnutrition is gradual, patients usually come to medical attention through an intercurrent infection or with severe diarrhea accompanied by fluid and electrolyte imbalance. Such secondary problems are associated with a high mortality rate. For this reason, appropriate fluid and antibiotic therapy deserves a higher immediate priority than realimentation. Signs which indicate a particularly bad prognosis include (a) body weight below 60 per cent of normal for height; (b) an age under six months at time of presentation; (c) intercurrent infection, especially measles, which is often fatal; (d) severe hypokalemia; and (e) marked liver enlargement.

Fluid and electrolyte therapy usually must include potassium as well as magnesium. Potassium deficiency is very common, and there is mounting evidence that body magnesium is also frequently diminished. Several successfully used multi-electrolyte regimens are half-isotonic and include sodium, potassium, and magnesium as well as glucose. Overhydration must be carefully avoided because heart failure is a common occurrence during early rehabilitation.

Oral feeding of *calories and proteins* should be initiated cautiously and increased very gradually during the first four days to one week. Initially, 1 g. protein per kg. and 80 to 100 calories per kg. per day are sufficient. This can be increased slowly to 4 g. protein per kg. and 150 to 180 calories per kg. per day. Milk must be used with caution or avoided among populations where lactose intolerance is common as, for example, in West Africa. Lactose-rich, milk-based feedings may aggravate diarrhea in affected individuals.

Animal protein (skim milk, eggs, and meat) can be used for brief periods, but economic and social factors usually dictate a return to a cereal source of protein when the child is at home. Cereal proteins generally lack sufficient lysine and, in some cases, also methionine or tryptophan or both to support optimal growth. The deficiencies in cereal proteins can be corrected by (a) the combination of two or more cereals of complementary amino acid composition to improve protein quality (this method is inexpensive but fails to achieve the growth-promoting quality of animal protein); (b) supplementation with inexpensive animal protein, such as casein or fish meal; and (c) the addition of deficient essential amino acids to cereal. The latter (c) has the greatest promise in the prevention of protein malnutrition, since the cost of synthetic amino acids is declining rapidly while that of fish and milk is rising. A product incorporating all of these features has been developed by the Institute of Nutrition of Central America and Panama (INCAP) and is marketed as "Incaparina."

Vitamin and mineral supplements are essential to the treatment of protein-calorie malnutrition. If none are included in the treatment regimen, deficiency of iron or folate or both is likely to develop within two weeks, and a lag in the production of hemoglobin is evident shortly thereafter. These deficiencies may not be apparent initially, since high serum iron or folate concentrations may result when iron- or folate-dependent synthesizing processes are compromised by a more severe lack of protein. The vitamin-mineral supplement should be adjusted according to what is known of local patterns of deficiency and should provide two to five times the estimated normal requirement for those vitamins and minerals suspected of being deficient. In the absence of precise nutritional data, it is wise to supply a broad vitamin-mineral supplement, since many trace nutrients are required in increased quantity to support the rapid tissue growth that is anticipated during recovery.

The period of recovery from severe protein-calorie malnutrition is a very prolonged one, sometimes requiring months of hospitalization. "Catch-up" growth is often striking and may result in an approach toward normal weight and height within a year. The increase in red cell mass is independent of the level of protein intake, between 2 and 5 g. per kg. However, lean body mass increases at a rate that remains proportional to protein intake within this range, a further indication of the "high priority" for hemoglobin synthesis.

Completeness of recovery in terms of linear growth and mental function is hard to assess. The likelihood of permanent residua undoubtedly depends on the severity and duration of the deficiency as well as on the age at which it occurred. The younger the patient, the greater the risk of long-term sequelae. Since patients return to the same environment that was responsible for their deficiency, the chances are great for suboptimal recovery or a relapse.

LEAD POISONING (140–146)

Although lead serves no known function in the body, increased ingestion and inhalation of lead have become unavoidable in our industrialized society and can cause a mild hypochromic, microcytic anemia as a consequence of the inhibition of many of the enzymes of heme synthesis.

Metabolism and Pathogenesis

Exposure to lead is extremely variable, but the highest incidence of toxicity is among urban slum dwellers, particularly in preschool children, from the ingestion of paint chips in poorly maintained housing. Prior to 1940, lead was a common ingredient in interior paints and is still used in some paints designated for outdoor use. Severe cases of lead poisoning are restricted almost entirely to children living in old tenements, whereas neighbors residing in new housing developments are spared. There is an increased incidence of lead poisoning in the summer, which has been attributed to a greater opportunity to ingest lead-containing outdoor paint. A less common cause of lead poisoning is the use of lead-glazed pottery or pewter from which lead can be leached, particularly by acidic foods or beverages.

Net absorption of ingested lead is about 10 per cent, whereas about 50 per cent of inspired lead is retained. The average urban child between two and three years of age, the period of peak incidence of lead intoxication, is estimated to ingest between 100 and 200 μg. of lead daily and to inhale 6 to 18 μg. Lead from the combustion of leaded gasolines (containing about 1 g. per gallon) is a source of exposure, particularly in enclosed places like tunnels and car garages, but also near freeways and on city streets with heavy traffic.

Much of the lead absorbed from the intestinal tract is removed by the liver and appears in the bile. What remains in the systemic circulation is carried primarily by the red blood cells. Tissue deposition of lead is evident by x-ray as transverse lines of increased opacity in the epiphyseal portions of growing bones. The highest concentration of lead is found in hair. Both the timing and duration of lead exposure can be surmised from the distance from the hair root of high lead concentration in the hair shaft. Because hair is easily sampled, this may prove to be a particularly informative screening procedure.

ASSOCIATION BETWEEN IRON DEFICIENCY AND LEAD POISONING. There seems to be a metabolic link between these two conditions that may explain their common association. Recent animal experiments show that either iron or calcium deficiency results in increased assimilation and tissue retention of ingested lead (147). This suggests the possibility that iron deficiency may predispose to lead intoxication in man. Another explanation proposed is that pica, a craving for unnatural articles of food, is a manifestation of malnutrition in general and of iron deficiency in particular. Other evidence indicates that pica is more closely related to social factors, i.e., lack of maternal supervision and an increased opportunity for environmental exposure.

Glucose-6-phosphate dehydrogenase deficiency in blacks is another condition that seems to predispose to high concentrations of blood lead. Lead concentrations are higher in the red cell and lower in the serum than in unaffected individuals with similar exposure. The mechanism for this response is unknown.

HEMATOLOGIC MANIFESTATIONS. Effects of lead intoxication on hemoglobin and red cell kinetics resemble those of iron, folate, and vitamin B_{12} deficiencies. There is a moderately decreased survival of circulating erythrocytes. Total production of hemoglobin in the marrow is increased, but it conforms to the pattern of ineffective erythropoiesis in that there is also increased intramedullary degradation of heme. Anemia is not always present. It may develop as a result of an insufficient number of red blood cells released into the circulation to compensate for the decreased survival. Red cells are moderately hypochromic, presumably as a result of subnormal heme as well as globin synthesis. Additional morphologic evidence of a relative block in utilization of iron for hemoglobin synthesis is provided by electron microscopy which shows ferritin accumulation in the mitochondria, the site of the reaction of iron with protoporphyrin that produces heme. A moderate reticulocytosis is often present. Basophilic stippling is present in about half the cases and is revealed by electron microscopy to represent abnormal aggregates of ribosomes.

SYSTEMIC MANIFESTATIONS. Lead can affect the concentration of heme proteins other than hemoglobin. Cytochrome *c*, in particular, is decreased in kidney mitochondria of lead-treated rats, an abnormality that may be responsible for the impaired oxidation and phosphorylation also observed in this tissue.

Children with lead intoxication almost invariably have *central nervous system manifestations;* abdominal complaints are also common. Indeed, many children ultimately recognized as having lead encephalopathy were first mistakenly treated for gastroenteritis. Early symptoms in children are usually nonspecific and include irritability, anorexia, and vomiting. Later manifestations, such as lassitude, headaches, strabismus, coma, and convulsions, are more likely to suggest the correct diagnosis. Unfortunately, these severely affected cases have a mortality rate as high as 40 per cent and a high incidence of long-term sequelae, such as mental retardation, behavioral abnormalities, and convulsions. For this reason, large-scale, periodic screening of preschool children in high-risk areas seems the best approach to prevention of severe disease.

The clinical and laboratory similarities between lead poisoning and the far rarer acute intermittent porphyria are intriguing. Unfortunately, there is little understanding in either disease of the basis for neurologic manifestations or abdominal symptomatology.

Diagnosis and Screening

The *blood lead determination* (148) is the most accepted single indicator of lead intoxication. Although it does not always correlate with clinical manifestations of lead intoxication, it remains the standard against which other methods are evaluated. "Normal" concentrations of lead in the blood range from 15 to 40 mg. per 100 ml., according to environmental circumstances. Blood levels in urban children average twice as high as those in rural children. A concentration above 40 mg. per 100 ml. is considered suspect, and concentrations above 80 mg. are usually associated with clinical findings. Micromethods for the determination of blood lead are under development and should facilitate screening in the future.

The effects of lead poisoning on *heme synthesis* (149) are best understood and most useful diagnostically. The accumulation of several substrates along the heme synthetic pathway suggests that lead incompletely blocks many of the enzymatic steps rather than only one or two. A decrease in the activity of *aminolevulinic acid (ALA) dehydrase* (150) is an early finding in lead intoxication. The assay can be performed on microsamples of blood, and pilot studies show it to be a useful screening procedure. Its specificity still remains to be substantiated. Lead poisoning also causes an accumulation of ALA, the substrate for ALA dehydrase, in the serum and urine. However, blood lead levels or clinical toxicity are more closely correlated with ALA dehydrase activity than with ALA concentrations.

Other promising diagnostic tests make use of the increased *protoporphyrin* in red cells (55). Protoporphyrin produces an intense fluorescence of red cells that is evident by fluorescence microscopy of a blood smear. Protoporphyrin can be roughly quantitated from extracts of red cells that are visually graded according to the intensity of fluorescence. The assay is easy to perform, inexpensive, and lends itself readily to mass screening. The previously cumbersome quantitative assay has also been improved and partially automated. Marked elevations of erythrocyte protoporphyrin are characteristic of lead poisoning, the levels being well correlated with concentrations of blood lead. Lesser elevations of erythrocyte protoporphyrin can be confusing, since they may be associated either with lead poisoning or with iron deficiency. Thus other studies, such as transferrin saturation and blood lead levels, are needed to distinguish the two conditions.

Another substrate in the heme synthetic pathway that has been tested for diagnostic purposes is type III coproporphyrin, which accumulates in the urine. However, it may be normal, even in the presence of lead poisoning. Other abnormalities in the heme synthetic pathway include increased uroporphyrin in the bone marrow and deficient ALA synthetase, but these are not of clinical usefulness at present.

Treatment and Prevention

Lead is gradually cleared from the body, even without medication. Therefore, the most important aspect of treatment is the cessation of exposure to lead. In asymptomatic cases with blood levels below 80 mg. per 100 ml., this is generally adequate. However, such cases should be followed periodically, since continued exposure to lead is common.

Modification of the environmental hazards in a slum environment is an important but difficult task. One approach has been the enforced repainting of run-down apartments where cases of lead poisoning are reported, as is now required by law in New York City. The expense of such a program is probably justified by the high incidence of lead poisoning in slum areas and by the high morbidity and mortality of the disease, but it is important that the effectiveness of the program be monitored.

Ethylenediaminetetraacetic acid (EDTA) is commonly used when blood lead levels range between 60 and 100 μg. per 100 ml. (151, 152). However, it is contraindicated when lead is still present in the intestine, since it facilitates its absorption. Salts of EDTA form a nontoxic chelate with lead that is excreted in the urine. EDTA is administered intravenously in 5 per cent glucose in water or isotonic saline over about a one-hour period twice a day for a course of three to five days. It is made up in a concentration of 1 g. per 200 ml. The total dose should not exceed 70 mg. per kg. per day or 35 mg. per kg. per infusion. Initially, the patient must be watched carefully for untoward reactions. This course may be repeated after two weeks if blood lead concentrations remain elevated. When the blood lead concentration exceeds 100 μg. per 100 ml., EDTA and BAL (2,3-dimercaptopropanol) are given in combination over a five-day period. BAL is given alone for a first dose of 4 mg. per kg. as a deep intramuscular injection. It is continued in this dose, administered simultaneously with EDTA, 12.5 mg. per kg. every 4 hours, using separate deep intramuscular sites.

The management of cerebral edema remains a major unresolved problem. Urea, mannitol, and corticosteroids have been used, but apparently with no great success.

Copper Poisoning

Sudden increments of unbound serum copper may attack the red cell and produce acute hemolysis, perhaps by inhibiting membrane and intracellular enzymes. The acute hemolytic anemia observed in enzootic disease in sheep and in children with Wilson's disease may be due to sudden release of copper from the liver into the blood stream (153, 154).

References

NUTRITIONAL ANEMIAS

General References

1. Nutritional anemias. WHO Tech. Rep. Ser. #503, 1972.
2. Fomon, S. J.: *Infant Nutrition.* Philadelphia, W. B. Saunders Co., 1967.
3. Mauer, A. M.: *Pediatric Hematology.* New York, McGraw-Hill Book Co., 1969.
4. Oski, F., and Naiman, J. L.: *Hematologic Problems in the Newborn.* Philadelphia, W. B. Saunders Co., 1972.
5. Pike, R. L., and Brown, M. L.: *Nutrition: An Integrated Approach.* New York, John Wiley & Sons, 1967.
6. Recommended Dietary Allowances, 7th Revised Edition: A Report of the Food and Nutrition Board. Natl. Acad. Sci. Natl. Res. Council, Publ. 1964, Washington D.C., 1968.
7. Nutritional anemias. Semin. Hematol. 7:2, 1970.
8. Harris, J. W., and Kellermeyer, R. W.: *The Red Cell.* Cambridge, Harvard University Press, 1970.

INTERPRETATION OF ANEMIA

Definition of Anemia and Derivation of Normal Values

9. Garby, L., and Killander, A.: Definition of anaemia, In *Symposia of the Swedish Nutrition Foundation. VI. Occurrence, Causes and Prevention of Nutritional Anaemias.* Stockholm, Almqvist & Wiksell, 1968, p. 9.
10. Viteri, F. E., deTuna, V., et al.: Normal haematological values in the Central American population. Br. J. Haematol. 23:189, 1972.
11. Sjölin, S., and Wranne, L.: Iron requirements during infancy and childhood, In *Symposia of the Swedish Nutrition Foundation. VI. Occurrence, Causes and Prevention of Nutritional Anaemias.* Stockholm, Almqvist & Wiksell, 1968, p. 148.
12. Hunter, R. E., and Smith, N. J.: Hemoglobin and hematocrit values in iron deficiency in infancy. J. Pediatr. *81*:710, 1972.

TOPICS OF GENERAL APPLICABILITY

Individual Variations in Dietary Requirements

13. Williams, R. J.: *Biochemical Individuality.* Austin, University of Texas Press, 1956, p. 135.
14. Beutler, E.: Effect of flavin compounds on glutathione reductase activity: In vivo and in vitro studies. J. Clin. Invest. *48*:1957, 1969.
15. Yoshimura, H.: Anemia during physical training (sports anemia). Nutr. Rev. 28:251, 1970.
16. Gontzea, I., and Sutzescu, P.: *Natural Antinutritive Substances in Foodstuffs and Forages.* Basel, S. Karger, 1968.
17. Rosenberg, L. E.: Inherited aminoacidopathies demonstrating vitamin dependency. New Engl. J. Med. *281*:145, 1969.

18. Whipple, G. H.: Hemoglobin and plasma proteins: Their production, utilization and interrelation. Am. J. Med. Sci. 203:477, 1942.

Permanent Sequelae

19. Chase, P. H., Dabiere, C. S., et al.: Intra-uterine undernutrition and brain development. Pediatrics 47:491, 1971.
20. Cravioto, J., and De Licardie, E. R.: Long-term consequences of protein-calorie malnutrition. Nutr. Rev. 29:107, 1971.
21. Dobbing, J.: Undernutrition and the developing brain. The relevance of animal models to the human problem. Am. J. Dis. Child. 120:411, 1970.
22. Eichenwald, H. F., and Fry, P. C.: Malnutrition and learning. Inadequate nutrition in infancy may result in permanent impairment of mental function. Science 163:644, 1969.
23. Winick, M.: Biological correlations of nutrition, growth and mental development. Am. J. Dis. Child. 120:416, 1970.
24. Stein, Z., Susser, M., et al.: Nutritional and mental performance. Prenatal exposure to the Dutch famine of 1944–45 seems not related to mental performance at age 19. Science 178:708, 1972.
24a. Webb, T. E., and Oski, F. A.: Iron deficiency anemia and scholastic achievement in young adolescents. J. Pediatr. 82:827, 1973.

IRON DEFICIENCY

General References

25. Bothwell, T. H., and Finch, C. A.: *Iron Metabolism*. Boston, Little, Brown & Co., 1962.
26. Brown, E. B.: Clinical aspects of iron metabolism. Semin. Hematol. 3:314, 1966.
27. Charlton, R. W., and Bothwell, T. H.: Iron deficiency anemia. Semin. Hematol. 7:67, 1970
28. Extent and Meanings of Iron Deficiency in the U.S.: Summary, Proceedings of a Workshop, March 8-9, 1971. Food and Nutrition Board, Natl. Acad. Sci., Washington, D.C.
29. Fairbanks, V. F., Fahey, J. I., et al.: *Clinical Disorders of Iron Metabolism*. New York, Grune & Stratton, 1971.
30. Finch, C. A.: Iron deficiency anemia. Am. J. Clin. Nutr. 22:512, 1969.
31. Hallberg, L., Harwerth, H. G., et al. (eds.), *Clinical Symposium on Iron Deficiency*. New York, Academic Press, 1970.
32. Harris, J. W., and Kellermeyer, R. W.: Iron metabolism and iron-lack anemia, In *The Red Cell*. Cambridge, Harvard University Press, 1970, p. 64.
33. Lowe, C. V., Coursin, D. B., et al.: Iron balance and requirements in infancy. Committee on Nutrition, American Academy of Pediatrics. Pediatrics 43:134, 1969.
34. Report of the Sixty-second Ross Conference on Pediatric Research: Iron nutrition in infancy. Ross Laboratories, Columbus, 1970.
35. Vahlquist, B.: Occurrence of nutritional anaemias in children, In *Symposia of the Swedish Nutrition Foundation. VI. Occurrence, Causes and Prevention of Nutritional Anaemias.* Stockholm, Almqvist & Wiksell, 1968, p. 66.

Metabolism and Pathogenesis

36. Weinfeld, A.: Storage iron in man. Acta Med. Scand. [Suppl. 427]:39, 1964.
37. Crichton, R. R.: Ferritin: structure, synthesis and function. New Engl. J. Med. 284:1413, 1971.
38. Dallman, P. R.: Tissue effects of iron deficiency, In *Iron in Biochemistry and Medicine.* Jacobs, A. (ed.), London, Academic Press, 1974.
39. Schulman, I., and Smith, C. H.: Studies on the anemia of prematurity. III. The mechanism of anemia. Am. J. Dis. Child. 88:582, 1954.
40. Crosby, W. H.: The control of iron balance by the intestinal mucosa. Blood 22:441, 1963.
41. Bothwell, T. H., and Charlton, R. W.: Absorption of iron. Ann. Rev. Med. 21:145, 1970.
42. Sheehan, R. G., and Frankel, E. P.: The control of iron absorption by the gastrointestinal mucosal cell. J. Clin. Invest. 51:224, 1972.
43. Garby, L., Sjölin, S., et al.: Studies on erythrokinetics in infancy. IV. The long-term behavior of radioiron in circulating foetal and adult haemoglobin and its faecal excretion. Acta Paediatr. Scand. 53:33, 1964.
44. Hoag, M. S., Wallerstein, R. O., et al.: Occult blood loss in iron deficiency anemia of infancy. Pediatrics 27:199, 1961.
45. Woodruff, C. W., and Clark, J. L.: The role of fresh cow's milk in iron deficiency I. Albumin turnover in infants with iron deficiency anemia. Am. J. Dis. Child. 124:18, 1972.
46. Woodruff, C. W., Wright, S. W., et al.: The role of fresh cow's milk in iron deficiency. II. Comparison of fresh cow's milk with a prepared formula. Am. J. Dis. Child. 124:26, 1972.
47. Moe, P. J.: Iron requirements in infancy: Longitudinal studies of iron requirements during the first year of life. Acta Paediatr. (Stockholm) [Suppl. 150]:1, 1963.
48. Kimber, C., and Weintraub, L. R.: Malabsorption of iron secondary to iron deficiency. New Engl. J. Med. 279:453, 1968.
49. Shahidi, N. T., Nathan, D. G., et al.: Iron deficiency anemia associated with an error of iron metabolism in two siblings. J. Clin. Invest. 43:410, 1964.

Diagnosis: The Stages of Iron Depletion

50. Conrad, M. E., and Crosby, W. H.: The natural history of iron deficiency induced by phlebotomy. Blood 20:173, 1962.
51. Bainton, D. F., and Finch, C. A.: The diagnosis of iron deficiency. Am. J. Med. 37:62, 1964.
52. Addison, G. M., Beamish, M. R., et al.: An immunoradiometric assay for ferritin in the serum of normal subjects and patients with iron deficiency and iron overload. J. Clin. Pathol. 25:326, 1972.
53. Jacobs, A., Miller, F., et al.: Ferritin in the serum of normal subjects and patients with iron deficiency and iron overload. Br. Med. J. 4:206, 1972.

53a. Siimes, M. A., Addiego, J. E., et al.: Ferritin in serum: The diagnosis of iron deficiency and iron overload in infants and children. Blood, 1974 (in press).

54. Robinson, S. H., and Koeppel, E.: Preferential hemolysis of immature erythrocytes in experimental iron deficiency anemia: Source of erythropoietic bilirubin. J. Clin. Invest. 50:1847, 1971.

55. Piomelli, S., Davidow, B., et al.: The FEP (free erythrocyte porphyrins) test: A screening micromethod for lead poisoning. Pediatrics 51:254, 1973.

56. MacDougall, L. G., Judisch, J. M., et al.: Red cell metabolism in iron deficiency anemia. J. Pediatr. 76:660, 1970.

57. Card, R. T., and Weintraub, L. R.: Metabolic abnormalities of erythrocytes in severe iron deficiency. Blood 37:725, 1971.

58. Beutler, E.: Tissue effects of iron deficiency, In Iron Metabolism. Gross, F. (ed.), Berlin, Springer-Verlag, 1964, p. 256.

59. Jacobs, A.: Tissue changes in iron deficiency. Br. J. Haematol. 16:1, 1969.

60. Naiman, J. L., Oski, F. A., et al.: The gastrointestinal effects of iron-deficiency anemia. Pediatrics 33:83, 1964.

61. Schubert, W. K., and Lahey, M. E.: Copper and protein depletion complicating hypoferric anemia of infancy. Pediatrics 24:710, 1959.

Treatment

62. Herbert, V.: Drugs effective in iron-deficiency and other hypochromic anemias, In The Pharmacologic Basis of Therapeutics. Goodman, L. S., and Gilman, A. (eds.), New York, Macmillan, 1970, p. 1397.

63. Melhorn, D. K., and Gross, S.: Relationships between iron-dextran and vitamin E in iron deficiency anemia. J. Lab. Clin. Med. 74:789, 1969.

64. Stevens, A. R.: The treatment of iron deficiency anemia, In Iron in Clinical Medicine. Wallerstein, R. O., and Mettier, S. R. (eds.), Berkeley, University of California Press, 1958.

65. Dallman, P. R., Sunshine, P., et al.: Intestinal cytochrome response with repair of iron deficiency. Pediatrics 39:863, 1967.

Prevention

66. The Ten State Nutrition Survey—A Pediatric Perspective. Am. Acad. Pediatr. Newsletter (Suppl.), January, 1973.

67. Owen, G. M., Lubin, A. H., et al.: Preschool children in the United States: Who has iron deficiency? J. Pediatr. 79:563, 1971.

68. Brown, K., Lubin, B., et al.: Prevalence of anemia among preadolescent and young adolescent urban black Americans. J. Pediatr. 81:714, 1972.

69. Andelman, M. B., and Sered, B. R.: Utilization of dietary iron by term infants. Am. J. Dis. Child. 3:45, 1966.

70. Council on Foods and Nutrition: Iron in enriched wheat flour, farina, bread, buns, and rolls. J.A.M.A. 220:855, 1972.

71. Finch, C. A., and Monsen, E. R.: Iron nutrition and the fortification of food with iron. J.A.M.A. 219:1462, 1972.

72. Gorten, M. K., and Cross, E. R.: Iron metabolism in premature infants. II. Prevention of iron deficiency. J. Pediatr. 64:509, 1964.

73. Layrisse, M., and Martinez-Torres, C.: Food iron absorption. Progr. Hematol. 7:137, 1971.

74. Pearson, H. A.: Iron-fortified formulas in infancy. J. Pediatr. 79:557, 1971.

75. Bullen, J. J., Rogers, H. J., et al.: Iron-binding proteins and infection. Br. J. Haematol. 23:389, 1972.

MEGALOBLASTIC ANEMIAS

General References

76. Chanarin, I.: The Megaloblastic Anemias. Oxford, Blackwell Scientific Publications, 1969.

77. Harris, J. W., and Kellermeyer, R. W.: Pernicious anemia and the non-Addison megaloblastic anemias, In The Red Cell. Cambridge, Harvard University Press, 1970, p. 334.

78. Herbert, V.: The Megaloblastic Anemias. New York, Grune & Stratton, 1959.

79. Herbert, V.: Drugs effective in megaloblastic anemias, In The Pharmacologic Basis of Medical Practice. 4th ed. Goodman, L. S., and Gilman, A. (eds.), New York, Macmillan, 1970, p. 1414.

80. Nixon, P. F., and Bertino, J. R.: Interrelationships of vitamin B_{12} and folate in man. Am. J. Med. 48:555, 1970.

81. Symposium on vitamin B_{12} and folate. Am. J. Med. 48:539, 1970.

Folate Deficiency

82. Herbert, V.: The diagnosis and treatment of folic acid deficiency. Med. Clin. N. Am. 46:1365, 1962.

83. Streiff, R. R.: Folic acid deficiency anemia. Semin. Hematol. 7:23, 1970.

84. Burland, W. L., Simpson, K., et al.: Response of low birthweight infants to treatment with folic acid. Arch. Dis. Child. 46:189, 1971.

85. Matoth, Y., Pinkas, A., et al.: Studies on folic acid in infancy. I. Blood levels of folic and folinic acid in healthy infants. Pediatrics 33:507, 1964.

86. Matoth, Y., Pinkas, A., et al.: Studies on folic acid in infancy. II. Folic and folinic acid blood levels in infants with diarrhea, malnutrition and infection. Pediatrics 33:694, 1964.

87. Matoth, Y., Pinkas, A., et al.: Studies on folic acid in infancy. III. Folates in breast-fed infants and their mothers. Am. J. Clin. Nutr. 16:356, 1965.

88. Roberts, P. M., Arrowsmith, D. E., et al.: Folate state of premature infants. Arch. Dis. Child. 44:637, 1969.

89. Shojania, A. M., and Gross, S.: Folic acid deficiency and prematurity. J. Pediatr. 64:323, 1964.

90. Chanarin, I., Dacie, J. V., et al.: Folic acid deficiency in haemolytic anaemia. Br. J. Haematol. 5:245, 1959.

91. Lindenbaum, J., and Klipstein, F. A.: Folic acid

deficiency in sickle cell anemia. New Engl. J. Med. 269:875, 1963.

92. Drugs and folic acid utilization. Nutr. Rev. 29: 34, 1971.

93. Herbert, V.: Experimental nutritional folate deficiency in man. Trans. Assoc. Am. Physicians 75:307, 1962.

94. Kamel, K., Waslien, E. I., et al.: Folate requirements in children. II. Response of children recovering from protein-calorie malnutrition to graded doses of parenterally administered folic acid. Am. J. Clin. Nutr. 25:152, 1972.

Vitamin B₁₂ Deficiency

95. Sullivan, C. W.: Vitamin B₁₂ metabolism and megaloblastic anemia. Semin. Hematol. 7:6, 1970.

96. McIntyre, O. R., Sullivan, L. W., et al.: Pernicious anemia in childhood. New Engl. J. Med. 272:981, 1965.

97. Miller, D. R., Bloom, G. E., et al.: Juvenile "congenital" pernicious anemia. New Engl. J. Med. 275:978, 1966.

98. Foroozan, P., and Trier, J. S.: Mucosa of the small intestine in pernicious anemia. New Engl. J. Med. 277:553, 1967.

99. Katz, M., Lee S. K., et al.: Vitamin B₁₂ malabsorption due to a biologically inert intrinsic factor. New Engl. J. Med. 287:425, 1972.

100. Hakami, N., Neiman, P. E., et al.: Neonatal megaloblastic anemia due to inherited transcobalamin II deficiency in two siblings. New. Engl. J. Med. 285:1163, 1971.

101. Gräsbeck, R., Gordin, R., et al.: Selective vitamin B₁₂ malabsorption and proteinuria in young people. Acta Med. Scand. 167:289, 1960.

102. Lampkin, B., Shore, N., et al.: Megaloblastic anemia of infancy secondary to maternal pernicious anemia. New Engl. J. Med. 274: 1168, 1966.

103. Pearson, H. A., Vinson, R., et al.: Pernicious anemia with neurologic involvement in childhood. J. Pediatr. 65:334, 1964.

104. Smith, L. H., Jr.: Pyrimidine metabolism in man. New Engl. J. Med. 288:764, 1973.

COPPER DEFICIENCY

105. Karpel, J. T., and Peden, V. H.: Copper deficiency in long-term parenteral nutrition. J. Pediatr. 80:32, 1972.

106. Cordano, A., Baertl, J. M., et al.: Copper deficiency in infancy. Pediatrics 34:324, 1964.

107. Gubler, C. J.: Copper metabolism in man. J.A.M.A. 161:530, 1956.

108. Cartwright, G. E., Markowitz, H., et al.: Studies on copper metabolism. Am. J. Med. 28:555, 1960.

109. Lahey, M. E., Gubler, C. J., et al.: Studies in copper metabolism. II. Hematologic manifestations of copper deficiency in swine. Blood 7:1053, 1952.

110. Frieden, E.: Ceruloplasmin, a link between copper and iron metabolism. Nutr. Rev. 28:87, 1970.

111. Roeser, H. P., Lee, G. R., et al.: The role of ceruloplasmin in iron metabolism. J. Clin. Invest. 49:2408, 1970.

112. Goodman, J. R., and Dallman, P. R.: Role of copper in iron localization in developing erythrocytes. Blood 34:747, 1969.

113. Danks, D. M., Campbell, P. E., et al.: Menkes's kinky hair syndrome, an inherited defect in copper absorption with widespread effects. Pediatrics 50:188, 1972.

VITAMIN E DEFICIENCY

114. Silber, R., and Goldstein, B. D.: Vitamin E and the hematopoietic system. Semin. Hematol. 7:40, 1970.

115. Roels, O. A.: Present knowledge of vitamin E, In *Present Knowledge in Nutrition.* New York, Nutrition Foundation, 1967, p. 84.

116. Lubin, B. H., Baehner, R. L., et al.: The red cell peroxide hemolysis test in the differential diagnosis of obstructive jaundice in the newborn period. Pediatrics 48:562, 1971.

117. Horwitt, M. K., Cent, B., et al.: Erythrocyte survival time and reticulocyte level after tocopherol depletion in man. Am. J. Clin. Nutr. 12:99, 1963.

118. Barness, L. A., Oski, F. A., et al.: Vitamin E response in infants fed a low-fat formula. Am. J. Clin. Nutr. 21:40, 1968.

119. March, B. E., Coates, V., et al.: Reticulocytosis in response to dietary antioxidants. Science 164:1398, 1969.

120. Hashim, S. A., and Asfour, R. H.: Tocopherol in infants fed diets rich in polyunsaturated fatty acids. Am. J. Clin. Nutr. 21:7, 1968.

121. Melhorn, D. K., Gross, S., et al.: The hydrogen peroxide fragility test and serum tocopherol level in anemias of various etiologies. Blood 37:438, 1971.

122. Oski, F. A., and Barness, L. A.: Hemolytic anemia in vitamin E deficiency. Am. J. Clin. Nutr. 21:45, 1968.

123. Panos, T. C., Stinnett, B., et al.: Vitamin E and linoleic acid in the feeding of premature infants. Am. J. Clin. Nutr. 21:15, 1968.

124. Ritchie, J. H., Fish, M. B., et al.: Edema and hemolytic anemia in premature infants. New Engl. J. Med. 279:1185, 1968.

125. Melhorn, D. K., Gross, S., et al.: Vitamin E–dependent anemia in the premature infant. I. Effects of large doses of medicinal iron, *and* II. Relationships between gestational age and absorption of vitamin E. J. Pediatr. 79:569, 581, 1971.

125a. Ehrlich, H. P., Tarver, H., et al.: Inhibitory effects of vitamin E on collagen synthesis and wound repair. Ann. Surg. 175:235, 1972.

PROTEIN DEFICIENCY

126. McCance, R. A., and Widdowson, E. M. (eds.), Calorie deficiencies and protein deficiencies. Proceedings of a colloquium held in Cambridge, April, 1967. Boston, Little, Brown & Co., 1968.

127. Munro, H. N., and Allison, J. B. (eds.), *Mammalian Protein Metabolism.* Vols. I-IV. New York, Academic Press, 1964, 1969.

128. Munro, H. N.: A general survey of techniques used in studying protein metabolism in whole animals and intact cells, In *Mam-*

malian Protein Metabolism. Vol. III. Munro, H. N. (ed.), New York, Academic Press, 1969, p. 237.

129. Scrimshaw, N. S., and Behar, M.: Malnutrition in underdeveloped countries. New Engl. J. Med. 272:137, 1965.

130. Scrimshaw, N. S., and Gordon, J. E. (eds.), *Malnutrition, Learning and Behavior.* Cambridge, The M.I.T. Press, 1968.

131. Waterlow, J. C.: The assessment of protein nutrition and metabolism in the whole animal, with special reference to man, In *Mammalian Protein Metabolism.* Vol. III. Munro, H. N. (ed.), New York, Academic Press, 1969, p. 326.

132. Waterlow, J. C., and Alleyne, G. A. O.: Protein malnutrition: Advances in the last ten years. Adv. Protein Chem. 25:117, 1971.

133. Winick, N., and Noble, A.: Cellular response in rats during malnutrition at various ages. J. Nutr. 89:300, 1966.

134. Whipple, G. H., Miller, L. L., et al.: Raiding of body tissue protein to form plasma protein and hemoglobin: What is premortal rise of urinary nitrogen? J. Exp. Med. 85:277, 1947.

135. Gomez, F., Santaella, J. V., et al.: Studies on the undernourished child. XII. Anemia in malnourished children. Am. J. Dis. Child. 87:673, 1954.

136. Viteri, F. E., Alvarado, J., et al.: Hematological changes in protein calorie malnutrition. Vitam. Horm. 26:573, 1968.

137. Viteri, F. E., and Alvarado, J.: The creatinine height index: Its use in the estimation of the degree of protein depletion and repletion in protein calorie malnourished children. Pediatrics 46:696, 1970.

138. Whitehead, R. G., and Dean, R. F. A.: Serum amino acids in Kwashiorkor. I. Relationship to clinical condition. Am. J. Nutr. 14:313, 1964.

139. The effects of malnutrition on specific amino acids in the serum. Nutr. Rev. 29:76, 1971.

LEAD POISONING

140. Acute and chronic childhood lead poisoning. Committee on Environmental Hazards and Subcommittee on Accidental Poisoning of Committee on Accident Prevention, American Academy of Pediatrics. Pediatrics 47:950, 1971.

141. Chisolm, J. J., Jr., and Kaplan, E.: Lead poisoning in childhood—comprehensive management and prevention. J. Pediatr. 73:942, 1968.

142. Guinee, V. F.: Lead poisoning. Am. J. Med. 52:283, 1972.

143. Harris, J. W., and Kellermeyer, R. W.: *The Red Cell.* Cambridge, Harvard University Press, 1970, p. 35.

144. Hazards from lead. Nutr. Rev. 30:82, 1972.

145. Lin-Fu, J. S.: Undue absorption of lead among children—A new look at an old problem. New Engl. J. Med. 286:702, 1972.

146. Medical aspects of childhood lead poisoning. Pediatrics 48:464, 1971.

147. Six, K. M., and Goyer, R. A.: The influence of iron deficiency on tissue content and toxicity of ingested lead in the rat. J. Lab. Clin. Med. 79:128, 1972.

148. Chisolm, J. J., Jr.: Screening techniques for undue lead exposure in children: Biological and practical consideration. Commentary. J. Pediatr. 79:719, 1971.

149. Goldberg, A.: Lead poisoning as a disorder of heme synthesis. Semin. Hematol. 5:424, 1968.

150. Weissberg, J., Lipschutz, F., et al.: δ-Aminolevulinic acid dehydratase activity in circulating blood cells. New Engl. J. Med. 284:565, 1971.

151. Chisolm, J. J., Jr.: The use of chelating agents in the treatment of acute and chronic lead intoxication in childhood. J. Pediatr. 73:1, 1968.

152. Silver, W., and Rodriguez-Torres, R. R.: Lead intoxication, In *Current Pediatric Therapy.* Vol. 5. Gellis, S. S., and Kagan, B. M. (eds.), Philadelphia, W. B. Saunders Co., 1971, p. 686.

153. Deiss, A., Lee, G. R., et al.: Hemolytic anemia in Wilson's disease. Ann. Intern. Med. 73:413, 1970.

154. Boulard, M., Blume, K. G., et al.: The effect of copper on red cell enzyme activities. J. Clin. Invest. 51:549, 1972.

Chapter 5

Aplastic and Hypoplastic Anemias

by Elias Schwartz

APLASTIC ANEMIA

Aplastic anemia is a term used to describe severe pancytopenia due to diminished production of red cells, granulocytes, and platelets by the bone marrow. Since all three marrow elements are usually involved, aplastic pancytopenia would be more accurate, but aplastic anemia has been firmly rooted as the accepted term since early in this century. Ehrlich described the common clinical and pathologic findings in a young woman in 1888; they included high fever, ulceration and bleeding of the mucous membranes, pancytopenia, and a fatty, acellular marrow (1). Although the cause of suppression of the marrow is not known in many patients with acquired aplastic anemia, a relationship to exposure to chemicals and drugs, excessive irradiation, viral illnesses, and immunologic tolerance has been demonstrated. In addition, a variety of the disorder first described by Fanconi in 1927 in three siblings is distinguished by its usual association with multiple congenital abnormalities (2).

The various forms of aplastic anemia are not common in childhood. It is unusual to see more than three or four new patients a year, even in the largest pediatric centers in the United States. Despite the uncommon nature of the disorder, its usually devastating course has stimulated a great deal of investigation of etiology, pathogenesis, and therapy. Fundamental understanding of the pathogenesis of aplastic anemia will depend upon detailed knowledge of the regulation of hemopoiesis, a subject beyond the scope of this chapter or of this book. The reader should consult an excellent recent text devoted to this area.*

Acquired Aplastic Anemia

Clinical Manifestations

It is difficult to obtain a clear picture of the clinical manifestations and course of aplastic anemia in childhood because of the probable bias toward a severe picture gained from the reports from major referral centers. It is likely that many children with mild or moderate pancytopenia due to hypoplasia of the bone marrow recover rapidly and do not come to the larger centers. The clinical manifestations in these children may be very mild, with pallor and excessive bleeding after trauma being the most prominent features. Children with severe aplastic anemia usually present a very different picture with symptoms due to marked thrombocytopenia, such as petechiae, bruises, spontaneous bleeding from the gums, and epistaxis, being the most prominent initially. Ulceration of the mouth, bacterial infection, and fever may result from granu-

---

*Metcalf, D., and Moore, M. A. S.: Haematopoietic cells, In *Frontiers of Biology.* Neuberger, A., and Tatum, E. L. (eds.), New York, American Elsevier Publishing Company, 1971.

locytopenia, while pallor and anemia may occur somewhat later because of erythroid hypoplasia and blood loss. There is usually a rapid progression of symptoms after the initial manifestations of the disease have appeared. Unless supportive transfusion therapy is provided, the blood counts continue to fall with an increase in severity of clinical symptoms.

Splenomegaly, hepatomegaly, and lymphadenopathy are not part of the usual manifestations of this disease. The presence of these findings should arouse suspicion of disorders such as leukemia or hypersplenism as a cause of the pancytopenia, and appropriate investigations should be initiated.

Hematologic Manifestations

The anemia is normochromic and frequently macrocytic, with a mean cell volume as high as 120 μ^3 in some patients. The absolute reticulocyte count (total reticulocytes per mm.^{3}) is decreased, but the reticulocytes may comprise more than 1 per cent of the diminished number of red cells early in the course of the disease. The percentage of reticulocytes usually remains very low, and frequently only occasional reticulocytes can be found on an entire peripheral blood smear.

The granulocyte count is decreased without a marked change in the proportion of band forms. The absolute lymphocyte count is also frequently low. The relationship of lymphopenia to primary bone marrow failure is not clear. The reduction in platelet count is usually progressive, and the count may fall below 10,000 per mm.^{3}

Serum iron is increased, with an almost fully saturated iron-binding capacity. A rise in serum iron is probably the most reliable early sign of interference with erythropoiesis, and it may be used to monitor the effects of drugs such as chloramphenicol on red cell production (3, 4). Ferrokinetic and red cell survival studies are usually not essential in children with this disorder for diagnostic purposes because the diagnosis may be readily established by other clinical studies. In adults with aplastic anemia and in the small number of children who have been studied, the clearance of ^{59}Fe from the

plasma is considerably prolonged. Red cell incorporation of ^{59}Fe is a good measure of total erythroid activity, and as such it may be more useful than a single bone marrow aspiration in determining degree of hypoplasia (5, 6). The use of studies of ^{59}Fe incorporation into red cells as a prognostic guide in children with aplastic anemia has not been determined. Scanning for localization of ^{59}Fe or ^{52}Fe has been used recently in studying total body erythroid activity in adults with various hematologic conditions (7, 8). As with ^{59}Fe incorporation studies, the value of this technique in prediction of outcome in children with aplastic anemia remains to be determined. Serum haptoglobin is normal, and ^{51}Cr survival in adults has been normal, indicating a normal red cell life span (9). In occasional patients, the red cell survival may be decreased, particularly after multiple transfusions.

Bone marrow examination is of major importance in establishing the diagnosis of aplastic anemia. A good sample may be difficult to obtain if severe hypoplasia is present. Spicules may not be seen grossly, although some fat may be present. On microscopic examination after staining, occasional hypocellular spicules may be found, surrounded by clear, round areas indicating the presence of fat cells. Megakaryocytes are usually absent or are rarely seen. In children with aplastic anemia, lymphocytes are frequently the predominant cells in the hypoplastic background. Histiocytes, plasma cells, and mast cells appear to be relatively more common than usual because of the decreased number of other elements. Myeloid and nucleated erythroid cells may be seen, and there may be rare groups of normoblasts (Figs. 5–1 and 5–2). If there are large numbers of normal cells, the diagnosis should be questioned, and further studies, including ^{59}Fe kinetics, should be done to clarify the diagnosis. Although patients with normal marrow morphology and pancytopenia in the peripheral blood have been reported, this finding is certainly not common in children (10). It may indicate the presence of a different disease (e.g., paroxysmal nocturnal hemoglobinuria) (11, 12), markedly ineffective erythropoiesis (^{59}Fe clearance should be rapid), or a pocket of normal erythropoiesis in an otherwise aplastic marrow. Marrow aspiration at one or two other sites may help to clarify the total picture. A clot should be saved and sections examined. If bone marrow spicules are not obtained after two or three attempts at aspiration, a marrow biopsy is advisable. When used properly, the Turkel needle will usually provide an adequate although small biopsy specimen from which the cellularity of the marrow in the site of biopsy can be determined (13). The Westerman-Jensen needles are rather long and are traumatic in small children (14), and the Turkel (13) or newer varieties of biopsy needles (15) are preferable. A small open biopsy may be done, but it is rarely necessary for establishing the diagnosis. In uncommon patients with acute leukemia, the initial bone marrow specimen may show hypoplasia somewhat similar to that in aplastic anemia (15). The response to corticosteroids (16) or a more intensive investigation (17) may be helpful in differentiating the conditions.

Pancytopenia due to marrow replacement by tumor or involvement by tuberculosis is uncommon in childhood. An adequate biopsy will detect the presence of neuroblastoma (18), embryonal rhabdomyosarcoma, or other malignant cells (19). In children with tuberculosis, there is almost always pulmonary involvement before extensive marrow infection. Granuloma may be found on biopsy, and positive cultures may be obtained if the marrow is involved. Pancytopenia due to marrow replacement in children may rarely be seen with extensive infection of the bones by pyogenic organisms. In such an instance, multiple bone marrow aspirations may yield only serosanguineous material, consisting mainly of autolyzing neutrophils and bacteria.

The absolute amount of fetal hemoglobin present in the blood has been claimed to be of value in determining the prognosis of children with aplastic anemia (20). A more recent evaluation of many of the same patients plus a new group indicates clearly that there is no significant relationship between the amount of fetal hemoglobin and the ability of the marrow to recover (21).

Erythropoietin levels are extremely high in this disorder, and are generally higher than in patients with thalassemia who have similar hemoglobin levels (22). It has been suggested that the unusually high levels in hypoplastic anemia result from decreased consumption of erythropoietin by the marrow, while in thalassemia the active erythroid marrow utilizes some of the erythropoietin which is produced (23).

Since aplastic anemia is relatively uncommon and the disease is frequently so relentless in its course and tragic in its outcome, each new patient should be fully evaluated in order to provide a body of information which may be of value in determining prognosis and need for intensive treatment. In particular, an accurate assessment of total initial erythroid activity by bone marrow aspiration and biopsy, ^{59}Fe clearance and incorporation into red cells, and scanning for sites of erythropoiesis may provide information of value which will be difficult to obtain in any single center because of the uncommon occurrence of the disease.

Pathophysiology

In at least one-half of children with acquired aplastic anemia, the etiology of the disease cannot be determined. There is a clear association of many cases with exposure to drugs, chemicals, irradiation, or viral illnesses, and it must be suspected that in those instances in which a definite exposure cannot be confirmed, an unusual susceptibility to some environmental agent existed. Agents which are potentially suppressive to the bone marrow are ubiquitous in the environment of children in our society, ranging from non-prescription medicines to model airplane glue to food additives. It is extremely important that a thorough, probing history be obtained from the family of a child with acquired aplastic anemia, and that a careful search of his environment be made with the purpose of removing any possible offending agents. Unfortunately, even in instances where the offending agent is clearly identified, prevention of further exposure may not favorably alter the course of the disease, possibly because of severe damage to the pool of hemopoietic precursor cells. An attempt to remove the offending agent should therefore be made as early as possible in the course of the disease.

(Text continued on page 157)

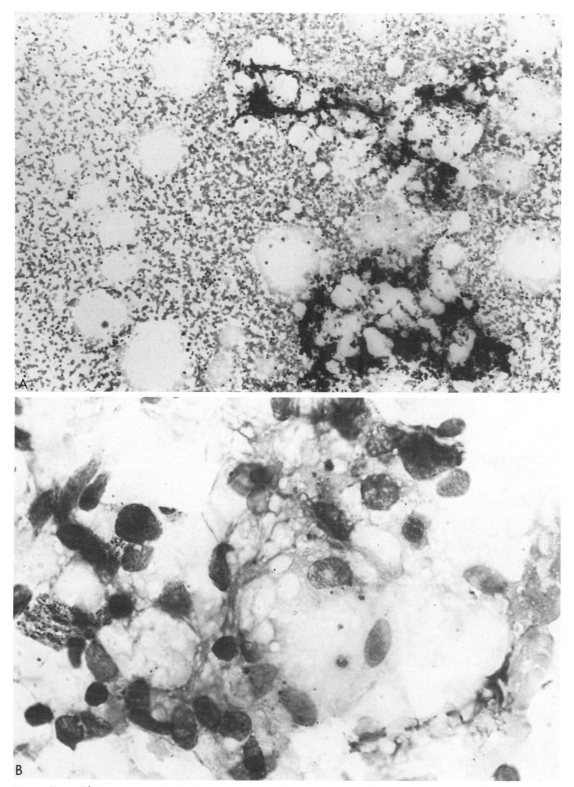

Figure 5–1. Photomicrographs of a bone marrow specimen obtained at the time of diagnosis of acquired aplastic anemia in an 8-year-old boy. The boy died after eight months of illness despite therapy with oxymetholone and prednisone and weekly platelet transfusions. *A,* Low-power view of extreme hypoplasia. *B,* High-power view of area containing many histiocytes.

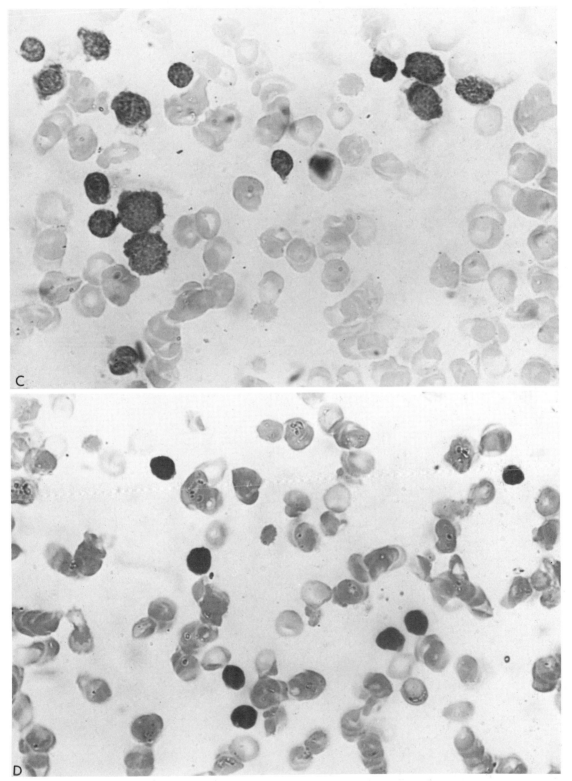

Figure 5–1 *Continued.* *C*, High-power view showing a focus of nucleated red blood cells. *D*, High-power view showing an area containing only lymphocytes.

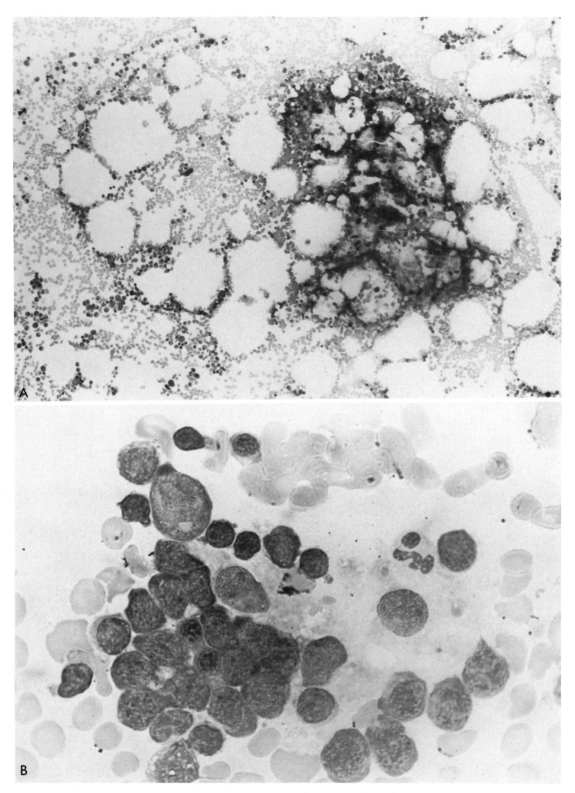

Figure 5–2. *See opposite page for legend.*

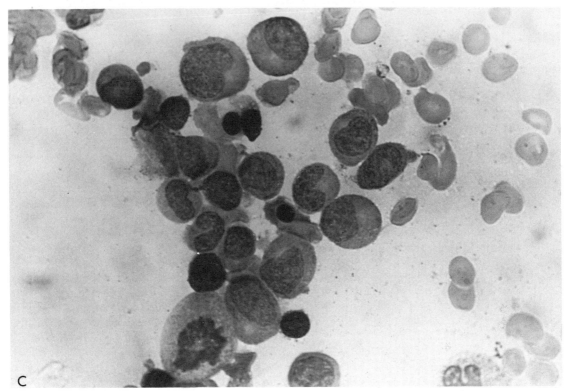

Figure 5–2. Photomicrographs obtained at the time of diagnosis from a 10-year-old girl with acquired aplastic anemia. The girl had improvement in her peripheral blood counts while taking oxymetholone and prednisone. She is presently doing well without drug therapy, although her blood counts have not completely returned to normal. *A*, Low-power view showing hypoplasia. *B*, High-power view showing a focus of nucleated red cells. *C*, High-power view of an area containing mainly nucleated white cells.

The most likely common pathway of injury which results in aplastic anemia is damage to a pluripotential stem cell. These cells have been defined as "primitive hematopoietic cells capable of extreme self-replication and endowed with a multiple differentiating capacity" (24). The study of these stem cells in animals by in vivo spleen colony and radioactive isotope techniques has provided a great deal of important information (25–29). The stem cells may be present in liver and spleen during fetal life, but after the newborn period they are found in the bone marrow. The pluripotential stem cell gives rise to unipotential committed cells which will differentiate into erythroid, myeloid, or thrombopoietic cell lines. The concept of pluripotential stem cells has received support from studies in irradiated rodents. If lethally irradiated animals are injected with bone marrow cells, isolated colonies of hemopoietic cells will appear in a short while in the spleen and elsewhere, presumably arising from single bone marrow cells (colony-forming units, CFU) (25). Each colony contains erythroid, myeloid, or thrombopoietic cells, with erythroid colonies being the most common in the spleen. Cells taken from any pure colony and injected into another irradiated animal will still produce colonies of all three cell lines (29). Some of the cells in each colony are thus presumed to remain pluripotential stem cells, while others become committed to develop as one type of blood cell, perhaps influenced by the local environment. The stem cell and early committed precursor cells have not been identified morphologically. The earliest recognizable cells in each line are the blast cells.

The control of differentiation and maturation of hemopoietic cells has not been completely clarified, but it is evident that humoral factors play an important, although probably not an exclusive, role. The actions of erythropoietin, a substance which stimulates erythropoiesis, have been extensively studied in humans and animals (30). Hypertransfused mice have no recognizable erythroid cells in the spleen. After injection of erythropoietin, the morphologic stages of erythroid development from early blast to reticulocyte can be seen to develop sequentially (31). Erythropoietin can thus act on the committed precursor cell, or perhaps even on the pluripotential stem cell, to initiate the differentiation and maturation of the erythroid line (32). Evidence for the existence of regulators of granulocyte (33) and thrombocyte (34) development has also been accumulated. In aplastic anemia, serum factors which stimulate hemopoiesis do not seem to be lacking (22), but rather there appears to be an absence of or malfunction of the pluripotential stem cell.

Drugs and Other Chemical or Physical Agents

A large number of drugs and chemicals have been associated with hypoplasia of the bone marrow and aplastic anemia. Many of the agents used to treat leukemia, lymphoma, and other malignancies will regularly suppress the bone marrow if given in sufficient dosage. Barring fatality due to pancytopenia or persistent infiltrates of malignant cells, the drug effect is usually reversible, and normal cellularity will be restored when the drug is discontinued or the dosage lowered.

The effect of radiation is similar to that of many antineoplastic drugs in that a sufficiently large exposure will result in bone marrow suppression and pancytopenia. The marrow will usually recover if the affected person does not die because of damage to other tissues or because of bleeding or infection. An analysis of the incidence of aplastic anemia other than that occurring soon after exposure in survivors of the atomic bomb explosions in Hiroshima and Nagasaki failed to implicate ionizing radiation in the pathogenesis of the disease (35). It is thus uncertain if there are long-term effects of irradiation which may lead to the development of aplastic anemia.

Many drugs which do not have a consistent pharmacologic effect in suppressing hemopoiesis have been associated with the occurrence of aplastic anemia. In most instances of presumed drug-induced aplasia of this type, pancytopenia has occurred in persons who had previously taken one or more medications in the usual pharmacologic dosages. The possible causal relationship between drug ingestion and subsequent bone marrow aplasia in these instances is tenuous, since extremely few people taking the drugs develop pancytopenia, and the mechanism of action or the reason for presumed susceptibility in affected persons is unknown. Since the taking of medicines is so common in our society, it would be expected that many adults or children developing aplastic anemia would have ingested some drugs within the preceding several months.

Despite the circumstantial nature of the evidence connecting certain drugs with the development of bone marrow aplasia, the association with several agents is frequent enough to warrant caution in their use. The chief offender in this group is chloramphenicol (35a). From 1953 to 1964, 408 cases of chloramphenicol-associated marrow suppression were reported to the American Medical Association Registry on Blood Dyscrasias (36). In 40 per cent of these patients, it had been the only drug taken in the preceding six months. In one study, the incidence of fatal aplastic anemia in persons who received chloramphenicol was about 1 in 25,000, 13 times the risk of the disease occurring without prior ingestion of the drug (37). The mechanism of action in causing aplasia is not known. Two different types of chloramphenicol-related suppression of bone marrow function have been observed. In one type, chloramphenicol interferes with erythropoiesis, as shown by a rise in serum iron and the appearance of vacuoles in nucleated red cells (38). This effect is reversible when the drug is stopped, and is related to dose. The suppression by the drug may result from inhibition of mitochondrial protein synthesis (39). There is no clear relationship between this action of the drug and the development of severe aplastic anemia in rare individuals weeks or months after the drug has been taken, presumably because of interference with the pluripotential stem cell (40). The occurrence of this second form of bone marrow suppression due to chloramphenicol is unrelated to dose. There may be a genetic susceptibility to the severe effects of the drug, as indicated by the occurrence of aplastic anemia after exposure to chloramphenicol in identical twins (40). The toxic effects of chloramphenicol in the newborn infants, which were related to blood levels of the drug and produced the "grey syndrome," were not due to suppression of hemopoiesis but rather to peripheral vasomotor collapse. Since numerous effective antibiotics are now available for most of the infections for which chloramphenicol had formerly been used, it is best to reserve its use only for those unusual instances in which there is no adequate alternative.

The occurrence of aplastic anemia in association with other drugs used in childhood is very low, particularly when the frequency of use of the drug is taken into account. The major drugs which have been noted are sulfonamides and their derivatives (sulfisoxazole, tolbutamide) and anticonvulsants (mephenytoin) (41, 42). With each of the drugs used in childhood besides chloramphenicol, the incidence of aplastic anemia is so low that the drug probably should not be avoided if there is a clear therapeutic indication for its use. With drugs used for long-term administration, such as anticonvulsant agents, it is helpful to follow blood counts and serum iron levels to detect early signs of toxicity. There is no evidence that the course of aplastic anemia in patients who will be severely affected will be altered by early detection of hematologic toxicity, but it is certainly prudent to stop the drug at the first indication of effect on the marrow in the hope that permanent damage may be avoided.

Certain chemicals which are common in our environment have been suggested as causes of aplastic anemia in children. The common feature to many of these is the presence of a benzene ring in the compound. Benzene and its derivatives are present in many solvents used in the home. Sufficient exposure to benzene may cause marrow hypoplasia (43, 44). In some patients, leukemia may develop after exposure to benzene, occasionally with an intervening period of marrow aplasia (45). DDT and other insecticides may also be toxic to the bone marrow, particularly with high exposure (46). Aplastic anemia has also oc-

curred in children who have been sniffers of model airplane glue, perhaps because of the effects of toluene (47).

Despite the many epidemiologic studies and investigations of the effects of individual chemical agents on the bone marrow, we are unable to clarify the etiology or basic tissue defect which leads to aplastic anemia in most affected children. The term "idiopathic aplastic anemia" is a sign of our lack of knowledge and the need for further intensive study.

Viral Hepatitis and Aplastic Anemia

In recent years it has become apparent that there is a much higher than chance association of viral hepatitis and severe aplastic anemia in both children and adults. At least 55 patients with this combination of disorders have been reported, most having severe aplastic anemia resulting in death (48–51). The hepatitis usually resolves fairly readily, to be followed by increasing pancytopenia. Only two children have been reported who have had recovery from the pancytopenia stage (49). The relationship of the viral infection to severe bone marrow depression is not clear, but the virus may infect the bone marrow as well as the liver, kidney, and other organs (52), causing damage to the hemopoietic stem cells. The possibility that the relationship is based on interference with detoxification of potential bone marrow poisons by the liver is less likely, since aplastic anemia does not seem to be associated with other common forms of liver disease.

Other Causes

Several children have been described with pancreatic insufficiency and bone marrow hypoplasia (53, 54). Three children were in one family, suggesting a genetic component to the syndrome. The children had normal sweat tests and were without respiratory disease, indicating that they did not have cystic fibrosis. Poor weight gain and abnormal stools were present from infancy. Neutropenia was the predominant hematologic abnormality, although anemia and thrombocytopenia were present at times in some patients. The pancytopenia was not relentlessly progressive, but waxed and waned. On bone marrow aspiration, hypocellularity was usually found. The hematologic abnormalities did not respond to oral replacement of pancreatic enzymes nor to hematinics.

The graft-versus-host (GVH) reaction, or runt disease, occurs in immunologically tolerant animals in whom there is a "take" of foreign hemopoietic tissue. The features of the syndrome are wasting, dermatitis, diarrhea, aplastic anemia, histocytosis, and death. Children have been described with a similar clinical syndrome after blood transfusions (55). Two children with progressive vaccinia necrosum, one with the Swiss type of agammaglobulinemia, received multiple transfusions of whole blood or leukocyte-rich plasma and subsequently died of pancytopenia. Associated findings of erythrodermia, hepatosplenomegaly, severe bone marrow hypoplasia, and diffuse histiocytic infiltration indicated that a GVH reaction had occurred in each child. This syndrome is becoming more common as the attempts at immunologic reconstitution and bone marrow transplantation increase, and it is important to anticipate situations in which appropriate early treatment for the GVH reaction with amethopterin and other agents might be instituted.

A 5-year-old boy with a benign thymoma and mild anemia developed severe aplastic anemia one month after thymectomy and died soon afterwards (56). The child had received chloramphenicol and sulfa drugs two months before thymectomy, but the initial presentation with anemia is unusual for drug-induced aplastic anemia. In adults with thymic tumors and hematologic problems, anemia is frequently the first (and only) sign of bone marrow hypoplasia (57).

It has been suggested that some cases of aplastic anemia may be due to defects of the sinusoidal microcirculation of the bone marrow rather than primary depletion of stem cells (58). The defect proposed by this hypothesis would explain why some human patients do not repopulate their marrows despite active foci of hemopoiesis when they are first seen. Ultrastructural studies of the bone marrow sinusoids in aplastic anemia have not revealed any abnormalities (58a).

Treatment

The management of a child with aplastic anemia is complex and is probably best carried out at a center with adequate facilities for replacement therapy with blood components and other specialized procedures. The emotional needs and problems of the family and the child are as diverse and as difficult to manage as those of children with leukemia and other malignancies. The child is best cared for when the thought and facilities used for his physical problem are equally matched by careful planning for emotional problems, including the help of social workers and child psychiatrists when indicated.

ANDROGENS. The value of therapy with drugs and other modalities can be determined only by comparison with the outcome of the disease in untreated children. Adequate data have been difficult to obtain, probably because of differences in severity of the disorder in different centers because of the local referral pattern of mild and severe cases.

In general, it is still not possible to determine on the basis of published reports whether therapy with drugs which stimulate the bone marrow has any effect on the outcome of this disease. The group of drugs which has offered the most promise has been the androgens. Testosterone was first noted to stimulate erythropoiesis in women with breast cancer (59). Testosterone and related androgens were first tried in children with aplastic anemia by Shahidi and Diamond at The Children's Hospital Medical Center in Boston (60, 61). It is of value to review the results of children managed at that hospital in order to point out the difficulties in evaluating the effect of therapy in this disorder. Of 40 patients with aplastic anemia seen between 1938 and 1958, only two had spontaneous remissions, and one of these relapsed within a year (61). Starting in 1958, children with the disease were treated with testosterone and corticosteroids. The corticosteroids were used to counteract the growth-accelerating effects of androgen, and not for any inherent property of stimulation of the marrow. By 1961, 17 patients with acquired disease had been treated, and nine had achieved sustained remissions (61). The medication was discontinued after remission was present. By 1965, a total of 45 patients had been treated on whom full data were available, with an additional two lost to follow-up. Fifteen of those patients were living by 1970, with a long-term survival of 33 per cent after testosterone therapy, a seeming major advance in the treatment of the disease when compared with the 1938-58 results (21). Eleven additional patients were seen between 1966 and 1970 who were treated with a variety of androgens, including oxymetholone (21). Each of the 11 patients died. It is difficult to explain this pattern observed for 32 years at one institution. The differences in response to androgens between 1958-65 and 1966-70 might have occurred by chance alone, but this is very unlikely. The nature of the disease may have changed, but reports of successful treatment from other institutions since 1966 do not bear this out (62–66). A possible explanation may involve the severity of disease in the patients referred in the different time periods, the patients with milder disease in recent years perhaps being cared for at local hospitals where facilities have improved and trained specialists are more common. The patients with milder disease may respond more readily to androgens or, equally likely, may have a greater potential for spontaneous improvement.

Studies reported since 1965 from other institutions, although equally lacking in adequate controls, have suggested that the effect of androgens on survival is not as great as originally believed (63, 67, 67a, 67b). On the other hand, several recent studies report major benefits from testosterone, oxymetholone, and nandrolone decanoate on the course of aplastic anemia (62, 64–66, 68). A most interesting recent paper by Heyn, Ertel, and Tubergen reported that 17 of 33 children at the University of Michigan Hospital survived without the use of androgens (69). It is very important in evaluating the results of all these studies to compare the clinical data available at the time of diagnosis. Patients with severe aplastic anemia usually have marked hypocellularity and pancytopenia when first seen. Children with normocellular or mildly hypocellular marrows may have a different disorder and prognosis. The percentage of lymphocytes in the first

marrow may be of importance in prognosis, and may thus serve as one criterion for evaluating the effects of future therapy (21, 69). The mortality appears to be considerably higher in patients with greater than 80 per cent lymphocytes than in those with fewer lymphocytes and more myeloid and erythroid cells.

Numerous forms of androgens have been used to treat aplastic anemia. Testosterone propionate (1 to 2 mg. per kg.) may be taken sublingually in order to avoid high concentrations of the drug in the liver and possible liver toxicity. Studies of the action of androgens on erythropoiesis in animals have indicated that certain compounds may be more effective than others (70, 71, 71a). Nandrolone decanoate, which is available at 100 mg. per ml. for intramuscular injections, may be given weekly at a dose of 5 mg. per kg. to thrombopenic patients if careful injection technique is utilized. The use of oxymetholone, a potent stimulator of erythropoiesis in children (2 to 6 mg. per kg.) and adults, has been accompanied by remissions in some reports (62, 64, 65) and by lack of effect in others (21). In high doses given for prolonged periods this methylated compound may cause severe liver disease or even hepatic tumors (71b).

It is difficult to decide whether to treat an individual child with androgens, since the efficacy of the therapy has not been clearly established. The side effects may be very disturbing, particularly in girls. Proponents claim that treatment for six months or longer may be needed before a response is observed. In the absence of parameters which can serve as an early guide to response to androgens and because of the severity of the disease, it may be best to offer each child a full trial of therapy. The therapy may be continued until a response occurs or for several months, unless toxicity or side effects make its use difficult. Estimations of bone age should be made by appropriate roentgenograms initially and every three to four months. Corticosteroids, such as prednisone (0.5 to 1.0 mg. per kg.), should be used to counteract the effect of androgens in accelerating maturation of growth centers in the bones. It is not certain whether intermittent corticosteroid dosage may be used to counteract the growth-promoting effects of androgens, but it is likely that they will be effective when used in this manner. Large dosages of corticosteroids may suppress bone marrow activity and should be avoided.

SUPPORTIVE THERAPY. Adequate supportive therapy is of major importance in maintaining the affected patient while waiting for spontaneous improvement or a response to therapy. Transfusions of blood components will usually be necessary in response to crisis situations or to maintain blood counts at adequate levels. The purpose of transfusion therapy should be to maintain the child at as normal a functional level as possible and to provide red cells, platelets, and granulocytes as they are needed.

It is useful to obtain complete typing for red cell antigens before the first red cell transfusion as an aid in choosing appropriate units for transfusion and in identifying antibodies to red cells which may occur later in the course of the disease. There is no evidence that maintaining a low red cell count in order to have a maximum erythropoietic stimulus is of value in hastening recovery. Accordingly, the hemoglobin concentration should be kept at a level necessary for a feeling of well-being and for maintaining reasonable activities. This level is usually above 7 g. per 100 ml. The red cell survival is normal if antibodies do not develop, and packed red cell transfusions are only needed every three to four weeks. If bleeding is present, more frequent transfusions may be needed.

The appropriate use of platelet transfusions in this disorder has not been clarified. Some groups use platelets only when needed to stop major bleeding, while others use them more liberally. Antibodies may develop in patients who have received multiple platelet transfusions, reducing the effectiveness of further transfusions (72, 73). In some patients splenectomy has been of help in restoring a previously noted beneficial effect of platelets, perhaps by lessening sequestration of antibody-coated platelets or by removing a major source of antibody production (73). Transfusion with platelets which have been found to be compatible by specialized typing techniques may also be used to raise the platelet count in sensitized patients (74). Since bleeding and infection are the major causes of mortality in this disease, it is important to try to maintain the effectiveness of trans-

fusion therapy needed to treat these complications.

In patients with marked thrombocytopenia, concern about severe bleeding may limit the child's activities to a major extent and accentuate the anxiety already present in the family. The continual appearance of fresh petechiae and bruises serves to heighten fears of episodes of major bleeding. Experience with frequent platelet transfusions suggests that in many patients it may be possible to maintain platelet levels which are high enough to prevent spontaneous hemorrhage (75, 76). The platelets are best obtained by plasmapheresis from close relatives in order to lessen the risk of sensitization, unless bone marrow transplantation will be attempted. We have been able to transfuse platelets into two children with aplastic anemia weekly as out-patients without clinically significant sensitization after several months of therapy. Petechiae and bruises usually do not occur until a few days after the platelet count falls below 10,000 per mm.[3], perhaps indicating a protective effect on the vessels which is not dependent on the immediate presence of platelets in the circulation. Further studies are necessary on the incidence of clinically significant platelet antibodies with various types of therapy and on the value of splenectomy and HL-A typing in platelet transfusion therapy. The capacity for increased activity and the partial removal of anxiety in children who are prevented from bleeding indicates that this treatment may be of value.

The brief life span of granulocytes in the circulation and the lack of adequate means of extracting them in sufficient quantity from normal donors in most hospitals make this form of replacement therapy the least satisfactory at present. Administration of 1×10^{10} to 1×10^{11} white cells per m.[2] of body surface to patients with granulocytopenia and fever resulting from proved or presumed bacterial infection has led to clinical improvement in many (77). The response is related to the number of granulocytes given, the availability of cells for repeated treatment, and the nature of the infection. Several methods of preparing granulocyte transfusions have been used. An adequate number of cells may be obtained by repeated plasmapheresis or continuous flow centrifugation of blood from adults with chronic myelogenous leukemia or myeloid metaplasia whose white blood cell counts are above 50,000 per mm.³ and who are neither infected nor being treated (77, 78). The NCI-IBM Cell Separator is capable of separating blood components from normal donors and yielding sufficient granulocytes from one to several donor for an effective transfusion. It is usually necessary to transfuse granulocytes daily for three to four days to overcome a severe septic episode (79). A less expensive method which may be of considerable value has recently been described in which repeated extractions of granulocytes from a single donor by the use of a commercially available filter will provide 1×10^{10} to 1×10^{11} cells within three to four hours (80). The use of a single normal donor lessens the chance of sensitization and increases the ease of obtaining granulocytes. A pilot model of a machine capable of conducting most of this procedure automatically has now been built, and its use is being evaluated. The in vitro functions of granulocytes prepared by this method are normal (80a). Because of their short survival time, granulocytes will probably not be used prophylactically in aplastic anemia. There is a great need, however, for an adequate means of providing cells for aid in treatment of infection, and recent advances in technology may soon meet this need.

Children with aplastic anemia are best treated as out-patients, unless severe bleeding episodes or infections occur. With proper planning and adequate facilities, the patient's time in the clinic may be minimized, even when repeated transfusions are needed. The in-patient service of the hospital may serve as a source of organisms which may be difficult to treat. When hospitalization does become necessary, it is probably best to keep the child in protective isolation, although there is little evidence that the usual method of isolation in the hospital is effective in decreasing the incidence of infection. Life islands are very good at separating a patient from the surrounding bacteriologic environment (81), but it would seem that the inability to even touch another person's hand in this type of isolation would be detrimental to a child's spirit and his general outlook. Laminar flow rooms appear to be much more suitable for keeping children protected from exogenous pathogens (82), but they

are very expensive and are not available in many large centers. Many infections may be initiated by organisms from the gastrointestinal tract, and, even with the most thorough isolation, endogenous pathogens may cause severe infections. Unusual organisms and sites of infections may be found in these children, and a thorough evaluation with adequate cultures should be obtained whenever fever occurs. Treatment with adequate levels of antibiotics should be instituted promptly in a patient with high fever and granulocytopenia after appropriate initial examination and cultures. Cephalothin (100 mg. per kg.) every six hours and gentamycin (5 mg. per kg.) every eight hours given intravenously are a good combination for initial therapy, with specific therapy to be substituted for these as soon as the offending organism or organisms are identified. The possibility of infections with fungi and unusual bacteria should be kept in mind, and appropriate culture techniques used. The most difficult problem in treating patients with aplastic anemia and high fever occurs when the cultures have not been successful in isolating a pathogen and there has been no response to antimicrobial and antifungal therapy. White cell transfusions may be of great benefit in such situations, but suitable donors or the proper equipment are frequently not available. Prophylactic treatment with antibiotics is not advisable (82a).

Children with aplastic anemia may play in the home and outside, but they should avoid activities which may result in even mild trauma to the head. Children receiving chronic platelet transfusions are able to engage safely in a wider range of activities than children who are not. It is difficult to decide whether children of school age should be allowed to attend classes. If bleeding manifestations are not prominent, the child is fairly safe at school, since the danger of acquiring a significant bacterial infection from classmates is slight.

It is best to avoid using a toothbrush to clean the teeth, since bleeding or introduction of bacteria into the blood stream may occur. Maintaining cleanliness of the teeth is important in order to avoid gum infections, and soft cotton wrapped on a flexible stick may be used for this purpose.

BONE MARROW TRANSPLANTATION. Bone marrow transplantation may offer some hope for treatment of children with severe aplasia of the bone marrow, but this therapy is still in the early stages of evaluation. In general, marrow transplants have been most successful in patients with immunologic deficiencies. Recent experiences have indicated that success may also be possible in animals and in patients with aplastic anemia if recipients are prepared properly. In rabbits with benezene-induced aplastic anemia, pregraft treatment of the recipients with horse antirabbit antilymphocytic globulin resulted in a high percentage of takes without graft-versus-host reactions (83). Treatment of aplastic anemia in eight humans with antilymphocytic serum and marrow infusions resulted in four takes of two to five months' duration (84). In four other patients, conditioning of the recipients with cyclophosphamide followed by marrow infusion from siblings who were compatible with the patients at the major histocompatibility loci resulted in four prompt takes (85). One patient subsequently died of a graft-versus-host reaction, while a second rejected the graft in one to two months. The two youngest patients, aged 12 and 16, continued to be well at four and seven months, respectively, after grafting. This experience has now been considerably expanded, and it appears that approximately 40 per cent of patients with severe aplastic anemia may respond favorably to marrow transplantation (85a, 85b). It is of importance that a potential recipient of a marrow graft for whom a matched donor is available be transfused as little as possible before the procedure to avoid inducing sensitivity to histocompatibility antigens. Family members should certainly be excluded as donors of red cells, platelets, or granulocytes. With the methods presently available, the donor must be histocompatible and nonreactive in the mixed lymphocyte reaction. Such donors are almost always siblings. An identical twin is the ideal donor (86). The identification of patients with severe disease early in their course before extensive transfusion therapy is difficult because of the lack of clear prognostic indicators. A high percentage of lymphocytes appears to be a bad prognostic sign, but even in this group, patients have recovered spontaneously from their disease (69). Posthepatitic aplastic anemia seems to be particularly lethal. Further studies are needed to improve methods of grafting and to determine how to select appropriate patients for marrow transplantation.

Constitutional Aplastic Anemia

Constitutional aplastic anemia is a disorder characterized by pancytopenia, a hypoplastic bone marrow, and evidence for a congenital or familial defect causing the disease. Most of the affected children have also had multiple congenital malformations. In 1927 Fanconi described three brothers with aplastic anemia and multiple congenital abnormalities (2), a syndrome to which is applied the eponym "Fanconi's aplastic anemia." About 200 additional children with the disorder have since been reported. Instances of familial occurrence without other congenital abnormalities have also been reported (87, 88). Other constitutional disorders involving the decreased production of blood cells, including congenital hypoplastic anemia (89) and radial-platelet hypoplasia (90), may be distinguished from this disorder by the limitation of involvement to one type of blood cell and the nature of the associated anomalies.

Clinical Manifestations

The hematologic manifestations of this disorder usually first become apparent between 4 and 12 years of age. Thrombocytopenia and granulocytopenia are usually first to appear, with anemia occurring subsequently. The clinical manifestations of pancytopenia will gradually progress in severity, necessitating red cell transfusions because of anemia and resulting in increasing susceptibility to bleeding and infection. In some children there may be bleeding with thrombocytopenia and decreased megakaryocytes in the first year of life, followed by pancytopenia later in the first decade (91). The ratio of affected males to females is about two to one (93).

The congenital abnormalities involve many systems (93). Some occur commonly, such as those involving the skin, skeleton, kidneys, eyes, and nervous system. Cardiovascular anomalies are rare.

Short stature and decreased bone age are frequently present (94). The cause for retarded growth has not been clarified, although deficiency of growth hormone has been demonstrated in a few instances (95, 96). Low birth weights are common. Despite problems with physical growth, mental age is usually normal, although retardation is found in 17 per cent of patients (93).

Hyperpigmentation of the skin due to increased melanin is common, with the face, hands, and feet usually spared. The areas of pigmentation may be patchy, with particularly intense areas occurring in skin folds. Café-au-lait spots are common. In "congenital dyskeratosis," a familial disorder occurring in childhood, a clinically similar hyperpigmentation occurs along with abnormalities of the nails and leukokeratosis in the mouth. The high incidence of hypoplasia of the bone marrow in association with congenital dyskeratosis (97–99) had led to the suggestion that the two disorders may be part of a spectrum of clinical manifestations associated with the same underlying congenital defect (97).

Abnormalities of the skeleton are common, especially those involving the thumb. The thumb may be absent or hypoplastic (Fig. 5–3), and there may be associated absence or abnormalities of the radius (94, 99a). When these abnormalities are present, they are usually bilateral. Absent radii with thumbs present, the characteristic skeletal abnormality in the radial-platelet hypoplasia syndrome (90), are not found in these children. The number of carpal bones is reduced in one-third of affected children (94).

Microphthalmia is frequently found. Hyperreflexia is present in most affected children and is the most common neurologic disorder (93). Other less common disorders involving the sensory organs and neurologic system include strabismus, ear abnormalities, and microcephaly.

Renal abnormalities may be fairly common, but they are usually not of major clinical significance. The anomalies which have been found include absence of a kidney, ectopic and horseshoe kidneys, and double ureters (100). An intravenous pyelogram

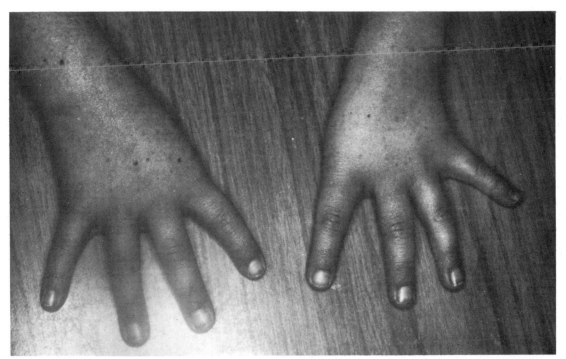

Figure 5–3. Photograph of the hands of a 6-year-old boy with constitutional aplastic anemia showing the absence of thumbs.

should be performed on every child with constitutional aplastic anemia in order to detect possible abnormalities.

Absent radial pulses appear to be a common anomaly, even in instances where the thumbs are present (101). Other abnormalities which have been noted but which occur less commonly involve the genital and cardiovascular systems.

Several families have been described in which two or more siblings have had aplastic anemia with associated congenital abnormalities (93, 102). Other families have been reported in which one sibling had the usual manifestations of Fanconi's aplastic anemia while another sibling had aplastic anemia without other congenital abnormalities (93, 102). It is also likely that some of the instances of familial occurrence of aplastic anemia without associated defects represent a constitutional rather than acquired form of the disease.

Hematologic Manifestations

The hematologic manifestations are similar in many respects to those found in acquired aplastic anemia. The pancytopenia is due to the reduced production of cells by the bone marrow. If an affected child is detected at an early stage because of a previously affected sibling or because of the presence of a typical group of congenital anomalies, the marrow will be cellular during the early stages of pancytopenia (93). In the absence of appropriate drug therapy, the cellularity will progressively decrease to the point of marked hypoplasia (Fig. 5–4). Red cell survival may be shortened in some instances (93). With marked hypoplasia, ferrokinetic studies show a prolonged clearance of ^{59}Fe from the plasma and a decreased incorporation of the isotope into red cells. Uncommonly, ^{59}Fe clearance may be increased, and the findings of ineffective erythropoiesis may be present (103).

The anemia is characteristically macrocytic, and the mean cell volume may be as high as 120 $\mu.^3$ The maturation of nucleated red cells in the marrow is not megaloblastic, although red cells with unusual maturation may be seen early in the course of the disease (61, 93). Folic acid and vitamin B_{12} levels are not decreased (61). In contrast to acquired aplastic anemia with severe aplasia, the percentage of reticulocytes may be normal, although the absolute number is usually decreased. Hb F levels are usually increased, and may comprise more than 10 per cent of the total hemoglobin before red cell transfusions are given (102). The distribution of Hb F among the red cells is not uniform, as indicated by examination of slides prepared by the Betke-Kleihauer technique (104). The elevation of Hb F has been noted to precede the onset of anemia in some children and may act as an early indication of a disturbance in red cell production (102). The level of Hb F may drop slightly after response to therapy, but the fall is not consistent, and the level usually does not return to normal, even after several years of therapy.

Chromosomal abnormalities are commonly found in constitutional aplastic anemia (105). Peripheral blood lymphocytes, bone marrow cells, and skin fibroblasts have a variety of chromosomal disturbances, including an increased frequency of breaks, chromatid exchanges, and endoreduplication (91, 92). The significance of the changes in bone marrow and fibroblasts has been disputed (106), but the variant findings may depend on conditions of culture. The marrow cells are cultured for only a few hours in vitro, while peripheral blood incubates for 48 to 72 hours before analysis. The decreased frequency of chromosome breaks in marrow cells compared to peripheral blood cells in constitutional aplastic anemia may reflect the incidence of breaks during in vitro culture (106a, 106b). Chromosome breaks may be found in normal persons in 0 to 2 per cent of peripheral blood lymphocytes, but in constitutional aplastic anemia as many as 10 to 50 per cent of the cultured lymphocytes may have breaks in one or more chromosomes (91). Similar findings have been noted in patients exposed to certain viral infections, cytotoxic agents, or irradiation, but these insults cannot explain the high incidence of abnormalities in this group of children. Some children with classical manifestations of the disease do not have chromosomal abnormalities (91), while others with familial aplastic anemia not associated with congenital abnormalities have an increased percentage of chromosome disturbances (88). A 7-month-old infant with severe growth retardation

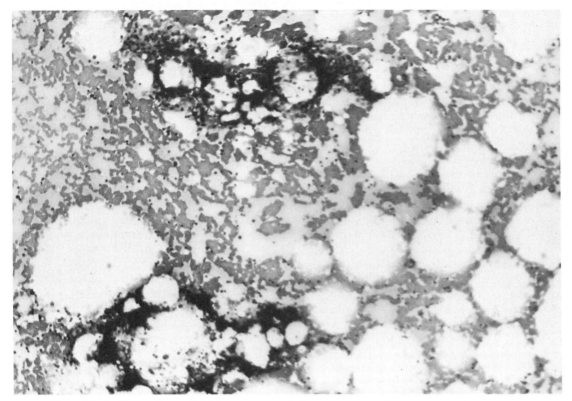

Figure 5–4.   Marked hypoplasia of the bone marrow before response to therapy in a 6-year-old boy with constitutional aplastic anemia and associated constitutional abnormalities.

and absence of the thumbs was found to have the chromosome anomalies usually associated with the syndrome, but without pancytopenia (107). As with elevation of Hb F, the chromosomal abnormalities may antedate the development of the full clinical syndrome. Children with acquired aplastic anemia usually do not have similar chromosomal abnormalities (91).

An affected child in a family with three children with the Fanconi type of constitutional aplastic anemia was also found to have paroxysmal nocturnal hemoglobinuria (108). A similar relationship occurs in acquired aplastic anemia (11). Appropriate studies to investigate this possibility should be done whenever excessive red cell destruction is suspected.

Pathophysiology

Most of the available evidence indicates that constitutional aplastic anemia is an inherited disorder with transmission as an autosomal recessive, but Fanconi has suggested that some manifestations may be present in the heterozygous state (93). Congenital anomalies or abnormal blood findings are unusual in the parents. There is an increased incidence of consanguinity in the families (109, 110). Several sibships contain two or more affected children (93, 102).

The relationship of the multiple congenital abnormalities to the hematologic disorder is not clear. It has been suggested that a similar period of embryonic development (25th to 34th day of fetal life) for the involved organ systems may allow a single defect to affect multiple systems (111), but the nature of such a defect is unknown. A similar unexplained relationship of hypoplasia of hematopoiesis and congenital abnormalities occurs in the inherited disorder, radial-platelet hypoplasia, in which a specific abnormality of the forearms is associated with hypomegakaryocytic thrombocytopenia (90). It is also difficult to explain the prolonged period of normal blood counts in these patients before onset of pancytopenia. It would be expected that a single genetic defect affecting other systems in utero would show earlier signs of affecting the hemopoietic stem cell.

The relationship of the chromosome abnormalities found in several varieties of cells to the clinical disorder is equally obscure. The breaks which occur may be spontaneous or may reflect an unusual susceptibility to breakage by common external agents, such as viruses. The findings are not specific for this type of inherited disorder, since they are also found in Bloom's syndrome, a disease in which there is stunted growth and photosensitivity of the skin (112, 113). Children with both of these disorders have an increased incidence of malignant disease. The high percentage of chromosome breaks may be an indication of increased mutability of the cell, since they are also seen in persons exposed to leukemogenic agents, such as irradiation and benzene. A tendency to produce unusual cell lines with chromosomal breaks might result in defective hemopoietic stem cells, but such a relationship is not based on any present evidence.

Certain inbred mice with hypoplastic anemia (Sl/Sl^d) appear to have a defective environment in their bone marrow for normal development of blood cell precursors, while another type of mouse (W/W^v) has pancytopenia due to defective stem cells (114). An abnormality similar to one of these defects might exist in constitutional aplastic anemia, but experiments to differentiate between these types of defects are not available.

Before drug therapy was available for this disorder, almost all patients eventually died from complications associated with pancytopenia. The use of androgens in stimulating production of blood cells in this disease has resulted in prolonged survival (61), but has also revealed an increased incidence of malignancies (115). Several patients have developed acute leukemia, including the unusual monocytic or myelomonocytic type (116). Solid tumors have been diagnosed in six young adults with constitutional aplastic anemia (115, 118). There also appears to be an increased incidence of death from malignant neo-

plasms in relatives and, in particular, in those relatives with a high likelihood of being heterozygotes for the disorder. The risk of a heterozygote dying from a malignancy has been estimated to be 0.48, a value approximately three times the normal risk (115). The incidence of heterozygotes for constitutional aplastic anemia in the general population may be 1 in 300 or higher. Using these figures, it may be calculated that 1 per cent of all deaths from malignancy may occur in these heterozygotes, and that about 1 in 20 patients dying of acute leukemia may also be heterozygotes for constitutional aplastic anemia (115, 119). There is also an increased prevalence of diabetes mellitus in relatives of patients with constitutional aplastic anemia, suggestive of an association of the genes for these two disorders (119a).

The basis for the unusual susceptibility for development of malignancies in homozygotes and heterozygotes is not clear, but it may be related to the reaction of fibroblasts from these patients to known oncogenic viruses. Cultured fibroblasts from patients with congenital aplastic anemia are more susceptible to transformation in vitro by SV40 (simian virus 40) than are cells from normal persons (117, 120, 120a). Other disorders with an increased incidence of malignancy and chromosome abnormalities, including Down's syndrome and Klinefelter's syndrome, show a similar ease of transformation (121, 122). Heterozygous relatives, who usually do not have visible chromosome abnormalities, may also have an increased susceptibility to transformation by SV40 (120), although this finding has been disputed (123). The laboratory findings of chromosome abnormalities and increased susceptibility of fibroblasts to transformation by oncogenic viruses is in accord with the increased incidence of malignancy in congenital aplastic anemia. The specific lesion which produces this predisposition, the congenital abnormalities, and the pancytopenia remains to be determined.

Treatment

The symptomatic treatment for pancytopenia in constitutional aplastic anemia is the same as that described for acquired aplastic anemia. Before 1959 transfusion was the only effective treatment for anemia, and most patients died as a result of thrombocytopenia or granulocytopenia. In 1959 and 1960 successful treatment of a few patients with androgens was reported (60, 124). In 1961 Shahidi and Diamond described the successful treatment with testosterone of several patients who had needed frequent blood transfusions (61). The percentage of reticulocytes increased in each patient, reaching a peak of 8 to 20 per cent in one to nine months after start of therapy. The hemoglobin rose in six of seven patients to levels above 9 g. per 100 ml. during the course of several months of treatment. There appeared to be a discrepancy between the reticulocyte response and the hemoglobin rise. This may have been due to decreased survival of the red cells, but survival of tagged cells was not measured. The one child who did not have a rise in hemoglobin had an unusual syndrome with amegakaryocytic thrombocytopenia at birth and pancytopenia first developing at 5 years of age and without the usual chromosomal abnormalities. The number of neutrophils rose in each patient to levels above 2500 per mm.^{3} during three to ten months of treatment. There was little effect on the platelet count, and a significant rise was only noted in one patient. When the medication was discontinued in some of the patients after several months of therapy, a prompt relapse occurred. It was possible to taper the dosage of testosterone to low maintenance levels in some patients.

The use of androgen therapy was a major advance in the treatment of these patients. There are insufficient data in the literature to compare the various forms of androgen. Testosterone propionate (1 to 2 mg. per kg.) may be taken sublingually, with an appropriate response in most patients. Occasional patients will not respond to therapy with testosterone, and other agents, such as oxymetholone, should be tried in these instances. Corticosteroids should be used to counteract the accelerated maturation of growth centers due to the androgen. Prednisone (0.5 to 1 mg. per kg.) is a suitable agent. The dosage of both of these drugs should be appropriately adjusted to obtain an optimal and continued response on the least possible amount of medication. A recent report indicates that oxymetholone (2 to 4 mg. per kg.) may be more effective than testosterone in some patients (124a).

Although most patients require continuing drug therapy, a prolonged remission may occasionally be sustained after discontinuing therapy. In two patients aged 16 and 20, remissions were still maintained 16 months and 33 months after cessation of testosterone treatment (101).

Despite the marked improvement in survival with drug therapy, the prognosis must still be guarded. Of the children treated with androgens at The Children's Hospital Medical Center in Boston, only 45 per cent were alive after seven to 11 years of therapy (21). Some of the deaths were due to malignancies. The occurrence of hepatocellular carcinoma in particular may be related to androgen therapy (71b). The continuing presence of thrombocytopenia in the patients is also a threat to their well-being.

Evaluation of the nature of the associated congenital anomalies and their correction where possible is of great importance. A few children have been shown to have growth hormone deficiency and to respond to the administration of growth hormone (95, 96). Appropriate studies for this deficiency in patients with short stature are indicated, and suitable therapy should be given if it is available. Orthopedic deformities should be corrected where necessary, particularly to provide an apposable digit in the hands when the thumb is absent or atrophic. Platelet transfusions may be needed to prevent bleeding during surgery. These children have complex problems, and their optimal care frequently involves several specialists and allied health personnel. Genetic counseling is of great importance. There is no published information about the possibility of making an in utero diagnosis on the basis of chromosomal abnormalities and susceptibility of fetal cells to transformation by virus.

PURE RED CELL APLASIA

Pure red cell aplasia is an uncommon disorder in childhood. In the absence of adequate knowledge of the etiologies of the various forms of this disease, the classification is based mainly on age of occurrence, chronicity of symptoms, and association with other hematologic disorders. Children who develop anemia early in infancy, usually before 4 to 6 months of age, are said to have congenital hypoplastic anemia. Acquired hypoplastic anemia usually occurs at an older age and may be transient or chronic. An acute, self-limited suppression of erythropoiesis is noted occasionally in children with chronic hemolysis and may result in severe anemia. Prompt and accurate diagnosis of these disorders is important because effective treatment is available in many instances.

Congenital Hypoplastic Anemia

Clinical Manifestations

In 1936 Josephs described a hypoplastic anemia with a failure of erythropoiesis in two children (125), and in 1938 Diamond and Blackfan reported four children with similar findings (126). About 100 further cases of young children with severe normochromic, normocytic anemia and isolated deficiency of red cell precursors in the bone marrow have been reported (89, 127, 128). In these children the levels of white blood cells and platelets are normal. Pallor is occasionally first noted at birth but most frequently has an insidious onset during the first six months of extrauterine life. There is no unusual incidence of prematurity or of problems during pregnancy. The infants become increasingly pale and lethargic, although the significance of early symptoms is frequently noted only in retrospect. If the pallor is overlooked, heart failure may occur because of severe anemia.

The physical findings early in the course of the disease are usually due to the effects of anemia. Pallor, tachycardia, and hemic murmurs are frequently noted. Enlargement of the liver and spleen occurs in many of the children, with return to normal size after transfusion therapy. Short stature is

found commonly, but it most frequently occurs as the result of chronic therapy with corticosteroids or blood transfusions rather than as an inherent manifestation of the disease. Congenital abnormalities of the heart, bones, or kidneys have been present in about 25 per cent of the patients, but there is no consistent pattern of anomalies such as is noted in congenital pancytopenia (Fanconi's anemia) (89, 99a, 127, 128). Five children have been described with congenital hypoplastic anemia and triphalangeal thumbs (89, 128a 128b, 128c). The association of these two rare disorders in five patients suggests that it may constitute a distinct form of congenital anemia.

In most patients, depression of erythropoiesis probably starts in the perinatal period. The effects of erythroid hypoplasia become noticeable clinically as the red cells formed during intrauterine life age and are removed from the circulation. Occasional patients have a delayed onset, with anemia first being noted past the first year of life (89, 127). Although these children are frequently described as having congenital hypoplastic anemia, in the absence of a demonstration of the precise biochemical and cellular abnormalities of this disease, it is not possible to determine whether this older group has a different, acquired disorder.

Hematologic Manifestations

The major hematologic findings in the peripheral blood are a normochromic, normocytic anemia with decreased or absent reticulocytes. Macrocytosis may occur. White blood cells and platelets are usually normal. The bone marrow has a normal or slightly decreased degree of cellularity, with a marked decrease in nucleated red cells (Fig. 5–5). The erythroid to myeloid ratio in 25 patients ranged from 1:5 to 1:240 (89). If the patient has not received corticosteroid therapy, the ratio will usually be less than 1:10, and frequently it is difficult to find more than an occasional nucleated erythrocyte. Megaloblastic changes are usually not present, although they have been noted in occasional patients (127). Increased amounts of iron are fre-

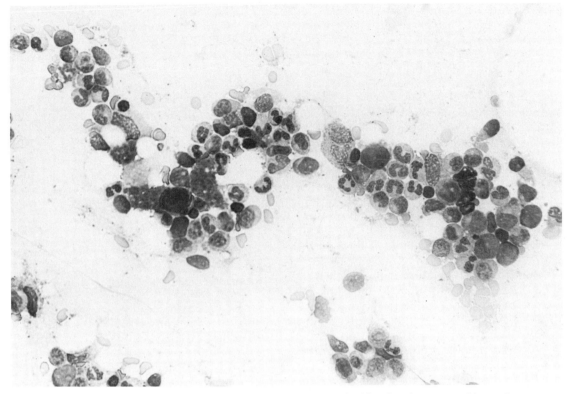

Figure 5–5.   Photomicrographs of the bone marrow from a 5-month-old girl with congenital hypoplastic anemia before treatment. Note the absence of nucleated red cells and the predominence of myeloid cells.

quently seen in the bone marrow, in contrast to the diminished iron stores in normal children after the first few months of life.

It is important not to confuse the hematologic findings in congenital hypoplastic anemia with the normal adjustments of bone marrow morphology which occur in infancy. There is normally a relative erythroid hypoplasia of the marrow starting at a week or two of age and sometimes persisting for two or three months. In premature infants in particular, anemia may develop which may be mistaken for congenital hypoplastic anemia. The relative hypoplasia of the marrow, the shortened red cell life span, and the suceptibility to hemolysis of red cells in the premature infant may combine to produce progressively severe anemia. In these infants the erythroid to myeloid ratio is usually greater than 1:10, and a mild reticulocytosis may be present. These findings in a small premature infant indicate an extreme physiologic process rather than the presence of congenital hy-poplastic anemia. Time will clarify the diagnosis in doubtful cases.

Red cell survival of transfused cells, as determined by the fall in hemoglobin in patients with severely depressed erythropoiesis, appears to be normal (89). Radioactive iron clearance is prolonged (128). Incorporation of ^{59}Fe into red cells is markedly decreased (128). Serum iron levels may be elevated or normal. Fetal hemoglobin levels have usually been appropriate for the affected infant's age.

Pathophysiology

Analysis of family data does not clearly indicate whether this disorder is inherited or congenitally acquired. In five of 28 families reported by Diamond, Allen, and Magill, there were two affected siblings, with consanguinity present in only one family of the 28 (89). The disease was not noted in members of affected families other than siblings. Approximately equal numbers of girls and boys are affected, while the male to female ratio in constitutional aplastic anemia is 2:1 (93).

Although abnormalities of tryptophan metabolism in this disorder, including excretion of excess amounts of anthranilic acid and kynurenine, have been reported on several occasions since 1953 (129–131), carefully controlled studies have failed to elicit a consistent abnormality. A study of 15 affected children failed to confirm the previous findings of excretion of increased amounts of anthranilic acid (132). After a loading dose of tryptophan, some of the affected children excreted more kynurenine and hydroxykynurenine, major metabolites of tryptophan, than did those of the control group. Studies of pyridoxine metabolites indicated that the abnormal tryptophan metabolism was not due to vitamin B_6 deficiency. Since abnormal trytophan metabolism may occur in other hematologic disorders and may possibly be due to the activity of the rate-limiting liver enzyme, tryptophan oxygenase, the occasional abnormal findings in congenital hypoplastic anemia may be a secondary effect of the disease and its therapy rather than an indicator of a primary lesion of the erythron.

Chromosomes have been normal, except in one patient with associated hypocalcemia (133).

Thymoma has been found in about 50 per cent of adults with acquired pure red cell aplasia (134). Thymic hyperplasia or tumor is very rare in children with congenital red cell aplasia (134a).

Erythropoietin levels are extremely high in this disease, indicating that there is an adequate stimulus for erythropoiesis but a lack of response of the marrow (135).

Antibodies which prevent the growth of red cell precursors have been found in some adults with acquired red cell aplasia (136–139, 139a). Five adult patients had remissions after treatment with immunosuppressive agents (139a, 140, 140a). In four cases, IgG antibody to erythroblast nuclei was found. Several patients did not respond to similar therapy. One patient did not respond to corticosteroids, cyclophosphamide, or splenectomy, but had an increase in red cell production on combined treatment with cyclophosphamide and horse antihuman thymocyte gamma globulin

(139). The response of many children with congenital hypoplastic anemia to corticosteroids (128, 141) and the occasional amelioration of the anemia by splenectomy (89) suggest a possible immunologic basis to the childhood disease. Smith has reported one child with blood group A cells with a prolonged persistence of a high anti-A titer (142). In most affected infants there is no major blood group incompatibility between mother and child (89). Search for immunoglobulins which suppress heme synthesis or which are specific for erythroblast nuclei has not been reported in children.

Treatment

CORTICOSTEROIDS. In 1951 Gasser described the successful treatment of this disorder with cortisone (143). Before that time effective treatment was limited mainly to frequent blood transfusions. Spontaneous remissions occasionally occurred in the disease, in perhaps one-fifth of the children. The remissions appear to occur more frequently after the start of adolescence. Remissions may even occur in late adolescence, after lifelong illness and several blood transfusions (89). The use of corticosteroids has been very beneficial in improving these results and allowing the discontinuance of transfusions in about 60 per cent of the children.

Administration of corticosteroids effects a reproducible and beneficial response in many patients (128, 141). A variety of drugs have been used, including prednisone, prednisolone, triamcinolone, cortisone, hydrocortisone, and corticotropin (ACTH). In responsive patients, the degree of reticulocytosis and duration of response are dependent on the drug dosage and duration of therapy. A good starting dose of prednisone is 2 mg. per kg. of body weight in divided doses daily. Reticulocytosis occurs by the fourth to eighth day, is maximal by 11 days, and is usually greater than 10 per cent in those patients who respond. In patients who do not respond by eight days, the prednisone dose may be doubled and continued for another ten days. Allen and Diamond have suggested giving as much as 30 mg. per day of prednisone to 1-month-old infants as a priming dose (141). None of their patients who responded failed to respond to this dosage. It is important that trials with dosages of corticosteroids this high be terminated promptly in the absence of a response.

The relationship between duration of therapy and height of reticulocyte response is clearly indicated in a study by Sjolin and Wranne (128). A patient was given 20 mg. of prednisone daily for two, four, or seven days, and the height of reticulocyte response was observed in each trial at nine or ten days after starting therapy. After a two-day treatment, the maximum reticulocytosis was 2.2 per cent, after a four-day treatment it was 5.2 per cent, and after seven days of therapy it was 15.4 per cent. If therapy is discontinued after an initial trial period, the reticulocytes and hemoglobin levels will usually fall to pretreatment levels. A subsequent course of treatment in responders will have results similar to those of the initial trial.

The dose of corticosteroid necessary for maintaining adequate hemoglobin concentrations (above 10 g. per 100 ml.) is usually much lower than the initial dose and may be extremely small. After an initial response, intermittent therapy may be tried and the dose adjusted according to hemoglobin and reticulocyte levels.

Since growth retardation has been a major side effect of this type of corticosteroid therapy in the past, it is very important to attempt to use intermittent therapy to allow maximal normal growth. The rate of change of height should be carefully followed in these children. Despite the use of intermittent therapy, it may be difficult to find a dose of prednisone which will allow normal growth and maintain an adequate hemoglobin level. The best dosage schedules tried so far appear to be treatment for two to four days a week or treatment for one week out of three.

Patients receiving corticosteroids may undergo remission. The remission may be sustained after stopping therapy, or a subsequent relapse may occur. On relapse, therapy with corticosteroids will again produce a response.

Many of the patients who do not respond adequately to corticosteroids have a brief or delayed rise in reticulocytes to 2 to 3 per cent. The rise is not consistent, and hemoglobin levels usually do not rise appropriately (128).

The mechanism of action of corticosteroids in this disorder is a mystery. The short, definite period needed for a response suggests that an immediate action on a primitive erythroid precursor, perhaps triggering it into cycle, is then amplified by the high levels of erythropoietin present. It is difficult to understand why maintenance therapy which provides corticosteroid levels only slightly higher than physiologic levels makes a critical difference in some patients.

TRANSFUSION. In patients who do not respond to corticosteroids, transfusions will usually be necessary to maintain adequate hemoglobin levels unless a spontaneous remission occurs. It seems best to keep the hemoglobin concentration above 8 to 9 g. per 100 ml. in order to allow full activity for the child. The choice of minimum level of hemoglobin must be made on a different basis from that in thalassemia major, since the marrow suppression afforded by high hemoglobin levels is not needed in congenital red cell aplasia. Precise comparisons of iron absorption at equivalent hemoglobin levels in these two conditions with markedly different erythroid activity in the bone marrow have not been reported.

Hemosiderosis develops in all of the patients requiring prolonged transfusion therapy (89). Skin pigmentation progressively increases, sexual maturation may be delayed or absent, osteoporosis and retardation of bone age may be present, and progressive cirrhosis may occur. Portal hypertension is present in some cirrhotic patients, with accompanying hypersplenism causing decreased platelet and granulocyte counts and shortened red cell survival. The portal hypertension does not usually cause demonstrable esophageal varices. It is interesting that blood group antibodies have not been found after multiple transfusions in children in this group, in contrast to the 20 per cent incidence in Cooley's anemia (89).

Chronic chelation therapy with deferoxamine is effective in removing a considerable amount of excess iron accumulated on the basis of transfusion therapy. A 5-year-old boy with congenital hypoplastic anemia and clinical evidence of iron overload was given 500 mg. of deferoxamine by injection once or twice daily for the next five years (144). The urinary iron loss increased considerably, and 30 per cent of the total iron administered in red cell transfusions during the period of therapy was removed by the chelating agent. At splenectomy after 41 months of chelation therapy, the spleen did not contain increased iron, but there was a large excess in the liver. The patient had an episode of congestive heart failure during the treatment period, suggesting that cardiac toxicity was not prevented. The value of chelation therapy in this disorder needs further study.

SPLENECTOMY. There is no direct relationship between splenectomy and induction of remission. Splenectomy is thus only indicated in this disorder for amelioration of significant problems secondary to hypersplenism. Overwhelming infection with pneumococci appears to occur frequently in the children with congenital hypoplastic anemia and accompanying hemosiderosis who have had their spleens removed (89).

OTHER DRUGS. The administration of various hematinics, including ferrous sulfate, crude liver extract, folic acid, riboflavin, vitamin B_{12}, testosterone, and oxymetholone, has failed to correct the anemia in these patients (89, 144).

Acquired Hypoplastic Anemia

Acquired hypoplastic anemia is an uncommon disorder in childhood. Patients in this category are usually past infancy and have anemia, reticulocytopenia, a marked decrease of red cell precursors in the marrow, normal white cells and platelets, and absence of an associated disease. The group is probably a collection of hypoplastic anemias of different etiologies. Anemia is not usually the first sign of pancytopenia occurring with acquired aplastic anemia. More than 40 per cent of adults with pure red cell aplasia have a thymoma (134), but this association is very rare in childhood (134a). Acute erythroid aplasia may occur in normal children (145), presumably with viral infections, but the duration is so brief that it is only of clinical importance in those children in whom there is also

shortened red cell survival, as described in the next section. Children described as having congenital erythroid hypoplasia with onset of symptoms past one or two years of age are probably best considered in the present category, since there is little evidence to indicate that their disorder is on a congenital or genetic basis. Four of the patients described by Diamond, Allen, and Magill were first noted to have anemia past the age of two [$2^{8}/_{12}$ to $3^{10}/_{12}$ years (89)]. Two of the children responded to corticosteroid therapy and two did not. Two of the children died, one at age 25 from transfusion hemosiderosis, and the other from pneumonia while on steroid therapy. A third child had a remission while taking steroids and was able to stop all therapy, while the fourth child still required transfusions at age 18. A boy described by O'Gorman Hughes with onset of anemia at 18 months had mild normoblastic erythroid hypoplasia requiring transfusions until a successful response to a first trial of prednisone at age 8 (127). At age 10 he still required steroid therapy to maintain a normal hemoglobin level.

A different type of hypoplastic anemia with transient erythroblastopenia and rapid remission has been described in four children aged 8 months to 4 years (146). Each child had a previously normal hemoglobin level, a marked decrease in erythroblasts in the bone marrow, hemoglobin levels at the time of illness of below 8 g. per 100 ml., and reticulocytes of 0 to 0.2 per cent. Serum iron levels were elevated, haptoglobin levels were normal, and Coombs' tests were negative. White cells and platelets were not affected. Spontaneous remission or improvement while on prednisone was rapid and was sustained without therapy.

Another variety of hypoplastic anemia with onset at infancy and rapid, although transient, recovery has been described (147). In a seven-year period, the child had two to three episodes a year of marked erythroblastopenia followed by spontaneous reticulocytosis and recovery. This disorder may be a variant of congenital hypoplastic anemia or an acquired anemia. Its etiology remains obscure.

The group of patients described above may present a misleading picture of the incidence and severity of acquired hypoplastic anemia, since most were children who were ill enough to go to large referral centers. If acquired hypoplastic anemia is more common than indicated by published reports, the period of erythroblastopenia is probably brief and not of major clinical significance.

Transient Red Cell Aplasia in Hemolytic Anemia

Periods of temporary erythroid aplasia occur in normal persons (145), and may even be fairly common, but their effect is usually only of importance in patients with shortened red cell survival. Owren first used the term "aplastic crisis" to describe the rapid drop in hemoglobin level which occurs in patients with hemolytic anemia and acute red cell aplasia (148). Aplastic crises in childhood have been reported in association with hereditary spherocytosis (149, 150), sickle cell disease (151, 152), and erythroblastosis fetalis (153), while association with additional disorders, including acquired hemolytic anemia (154) and paroxysmal nocturnal hemoglobinuria (155), has been described in adults. It is apparent that red cell aplasia of several days' duration will cause a major drop in hemoglobin level in any form of hemolytic anemia encountered in children.

Clinical and Hematologic Manifestations

Rapidly increasing pallor and listlessness without a parallel increase in severity of jaundice in a child with hemolytic anemia suggests the presence of red cell aplasia. The red cell morphology is characteristic of the type of hemolytic anemia which is present, and reticulocytes are markedly lower than the usual level associated with the degree of hemolysis and frequently are below 1 per cent. If jaundice was present before the onset of aplasia, the yellow color may become lighter as the hemoglobin drops and a smaller number of red cells are broken down each day. The bone marrow morphology depends on the stage in the episode when a sample is obtained. Although a complete absence of recognizable red cell precursors may occur at the beginning of an aplastic episode, a marrow aspirate is usually not obtained until the fall in red cell count is noticed clinically. Frequently the marrow is beginning to recover by this stage, so that most of the nucleated red cells may appear to be at one stage, either proerythroblasts, basophilic erythroblasts, or more mature nucleated cells. Reticulocytes begin to increase in the peripheral blood on the day or two following the appearance of large numbers of eosinophilic erythroblasts in the marrow. A peak reticulocytosis of 50 per cent or more may be present in the week after the onset of recovery, and the hemoglobin concentration will rapidly rise to precrisis levels. There may occasionally be rapid changes in granulocyte and platelet levels as well, but the decline and rise of the red cell count is usually the most dramatic. The findings of an unusually low hemoglobin level and an uncommonly high level of reticulocytes in a patient with chronic hemolytic anemia should arouse suspicion of a previous aplastic crisis which is in the recovery phase. The direction of change of hematocrit, reticulocytes, and bilirubin during the following days should indicate whether increased hemolysis or previous aplasia was present.

Pathogenesis

Since the course of aplastic crises in hemolytic anemia is usually brief and the occurrence of clinically significant episodes are uncommon, it has been difficult to establish the etiology of these crises. The episodes are frequently preceded or accompanied by an upper respiratory infection, and they occasionally occur within a brief time period in two siblings with hemolytic anemia (150). Viral illness is thus suspected as a major cause of these episodes. Coxsackie virus infections cause aplastic crises in mice which are similar to those in humans (156). Folic acid deficiency may be present in some patients with aplastic crisis, but it is usually difficult to determine a cause-and-effect relationship between mild folate deficiency and the onset of an aplastic crisis. Frank megaloblastosis is rarely seen.

It is important to distinguish the morphologic changes present in active erythroid marrows ("megaloblastoid") or marrows with young proerythroblasts from those seen in megaloblastosis.

Treatment

The aplastic episodes are usually short in duration, followed by a rapid and adequate erythroid response of the marrow. If the red cell life span is very short, the hemoglobin level may fall rapidly, necessitating a red cell transfusion to prevent heart failure. Children with aplasia who are awaiting a clinical response should be kept at bed rest or allowed only light activity in order in reduce the load on the heart and avoid transfusion.

SECONDARY ANEMIAS

Anemia frequently occurs in association with a variety of chronic diseases, including infections, rheumatoid arthritis, cancer, renal failure, and endocrine deficiencies. The anemia in these disorders may be due to one of several causes, including hemolysis, hemorrhage, invasion or infection of the bone marrow, iron deficiency, drug toxicity, hormone deficiencies, poor utilization of iron, or a combination of any of these. This section will deal with those secondary anemias which primarily result from inadequate erythropoiesis due to a variety of chronic diseases. Although these anemias are probably second only to iron deficiency as a cause of anemia in childhood, investigation of their pathogenesis in this age group has been limited. Some of the following discussion will thus be based on results of studies in adults, which may not be entirely applicable to children with related disorders.

Anemia of Chronic Disorders

In most chronic disorders accompanied by infection or inflammation, a mild anemia will usually develop within one to two months after the onset of the disease. The characteristic features of this anemia in adults are decreased serum iron levels, decreased iron-binding capacity, decreased bone marrow sideroblasts, and the presence of normal or increased amounts of iron in reticuloendothelial cells in the marrow (157). The latter two findings are variable in childhood, since iron stores may normally be absent after the newborn period. The term "anemia of chronic disorders" is vague and does not indicate any precise characteristics of the disease process, but it has been generally accepted to denote the specific form of anemia with the characteristics outlined above. The prominence of chronic infections in the group of disorders associated with this form of anemia has decreased markedly with the use of modern antibiotic therapy, but subacute bacterial endocarditis, chronic osteomyelitis, tuberculosis, and chronic infections following surgery still frequently result in this type of anemia. Rheumatoid arthritis is the most common of the chronic inflammatory diseases in childhood causing this anemia. The anemia is also found in other collagen diseases, ulcerative colitis and regional enteritis. Many types of malignant tumors and lymphomas will have a similar form of anemia in the absence of bone marrow invasion. In each of the conditions mentioned, the mild anemia characterized by low serum levels of iron and iron-binding capacity may be intensified by bleeding, nutritional problems, and other causes of anemia, so that a "pure" picture of the anemia of chronic disorders may frequently be blurred by anemia due to multiple other causes.

Clinical and Hematologic Manifestations

This type of anemia is rarely of sufficient degree to cause major clinical symptoms, especially with the usual limitation of activity due to the primary disease. A moderate amount of pallor may be present. Enlargement of the liver and spleen are usually not associated with this form of anemia, although splenomegaly may be present in young children in particular because of the response of lymphoid tissue to the primary disease.

The hemoglobin level falls gradually for a month or two after the onset of illness, usually reaching a plateau between 7 to 11 g. per 100 ml. The absolute reticulocyte count (reticulocytes per mm.^{3}) is normal or only slightly elevated. The morphology of the red cells may be normal, but mild hypochromia and microcytosis are frequently found. The mean corpuscular hemoglobin concentration (MCHC) frequently decreases before any change is present in the mean cell volume (MCV).

The plasma iron level is decreased, with a mean of 30 μg. per 100 ml. and a range of 10 to 70 μg. per 100 ml. in adults with this disorder (157). A comparable drop is seen in children. The iron-binding capacity is also decreased, with a mean of 200 μg. per 100 ml. and a range from 100 to 300 μg per 100 ml., a level considerably lower than that found in children with decreased serum iron due to iron deficiency. The fall in iron is rapid at the onset of the disease process, frequently occurring within a day or two (158), while the iron-binding capacity drops more slowly. The difference is probably related to the brief half-life of iron in the plasma (60 to 120 minutes) compared to the longer half-life of transferrin (8 to 12 days). The abrupt fall in serum iron is also noted with any major tissue damage such as occurs in surgical operations (159). At the onset of an infection, the decreased serum iron and normal iron-binding capacity with a low percentage of saturation of transferrin may suggest iron deficiency, but within 5 to 10 days the fall in transferrin will also become apparent if the infection continues.

Bone marrow examination is not as helpful in establishing the diagnosis in children with this disorder as it is in adults. Erythroid morphology and cellularity are usually normal. Sufficient iron is present in the bone marrow of normal adults, so as to be readily visible after staining with Prussian Blue as large blue granules (hemosiderin) inside and adjacent to histiocytic (reticuloendothelial) cells, and as small granules in about 40 per cent of nucleated red cells (sideroblasts). In the anemia of chronic disorders in adults, sideroblasts are decreased in number, and the amount of reticuloendothelial iron is increased (157). Although a variable number of sideroblasts may be found in most children, the larger deposits of iron in reticuloendothelial cells are frequently absent in children of both sexes after the newborn period until 8 to 12 years of age. In girls, the absence of large, visible iron deposits may continue throughout adolescence because of the loss of iron with menstrual flow. An absence of, or markedly decreased number of, sideroblasts and the presence of reticuloendothelial iron help support the diagnosis of anemia of chronic disorders in children, but the absence of reticuloendothelial iron does not rule out this form of anemia.

It has been recommended that iron deficiency may be detected in the presence of the anemia of chronic disorders following the response to the administration of oral iron. After therapy the bone marrow will have the expected depression of sideroblasts and normal or increased amounts of hemosiderin in histiocytic cells. A similar therapeutic-diagnostic trial may be successful in children without significant iron stores, but the prolonged period needed to restore bone marrow hemosiderin makes it of little practical value.

The study of iron kinetics in this form of anemia helps to clarify the pathogenesis but is not very helpful clinically. Clearance of injected ^{59}Fe from the plasma is unusually rapid (160). Incorporation of injected iron into red cells is normal, indicating effective erythropoiesis. Plasma iron turnover is normal or only slightly increased. Utilization of ^{59}Fe in injected red cells or hemoglobin solution is markedly decreased, indicating poor iron reutilization (158, 161).

Free erythrocyte protoporphyrin is usually elevated, as it is in iron deficiency (157). Bilirubin is usually normal. Plasma copper may be elevated. Elevation of the white cell count and rapidity of the erythrocyte sedimentation rate are dependent on the nature and activity of the primary disease process.

Pathophysiology

On the basis of studies in adults and in experimental animals, three major factors have been implicated in the pathogenesis of this anemia: decreased erythrocyte survival, inadequate response in erythropoietin levels to the degree of anemia, and disturbed utilization of iron. The survival of normal donor red cells in the patients is mildly reduced, while the survival of patients' red cells in normal recipients is normal, indicating an extracorpuscular defect (157). The cause of the increased red cell destruction is uncertain, but it may be related to a generalized hyperactivity of the reticuloendothelial system (162), fever (163), or local disturbances in infectious or inflammatory foci.

In the presence of anemia due to hemolysis, there is usually a stimulus to produce increased amounts of erythropoietin, followed by reticulocytosis. The full sequence is not present in this anemia, as indicated by the lack of significant reticulocytosis and the normal or only slightly increased rate of iron turnover. The defect is in the failure to elicit increased levels of erythropoietin and not in the ability of the marrow to respond to erythropoietin (164). In addition, erythropoietin release can be stimulated by hypoxia and cobalt in this disorder (165), suggesting that the primary defect is a deficiency in the information flow necessary for erythropoietin release in anemia.

The findings related to disturbances in iron in the bone marrow and blood and the demonstrated deficiency in reutilization of iron indicate that there is a block in the transfer of iron from the reticuloendothelial system to nucleated red cells. The decreased MCHC and MCV and elevated free erythrocyte protoporphyrin are the results of this iron-deficient type of erythropoiesis.

Treatment

The mild anemia seen with many chronic disorders seems to have a common pathogenesis and clinical manifestations, and may be a protective reaction by the body to conserve resources for other uses. It is rarely of major significance to the well-being of the affected patient, and the therapeutic efforts should be concentrated on treatment of the primary disease. Transfusion is not indicated for this mild anemia, although the presence of additional causes of anemia may increase the severity and occasionally necessitate transfusion. If iron deficiency is also felt to be present, a trial of iron therapy may be instituted in order to correct that component of the anemia. The administration of erythropoietin would probably increase red cell production, but the resultant cells might be increasingly hypochromic because of the block of iron reutilization. There is not enough purified erythropoietin available at present for such a trial, and the necessity for such therapy is not clear. Cobalt stimulates erythropoietin production, but its side effects make it an undesirable agent for use. The treatment of this mild anemia is not as important as the recognition of its characteristics and significance as an indicator of the presence of major primary disease.

Anemia of Chronic Renal Disease

Anemia is present in many types of renal disease in childhood. In acute glomerulonephritis, the mild anemia frequently is due in large part to a dilutional effect of the increased plasma volume. In the hemolytic-uremic syndrome, there is brisk hemolysis due to an extracorpuscular factor, perhaps microangiopathy, with associated thrombocytopenia and other clotting disturbances (166). This section will deal with the anemia seen in association with chronic renal failure, which results from a combination of causes, including depressed erythropoiesis, shortened red cell life span, and bleeding.

Clinical and Hematologic Manifestations

The clinical features of patients with renal failure depend primarily on the disease process which involves the kidney. Pallor due to anemia is frequently found and may occasionally be the first physical sign of kidney disease. Purpura becomes more common as the degree of uremia increases. It is usually due to abnormal platelet function (167), although other clotting disorders may also be found.

The anemia is usually normochromic and normocytic. If there has been sufficient bleeding to cause iron deficiency, hypochromia and microcytosis may be present. If the primary renal disease is associated with significant infection or inflammation, red cell indices may be decreased because of the presence of anemia of chronic disease. Abnormally shaped red cells, including burr cells with multiple spicules, and schistocytes resulting from burst blebs, are frequently found on the peripheral blood smear of adults and less commonly in children. A mild reticulocytosis is common, particularly in patients with reduced red cell survival (168). The white cells and platelets are usually normal, but the platelet count may be somewhat decreased in severe disease. The bone marrow is usually normocellular or slightly hypercellular without the specific increase in erythropoiesis which would be expected as a response to anemia. In some patients with severe chronic disease there may be marked erythroid hypoplasia.

Red cell survival measured with radioactive chromium is shortened in about one-half of the patients, with the half-life in a small number dropping as low as 10 to 15 days (normal, above 24 days) (169, 170). The clearance of injected radioactive iron is normal, unless iron deficiency is present, causing rapid clearance. Patients with anemia frequently have somewhat decreased incorporation of ^{59}Fe into their red cells, indicating ineffective erythropoiesis (171). The iron turnover is usually normal, indicating that there is an inadequate response to the stimulus of anemia. The serum iron and iron-binding capacity may be normal, but they are frequently outside of the normal range because of the additional effects of iron deficiency and the anemia of chronic disorders.

Pathophysiology

The shortened survival of red cells in patients with uremia appears to be due to an extrinsic defect, since normal red cells frequently have a shortened life span in these patients (172). The shortened survival is corrected at least partially by dialysis (173). The cause of the decreased survival is not clear, but it is probably related to acquired metabolic defects due to uremia and mechanical damage of red cells in the vessels of the renal circulation. The degree of spontaneous autohemolysis in vitro is closely correlated with the half-life of chromium-labeled red cells (174). In most patients, levels of several red cell glycolytic enzymes are normal, including glucose-6-phosphate dehydrogenase (G6PD) and lactate dehydrogenase (175). Significant hemolysis in some uremic patients may be due to a plasma factor which depresses hexose monophosphate shunt activity but does not affect G6PD (176). The effect may be potentiated by trace metals in dialysis fluids. Hemolysis may be accentuated in these patients by the use of drugs with oxidant properties. Hyperphosphatemia in uremic plasma affects red cell glycolysis by increasing glucose utilization, lactate production, and adenosine triphosphate (ATP) levels (177). Membrane adenosine triphosphatase (ATPase) is normal. The red cell 2,3-diphosphoglycerate (2,3-DPG) levels are elevated, especially in anemic subjects (177). The metabolic error responsible for the increased autohemolysis does not seem to lie in the glycolytic pathway, but, at least in some patients, the hexose monophosphate shunt or membrane transport of ions (178) may be defective.

The lack of adequate response to anemia in patients with uremia is due to ineffective erythropoiesis, reduced responsiveness to erythropoietin, and impaired release of erythropoietin. Ferrokinetic data indicate a mild to moderate degree of ineffective erythropoiesis in many uremic patients (171). The response to administration of erythropoietin to uremic rats and man is suboptimal and related to the severity of uremia (179, 180). Erythropoietin is probably produced, stored, or activated in the kidney, the rate of release possibly controlled by the level of hypoxia in the renal tissue. Severe renal disease probably destroys the capacity of the kidney to release erythropoietin, and this lack cannot be corrected by dialysis (181).

The study of patients subjected to bilateral nephrectomy and dialysis in preparation for renal transplantation has provided evidence for residual erythropoiesis in the absence of kidney erythropoietin (182–184). The hemoglobin levels are maintained at about 7 to 9 g. per 100 ml., perhaps regulated by extrarenal erythropoietin or endogenous bone marrow control.

The transfusion requirement rises in many patients on regular hemodialysis following bilateral nephrectomy, suggesting that erythropoietic activity may be present, even in severely atrophic kidneys (185).

Among the other causes of anemia in patients with chronic renal disease, iron deficiency is one of the most common. Iron may be lost by epistaxis, gastrointestinal bleeding, and repeated phlebotomy for studies or during dialysis (186). The average rate of loss of iron in patients on regular dialysis is more than five times the loss in nondialyzed patients with severe chronic renal disease (187). Folic acid deficiency causing megaloblastic erythropoiesis may also occur in patients with chronic renal disease, particularly those on hemodialysis.

Treatment

Unlike the anemia of chronic diseases, the anemia of renal disease may become severe enough to necessitate therapy. Iron and folic acid deficiencies should be sought and treated if present, especially in patients on chronic hemodialysis. Red cell transfusions may be helpful, but the hemoglobin level at which transfusion is needed varies between children. In general, children will be able to maintain optimal activity at hemoglobin levels above 7 or 8 g. per 100 ml. In many children below this level, unless activity is markedly restricted by the primary disease, anemia will cause lassitude, a limitation of physical activity, and a tendency to tire easily. In these children, red cell transfusions may be administered at first on a trial basis to see if there is an improvement in well-being. If successful in correcting symptoms of fatigue, transfusions may be given when symptoms begin to reappear as hemoglobin levels fall. Some children will not have significant symptoms of anemia, even at levels of hemoglobin below 7 g. per 100 ml.

Other forms of therapy have been suggested, but they have not been used in children and have had only equivocal success in adults. Splenectomy has been successful in improving red cell survival and decreasing the transfusion requirement in patients with a marked reduction in red cell survival (188). Most patients will probably not benefit sufficiently to warrant the surgery, and it is to be particularly avoided in children because of the increased danger of infection following surgery. A satisfactory response to weekly injections of testosterone enanthate has been noted in fifteen men in a maintenance dialysis program (189). The need for transfusions was eliminated in most of the treated patients. In two iron-deficient patients, response to testosterone did not occur until after adequate iron replacement. The men had improved appetites and a sense of well-being. The side effects included acne, jaundice, and hematomas at injections sites. In another study of the effect of oxymetholone on six uremic men with high blood urea nitrogen levels (190), there was no response to therapy. The use of testosterone in children with renal disease would produce side effects disturbing to patients and their families, and it probably should only be attempted if anemia becomes a severe problem.

Anemia of Endocrine Disease

Anemia is found in association with deficiency of function of the pituitary, thyroid, and adrenal glands.

Hypopituitarism

The anemia seen in patients with pituitary insufficiency is normochromic and normocytic. It is due to bone marrow hypoplasia. The anemia is probably mainly related to a combined deficiency of thyroid, adrenal, and gonadal hormones, and it is corrected by administration of these hormones (191).

Hypothyroidism

The anemia which commonly accompanies hypothyroidism and cretinism is normochromic and normocytic. The appearance of the red cells may be modified by the presence of factors in addition to hypothyroidism. The cells in the young cretin are large, as is usual in the newborn period. In the presence of iron deficiency, the cells in hypothyroidism are microcytic, while with deficiencies of folate or vitamin B_{12}, the cells are macrocytic (192). The presence of small numbers of irregularly contracted red cells, or burr cells, has been described in 15 of 23 adults with untreated hypothyroidism (193). The finding awaits confirmation in children. The hemoglobin level is usually no lower than 8 g. per 100 ml. The anemia is due to mild bone marrow hypoplasia. There is a decrease in total red cell mass (194). Red cell survival is normal (195). Plasma clearance of radioactive iron is normal, as is incorporation of ^{59}Fe into red cells. The plasma iron turnover is decreased. The results of ferrokinetic studies indicate decreased red cell production without ineffective erythropoiesis.

Red cell levels of glucose-6-phosphate dehydrogenase are decreased in children with hypothyroidism of hypopituitarism before treatment and they increase with therapy (196). This finding may reflect degree of reticulocytosis and mean cell age rather than a direct effect of hormones on enzyme levels. Thyroid hormone does affect red cell metabolism directly by increasing the concentration of 2,3-DPG (197). In hyperthyroidism there is decreased affinity of hemoglobin for oxygen due to elevated levels of 2,3-DPG (198). It would be expected that oxygen affinity of hemoglobin would be increased and 2,3-DPG would be decreased in hypothyroidism, but adequate data are not available.

The anemia of hypothyroidism is corrected by adequate treatment with thyroid hormone.

Hypoadrenalism

A normochromic, normocytic anemia may be seen in Addison's disease (199). The reduction in red cell mass may be greater than indicated by the mild degree of anemia because of the usual decrease in plasma volume in this disease. Treatment with ACTH or adrenal hormones corrects the anemia.

LEUKOERYTHROBLASTIC ANEMIA

Leukoerythroblastic anemia, or myeloid metaplasia, is rare in childhood. The disorder is characterized by the presence of anemia and of nucleated red cells and immature white cells in the peripheral blood, usually on the basis of hemopoiesis in the spleen and liver and impairment of production of blood cells in the marrow. There are frequently giant platelets in the blood and

a considerable degree of poikilocytosis. Splenic and hepatic hemopoiesis are present in fetal life, and newborn infants may have a leukoerythroblastic blood picture, with immature white cells and nucleated red cells for a short period after birth, usually no longer than a week. A similar blood response may be seen during the course of leukemia or lymphoma or with invasion of the marrow by a malignant tumor. Several unusual instances of leukoerythroblastic anemia not associated with the above causes will be summarized below. A photomicrograph of leukoerythroblastosis may be found on Color Plate I.

Osteopetrosis

Osteopetrosis is a rare inherited disease characterized by increased thickening of the cortex of the bones (200). The marrow spaces are reduced in volume. The bones are brittle, and radiographic studies of a fracture may suggest the diagnosis. Growth is usually retarded.

Enlargement of the liver and spleen is common, with extramedullary hemopoiesis occurring in these organs. Anemia is common, frequently accompanied by nucleated red cells and immature white cells in the peripheral blood. Although in some patients hemolysis may contribute to the anemia (201), perhaps on the basis of hypersplenism or defective red cells produced in extramedullary sites, other patients have no evidence of a shortened red cell survival (202). Thrombocytopenia is common, and the white cell count may be high. Adequate bone marrow samples are very difficult to obtain by aspiration.

The hematologic problems appear to be primarily due to limitation of the marrow space by excessive calcification and, secondarily, to the effects of hypersplenism in some patients. The process may begin during intrauterine life, producing anemia and other blood abnormalities at birth (202).

The prognosis depends on the severity of the bone disease, some infants dying as early as three months of age (202). Treatment for the blood disorder consists of replacement therapy when indicated for anemia or bleeding due to thrombocytopenia. The decision to perform splenectomy because of evidence of hypersplenism is as difficult to make in this disease as it is in adults with idiopathic myeloid metaplasia. The spleen may be a major source of red cell production in these children, and the effects of removal of that source must be balanced against the severity of hemolysis and thrombocytopenia. Radioisotope studies may be of help in evaluating the necessity for removing the spleen. Splenectomy has resulted in improvement of anemia, thrombocytopenia, and red cell survival in some patients (201).

Myelofibrosis

Myelofibrosis is primarily a disorder of adults, the most common age of onset being in the sixth decade (203). Although several hundred cases have been reported in adults, only about ten have been described in children. The children have had anemia, leukoerythroblastosis, and hepatosplenomegaly (204). A possible early stage of myeloid metaplasia without myelofibrosis has been described in a few children. The presence of fibrous tissue in the marrow may indicate a late stage in the disease. The pediatric cases have occurred in girls ranging from four months of age to ten years at clinical onset. The early clinical signs were usually pallor, easy fatigability, anemia, and splenomegaly. Roentgenographic examination of the bones is usually normal. The peripheral blood contains nucleated red cells, metamyelocytes, myelocytes, and poikilocytes. The white blood count is elevated, but thrombocytopenia is not common in affected children, although it does occur in adults (204). Bone marrow aspiration usually is not adequate in patients with this disorder, and a bone marrow biopsy should be done to confirm the diagnosis.

The etiology of the disorder is not known. Fibrosis of the marrow may occur after exposure to toxic substances or in association with leukemia. Many adult patients develop acute granulocytic leukemia during the course of the disease (205), but this may be related to therapy in some instances.

The finding of many immature white cells in the peripheral blood may suggest the diagnosis of chronic myelogenous leukemia (CML). The two conditions may usually be easily distinguished, particularly the infantile form of CML in which there are very high fetal hemoglobin levels.

Leukocyte alkaline phosphatase is usually markedly decreased in the common type of CML (206), while it is variable in myelofibrosis in adults. Examination of the bone marrow will usually be the best way to confirm either diagnosis. The presence of a Ph[1] chromosome in 90 per cent of patients with the common type of CML will also help to make the differentiation (207).

The prognosis in adults is poor, most patients dying within five years after onset. The outlook in children appears to be equally bad. Supportive therapy consists mainly of red cell transfusions. Splenectomy should be avoided except in some patients with a marked decrease in red cell survival. Therapy with androgens has been of some benefit in adults, but there are no reported trials of therapy in affected children.

An unusual child with the McCune-Albright syndrome (polyostotic fibrous dysplasia, abnormal skin pigmentation, advanced skeletal maturation, precocious puberty, hyperthyroidism) and myelofibrosis has been described (208). The child developed a huge spleen with a shortened red cell survival. The enlarged spleen also caused considerable physical discomfort. Splenectomy resulted in a return of red cell survival to normal and a temporary improvement in clinical status. However, the hemoglobin level fell progressively during the postoperative six months, and the platelet count was also decreased.

Myeloproliferative Disease

A family with nine children with a peculiar myeloproliferative disease is perhaps a unique instance of possible inheritance of this type of disorder (209). There were marked hepatosplenomegaly and leukocytosis in the affected children, with anemia, immature granulocytes in the peripheral blood, and thrombocytopenia. Extramedullary erythropoiesis was present in liver and spleen. Three children died with the disorder, but two others appeared to recover completely during adolescence.

A marked myeloproliferative reaction occurs in some children with Down's syndrome in infancy. The extreme proliferation of granulocytes, which may be confused with acute leukemia, usually subsides spontaneously. There does not appear to be a direct connection between this transient disorder and the propensity for leukemia occurring somewhat later in life in children with Down's syndrome (210).

A myeloproliferative syndrome has been described in a 5½-month-old child with an absent C-group chromosome in the bone marrow (211). Massive hepatosplenomegaly was present, as well as anemia, thrombocytopenia, leukocytosis, and nucleated red cells and immature white cells in the peripheral blood. The progression of bone marrow findings to 51 months of age was suggestive of preleukemia, but overt leukemia was not present.

References

1. Ehrlich, P.: Über einen Fall von Anaemie mit Bemerkungen über regenerative Veränderungen des Knochenmarkes. Charité-Ann. *13*:300, 1888.
2. Fanconi, G.: Familiäre infantile perniziosaartige Anämie (perniziöses Blutbild und Konstitution). Jb. Kinderheilk. *117*:257, 1927.
3. Rubin, D., Weisberger, A. S., et al.: Early detection of drug-induced erythropoietic depression. J. Lab. Clin. Med. *56*:453, 1960.
4. McElfresh, A. E., and Huang, N. N.: Bone marrow depression resulting from the administration of methicillin: With a comment on the value of the serum iron determination. New Engl. J. Med. *266*:246, 1962.
5. Gurwitz, M. R., and Berlin, N. J.: Erythrokinetic studies in severe bone marrow failure of diverse etiology. Blood *18*:637, 1961.
6. Viala, J. J., Barbier, Y., et al.: Confrontation entre histologie médullaire et métabolisme du fer radio-actif dans les insuffisances médullaires et valeur pronostique de ce dernier examen. Nouv. Rev. Fr. Hématol. *9*:841, 1969.
7. Van Dyke, D. C., Shkurkin, C., et al.: Differences in distribution of erythropoietic and reticuloendothelial marrow in hematologic disease. Blood *30*:364, 1967.
8. Ronai, P., Winchell, H. S., et al.: Whole body scanning of ^{59}Fe for evaluating body distribution of erythropoietic marrow, splenic sequestration of red cells and hepatic deposition of iron. J. Nucl. Med. *10*:469, 1969.
9. Mohler, D. N., and Leavell, B. S.: Aplastic anemia: An analysis of 50 cases. Ann. Intern. Med. *49*:326, 1958.
10. Hathaway, W. E., and Githens, J. H.: Pancytopenia with hyperplastic marrow. Am. J. Dis. Child. *10*:389, 1961.
11. Lewis, S. M., and Dacie, J. V.: The aplastic anaemia–paroxysmal nocturnal haemoglobinuria syndrome. Br. J. Haematol. *13*:236, 1967.

12. Miller, D. R., Baehner, R. L., et al.: Paroxysmal nocturnal hemoglobinuria in childhood and adolescence. Clinical and erythrocyte metabolic studies. Pediatrics *39*:675, 1967.
13. Tarrow, A. B., Turkel, H., et al.: Infusions via the bone marrow and biopsy of the bone and bone marrow. Anesthesia *13*:501, 1952.
14. Ellis, L. D., Jensen, W. N., et al.: Needle biopsy of bone and marrow. An experience with 1,445 biopsies. Arch. Intern. Med. *114*:213, 1964.
15. Jamshidi, K., and Swaim, W. R.: Bone marrow biopsy with unaltered architecture: A new biopsy device. J. Lab. Clin. Med. *77*:335, 1971.
16. Melhorn, D. K., Gross, S., et al.: Acute childhood leukemia presenting as aplastic anemia. The response to corticosteroids. J. Pediat. *77*:647, 1970.
17. Sturgeon, P.: Idiopathic aplastic anemia in children: Its early differentiation from aleukemic leukemia by bone marrow aspiration. Pediatrics *8*:216, 1951.
18. Gaffney, P. D., Hausman, C. F., et al.: Experience with smears of aspirates from bone marrow in the diagnosis of neuroblastoma. Am. J. Clin. Pathol. *31*:213, 1959.
19. Delta, B. G., and Pinkel, D.: Bone marrow aspiration in children with malignant tumours. J. Pediat. *64*:542, 1964.
20. Bloom, G. E., and Diamond, L. K.: Prognostic value of fetal hemoglobin levels in acquired aplastic anemia. New Engl. J. Med. *278*:304, 1968.
21. Li, F. P., Alter, B. P., et al.: The mortality of acquired aplastic anemia in children. Blood *40*:153, 1972.
22. Hammond, G. D., Ishikawa, A., et al.: Relationship between erythropoietin and severity of anemia in hypoplastic and hemolytic states, In *Erythropoiesis*. Jacobson, L. O., and Doyle, M. (eds.), New York, Grune & Stratton, 1962, p. 351.
23. Stohlman, F., Jr.: Erythropoiesis. New Engl. J. Med. *267*:392, 1962.
24. Metcalf, D., and Moore, M. A. S.: *Haemopoietic Cells: Their Origin, Migration and Differentiation.* (Frontiers of Biology Ser., No. 24). Amsterdam, North-Holland Publishing Company, 1971.)
25. Lewis, J. P., and Trobaugh, F. E., Jr.: Haematopoietic stem cells. Nature (Lond.) *204*:589, 1964.
26. Becker, A. J., McCulloch, E. A., et al.: The effect of differing demands for blood cell production on DNA synthesis by hemopoietic colony-forming cells of mice. Blood *26*:296, 1965.
27. Porteous, D. D., and Lajtha, L. G.: On stem cell recovery after irradiation. Br. J. Haematol. *12*:177, 1966.
28. Wu, A. M., Till, J. E., et al.: A cytological study of the capacity for differentiation of normal hemopoietic colony-forming cells. J. Cell. Physiol. *69*:177, 1967.
29. Curry, J. L., and Trenton, J. J.: Hemopoietic spleen colony studies. I. Growth and differentiation. Dev. Biol. *15*:395, 1967.

30. Krantz, S. B., and Jacobson, L. O.: *Erythropoietin and the Regulation of Erythropoiesis.* Chicago, University of Chicago Press, 1970.

31. Filmanowicz, E., and Gurney, C. W.: Studies on erythropoiesis. XVI. Response to a single dose of erythropoietin in the polycythemic mouse. J. Lab. Clin. Med. 57:65, 1961.

32. Erslev, A. J.: The effect of anemia anoxia on the cellular development of nucleated red cells. Blood 14:386, 1959.

33. Chan, S. H., Metcalf, D., et al.: Stimulation and inhibition by normal human serum of colony-formation *in vitro* by bone marrow cells. Br. J. Haematol. 20:329, 1971.

34. Abilgaard, C. F., and Simone, J. V.: Thrombopoiesis. Semin. Hematol. 4:424, 1967.

35. Kirshbaum, J. D., Matsuo, T., et al.: A study of aplastic anemia in an autopsy series with special reference to atomic bomb survivors in Hiroshima and Nagasaki. Blood 38:17, 1971.

35a. Yunis, A. A.: Chloramphenicol-induced bone marrow suppression. Semin. Hematol. 10: 225, 1973.

36. Best, W. R.: Chloramphenicol-associated blood dyscrasias. A review of cases submitted to the American Medical Association Registry. J.A.M.A. 201:181, 1967.

37. Wallerstein, R. D., Condit, P. K., et al.: Statewide study of chloramphenicol therapy and fatal aplastic anemia. J.A.M.A. 208:2045, 1969.

38. Saidi, P., Wallerstein, R. D., et al.: Effect of chloramphenicol on erythropoiesis. J. Lab. Clin. Med. 57:247, 1961.

39. Yunis, A. A., Smith, U. S., and Restrepo, A.: Reversible bone marrow suppression from chloramphenicol. Arch. Intern. Med. 126: 272, 1970.

40. Nagao, T., and Mauer, A. M.: Concordance for drug-induced aplastic anemia in identical twins. New Engl. J. Med. 281:7, 1969.

41. Erslev, A. J.: Drug-induced blood dyscrasias. J.A.M.A. 188:531, 1964.

42. Robins, M. M.: Aplastic anemia secondary to anticonvulsants. Am. J. Dis. Child. 104:614, 1962.

43. Aksoy, M., Dinçol, K., et al.: Clinical and laboratory observations in 32 patients with aplastic anemia and two with acute myeloblastic leukemia due to chronic benzene poisoning. Abstracts XIII Int. Congr. Hematol., 1970, p. 134.

44. Roxman, C., Ribas, M. M., et al.: Estudio clinico hematologica de 43 casos de anemia aplastica con particular atencion a las de origin benzolico (20 casos). Med. Clin. 44:10, 1965.

45. DeGowin, R. L.: Benzene exposure and aplastic anemia followed by leukemia fifteen years later. J.A.M.A. 185:748, 1963.

46. Sanchez-Medal, L., Castanedo, J. P., et al.: Insecticides and aplastic anemia. New Engl. J. Med. 269:1365, 1963.

47. Powars, D.: Aplastic anemia secondary to glue sniffing. New Engl. J. Med. 273:700, 1965.

48. Levy, R. N., Sawitsky, A., et al.: Fatal aplastic anemia after hepatitis. New Engl. J. Med. 273:1118, 1965.

49. Schwartz, E., Baehner, R. L., et al.: Aplastic anemia following hepatitis. Pediatrics 37: 681, 1966.

50. Rubin, E., Gottlieb, C., et al.: Syndrome of hepatitis and aplastic anemia. Am. J. Med. 45:88, 1968.

51. Rosner, F.: Aplastic anemia and viral hepatitis. Lancet 2:1080, 1970.

52. Conrad, M. E., Schwartz, F. D., et al.: Infectious hepatitis—a generalized disease. Am. J. Med. 37:789, 1964.

53. Schwachman, H., Diamond, L. K., et al.: The syndrome of pancreatic insufficiency and bone marrow dysfunction. J. Pediatr. 65: 645, 1964.

54. Mozziconacci, P., Boisse, J., et al.: Hypoplasie du pancreas exocrine avec troubles hématologiques. Arch. Fr. Pédiatr. 24:741, 1967.

55. Hathaway, W. E., Githens, J. H., et al.: Aplastic anemia, histiocytosis and erythroderma in immunologically deficient children. Possible runt disease. New Engl. J. Med. 273:953, 1965.

56. Talerman, A., and Amigo, A.: Thymoma associated with aregenerative and aplastic anemia in a five-year old child. Cancer 21:1212, 1968.

57. Hirst, E., and Robertson, T. I.: Thymoma and erythroblastopenia. Medicine (Baltimore) 46: 225, 1967.

58. Knospe, W. H., and Crosby, W. H.: Aplastic anemia: A disorder of the bone-marrow sinusoidal microcirculation rather than stem-cell failure? Lancet 1:20, 1971.

58a. Samson, J. P., Hulstaert, C. E., et al.: Fine structure of the bone marrow sinusoidal wall in idiopathic and drug-induced panmyelopathy. Acta Haematol. 48:218, 1972.

59. Kennedy, B. J., and Gilbertson, A. S.: Increased erythropoiesis induced by androgenic-hormone therapy. New Engl. J. Med. 256:719, 1953.

60. Shahidi, N. T., and Diamond, L. K.: Testosterone-induced remission in aplastic anemia. A.M.A. J. Dis. Child. 98:293, 1959.

61. Shahidi, N. T., and Diamond, L. K.: Testosterone-induced remission in aplastic anemia of both acquired and congenital types. New Engl. J. Med. 264:953, 1961.

62. Allen, D. M., Fine, M. H., et al.: Oxymetholone therapy in aplastic anemia. Blood 32:83, 1968.

63. Killander, A., Lundmark, K., et al.: Idiopathic aplastic anemia in children. Acta Paediatr. Scand. 58:10, 1969.

64. McCredie, K. B.: Oxymetholone in refractory anemia. Br. J. Haematol. 17:265, 1969.

65. Sanchez-Medal, L., Gomez-Leal, A., et al.: Anabolic androgenic steroids in the treatment of acquired aplastic anemia. Blood 34:283, 1969.

66. Daiber, A., Heruvé, L., et al.: Treatment of aplastic anemia with nandrolone decanoate. Blood 36:748, 1970.

67. Davis, S., and Rubin, A. D.: Treatment and prognosis in aplastic anemia. Lancet 1:871, 1972.

67a. O'Gorman Hughes, D. W.: Bone-marrow depression in childhood. Med. J. Aust. 1:357, 1973.

67b. Najean, Y., Laprevotte, I., et al.: Évolution à long terme des insuffisances médullaires traitées initialement avec suceès par les androgènes. Nouv. Press Méd. 2:359, 1973.

68. Desposito, F., Akatsuka, J., et al.: Bone marrow failure in pediatric patients. J. Pediatr. 64:683, 1964.

69. Heyn, R. M., Ertel, I. J., et al.: Course of acquired aplastic anemia in children treated with supportive care. J.A.M.A. 208:1372, 1969.

70. Duarte, L., Sanchez-Medal, L., et al.: The erythropoietic effects of anabolic steroids. Proc. Soc. Exp. Biol. Med. 125:1030, 1967.

71. Gorshein, D., Murphy, S., et al.: Comparative study on the erythropoietic function of androgens and their mode of action in mice. Clin. Res. 18:405, 1970.

71a. Besa, E. L., Gorshein, D., et al.: Effective erythropoiesis induced by 5β-pregnane-3β-hydroxy-20-one in squirrel monkeys. J. Clin. Invest. 52:2278, 1973.

71b. Johnson, F. L., Teagler, J. R., et al.: Association of androgenic anabolic steroid therapy with development of hepatocellular carcinoma. Lancet 2:1273, 1972.

72. Freireich, E. J., Klinman, A., et al.: Response to repeated platelet transfusions from the same donor. Ann. Intern. Med. 59:227, 1963.

73. Flatow, F., and Freireich, E. J.: Effect of splenectomy on the response to platelet transfusion in three patients with aplastic anemia. New Engl. J. Med. 274:242, 1966.

74. Yankee, R. A., Grumet, F., et al.: Platelet transfusion therapy. The selection of compatible platelet donors for refractory patients by lymphocyte HL-A typing. New Engl. J. Med. 281:1208, 1969.

75. Bellanti, J. A., and Pinkel, D.: Idiopathic aplastic anemia treated with methyltestosterone and fresh platelets. J.A.M.A. 178:70, 1961.

76. Lovin, R. H., Baieh, F. H. D., et al.: Platelet therapy and red cell defect in aplastic anemia. Arch. Intern. Med. 114:278, 1964.

77. Yankee, R. A., Friereich, E. J., et al.: Replacement therapy using normal and CML leukocytes. Blood 24:844, 1964.

78. Buckner, D., Graw, R. G., Jr., et al.: Leukapheresis by continuous flow centrifugation in patients with chronic myelocytic leukemia. Blood 33:353, 1969.

79. Graw, R. G., Jr., Herzig, G., et al.: Granulocyte transfusion therapy: Septicemia due to gram-negative bacteria. New Engl. J. Med. 287:367, 1972.

80. Djerassi, I., Kim, J. I., et al.: Continuous flow filtration leukophoresis. Transfusion 12:75, 1972.

80a. Harris, M. B., Djerassi, I., et al.: Granulocytes (PMN) for transfusion: Viability and function. Pediat. Res. 7:352, 1973 (abstract).

81. Levitan, A. A., and Perry, S.: The use of an isolator system in cancer chemotherapy. Am. J. Med. 44:234, 1968.

82. Burke, J. F.: A new approach to isolation. Hosp. Practice 2:23, 1967.

82a. Rykner, G., Francoual, C., et al.: La flore bactérienne des aplastiques. Nouv. Presse Méd. 2:1823, 1973.

83. Speck, B., and Kissling, M.: Successful bone marrow grafts in experimental aplastic anemia using antilymphocytic serum for conditioning. Rev. Eur. Etud. Clin. Biol. 15:1047, 1971.

84. Mathé, G., Amiel, J. L., et al.: Bone marrow grafts in man after conditioning by antilymphocytic serum. Br. Med. J. 2:131, 1970.

85. Thomas, E. D., Buckner, C. D., et al.: Aplastic anemia treated by marrow transplants. Lancet 1:284, 1972.

85a. Buckner, C. D., Clift, R. A., et al.: Aplastic anemia treated by marrow transplantation. Transplantation Proc. 5:913, 1973.

85b. Storb, R., Thomas, E. D., et al.: Allogeneic marrow grafting for treatment of aplastic anemia. Blood 43:157, 1974.

86. Robins, M. M., and Noyes, W. D.: Aplastic anemia treated with bone marrow transfusion from an identical twin. New Engl. J. Med. 265:974, 1961.

87. Estren, S., and Dameshek, W.: Familial hypoplastic anemia of childhood. Am. J. Dis. Child. 73:671, 1947.

88. Zaizov, R., Mathoth, Y., et al.: Familial aplastic anaemia without congenital malformations. Acta. Paediatr. Scand. 58:151, 1969.

89. Diamond, L. K., Allen, D. M., et al.: Congenital (erythroid) hypoplastic anemia. Am. J. Dis. Child. 102:403, 1961.

90. Hall, J. G., Levin, J., et al.: Thrombocytopenia with absent radius (TAR). Medicine (Baltimore) 48:411, 1969.

91. Bloom, G. E., Warner, S., et al.: Chromosome abnormalities in constitutional aplastic anemia. New Engl. J. Med. 274:8, 1966.

92. Swift, M. R., and Hirschhorn, K.: Fanconi's anemia. Inherited susceptibility to chromosome breakage in various tissues. Ann. Intern. Med. 65:496, 1966.

93. Fanconi, G.: Familial constitutional panmyelocytopathy, Fanconi's anemia. I. Clinical aspects. Semin. Hematol. 4:233, 1967.

94. Juhl, J. H., Wesenberg, R. L., et al.: Roentgenographic findings in Fanconi's anemia. Radiology 89:646, 1967.

95. Pochedly, C., Collipp, P. J., et al.: Fanconi's anemia with growth hormone deficiency. J. Pediatr. 79:93, 1971.

96. Zachman, M., Illig, R., et al.: Fanconi's anemia with isolated growth hormone deficiency. J. Pediatr. 80:159, 1972.

97. Barrière, H.: Dyskératose congenitale avec thrombopenie. Ses relations avec l'anemie de Fanconi. Sem. Hop. Paris 46:3083, 1970.

98. Van Voolen, G. A., Sterrer, W., et al.: Dyskeratosis congenita: Relationship to Fanconi's anemia (abstract). Am. Soc. Hematol. 14th Annual Meeting. San Francisco, Calif., Dec., 1971.

99. Ortega, J. A., Swanson, V., et al.: Aplastic anemia associated with congenital dyskeratosis and thymic dysplasia (abstract). Am. Soc. Hematol. 14th Annual Meeting. San Francisco, Calif., Dec., 1971.

99a. Minagi, H., and Steinbach, H. L.: Roentgen appearance of anomalies associated with hypoplastic anemias of childhood: Fanconi's anemia and congenital hypoplastic anemia (erythrogenesis imperfecta). Am. J. Roentgenol. 97:100, 1966.

100. Pochedly, C.: Fanconi's anemia: Clues to early recognition. Clin. Pediatr. 11:20, 1972.

101. McDonald, R., and Mibashan, R. S.: Prolonged remission in Fanconi type anemia. Helv. Paediatr. Acta 23:566, 1968.

102. Shahidi, N. T., Gerald, P. S., et al.: Alkali-resistant hemoglobin in aplastic anemia of both acquired and congenital types. New Engl. J. Med. 266:117, 1962.

103. Sjolin, S., and Wranne, L.: Erythropoietic dysfunction in a case of Fanconi's anaemia. Acta Haematol. (Basel) 28:230, 1962.

104. Betke, K., and Kleihauer, E.: Fetaler und bleibender Blutfarbstoff in Erythrozyten und Erythroblasten von menschlichen Feten und Neugeborenen. Blut 4:241, 1958.

105. Schroeder, T. M., Anschutz, F., et al.: Spontane Chromosomenaberrationen bei familiärer Panmyelopathie. Humangenetik 1:194, 1964.

106. Schmid, W.: Familial constitutional panmyelocytopathy, Fanconi's anemia. II. Discussion of the cytogenetic findings in Fanconi's anemia. Semin. Hematol. 4:241, 1967.

106a. Walman, S. R., and Swift, M.: Bone marrow chromosomes in Fanconi's anemia. J. Med. Genet. 9:473, 1972.

106b. Shahid, M. J., Khouri, F. P., et al.: Fanconi's anemia: Report of a patient with significant chromosomal abnormalities in bone marrow cells. J. Med. Genet. 9:474, 1972.

107. Varela, M. A., and Sternberg, W. H.: Preanemic state in Fanconi's anemia. Lancet 2:566, 1967.

108. Dacie, J. U., and Gilpin, A.: Refractory anaemia (Fanconi's type). Its incidence in three members of one family, with in one case a relationship to chronic haemoglobinuria (Marchiafava-Micheli disease of "nocturnal haemoglobinuria"). Arch. Dis. Child. 19:155, 1944.

109. Boivin, P., Bousser, J., et al.: Pancytopénie avec malformations multiples (syndrome de Fanconi). Présentation de 3 nouveaux cas et revue de la littérature. Arch. Fr. Pédiatr. 15:1289, 1958.

110. Nilsson, L. R.: Chronic pancytopenia with multiple congenital abnormalities (Fanconi's anemia). Acta Paediatr. (Stockholm) 49:518, 1960.

111. Althoff, H.: Zur Panmyelopathie Fanconi als Zustandsbild multipler Abartungen. Z. Kinderheilkd. 72:267, 1953.

112. German, J., Archibald, R., et al.: Chromosomal breakage in a rare and probably genetically determined syndrome of man. Science 148:506, 1965.

113. Schroeder, T. M., and Kurth, R.: Spontaneous chromosomal breakage and high incidence of leukemia in inherited disease. Blood 37:96, 1971.

114. Bernstein, S. E., Russell, E. S., et al.: Two hereditary mouse anemias (Sl/Sl^d and W/W^v) deficient in response to erythropoietin. Ann. N. Y. Acad. Sci. 149:475, 1968.

115. Swift, M.: Fanconi's anemia in the genetics of neoplasia. Nature (Lond.) 230:370, 1971.

116. Garriga, S., and Crosby, W. H.: The incidence of leukemia in families of patients with hypoplasia of the marrow. Blood 14:1008, 1959.

117. Dosik, H., Hsu, L. Y., et al.: Leukemia in Fanconi's anemia: Cytogenetic and tumor virus susceptibility studies. Blood 36:341, 1970.

118. Bernstein, M. S., Hunter, R. L., et al.: Hepatoma and peliosis hepatitis developing in a patient with Fanconi's anemia. New Engl. J. Med. 284:1135, 1971.

119. Miller, R. W., and Todaro, G. J.: Viral transformations of cells from persons at high risk of cancer. Lancet 1:81, 1969.

119a. Swift, M., Sholman, L., et al.: Diabetes mellitus and the gene for Fanconi's anemia. Science 178:308, 1972.

120. Todaro, G. J., Green, M., et al.: Susceptibility of human diploid fibroblast strains to transformation by SV40 virus. Science 153:1252, 1966.

120a. Beard, M. E. J., Young, D. E., et al.: Fanconi's anemia. Quart. J. Med. 42:403, 1973.

121. Todaro, G. J., and Martin, G. M.: Increased susceptibility of Down's syndrome fibroblasts to transformation by SV40. Proc. Soc. Exp. Biol. Med. 124:1232, 1967.

122. Muckerjee, D., Bowen, J., et al.: Simian papovavirus 40 transformation of cells from cancer patients with XY/XXY mosaic Klinefelter's syndrome. Cancer Res. 30:1769, 1970.

123. Young, D.: S.V. 40 transformation of cells with Fanconi's anemia. Lancet 1:294, 1971.

124. McDonald, R.: Treatment of Fanconi's anaemia. Lancet 2:1146, 1960.

124a. Krawitz, S., Altman, H., et al.: Oxymetholone therapy in children with aplastic and other refractory anemias. S. Afr. Med. J. 47:1864, 1973.

125. Josephs, W. H.: Anemia of infancy and early childhood. Medicine (Baltimore) 15:307, 1936.

126. Diamond, L. K., and Blackfan, K. D.: Hypoplastic anemia. Am. J. Dis. Child. 56:464, 1938.

127. O'Gorman Hughes, D. W.: Hypoplastic anaemia in infancy and childhood: Erythroid hypoplasia. Arch. Dis. Child. 36:349, 1960.

128. Sjolin, S., and Wranne, L.: Treatment of congenital hypoplastic anaemia with prednisone. Scand. J. Haematol. 7:63, 1970.

128a. Aase, J. M., and Smith, D. W.: Congenital anemia and triphalangeal thumbs: A new syndrome. J. Pediatr. 74:471, 1969.

128b. Murphy, S., and Lubin, B.: Triphalangeal thumbs and erythroid hypoplasia: Report of a case with unusual features. J. Pediatr., 81:987, 1972.

128c. Jones, B., and Thompson, H.: Triphalangeal thumbs associated with hypoplastic anemia. Pediatrics 52:609, 1973.

129. Altman, K. I., and Miller, G.: A disturbance of tryptophan metabolism in congenital hypoplastic anemia. Nature (Lond.) 172:868, 1953.

130. Pearson, H. A., and Cone, T. E., Jr.: Congenital hypoplastic anemia. Pediatrics 19:192, 1957.

131. Marver, H. S.: Studies on tryptophan metabolism. I. Urinary tryptophan metabolites in hypoplastic anemias and other hematologic disorders. J. Clin. Lab. Med. 58:425, 1961.

132. Price, J. M., Brown, R. R., et al.: Excretion of urinary tryptophan metabolites by patients with congenital hypoplastic anemia (Diamond-Blackfan syndrome). J. Lab. Clin. Med. 75:316, 1970.

133. Tartaglia, A. P., Propp, S., et al.: Chromosome abnormality and hypocalcemia in congenital erythroid hypoplasia (Blackfan-Diamond syndrome). Am. J. Med. 41:990, 1966.

134. Hirst, E., and Robertson, T. I.: The syndrome of thymoma and erythroblastopenic anemia. Medicine (Baltimore) 46:225, 1967.

134a. Talerman, A., and Amigo, A.: Thymoma associated with aregenerative and aplastic anemia in a five-year-old child. Cancer 21:1212, 1968.

135. Hammond, D., Shore, N., et al.: Production, utilization and excretion of erythropoietin. I. Chronic anemias. II. Aplastic crises. III. Erythropoietic effect of normal plasma. Ann. N. Y. Acad. Sci. 149:516, 1968.

136. Jepson, J. H., and Lowenstein, L.: Inhibition of erythropoiesis by a factor present in the plasma of patients with erythroblastopenia. Blood 27:425, 1966.

137. Krantz, S. B., and Kao, V.: Studies on red cell aplasia. I. Demonstration of a plasma inhibitor to heme synthesis and an antibody to erythroblast nuclei. Proc. Nat. Acad. Sci. USA 58:493, 1967.

138. Safdar, S. H., Krantz, S. B., et al.: Successful immunosuppressive treatment of erythroid aplasia appearing after thymectomy. Br. J. Haematol. 19:435, 1970.

139. Krantz, S. B.: Studies on red cell aplasia. III. Treatment with horse antihuman thymocyte gamma globulin. Blood 39:347, 1972.

139a. Krantz, S. B., Moore, W. H., et al.: Studies on red cell aplasia. V. Presence of erythroblast cytotoxicity in γG-globulin fraction of plasma. J. Clin. Invest. 52:324, 1973.

140. Krantz, S. B., Kao, V., et al.: Treatment of red cell aplasia with immunosuppressive drugs. J. Clin. Invest. 48:46a, 1969.

140a. Vilan, J., Rhyner, K., et al.: Pure red cell aplasia: Successful treatment with cyclophosphamide. Blut 26:27, 1973.

141. Allen, D. M., and Diamond, L. K.: Congenital (erythroid) hypoplastic anemia. Cortisone treated. Am. J. Dis. Child. 102:162, 1961.

142. Smith, C. H.: Chronic congenital aregenerative anemia (pure red-cell anemia) associated with iso-immunization by the blood group factor "A." Blood 4:697, 1949.

143. Gasser, C.: Aplastiche Anämie (chronische Erythroblastophthisie) und Cortison. Schweiz. Med. Wochenschr. 81:1241, 1951.

144. Lukens, J. N., and Neuman, L. A.: Excretion and distribution of iron during chronic deferoxamine therapy. Blood 38:614, 1971.

145. Gasser, C.: Akute Erythroblastopenie: 10 Fälle aplasticher Erythroblastenkrisen mit risen Proerythroblasten bei allergisch-taxischen Zustands Bildern. Helv. Paediatr. Acta 4: 107, 1949.

146. Wranne, L.: Transient erythroblastopenia in infancy and childhood. Scand. J. Haematol. 7:76, 1970.

147. Gordon, R. R., and Varad, S.: Congenital hypoplastic anaemia (pure red-cell anaemia) with periodic erythroblastopenia. Lancet 1:296, 1962.

148. Owren, P. A.: Congenital hemolytic jaundice: The pathogenesis of the "hemolytic crisis." Blood 3:231, 1948.

149. Dameshek, W., and Bloom, M. L.: The events of hemolytic crisis of hereditary spherocytosis with particular reference to the reticulocytopenia, pancytopenia and abnormal splenic mechanism. Blood 3:1381, 1948.

150. Greig, H. B., Metz, J., et al.: The familial crisis in hereditary spherocytosis: Report of five cases. S. Afr. J. Med. Sci. 23:17, 1958.

151. Singer, K., Motulsky, A. G., et al.: Aplastic crisis in sickle cell anemia: A study of its mechanism and its relationship to other types of hemolytic crisis. J. Lab. Clin. Med. 35:721, 1950.

152. MacIver, J. E.: The aplastic crises in sickle cell anemia. Lancet 1:1086, 1961.

153. Hurdle, A. D. F., and Walker, A. G.: Bone marrow hypoplasia in the course of haemolytic disease of the newborn. Br. Med. J. 1:518, 1963.

154. Miesch, D. C., Baxter, R., et al.: Acute erythroblastopenia: Pathogenesis, manifestations and management. A.M.A. Arch. Intern. Med. 99:461, 1957.

155. Crosby, W. H.: Paroxysmal nocturnal haemoglobinuria: Report of a case complicated by an aregenerative (aplastic) crisis. Ann. Intern. Med. 39:1107, 1953.

156. Fikrig, S. M., and Berkovich, S.: Virus induced aplastic crisis in mice. Blood 33:589, 1969.

157. Cartwright, G. E., and Lee, G. R.: The anaemia of chronic disorders. Br. J. Haematol. 2:147, 1971.

158. Haurani, F. I., Burke, W., et al.: Defective reutilization of iron in the anemia of inflammation. J. Lab. Clin. Med. 65:560, 1965.

159. Erslev, A. J., and McKenna, P. J.: Effect of splenectomy on red cell production. Ann. Intern. Med. 65:5, 1967.

160. Bush, J. A., Ashenbrucker, H., et al.: The anemia of infection. XX. The kinetics of iron metabolism in the anemia associated with chronic infection. J. Clin. Invest. 35:89, 1956.

161. Freireich, E. M., Miller, A., et al.: The effect of inflammation on the utilization of erythrocyte and transferrin-bound radio-iron for red cell production. Blood 12:972, 1957.

162. Karle, H.: The site of abnormal erythrocyte destruction during experimental fever. Br. J. Haematol. 15:475, 1968.

163. Karle, H.: Effect on red cells of a small rise in temperature: In vitro studies. Br. J. Haematol. 16:409, 1969.

164. Ward, H. P., Kurnick, J. E., et al.: Serum level of erythropoietin in anemias associated with chronic infection, malignancy and primary

hematopoietic disease. J. Clin. Invest. 50: 332, 1971.

165. Robinson, J. C., James, G. W., III, et al.: The effect of oral therapy with cobaltous chloride on the blood of patients suffering with chronic suppurative infection. New Engl. J. Med. 240:749, 1949.

166. Brain, M. C.: Microangiopathic hemolytic anemia. Ann. Rev. Med. 21:133, 1970.

167. Castaldi, P. A., Rozenberg, M. C., et al.: The bleeding disorder of uremia: A qualitative platelet defect. Lancet 2:66, 1966.

168. Shaw, A. B., and Scholes, M. C.: Reticulocytosis in renal failure. Lancet 1:7494, 1967.

169. Stewart, J. H.: Haemolytic anaemia in acute and chronic renal failure. Quart. J. Med. 36:85, 1967.

170. Erslev, A. J.: Anemia of chronic renal disease. Arch. Intern. Med. 126:774, 1970.

171. Magid, E., and Hilden, M.: Ferrokinetics in patients suffering from chronic renal disease and anemia. Scand. J. Haematol. 4:33, 1967.

172. Ragen, P. A., Hagedorn, A. B., et al.: Radioisotope study of anemia in chronic renal disease. A.M.A. Arch. Intern.Med. 105:518, 1960.

173. Berry, E. R., Rambach, W. A., et al.: Effect of peritoneal dialysis on erythrokinetics and ferrokinetics of azotemic anemia. Trans. Am. Soc. Artif. Intern. Organs 10:415, 1965.

174. Giovannetti, S., Giagnoni, P., et al.: Red cell survival in chronic uraemia: Its relationship with the spontaneous in vitro autohemolysis and with the degree of anaemia. Experientia 22:739, 1966.

175. Stuart, J., Skowron, P. N., et al.: Erythroid-cell enzyme activity in chronic renal failure. Lancet 2:297, 1968.

176. Yawata, Y., Howe, R., et al.: Mechanism of uremic hemolytic anemia: Acquired hexosemonophosphate shunt deficiency. J. Clin. Invest. 54:105a, 1972.

177. Lichtman, M. A., and Miller, D. R.: Erythrocyte glycolysis, 2,3-diphosphoglycerate, and adenosine triphosphate concentration in uremic subjects: Relationship to extracellular phosphate concentration. J. Lab. Clin. Med. 76:267, 1970.

178. Villamil, M. F., Rettori, V., et al.: Sodium transport by red blood cell in uremia. J. Lab. Clin. Med. 72:308, 1968.

179. Van Dyke, D., Keighley, G., et al.: Decreased responsiveness to erythropoietin in a patient with anemia secondary to chronic uremia. Blood 22:838, 1963.

180. Larsen, O. A., Josephsen, P., et al.: Nefrogen anaemi behandlet med erythropoietin. Ugeskr. Laeger 125:435, 1963.

181. Mirand, E. A., Murphy, G. P., et al.: Erythropoietin activity in anephric allotransplanted, unilaterally nephrectomized and intact man. J. Lab. Clin. Med. 73:121, 1969.

182. Nathan, D. G., Schupack, E., et al.: Erythropoiesis in anephric man. J. Clin. Invest. 43:2158, 1964.

183. Naets, J. P., and Wittek, M.: Erythropoiesis in anephric man. Lancet 1:941, 1968.

184. Erslev, A. J., McKenna, P. J., et al.: Rate of red cell production in two nephrectomized patients. Arch. Intern. Med. 22:230, 1968.

185. van Ypersele de Strihou, C., and Stragier, A.: Effect of bilateral nephrectomy on transfusion requirements of patients undergoing chronic dialysis. Lancet 2:7623, 1969.

186. Edwards, M. S., Pegrum, G. D., et al.: Iron therapy in patients on maintenance haemodialysis. Lancet 2:481, 1970.

187. Lawson, D. H., Boddy, K., et al.: Iron metabolism in patients with chronic renal failure on regular dialysis treatment. Clin. Sci. 41:345, 1971.

188. Hartley, L. C. J., Innis, M. D., et al.: Splenectomy for anemia in patients on regular haemodialysis. Lancet 2:1343, 1971.

189. Richardson, J. R., Jr., and Weinstein, M. B.: Erythropoietic response of dialyzed patients to testosterone administration. Ann. Intern. Med. 73:403, 1970.

190. McCredie, K. B.: Oxymetholone in refractory anaemia. Br. J. Haematol. 17:265, 1969.

191. Daughaday, W. H.: The adenohypophysis, In Textbook of Endocrinology. 5th ed. Williams, R. H. (ed.), Philadelphia, W. B. Saunders Co., 1974, p. 57.

192. Tudhope, G. R., and Wilson, G. M.: Anemia in hypothyroidism: Incidence, pathogenesis and response to treatment. Quart. J. Med. 29:513, 1960.

193. Wardrop, C., and Hutchinson, H. E.: Red-cell shape in hypothyroidism. Lancet 1:1243, 1969.

194. Muldowney, F. R., Crooks, J., et al.: The total red cell mass in thyrotoxicosis and myxedema. Clin. Sci. 16:311, 1957.

195. Keily, J. M., Purnell, D. C., et al.: Erythrokinetics in myxedema. Ann. Intern. Med. 67:533, 1967.

196. Root, A. W., Oski, F. A., et al.: Erythrocyte glucose-6-phosphate dehydrogenase activity in children with hypothyroidism and hypopituitarism. J. Pediatr. 70:369, 1967.

197. Snyder, L. M., and Reddy, W. J.: Thyroid hormone control of erythrocyte 2,3-diphosphoglyceric acid concentrations. Science 169:879, 1970.

198. Miller, W. W., Delivoria-Papadopoulos, M., et al.: Oxygen releasing factor in hypothyroidism. J.A.M.A. 211:1824, 1970.

199. Baez-Villasenor, J., Rath, C. E., et al.: The blood picture in Addison's disease. Blood 3:769, 1948.

200. McCune, D. J., and Bradley, C.: Osteopetrosis (marble bones) in an infant. Am. J. Dis. Child. 48:949, 1934.

201. Gamsu, H., Lorber, J., et al.: Hemolytic anemia in osteopoetrosis: A report of two cases. Arch. Dis. Child. 36:494, 1961.

202. Solcia, E., Rondini, G., et al.: Clinical and pathological observations on a case of newborn osteopetrosis. Helv. Paediatr. Acta 23:650, 1968.

203. Silverstein, M. N., Gomes, M. R., et al.: Agnogenic myeloid metaplasia. Arch. Intern. Med. 120:546, 1967.

204. Say, B., and Burkel, I.: Idiopathic myelofibrosis in an infant. J. Pediatr. 64:580, 1964.

205. Silverstein, M. N., and Linman, J. W.: Causes of death in agnogenic myeloid metaplasia. Mayo Clin. Proc. 44:36, 1969.

206. Tanaka, K. R., Valentine, W. N., et al.: Diseases or clinical conditions associated with low leukocyte alkaline phosphatase. New Engl. J. Med. 262:912, 1960.

207. Sandberg, A. A., Ishihara, T., et al.: Comparison of chromosome constitution in chronic myelocytic leukemia and other myeloproliferative disorders. Blood 20:393, 1962.

208. Samuel, S., Gilman, S., et al.: Hyperthyroidism in an infant with McCune-Albright syndrome: Report of a case with myeloid metaplasia. J. Pediatr. 80:275, 1972.

209. Randell, D. L., Reiquam, C. W., et al.: Familial myeloproliferative disease. A new syndrome closely simulating myelogenous leukemia in childhood. Am. J. Dis. Child. 110:479, 1965.

210. Miller, R. W.: Down's syndrome (mongolism), other congenital malformations and cancers among the sibs of leukemic children. New Engl. J. Med. 268:393, 1963.

211. Humbert, J. R., Hathaway, W. E., et al.: Preleukemia in children with missing bone marrow C chromosome and a myeloproliferation disorder. Br. J. Haematol. 21:705, 1971.

Red Cell Destruction: Disorders of Membrane and Metabolism

Chapter 6

The Red Blood Cell Membrane and Mechanisms of Hemolysis

by Stephen B. Shohet and Samuel E. Lux

INTRODUCTION

Hemolysis, by definition, is membrane failure. Basing our discussion on this precept, in this chapter we examine the pathophysiology of various hemolytic anemias in relation to known modes of red cell membrane failure. We first discuss the structure of the red cell membrane, with special emphasis on recent evidence concerning the dynamic and asymmetric aspects of membrane organization. Second, we describe three processes (fragmentation, whole cell lysis, and filtration and entrapment) which can lead to membrane failure. Finally, selected disease states which illustrate these mechanisms are discussed. Other related diseases are presented in subsequent chapters.

THE ANATOMY OF THE ERYTHROCYTE MEMBRANE

In the nearly four decades since the introduction of the paucimolecular model of membrane structure by Danielli and Davson (1), a variety of membrane models have been cast. These are reviewed and compared in a number of recent articles (2–6). Current views of membrane architecture retain the lipid bilayer as a cornerstone but differ substantially from the original construct, especially in regard to the disposition of membrane proteins (see p. 199). In particular, recent studies of both artificial and natural membranes emphasize the mobility and asymmetrical distribution of the protein and lipid components, presenting a much more dynamic picture of membrane structure than previously realized (7).

Membrane Lipid Composition and Renewal Pathways

Lipids compose about 50 per cent by weight of the red cell membrane. Phospholipids and unesterified cholesterol predominate and are present in nearly equal proportions (cholesterol/phospholipid molar ratio $\simeq 0.80$) (8, 9, 11). Small amounts of glycolipids, principally GL-4 (Fig. 6–1), are also present (9). One can calculate that the average red cell contains about 240 million phospholipid molecules, 190 million cholesterol molecules, 12 million glycolipid molecules, and 4 to 5 million protein molecules (see below) in a membrane whose total surface area is about 167 μ^2 (10). Phosphatidyl choline (PC) (28 per cent), phosphatidyl ethanolamine (PE) (26 per cent), sphingomyelin (SM) (25 per cent), and phosphatidyl serine (PS) (13 per cent) are the preponderant phospholipids (11). Their structures are shown in Figure 6–1. Small amounts of phosphatidic acid (PA) (2 per cent), phosphatidyl inositol (PI) (1 per cent), and lysophospholipids are also present (11, 12). It is notable that, at physiologic pH's, PS, PA, and PI have a net negative charge, while the other phospholipids are electrically neutral. With the exception of SM, these lipids have two fatty acids attached to a glycerol backbone. These are usually in ester linkage, although occasionally (particularly in PE) the fatty acids are in vinyl ether or plasmalogen linkage.

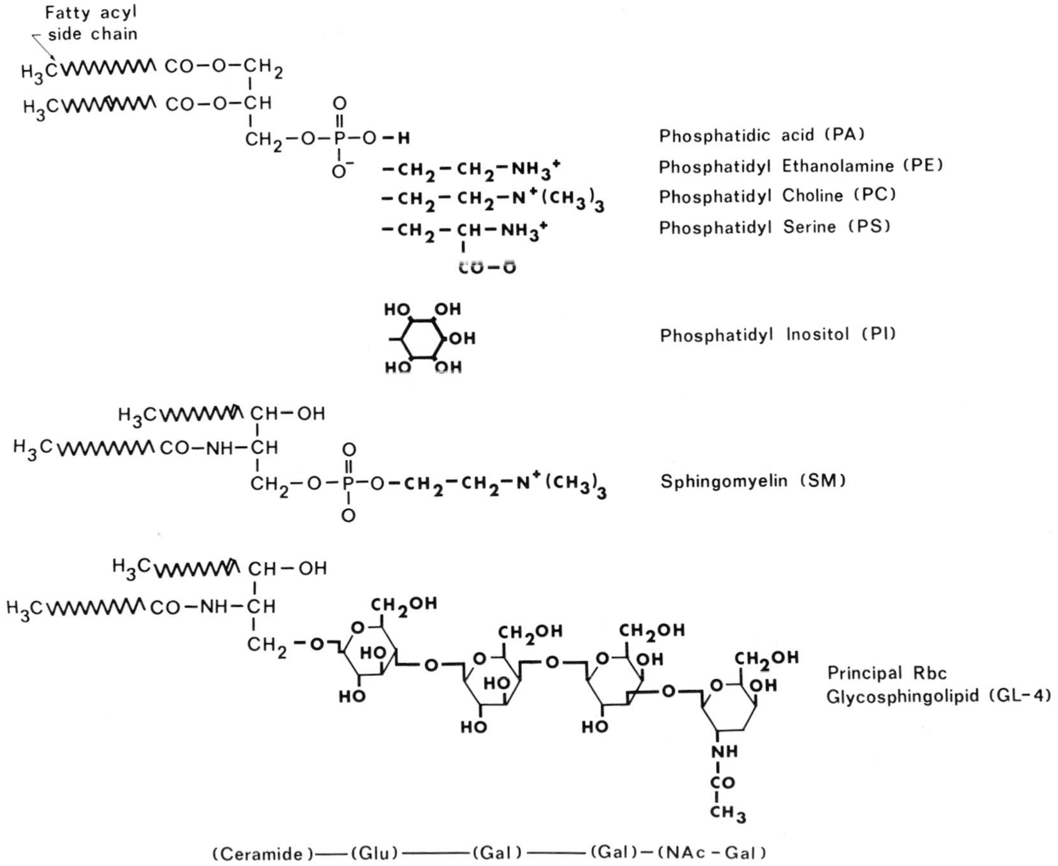

Figure 6–1. Chemical structures of the major phospholipids and the principal glycosphingolipid of the red cell membrane. Note that PC and SM share the same polar moiety (choline) and that SM and GL-4 share the same nonpolar moiety (ceramide).

The lysophospholipids have only one fatty acid and are named for their strong detergent qualities (13). The large mass of fatty acyl side chains in membrane phospholipids probably influences the physical characteristics of the membrane in a major way, and changes in their composition may be expected to effect changes in those physical characteristics. In particular, an increase in either the chain length or the saturation of the hydrocarbon chains would tend to decrease membrane lipid mobility (see below) in comparison with membranes with shorter or more unsaturated fatty acids (14). As noted below, however, the large amount of cholesterol in the red cell membrane may equalize these differences to a certain degree.

The fatty acids of PC, PE, and probably other red cell phospholipids can be renewed in the mature circulating erythrocyte by means of an acylation system which requires ATP and coenzyme A (Fig. 6–2) (15–20). This system utilizes endogenous or plasma lysophospholipids together with plasma free fatty acids as substrates. This process may be important to the cell for several reasons: first, it enables both replacement and renewal of lost or damaged phospholipid fatty acids; second, it accomplishes this at very little metabolic cost (only one ATP molecule is required to, in effect, entrap a large lipid molecule) (17); and third, it serves to prevent the accumulation of deleterious lysophospholipids within the membrane.

In addition to this active pathway for individual phospholipid renewal, a significant fraction of complete, preformed, red cell membrane phospholipids can be replaced by passive exchange with the phospholipids of plasma lipoproteins (20, 21). This fraction is, in large part, metabolically distinct from the actively renewed fraction (20) and may eventually reflect plasma lipid changes induced by diet or disease (22). These two mechanisms of phospholipid renewal are especially important to the circulating red cell, since no mechanisms for the *de novo* synthesis of fatty acids or phospholipids are present in mature erythrocytes (23).

The remaining major lipid component of the red cell membrane is *unesterified* (free) cholesterol (8, 9, 12). This component exchanges readily with the free cholesterol

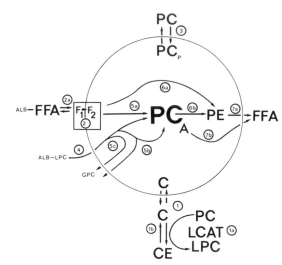

Figure 6–2. Proposed fatty acid renewal pathways and lipid exchange pathways in the human erythrocyte. (1) Passive exchange of red cell and plasma free cholesterol. (1a) Lecithin:cholesterol acyltransferase (LCAT) regulation of free cholesterol and esterified cholesterol levels in plasma. (1b) Regeneration of free cholesterol in the plasma by cholesteryl ester hydrolase. (2a) Passive exchange of free fatty acid (FFA) between plasma albumin and the red cell membrane. (2b) Active transport of FFA through membrane pools (F_1 and F_2) to membrane site for incorporation of FA into membrane phospholipids. (3) Passive exchange of preformed plasma phosphatidyl choline (PC) and passively derived membrane PC pool (PC_p). (4) Passive exchange of plasma and membrane lysophosphatidyl choline (LPC). (5a) Assembly of LPC and FFA to form actively generated pool of membrane PC (PC_a). (5b) Transacylation of LPC to form PC and glycerophosphoryl choline (GPC). (5c) Lysophospholipase mediated catabolism of LPC to GPC. (6a) Assembly of lysophosphatidyl ethanolamine and FFA to form phosphatidyl ethanolamine. (6b) Assembly of lysophosphatidyl ethanolamine and FA derived from PC_a to form phosphatidyl ethanolamine. (7a,b) Release of phospholipid FA as FFA from cell to plasma. (Modified from Shohet, S. B.: New Engl. J. Med. 286:577, 1972.)

in plasma lipoproteins (24). In the plasma, free cholesterol may be converted to *esterified* cholesterol by the action of LCAT (lecithin:cholesterol acyltransferase) (Fig. 6–2) (25). Since the newly formed cholesteryl ester cannot return to the red cell membrane (there is virtually no esterified cholesterol in the membrane), LCAT provides a unidirectional pathway which tends to deplete the membrane of cholesterol and decrease its surface area. Conversely, if LCAT is absent or inhibited, excess membrane free cholesterol accumulates, expanding the membrane surface area (26).

There is now substantial evidence that the major portion of the phospholipids in a variety of intact membranes are in the bilayer form. For example, differential scanning calorimetry of intact *Mycoplasma* or of isolated *Mycoplasma* membranes indicates that approximately 70 per cent of the fatty acid side chains of the membrane phospholipids exhibit a transition from a gel to a liquid-crystalline state at the same temperature as the fatty acid side chains of the extracted membrane phospholipids dispersed as bilayers in water (27). The erythrocyte membrane is no exception. X-ray diffraction (28) and spin-label (29) studies indicate extensive regions of phospholipid bilayer structure within the red cell membrane. However, the possibility that other phospholipid organizations may be present in special loci has not been excluded. One of these, the H_{II} hexagonal phase (30, 31), is of special interest since in this configuration the phospholipid head groups could form membrane-spanning aqueous channels. In addition, in the erythrocyte and other membranes, approximately 20 to 30 per cent of the membrane phospholipids do not exhibit the cooperative, fluid properties of a bilayer and are inaccessible to enzymatic degradation by phospholipase C (27, 32, 33). Probably, many of these "cryptic" phospholipids are excluded from the bilayer domain because they are tenaciously bound to certain amphipathic membrane proteins. Jost has recently shown that in the cytochrome oxidase membrane each mole of cytochrome oxidase immobilizes 47 moles of phospholipid, an amount just sufficient to form a single layer of phospholipid around the protein (34).

Lipid Motions

A variety of optical and magnetic spectroscopic probes have been used to monitor the structure of both phospholipid bilayers and natural membranes.* These studies emphasize that lipid components in a bi-

layer are constantly moving in a variety of ways.

FATTY ACID "WAGGLE." Purified phospholipids exhibit discrete, liquid-crystalline to gel phase transitions which are dependent on the length and degree of unsaturation of their fatty acids (40). Above this transition, the fatty acid side chains waggle very rapidly (10^8 to 10^9 times per second) from side to side, with progressively greater excursions as one proceeds from the glycerol ester linkage to the terminal methyl group (41–43). This "flexibility gradient" is not uniform. The hydrocarbon chains are relatively tightly packed and ordered for the first eight to ten carbons, after which their mobility rapidly increases (41–43). The presence of a double bond in the fatty acid increases the disorder between the double bond and the terminal methyl group but has little effect on the ordering of the side chain proximal to the double bond (44). Below the liquid-crystalline transition temperature, the fatty acid side chains are much more ordered and are more nearly solid than liquid.

Membrane cholesterol molecules are intercalated between the phospholipids with their hydroxyl groups at the aqueous interface and with their long axes perpendicular to the plane of the membrane (45). Spin-label studies indicate that, above the gel to liquid-crystalline phase transition, cholesterol molecules tend to immobilize the fatty acid side chains of the phospholipids, particularly the proximal six to eight carbons (41), while below this transition they tend to disrupt the ordering of the fatty acids, in effect preserving membrane fluidity (46). The net result is that cholesterol tends to abolish the gel to liquid-crystalline transition and create an intermediate fluid condition in which the proximal end of the phospholipid hydrocarbon chains are extended and relatively rigid, and the distal ends are more disordered and fluid. Rothman and Engelman have analyzed the phospholipid-cholesterol interaction using molecular models and observed that cholesterol tends to equalize the differences between fatty acids of different chain length and saturation (47). They argue that in a cell such as the erythrocyte, which is exposed to an environment whose lipid composition continually varies, cholesterol would serve to stabilize the membrane

---

*Several good reviews of the application of electron spin resonance spectroscopy (ESR) and nuclear magnetic resonance spectroscopy (NMR) to the study of membrane structure are now available (35–39).

against changes in its physical properties that would otherwise result from lipid exchange reactions, such as those described in Figure 6–2.

LATERAL DIFFUSION. Using spin-labeled phospholipids, Kornberg, Deveaux, and McConnell observed that PC molecules move about rapidly within the plane of the bilayer (48, 49). From their measured diffusion constant (1.8×10^{-8} cm.² per second) (49), one can calculate that, on the average, a phospholipid molecule exchanges places with a neighboring phospholipid every 10^{-7} seconds. Cholesterol decreases the lateral diffusion of phospholipid molecules (49), presumably secondary to the restrictions it imposes on the mobility of the fatty acid side chains. In accord with this, recent evidence suggests that lateral diffusion in the cholesterol-rich erythrocyte membrane may be at least an order of magnitude slower than in phospholipid bilayers (50).

PHOSPHOLIPID FLIP-FLOP. Phospholipid "flip-flop" refers to the translocation of a phospholipid molecule from the inside to the outside of the bilayer and vice versa. This is by far the slowest of the observed lipid motions. On the average, in model bilayers, a particular phospholipid flips (or flops) only once every 10^4 to 10^5 seconds (51). As with lateral diffusion, this rate may well be much slower in the erythrocyte membrane.

These membrane lipid motions must have profound implications for biological membrane functions. It is evident that lipid-soluble drugs can traverse a membrane more readily when it is in a fluid state. Less obviously the passage of small polar molecules due to transient discontinuities in the nonpolar membrane barrier will also be enhanced by increased membrane fluidity. Many other poorly understood membrane functions, such as transport by "carrier" proteins, pinocytosis, phagocytosis, and amoeboid movement, are also likely to be dependent, at least in part, on membrane fluidity. Similarly it is reasonable to expect that the function of certain membrane-bound enzymes might be profoundly influenced by the state of the lipid "solution" in which they reside.

Such correlations of membrane lipid motions and membrane function are now under active investigation in many laboratories.

So far only the influence of hydrocarbon side chain motion has received much attention, principally because methods for monitoring lateral diffusion and phospholipid flip-flop in intact membranes or living cells are only beginning to be described (50). As anticipated, there is increasing evidence from studies in bacterial systems that membrane transport, the function of membranous enzymes, and even cell survival depend critically on the ability of an organism to maintain its fatty acid side chains in a fluid state at a particular environmental temperature (43, 52–54). Undoubtedly many red cell membrane functions will also be found to be critically dependent on the fluidity of the membrane. For example, membrane deformability, a property of primary importance for the survival of the circulating erythrocyte, must be closely related to lipid mobility. The relationship of changes in membrane lipid dynamics to this and other aspects of the pathophysiology of diseases associated with alterations in the content of membrane cholesterol, phospholipid polar groups, or hydrocarbon chains (e.g., see sections on Chemical Agent Damage, High Phosphatidyl Choline Hemolytic Anemia, Acanthocytosis, Liver Disease, and LCAT Deficiency) should prove a particularly fruitful area of future scientific inquiry.

Lipid Asymmetry

There is scant but increasing evidence that membrane lipids, like membrane proteins (see below), are asymmetrically distributed within (*cis asymmetry*) and across (*trans asymmetry*) the bilayer. Studies in model systems have established that mixtures of phospholipids or phospholipids and cholesterol form complex phases containing both fluid and solid components. These segregate by lateral diffusion, producing separate regions of fluid and solid lipids within each bilayer plane (55), a form of cis asymmetry. There is also evidence from model studies that lateral phase separations and cis asymmetry can be induced by divalent cations in bilayers containing mixtures of neutral and anionic phospholipids. For example, Ohnishi and Ito found, in mixtures of PC and PS, that calcium ions bind the negatively charged PS molecules into rigid aggregates, leaving the excluded, neutral PC in fluid clusters (56). Possibly this may explain, at least in part, the capacity of membrane-bound calcium to stiffen red cell membranes and decrease cell deformability (see section ATP-Depleted Cells). A third example of cis asymmetry noted above is the segregation of protein-bound lipids from the remainder of the bilayer pool (34).

There is also recent evidence for a trans asymmetry of phospholipids in the red cell membrane. Bretscher (57, 58) and more recently Gordesky and Marinetti (59) have examined the accessibility of PE and PS to alkylating agents which react with primary amino groups but do not readily penetrate the membrane. In the intact erythrocyte, only about one-third of the PE and essentially none of the PS were alkylated. These phospholipids were much more reactive in red cell ghosts and were completely reactive in extracted membrane lipids. Both groups have concluded that PS and PE are preferentially localized to the inner membrane surface (although the possibility that the relative unreactivity of these phospholipids might also be due to an intimate association with membrane proteins has not been completely excluded). By difference, PC and SM must predominate in the outer half of the membrane. Since phospholipid flip-flop is a very slow process, there is probably little interchange of phospholipids between the two membrane halves. This proposed asymmetry of phospholipid organization provides a logical explanation why PE and PS exchange much more slowly between the red cell membrane and plasma lipoproteins than do PC and SM (21).

These conclusions about phospholipid trans asymmetry are indirectly supported by studies of the interaction of phospholipases with intact erythrocytes (57, 60, 61). These enzymes are valuable tools for evaluating the contribution of phospholipid components to membrane stability and function (61–67), but their effects are complex and beyond the scope of the present chapter.

Membrane Protein Composition

Unlike their lipid neighbors, membrane proteins have, until lately, stubbornly resisted analysis. As recently as 1968, it was widely believed that the matrix of the red cell (68, 69) and other membranes (70) contained a single "structural" protein, characterized by its recalcitrant insolubility in aqueous media. We now know that this concept was erroneous and that the red cell membrane contains many diverse proteins (71, 72).

It is important to realize that precise enumeration of all membrane proteins will probably never be achieved because the erythrocyte membrane is so hard to define. The membrane is not abruptly discontinuous but extends its influence into the adjacent plasmic and cytoplasmic spaces. Proteins which reside in the latter compartments may normally be oriented by the influence of the membrane electrostatic field or be bound to the membrane by forces which are too weak to withstand some isolation procedures. Whether such proteins are true membrane residents or adventitious intruders depends on the point of view of each investigator and the methods he employs to isolate and thereby "define" the red cell membrane. Since minor differences in isolation procedures can produce conspicuous alterations in the membrane product (73), interlaboratory comparisons, particularly of membrane function and enzymology, can be quite difficult.

At the present time, the red cell membrane is usually defined by the isolation procedure of Dodge, Mitchell, and Hanahan (74), and the membrane proteins identified by polyacrylamide gel electrophoresis in sodium dodecyl sulfate (SDS-PAGE), which separates them principally according to their molecular weights.

Eight major protein bands are regularly seen in SDS-PAGE of human red cell membranes (Fig. 6–3, B) (75). Up to ten other bands can be discerned in heavily loaded gels. In addition, one major (PAS-1) and two minor glycoprotein bands stain poorly with protein stains but are easily visualized with a periodic acid–Schiff (PAS) stain (Fig. 6–3, A) (75).

Through the ingenious efforts of a number of investigators (61, 76–85), we now know where many of these proteins are located in the membrane. In general, the strategy has been to selectively modify one side of the membrane with a protein (e.g., trypsin, neuraminadase, lactoperoxidase-mediated iodination, specific antibodies) or

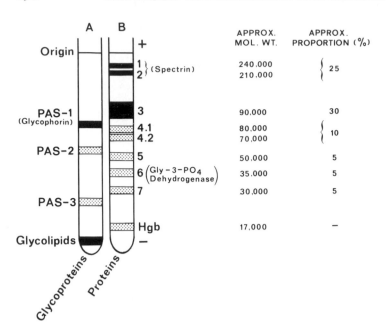

Figure 6–3. SDS-PAGE patterns (5 per cent acrylamide gels) of the major proteins (B) and glycoproteins (A) of the erythrocyte membrane.

a nonpenetrating alkylating reagent and then monitor the alteration by SDS-PAGE. By determining which membrane proteins are modified in intact red cells and resealed ghosts and which are modified in unsealed ghosts and inside-out membrane vesicles (86), one can localize a protein to the exterior or cytoplasmic face of the membrane* (Fig. 6–4).

These studies strongly suggest that red cell membrane proteins are anisotropically exposed on the two membrane surfaces (trans asymmetry). The glycoproteins and glycolipids are all confined to the outer membrane surface, while the remaining major proteins address the inner membrane face. Surprisingly, all the major glycoproteins seem to span the membrane barrier (Fig. 6–4).

Specific Protein Components

BANDS 1, 2, AND 5.   These three proteins are easily extracted from the red cell membrane by low ionic strength, slightly alkaline solutions, particularly in the presence of EDTA (72, 76, 88–90). This extract was originally named *spectrin* (i.e., "derived from ghosts") (90a), but in most cases this term now refers to just bands 1 and 2 (88–

90). These two bands are asymmetrical, high molecular weight proteins which are located on the cytoplasmic membrane surface. Together with band 5 they account for 25 to 35 per cent of the erythrocyte membrane protein (75, 88). Cross-linking studies suggest that bands 1 and 2 are closely associated in the intact membrane (77, 90), but their physical relationship, if any, to band 5 is still poorly defined.

Despite the loose association implied by their easy extraction, one or more of these proteins may play a structural role, since the membrane undergoes vesiculation upon their removal (89). This speculation is furthered by the observation that these three proteins are superficially similar to actomyosin subunits in size and composition (91) and form coiled fibrils morphologically similar to F-actin filaments on incubation with divalent cations (89). Apparently identical filaments are present on the cytoplasmic membrane surface before, but not after, extraction of bands 1, 2, and 5 (89, 92). Band 2 (and possibly band 1) is phosphorylated by [γ-^{32}P]-ATP in the presence of magnesium (93–95), and this phosphorylation is stimulated by cyclic AMP and inhibited by calcium (94, 95). Interestingly, a preliminary report indicates that in hereditary spherocytosis spectrin phosphorylation is markedly diminished (95a). These observations suggest that spectrin participates in some energy-related biochemical process — possibly the maintenance of erythrocyte shape and deformability.

---

*Some investigators (61, 87) argue that this approach does not permit an unambiguous differentiation of membrane "sidedness." They contend the differences in reactivity of membrane proteins in intact red cells and ghosts might also be explained by changes in membrane protein organization induced by hemolysis (73).

Figure 6–4. Schematic illustration of the organization of the major erythrocyte membrane apoproteins deduced from chemical and enzymatic analysis of intact, inside-out, and right side–out membranes (76–85). The specific proteins are not drawn to scale. Proteins whose properties are consistent with "integral proteins" (see text) are shown partially or completely penetrating the lipid bilayer. "Peripheral proteins" are depicted as just touching the membrane surface. Bands 1 and 2 are shown extending into the cytoplasm, as suggested by electron micrographs (89, 92). However, recent evidence suggests that Bands 1 and 2 (spectrin) may instead lie *parallel* to the cytoplasmic membrane face and form a meshwork crosslinking proteins exposed at that surface (169, 378).

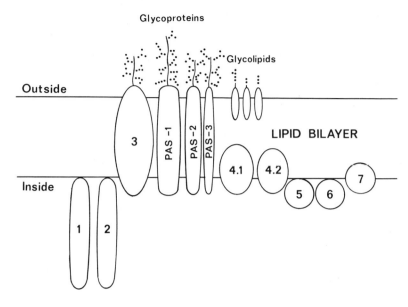

BAND 3. Although this band represents one of the two major fractions of the red cell membrane protein, it has been difficult to isolate and characterize because of its hydrophobic nature. In general, purification has been approached by attempting to solubilize all of the major proteins except the major band 3 component (85, 96, 97). Analyses indicate that this component contains a small amount (7 per cent) of carbohydrate (85), including a binding site for concanavalin A (98). Recently, Guidotti and his co-workers have utilized this affinity to purify the major band 3 protein on columns containing immobilized concanavalin A (98a). Different portions of this glycoprotein are accessible to chemical modification and proteolytic attack at the inner and outer membrane surface, suggesting it spans the membrane barrier (76, 78, 79). This has led to speculation that it may serve a transport function. Interestingly, preliminary reports indicate that amino-reactive inhibitors of erythrocyte phosphate, chloride, and sulfate permeability almost selectively label this band (98, 99). Further, incorporation of the major band 3 protein into phospholipid liposomes markedly increases their permeability to phosphate (98), and this potentiation is abolished by inhibitors of anion transport (98). These results indicate this protein is integral to red cell anion transport, perhaps serving as an anion transport channel.

There is increasing evidence that band 3 is nonhomogeneous and contains several compounds other than the "anion transport"

protein. One of these is erythrocyte acetylcholinesterase, a glycoprotein located on the outer membrane surface which is easily purified by affinity chromatography (100–102). Another is a protein which may be a component of the red cell's glucose transport system, since it is labeled by a glucose analogue known to interfere with glucose transport and the labeling is inhibited by D-glucose (103). A third is a protein which is phosphorylated by $[\gamma\text{-}^{32}P]$-ATP (93, 104). The phosphorylation of this protein is stimulated by sodium, and its dephosphorylation is stimulated by potassium and inhibited by ouabain, implying that it may be the phosphorylated intermediate of the Na^+- and K^+-activated ATPase involved in red cell sodium and potassium transport (104). Since the activity of Na^+- and K^+-activated ATPase in the erythrocyte membrane is among the lowest of any membrane known to possess this activity (it is estimated that a single red cell may contain only 200 Na^+-K^+ pump sites or <0.3 mg. per liter of red cells) (105), it is clear that this intermediate is only a minor component of band 3.

BAND 4 PROTEINS. This molecular weight class contains two discrete proteins (bands 4.1 and 4.2) and several additional, poorly resolved, minor components which migrate in the region between bands 4.2 and 5 on SDS-PAGE. Bands 4.1 and 4.2 are accessible to proteolytic and chemical modification only at the cytoplasmic membrane surface (Fig. 6–4) (76, 79, 81, 82, 84) and are solubilized at high pH (107). Preliminary evidence suggests that band 4.2 may be associated with band 3 in the intact membrane (105a). Neither band 4.1 nor 4.2 has been purified or functionally characterized.

The band 4 region also contains one or more poorly characterized glycoproteins. Unlike the membrane sialoglycoproteins (see below), these glycoproteins do not stain with PAS and are not labeled when red cell sialic acids are tritiated (107). However, they are identified when intact red cells are modified by a method which specifically labels surface galactose and galactosamine residues (105b, 107).

An interesting minor component in the region between bands 4.2 and 5 seems to be the preferred substrate of an erythrocyte protein kinase when cyclic AMP is present. Bands 2, 3, and, possibly, 1 are also phosphorylated by this protein kinase(s) (93–95a), and the phosphorylation of each is enhanced by cyclic AMP (95). The physiologic significance of this kinase(s) is unclear, since mature human erythrocytes reportedly lack a hormone-sensitive adenylate cyclase (94).

BANDS 6 AND 7. These two proteins, like the other membrane proteins which lack carbohydrate, are confined to the cytoplasmic membrane surface (Fig. 6–4). Their association with the membrane varies: band 6 is easily eluted at high ionic strength (75, 106), while band 7 can only be solubilized with strong dissociating agents (107). Tanner and Gray (106) have shown that band 6 has the N-terminal sequence and enzymatic activity of glyceraldehyde-3-phosphate dehydrogenase (G3PD). This enzyme binds to specific sites [perhaps on a band 3 protein component (105a)] on the inner membrane surface (108). This binding is modulated by several metabolites related to the action of G3PD, suggesting that in vivo the relationship of G3PD to the red cell membrane may vary with changes in the metabolic and ionic microenvironment (108).

PAS-1, -2, AND -3. These sialoglycoproteins and all the glycolipids are exposed on the outer surface of the membrane (76, 78–84). PAS-1 or *glycophorin* is the best characterized of all the erythrocyte membrane proteins, largely because of the elegant work of Winzler, Bloomenfeld, Marchesi, Segrest, and their coworkers (80, 109–112). It has a molecular weight of about 25,000 to 30,000 (113) but runs anomalously on SDS-PAGE (Fig. 6–3), because the large proportion of carbohydrate (60 per cent) interferes with SDS binding (114). This unusual protein contains three distinct domains linked together in a single polypeptide chain which spans the membrane barrier (Fig. 6–5). The receptor domain at the N-terminal end of the molecule contains many of the membrane antigens, including the A, B, M, and N antigens, as well as phytohemagglutinin, influenza, and wheat germ agglutinin-binding sites (109, 111). This portion contains all of the carbohydrate and is external to the membrane surface (80, 109, 111). The C-terminal end of glycophorin resides on the cytoplasmic membrane surface (80). Sandwiched between these hydrophilic extremities is the intramembranous domain which contains a sequence of 23 hydrophobic and neutral amino acids, believed to be coiled in a helix

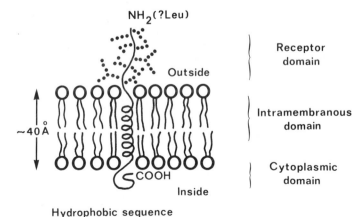

Figure 6–5. Proposed organization of erythrocyte membrane glycophorin based on studies of Winzler (111) and Marchesi, Segrist and their co-workers (80, 109, 110). The amino acid sequence of a hydrophobic peptide which is thought to be a part of the intramembranous domain (110) is shown at the bottom.

and specifically associated with lipid side chains in the membrane interior (111) (Fig. 6–5).

Glycophorin may be abnormal in paroxysmal nocturnal hemoglobinuria (PNH) (see also p. 217 and Ch. 8). Righetti and his co-workers (115) have found that the apparent molecular weight of PNH glycophorin is slightly less than normal, and that this alteration is also present in "pseudo-PNH" cells produced by treating normal red cells with 2-amino-ethyl-thiouronium bromide.

PAS-2 and PAS-3 are less well characterized than PAS-1. Proteolytic digestion experiments suggest that they, like PAS-1 and the major band 3 glycoprotein, span the membrane (Fig. 6–4) (76). Analyses of partially purified PAS-1, -2, and -3 indicate that blood group antigen M is primarily associated with PAS-1, and antigens A, I, and S are primarily associated with PAS-3 (116). N antigen activity is equally strong in all three glycoproteins (116).

In addition to these major components, it must be emphasized that the erythrocyte membrane also contains many additional protein antigens, enzymes, receptors, and other proteins which are omitted from discussion in this brief survey, either because they constitute less than 3 per cent of the membrane protein or because they are incompletely characterized. A list of some of the enzymes closely associated with the red cell membrane is presented in Table 6–1.

Peripheral and Integral Proteins

There is a tendency to broadly classify membrane proteins into two categories: *peripheral* (or *extrinsic*) and *integral* (or *intrinsic*) (6, 7). While this is undoubtedly an oversimplification, it may serve a useful purpose in emphasizing two extreme situations. By these criteria, peripheral proteins require only mild conditions to disengage them from the membrane. They dissociate free of lipids and are relatively soluble in aqueous media in the dissociated state. They are presumably attached to the surface of the membrane, perhaps by electrostatic interactions. Spectrin (bands 1 and 2) and glyceraldehyde-3-phosphate dehydrogenase (band 6) are examples of this class of membrane proteins.

In contrast, integral proteins require surfactants, organic solvents, or other dis-

TABLE 6–1. ENZYMES ASSOCIATED WITH THE HUMAN ERYTHROCYTE MEMBRANE

Acetylcholinesterase (102)
Acyl-CoA: acylglycerophosphorylacyltransferase (15, 17)
Adenosine deaminase (117)
Adenosine kinase (117, 118)
Adenosine monophosphate deaminase (119)
Adenylate kinase (120)
Aldolase (121, 122)
Ca^{2+}-dependent Mg^{2+} adenosine triphosphatase (123, 124)
Cyclic AMP–dependent protein kinase (94, 95, 125)
Diglyceride kinase (126, 127)
Glyceraldehyde-3-phosphate dehydrogenase (106, 121, 122, 128, 129)
K^+-activated phosphatase° (130, 131)
Na^+-, K^+-dependent Mg^{2+} adenosine triphosphatase (132)
NAD (P) H: glycohydrolase (133)
NADH: (acceptor) oxidoreductase (134)
NAG: transferase (135)
Phosphatidylinositol kinases (126, 136)
3-phosphoglycerate kinase (128, 129)
Protease (137)
Triphosphoinositide phosphomonoesterase (138)

°Associated with Na^+-, K^+-dependent Mg^{++} adenosine triphosphatase (24).

sociating agents to release them from membranes and maintain solubility during subsequent purification. They may dissociate as lipoproteins, and, when delipidated, tend to form recalcitrant, insoluble aggregates in aqueous media. They are inferred to be amphipathic or bimodal proteins with one or more hydrophilic ends exposed at the membrane surfaces and a lipophilic region intruding into the membrane interior. Their tenacious membrane attachment is believed to result from hydrophobic interactions between the lipophilic domain on the protein and surrounding membrane phospholipids. Glycophorin (PAS-1) is the paradigm of this protein class.

Membrane Architecture

HISTORICAL. Since its introduction by Gorter and Grendel in 1925 (139), the lipid bilayer has been the cornerstone of membrane architecture. This basic concept was first embellished by the addition of surface layers of globular protein by Danielli and Davson (1) and later refined by Robertson into the unit membrane hypothesis (140) (Fig. 6–6, *A*). Besides the lipid bilayer, the key features of this hypothesis, at least in its early representations, were that the

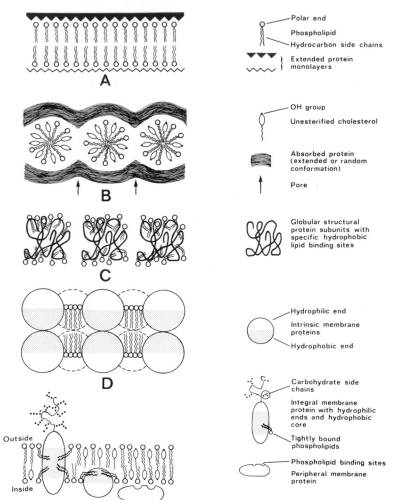

Figure 6–6. Some examples of different membrane models. A, Unit membrane hypothesis (140). B, Micellar lipid subunit hypothesis (145). C, Lipoprotein subunit model (150). D, Protein-crystal model (152). E, Current working model for the erythrocyte membrane, the fluid-mosaic model (7). It should be noted that a number of features discussed in the text, including lipid asymmetry, the many specific proteins portrayed in Figures 6–3 and 6–4, and the various lipid and protein motions have been omitted from this latter model for the sake of clarity.

membrane protein was confined to the outside of the lipid bilayer, that the lipid-protein interaction was predominately electrostatic, and that the membrane protein was in an extended or β-conformation. Allowances were made for differences in the proteins at the inner and outer membrane surfaces. The model suffered in that it did not account for many of the specialized functions of biologic membranes, especially selective permeability, and it did not agree with subsequent freeze-fracture electron microscopic (141) and spectroscopic (142, 143) observations, which indicated that some of the membrane proteins penetrated or spanned the bilayer core and that membrane proteins contained little or no β-structure.

During the middle 1960's, alternatives to the unit membrane hypothesis appeared, which suggested that membranes were composed of more or less globular subunits arranged in a two dimensional mosaic. Based on work in nonphysiologic systems, which showed that mixtures of phospholipids and cholesterol could form stable structures other than bilayers (30, 144), Lucy (145) proposed that membranes might be composed of hexagonally arranged lipid micelles sandwiched between monolayers of protein (Fig. 6–6, B). Recent x-ray diffraction evidence (28) refutes the general applicability of this proposal, but does not exclude the possibility that membrane lipids may assume nonbilayer configurations, either micellar or cylindrical, in selected loci.

Other proposals at about this time emphasized the membrane proteins rather than lipids. A unifying hypothesis was advanced, primarily by Green and his collaborators (146), that all membranes were composed of similar lipoprotein structural subunits to which various membrane-specific functional subunits were attached. This concept evolved from (a) evidence for hydrophobic interactions between lipids and proteins (147), (b) electron microscopic evidence suggesting membrane subunits (148), (c) spectroscopic evidence favoring a globular structure for membrane proteins (142, 143), and (d) reports of the purification and characterization of a so-called "structural protein" from a variety of different membranes (149). A general model of this type proposed by Benson (150) is shown in Figure 6–6, *C*. The credibility of these subunit models was particularly damaged by the application of SDS-PAGE and physical techniques, such as magnetic resonance spectroscopy, to the study of membranes. These new methodologies proved that most membranes contained a heterogeneous collection of proteins, that there was no common "structural" protein, and that the lipid bilayer was the predominant lipid structure (29, 45, 75, 151). A variation of this model which accounts for some of these discrepancies has recently been proposed by Vanderkooi and Green and dubbed "the protein crystal model" (6, 152) (Fig. 6–6, *D*). It depicts the membrane as an orderly array of bimodal, integral proteins organized by protein-protein interactions. The spaces between these proteins are occupied by small lipid bilayer pools. Peripheral proteins are attached to the surface of the integral protein "crystal" (not shown). This model is an example of a "protein matrix" as opposed to a "lipid matrix" (see below).

THE FLUID-MOSAIC MODEL OF THE MEMBRANE. The evidence advanced so far in this chapter leads us to a picture of the erythrocyte membrane as a mosaic of lipoproteins (the integral membrane proteins and their complement of tightly bound lipids), interspersed with regions of viscous, motile lipids organized in a bilayer (Fig. 6–6, *D* or *E*). Various peripheral proteins are disposed on both membrane faces (particularly the cytoplasmic face). Presumably some are associated with specific integral proteins, while others are attracted to lipid polar groups. Both proteins and lipids are asymmetrically but specifically ordered on the inner and outer membrane surfaces.

One of the key questions engendered by this lipoprotein-lipid bilayer-mosaic model is whether the membrane matrix (the element that holds the membrane together) is primarily lipid or protein (7). A protein matrix (Fig. 6–6, *D*) implies that the organization of the membrane results from protein-protein interactions. This would impose a regular (nonrandom) order to the integral membrane proteins and would not favor lateral diffusion of these protein molecules, since many noncovalent protein-protein bonds would have to be simultaneously broken for diffusion to occur. In contrast, in a lipid matrix (Fig. 6–6, *E*) there should be no long-range order of membrane proteins, and lateral diffusion would occur at a rate dependent on the fluidity of the lipid matrix. It should be noted that a lipid matrix does not preclude short-range protein-protein interactions leading to specific protein complexes or clusters, but does predict that such aggregates, like single protein molecules, would be randomly distributed in the membrane plane. This lipid matrix concept has been formalized in the fluid-mosaic membrane model (7) (Fig. 6–6, *E*). Its key features were proposed independently in 1966 by Wallach and Zahler (142) and Lenard and Singer (143), and subsequently have been elaborated by Singer (7).

Protein Motions: Lateral Mobility

SURFACE ANTIGENS. Evidence that membrane proteins are indeed laterally mobile has come from several quarters. In a particularly illustrative study, Frey and Edidin followed the migration of human and mouse membrane antigens on the surface of cell-cell hybrids by fluorescence microscopy (153) (Fig. 6–7). They labeled antigens on the human and mouse halves of the heterokaryon membrane with specific antibodies, and then relabeled these antibodies with different-colored fluorescent-tagged anti-γ-globulins (red for human and green for mouse). At ten minutes after fusion most hybrids showed distinct red and green halves, but within 40 minutes the colors were completely mixed. The process

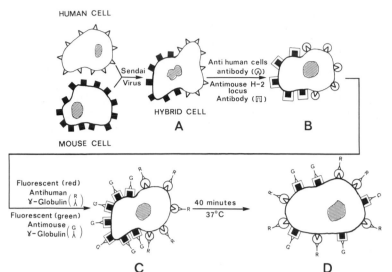

Figure 6–7. Schematic illustration of the experiment of Frye and Edidin (153), which showed that membrane proteins have lateral mobility. Heterokaryons of human and mouse cell lines were produced (*A*), labeled with antibodies specific for either mouse or human cell membrane antigens (*B*), and relabeled with species-specific, fluorescent antigammaglobulins (*C*). The human and mouse antigens, initially segregated, were observed to intermix during subsequent incubation (*D*).

was not affected by inhibitors of protein synthesis or oxidative phosphorylation, but it ceased dramatically at temperatures below 15°C (presumably because of a phase transition of the membrane lipids). It was calculated that this high rate of lateral diffusion was consistent with the movement of molecules 200 Å in diameter in a medium with the viscosity of castor oil (153). Subsequent experiments in lymphocytes (154) and a variety of other cell types (155) have shown that surface antigens labeled with fluorescent antibodies or lectins pool (or "cap") under appropriate conditions, suggesting that lateral mobility of plasma membrane proteins may be a generalized property of all cells. To date, however, membrane "capping" has not been observed in intact erythrocytes, nor has it been proven that integral, and not merely peripheral, proteins are capable of being capped in those cells, such as lymphocytes, which exhibit the capping phenomenon.

FREEZE-CLEAVE ELECTRON MICROSCOPY. Additional evidence for lateral mobility of membrane proteins comes from freeze-cleave electron microscopy of erythrocytes. In this technique, packed red cells are rapidly frozen, and the frozen specimen cleaved at low temperatures with a razor blade. The two fracture faces are then coated ("replicated") with carbon and platinum, and the replicas removed and examined in a transmission electron microscope. It is now well established that the

fracture plane produced by this technique often passes along the center of the membrane bilayer, exposing two surfaces which normally face each other inside the membrane (141, 156). In freeze-cleave studies of lipid bilayers, these surfaces are completely smooth, but in functionally active membranes, such as the red cell, both surfaces are studded with 80- to 100-Å particles (Fig. 6–8). The surface, with acyl chains facing the extracellular space (the inner segment of the bilayer, "surface A"), has four to five times as many particles as the surface with acyl chains facing the cytoplasmic compartment (the outer segment of the bilayer, "surface B"). Several lines of evidence indicate that the particles are made of protein (157) which, from the arguments above, must intrude deeply into the membrane interior or even span the membrane.

In red cell ghosts the particles are randomly dispersed, but under conditions which favor the precipitation of spectrin they move laterally and aggregate (158, 158a) (Fig. 6–9). In intact red cells the intramembranous particles are less mobile but do aggregate under certain circumstances (158b, 162).

Recent work indicates the intramembranous particles are somehow intimately associated with both glycophorin and the major band 3 protein. If the carbohydrate-rich receptors of glycophorin are tagged with ferritin-labeled antibodies or influenza viruses so that their position on the outer

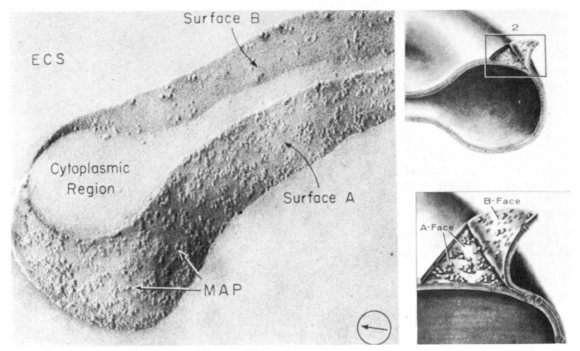

Figure 6–8. Freeze-cleave electron microscopy of a human red cell ghost. (From Weinstein, R. S., and Koo, V. M.: Proc. Soc. Exp. Biol. Med. *128*:353, 1968.) As shown in the drawing on the right, it is now well established that the fracture plane frequently passes through the membrane interior, exposing two new surfaces: the A-face (acyl chains directed outward), and the B-face (acyl chains directed inward). These faces are shown in the electron micrograph at the left. They are randomly covered with clusters of 100 Å membrane-associated particles (MAP). Surface A, which faces the extracellular space (ECS), has more particles than surface B. The encircled arrow shows the direction of platinum shadowing. (From Weinstein, R. S., and McNutt, N. S.: Ultrastructure of red cell membranes. Semin. Hematol. 7:259–274, 1970, by permission of Grune & Stratton.)

membrane surface can be identified, one observes that the location and distribution of glycophorin and the intramembranous particles correspond (109, 159, 160) (Fig. 6–10). Similarly, the major band 3 protein, tagged with ferritin-labeled concanavalin A, aligns with the intramembranous particles (98). Estimates of the numbers of these particles (~600,000 per red cell) and the numbers of glycophorin and band 3 molecules also agree (109). However, since the particles are larger than either of these proteins alone, their exact relationship remains a mystery.

The lateral movement and distribution of the intramembranous particles are also influenced by events at the cytoplasmic membrane surface. As shown in Figure 6–11, the covalent attachment of clumps of denatured hemoglobin (Heinz bodies) to the inner membrane surface (161) causes the intramembranous particles to cluster over the sites of attachment (162). We do not yet know which protein(s) on the cytoplasmic membrane surface (see Fig. 6–4) are bound to the Heinz bodies.

These observations suggest that the intramembranous particles either span the membrane or interact with integral membrane proteins facing both membrane surfaces. Since they are larger than all but the largest membrane proteins (bands 1 and 2), the possibility exists that they may be complexes of one or several membrane protein species (e.g., a combination of both glycophorin and the major band 3 protein). Singer (163) has postulated that transport channels would likely be formed of such protein complexes. In addition to the relationships between anion transport, band 3, and the intramembranous particles discussed above, other recent evidence suggests that, at least at very low temperatures, the passage of water across the membrane occurs through or adjacent to the intramembranous particles (164).

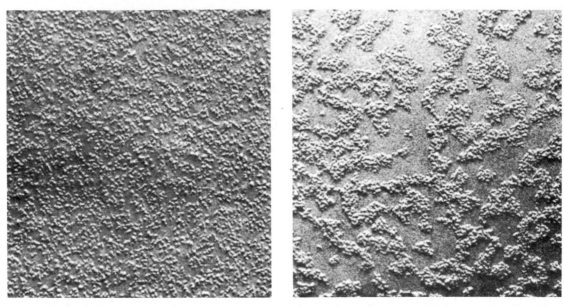

Figure 6–9.   Fracture faces (A-face) of red cell ghost membrane exposed to pH 7.5 (left) or pH 5.5 (right) before freeze-fracture. The intense aggregation of the intramembranous particles evident at low pH was rapid (occurred in less than two minutes), was reversible on return to neutral pH, and could be prevented by prefixation with glutaraldehyde at pH 7.5 or by media of high ionic strength. (From Pinto DaSilva, P.: J. Cell. Biol. 53:777, 1972.)

Protein Topography

The lipid matrix concept predicts that membrane proteins, as well as being laterally mobile, will be randomly distributed in the plane of the membrane. Nicolson and Singer have provided strong support for this supposition with a technique they developed for observing the topographical distribution of ferritin conjugates on membrane surfaces (165–167). The cells are labeled with an antibody to a specific membrane component, lysed, mounted flat on an electron microscope grid, and counterstained with ferritin-conjugated anti-γ-globulin (Fig. 6–12). Only the top surface of the flattened ghost is ferritin-labeled, since the surface attached to the grid is inaccessible to the ferritin antibodies. A topographical distribution of the protein of interest is obtained from the clusters of ferritin which mark each antigenic site.

These studies confirm the random topography of membrane proteins. Some, like the Rh_0 antigen, are solitary (166) (Fig. 6–13), while others, like the $H-2^b$ histocompatibility sites on mouse red cells, are clustered in randomly distributed patches of variable size (167) (Fig. 6–14). Since the Rh_0 antigen exhibits the properties of an integral protein (168), these studies of protein topography argue for the lipid matrix concept. However, as noted above, recent evidence suggests that the lateral mobility of membrane proteins exposed at the cytoplasmic surface may be inhibited by interactions with an underlying network of spectrin (158a), a feature more compatible with a protein matrix. Accordingly, the question of whether the matrix of the native red cell is more nearly "lipid" or "protein" remains unanswered.

Finally, using a variation of this technique, Nicolson has recently presented evidence that alterations in the distribution of a membrane component on the inner membrane surface may be communicated to the outer membrane surface by penetrating proteins, such as glycophorin or band 3. By incorporating antispectrin into resealed erythrocyte ghosts, he was able to show that the antibody-induced aggregation of spectrin was reflected at the plasmic surface by aggregation of the normally dispersed glycophorin molecules (169). This "trans-perturbation" experiment illustrates how mem-

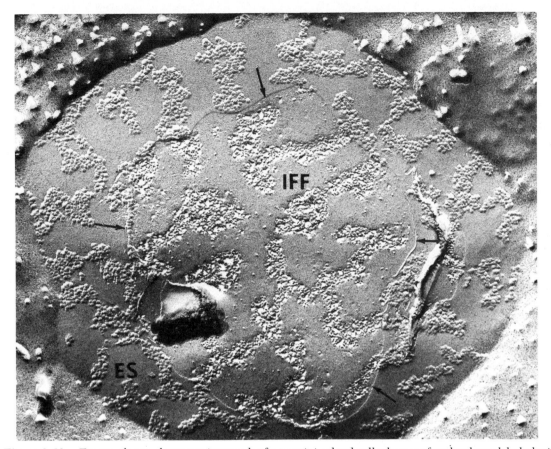

Figure 6-10. Freeze-cleave electron micrograph of a trypsinized red cell whose surface has been labeled with ferritin-conjugated phytohemagglutin (PHA). The preparation has been "etched" (i.e., surface ice removed by sublimation) following freeze-fracture to expose the external surface (ES) of the red cell. Arrows mark the junction between the inner fracture face (IFF, A-face) and the external surface. The intramembranous particles on the inner fracture face are aggregated secondary to the trypsin treatment. There is a remarkable correspondence between the distribution of these particles and the distribution of the ferritin-PHA particles on the external surface. The aggregates of intramembranous particles appear continuous across the cleavage line with the aggregates of ferritin-PHA. Furthermore, the aggregates of intramembranous particles are depressed into the inner fracture face by the overlying ferritin-PHA. The latter are thought to be attached to PHA receptors on the glycophorin molecule (× 73,000). (From Tillack, T. W., Scott, R. E., et al.: J. Exp. Med. *135*:1209, 1972.)

brane-spanning proteins might allow external modulators of cell metabolism (e.g., hormones) or internal events which affect cell surface properties (e.g., malignant transformation) to mediate their effects across an impenetrable membrane barrier.

Two caveats should be noted, however. First, the final molecular mechanism of cell destruction is rarely known, and second, even these broad categories of hemolytic mechanisms are frequently combined in a given hemolytic disorder.

MODES OF MEMBRANE DESTRUCTION

Fragmentation, whole cell lysis, and cellular entrapment are broad classifications of the mechanisms of cell destruction operative in most hemolytic conditions.

Fragmentation

Cell fragmentation can result from direct intravascular trauma. Although the membrane is remarkably flexible and resilient to bending forces which act *across* the plane of the membrane, it has comparatively little elasticity *within* the membrane plane and

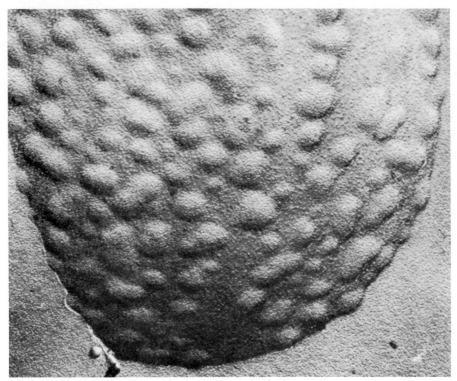

Figure 6–11. Freeze-cleave electron micrograph of a Heinz body–laden red cell. The picture shows the A-face. The impressions of the underlying Heinz bodies, attached to the cytoplasmic membrane surface, are clearly evident. The intramembranous particles are clustered over the sites of Heinz body attachment, and are relatively sparse in the "valleys" between. (From Lessin, L. S.: Nouv. Rev. Fr. Hematol. *12*:871, 1972.)

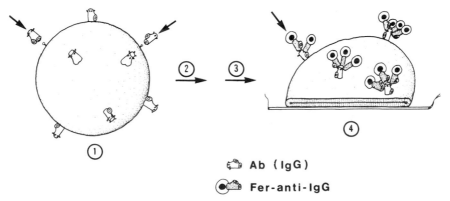

Figure 6–12. Diagram of the indirect staining technique used to determine the topographic distribution of specific red cell membrane components. *1*, The intact red cell is maximally labeled with antibodies to a specific membrane component. *2*, The cell is lysed at an air-water interface, which causes its membrane to spread out flat. *3*, The flattened ghost is picked up on an electron microscope grid. *4*, The mounted membrane is counter-stained with ferritin-labeled anti–gamma globulins and washed. Only half of the membrane stains with the ferritin antibodies, since the surface next to the grid is inaccessible to the counter-stain. Each of the clusters of ferritin marks the position of one antigenic site. (From Nicolson, G. L., and Singer, S. J.: Ann. N. Y. Acad. Sci. *195*:368, 1972.)

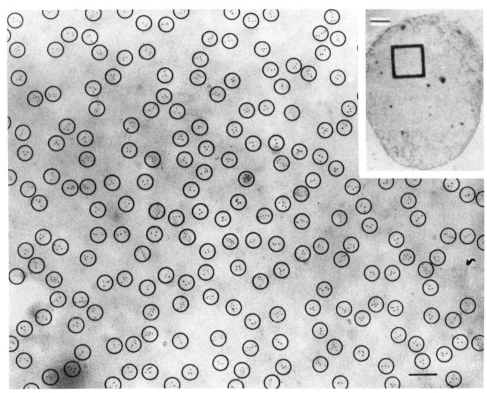

Figure 6-13. Topographic distribution of the Rh_0 (D) antigen on the human erythrocyte membrane. Each Rh_0 (D) antigenic site is marked by an encircled cluster of two to eight ferritin antibodies. There are approximately 10,000 such sites per Dd red cell. Bar equals 0.1 μm.; inset bar equals 1 μm. (From Nicolson, G. L., et al.: Proc. Natl. Acad. Sci. USA 68:1416, 1971.)

can probably tolerate less than a 15 per cent increase in area without rupture and hemolysis (170). Apparently, intramembrane tensions produced by shearing forces in turbulent vascular flow are adequate to cause this slight stretching of the membrane and result in its disruption (171). Such turbulence is usually the result of some defect of the vessel wall, and may be produced in "vessels" as large as the heart (with a Teflon patch graft surface) (172) or as small as an arteriole (with transverse fibrin strand obstructions) (173). If the shear forces are momentary, re-formation of membranes is possible, but frequently some hemoglobin is lost, or the re-formed membranes are only fragments of the complete cell. These fragments are thereafter especially susceptible to further circulatory difficulties, as noted below, and are probably rapidly cleared.

Finally, it is possible that damage to selected membrane proteins could sufficiently alter membrane stability so that even the normal circulatory sojourn would imperil the red cell's survival. Unfortunately we still know so little about the function of the various erythrocyte membrane proteins that we can only speculate about which proteins might be defective in disorders such as hereditary spherocytosis (174) or the hemolysis associated with burns (175), in which diminished membrane stability and fragmentation seem to play a role in the cell's demise.

Whole Cell Lysis

In contrast to partial cell fragmentation, erythrocytes may be totally destroyed within the circulation. This whole cell lysis usually results from severe chemical or immunologic damage to normal membrane constituents. Rarely it can be due to a primary failure of the membrane's capacity to handle ionic gradients due to an inherited

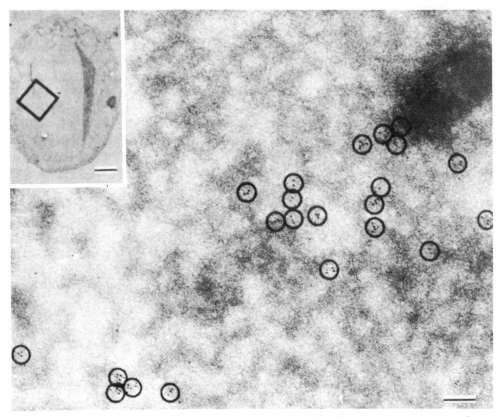

Figure 6–14. Topographic distribution of the H2^b histocompatibility alloantigen on murine erythrocyte membranes. The ferritin clusters are present in randomly spaced "patches" of variable size on the membrane surface. Bar equals 0.1 μm.; inset bar equals 1 μm. (From Nicolson, G. L., et al.: J. Cell Biol. *50*:905, 1971.)

defect in the cation barrier (176, 177). Chemical attacks can involve destruction of either membrane proteins or lipids or both. The offending agents may be either in the plasma (e.g., phospholipases and proteases) (178–180) or within the cell itself (e.g., denatured hemoglobin, intracellular oxidants, or drugs) (181). The immunologic attacks which result in whole cell lysis usually involve complement fixation to the membrane, and the associated production of a defect which has the morphologic appearance of a small "hole" (182) or "pit" (183). In both of these circumstances, final cell lysis probably occurs because of massive permeability changes which overwhelm the capacity of the cell's cation pump. Water rushes into the cell, attempting to equalize the cell to plasma colloid osmotic gradient; the cell swells, and, unable to stretch, bursts.

Filtration and Entrapment

Cells which are rheologically abnormal owing to increased agglutinability, unusual shape, inadequate cytoplasmic deformability, inadequate membrane flexibility, or clumsy cytoplasmic inclusions (181) may be filtered by the RE system (184). This process is accomplished primarily in the spleen and the liver. Because of its unique circulation, the spleen is the most sensitive organ to detect minimally defective erythrocytes (185) (see Fig. 7–1, Chapter 7). Because of its size and blood supply, the liver, though less sensitive, is capable of entrapping more cells than the spleen if it can recognize them (186). Once a cell is caught in either organ, it may be digested by phagocytosis within littoral reticuloendothelial cells. The relatively high concentration of phospholipase within the spleen suggests that this may be an important process in that organ (187). Alternatively, the trapped cell may be "starved" to death in a hostile static environment of low pH, hypoglycemia, and anoxia (188, 189). There its metabolic machinery may fail, with eventual collapse of membrane renewal processes and loss of resistance to cation gradients, finally resulting in local colloid osmotic lysis.

Splenic entrapment with only a temporary sojourn in the spleen may result in cell membrane fragmentation similar to that previously described. Sometimes offending cellular inclusions may be specifically removed from the cell during this process (190, 191) (Fig. 6–15). Under these circumstances, it appears that the cells may be able to tear themselves away from the meshwork of littoral cells if they can be freed of their indeformable cytoplasmic baggage. How-

ever, either membrane resealing is not perfect or excess membrane is lost in comparison to cellular contents during this process, since the resultant spherocytes which manage to emerge from the spleen are at high risk for entrapment and complete destruction on the next circulation through that organ. Healthy reticulocytes which spend their first few days following release from the marrow in the spleen may be normally remodeled in this fashion (193, 194).

DISORDERS PRIMARILY DUE TO FRAGMENTATION

Traumatic Hemolysis

Hemolytic anemia can occur by direct physical trauma to the cell membrane in a

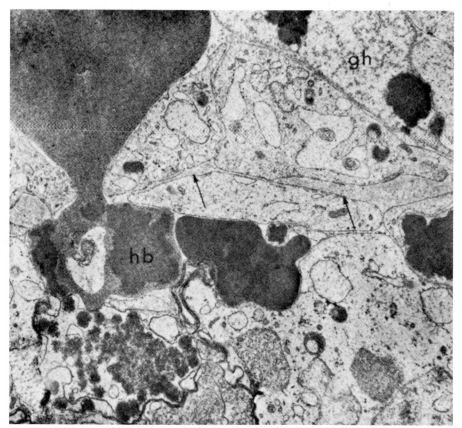

Figure 6–15.   Electron micrograph of a portion of a red cell burdened by a Heinz body (hb) entrapped within the spleen. The red cell appears to be impeded in its passage through a slit in the basement membrane (arrows) separating a splenic cord (below) from an adjacent sinusoid (above). These slits between endothelial cells are shown diagrammatically in Chapter 7, Figure 7–1. A heinz body containing ghost (gh) lies in the splenic sinusoid. (From Rifkind, R. A.: Heinz body anemia: An ultrastructural study. II. Red cell sequestration and destruction. Blood 26 :433–448, 1965, by permission of Grune & Stratton.)

variety of disorders. These are described in detail in Chapter 7 and are only briefly noted here. The hallmark of these disorders is the production of fragments and pieces of the traumatized cells (Fig. 6–16). These fragments are seen often as small, triangular "schistocytes" or tiny microspherocytes and occasionally as teardrop cells. In all these disorders, characteristic schistocytes may be seen on the smear. Hemolysis in these disorders is intravascular. Hemoglobin is liberated directly into the plasma, where it is bound by haptoglobin and hemopexin. These hemoglobin complexes are rapidly cleared by the reticuloendothelial system. As a result the concentrations of both haptoglobin and hemopexin are both frequently diminished (196). Free hemoglobin is only rarely found in the plasma. However, during hemolytic episodes some free hemoglobin is filtered, pinocytized by urinary tract cells, and converted to hemosiderin (197). Since these cells are subsequently shed, an iron stain of the urinary sediment is a valuable tool in the diagnosis of traumatic hemolysis and other disorders characterized by intravascular destruction of red cells.

Various disorders within this group can be separated on the basis of the cause of the trauma, but the mechanism and signs are similar for all. Thus, in the "Waring blender syndrome" following the insertion of valvular or other intracardiac prosthesis (198), hemolysis is usually due to the high speed percussion of a regurgitant jet stream of red cells against an unyielding plastic foreign body. The resultant shear stress upon the red blood cell membrane (199) simply tears the cells apart. Rarely, in this disorder other subtle defects can be introduced in the membrane, producing a bizarre, unexplained positive Coombs' test in addition to fragmentation (200). Elimination of the defective prosthesis or the regurgitant jet usually controls the hemolysis in either case.

March Hemoglobinuria

In the syndrome of "march hemoglobinuria" found in certain unusual patients, repeated pounding of red cells in the small vessels of the feet during sustained marching can produce hemolysis (201). Heavy socks or softer shoe soles have frequently

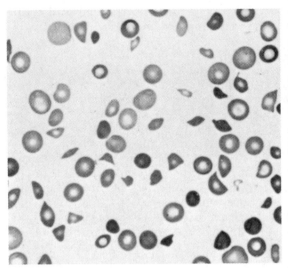

Figure 6–16. Photomicrograph of the peripheral smear of blood from a child with chronic microangiopathic hemolytic anemia. Note the numerous fragmented cells and dense microspherocytes. (From Dacie, J. V.: Secondary or symptomatic haemolytic anemias. Part III of *The Haemolytic Anemias, Congenital and Acquired.* London, J. & A. Churchill, Ltd., 1967.)

eliminated the problem (202). All marchers are not similarly susceptible, however, and efforts to experimentally reproduce the hemolysis with percussion alone have not always been successful. There probably are other unknown factors beyond simply trauma involved in the genesis of this disorder.

Burn Hemolysis

Similar hemolysis and cell fragmentation occurs with direct thermal injury to cells following major cutaneous burns. Immediately following the burn (or after in vitro heating to 44 to 48°C), the red cell membrane becomes irregular, and small bubbly extensions of the membrane form which eventually fall off (Fig. 6–17) (203, 204). Red cell fragments and microspherocytes transiently circulate and can be seen in peripheral blood smears. The hemolysis can be major, depending upon the extent and degree of the burn. Hemoglobinemia and hemoglobinuria may precipitate acute renal

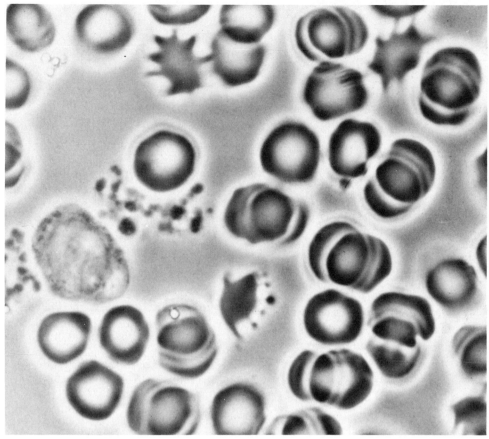

Figure 6–17. Phase photomicrograph of erythrocytes heated to 46°C for 30 minutes. Note the small, bubbly excrescences beginning to form. The cells eventually become spherocytic, and small vesicles of lipid-rich "blood dust" can be isolated from the suspending medium by ultracentrifugation.

failure in such cases, even without antecedent hypotension. A rare variety of this disorder has been reported following the use of red cells which were inadvertently overheated in vitro in an operating room microwave preheater prior to transfusion (205).

Microangiopathic Anemias

Microangiopathic hemolytic anemia is the small vessel analog of the Waring blender syndrome (206). It may occur in any disorder in which the small vessels develop roughened or irregular endothelial surfaces. Renal vascular hypertension (207), thrombotic thrombocytopenic purpura (208), and generalized vasculitis (195) are some examples. A more complete classification is presented in Chapter 7. Though the flow

through these roughened small vessels may be much less than in the regurgitant jets of the cardiac prosthesis, the shearing forces, which are exponentially related to the inverse of vessel diameter, may be as great or greater. The hemolysis is controlled in these disorders only by successful treatment of the underlying disease.

DISSEMINATED INTRAVASCULAR COAGULATION (see also Chapter 7). Disseminated intravascular coagulation (DIC) or consumption coagulopathy is a special case of microangiopathic anemia which deserves individual classification, since the hemolysis is an incidental part of a more general process in which incoagulability and hemorrhage frequently predominate over the hemolysis (209). In this disorder, fibrin and platelet microthrombi are formed in the small vessels secondary to activation of the clotting sequence by a variety of underlying disorders. These include severe sepsis, disseminated malignancy, several leukemias (especially promyelocytic leukemia), heat stroke, marked dehydration, and perhaps thrombotic thrombocytopenic purpura (209–214).

The circulating red cells encounter these fibrin microthrombi and become momentarily entrapped within them. If the blood flow and pressure are adequate, they may then escape from the meshwork, but in doing so they are cut and torn by the thin fibrin strands, much like "pancakes hurled at a clothesline" (Fig. 6–18). The resulting fragments are especially susceptible to entrapment by the RE system. Though simplistic, this explanation is supported by elegant scanning electron micrographs and cine photographs in model systems which show just such changes in vitro (173).

The diagnosis of disseminated intravascular coagulation is one of the most difficult in clinical hematology (208). Ideally, progressive hemolytic anemia, thrombocytopenia, and depletion of procoagulant clotting factors (fibrinogen, factors V, VII, and VIII) are expected, together with the production of fibrin split-products by a secondary activation of fibrinolysis. Unfortunately, only a portion of the complete picture is usually present, the clinical situation is unstable, and hemorrhage frequently predominates over hemolysis. Thus the necessity for therapy of the underlying disorder which precipitates the syndrome is urgent. In certain cases, therapy with heparin in the minimal effective dose is useful. A detailed description of the treatment of DIC is offered in Chapter 20.

LOCALIZED INTRAVASCULAR COAGULATION.   In the past few years, some evidence has been presented for "localized" intravascular coagulation and hemolysis occurring in renal vessels in the hemolytic uremic syndrome, renal graft rejection, and some forms of both acute and chronic glomerulonephritis (215–218). A similar process probably accounts for the thrombocytopenia associated with some cavernous hemangiomas (Kasabach-Merritt syndrome) (219, 220). Theoretically, the clotting abnormalities of disseminated intravascular coagulation should be evident in the localized analog. However, interpretation of the data is even more difficult because of the circumscribed nature of the process and the

dilution effect of the normal part of the circulation. Although poorly controlled, there are sporadic but somewhat encouraging reports on the effectiveness of heparin and other anticoagulant therapy in these conditions (221–223).

"Stress Reticulocyte" Fragmentation

Finally, a discussion of disorders of fragmentation should include mention of "stress reticulocyte" hemolysis. Stress reticulocytes are the unusually large reticulocytes which are released from the marrow following repeated severe hemorrhage (224). They have an apparently short survival (225), and hypotheses for both premature whole cell destruction (226) and partial cell fragmentation (227) have been advanced to explain this. Though explicit data in man are lacking at present, in a rat experimental model, it appears that these cells lose membrane-rich fragments containing hemoglobin during the first few days of their circulation (228, 229). Studies with cohorts of these cells, doubly labeled in both their hemoglobin and their membrane, show that much more membrane than hemoglobin is lost during this process (229). Hence some remodeling of the reticulocyte membrane appears to occur by fragmentation of the surface of these cells. Removal of the spleen markedly slows this effect, so the RE system is probably an important effector in the process.

Even normal reticulocytes spend approximately the first two days of the extramedullary life in the spleen (193). They become smaller and lose considerable lipid in the process (194). Perhaps, then, fragmentation is also a mechanism for remodeling normal red cells in their first few days of life.

DISORDERS PRIMARILY DUE TO WHOLE-CELL LYSIS

The final event of whole cell hemolysis is usually colloid osmotic hemolysis. Hence hemolyzing cells may reveal failure of membrane barrier function, with ingress of water and dilution of the cell's interior

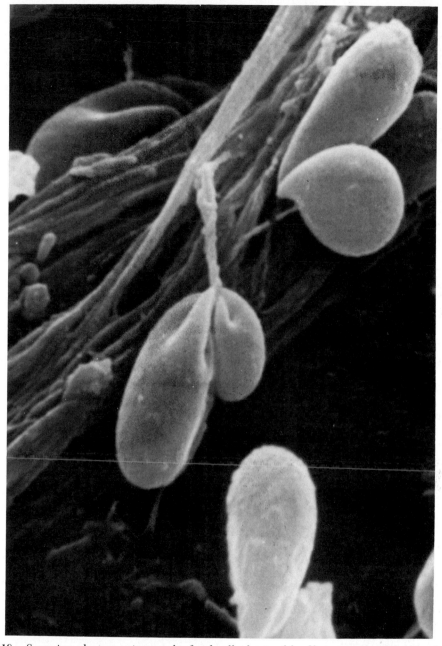

Figure 6–18.   Scanning electron micrograph of red cells detained by fibrin strands. If the blood pressure and flow were adequate, these red cells might escape from the fibrin meshwork but would likely be cut or torn in the process. (From Bull, B. S., and Kuhn, I. N.: The production of schistocytes by fibrin strands (a scanning electron microscope study). Blood 35:104–111, 1970, by permission of Grune & Stratton.)

electrolytes and hemoglobin. The resultant "hydrocyte" may be recognized by an increased mean cell volume and increased absolute amounts of water per cell (177). In contrast to "dessicytes" due to cell dehydration (which will be described below under destruction by filtration and entrapment), these hydrocytes may have low cell viscosity and pass through fine filters even more readily than normal cells.

Direct attack on the cell membrane by bacterial, chemical, or immunologic processes in the plasma can induce the events which lead to whole cell lysis.

Natural Product--Mediated Membrane Damage

Clostridial sepsis is a prime example of this process. It is occasionally associated with fulminant hemolysis, with hematocrits dropping from 40 to 0 in eight hours (230). This rapid and lethal complication is probably due to the release of lytic toxins from the bacteria. The toxin is a strong source of phospholipase C, which can cleave the phosphoryl bases from membrane phospholipids. Since phospholipids are major structural constituents of membranes, this could be the basis of clostridial hemolysis (231). However, in vitro treatment of red cells with phospholipase C produces shrunken but otherwise intact cells (32). Furthermore, cells of a patient with massive hemolysis due to *Clostridium welchii* septicemia were found to have profound protein compositional and structural changes without significant lipid alterations (232). This suggests that proteolytic rather than lipolytic bacterial toxins may be responsible for the cell destruction. Marked hemolysis also occurs following certain rattlesnake and cobra venom bites. Again, though these venoms often contain phospholipases (frequently phospholipase A_2), the possibility of proteolytic factors operating independently or in concert with the phospholipase has been suggested by in vitro studies (180).

Recognition of the danger of these hemolytic catastrophes should be obvious from the history and clinical situation. An early sign of impending hemolysis may be a rapid rise in the serum potassium due to the prelytic leak of this ion from the red cells. Once hemolysis is established, therapy other than transfusion is usually of little use. Antibiotic therapy and hyperbaric oxygen have been occasionally used with success for hemolytic *C. welchii* septicemias (233). In the case of snake bites, localization or drainage of the venom and prompt administration of antitoxin can be lifesaving.

Chemical Agent Damage

In addition to complex bacterial toxins, simple chemical agents may produce whole cell lysis. In this case, again, there may be a mixed attack on membrane lipid and protein. Hydrogen peroxide (H_2O_2)–mediated hemolysis of vitamin E–deficient erythrocytes is a good example of this circumstance and may be a useful model of other clinically relevant types of oxidative hemolysis [e.g., dapsone-induced hemolytic anemia (234, 235)]. In vitro exposure of vitamin E–deficient erythrocytes to H_2O_2 results in peroxidation of both membrane unsaturated fatty acids and membrane sulfhydryl-containing proteins (178). Lipid peroxidation stimulates a membrane repair process, which replaces peroxidation-prone unsaturated fatty acids with peroxidation-resistant saturated fatty acids and eventually produces a marked change in membrane fatty acid composition (236). This, in turn, may make the cell less deformable and profoundly influence its rheology. As discussed below, in vivo such a cell would be especially susceptible to splenic entrapment. Peroxide-damaged cells also exhibit marked hyperpermeability and impairment of the ATPase-mediated cation pump (237). These combined and synergistic defects conspire to produce rapid in vitro hemolysis, even in the absence of splenic filtration, and this phenomenon is used as the basis of a sensitive test for vitamin E deficiency in the infant with prematurity or biliary atresia (238).

It is uncertain whether the hemolysis which does occur in vitamin E–deficient premature infants (239) [and perhaps in some normal men exposed to hyperbaric oxygen (240)] is due to H_2O_2 or to some other intracellularly produced peroxidant. Practically, however, the hemolysis abates with vitamin E replacement (241). This lipid-soluble vitamin, which is normally dissolved within all lipid membranes, acts as an efficient free radical trap, and thereby prevents peroxides from ever reaching the sensitive lipid double bonds and protein sulfhydryl groups (242).

Heavy metal excess resulting in hemolysis is best exemplified by the problem of lead and copper poisoning described in Chapter 4.

Chemically induced damage in the membrane does not have to originate from the external environment. The cell contents themselves may become deleterious for the membrane. In particular, as described in detail in Chapters 13 and 15, many unstable hemoglobins appear to injure the membrane. In most of these cases, the molecular defect is an amino acid substitution or deletion in the vicinity of the heme group, which diminishes the avidity of the globin for the heme (e.g., Hb Köln or Gun Hill) (181). Less often, a substitution in the critical contact region between alpha and beta chains occurs (e.g., Hb Philly) (243). In either case, the resulting globin is unstable and rapidly dissociates and precipitates to form Heinz bodies which affix to the membrane. In the process, membrane proteins are damaged [among other events, membrane sulfhydryl groups are oxidized (244)], and major permeability defects are produced. This cell is in double jeopardy. It may suffer intravascular whole cell hemolysis due to the permeability defect, or it may survive only to be trapped in the spleen because of its cumbersome Heinz body baggage (245).

Primary Disorders of Cation Permeability I

HYDROCYTOSIS AND STOMATOCYTOSIS. A number of conditions characterized by mild to moderate hemolytic anemia and excessive red cell sodium and water content have been recently described (176). The normal balance of cations is discussed in Chapter 1 and in an elegant review by Parker and Welt (177). The first two examples of these rare inherited disorders of the membrane generate red cell "hydrocytes," which are probably destroyed in large part by whole cell hemolysis (246, 247). In both instances, the membranes of the cells were found to be highly permeable to cations, and the cells accumulated sodium and water in excess of potassium loss. The cation pump response of the cells to the excess sodium influx differed in these kindreds. In the first case, the ouabain-inhibitable sodium pump was so rapid that it could not be accurately measured, but approached 30 mEq. per liter of cells per hour (246). This undoubtedly included both net transport and ouabain-inhibitable sodium-sodium exchange. In the second case, the activity of the sodium pump decreased with cell age, so that the older cells contained much more sodium and water than the younger cells (247). In both instances, the demand upon glycolysis for driving the cation pump was markedly increased.

Since these patients were reported a number of similar cases have been described, most of which have in common increased cell cations and moderate hemolytic anemia (176, 177). In one large family study performed by Miller and his co-workers (248), and in the study reported by Oski and his collaborators (247), the disorder seemed to be transmitted by a dominant gene. In this group of disorders, the cells in dried smears may have a central slit ("stoma") and are termed stomatocytes (see Red Cell Morphology, Fig. 1, 7). In wet preparations, the cells are bowl-shaped. The clinical presentations vary from no anemia (249) to severe hemolysis controlled but not cured by splenectomy and transfusion (176, 177). This suggests that the morphologically and chemically similar cells must represent several distinct disorders.

In some of these cases the combination of a very high pump rate and extraordinary sodium permeability makes the cell especially susceptible to the slightest metabolic inhibition of the pumping process. Acidosis secondary to systemic infection is sometimes associated with brisk hemolysis, and splenectomy may be helpful since the spleen is a major circulatory cul-de-sac where acidosis and hypoglycemia combine to inhibit glycolysis. Splenectomy may also be helpful in that the normal membrane lipid removal function of the spleen, mentioned above under membrane fragmentation, is eliminated, allowing the cell more membrane reserve to tolerate hydrocytosis. No abnormalities of cell lipids have been detected in stomatocyte membranes, so that the permeability defects are assumed, for the time being, to be due to some inherited defect of a membrane protein.

HIGH PHOSPHATIDYL CHOLINE HEMOLYTIC ANEMIA. This rare disorder, described in a family from the Dominican Republic, is also associated with major abnormalities of membrane cation permeability. In these patients, however, imbalances in membrane phospholipid content (phosphatidyl choline elevated, phosphatidyl ethanolamine depressed) are present (250–252). Though unequivocal proof is lacking, by analogy with model lipid bilayer systems, these lipid changes appear to be responsible for the cation permeability abnormalities.

The lipid abnormalities are probably secondary to an enzymatic defect in the transfer of fatty acids among phospholipid classes in the erythrocyte membrane (Fig. 6–19) (252). As in stomatocytosis, the cation permeability defect(s) is counteracted by increased activity of the membrane cation pump, and the cell is therefore endangered by environmental conditions in which glycolysis is depressed (253). Mild metabolic stress in vitro, such as brief storage at 4°C, causes marked abnormalities of the cation contents of these cells (251).

The hemolysis in patients with high phosphatidyl choline hemolytic anemia worsens during intercurrent disease or physiologic stress. As in other hemolytic anemias, gallstones and biliary tract disease have also been associated problems; however, in general the patients have not been debilitated by the disease. Splenectomy, again, would seem to be a reasonable protective measure for these patients.

Immune Processes I

"AUTOIMMUNE" HEMOLYTIC ANEMIA. Immunologic membrane damage can cause red cell death by whole cell hemolysis, filtration and entrapment (see Immune Processes II), or both. These disorders are discussed in depth in Chapter 8. With the clinically important exception of transfusion reactions, the major causes of these types of membrane damage are nonhematologic diseases which evoke so-called "autoantibodies" that only incidentally stick to the red cells. The presence of "warm" antibodies, mainly IgG, can give rise to severe hemolytic anemia. These antibodies can be detected in vitro at 37°C. They may be idiopathic or found in association with lymphomas, systemic lupus erythematosus, ovarian teratomas, or certain drugs. Sometimes the autoantibodies are of the IgM or "cold" type, which are detected in vitro after chilling the blood. One can distinguish both a "cold" hemagglutinin syndrome associated with an IgM antibody (sometimes secondary to *Mycoplasma pneumoniae* infection, infectious mononucleosis, or lymphomas), and a paroxysmal cold hemoglobinuria syndrome associated with an IgG antibody (the Donath-Landsteiner antibody) by elution of the antibody from the red cells, followed by electrophoresis against immunospecific antisera, by immunospecific Coombs' tests, or by specific temperature requirements for the antibody fixation (254).

The abnormal IgG and IgM immunoglobulins which cause whole cell lysis usually fix complement to the membrane in the process. The complement, if activated to its late stages, in turn disrupts the membrane architecture (255). In the case of the Donath-Landsteiner antibody, warming the cell-antibody complex is necessary for the activation. The mechanism of this final insult is not known, but elegant model studies which show this effect with purified erythrocyte membrane lipids (256) suggest that the process does not depend upon either chemical changes in the lipid or specific attack on the membrane proteins (257). Instead, physical rearrangements in the lipid arrays of the membrane apparently occur which disrupt permeability resistance in the model system. Perhaps complement acts as a detergent-like molecular "wedge," which insinuates itself between crucial

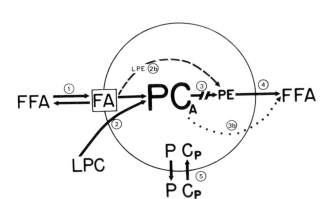

Figure 6–19. Block in transfer of fatty acid from PC to PE in the red cell membranes of a patient with high phosphatidyl choline hemolytic anemia (reaction 3). This results in the accumulation of PC in these cells. Compare with Figure 6–2 (reaction 6b). (From Shohet, S. B., Livermore, B. M., et al.: Hereditary hemolytic anemia associated with abnormal membrane lipids: Mechanism of accumulation of phosphatidyl choline. Blood 38:445–456, 1971, by permission of Grune & Stratton.)

structural elements or which causes phase state changes within the membrane (258).

If a transfusion reaction is suspected, the diagnosis should be obvious from the history, and immediate cessation of the transfusion, coupled with efforts to maintain renal function by osmotic diuresis, is the therapy of choice. Diagnosis of other antibody-mediated disorders producing whole cell hemolysis depends upon the demonstration of intravascular hemolysis (elevated plasma hemoglobin, reduced haptoglobins, and the presence of urinary hemosiderin) and the classic in vitro demonstration of a specific complement-fixing antibody in the patient's plasma or upon his cells (indirect and direct Coombs' tests).

In comparison to the conventional antiglobulin Coombs' test, marked increase in sensitivity for detecting these antibodies has been recently developed by the use of Polybrene. This agent, which neutralizes cell surface charges, allows cell agglutination to occur with miniscule amounts of antibody. In addition, the thermal resistance of the resulting cell to cell bonds appears to have specificity in terms of the type of antibody involved (259).

Therapy of these disorders is usually aimed at resolving the underlying disease in the hope that the antibody level will fall. Direct immunosuppression is probably futile in the long run (260). Some clinical usefulness of steroids and antimetabolites has been claimed (261, 262), but the mechanism of these effects is not clear, and many of these studies are not controlled (260). Occasionally, spontaneous remissions occur. These may be due to decrease in host complement levels or to spontaneous loss of the antibody synthesis.

PAROXYSMAL NOCTURNAL HEMOGLOBINURIA (see also Chapter 8). In paroxysmal nocturnal hemoglobinuria (PNH), no specific antibody is present. Instead, the PNH erythrocyte, through an acquired mutation, becomes an especially sensitive complement receptor (263) which, even without apparent antibody, fixes complement. Minimal acidosis and reduced ionic strength further accelerate this process (255, 264, 265). Hence, hemolysis classically occurs nocturnally (266) when the pH normally falls because of respiratory changes (267); the Ham acid hemolysis test and the hypotonic sucrose-water test (265) can be used in vitro to diagnose the disorder. The specific membrane defect in PNH is unknown, but the final effects are identical to those of other complement-mediated hemolytic processes: the membrane is disrupted, with the production of morphologically distinctive defects which may act like holes (182): water rushes in to balance colloid osmotic gradients, the cell swells to the limits of its excess membrane, and lysis ensues. Although hemolysis is a major part of the symptomatology, patients often succumb to aplastic anemia or leukemia as this disorder evolves (268, 269). These untoward sequelae support the concept that this disorder is the result of an underlying mutation in marrow proliferative cells (270).

Water Dilution Hemolysis

For the purpose of completeness, the rare occasion of water dilution hemolysis should also be included as a cause of whole cell hemolysis. If, because of near drowning in fresh water or by technical error, a patient receives a rapid infusion of distilled water, colloid osmotic hemolysis may occur because of the momentarily increased osmotic gradient between the cells and the plasma. One notable occasion where this tended to occur in the past was the use of distilled water irrigations during lower urinary tract surgery (271). Fortunately, the dangers of this practice are now recognized, and it has fallen into disuse.

DISORDERS PRIMARILY DUE TO ERYTHROCYTE FILTRATION AND ENTRAPMENT

Hemolysis may occur following entrapment of erythrocytes in the organs of the reticuloendothelial (RE) system, particularly the spleen. The rich supply of phagocytic cells and digestive enzymes together with the deleterious conditions of stasis within those organs makes them ideal sites for such "extravascular" erythrocyte destruction. Erythrocytes may be recognized and filtered by the RE tissue because of abnormalities of their surface, their shape, or their contents.

Red Blood Cell Surface Defects

IMMUNE PROCESSES II (see also Chapter 8). Immunologic processes are the primary mediators of surface abnormalities responsible for much of the reticuloendothelial red cell destruction. As opposed to the immunologic disorders which produce whole cell hemolysis, the antibodies involved here often do not fix complement in vitro and only rarely induce direct cell lysis in vivo. Instead, they are usually "autoantibodies" of the IgG_1 or IgG_3 type, which either induce increased intracellular erythrocyte aggregation or, like a bacterial opsonin, prepare the cell for reticuloendothelial phagocytosis (272). This specificity may relate to specific monocyte receptors for C3 (273), IgG_1, and IgG_3 (272, 274).

Disorders which produce hemolysis by this mechanism include many drug-induced Coombs'-positive hemolytic anemias (275) and some hemolytic conditions associated with systemic lupus erythematosus (276), lymphomas (277), and other lymphoproliferative disorders (278). The usual site of cell entrapment is the liver (186), since aggregated cells are readily picked up by that organ, and it receives a large percentage of the circulating blood volume. However, the spleen, because of the slow blood flow in the pulp and the rich supply of reticuloendothelial cells, can become an active site of destruction as well. Therapy is aimed at treatment of the underlying disease. As with immunologic processes producing whole cell hemolysis, therapy often includes the use of steroids and antimetabolites. Again, the studies are mostly uncontrolled, and the results are similarly equivocal (260).

HEREDITARY SPHEROCYTOSIS.* Hereditary spherocytosis (HS) is the archetype of a hemolytic disease in which the cell shape abnormality leads to reticuloendothelial (primarily splenic) entrapment and eventual hemolysis. In this autosomal dominant disorder, the characteristic cell is a dense (high MCHC) spherocyte with abnormally reduced amounts of membrane (see Red Cell Morphology, Fig. 1, *1*). Prior to splenectomy, the morphology of the peripheral blood is frequently heterogeneous, characterized by large polychromatophilic reticu-

locytes and smaller dense spherocytes. Following splenectomy, the morphology is more uniform. Reticulocytes are present in either normal or only slightly increased numbers. Most of the cells are spherocytes of normal volume, but with increased mean corpuscular hemoglobin concentration. A few small microspherocytes are almost always present.

Spherocytosis is, by definition, a condition in which marked reduction of membrane surface area relative to cell volume occurs. Hence it is to be expected that the content of membrane per cell must be reduced in hereditary spherocytosis. This could be accomplished by loss of membrane protein(s), membrane lipid(s), or both. The actual situation is unknown, since accurate measurements of the membrane protein content of HS cells have not been made. Membrane lipid analyses reveal a symmetrical reduction of all membrane lipids in HS cells prior to splenectomy (281). Lipid content per cell is reduced when compared with reticulocyte-rich blood from patients with other forms of hemolytic anemia. Following splenectomy, the lipid content of HS cells is equal to the lipid content of cells observed in normal individuals with intact spleens. It is considerably lower than the lipid content of the red cells of patients splenectomized for other disorders, including trauma and idiopathic thrombocytopenic purpura. These results indicate that some "polishing" function of the spleen reduces the lipid content of normal cells, and that excessive lipid loss occurs from the surface of HS cells, even when the spleen is absent. The "normal" value of membrane lipids in HS cells following splenectomy may be more apparent than real. The measurement of red cell lipids involves complete extraction from intact cells. There is now evidence that under certain deleterious circumstances a considerable amount of surface membrane may be internalized in red cells (282). Therefore, the measurement of total lipid in HS cells may overestimate the amount actually present in the surface membrane of the cell.

HS membranes are "unstable." Demonstration of this instability in vitro requires unusual incubation conditions. When HS cells are incubated at low hematocrit, at a normal pH, and with glucose and phosphate in the medium sufficient to maintain gly-

---

*Comprehensive recent reviews include those by Jandl (279) and Jandl and Cooper (280).

colysis, membrane loss is not observed. However, if the pH is permitted to fall, or if glucose becomes exhausted, HS cells fragment (174) and symmetrically lose lipid (and possibly membrane protein) more rapidly than normal cells under similar incubation conditions (283–285). Thus it may be inferred that splenic entrapment of HS cells and prolonged stasis in that organ may lead to relatively rapid membrane loss and further spherocytosis (286). This "conditioning" effect of the spleen has been demonstrated by measurement of the osmotic fragility of HS cells derived from peripheral vein, splenic vein, and splenic pulp samples (188, 287, 288), as shown in Figure 6–20. In addition, Griggs, Weisman, and Harris (289) have shown that HS cells derived from the spleen have a considerably shorter survival than do HS cells from peripheral blood.

The metabolic basis of membrane instability in HS cells has been the subject of intensive inquiry. Since membrane renewal is at least partially dependent on cell ATP metabolism, several measurements of glycolysis and ATP renewal in HS cells have been performed (283, 290–293). None of these studies has revealed an important primary disorder. Although the level of aldolase activity has been found to be somewhat lower than expected in certain samples of HS cells (294), this probably represents an artifact of cell shape and water content (295) and cannot be critical, since spherocytosis is not observed in severe homozygous red cell aldolase deficiency (296). The rate of glycolysis in HS cells prior to splenectomy is increased, consistent with the young age of red cells in any hemolytic anemia. Even following splenectomy, the glycolytic rate of HS cells is actually somewhat increased above that observed in normal cells (297). This small increase may be partially explained by the fact that the mean age of HS cells following splenectomy may be slightly younger than normal cells (298, 299). Although splenectomy largely abolishes the hemolytic anemia, some slight shortening of the mean cell life span does persist. In addition, the rate of sodium pumping in HS cells is somewhat increased (297). This increased cation pumping activity contributes to the observed increase in HS cell glycolysis, much of which is reduced by ouabain inhibition

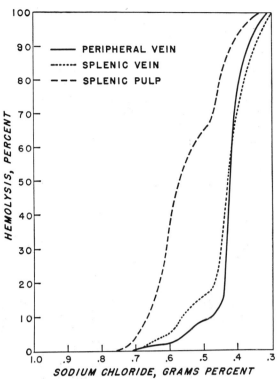

Figure 6–20. Influence of the spleen on the osmotic fragility of hereditary spherocytes. The majority of the red cells in the peripheral blood (solid line) were only slightly more spherical (i.e., more osmotically fragile) than normal. However, a small proportion (about 10 per cent) are decidedly more spherical and produce a "tail" on the osmotic fragility curve. A somewhat higher proportion of spherical cells were present in the splenic vein (dotted line), while in the splenic pulp (dashed line) the majority of the red cells were highly spherical. [From Jandl, J. H., and Cooper, R. A., In *The Metabolic Basis of Inherited Disease*, Stanbury, J. B., Wyngaarden, J. B., and Fredrickson, D. S. (eds.), New York, McGraw-Hill, 1972, p. 1323.]

of the ATPase required for sodium pumping (297).

Since a primary defect in energy metabolism has not been detected in HS cells, attention has been focused on the membrane itself in the search for a molecular basis of the disorder. Although a number of interesting abnormalities of membrane function have been detected, understanding of the primary basis of the disease remains elusive. HS cells (297, 300) and elliptocytes as well (301) (see below) have a somewhat increased permeability to sodium and normal permeability to potassium. Associated with the increased sodium permeability, there is increased sodium pumping. The renewal of phosphorous in the phospholipids of HS cells is also increased (302). Although the increased permeability to sodium was thought at one time to be causally related to the membrane instability (303), subsequent studies have shown that this is not the case. In fact, patients with inherited abnormalities of sodium metabolism associated with sodium permeability and pump-defects vastly in excess of that observed in HS have no evidence of spherocytosis (246, 247), and it is now believed that the error in sodium metabolism observed in HS cells represents an epiphenomenon secondary to the membrane defect, and is not the primary cause of the membrane instability (304).

Various authors have suggested that the primary defect in HS is in one of the membrane proteins (174, 303, 305–308). Immuno-electrophoretic studies disclose no differences between HS and normal membranes (309), but two analyses of HS membrane proteins by polyacrylamide gel electrophoresis suggest that some of the proteins may be abnormal or missing (305, 306). These studies are difficult to interpret because the protein bands in question were not identified or related to proteins visualized by the widely used SDS gel electrophoresis technique. In addition, in one study (305) the protein abnormality was variably present, even in the same patient, while in the other (306) the altered protein electrophoretic pattern was not unique, but was observed in autoimmune hemolytic anemias as well as in HS.

Recently Jacob and his co-workers noted that solubilized but unfractionated HS membrane proteins aggregated less than unfractionated normal membrane proteins in the presence of calcium or vinblastine (307). In a subsequent study they found that many of the characteristics of HS cells could be induced in normal cells by treatment with vinblastine, colchicine, and strychnine (308). Since these three drugs and calcium share the common attribute of precipitating a heterogeneous and poorly characterized group of proteins termed "microfilamentous proteins" (310), the authors hypothesize that "hereditary spherocytosis might result from genetically defective microfilaments in erythrocyte membranes" (308). These studies, while of

great interest, are limited by the failure to identify which of the many red cell membrane proteins is responsible for the altered precipitability. Furthermore, the existence of "microfilamentous proteins" in normal red cell membranes has not been proved, although conceivably spectrin, which forms fibrils under certain conditions, could be considered a candidate for this appellation. Seeman and his co-workers note that vinblastine and strychnine, like other nonspecific lipid soluble drugs, expand the erythrocyte membrane (311). They contend that the concentrations of these drugs used in some of the experiments of Jacob et al. (308) overexpand the membrane and could produce the observed membrane invagination, lipid loss, sodium leakage, and hemolysis independent of any effect they may have on the hypothetical microfilamentous proteins.

Preliminary observations by Greenquist and Shohet (95a) suggest another explanation for the membrane defect in hereditary spherocytosis. As noted earlier, recent evidence indicates that several membrane proteins, including spectrin and one or more of the band 3 proteins (Fig. 6–3, B), are phosphorylated by a membrane-bound protein kinase (93–95). This enzyme is stimulated by magnesium and cyclic AMP and inhibited by calcium. It meets many of the criteria that would be required for a process involved in the maintainence of red cell shape and pliability, including energy dependence; continuous turnover; sensitivity to cell shape perturbants, such as sulfhydryl reagents and calcium; and interaction with major membrane components, such as spectrin. Preliminary results in four patients indicate that phosphorylation of both spectrin and a band 3 polypeptide is decreased in hereditary spherocytosis (95a). This suggests that the primary membrane defect may reside in the kinase enzyme and that the observed morphologic and transport defects may result, secondarily, from failure of one of the unphosphorylated protein substrates to assume a required conformation.

Together these studies reinforce the suspicion that HS is due to defective membrane protein(s), but the specific molecular defect(s) remains elusive. Further detailed dissection and examination of HS membranes will be required to conclusively identify faulty or deficient proteins and establish their relation to the spherocyte's demise.

Despite our lack of knowledge of the precise molecular pathogenesis of hereditary spherocytosis, knowledge of the interaction of the spleen and the spherocyte is fairly complete.

The unique anatomy of the spleen, which demands that a small percentage of red cells passing through it must navigate 3- to 4-μ fenestrations between the cords and the sinuses (185) (see Fig. 7–1, Chapter 7), makes this organ an ideal filter for such indeformable spherocytes. Although correlation of the activity of the disease and the extent of spheroidicity is poor (312), the major clinical and laboratory characteristics of this disorder can be explained on the basis of the spherocytosis alone. Hence, increased osmotic fragility due to the absence of reserve membrane is the laboratory hallmark of this disease (188). Likewise, the usually compensated hemolytic anemia of most patients is strikingly ameliorated by splenectomy (313). Moreover, the spleens, when removed, are large and show evidence of congestion and "work hypertrophy" from their major role in the clearance of spherocytes. In patients with this disorder, any intercurrent process which stimulates the activity of the spleen [such as bacterial infection (314)] is frequently associated with increased clearance of spherocytes and results in the so-called "hemolytic crisis," with a rapid fall in hematocrit and rise in indirect bilirubin. Recurrence of symptoms after splenectomy is almost always associated with hypertrophy of small accessory spleens or splenic remnants left behind during the original surgery.

In confirmation of the importance of the role of reduced membrane surface area in the pathophysiology of the hemolysis, intracurrent obstructive liver disease, which tends to increase membrane lipid and surface area, has been noted to decrease indirect bilirubinemia and hemolysis in patients with hereditary spherocytosis (315). In elegant experiments confirming these clinical observations, chromium-labeled HS cells transfused into patients with obstructive jaundice developed decreased osmotic fragility and produced more nearly normal chromium survival patterns (281).

A unique feature of the anemia of hereditary spherocytosis is the relatively low level of HS erythrocyte 2,3-DPG (316). This paradoxical failure of a normal physiologic response to anemia is not due to any deficiency of glycolysis in HS cells as they are studied in vitro. It is thought that prolonged sequestration of HS cells in the spleen may be responsible for the reduction of 2,3-DPG, for in that acidic environment glycolysis may be sufficiently embarrassed to require the consumption of this glycolytic intermediate, which represents a "storage" source of ATP. Despite the reduced level of 2,3-DPG in HS erythrocytes, the oxygen saturation curve is not shifted to a higher state of oxygen affinity (316). This is probably because the high concentration of hemoglobin in spherocytes tends to shift the curve to a lower affinity state. Hence the combination of low 2,3-DPG and high MCHC allows the HS cell oxygen saturation curve to remain at a normal position.

Clinical Manifestations of Hereditary Spherocytosis. Hereditary spherocytosis is characterized by anemia, jaundice, and splenomegaly (317). The severity of the disease is extremely variable. It varies from family to family, but not usually within families. In at least 25 per cent of the cases, the disease appears to be spontaneous, and no evidence of the usual dominant transmission can be detected. At birth, infants with HS may be severely jaundiced and anemic, and their hyperbilirubinemia may be so severe as to require exchange transfusion. Following the newborn period, the disease is usually considerably milder, and compensated hemolysis ensues. Rarely is there need for a red cell transfusion. In most patients, the hemoglobin stabilizes between 8 and 11 g. per 100 ml., with a reticulocyte count between 7 and 20 per cent and an MCHC greater than 35 g. per 100 ml. The average reticulocyte count is 10 per cent. Jaundice may or may not be present, and is characterized by indirect hyperbilirubinemia without bilirubinuria.

The osmotic fragility test remains the classical laboratory procedure by which the diagnosis of HS and other forms of spherocytosis is determined. Since spherocytes have a reduction of the ratio of membrane surface area to volume, they cannot tolerate the small introduction of free water which occurs when they are placed in solutions of low osmolarity. The more spheroidal the cells, the more apt they are to hemolyze at solute concentrations slightly below isotonicity. If only a small population of cells in the blood are spheroidal, only a few cells hemolyze, and if they have an intermediary ratio of surface to volume, they will only hemolyze at somewhat lower salt concentrations. This provides the well-known "tail" of the osmotic fragility curve, which suggests the diagnosis of HS. Since freshly drawn HS cells may not exhibit a marked shift in the osmotic fragility curve, the incubation osmotic fragility test has been adopted as a further laboratory evaluation. Here, HS cells are incubated under adverse conditions for 24 hours, in the absence of added glucose or careful buffering. Under these circumstances, they lose membrane and hence surface area more rapidly than normal cells, and the osmotic fragility curve is much more radically shifted toward osmotic sensitivity than is the case with normal cells. In contrast, cells with a high membrane surface area to volume ratio, such as the red cells of iron deficiency, thalassemia, or liver disease, have increased resistance to hypotonic lysis, and therefore are characterized as cells with increased osmotic resistance.

The presence of spherocytes and increased osmotic fragility certainly suggests the diagnosis of HS, but several other hematologic conditions are associated with spherocytosis. These include immune hemolysis, burns, liver disease with portal hypertension, and hypersplenism of any cause. Thus the diagnosis of HS must be based on careful clinical and laboratory examinations, and family studies.

The spleen in HS is usually palpable 2 or 3 cm. below the left costal margin. It may grow to an impressively large size, but it is usually only about 2 to 3 times normal. In our experience, most children with HS have a fairly uncomplicated clinical course, and splenectomy may be delayed until the age of five. In some, however, a major complication of chronic hemolytic anemia, the "aplastic crisis," occurs with such frequency that splenectomy is desirable much earlier. Decreased production of red cells probably occurs normally during many acute viral infections. In patients with chronic hemolytic anemia, such interruption of erythropoiesis may lead to sudden and profound anemia that may result in acute congestive heart failure. In fact, lessening of icterus in

a patient with HS, which is often welcomed by parents, usually implies an acute decrease in red cell production due to aplastic crisis and warrants careful investigation. Ordinarily, aplastic crises are self-limited, and patients recover without a need for transfusion. However, if the episodes are frequent and severe enough, early splenectomy should be seriously considered despite its hazards (see below).

Since patients with HS may have mild compensated hemolytic anemia, permanent avoidance of splenectomy is sometimes considered. We are not in favor of such a policy. Although patients with HS may certainly live quite comfortably well into their seventies, the incidence of gallstone-induced biliary tract disease is high enough to recommend splenectomy for all of these patients. It should be noted that the osmotic fragility curve does not normalize following splenectomy, and on occasion may even worsen, since spherocytes remain in the circulation following the procedure.

One note of caution should be mentioned concerning splenectomy in very young children. There is considerable evidence that in early life the spleen is a major part of the host's bacterial defense system (318). This may be related to the spleen's role as a simple filter or to its role as a major site of antigen recognition and antibody production in the young child (319, 320). In any event, splenectomy before the age of four should be avoided if possible, since fulminant pneumococcal sepsis and death have been observed in patients splenectomized in early life (321). If splenectomy is mandatory for patients in this age group, they should be followed very closely for any signs of sepsis or bacteremia. If, as is often the case, such follow-up seems impractical or impossible, the prophylactic use of penicillin may be indicated (322). Though controlled studies are not yet available, the use of this drug seems reasonable in view of the specific sensitivity of the pathogens which are most often responsible for explosive sepsis in these patients.

HEREDITARY ELLIPTOCYTOSIS. Hereditary elliptocytosis is a disorder allied to hereditary spherocytosis which has a similar clinical presentation and genetic pattern. As implied by the name, the cells are typically elliptical on smears (see Red Cell Morphology, Fig. 1, 9). In normal individuals up to 15 per cent of the red cells on peripheral blood smears may be elliptical (323), whereas in patients with hereditary elliptocytosis, at least 25 per cent and frequently more than 75 per cent of the cells are normocytic, normochromic elliptocytes (324, 325). There is some evidence for localization of cholesterol at the apical ends of the ellipse (326), but the cells are normal in overall lipid composition and content. In most cases, the red cell survival is normal or only minimally decreased, and the disorder is nothing more than a morphologic curiosity (327). However, in 10 to 15 per cent of the patients, a distinct hemolytic anemia occurs which is similar in all respects — and probably in pathophysiology — to that of hereditary spherocytosis. Increased osmotic fragility, glucose consumption, sodium leak, lipid loss, and splenic sequestration may all be present (301). Although the elliptocytes are morphologically identical in both the mild and severe cases, patients with hemolysis may sometimes be distinguished by the presence of microovalocytes, bizarre-shaped red cells, and red cell fragments (325, 327). The degree of hemolysis does not correlate with the percentage of elliptocytes (327). In some but not all families, the gene for hereditary elliptocytosis is linked with the gene for Rh blood type (324, 328). In general the kindreds with hemolysis do not show this linkage (329, 330).

The diagnosis is usually evident from the morphology and family history. Elliptic cells also occur in thalassemia, iron deficiency anemia, myelophthisic anemias, sickle cell disease, and megaloblastic anemias, but these disorders are usually distinguishable on other grounds. If significant hemolysis is present, splenectomy is useful (325). By analogy with hereditary spherocytosis, the defect in elliptocytosis may possibly be a primary abnormality in a membrane protein or proteins.

ACANTHOCYTOSIS. Acanthocytes, or thorny cells (Fig. 6–21 and Red Cell Morphology, Fig. 1, 6), are classically found in abetalipoproteinemia (Bassen-Kornzweig syndrome) (331). In this disorder, progressive ataxic neurologic disease, retinitis pigmentosa, malabsorption, and abetalipoproteinemia are associated with the usual red cells. The membrane lipid of these cells contains decreased lecithin and increased sphingomyelin and cholesterol, and the plasma has decreased lecithin and probably decreased lecithin:cholesterol acyltransferase (LCAT) activity (332–334). Unequivocal proof that the morphologic abnormality is due to the cell lipid abnormalities is lacking, but it seems likely in view of the similar morphologic abnormalities associated with membrane lipid abnormalities which are occasionally observed in very severe liver disease (see below) or following severe lipid starvation (334). Surprisingly, the hemolysis in acanthocytosis is mild to minimal (335), and it may be confined to a subtle shortening of ^{51}Cr red cell survival. Hence the cell, though very bizarre in appearance and rheologically abnormal in vitro (334), must usually be sufficiently deformable in vivo to avoid excessive entanglement and entrapment in the microcirculation. Treatment of the hemolytic process is not usually required, though parenteral vitamin E to replace its deficiency secondary to the malabsorption seems reasonable in order to prevent lipid peroxidation (336). The prognosis of this disorder is related much more to its neurologic sequelae than to its hematologic manifestations.

LIVER DISEASE, TARGET CELLS, AND SPUR CELL ANEMIA. Anemia in liver disease is of complex etiology. Common causes include blood loss, hypersplenism, iron deficiency, folic acid deficiency, and marrow suppression from alcohol, hepatitis virus, and other poorly understood factors (337, 338). In addition, acquired abnormalities of the red cell membrane may contribute to the anemia. Two morphologic syndromes are recognized. In one, target cells and spherocytes predominate (338), the latter presumably because of sequestration of red cells for prolonged periods in the spleen. Target cells are particularly characteristic of biliary obstruction (339) but also occur in other types of liver disease. Less commonly, a syndrome of brisk hemolysis in association with "spur" cells develops in patients with severe hepatocellular disease (340–342). Spur cells are morphologically identical to acanthocytes (Fig. 6–22) but differ in lipid composition (see below).

Both of these morphologic entities are acquired abnormalities of membrane lipids and can be produced in vitro or in vivo by

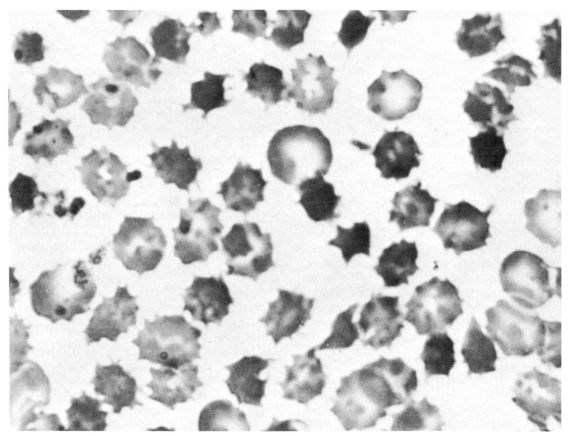

Figure 6-21. Acanthocytes from the original patient with abetalipoproteinemia. Note the irregular, "thorny" projections of the cell membranes. (From Bassen, F. A., and Kornzweig, A. L.: Malformation of the erythrocytes in a case of atypical retinitis pigmentosa. Blood 5:381–387, 1950, by permission of Grune & Stratton.)

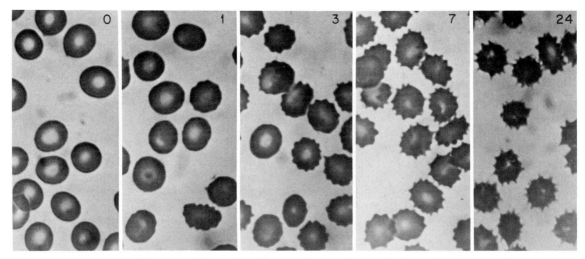

Figure 6-22. Acquired "spur cells" produced by incubation of normal cells in heated serum from a patient with severe liver disease. The hours of incubation are shown in the upper right-hand corner of each photomicrograph. Note the similarity of the 24-hour incubation sample with the acanthocytes in Figure 6–21. (From Cooper, R. A.: J. Clin. Invest. 48:1820, 1969.)

incubation of normal cells in the respective pathologic sera (Fig. 6–22) (339, 340, 342). Target cells are characterized by a balanced increase in both free cholesterol and phospholipid, whereas in spur cell membranes the free cholesterol content is greatly increased, but the phospholipid content is nearly normal (Fig. 6–23) (343). Thus the free cholesterol-phospholipid ratio of spur cells is markedly increased, while it tends to be normal in target cells. The abnormal lipids and morphology of target cells are reversible upon incubation in normal plasma (339). In contrast, on incubation in normal serum, spur cells lose their excess cholesterol but are converted into osmotically fragile spherocytes rather than biconcave disks (342). This probably occurs because the poorly deformable (334, 342) spur cells have lost membrane fragments during their circulatory life span and cannot tolerate the additional loss of membrane surface area which accompanies the removal of excess free cholesterol. Target cells are normally deformable and are not threatened by fragmentation.

The pathogenesis of lipid accumulation in these cells is not entirely clear. Three mechanisms have been suggested. First, since red cell membrane lipids exchange in part with the lipids of serum lipoproteins (19, 20, 23), the membrane lipid abnormalities may simply reflect a corresponding abnormality of serum lipoprotein composition. This mechanism is supported by recent studies of Cooper and his co-workers (343), who found a close correlation between the cholesterol-phospholipid ratios of spur cells, target cells, and their respec-

tive serum lipoproteins, particularly for low density lipoprotein (LDL). It is known that in obstructive liver disease a unique, abnormal lipoprotein, called LpX, accumulates in the LDL density class (344, 345). LpX appears to be a lipid bilayer vesicle containing approximately equimolar amounts of free cholesterol and phospholipid in addition to a small amount of protein (346). Since the production of target cells is associated with the accumulation of approximately equimolar amounts of free cholesterol and phospholipid, it would be interesting to know the relationship between LpX production and target cell formation.

A second proposed mechanism for the red cell lipid abnormalities in liver disease relates to the plasma enzyme lecithin: cholesterol acyltransferase (LCAT). As noted earlier, by controlling the esterification of free cholesterol in plasma lipoproteins, LCAT may be indirectly responsible for controlling the free cholesterol content of red cell membranes (24). Since LCAT activity is often decreased in patients with liver disease, it has been suggested that LCAT deficiency is primarily responsible for the red cell membrane lipid abnormalities observed in these patients (341, 347, 348) and that the enzyme deficiency is the result of inhibition by increased levels of certain bile acids (339). However, the levels of bile acids found in patients with liver disease are only 5 to 10 per cent of those required for LCAT inhibition (339, 349), and recent investigations by Cooper and his co-workers (343) reveal a poor correlation between LCAT activity and red cell choles-

Figure 6–23. The cholesterol and phospholipid content of target (●) and spur (△) cells. Note that target cells tend to have a balanced increase in cholesterol and phospholipid, while spur cells are usually selectively enriched in cholesterol. (From Cooper, R. A., Dilay-Puray, M., et al.: J. Clin. Invest. 51;3182, 1972.)

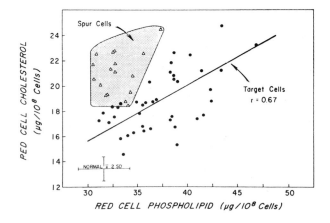

terol in patients with target cells or those with spur cells. Hence the role of LCAT in these disorders is still problematic.

The third proposed mechanism seeks to relate the changes in the serum concentration of specific bile acids in liver disease with the genesis of target and spur cells. Cooper's studies reveal significant variations in the bile acid composition of spur cell and target cell sera (343). In particular, the presence of spur cells was correlated with a relative increase in the amount of chenodeoxycholic acid. Lithocholic acid, a derivative of chenodeoxycholate, can induce spur cell formation in vivo (350), but unfortunately, in the reported study, no lithocholic acid was detected in spur cell patients despite the increased chenodeoxycholic acid levels (343).

FAMILIAL LECITHIN:CHOLESTEROL ACYLTRANSFERASE (LCAT) DEFICIENCY. Familial LCAT deficiency is characterized by anemia, corneal opacities, and renal disease (26). All the reported patients have had a moderate normochromic anemia, with prominent target cell formation. There is evidence for both hemolysis and decreased erythropoiesis in the pathogenesis of the anemia (26), but interpretation of this evidence is complicated by the coexisting renal disease. As expected from the near absence of LCAT activity, there is a pronounced decrease in cholesteryl esters and an increase in free cholesterol in the plasma lipoproteins (26). The red cell membranes are also overloaded with free cholesterol (17.5 to 20.6 μg per 10^8 cells; compare with Fig. 6–23), but their total membrane phospholipid content is normal (PC is increased, but this is balanced by decreased PE and SM). Hence the red cells in these patients resemble target cells morphologically but spur cells chemically. It is clear from these and other studies (Table 6–2) that the relationship of red cell morphology to plasma and membrane lipid composition and LCAT activity is complex and incompletely understood.

Primary Disorders of Cation Permeability II: Desiccytosis

The opposite of the hydrocyte, previously described, is the desiccyte: a shrunken, dehydrated red cell (176). Such cells result from excessive loss of intracellular potassium unbalanced by sodium gain. An obligatory decrease in cell water follows. Desiccytosis may be secondary to red cell defects, such as pyruvate kinase deficiency (353) and sickle cell anemia (354), or it may be the result of a primary defect in membrane permeability as in the kindred recently described by Glader and his co-workers (355). In the latter family, the defect was manifest in two generations as a severe congenital hemolytic anemia with hepatosplenomegaly. The erythrocyte morphology was bizarre. Shrunken, spiculated cells and cells in which the hemoglobin appeared to be "puddled" on one side of the cell were particularly striking (Fig. 6–24). The membranes of these red cells were highly permeable to cations, and the cells lost potassium and water in excess of sodium gain. In older red cells, cellular potassium approached half-normal levels. The accompanying dehydration was reflected by their very high MCHC, increased resistance to osmotic stress, and poor filterability. Splenectomy was performed in one of the two affected family members, but did not alter the course of the disease, presumably because the defective red cells were so compromised that they were detected and eliminated in other areas of the reticuloendothelial system. The specific membrane abnormality responsible for these progeric red cells is unknown.

Cell Content Abnormalities

Abnormalities in cellular content may have secondary effects upon the red cell membrane which result in entrapment by the reticuloendothelial system and hemolysis. These include disorders in which inadequate ATP is produced to maintain membrane function.

SICKLE CELL ANEMIA. Sickle cell anemia, which is discussed in depth in Chapter 14, should, of course, be mentioned as a cell content abnormality which leads to splenic and microvascular entrapment. While the morphologically sickled form is clearly dependent upon the abnormal physical characteristics of the sickle hemoglobin, damage to the membrane of sickle cells is probably crucial in the entrapment process which is central to the patho-

TABLE 6–2. RELATIONSHIP OF SOME PLASMA AND MEMBRANE LIPIDS AND LCAT ACTIVITY IN VARIOUS DISORDERS

Disorder	LCAT Activity	Plasma			Red Cell			Morphology
		Free Cholesterol	Total Phospholipids	% Lecithin°	Free Cholesterol	Total Phospholipids	% Lecithin°	
Spur cell anemia (343)	↓↓	↑	N	↓	↑↑	N	↑	Acanthocytes
Liver disease with target cells (343)	↓	±↑	N	N	↑	↑	↑↑	Target cells
Abetalipoproteinemia (332, 333, 351)	↓	↓↑	↓↑	↓↑	±↑	N	↓↑	Acanthocytes
Analphalipoproteinemia (Tangier disease) (351, 352)	↓	↓	↓	N	N	N	±↑	Normal
Familial LCAT deficiency (26)	Absent	↑↑	↑	↑↑	↑↑	N	↑↑	Target cells

°Lecithin is synonymous with phosphatidyl choline (Fig. 6–2).

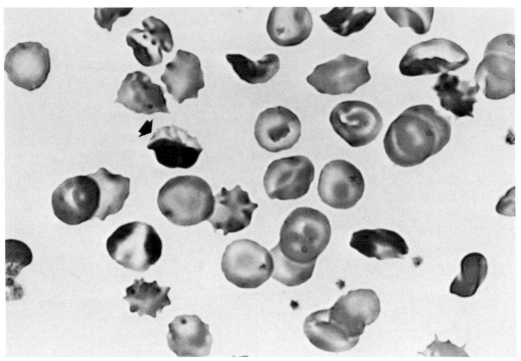

Figure 6–24. Peripheral blood smear from a patient with low potassium red cells ("desiccytosis") described by Glader et al., (355). Target cells and shrunken, spiculated cells predominate. In occasional cells the hemoglobin appears to be "puddled" on one side of the cell (arrow).

physiology of this disorder. Filtration studies (356, 357) and cine photographs of sickled cells passing through capillary beds show that, although sickled cells are much more rigid than normal cells in vitro, they are still surprisingly deformable and manage to navigate the interstices of the microcirculation in vivo with some success despite their abnormal shape. It is primarily when the cells are "irreversibly sickled" (358) that they develop serious rheologic liabilities (359) and stasis begins to occur. Electron micrographic studies indicate that this state of "irreversible sickling" is a membrane phenomenon; that is, the hemoglobin can be in the amorphous, nonsickled state despite a sickled membrane form (360).

Two observations may partially explain this unexpected finding and offer approaches to therapy. First, irreversibly sickled cells may have considerably less lipid per cell than reversibly sickled cells (361). Second, as noted above, irreversibly sickled cells have a permanently reduced content of cations and water and, hence, behave as excessively viscous "desiccytes."

This phenomenon may be an exaggeration of the excess cation loss across sickle membranes which occurs during the sickling process (354). Both these phenomena suggest that therapy designed to stabilize sickle cell membrane lipids (362) or to prevent sickle cell cation loss might prevent the accumulation of irreversibly sickled cells and thereby ameliorate the disease.

INCLUSION-BEARING CELLS. Cells with inclusions due to unstable hemoglobins (Chapters 13 and 15) have already been discussed in terms of the whole cell hemolysis which may occur because of secondary effects of the unstable globin precipitates on membrane permeability. As noted, however, if these cells are not lysed in the circulation, they are still likely to be trapped in the spleen because of their burdensome inclusions (192, 245).

Similar inclusions are produced in cells which are unable to accommodate oxidative threats due to defects in their glycolytic pathways—the so-called "Heinz body" hemolytic anemias (363) (Chapter 11). Likewise, cellular inclusions are produced in the various thalassemias (364) (Chapter 15), in which excess globin chains of one type are present because of a defect in the synthesis of the complementary type (365). These excess unpaired chains are unstable and form similar precipitate inclusions.

Apparently the presence of the inclusions in all these disorders makes the cell particularly vulnerable to splenic entrapment (Fig. 6–15). The precise membrane damage that results in hemolysis following entrapment is not known. The cell may be directly phagocytized and digested or destroyed by a variety of physical (e.g., shearing) and chemical (e.g., phospholipase) attacks, coupled with inhibition of the cell's metabolic defenses in the harsh splenic environment. If the cells are not actually destroyed in the spleen, they then emerge markedly weakened and susceptible to whole cell hemolysis due to newly acquired permeability defects or to re-entrapment and final digestion within the spleen.

As expected, splenectomy may be of some value in ameliorating these disorders. However, results are not nearly as dramatic as in hereditary spherocytosis, since other parts of the RE system—notably the liver and the marrow itself—are often capable of recognizing many inclusion-bearing cells. Following splenectomy, these organs may hypertrophy and become the graveyard for such overburdened cells. In fact, in some thalassemias the marrow seems so advanced in this role (366) that large proportions of intramedullary hemolysis can be detected by abnormal bilirubin turnover, even in patients with thalassemia trait (367).

The ideal therapy of these disorders would be to prevent inclusion formation. This may be achieved in patients with Heinz body hemolytic anemias by prohibiting exposure to oxidative drugs. Successful therapy of the thalassemias and unstable hemoglobinopathies, however, will probably await development of genetic or molecular-biologic methods for the control of hemoglobin chain production (368).

ATP-DEPLETED CELLS. Disorders in which cellular ATP generation is defective form a final theoretical classification of disorders in which reticuloendothelial entrapment would be expected. When ATP levels fall sufficiently, several consequences may result: the maintenance of cell cation gradients may fail (369), membrane lipid renewal may decline (370, 371), and, most importantly, calcium may bind to the membrane and its cellular contents (372). The latter phenomenon is apparently due to the loss of the normal chelating activity of ATP for calcium. When calcium does bind to the cell contents, gel-sol transformations occur, and the cell membrane and cytoplasm become extremely stiff and indeformable (372, 373). Splenic entrapment follows. While this mechanism for generating "stiff" cells has been convincingly demonstrated in vitro, it is difficult to unequivocally demonstrate in vivo. However, in the hemolytic anemias of phosphoglycerokinase deficiency and pyruvate kinase deficiency in which ATP generation is impaired, splenic erythrocyte sequestration is observed, and populations of relatively stiff, indeformable cells have been found (374, 375). The rare hemolysis which has been observed with phosphate depletion (and, secondarily, ATP depletion) may also occur via this mechanism (376).

SUMMARY

Hemolysis is membrane failure. Since the erythrocyte membrane consists of a complex combination of lipid and protein molecules, and since that membrane travels through a complex series of changing environments, it is not surprising that many different mechanisms of membrane failure can occur. Fragmentation, whole cell hemolysis, and cellular entrapment can all serve as mechanisms for red cell destruction. Defects in the membrane, combined with interactions between the membrane and the environment, are frequently responsible for this destruction.

Dr. Shohet is the recipient of NIH grant A.M.–16095 and Career Development Award A.M.–37237.

References

1. Danielli, J. F., and Davson, H. A.: A contribution to the theory of the permeability of thin films. J. Cell. Comp. Physiol. 9:89, 1936.
2. Stoeckneius, W., and Engelman, D. M.: Current models for the structure of biological membranes. J. Cell. Biol. 42:613, 1969.

3. Hendler, R. W.: Biological membrane ultrastructure. Physiol. Rev. 51:66, 1971.

4. Shohet, S. B.: Hemolysis and changes in erythrocyte membrane lipids. New Engl. J. Med. 286:577, 1972.

5. Robertson, J. D.: The structure of biological membranes. Current status. Arch. Intern. Med. 129:202, 1972.

6. Vanderkooi, G.: Molecular architecture of biological membranes. Ann. N.Y. Acad. Sci. 195:6, 1972.

7. Singer, S. J., and Nicolson, G. L.: The fluid mosaic model of the structure of cell membranes. Science 175:720, 1972.

8. Ways, P., and Hanahan, D. J.: Characterization and quantification of red cell lipids in normal man. J. Lipid Res. 5:318, 1964.

9. Sweeley, C. C., and Dawson, G.: Lipids of the erythrocyte, In Red Cell Membrane Structure and Function. Jamieson, G. A., and Greenwalt, T. J. (eds.), Philadelphia, J. B. Lippincott, 1969, p. 172.

10. Houchin, D. N., Munn, J. I., et al.: A method for the measurement of red cell dimension and calculation of mean corpuscular values and surface area. Blood 13:1185, 1958.

11. Turner, J. D., and Rouser, G.: Precise quantitative determination of human blood lipids by thin layer and triethylaminoethyl cellulose column chromatography. Anal. Biochem. 38:423, 1970.

12. Cooper, R. A.: Lipids of human red cell membrane: Normal composition and variability in disease. Semin. Hematol. 7:296, 1970.

13. Bishop, D. G.: Topical metabolism, In Biochemistry and Methodology of Lipids. Johnson, A. R., and Davenport (eds.), New York, Wiley-Interscience, 1971, p. 397.

14. Dowben, R. M.: Composition and structure of membranes, In Biological Membranes. Dowben, R. M. (ed.), Boston, Little, Brown and Co., 1969, p. 1.

15. Oliveira, M. M., and Vaughan, M.: Incorporation of fatty acids into phospholipids of erythrocyte membranes. J. Lipid Res. 5:156, 1964.

16. Tarlov, A. R.: Lecithin and lysolecithin metabolism in rat erythrocyte membranes. Blood 28:990, 1966.

17. Shohet, S. B., Nathan, D. G., et al.: Stages in the incorporation of fatty acids into red blood cells. J. Clin. Invest. 47:1096, 1968.

18. Donabedian, R. K., and Karmen, A.: Fatty acid transport and incorporation into human erythrocytes in vitro. J. Clin. Invest. 46:1017, 1967.

19. Mulder, E., and Van Deenen, L. L. M.: Metabolism of red-cell lipids. I. Incorporation in vitro of fatty acids into phospholipids from mature erythrocytes. Biochim. Biophys. Acta 106:106, 1965.

20. Shohet, S. B.: Release of phospholipid fatty acid from human erythrocytes. J. Clin. Invest. 49:1668, 1970.

21. Reed, C. F.: Phospholipid exchange between plasma and erythrocytes in man and the dog. J. Clin. Invest. 47:749, 1968.

22. De Gier, J., and Van Deenen, L. L. M.: A dietary investigation on the variations in phospho-lipid characteristics of red-cell membranes. Biochim. Biophys. Acta 84:294, 1964.

23. Weir, G. C., and Martin, D. B.: Fatty acid biosynthesis in the erythrocyte. II. Evidence in immature erythrocytes for the presence of acetyl coenzyme A carboxylase. J. Lab. Clin. Med. 81:37, 1973.

24. Quarfordt, S. H., and Hilderman, H. L.: Quantitation of the in vitro free cholesterol exchange of human red cells and lipoproteins. J. Lipid Res. 11:528, 1970.

25. Glomset, J. A.: The plasma lecithin:cholesterol acyltransferase reaction. J. Lipid Res. 9:155, 1968.

26. Norum, K. R., Glomset, J. A., et al.: Familial lecithin-cholesterol acyltransferase deficiency, In The Metabolic Basis of Inherited Disease. Stanbury, J. B., Wyngaarden, J. B., and Fredrickson, D. S. (eds.), New York, McGraw-Hill, 1972, p. 531.

27. Stein, J. M., Tourtellotte, J. C., et al.: Calorimetric evidence for the liquid-crystalline state of lipids in a biomembrane. Proc. Natl. Acad. Sci. USA 63:104, 1969.

28. Wilkins, M. H. F., Blaurock, A. E., et al.: Bilayer structure in membranes. Nature [New Biol.] 230:72, 1971.

29. Hubbell, W. L., and McConnell, H. M.: Orientation and motion of amphiphilic spin labels in membranes. Proc. Natl. Acad. Sci. USA 64:20, 1969.

30. Luzzati, V., and Husson, F.: The structure of the liquid-crystalline phases of lipid-water systems. J. Cell Biol. 12:207, 1962.

31. Tinker, D. O., and Pinteric, L.: On the identification of lamellar and hexagonal phases in negatively stained phospholipid-water systems. Biochemistry 10:860, 1971.

32. Glaser, N., Simpkins, H., et al.: On the interactions of lipids and proteins in the red blood cell membrane. Proc. Natl. Acad. Sci. USA 65:721, 1970.

33. McFarland, B. G.: The molecular basis of fluidity in membranes. Chem. Phys. Lipids 8:303, 1972.

34. Jost, P. C., Griffith, O. H., et al.: Evidence for boundary lipid in membranes. Proc. Natl. Acad. Sci. USA 70:480, 1973.

35. Griffith, O. H., and Waggoner, A. S.: Nitroxide free radicals: Spin labels for probing biomolecular structure. Accounts Chem. Res. 2:17, 1969.

36. Hubbell, W. L., and McConnell, H. M.: Molecular motion in spin-labeled phospholipids and membranes. J. Am. Chem. Soc. 93:2, 1971.

37. Mehlhorn, R. J., and Keith, A. D.: Spin labeling of biological membranes, In Membrane Molecular Biology. Fox, C. F., and Keith, A. D. (eds.), Stamford, Conn., Sinauer Assoc., Inc., 1972, p. 192.

38. Horwitz, A. F.: Nuclear magnetic resonance studies on phospholipids and membranes, In Membrane Molecular Biology. Fox, C. F., and Keith, A. D. (eds.), Stamford, Conn., Sinauer Assoc., Inc., 1972, p. 164.

39. Chapman, D.: Nuclear magnetic resonance spectroscopic studies of biological membranes. Ann. N.Y. Acad. Sci. 195:179, 1972.

40. Chapman, D., and Wallach, D. F. H.: Recent physical studies of phospholipids and natural membranes, In *Biological Membranes, Physical Fact and Function*. Chapman, D. (ed.), New York, Academic Press, 1968, p. 125.

41. McConnell, H. M., and McFarland, B. G.: The flexibility gradient in biological membranes. Ann. N.Y. Acad. Sci. *195*:207, 1972.

42. Levine, Y. K., Birdsall, N. J. M., et al.: ^{13}C nuclear magnetic resonance relaxation measurements of synthetic lecithins and the effect of spin-labeled lipids. Biochemistry *11*:1416, 1972.

43. Seelig, J., and Hasselbach, W.: A spin label study of sarcoplasmic vesicles. Eur. J. Biochem. *21*:17, 1971.

44. Eletr, S., and Keith, A. D.: Spin-label studies of dynamics of lipid alkyl chains in biological membranes: Role of unsaturated sites. Proc. Natl. Acad. Sci., USA *69*:1353, 1972.

45. Hubbell, W. L., and McConnell, H. M.: Motion of steroid spin labels in membranes. Proc. Natl. Acad. Sci. USA *63*:16, 1969.

46. Oldfield, E., and Chapman, D.: Effects of cholesterol and cholesterol derivatives on hydrocarbon chain mobility in lipids. Biochem. Biophys. Res. Commun. *43*:610, 1971.

47. Rothman, J. E., and Engelman, D. M.: Molecular mechanism for the interaction of phospholipid with cholesterol. Nature [New Biol.] *237*:42, 1972.

48. Kornberg, R. D., and McConnell, H. M.: Lateral diffusion of phospholipids in a vesicle membrane. Proc. Natl. Acad. Sci. USA *68*:2564, 1971.

49. Deveaux, P., and McConnell, H. M.: Lateral diffusion in spin-labeled phosphatidylcholine multibilayers. J. Am. Chem. Soc. *94*:4475, 1972.

50. Lee, A. G., Birdsall, N. J. M., et al.: Measurement of lateral diffusion of lipids in vesicles and in biological membranes by ^{1}H nuclear magnetic resonance. Biochemistry *12*:1650, 1973.

51. Kornberg, R. D., and McConnell, H. M.: Inside outside transitions of phospholipids in vesicle membranes. Biochemistry *10*:1111, 1971.

52. Raigon, J. K., Lyons, J. M., et al.: Temperature-induced phase changes in mitochondrial membranes detected by spin-labeling. J. Biol. Chem. *246*:4036, 1971.

53. Tourtellotte, M. E.: Mycoplasma membranes: structure and function, In *Membrane Molecular Biology*, Fox, C. F., and Keith, A. D. (eds.), Stamford, Conn., Sinauer Assoc., Inc., 1972, p. 439.

54. Esfahani, M., Crowfoot, P. D., et al.: Molecular organization of lipids in *E. coli* membranes. II. Effect of phospholipids on succinicubiquinone reductase activity. J. Biol. Chem. *247*:7251, 1972.

55. Shimshick, E. J., and McConnell, H. M.: Lateral phase separation in phospholipid membranes. Biochemistry *12*:2351, 1973.

56. Ohnishi, S., and Ito, T.: Clustering of lecithin molecules in phosphatidylserine membranes induced by calcium ion binding to phosphatidylserine. Biochem. Biophys. Res. Commun. *51*:132, 1973.

57. Bretscher, M.: Asymmetrical lipid bilayer structure for biological membranes. Nature [New Biol.] *236*:11, 1972.

58. Bretscher, M.: Phosphatidyl-ethanolamine: Differential labeling in intact cells and cell ghosts of human erythrocytes by a membrane-impermeable reagent. J. Mol. Biol. *71*:523, 1972.

59. Gordesky, S. E., and Marinetti, G. V.: The asymmetric arrangement of phospholipids in the human erythrocyte membrane. Biochem. Biophys. Res. Commun. *50*:1027, 1973.

60. Colley, C. M., Zwaal, R. F., et al.: Lytic and nonlytic degradation of phospholipids in mammalian erythrocytes by pure phospholipases. Biochim. Biophys. Acta *307*:74, 1973.

61. Zwaal, R. F. A., Roelofsen, B., et al.: Localization of red cell membrane constituents. Biochim. Biophys. Acta *300*:159, 1973.

62. Roelofsen, B., Zwaal, R. F. A., et al.: Action of pure phospholipase A_2 and phospholipase C on human erythrocytes and ghosts. Biochim. Biophys. Acta *241*:925, 1971.

63. Gul, S., and Smith, A. D.: Haemolysis of washed human red cells by the combined action of *Naja Naja* phospholipase A_2 and albumin. Biochim. Biophys. Acta *288*:237, 1972.

64. Simpkins, H., Tay, S., et al.: Changes in the molecular structure of axonal and red blood cell membranes following treatment with phospholipase A_2. Biochemistry *10*:3579, 1971.

65. Lenard, J., and Singer, S. J.: Structure of membranes: Reaction of red blood cell membranes with phospholipase C. Science *159*: 738, 1968.

66. Coleman, R., Finean, J. B., et al.: A structural study of the modification of erythrocyte ghosts by phospholipase C. Biochim. Biophys. Acta *219*:81, 1970.

67. Kahlenberg, A., and Banjo, B.: Involvement of phospholipids in the D-glucose uptake activity of isolated human erythrocyte membranes. J. Biol. Chem. *247*:1156, 1972.

68. Bakerman, S., and Wasemiller, G.: Studies on structural units of human erythrocyte membrane. I. Separation, isolation and partial characterization. Biochemistry *6*:1100, 1967.

69. Schneiderman, L. J., and Junga, I. G.: Isolation and partial characterization of structural protein derived from human red cell membranes. Biochemistry *7*:2281, 1968.

70. Criddle, R. S., Edwards, D. L., et al.: Chemical studies on the homogeneity of the structural protein from mitochondria. Biochemistry *5*:578, 1966.

71. Maddy, A. H.: Erythrocyte membrane proteins. Semin. Hematol. *7*:275, 1970.

72. Steck, T. L., and Fox, C. F.: Membrane proteins, In *Membrane Molecular Biology*, Fox, C. F., and Keith, A. D. (eds.), Stamford, Conn., Sinauer Assoc., Inc., 1972, p. 27.

73. Hanahan, D. J., Ekholm, J., et al.: Biochemical variability of human erythrocyte membrane preparations as demonstrated by sodium-potassium-magnesium and calcium adenosine triphosphatase activities. Biochemistry *12*:1374, 1973.

74. Dodge, J. T., Mitchell, C., et al.: The prepara-

tion and chemical characteristics of hemo-globin-free ghosts of human erythrocytes. Arch. Biochem. Biophys. *100*:119, 1963.

75. Fairbanks, G., Steck, T. L., et al.: Electrophoretic analysis of the major polypeptides of the human erythrocyte membrane. Biochemistry *10*:2606, 1971.

76. Steck, T. L., Fairbanks, G., et al.: Disposition of the major proteins in the isolated erythrocyte membrane. Proteolytic dissection. Biochemistry *10*:2617, 1971.

77. Steck, T. L.: Cross-linking the major proteins of the isolated erythrocyte membrane. J. Mol. Biol. *66*:295, 1972.

78. Bretscher, M. S.: Major human erythrocyte glycoprotein spans the cell membrane. Nature [New Biol.] *231*:229, 1971.

79. Bretscher, M. S.: Human erythrocyte membranes: Specific labeling of surface proteins. J. Mol. Biol. *58*:775, 1971.

80. Segrest, J. P., Kahane, I., et al.: Major glycoprotein of the human erythrocyte membrane: Evidence for an amphipathic molecular structure. Arch. Biochem. Biophys. *155*:167, 1973.

81. Berg, H. C.: Sulfanilicacia diazonium salt: A label for the outside of the human erythrocyte membrane. Biochim. Biophys. Acta *183*:65, 1969.

82. Triplett, R. B., and Carraway, K. L.: Proteolytic digestion of erythrocytes, resealed ghosts, and isolated membranes. Biochemistry *11*:2897, 1972.

83. Nicholson, G. L., and Singer, S. J.: Ferritin-conjugated plant agglutinins as specific saccharide stains for electron microscopic application to saccharides bound to cell membranes. Proc. Natl. Acad. Sci. USA *68*:942, 1971.

84. Phillips, D. R., and Morrison, M.: Exposed protein on the intact human erythrocyte. Biochemistry *10*:1766, 1971.

85. Tanner, M. J. A., and Boxer, D. H.: Separation and some properties of the major proteins of the human erythrocyte membrane. Biochem. J. *129*:333, 1972.

86. Kant, J. A., and Steck, T. L.: Cation-impermeable inside-out and right-side-out vesicles from human erythrocyte membranes. Nature [New Biol.] *240*:26, 1972.

87. Schmidt-Ullrich, R., Knüfermann, H., et al.: The reaction of 1-dimethylaminonaphthalene-5-sulfonyl chloride (Dansel) with erythrocyte membranes. A new look at "Vectorial" membrane probes. Biochim. Biophys. Acta *307*:353, 1973.

88. Marchesi, S. L., Steers, E., et al.: Physical and chemical properties of a protein isolated from red cell membranes. Biochemistry *9*:50, 1970.

89. Marchesi, V. T., Steers, E., et al.: Some properties of spectrin. A fibrous protein isolated from red cell membranes, In *Red Cell Membrane Structure and Function.* Jamieson, G. A., and Greenwalt, T. J., (eds.), Philadelphia, J. B. Lippincott, 1969, p. 117.

90. Clarke, M.: Isolation and characterization of a water-soluble protein from bovine erythro-cyte membranes. Biochem. Biophys. Res. Commun. *45*:1963, 1971.

90a. Marchesi, V. T., and Steers, E., Jr.: Selective solubilization of a protein component of the red cell membrane. Science *159*:203, 1968.

91. Guidotti, G.: The composition of biological membranes. Arch. Intern. Med. *129*:194, 1972.

92. Rosenthal, A. S., Kregenow, F. M., et al.: Some characteristics of a Ca^{2+}-dependent ATPase activity associated with a group of erythrocyte membrane proteins which form fibrils. Biochim. Biophys. Acta *196*:254, 1970.

93. Williams, R. P.: The phosphorylation and isolation of two membrane proteins *in vitro.* Biochem. Biophys. Res. Commun. *47*:671, 1972.

94. Guthrow, C. E., Jr., Allen, J. E., et al.: Phosphorylation of an endogenous membrane protein by endogenous, membrane-associated cyclic adenosine 3',5'-monophosphate-dependent protein kinase in human erythrocyte ghosts. J. Biol. Chem. *247*:8145, 1972.

95. Roses, A. D., and Appell, S. H.: Erythrocyte protein phosphorylation. J. Biol. Chem. *248*:1408, 1973.

95a. Greenquist, A., and Shohet, S. B.: ATP-dependent phosphorylation of a membrane protein in normal and hereditary spherocytosis red cells. Blood *42*:997, 1973.

96. Juliano, R. L., and Rothstein, A.: Properties of an erythrocyte membrane lipoprotein fraction. Biochim. Biophys. Acta *249*:227, 1971.

97. Steck, T.: Selective solubilization of red cell membrane proteins with guanidine hydrochloride. Biochim. Biophys. Acta *255*:553, 1972.

98. Guidotti, G.: Personal communication.

98a. Findlay, J., and Guidotti, G.: Personal communication.

99. Cabantchik, Z. I., and Rothstein, A.: The location of an anion modifying agent in proteins of the red cell membrane. Fed. Proc. *32*:288a, 1973.

100. Bellkorn, M. B., Blumenfeld, O. O., et al.: Acetylcholinesterase of the human erythrocyte membrane. Biochem. Biophys. Res. Commun. *39*:267, 1970.

101. Berman, J. D., and Young, M.: Rapid and complete purification of acetylcholinesterases of electric eel and erythrocyte by affinity chromatography. Proc. Natl. Acad. Sci. USA *68*:395, 1971.

102. Ciliv, G., and Ozand, P. T.: Human erythrocyte acetylcholinesterase. Purification, properties, and kinetic behavior. Biochim. Biophys. Acta *284*:136, 1972.

103. Taverna, R. D., and Langdon, R. G.: D-Glucosyl isothiocyanate, an affinity label for the glucose transport proteins of the human erythrocyte membrane. Biochem. Biophys. Res. Commun. *54*:593, 1973.

104. Avruch, J., and Fairbanks, G.: Demonstration of a phosphopeptide intermediate in the Mg^{++}-dependent, Na^+- and K^+-stimulated adenosine triphosphatase reaction of the erythrocyte membrane. Proc. Natl. Acad. Sci. USA *60*:1216, 1972.

104a. Greenquist, A., and Shohet, S. B.: Unpublished observations.

105. Dunham, P. B., and Hoffman, J. F.: Partial purification of the ouabain-binding component and of Na, K-ATPase from human red cell membranes. Proc. Natl. Acad. Sci. USA 66: 936, 1970.

105a. Yu, J., and Steck, T. L.: Selective solubilization, isolation, and characterization of a predominant polypeptide from human erythrocyte membranes. J. Cell. Biol. 59:374a, 1973.

105b. Gahmberg, C. G., and Hakomori, S.: External labeling of cell surface galactose and galactosamine in glycolipid and glycoprotein of human erythrocytes. J. Biol. Chem. 248:4311, 1973.

106. Tanner, M. J. A., and Gray, W. R.: Isolation and functional identification of a protein from the human erythrocyte "ghost." Biochem. J. 125:1109, 1971.

107. Steck, T. L.: The organization of proteins in the red cell membrane, In Membrane Research. Fox, C. F. (ed.), New York, Academic Press, 1972, p. 71.

108. Kant, J. A., and Steck, T. L.: Specificity in the association of glyceraldehyde 3-phosphate dehydrogenase with isolated human erythrocyte membranes. J. Biol. Chem. 248:8457, 1973.

109. Marchesi, V. T., Tillack, T. W., et al.: Chemical characterization and surface orientation of the major glycoprotein of the human erythrocyte membrane. Proc. Natl. Acad. Sci. USA 69:1445, 1972.

110. Segrist, J. P., Jackson, R. L., et al.: Red cell membrane glycoprotein: Amino acid sequence of an intramembranous region. Biochem. Biophys. Res. Commun. 49:964, 1972.

111. Winzler, R. J.: A glycoprotein in human erythrocyte membranes, In Red Cell Membrane Structure and Function. Jamieson, G. A., and Greenwalt, T. J., (eds.), Philadelphia, J. B. Lippincott, 1969, p. 157.

112. Zvilichovsky, B., Gallop, P. M., et al.: Isolation of a glycoprotein-glycolipid fraction from human erythrocyte membranes. Biochem. Biophys. Res. Commun. 44:1234, 1971.

113. Kobylka, D., Khettry, A., et al.: Proteins and glycoproteins of the erythrocyte membrane. Arch. Biochem. Biophys. 148:475, 1972.

114. Segrist, J. P., Jackson, R. L., et al.: Human erythrocyte membrane glycoprotein: A re-evaluation of the molecular weight as determined by SDS polyacrylamide gel electrophoresis. Biochem. Biophys. Res. Commun. 44:390, 1971.

115. Righetti, P. G., Perrella, M., et al.: The membrane protein abnormality of the red cell in paroxysmal nocturnal haemoglobinuria. Nature (Lond.) 245:273, 1973.

116. Hamaguchi, H., and Clive, H.: Solubilization of human erythrocyte membrane glycoproteins and separation of the MN glycoprotein from a glycoprotein with I, S, and A activity. Biochim. Biophys. Acta 278:271, 1972.

117. Schrader, J., Berne, R. M., et al.: Uptake and metabolism of adenosine by human erythrocyte ghosts. Am. J. Physiol. 223:159, 1972.

118. Lerner, M. H., and Rubinstein, D.: The role of adenine and adenosine as precursors for adenine nucleotide synthesis by fresh and preserved human erythrocytes. Biochim. Biophys. Acta 224:301, 1970.

119. Rao, S. N., Hara, L., et al.: Alkali cation-activated AMP diaminase of erythrocytes: Some properties of the membrane-bound enzyme. Biochim. Biophys. Acta 151:651, 1968.

120. Nilsson, O., and Ronist, G.: Enzyme activities and ultrastructure of a membrane fraction from human erythrocytes. Biochim. Biophys. Acta 183:1, 1969.

121. Shin, B. C., and Carraway, K. L.: Association of glyceraldehyde 3-phosphate dehydrogenase with the human erythrocyte membrane. Effect of detergents, trypsin, and adenosine triphosphate. J. Biol. Chem. 248:1436, 1973.

122. Duchon, G., and Collier, H. B.: Enzyme activities of human erythrocyte ghosts: Effects of various treatments. J. Memb. Biol. 6:138, 1971.

123. Dunham, E. T., and Glynn, I. M.: Adenosine triphosphatase activity and the active movements of alkali metal ions. J. Physiol. (Lond.) 156:274, 1961.

124. Hoffman, J. F.: Cation transport and structure of the red cell plasma membrane circulation. 26:1201, 1962.

125. Rubin, C. S., and Rosen, O. M.: The role of cyclic AMP in the phosphorylation of proteins in human erythrocyte membranes. Biochem. Biophys. Res. Commun. 50:421, 1973.

126. Redman, C. M.: Phospholipid metabolism in intact and modified erythrocyte membranes. J. Cell Biol. 49:35, 1971.

127. Hokin, L. E., and Hokin, M. R.: The incorporation of ^{32}P from triphosphate into polyphosphoinositides $[\gamma\text{-}^{32}P]$, adenosine, and phosphatidic acid in erythrocyte membranes. Biochim. Biophys. Acta 84:563, 1964.

128. Schrier, S. L.: ATP synthesis in human erythrocyte membranes. Biochim. Biophys. Acta 135:591, 1967.

129. Parker, J. C., and Hoffman, J. F.: The role of membrane phosphoglycerate kinase in the control of glycolytic rate by active cation transport in human red blood cells. J. Gen. Physiol. 50: 893, 1967.

130. Jadah, J., Ahmed, K., et al.: Ion transport and phosphoproteins of human red cells. Biochim. Biophys. Acta 65:472, 1962.

131. Heller, M., and Hanahan, D. J.: Erythrocyte membrane-bound enzymes:ATPase, phosphatase and adenylate kinase in human bovine and porcine erythrocytes. Biochim. Biophys. Acta 255:239, 1972.

132. Post, R. L., Merritt, C. R., et al.: Membrane adenosine triphosphatase as a participant in the active transport of sodium and potassium in the human erythrocyte. J. Biol. Chem. 235:1796, 1960.

133. Frischer, H., Nelson, R., et al.: NAD(P) glycohydrolase deficiency in human erythrocytes and alteration of cytosol NADH-methemoglobin diaphorase by membrane NAD-glycohydrolase activity. Proc. Natl. Acad. Sci. USA 70:2406, 1973.

134. Zamudio, I., Cellino, M., et al.: The relation between membrane structure and NADH: (acceptor) oxidoreductase activity of erythrocyte ghosts. Arch. Biochem. 129:336, 1969.

135. Kin, Y. S., Perdomo, J., et al.: N-acetyl-D-galacto-saminyl- transferase in human serum and erythrocyte membranes. Proc. Natl. Acad. Sci. USA 68:1753, 1971.

136. Schneider, R. P., and Kirscher, L. B.: Di and triphosphoinositide metabolism in swine erythrocyte membranes. Biochim. Biophys. Acta 202:283, 1970.

137. Moore, G. L., Kocholaty, W. F., et al.: A proteinase from human erythrocyte membranes. Biochim. Biophys. Acta 212:126, 1970.

138. Salway, J. G., Kai, M., et al.: Triphosphoinositide phosphomonoesterase activity in neural cell bodies, neuroglia and subcellular fractions from whole rat brain. J. Neurochem. 14:1013, 1967.

139. Gorter, E., and Grendel, F.: Bimolecular layers of lipoids on the chromocytes of the blood. J. Exp. Med. 41:439, 1925.

140. Robertson, J. D.: New observations on the ultrastructure of the membranes of frog peripheral nerve fibers. J. Biophys. Biochem. Cytol. 3:1043, 1957.

141. Weinstein, R. A., and McNutt, N. S.: Ultrastructure of red cell membranes. Semin. Hematol. 7:259, 1970.

142. Wallach, D. F. H., and Zahler, P. H.: Protein conformations in cellular membranes. Proc. Natl. Acad. Sci. USA 56:1552, 1966.

143. Lenard, J., and Singer, S. J.: Protein conformation in cell membrane preparations as studied by optical rotatory dispersion and circular dichroism. Proc. Natl. Acad. Sci. USA 56:1828, 1966.

144. Lucy, J. A., and Glauert, A. M.: Structure and assembly of macromolecular lipid complexes composed of globular micelles. J. Mol. Biol. 8:727, 1964.

145. Lucy, J. A.: Globular lipid micelles and cell membranes. J. Theor. Biol. 7:360, 1964.

146. Green, D. E., and Perdue, J. F.: Membranes as expressions of repeating units. Proc. Natl. Acad. Sci. USA 55:1295, 1966.

147. Lenaz, G., Sechi, A. M., et al.: Nonionic interactions between proteins and lipids in mitochondrial membranes. Biochem. Biophys. Res. Comm. 34:392, 1969.

148. Sjöstrand, F. S.: A new ultrastructural element of the membranes in mitochondria and some cytoplasmic membranes. J. Ultrastruct. Res. 9:340, 1963.

149. Green, D. E., Haard, N. E., et al.: On the noncatalytic proteins of membrane systems. Proc. Natl. Acad. Sci. USA 60:277, 1968.

150. Benson, A. A.: On the orientation of lipids in chloroplast and cell membranes. J. Am. Oil Chem. Soc. 43:265, 1966.

151. Schnaitman, C.: Comparison of rat liver mitochondrial and microsomal proteins. Proc. Natl. Acad. Sci. USA 63:412, 1969.

152. Vanderkooi, G., and Green, D. E.: Biological membrane structure. I. The protein crystal model for membranes. Proc. Natl. Acad. Sci. USA 66:615, 1970.

153. Frye, L. D., and Edidin, M.: The rapid intermixing of cell surface antigens after formation of mouse-human heterokaryons. J. Cell. Sci. 7:319, 1970.

154. Edelman, G. M., Yahara, I., et al.: Receptor mobility and receptor-cytoplasmic interactions in lymphocytes. Proc. Natl. Acad. Sci. USA 70:1442, 1973.

155. Sundquist, K. G.: Redistribution of surface antigens—a general property of animal cells? Nature [New Biol.] 239:147, 1972.

156. Pinto DaSilva, P., and Branton, D.: Membrane splitting in freeze-etching: Covalently bound ferritin as a membrane marker. J. Cell Biol. 45:598, 1970.

157. Tourtellotte, M. E., and Zupnik, J. S.: Freeze-fractured Acholeplasma laidlawii membranes: Nature of particles observed. Science 179:84, 1973.

158. Pinto DaSilva, P.: Translational mobility of the membrane intercalated particles of human erythrocyte ghosts. J. Cell Biol. 53:777, 1972.

158a. Elgsaeter, A., Shotton, D., et al.: Control of protein distribution in the erythrocyte membrane. J. Cell Biol. 59:89a, 1973.

158b. Karnovsky, M. J.: Personal communication.

159. Pinto DaSilva, P., Douglas, S. D., et al.: Localization of A antigen sites on human erythrocyte ghosts. Nature (London) 232:194, 1971.

160. Tillack, T. W., Scott, R. E., et al.: The structure of erythrocyte membranes studied by freeze-etching. II. Localization of receptors for phytohemagglutinin and influenza virus to the intramembranous particles. J. Exp. Med. 135:1209, 1972.

161. Jacob, H. S.: Mechanisms of Heinz body formation and attachment to red cell membrane. Semin. Hematol. 7:341, 1970.

162. Lessin, L. S.: Membrane ultrastructure of normal, sickled and Heinz-body erythrocyte by freeze-etching. Nouv. Rev. Fr. Hematol. 12:871, 1972.

163. Singer, S. J.: Architecture and topography of biologic membranes. Hosp. Practice 8:81, 1973.

164. Pinto DaSilva, P.: Membrane intercalated particles in human erythrocyte ghosts: Sites of preferred passage of water molecules at low temperatures. Proc. Natl. Acad. Sci. USA 70:1339, 1973.

165. Nicolson, G. L., and Singer, S. J.: Ferritin-conjugated plant agglutinins as specific saccharide stains for electron microscopy: Application to saccharides bound to cell membranes. Proc. Natl. Acad. Sci. USA 68:942, 1971.

166. Nicolson, G. L., Masouredis, S. P., et al.: Quantitative two-dimensional ultrastructural distribution of Rh₀ (D) antigenic sites on human erythrocyte membranes. Proc. Natl. Acad. Sci. USA 68:1416, 1971.

167. Nicolson, G. L., and Singer, S. J.: Electron microscopic localization of macromolecules on membrane surfaces. Ann. N.Y. Acad. Sci. 195:368, 1972.

168. Green, F. A.: Phospholipid requirement for Rh antigenic activity. J. Biol. Chem. 243:5519, 1968.

169. Nicolson, G. L., and Painter, R. G.: Anionic sites of human erythrocyte membranes. II. Antispectrin-induced transmembrane aggregation of the binding sites for positively charged colloidal particles. J. Cell Biol. 59:395, 1973.

170. LaCelle, P. L.: Alterations of membrane deformability in hemolytic anemias. Semin. Hematol. 7:355, 1970.

171. Schrier, S. L., Godin, D., et al.: Characterization of microvesicles produced by shearing of human erythrocyte membranes. Biochim. Biophys. Acta 233:26, 1971.

172. Sigler, A. T., Forman, E. N., et al.: Severe intravascular hemolysis following surgical repair of endocardiac cushion defects. Amer. J. Med. 35:467, 1963.

173. Bull, D. S., and Kuhn, I. N.: The production of schistocytes by fibrin strands (a scanning electron microscope study). Blood 35:104, 1970.

174. Weed, R. I., and Bowdler, A. J.: Metabolic dependence of the critical hemolytic volume of human erythrocytes: Relationship to osmotic fragility and autohemolysis in hereditary spherocytosis and normal red cells. J. Clin. Invest. 45:1137, 1966.

175. Ham, T. H., Shen, S. C., et al.: Studies on the destruction of red blood cells. IV. Thermal injury: Action of heat in causing increased spheroidicity, osmotic and mechanical fragilities and hemolysis of erythrocytes. Observations on the mechanisms of destruction in such erythrocytes in dogs and in a patient with a fatal thermal burn. Blood 3:373, 1948.

176. Nathan, D. G., and Shohet, S. B.: Erythrocyte ion transport defects and hemolytic anemia: "Hydrocytosis and desiccytosis." Semin. Hematol. 7:381, 1970.

177. Parker, J. C., and Welt, L. G.: Pathologic alterations of cation movements in red blood cells. Arch. Intern. Med. 129:320, 1972.

178. Jacob, H. S., and Lux, S. E., IV: Degradation of membrane phospholipids and thiols in peroxide hemolysis: Studies in vitamin E deficiency. Blood 32:549, 1968.

179. Boulard, M., Blume, K. G., et al.: The effect of copper on red cell enzyme activity. J. Clin. Invest. 51:459, 1972.

180. Condrea, E., Mammon, Z., et al.: Susceptibility of erythrocytes of various animal species to the hemolytic and phospholipid splitting action of snake venom. Biochim. Biophys. Acta 84:365, 1964.

181. Jacob, H. S.: Mechanisms of Heinz body formation and attachment to red cell membrane. Semin. Hematol. 7:341, 1970.

182. Rosse, W. F., and Dacie, J. V.: Complement and the paroxysmal nocturnal haemoglobinuria red cell, In Wolstenholme, G. E. W., and Knight, J. (eds.), Complement, Ciba Foundation Symposium. London, J. & A. Churchill, 1965, p. 343.

183. Seeman, P., and Iles, G. H.: Pits in the freeze-cleavage plane of normal erythrocyte membranes; and ultrastructure of membrane lesions in immune lysis. Nouv. Rev. Fr. Hematol. 12:889, 1972.

184. Weed, R. I.: Disorders of red cell membrane: History and perspectives. Semin. Hematol. 7:372, 1970.

185. Weiss, L., and Tavassoli, M.: Anatomical hazards to the passage of erythrocytes through the spleen. Semin. Hematol. 7:372, 1970.

186. Jandl, J. H., Jones, A. R., et al.: Destruction of red cells by antibodies in man. I. Observations on the sequestration and lysis of red cells altered by immune mechanisms. J. Clin. Invest. 36:1428, 1957.

187. Gallai-Hatchard, J. J., and Thompson, R. H.: Phospholipase-A activity of mammalian tissues. Biochim. Biophys. Acta 98:128, 1965.

188. Emerson, C. P., Jr., Shen, S. C., et al.: Studies on the destruction of red blood cells. IX. Quantitative methods for determining the osmotic and mechanical fragility of red cells in the peripheral blood and splenic pulp; the mechanism of increased hemolysis in hereditary spherocytosis (congenital hemolytic jaundice) as related to the function of the spleen. Arch. Intern. Med. 97:1, 1956.

189. Jandl, J. H., and Aster, R. H.: Increased splenic pooling and the pathogenesis of hypersplenism. Am. J. Med. Sci. 253:383, 1967.

190. Crosby, W. H.: Normal function of the spleen relative to red blood cells: A review. Blood 14:399, 1959.

191. Weed, R. I., and Weiss, L.: The relationship of red cell fragmentation occurring within the spleen to cell destruction. Trans. Assoc. Am. Physicians 79:426, 1966.

192. Rifkind, R. A.: Heinz body anemia: An ultrastructural study. II. Red cell sequestration and destruction. Blood 26:433, 1965.

193. Jandl, J. H.: The agglutination and sequestration of immature red cells. J. Lab. Clin. Med. 55:663, 1960.

194. Winterbourn, C. C., and Batt, R. D.: Lipid composition of human red cells of different ages. Biochim. Biophys. Acta 202:1, 1970.

195. Dacie, J. V.: Secondary or Symptomatic Haemolytic Anemias, In Part III of The Haemolytic Anemias, Congenital and Acquired. London, J. & A. Churchill, Ltd., 1967.

196. Sears, D. A.: Plasma heme binding in patients with hemolytic disorders. J. Lab. Clin. Med. 71:484, 1967.

197. Fyster, E.: Traumatic hemolysis with hemoglobinuria due to ball valve variance. Blood 33:391, 1969.

198. Marsh, G. W., and Lewis, S. M.: Cardiac hemolytic anemia. Semin. Hematol. 6:133, 1969.

199. Nevaril, C. G., Lynch, E. C., et al.: Erythrocyte damage and destruction induced by shearing stress. J. Lab. Clin. Med. 71:784, 1968.

200. Pirofsky, B.: Hemolysis in valvular heart disease. Ann. Intern. Med. 65:373, 1966.

201. Davidson, R. J. L.: March or exertional hemoglobinuria. Semin. Hematol. 6:150, 1969.

202. Davidson, R. J. L.: Exertional haemoglobinuria: A report on three cases with studies of the haemolytic mechanism. J. Clin. Path. 17:536, 1964.

203. Ponder, E.: Hemolysis and Related Phenomena. New York, Grune & Stratton, 1948 (reprinted 1971), p. 323.

204. Ham, T. H., Shin, S. C., et al.: Studies on the destruction of red blood cells. IV. Thermal injury. Blood 3:373, 1948.

205. McCollough, J., Polesky, H. F., et al.: Iatrogenic hemolysis: A complication of blood warmed by a microwave device. Anesth. Analg. (Cleve.) 51:102, 1972.

206. Brain, M. C, Dacie, J. V., et al.: Microangiopathic haemolytic anaemia: The possible role of

vascular lesions in pathogenesis. Br. J. Haematol. 8:358, 1962.

207. Hensley, W. J.: Haemolytic anaemia in acute glomerulonephritis. Aust. Ann. Med. 1:180, 1952.

208. Colman, R. W., Robboy, S. J., et al.: Disseminated intravascular coagulation (DIC)—an approach. Am. J. Med. 52:679, 1972.

209. Amorosi, E. L., and Ultman, J. E.: Thrombotic thrombocytopenic purpura. Report of 16 cases and review of the literature. Medicine (Baltimore) 45:139, 1966.

210. Corrigan, J. J., Jr., Roy, W. L., et al.: Changes in the blood coagulation system associated with septicemia. New Engl. J. Med. 279:85, 1968.

211. Didisheim, P., Trombold, J. S., et al.: Acute promyelocytic leukemia with fibrinogen and factor V deficiencies. Blood 23:717, 1964.

212. Shibolet, S., Coll, R., et al.: Heatstroke. Its clinical picture and mechanism in 36 cases. Quart. J. Med. 36:525, 1967.

213. Joseph, R. R., Day, J. J., et al.: Microangiopathic haemolytic anemia associated with consumption coagulopathy in a patient with disseminated carcinoma. Scand. J. Haematol. 4:271, 1967.

214. Taub, R. N., Rodriguez, E., et al.: Intravascular coagulation. The Schwartzman reaction and the pathogenesis of T.T.P. Blood 24:775, 1964.

215. Brain, M. C.: The hemolytic-uraemic syndrome. Lancet 2:1394, 1968.

216. Clarkson, A. R., Morton, J. B., et al.: Urinary fibrin/fibrinogen degradation products after renal transplantation. Lancet 2:1220, 1970.

217. Stiehm, E. R., and Trystad, C. W.: Split products of fibrin in human renal disease. Am. J. Med. 46:774, 1969.

218. Chirawang, P., Nanra, R. S., et al.: Fibrin degradation products and the role of coagulation in "persistent" glomerulonephritis. Ann. Intern. Med. 74:859, 1971.

219. Kasabach, H. H., and Merritt, K. K.: Hemangioma with extensive purpura. Am. J. Dis. Child. 59:1063, 1940.

220. Shin, W. K. T.: Hemangiomas of infancy complicated by thrombocytopenia. Am. J. Surg. 116:896, 1968.

221. Gilchrest, G. S., Lieberman, E., et al.: Heparin therapy in the hemolytic uremic syndrome. Acta Paediatr. Scand. 56:436, 1967.

222. Arieff, A. I., and Pinggera, W. F.: Rapidly progressive glomerulonephritis treated with anticoagulants. Arch. Intern. Med. 129:77, 1972.

223. Kinkaid-Smith, P., Louer, M. C., et al.: Dipyridamole and anticoagulants in renal disease due to glomerular and vascular lesions: A new approach to therapy. Med. J. Aust. 1:145, 1970.

224. Brecher, G., and Stohlman, F., Jr.: Reticulocyte size and erythropoietin stimulation. Proc. Soc. Exp. Biol. Med. 107:887, 1961.

225. Berlin, N. I., and Lotz, C.: Life span of the red cell of the rat following acute hemorrhage. Proc. Soc. Exp. Biol. Med. 78:788, 1951.

226. Stohlman, F., Jr.: Erythropoiesis. New Engl. J. Med. 267:342, 1962.

227. Ganzoni, A., Hillman, R. S., and Finch, C. A.: Maturation of the macroreticulocyte. Br. J. Haematol. 16:119, 1969.

228. Shattil, S. J., and Cooper, R. A.: Maturation of macroreticulocyte membranes in vivo. J. Lab. Clin. Med. 79:215, 1972.

229. Come, S. E., Shohet, S. B., et al.: Surface remodelling of reticulocytes produced in response to erythroid stress. Nature [New Biol.] 236:157, 1972.

230. Dean, H. M., Decker, C. L., et al.: Temporary survival in clostridial hemolysis with absence of circulating red cells. New Engl. J. Med. 277:700, 1967.

231. Furr, W. E., Jr., Bourdeau, R. V., et al.: In vivo effects of Clostridium welchii lecithinase. Surg. Gynecol. Obstet. 95:465, 1952.

232. Simpkins, H., Kahlenberg, A., et al.: Structural and compositional changes in the red cell membrane during Clostridium welchii infection. Br. J. Haematol. 21:173, 1971.

233. Irvin, T. T., Moir, E. R. S., et al.: Treatment of Clostridium welchii infection with hyperbaric oxygen. Surg. Gynecol. Obstet. 127:1058, 1968.

234. Glader, B. E., and Conrad, M. E.: Hemolysis by diphenylsulfones: Comparative effects of DDS and hydroxylamine-DDS. J. Lab. Clin. Med. 81:267, 1973.

235. Rasbridge, M. R., and Scott, G. L.: The haemolytic action of dapsone: Changes in the red-cell membrane. Br. J. Haematol. 24:183, 1973.

236. Lubin, B. H., Shohet, S. B., et al.: Changes in fatty acid metabolism after erythrocyte peroxidation, stimulation of a membrane repair process. J. Clin. Invest. 51:338, 1972.

237. Lubin, B. H., and Shohet, S. B.: Unpublished observations.

238. Lubin, B. H., Baehner, R. I., et al.: The red cell peroxide hemolysis test in the differential diagnosis of obstructive jaundice in the newborn period. Pediatrics 48:562, 1971.

239. Oski, F. A., and Barness, L. A.: Vitamin E deficiency: A previously unrecognized cause of hemolytic anemia in the premature infant. J. Pediatr. 70:211, 1967.

240. Mengel, E. E., Kahn, H. E., Jr., et al.: Effects of in vitro hyperoxia on erythrocytes. II. Hemolysis in a human after exposure to oxygen under high pressure. Blood 25:822, 1965.

241. Panos, T. C., Stinnett, B., et al.: Vitamin E and linoleic acid in the feeding of premature infants. Am. J. Clin. Nutr. 21:15, 1968.

242. Tappel, A. L.: Vitamin E as the biological lipid antioxidant. Vitam. Horm. 20:493, 1962.

243. Rieder, R. F., Oski, F. A., et al.: Hemoglobin Philly (β^{35} tyrosine–phenylatanine): Studies in the molecular pathology of hemoglobin. J. Clin. Invest. 48:1627, 1969.

244. Jacob, H. S., Brain, M. C., et al.: Altered sulfhydryl reactivity of hemoglobins and red cell membranes in congenital Heinz body hemolytic anemia. J. Clin. Invest. 47:2664, 1968.

245. Nathan, D. G.: Rubbish in the red cell (editorial). New Engl. J. Med. 281:558, 1969.

246. Zarkowsky, H. S., Oski, F. A., et al.: Congenital hemolytic anemia with high-sodium, low-potassium red cells. I. Studies of membrane permeability. New Engl. J. Med. 278:573, 1968.

247. Oski, F. A., Naiman, J. L., et al.: Congenital hemolytic anemia with high-sodium, low-potassium red cells, studies of three generations of a family with a new variant. New Engl. J. Med. 280:909, 1969.

248. Miller, D. R., Rickles, F. R., et al.: A new variant of hereditary hemolytic anemia with stomatocytosis and erythrocyte cation abnormality. Blood 38:184, 1971.

249. Muir-Jackson, J., and Knight, D.: Stomatocytosis in migrants of Mediterranean origin. Med. J. Aust. 1:939, 1969.

250. Jaffé, E. R., and Gottfried, E. L.: Hereditary nonspherocytic hemolytic disease associated with an altered phospholipid composition of the erythrocytes. J. Clin. Invest. 47:1375, 1968.

251. Shohet, S. B., Nathan, D. G., et al.: Abnormal RBC cation flux in familial hemolytic anemia associated with abnormal membrane lipids. Blood 36:858, 1970.

252. Shohet, S. B., Livermore, B. M., et al.: Hereditary hemolytic anemia associated with abnormal membrane lipids: Mechanism of accumulation of phosphatidyl choline. Blood 38:445, 1971.

253. Segal, G., Feig, S., et al.: Abnormal cation fluxes in human erythrocytes. Relation to ATP, In Proceedings 2nd Int. Symposium on the Metabolism and Membrane Permeability of Erythrocytes, Thrombocytes and Leukocytes. Moser, K. (ed.), Vienna, Verlag Wiener Medizinidren Akademia, 1972 (in press).

254. Donath, J., and Landsteiner, K.: Uber paroxysmale haemoglobinuria. Munch. Med. Wochenschr. 512:590, 1904.

255. Müller-Eberhard, H. J.: Chemistry and reaction mechanisms of complement, In Advances in Immunology. Dixon, F., and Kunkel, H. (eds.), New York, Academic Press, 1968, p. 1.

256. Kinsky, S. C.: Antibody-complement interactions with lipid model membranes. Biochim. Biophys. Acta 203:1, 1972.

257. Inoue, K., and Kinsky, S. C.: Fate of phospholipids in liposomal model membranes damaged by antibody and complement. Biochemistry 9:4767, 1970.

258. Lucy, J. A.: The fusion of biological membranes. Nature (Lond.) 227:815, 1970.

259. Lalezari, P., and Oberhardt, B.: Temperature gradient dissociation of red cell antigen-antibody complexes in the polybrene technique. Br. J. Haematol. 21:131, 1971.

260. Skinner, M. D., and Schwartz, R. S.: Immunosuppressive therapy. New Engl. J. Med. 287:221, 1972.

261. Worlledge, S. M., Brain, M. C., et al.: Immunosuppressive drugs in the treatment of autoimmune haemolytic anemia. Proc. R. Soc. Med. 61:1312, 1968.

262. Schwartz, R. A., and Damashek, W.: The treatment of autoimmune hemolytic anemia with 6-mercaptopurine and thioguanine. Blood 19:485, 1962.

263. Rosse, W. F., and Dacie, J. W.: Immune lysis of normal human and paroxysmal nocturnal hemoglobinuria (PNH) red blood cells. I. The sensitivity of PNH red cells to lysis by complement and specific antibody. J. Clin. Invest. 45:736, 1966.

264. Hizmans VandenBergh, A. A.: Ictére hémolytique quec crises hémoglobinuriques. Fragilité globulaire. Rev. Med. 31:63, 1911.

265. Hartman, R. C., and Jenkins, D. E., Jr.: The "sugar-water" test for paroxysmal nocturnal hemoglobinuria. New Engl. J. Med. 275:155, 1966.

266. Strübing, P.: Paroxysmale hemoglobinurie. Dtsch. Med. Wochenschr. 8:1, 1882.

267. Blum, S. F., Sullivan, J. N., et al.: The exacerbation of hemolysis in paroxysmal nocturnal hemoglobinuria by strenuous exercise. Blood 30:515, 1967.

268. Dacie, J. V., and Lewis, S. M.: Paroxysmal nocturnal haemoglobinuria: Variation in clinical severity and association with bone-marrow hypoplasia. Br. J. Haematol. 7:442, 1961.

269. Ham, T. H., and Dingle, J. H.: Studies on destruction of red blood cells. II. Chronic hemolytic anemia with paroxysmal nocturnal hemoglobulinuria: Certain immunological aspects of the hemolytic mechanism with special reference to serum complement. J. Clin. Invest. 18:657, 1939.

270. Damashek, W.: A proposal for considering paroxysmal nocturnal hemoglobinuria (PNH) as a "candidate" myeloproliferative disorder. Blood 33:263, 1969.

271. Landsteiner, E. K., and Finch, C. A.: Hemoglobinemia accompanying transurethral resection of the prostate. New Engl. J. Med. 237:310, 1947.

272. Lo Buglio, A. F., Cotran, R. S., et al.: Red cells coated with immunoglobulin G: Binding and sphering by mononuclear cells in man. Science 158:1582, 1967.

273. Huber, H., Polley, M. J., et al.: Human monocytes. Distinct receptor sites for the third component of complement and for immunoglobulin G. Science 162:1281, 1965.

274. Abramson, N., Lo Buglio, A. F., et al.: The interaction between human monocytes and red cells. Binding characteristics. J. Exp. Med. 132:1191, 1970.

275. Worlledge, S. M.: Immune drug induced haemolytic anemia. Semin. Hematol. 6:181, 1969.

276. Schubothe, H.: The cold hemagglutinin disease. Semin. Hematol. 3:27, 1966.

277. Videback, A.: Autoimmune hemolytic anemia in systemic lupus erythematosus. Acta Med. Scand. 171:187, 1962.

278. Swisher, S. N., Trobold, N., et al.: Clinical correlations of the direct antiglobulin reaction. Ann. N.Y. Acad. Sci. 124:441, 1965.

279. Jandl, J. H.: Hereditary spherocytosis, In Hereditary Disorders of Erythrocyte Metabolism. Beutler, E. (ed.), New York, Grune and Stratton, 1968, p. 209.

280. Jandl, J. H., and Cooper, R. A.: Hereditary spherocytosis, In The Metabolic Basis of Inherited Disease. Stanbury, J. B., Wyngaarden, J. B., and Fredrickson, D. S. New York, McGraw-Hill, 1972, p. 1323.

281. Cooper, R. A., and Jandl, J. H.: The role of membrane lipids in the survival of red cells in hereditary spherocytosis. J. Clin. Invest. 48:736, 1969.

282. Ben-Bassat, I., Bensch, K. G., et al.: Drug-induced erythrocyte membrane internalization. J. Clin. Invest. 51:1833, 1972.

283. Prankerd, T. A. J.: Studies on the pathogenesis of haemolysis in hereditary spherocytosis. Quart. J. Med. 24:199, 1960.

284. Reed, C. F., and Swisher, S. N.: Erythrocyte lipid loss in hereditary spherocytosis. J. Clin. Invest. 45:777, 1966.

285. Murphy, J. R.: The influence of pH and temperature on some physical properties of normal erythrocytes and erythrocytes from patients with hereditary spherocytes. J. Lab. Clin. Med. 69:758, 1967.

286. Young, L. E., Platzer, R. F., et al.: Hereditary spherocytosis. II. Observations on the role of the spleen. Blood 6:1099, 1951.

287. Emerson, C. P., Jr., Shen, S. C., et al.: The osmotic fragility of the red cells of the peripheral and splenic blood in patients with congenital hemolytic jaundice transfused with normal red cells. J. Clin. Invest. 25:922, 1946.

288. Emerson, C. P., Jr., Shen, S. C., et al.: The mechanism of blood destruction in congenital hemolytic jaundice. J. Clin. Invest. 26:1180, 1947.

289. Griggs, R. C., Weisman, R., Jr., et al.: Alterations in osmotic and mechanical fragility related to in vivo erythrocyte aging and splenic sequestration in hereditary spherocytosis. J. Clin. Invest. 39:89, 1960.

290. Selwyn, J. G., and Dacie, J. V.: Autohemolysis and other changes resulting from the incubation in vitro of red cells from patients with congenital hemolytic anemia. Blood 9:414, 1954.

291. Dunn, I., Ibsen, K. H., et al.: Erythrocyte carbohydrate metabolism in hereditary spherocytosis. J. Clin. Invest. 42:1535, 1963.

292. Loder, P. B., Babarczy, G., et al.: Red cell metabolism in hereditary spherocytosis. Br. J. Haematol. 13:95, 1967.

293. Pohl, A., and Moser, K.: Abnormal metabolic regulation of lysolecithin conversion in red blood cells in hereditary spherocytosis, In Erythrocytes, Thrombocytes, Leukocytes: Recent Advances in Membrane and Metabolic Research. Gerlach, E., Moser, K., et al. Stuttgart, Georg Thieme, Publishers, 1973, p. 25.

294. Chapman, R. G.: Red cell aldolase deficiency in hereditary spherocytosis. Br. J. Haematol. 16:145, 1969.

295. Hanes, T. E., Patterson, J., et al.: Red cell aldolase and other enzyme activities in hereditary spherocytosis. J. Lab. Clin. Med. 75:654, 1970.

296. Beutler, E., Scott, S., et al.: Red cell aldolase deficiency and hemolytic anemia: A new syndrome. Clin. Res. 21:727, 1973.

297. Jacob, H. S., and Jandl, J. H.: Cell membrane permeability in the pathogenesis of hereditary spherocytosis (HS). J. Clin. Invest. 43:1704, 1964.

298. Chapman, R. G.: Red cell life span after splenectomy in hereditary spherocytosis. J. Clin. Invest. 47:2263, 1968.

299. Baird, R. N., McPherson, A. S., et al.: Red-blood-cell survival after splenectomy in congenital spherocytosis. Lancet 1:1060, 1971.

300. Bertles, J. E.: Sodium transport across the surface membrane of red blood cells in hereditary spherocytosis. J. Clin. Invest. 36:8116, 1957.

301. Peters, J. C., Rowland, M., et al.: Erythrocyte sodium transport in hereditary elliptocytosis. Can. J. Physiol. Pharmacol. 44:817, 1966.

302. Jacob, H. S., and Karnovsky, M. L.: Concomitant alterations of sodium flux and membrane phospholipid metabolism in red blood cells: Studies in hereditary spherocytosis. J. Clin. Invest. 46:173, 1967.

303. Jacob, H.S.: Dysfunction of the red blood cell membrane in hereditary spherocytosis. Br. J. Haematol. 14:99, 1968.

304. Zipursky, A., and Israels, L. G.: Significance of erythrocyte sodium flux in the pathophysiology and genetic expression of hereditary spherocytosis. Pediatr. Res. 5:614, 1971.

305. Kimber, G. K., Davis, R. F., et al.: Acrylamide gel electrophoretic studies of human erythrocyte membrane. Blood 36:111, 1970.

306. Gomperts, E. D., Metz, J., et al.: A red cell membrane protein abnormality in hereditary spherocytosis. Br. J. Haematol. 23:363, 1972.

307. Jacob, H. S., Ruby, A., et al.: Abnormal membrane protein of red blood cells in hereditary spherocytosis. J. Clin. Invest. 50:1800, 1971.

308. Jacob, H., Amsden, T., et al.: Membrane microfilaments of erythrocytes: Alteration in intact cells reproduces the hereditary spherocytosis syndrome. Proc. Natl. Acad. Sci. USA 69:471, 1972.

309. Gomperts, E. D., Metz, J., et al.: Immunological homogeneity of membrane proteins from hereditary spherocytic, hereditary elliptocytic and normal red cells. Br. J. Haematol. 20:443, 1971.

310. Wilson, L., Bryan, J., et al.: Precipitation of proteins by vinblastine and calcium ions. Proc. Natl. Acad. Sci. USA 66:807, 1970.

311. Seeman, P., Chau-Wong, M., et al.: Membrane expansion by vinblastine and strychnine. Nature [New Biol.] 241:22, 1973.

312. Harris, J. W., and Kellermeyer, R. W.: The Red Cell. Cambridge, Harvard University Press, 1970, p. 553.

313. Emerson, C. P.: Influence of the spleen on the osmotic behavior and the longevity of red cells in hereditary spherocytosis (congenital hemolytic jaundice): A case study. Boston Med. Quart. 5:65, 1954.

314. Gasser, C.: Erythroblastopénie argue dans les anémies hemolytiques. Sang 21:237, 1950.

315. Diamond, L. K.: Personal communication.

316. Fernandez, L. A., and Erslev, A. J.: Oxygen affinity and compensated hemolysis in hereditary spherocytosis. J. Lab. Clin. Med. 80:780, 1972.

317. Krueger, H. C., and Burgert, E. O.: Hereditary spherocytosis in 100 children. Mayo Clin. Proc. 41:821, 1966.

318. Shinefield, H. R., Steinberg, C. R., et al.: Effect of splenectomy on the susceptibility of mice inoculated with Diplococcus pneumoniae. J. Exp. Med. 125:777, 1966.

319. Pearson, H. A., Cornelius, E. A., et al.: Trans-

fusion-reversible functional asplenia in young children with sickle cell anemia. New Engl. J. Med. 283:334, 1970.

320. Taliaferro, W. H., and Taliaferro, L. G.: The dynamics of hemolysis formation in intact and splenectomized rabbits. J. Infect. Dis. 87:37, 1950.

321. Ellis, E. F., and Smith, R. T.: The role of the spleen in immunity (with special reference to the post-splenectomy problems in infants). Pediatrics 37:111, 1966.

322. Diamond, L. K.: Splenectomy in childhood and the hazard of overwhelming infection. Pediatrics 43:886, 1969.

323. Florman, A. L., and Wintrobe, M. M.: Human elliptical red corpuscles. Bull. Johns Hopkins Hosp. 63:209, 1938.

324. Bannerman, R. M., and Renwick, J. H.: The hereditary elliptocytoses: Clinical and linkage data. Ann. Hum. Genet. 26:23, 1962.

325. Lipton, E. L.: Elliptocytosis with hemolytic anemia: The effects of splenectomy. Pediatrics 15:67, 1955.

326. Murphy, J. R.: Erythrocyte metabolism. VI. Cell shape and the location of cholesterol in the erythrocyte membrane. J. Lab. Clin. Med. 65:756, 1965.

327. Dacie, J. V.: Hereditary elliptocytosis, In The Hemolytic Anemias, Congenital and Acquired. Part I. The Congenital Anemias. New York, Grune and Stratton, 1960.

328. Morton, N. E.: The detection and estimation of linkage between the genes for elliptocytosis and the Rhesus blood type. Am. J. Hum. Genet. 8:80, 1956.

329. Cutting, H. O., McHugh, W. J., et al.: Autosomal dominant hemolytic anemia characterized by ovalocytosis. Am. J. Med. 39:21, 1965.

330. Geerdink, R. A., Helleman, P. W., et al.: Hereditary elliptocytosis and hyperhaemolysis. A comparative study of 6 families with 145 patients. Acta Med. Scand. 179:715, 1966.

331. Bassen, F. A., and Kornzweig, A. L.: Malformation of the erythrocytes in a case of atypical retinitis pigmentosa. Blood 5:381, 1950.

332. Ways, P., Reed, C. F., et al.: Red cell and plasma lipids in acanthocytosis. J. Clin. Invest. 42:1248, 1963.

333. Cooper, R. A., and Gulbrandsen, C. L.: The relationship between serum lipoproteins and red cell membranes in abetalipoproteinemia: Deficiency of lecithin:cholesterol acyltransferase. J. Lab. Clin. Med. 78:323, 1971.

334. McBridge, J. A., and Jacob, H. S.: Abnormal kinetics of red cell membrane cholesterol in acanthocytes: Studies in genetic and experimental abetalipoproteinaemia and in spur cell anaemia. Br. J. Haematol. 18:383, 1970.

335. Simon, E. R., and Ways, P.: Incubation hemolysis and red cell metabolism in acanthocytosis. J. Clin. Invest. 43:1311, 1964.

336. Dodge, J. T., Cohen, G., et al.: Peroxidase hemolysis of red blood cells from patients with lysis of red blood cells from patients with abetalipoproteinemia (acanthocytosis). J. Clin. Invest. 46:357, 1967.

337. Kimber, C. D., Deller, J., et al.: The mechanism of anaemia in chronic liver disease. Quart. J. Med. 34:33, 1965.

338. Jandl, J. H.: The anemia of liver disease: Observa-

tions on its mechanism. J. Clin. Invest. 34:390, 1955.

339. Cooper, R. A., and Jandl, J. H.: Bile salts and cholesterol in the pathogenesis of target cells in obstructive jaundice. J. Clin. Invest. 47:809, 1968.

340. Smith, J. A., Lonergan, E. T., et al.: Spur cell anemia, hemolytic anemia with red cells resembling acanthocytes in alcoholic cirrhosis. New Engl. J. Med. 276:396, 1964.

341. Silber, R., Amorosi, E., et al.: Spur-shaped erythrocytes in Laennec's cirrhosis. New Engl. J. Med. 275:639, 1966.

342. Cooper, R. A.: Anemia with spur cells. A red cell defect acquired in serum and modified in the circulation. J. Clin. Invest. 48:1820, 1969.

343. Cooper, R. A., Diloy-Puray, M., et al.: An analysis of lipoproteins, bile acids, and red cell membranes associated with target cells and spur cells in patients with liver disease. J. Clin. Invest. 51:3182, 1972.

344. Switzer, S.: Plasma lipoproteins in liver disease. I. Immunologically distinct low-density lipoproteins in patients with biliary obstruction. J. Clin. Invest. 46:1855, 1967.

345. Seidel, D., Alaupovic, P., and Furman, R. H.: A lipoprotein characterizing obstructive jaundice. I. Method for quantitative separation and identification of lipoproteins in jaundiced subjects. J. Clin. Invest. 48:1211, 1969.

346. Hamilton, R. L., Havel, R. J., et al.: Cholestasis: Lamellar structure of the abnormal human serum lipoprotein. Science 172:475, 1971.

347. Gjone, E., and Norum, K. R.: Plasma lecithin: cholesterol acyltransferase and erythrocyte lipids in liver disease. Acta Med. Scand. 187:153, 1970.

348. Simon, J. B., and Scheig, R.: Serum cholesterol esterification in liver disease. Importance of lecithin:cholesterol acyltransferase. New Engl. J. Med. 283:841, 1970.

349. Jones, D. P., Sosa, F. R., et al.: Serum cholesterol esterifying and cholesterol ester hydrolyzing activities in liver diseases: Relationships to cholesterol, bilirubin, and bile salt concentrations. J. Clin. Invest. 50:259, 1971.

350. Cooper, R. A., Garcia, F. A., et al.: The effect of lithocholic acid on red cell membranes in vivo. J. Lab. Clin. Med. 79:7, 1972.

351. Fredrickson, D. S., Gotto, A. M., Jr., et al.: Familial lipoprotein deficiency (abetalipoproteinemia, hypobetalipoproteinemia, and Tangier disease), In The Metabolic Basis of Inherited Disease, Stanbury, J. B., Wyngaarden, J. B., and Fredrickson, D. S., (eds.), New York, McGraw-Hill, 1972, p. 493.

352. Levy, R. I., and Fredrickson, D. S.: Personal communication.

353. Mentzer, W. C., Baehner, R. L., et al.: Metabolic vulnerability of reticulocytes in pyruvate kinase (PK) deficiency. Blood 34:861, 1969.

354. Tosteson, D. C., Carlsen, E., et al.: The effects of sickling on ion transport. I. Effect of sickling on potassium transport. J. Gen. Physiol. 39:31, 1955.

355. Glader, B. E., Fortier, N., et al.: Desiccytosis associated with RBC potassium loss: A new congenital hemolytic syndrome. Pediatr. Res. 7:350, 1973.

356. Messer, M. J., and Harris, J. W.: Filtration char-

acteristics of sickle cell: Rates of alteration of filterability after deoxygenation and reoxygenation and correlations with sickling and unsickling. J. Lab. Clin. Med. 76:537, 1970.

357. Goldstone, G.: Personal communication.

358. Bertles, J., and Döbler, J.: Reversible and irreversible sickling: A distinction by electron microscopy. Blood 33:884, 1969.

359. Chien, S., Asami, S., et al.: Abnormal rheology of oxygenated blood in sickle cell anemia. J. Clin. Invest. 49:623, 1970.

360. Jensen, W. N., Bromberg, P. A., et al.: Membrane deformation: A cause of the irreversibly sickled cell (ISC). Clin. Res. 17:464, 1969.

361. Shohet, S. B., Jensen, M. C., et al.: Unpublished observations.

362. Devenuto, F., Ligon, D. F., et al.: Human erythrocyte membrane: Uptake of progesterone and chemical alterations. Biochim. Biophys. Acta 193:36, 1969.

363. Jandl, J. H.: The Heinz body hemolytic anemias. Ann. Intern. Med. 58:702, 1963.

364. Fessas, P.: Inclusions of hemoglobin in erythroblasts and erythrocytes of thalassemia. Blood 21:21, 1963.

365. Nathan, D. G., and Gunn, R. B.: Thalassemia: The consequences of unbalanced hemoglobin synthesis. Am. J. Med. 41:815, 1966.

366. Sturgeon, P., and Finch, C. A.: Erythro-kinetics in Cooley's anemia. Blood 12:64, 1957.

367. Robinson, S., Vanier, T., et al.: Jaundice in thalassemia minor. A consequence of "ineffective erythropoiesis." New Engl. J. Med. 267:523, 1962.

368. Tatum, E. L.: In Reflections on Research and the Future of Medicine. Lyght, C. E. (ed.), New York, McGraw-Hill, 1967, p. 21.

369. Feig, S. A., Segal, G. B., et al.: Energy metabolism in human erythrocytes. II. Effects of glucose depletion. J. Clin. Invest. 51:1547, 1972.

370. Shohet, S. B., Anderson, H. M., et al.: The source of ATP for erythrocyte (RBC) membrane lipid renewal. Blood 38:833, 1971.

371. Shohet, S. B., and Haley, J. E.: Red cell membrane shape and stability: Relation to cell lipid renewal pathways and cell ATP. Nouv. Rev. Fr. Hematol. 12:761, 1972.

372. Weed, R. I., LaCelle, P. L., et al.: Metabolic dependence of red cell deformability. J. Clin. Invest. 48:795, 1970.

373. LaCelle, P. L.: Alteration of membrane deformability in hemolytic anemias. Semin. Hematol. 7:355, 1970.

374. Valentine, W. N., Hsieh, H. S., et al.: Hereditary hemolytic anemia: Association with phosphoglycerate kinase deficiency in erythrocytes and leukocytes. New Engl. J. Med. 280:528, 1969.

375. Mentzer, W. C., Baehner, R. L., et al.: Selective reticulocyte destruction in erythrocyte pyruvate kinase deficiency. J. Clin. Invest. 50:688, 1971.

376. Jacob, H. S., and Amsden, T.: Acute hemolytic anemia with rigid red cells in hypophosphatemia. New Engl. J. Med. 285:1446, 1971.

Chapter 7

Destruction of Red Cells by the Vasculature and the Reticuloendothelial System

by Michael C. Brain

INTRODUCTION

The life span of the red cell is spent within the circulation, which it enters as a reticulocyte and from which it is removed when effete by the phagocytic cells of the reticuloendothelial system. Hemolytic anemia implies shortened survival in the circulation, whether due to an intrinsic defect in the red cell or due to external factors, including abnormalities in the vascular environment through which the red cell circulates. To survive normally the red cell must be able to withstand the physical stresses to which it is subjected during the phases of rapid flow within the heart and blood vessels, and must also be able to undergo repetitive deformation to pass through the capillaries of the microcirculation. Shortened red cell survival can result from abnormalities in the heart and blood vessels which may subject the red cells to damaging physical stresses. Conversely, changes in the red cell can result in loss of deformability and can impair passage through the microcirculation, especially within the microcirculation of the spleen, in which both the nature of the circulation and the presence of reticuloendothelial cells lining the vascular channels can bring about retention and phagocytosis of abnormal and effete red cells. Thus changes in the vascular system, whether in the heart or major blood vessels, in the microcircu-

lation, or in the specialized portions of the circulation lined by reticuloendothelial cells, can play an important role in either shortening the survival of normal red cells or by removing abnormal red cells from the circulation.

THE RETICULOENDOTHELIAL SYSTEM

The reticuloendothelial system carries out a number of important physiologic functions in relation to the red cell and the hemopoietic system, some of which are greatly increased in hemolytic anemia. These functions include the removal of the effete normal red cells from the circulation at the end of their life span, and the phagocytosis, lysis, and proteolytic digestion of red cells within phagocytic vacuoles to yield amino acids, iron, and bilirubin. The amino acids and iron are returned to their respective metabolic pools. The bilirubin is returned to the circulation for transport to the liver, where it undergoes conjugation and excretion in the bile. The latter functions are dependent on normal hepatic function. In the newborn, although there is evidence that reticuloendothelial function may be impaired (*vide infra*), hepatic function is much less capable of handling the

241

bilirubin load, and this leads to raised levels of unconjugated bilirubin in the circulation and the risk of development of kernicterus in neonatal jaundice.

In hemolytic anemias, when the survival of red cells in the circulation may be markedly shortened, the function of the reticuloendothelial system in removing and breaking down the abnormal red cells is correspondingly greatly increased.

In addition to the enhancement of the physiologic response of the reticuloendothelial system in hemolytic anemia, in certain diseases of the reticuloendothelial system, especially those associated with enlargement of the spleen, increased sequestration and destruction of apparently normal red cells can take place, resulting in both anemia and shortened red cell survival.

In addition to those functions of the reticuloendothelial system which can be specifically related to the removal and destruction of normal and abnormal red cells from the circulation, components of the reticuloendothelial system play an important role in the humoral immune response through the recognition of antigenically foreign, or antibody-coated, cells and through the initiation of antibody formation. Furthermore, the reticuloendothelial system plays an important role in the body's defenses against disease by the clearance of bacteria and other organisms from the circulation and their subsequent phagocytic destruction.

An understanding of the role of the reticuloendothelial system in hemolytic anemia necessitates a brief general description of the distribution and function of the reticuloendothelial system, and consideration of those factors which predispose both normal and abnormal red cells to selective sequestration and destruction.

Distribution

The reticuloendothelial system can be regarded as a specialized component of the blood and lymphatic vascular systems, in which the endothelial cells lining the vessels have the capability of phagocytic ingestion of particulate material. The reticuloendothelial system was originally recognized and its distribution defined by the uptake by endothelial cells of dyes and particulate material injected into the blood or tissues. The injection of such foreign material demonstrated the widespread distribution of phagocytic endothelial cells lining certain blood and lymphatic vessels. It was further recognized that these phagocytic endothelial cells had the property of forming reticulum-like fibers which stained with silver—hence the name reticuloendothelial cells and system. Phagocytic endothelial cells are present in many organs, notably the spleen, liver, bone marrow, lymph nodes, adrenal cortex, and anterior lobe of the pituitary. However, only the reticuloendothelial cells of the spleen, liver, and bone marrow play a role in the removal and destruction of red cells. The many and diverse functions of, and the distribution of, the reticuloendothelial system have been reviewed in detail by Stuart (1).

Red Cell Destruction

The removal of effete normal red cells from the circulation at the end of their life span is principally carried out by the spleen (2), although the reticuloendothelial cells of the bone marrow may also perform this function (3). In hemolytic anemia there is much evidence that the spleen, when present, is often the predominant site of red cell destruction. Furthermore, in certain hemolytic anemias, notably hereditary spherocytosis, the spleen plays a highly important role in the hemolytic process, since removal of the spleen corrects or greatly improves red cell survival despite the persistence of abnormal red cells within the circulation after splenectomy. In other disorders the spleen plays a more passive role, and although improvement may take place after splenectomy, hemolysis persists, and other components of the reticuloendothelial system undertake the removal of the abnormal cells from the circulation. The particular role of the spleen in the removal of normal and abnormal red cells from the circulation, and the evidence that sequestration of red cells within the spleen exposes them to an adverse environment for their survival necessitates detailed consideration of the peculiar anatomy and function of the spleen in relation to hemolytic anemia.

THE SPLEEN

The spleen has long been recognized as playing a major role in red cell destruction in hemolytic anemia, as evidenced by the response to splenectomy in hereditary spherocytosis. The introduction of radioactive chromium as a label of red cell survival not only permitted the accurate measurement of red cell life span (4–7), but also, by the use of surface counting over the spleen, liver, and heart, enabled the selective sequestration of red cells within the spleen to be demonstrated (8, 9). In patients with splenomegaly without overt hemolytic anemia, the injection of ^{51}Cr-labeled normal red cells combined with continuous monitoring of radioactivity over the spleen demonstrated the presence of rapid-mixing and slow-mixing pools of red cells within the spleen (10–12). The gradual accumulation of radioactivity within the spleen after the rapid mixing phase had been achieved was indicative of the sequestration of red cells within a slowly mixing compartment (10–12). The demonstration of more than one vascular compartment within the spleen in vivo has been borne out by the rate at which red cells can be recovered from the splenic vein or perfusion of the splenic artery from animal spleens removed surgically (13). Studies on spleens removed surgically from patients with hereditary spherocytosis demonstrated that the red cells were flushed out with difficulty and were more spherocytic than the red cells obtained from the peripheral blood at the time of operation, an indication of both the selective retention of abnormal cells within the spleen and an effect of the spleen on red cells sequestered within it (14–16).

Histologic and electron microscopic studies of human and animal spleens have provided an anatomic basis for the selective sequestration of abnormal red cells (17–21). The spleen comprises two distinct but closely related elements: the white pulp, comprising histiocytic macrophages, lymphocytes, and plasma cells of the germinal centers; and the Billroth cords and splenic sinuses of the red pulp, both of which are supported by fibrous trabeculae, through which the arteries gain access to both components, and the veins return to the splenic vein. Blood entering the spleen by the splenic arteries enters the white pulp by central arteries. The central arteries give off a number of right angle branches as they pass down the white pulp. The shape of these arterial branches may facilitate plasma skimming with the selective retention of plasma and small particles within the germinal center, a process which may facilitate the localization of antigenically foreign proteins and small particles within the germinal centers, an important site of antibody formation. The later branches of the central artery, in which the hematocrit has been increased by plasma skimming, enter the red pulp. The red pulp can be regarded, in essence, as a distensible and contractile filter bed, in which cells come into close contact with phagocytic endothelial cells. The red pulp is made up of two components; tortuous, tubular-shaped, endothelial-lined sinuses ultimately joining together to form trabecular veins, by which blood is returned to the splenic veins, and the splenic or Billroth cords, partitioning structures between the splenic sinuses. The cords are supplied by terminating arterioles.

The circulation through the red pulp, although greatly clarified by the recent histologic and electron microscopic studies (17–21), is still incompletely understood physiologically. However, of greater importance is the nature of this circulation and the appreciation that it can vary in disease. Blood entering the red pulp from the white pulp can gain direct access to the splenic sinuses either via capillaries in the marginal zone between the white pulp and red pulp or by passage through the Billroth cords. Although the terms "Billroth cord" and "splenic sinus" might appear to suggest that these are two independent structures, they are, in fact, very closely related to each other, the endothelial cells lining the splenic sinus being contiguous with the endothelial cells comprising the cords. Furthermore, the sinus endothelial cells are incompletely covered by basement membrane, being supported by filamentous fibers extending in from the trabeculae (Fig. 7–1). The lack of continuity of the basement membrane over the sinus endothelial cells permits the margins of the endothelial cells to move relative to each other, with the formation of inter-endothelial clefts or slits between the Billroth cords

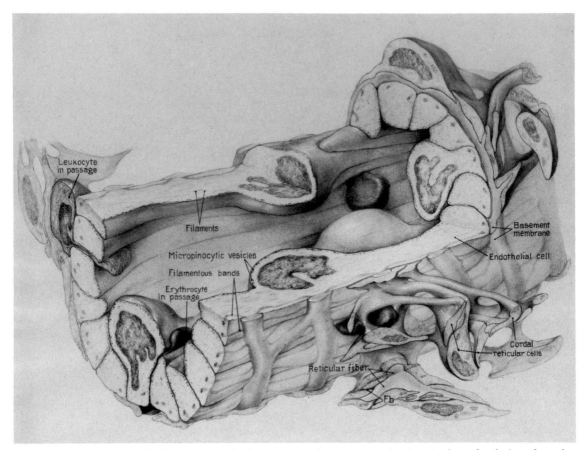

Figure 7–1. Diagram of splenic sinus, which represents the structure of a sinus in the red pulp based on electron microscopic observations. The sinus wall consists of a single layer of endothelial cells, a basement membrane, and adventitial cells which partially cover the cordal surface of both the basement membrane and the endothelium. The sinus is cut transversely and longitudinally. The endothelial cells running parallel to the longitudinal axis of the sinus are partially covered by ring and longitudinal components of basement membranes and by the adventitial cells. The adventitial cells branch into the cords and are part of the cordal reticulum. Most of the adventitial cells are omitted in this diagram in order to depict the basement membrane and filamentous bands in the basal portions of the endothelial cells. In reality the basement membrane is completely covered by the endothelial cells and adventitial cells, and the reticular fibers by the reticular cells. The basement membrane is continuous with the reticular fibers of the cords. The endothelial cells contain three distinctive structures: micropinocytotic vesicles, and two types of cytoplasmic filaments loosely organized and tightly aligned into arching bands. The filamentous bands depicted through the plasmalemma and in cross and longitudinal sections lie in the basal portions of the endothelial cells. The bands arch between the ring components of basement membrane, running perpendicular to the ring and, therefore, parallel to the long axis of the sinuses and their endothelial cells. The filaments of the filamentous bands are inserted into the plasmalemma. Blood cells are frequently present in passage through the slits of the sinus wall. They are tightly constricted. Filamentous bands (Fb) are also present in cordal reticular cells. Here, however, the bands do not have the orientation or arrangement they have in the sinus endothelium. (From Chen, L-T., and Weiss, L.: Am. J. Anat. *134*:425, 1972.)

and splenic sinus surfaces, through which cells within the Billroth cord can pass to reenter the splenic sinus (21). The endothelial cells lining both the splenic sinus and the Billroth cords lacking basement membrane have projections which extend into their respective vascular channels, and the cells contain pinocytic vacuoles. The potential clefts between the endothelial cells

provide an effective filtration system, through which red cells and white cells in the Billroth cords have to pass to regain the splenic sinuses and reenter the venous circulation (Fig. 7–1). Spherocytic red cells would be handicapped or prevented from passing between the endothelial cells and would thus become retained within the Billroth cords, which become distended and congested with abnormal red cells. Distention of the Billroth cords will also disturb the flow down the splenic sinuses, which, because of their shape and the nature of the endothelial cell projections lining the sinus, will retain and phagocytose abnormal red cells within the sinus. Thus both structures can contribute to splenic sequestration and destruction of abnormal red cells.

The interendothelial slits between the Billroth cords and splenic sinuses may play a particular role in splenic "pitting," or the removal of intracellular inclusions. The arrest of a red cell at such a barrier, combined with the phagocytic properties of the endothelial cells, would appear to provide the means by which intracellular inclusions, such as Howell-Jolly bodies, siderotic granules, denatured or unstable hemoglobin (such as Heinz bodies), and hemoglobin H ($\beta 4$) inclusions, are selectively removed from the red cell with or without the portion of the red cell membrane to which they may be attached (22–24). The removal of such inclusions appears to be a function primarily undertaken by the spleen. Although other components of the reticuloendothelial system remove intact red cells from the circulation after splenectomy, they seem less effective in removing intracellular inclusions. Thus, following splenectomy, there is an increase in intracellular inclusions, Howell-Jolly bodies, siderotic granules, and Heinz bodies in normal subjects, and a great increase in hemoglobin inclusions following splenectomy in patients with unstable hemoglobins or hemoglobin H disease (alpha thalassemia).

The removal of intracellular inclusions from the red cells by the spleen appears to be accomplished without detectable membrane damage. However, after removal of the spleen, surface abnormalities of the red cell membrane can be seen by interference contrast microscopy in patients with persistent hemolytic anemia and the presence of red cell inclusions (25).

Splenomegaly

When red cells are destroyed at a rapid rate within the spleen, the organ enlarges and may on occasion cause abdominal discomfort, as well as sequestration of granulocytes and platelets. The cellular basis of this enlargement has been amplified by the studies of Jacob, MacDonald, Jandl, and their co-workers (26, 27), who found that the injection of injured red cells causes rapid stimulation of the growth of intact spleen and explanted spleen in the rodent. This rapid growth is preceded by increased DNA synthesis in splenic phagocytes and littoral cells, particularly in splenic marginal zones which are the initial sites of red cell sequestration. The proliferation of phagocytes and littoral cells, together with the increased quantity of sequestered red cells, accounts for the observed enlargement of the organ.

Absence of the Spleen and Impaired Splenic Function

Absence of the spleen is a well recognized accompaniment to a variety of congenital malformations of the heart (28–31). Absence of the spleen can be suspected by the finding of Howell-Jolly bodies. In premature infants, in the absence of congenital malformations, there may be an increase in both Howell-Jolly bodies and the number of red cells showing "pocking" of the membrane surface, such as are observed normally only after splenectomy (32, 33).

Hyposplenism is also a feature of celiac disease, and the finding of a macrocytic anemia in association with Howell-Jolly bodies may provide supportive evidence for the diagnosis of celiac disease in a child, or idiopathic steatorrhea in an adult (34). Reduced splenic function can be confirmed by demonstrating the impaired clearance of ^{51}Cr-labeled, heat-damaged red cells from the circulation in such patients (35).

Hyposplenism can be demonstrated in children with sickle cell disease, even in the presence of enlargement of the spleen (36, 37) (see Chapter 14).

The Role of the Spleen in Red Cell Destruction

The spleen contributes to red cell destruction in a number of ways. The spleen sequesters immature cells, including reticulocytes, old cells at the end of their life spans, and abnormal red cells. Furthermore, the retention of normal and, more importantly, abnormal cells within a congested red pulp subjects the red cell to a deleterious metabolic environment with respect to glucose concentration, pH (which falls because of lactic acid formation), and low oxygen tension; any or all of these factors may contribute to metabolic embarrassment of normal or abnormal red cells, as will be discussed below.

Splenic Sequestration

The retention of red cells within the red pulp of the spleen is determined by two main mechanisms which are not mutually exclusive. The first is an alteration in surface properties of the red cell. The presence of immunoglobulin on the red cell surface predisposes the cell to splenic sequestration, presumably through the adherence of immunoglobulin-coated cells to the phagocytic endothelial cells; however, when large amounts of immunoglobulin are present, hepatic as well as splenic sequestration takes place (38) (see Chapter 8). The phenomenon of adherence of immunoglobulin-coated cells to phagocytic monocytes in vitro and their subsequent phagocytosis is well recognized (39, 40). The sequestration of reticulocytes within the spleen may also be due to a change in surface properties because of the presence of physiologic proteins, such as transferrin, attached to their membranes. It has also been shown that removal of sialic acid from the red cell surface through the action of neuraminidase predisposes the red cell to splenic sequestration, possibly as a direct consequence of loss of surface charge. Thus the diminution of surface charge which takes place with aging of the normal red cell may be a contributory factor in its splenic sequestration (41). The metabolic changes that take place in cell aging, with consequent changes in cation and water content and in red cell deformability, may be more significant factors in the removal of the effete normal red cell from the circulation. Apart from the presence of immunoglobulins or complement on the red cell surface, the most important factor leading

to splenic sequestration of red cells in hemolytic anemia is a change in red cell deformability.

The importance of red cell deformability to red cell survival and splenic sequestration has been recognized through in vitro studies of red cell filtration through filter paper and other membranes (42, 43). These techniques have shown that impaired filterability, often accompanied by increased viscosity of whole blood, can result from disorders of the red cell membrane, of red cell metabolism, or of the constitution or stability of the hemoglobin within the cell (Table 7–1).

Loss of red cell membrane, whether due to the as yet incompletely understood defect of the membrane in hereditary spherocytosis, or to mechanical fragmentation, or to partial phagocytosis of antibody-coated cells, results in the loss of surface relative to volume, with the formation of a spherocyte. This change in shape results in a marked loss of deformability and filterability when compared to the highly deformable, normal, disc-shaped red cell; moreover, it impedes its passage through the endothelial slits between the Billroth cord and splenic sinuses. Loss of deformability without surface area occurs with the transformation of a disc to a crenated sphere or ecchinocyte, with energy depletion and a fall in red cell ATP levels in normal red cells (44). Furthermore, loss of intracellular potassium and concomitant intracellular water on ATP depletion will increase red cell viscosity. Both these changes are liable to take place through impairment of cell metabolism, either as a consequence of

TABLE 7–1. DISORDERS ASSOCIATED WITH DIMINISHED RED CELL DEFORMABILITY

1. *Abnormalities of hemoglobin structure or stability*
   Sickle cell anemia (Hb SS)
   Sickle cell trait (Hb SA)
   Hemoglobin C disease (Hb CC)
   Heinz body formation

2. *Abnormalities of red cell membrane or metabolism*
   Hereditary spherocytosis
   Acanthocytosis (abetalipoproteinemia)
   ACD-stored red cells
   Heinz body formation

cell age or as a result of an enzyme deficiency in the glycolytic pathway (45). Such changes are likely to predispose an effete normal cell or a metabolically abnormal cell to sequestration within the spleen.

Changes in the constitution or stability of hemoglobin within the red cell will also impair red cell filterability and increase red cell viscosity (46). The most obvious abnormality is that associated with hemoglobin S, when, in the homozygous sickle cell anemia, the obstruction to the splenic circulation leads to splenic infarction or ischemic splenic atrophy. Diminished filterability has been demonstrated in hemoglobin S disease and in hemoglobin C disease (46, 47). Similar changes in red cell filterability and enhanced splenic sequestration take place as a result of instability of the hemoglobin or of globin peptide chains. Heinz bodies may result from the presence of an unstable hemoglobin, or through oxidative denaturation of hemoglobin on exposure to oxidant drugs due to enzyme deficiencies in the pentose phosphate pathway or the related enzymes responsible for the synthesis or regeneration of reduced glutathione (22–24). The degree of splenic sequestration will be dependent on the extent of hemoglobin denaturation and on the consequences of hemoglobin precipitation on membrane function. In many of the hemolytic anemias due to unstable hemoglobins, the principal role of the spleen involves its pitting function and consequent removal of the intracellular inclusions, and splenectomy may or may not lessen the hemolytic process.

Imbalance of globin chain synthesis results in the formation of red cell inclusions in both alpha and beta thalassemia. In beta thalassemia, the Hb H (β_4) inclusions removed by the spleen by the process of splenic pitting are much more numerous after splenectomy (22–25). In beta thalassemia major, the excess α chains are so unstable that they precipitate within red cell precursors within the bone marrow. The complete or partial phagocytosis of the red cells by bone marrow reticuloendothelial cells contributes to both the degree of ineffective erythropoiesis and the release of deformed red cells into the circulation (25). Splenic pitting and destruction also take place as splenectomy increases both the proportion of abnormally shaped red cells and the incidence of intracellular inclusions in circulating red cells (25).

The Adverse Splenic Environment and Hypersplenism

The sluggish circulation through the congested red pulp of the spleen in hemolytic anemia brings about a fall in glucose content and a fall in pH due to lactic acid formation (48, 49). Both these factors will result in a reduction in red cell metabolism, which may further embarrass an abnormal red cell with increased energy requirements due to abnormal cation content. Thus the hereditary spherocytic red cell undergoes accelerated membrane loss and disturbance of cation content, making it less able to traverse the splenic filter bed. Splenectomy in hereditary spherocytosis is beneficial in that it removes an adverse environment as well as a site for sequestration of the spherocytic red cell.

The adverse environment for red cell glycolysis, to which hereditary spherocytic red cells are peculiarly susceptible, may account for the shortened survival of normal red cells in children with massive splenomegaly due to portal hypertension or with infiltrative splenomegaly. Furthermore, massive splenomegaly, in addition to shortening the survival of normal or transfused red cells, contributes to anemia by the sequestration of a considerable proportion of the total circulating red cells, thereby lowering the venous to whole body hematocrit ratio (11, 12). Although massive splenomegaly may contribute to anemia through both these mechanisms, it is unusual for these factors alone to justify splenectomy unless alternative, more specific treatment of the causes of splenomegaly is unsuccessful or impractical, or unless blood transfusion requirements or anemia become a comparable or greater hazard to health than the risks of surgical removal of the spleen. Although removal of the spleen may successfully reduce the transfusion requirements of children with thalassemia major (50, 51) or with other disorders of red cell formation or hemoglobin synthesis, the operation is not without risk, may be of transient benefit, and increases the risk of transfusional hemosiderosis of the liver and other organs unless measures are taken to enhance the excretion of iron in the urine.

Splenectomy in Hemolytic Anemia (Table 7-2)

The indication for splenectomy in hemolytic anemia depends primarily upon the recognition and, where possible, the demonstration that the spleen is playing a major role in the shortened survival of the abnormal red cells. In hereditary spherocytosis the role of the spleen in shortening red cell survival is indisputable, and the decision when to carry out splenectomy is primarily determined by the severity of the hemolysis and the age of the child (*vide infra*). In pyruvate kinase deficiency the anemia may be improved by splenectomy; however, it should be borne in mind that anemia per se should not be regarded as a sufficient indication for splenectomy, as the high level of 2,3-diphosphoglycerate in the pyruvate kinase–deficient red cell greatly enhances tissue oxygen delivery despite the anemia. In other congenital hemolytic anemias, the response to splenectomy may not always be predictable, and it is desirable to have evidence of significant splenic sequestration using surface counting after reinjection of the patient's red cells labeled with ^{51}Cr before the operation is carried out.

Splenectomy may have to be considered in children with severe autoimmune hemolytic anemia, in whom hemolytic anemia is life threatening, who cannot be transfused with compatible blood and who have failed to respond to treatment with corticosteroids or ACTH or both in full doses.

Hazards of Splenectomy

The removal of the spleen from infants and young children is recognized to be associated with an increased risk of severe and sometimes fatal bacterial infections (52). The risk of infection is greatest when the splenectomy is associated with a severe and continuing disease, such as thalassemia major, and it is minimal in children with hereditary spherocytosis or in those without persistent disease process (53, 54) (Table 7–3). Nevertheless, it would appear ad-

TABLE 7–2. INDICATIONS FOR SPLENECTOMY IN HEMOLYTIC ANEMIA

1. *Probable or predictable improvement in anemia*
   Hereditary spherocytosis
   Hereditary elliptocytosis
   Pyruvate kinase deficiency
   Hexokinase deficiency

2. *Possible or unpredictable benefit*
   Acquired idiopathic autoimmune hemolytic anemia (corticosteroid-unresponsive)
   Phosphohexose isomerase deficiency

visable to postpone splenectomy until age 4 years unless there are clear-cut and pressing indications.

It has recently been recognized that splenectomy, in addition to removing an important component of the reticuloendothelial system responsible for the clearance and phagocytosis of bacteria which may enter the blood, is followed by a fall in the levels of serum IgM immunoglobulins (55). Since the IgM immunoglobulins play an important role in the resistance to bacterial infections, a reduction in the levels of IgM following splenectomy appears likely to be a contributing factor in the tendency of these children to develop

TABLE 7–3. COMPLICATIONS OF SPLENECTOMY IN CHILDHOOD: ANALYSIS OF 1413 CASES*

MORTALITY
1. *Postoperative*

Congenital hemolytic anemia	1 of 395
Idiopathic thrombocytopenic purpura	3 of 265
Trauma to spleen	6 of 348
Thalassemia	0 of 48
Other diseases (lymphoma, etc.)	27 of 360

2. *Death from primary disease after splenectomy*

Congenital hemolytic anemia	4 of 394
Idiopathic thrombocytopenic purpura	12 of 262
Trauma	4 of 342
Thalassemia	9 of 45
Other diseases	83 of 323

SEVERE INFECTIONS
1. *Low risk*

Congenital hemolytic anemia	2 of 394
Idiopathic thrombocytopenic purpura	7 of 262
Trauma	3 of 342

2. *High risk*

Thalassemia	2 of 45
Other disorders	20 of 323

*Modified from Eraklis, A. J., and Filler, R. M.: Splenectomy in childhood. A review of 1413 cases. J. Pediatr. Surg. 7:382–388, 1972, by permission of Grune & Stratton.

overwhelming bacterial infections, commonly by *Diplococcus pneumoniae* or *Hemophilus influenzae*. The levels of immunoglobulins should be measured in children both before and at intervals after splenectomy in order to recognize those children who may have impaired resistance to infection due to IgM deficiency.

In children with persistent anemia or complicating diseases, it would appear advisable to maintain the child on prophylactic penicillin for two or more years. Whenever splenectomy has been carried out, it is advisable to warn the parents of the increased risk from bacterial infections, and that advice should be sought and appropriate antibiotic treatment given for mild infections without delay.

In tropical areas where malaria is endemic, splenectomy can predispose the child to subsequent severe or fatal malarial infections, or result in an exacerbation of a previously quiescent chronic malarial infection.

THE LIVER AND BONE MARROW

The reticuloendothelial system in the liver and bone marrow is responsible for the removal of abnormal cells from the circulation in hemolytic anemias not corrected by splenectomy. In certain acquired autoimmune hemolytic anemias, surface counting may demonstrate that a proportion of the red cells are undergoing sequestration in the liver as well as the spleen (38). The role of the bone marrow in red cell destruction in hemolytic anemia is difficult to measure, although it may be important. The reticuloendothelial cells in the bone marrow play a major role in the removal of abnormal cells, or the prevention of their entering the circulation in disorders associated with ineffective erythropoiesis, such as the thalassemias (56).

HEMOLYTIC ANEMIA AND DISORDERS OF THE HEART AND BLOOD VESSELS

Hemolytic anemia, characterized by the presence of red cell fragments, spherocytes (Fig. 7–2), and evidence of intravascular

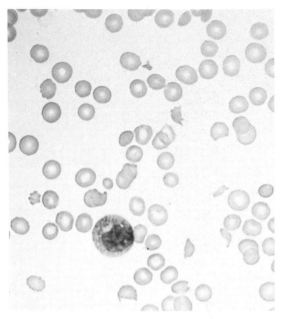

Figure 7–2. Peripheral blood smear of a patient with acute hemolytic uremic syndrome. Note fragmented erythrocytes and microspherocytes.

hemolysis, may occur in association with congenital and acquired valvular heart disease following the surgical repair of intracardiac defects or the insertion of prosthetic heart valves, or in association with a variety of disorders of the microcirculation (Table 7–4). The mechanism of the hemolysis in all these situations can be most readily explained by the interaction between circulating red cells and an abnormal hemodynamic or physical environment within the heart or blood vessels. A detailed consideration of the pathogenesis of hemolysis will follow the clinical descriptions.

Cardiac Hemolytic Anemia

Although mild hemolytic anemia has been recognized in association with congenital or acquired disease of the heart valves or aorta (57–61), the recognition of cardiac hemolytic anemia followed the introduction of open heart surgery and the repair of intracardiac defects and the insertion of prosthetic heart valves, initially in experimental animals and subsequently in man (62).

The success of open heart surgery in the repair of congenital cardiac defects and in the replacement of malfunctioning and dis-

TABLE 7–4.   ACQUIRED HEMOLYTIC
ANEMIA WITH RED CELL
FRAGMENTATION

---

1. *Macroangiopathic hemolytic anemia*
    Congenital heart disease
    Surgical repair of valvular defects
    Insertion of prosthetic heart valves
    Prosthetic repair of septal defects

2. *Microangiopathic hemolytic anemia*
    Hemolytic uremic syndrome
    Thrombotic thrombocytopenic purpura
    Cavernous hemangioma
    Renal or hepatic transplant rejection
    Metastatic carcinoma

---

eased heart valves was followed by the publication of a large number of accounts of postoperative hemolytic anemia, characterized by the presence of fragmented, distorted, and spherocytic red cells, hemoglobinemia, hemoglobinuria, or hemosiderinuria.

Although the successful insertion of a prosthetic heart valve is often followed by a mild, compensated hemolytic anemia with shortened red cell survival and lowering of serum haptoglobin levels, the incidence of frank hemolytic anemia has, with improved surgical techniques and improvement in design of prosthetic heart valves, become relatively uncommon and rarely exceeds 5 per cent of successful cardiac operations. It was recognized early that cardiac hemolytic anemia was often associated with the persistence of a postoperative hemodynamic abnormality. Incomplete repair of an intracardiac defect, abnormal function of the prosthetic valve, or more frequently defective attachment of the base of the prosthetic valve to the adjacent cardiac tissue may cause a regurgitant jet of blood to flow past the valve or impinge on an unendothelialized prosthetic surface. Although the persistent, postoperative hemodynamic abnormality may be detected clinically, not infrequently the hemolytic anemia may be severe in the absence of abnormal cardiac physical signs apart from those related to anemia. The presence of a hemodynamic disorder may be demonstrated by cineangiography or only be detected at reoperation. The successful repair of a postoperative defect or replacement of a malfunctioning prosthetic valve or its attachment or re-

attachment to the cardiac tissue can produce dramatic relief of the hemolysis.

Pathogenesis

The association of cardiac hemolytic anemia with replacement of the aortic valve or with hemodynamic defects connected with a high pressure gradient within the heart has reasonably suggested that the red cells were damaged by the high shear forces produced by turbulent blood flow. Indeed, studies of red cells in cone-plate viscometers demonstrated that red cells were damaged and hemolysis took place when the shear forces exceeded 3000 dynes per cm.[2] (63). Shear forces of this magnitude would be generated within the heart by the pressure gradient between the aorta and left ventricle, or left ventricle and left atrium. However, the hypothesis that the red cell damage is produced by shear forces within turbulent jets has been questioned by the demonstration that red cells can withstand shear forces of up to 15,000 dynes per cm.[2] without hemolysis when such forces are generated at a fluid-fluid interface (64). Shear forces of this magnitude far exceed those calculated to be encountered within the heart or circulation. It thus seems probable that red cell damage and hemolysis observed in cardiac hemolytic anemia are more likely to result from the interaction of red cells with abnormal surfaces within the heart or major blood vessels rather than from the turbulence produced by a jet of blood. The hemolysis produced in a cone-plate viscometer at 3000 dynes per cm.[2] may, in fact, be due to the interaction of the moving red cells and the stationary surface once a critical force has been exceeded rather than to the shear forces acting in the fluid medium. This conclusion is supported by reports of cessation of hemolysis which have followed the covering of an abnormal intracardiac prosthetic surface with endothelium (62).

The importance of hemodynamic factors in the pathogenesis of the hemolytic anemia is, nevertheless, borne out by the increase in the rate of hemolysis which accompanies a rise in cardiac output on exercise or with anemia (65). The loss of hemoglobin in the urine is diurnal, being greatest during the day in the ambulatory patient and least during the night (65). Hemoglobinuria also lessens with the fall in cardiac output resulting from the temporary correction of anemia by blood transfusion.

Diagnosis and Treatment

The diagnosis of postoperative cardiac hemolytic anemia presents little difficulty and should be suspected in any patient who develops hemolytic anemia after open heart surgery. The onset may immediately follow a cardiac operation, or it may be a late complication due to defective function of a prosthetic heart valve, although this is now less common with improvements in design and construction of prosthetic valves. The diagnosis is supported by the finding of distorted, fragmented, and spherocytic red cells in the peripheral blood, the presence of intravascular hemolysis with free hemoglobin in the plasma and urine, the absence of serum haptoglobin, and the demonstration of hemosiderin in the urinary deposit. The intravascular hemolysis is accompanied by release of the red cell enzyme, lactic dehydrogenase, into the plasma. The measurement of serum lactate dehydrogenase activity has been found to correlate very closely with the shortened ^{51}Cr-labeled red cell survival in patients with cardiac hemolytic anemia (66). Although a positive direct Coombs' test may occasionally follow cardiac surgery and be accompanied by hemolysis, the direct and indirect Coombs' tests are usually negative (62).

The hemolytic anemia may lessen in the first few weeks after surgery; however, it usually persists and becomes more severe as the patient becomes ambulatory and the cardiac output rises. The anemia may be of such severity as to necessitate frequent blood transfusions, and the loss of hemoglobin in the urine and of hemosiderin can result in iron deficiency (65, 67). Iron and folic acid should be prescribed to achieve a maximal erythropoietic response, but this may be insufficient to compensate for the hemolysis.

The only effective treatment is the surgical correction of the underlying hemodynamic abnormality. The decision to reoperate can often be delayed for weeks or months, depending on the severity of the hemolysis and the hemodynamic status of the patient, in the hope that hemolysis may lessen or become trivial. The hemolytic anemia itself is a valuable indicator of a hemodynamic abnormality which may not be detectable clinically and only with difficulty by cineangiography following the injection of contrast media.

The hemolytic anemia, if severe and requiring frequent blood transfusions, can itself be a sufficient indication for reoperation, and successful surgical correction of a small and hemodynamically trivial defect can result in dramatic cessation of hemolysis and the correction of anemia. In mild cases of postoperative cardiac hemolytic anemia, the risks of operation may outweigh the problems associated with a compensated hemolytic anemia.

Microangiopathic Hemolytic Anemia (68)

The term microangiopathic hemolytic anemia was first used as a descriptive title for thrombotic thrombocytopenic purpura. The term was subsequently broadened to describe the association of hemolytic anemia, characterized by red cell fragmentation, with a variety of diseases of the small blood vessels of differing pathogenesis (69). Although the initial hypothesis that small blood vessel disease could bring about red cell damage, resulting in red cell fragmentation and hemolysis, was tentative, subsequent experimental studies and clinical observations have lent support to the concept. It has become apparent that a wide variety of disorders of small blood vessels can give rise to microangiopathic hemolytic anemia; these include hemangioma, vascular tumors, the hemolytic uremic syndrome, and malignant hypertension. The pathogenesis and mechanism of microangiopathic hemolysis will be described and followed by the clinical syndromes with which microangiopathic hemolytic anemia is associated.

Pathogenesis and Mechanism

The original description of microangiopathic hemolytic anemia suggested that red cell damage, with consequent intravascular hemolysis and the formation of distorted red cell fragments, was brought about by red cells passing through partially obstructed blood vessels or infiltrating the abnormal blood vessel wall and escaping into the circulation again (69). The suggestion that an abnormal microvascular environment might cause red cell destruction had been originally suggested in a study of the tissues obtained at necropsy from adult patients dying from thrombotic thrombocytopenic purpura (70).

Studies in experimental animals have confirmed that obstruction of small blood vessels by platelet and fibrin thrombi produced by intravascular coagulation (71), and by alterations in blood vessel wall as a result of malignant hypertension (72), can induce both intravascular hemolysis and red cell fragmentation. The pathophysiology of disseminated intravascular coagulation is discussed in Chapter 19 and will not be further described here. That red cell fragmentation can be produced by passage of red cells through an abnormal microenvironment has been demonstrated in vitro (73). The forceful passage of red cells through fibrin strands results in the adherence of red cells to these strands and in their fragmentation, with the formation of abnormally shaped red cell fragments. The size and shape of the red cell fragments are related to the position in which the red cell becomes arrested, the proportion of the membrane lost, and the amount of hemoglobin retained within the red cell fragments so formed. The formation of red cell fragments has been elegantly illustrated by stereoscan electron microscopy (74). In primary disorders of the blood vessels, such as in malignant hypertension, it seems probable that red cell damage is sustained by partial entrapment of red cells within the disrupted endothelium (72). In these circumstances mechanical damage to the red cells seems the most likely explanation of membrane loss, but the local release of proteolytic enzymes may also contribute to membrane damage.

It seems likely in human disease that more than one of the possible mechanisms may be present, and the techniques used in production of experimental microangiopathic hemolytic anemia may have provided an oversimplification of the pathogenesis and of the therapeutic implications. Nevertheless, however microvascular disease is brought about, once it is of sufficient severity to produce localized intravascular hemolysis, it seems probable that the endothelial damage or the release of ADP and thromboplastin from the red cell is likely to result in further platelet deposition and fibrin formation. Although the hemolytic anemia may be dramatic in onset and result in severe anemia, the organ and tissue dysfunction which accompany the microangiopathy are of greater significance clinically in the treatment and prognosis of the patient. Thus the recognition of microangiopathic hemolytic anemia may provide an invaluable indication of localized or generalized microvascular disease, which, if it does not remit or respond to treatment, can result in permanent organ dysfunction. This situation is, perhaps, most obvious and relevant in the hemolytic uremic syndrome, the commonest cause of microganiopathic hemolytic anemia in children.

The Hemolytic Uremic Syndrome

The term hemolytic uremic syndrome was first used by Gasser and his colleagues (75) to describe the association of acute hemolytic anemia and thrombocytopenia with fatal oliguric or anuric renal failure in infants and young children. The hemolysis was noted to be intravascular and accompanied by striking distortion and contraction of red cells in the peripheral blood. At necropsy the children were found to have a patchy or complete symmetrical renal cortical necrosis and an associated microangiopathy.

This first and very complete account of the syndrome has been followed by many reports in which several aspects of the hemolytic uremic syndrome have been studied. Despite these detailed studies, the etiology remains obscure and the treatment uncertain, and the disease is accompanied by a considerable mortality and morbidity. The hemolytic uremic syndrome has been the subject of extensive reviews (76, 77).

Clinical Features

The disorder characteristically affects healthy, well-nourished infants and children. There is often a history suggestive of a preceding infection, which may be mild or severe, associated with a gastrointestinal disorder, such as vomiting and diarrhea, or resembling an upper respiratory tract infection. This initial episode is followed either immediately or after an interval of a few days by the onset of pallor and oliguria. The latter development usually results in medical attention being sought and the patient admitted to the hospital. At this time the child is clinically anemic and may have a mild hemorrhagic diathesis in the form of purpura or frank or occult hemorrhage; the urine is usually found to contain protein, red cells, and cellular casts. Laboratory investigation reveals a microangiopathic hemolytic anemia, thrombocytopenia, and biochemical evidence of renal disease. Hypertension may be present at the outset or develop during the course of the illness. The renal disease can vary in severity from complete anuria without recovery to a transient proteinuria and oliguria from which recovery takes place, with or without evidence of residual impairment of renal function. The incidence, etiology, pathogenesis, pathology, treatment, and prognosis of the disorder will be discussed in detail.

Incidence and Epidemiology

In temperate climates the disease appears to be sporadic in incidence, although occasionally epidemics in which severe and mild cases have occurred have been described. In warmer climates the disease may be endemic, and large series of cases have been reported from Buenos Aires, Johannesburg, and Los Angeles. The increased incidence of the syndrome in certain centers is currently unexplained.

The disease characteristically affects infants between the ages of 4 to 12 months, is not uncommon in children between 1 and 2 years, is less common in older children, and is rare but well documented in adults (76, 77).

The syndrome has been described in members of one family, both affecting related siblings and unrelated adopted siblings, and occasionally members of one family have developed and died from the disease over an interval of months or years.

The epidemic, endemic, and familial occurrence of the syndrome suggests that an infective agent(s) is responsible; however, detailed bacteriologic and viral studies have failed to reveal a single causative agent, although the relationship of the hemolytic uremic syndrome to certain virus infections appears well established.

Etiology

Attempts to incriminate a specific bacterial infection have proved disappointing, although in particular cases pathogenic bacteria have been isolated from blood, urine, and stools.

The analogy between the hemolytic uremic syndrome and the generalized Shwartzman reaction (vide infra) has suggested that the hemolytic uremic syndrome may be due to sequential bacterial infections or to the entry of bacterial endotoxins into the blood; however, attempts to demonstrate endotoxins in the blood have been unsuccessful (78).

Virologic studies have been more rewarding, as not only have viruses been isolated but also a rise in antiviral antibodies has been demonstrated in affected children, and in some instances neutralizing antibodies have been demonstrated in unaffected members of the family (79). Although viruses appear to be the causal agents in certain cases, a wide variety of viruses appears to be incriminated, including Coxsackie, ECHO, myxovirus, Asian influenza, and, in Buenos Aires, an unspecific arbor virus (76, 77). In the extensively studied Buenos Aires cases, the sera from affected children cross-reacted with the virus of Argentinian hemorrhagic fever (80). Despite these positive viral studies, equally detailed and competent studies in other centers have failed to isolate a virus (81). Thus, at the present time, it seems likely that the primary etiologic agent may be a virus infection, but by the time the child is admitted to the hospital it may not be possible to isolate the virus responsible; in other children, a bacterial infection may be responsible; in yet others, no pathogen has been isolated.

In a number of children the hemolytic uremic syndrome appears to have followed prophylactic inoculations, including triple vaccine (tetanus, diphtheria, and pertussis), measles, polio, and smallpox vaccination.

Such an association may be coincidental, as the maximum incidence of the hemolytic uremic syndrome is at the age at which immunization regimens would normally be carried out. Nevertheless, in a few instances the temporal association is so clear-cut that it has been suggested that there was, indeed, a causal link between the antigenic stimulus and the development of the syndrome.

Although the hemolytic uremic syndrome characteristically affects apparently healthy children, the disorder has been described in children with diseases in which the immunologic response was defective or therapeutically suppressed. Thus the hemolytic uremic syndrome has been described in thymic lymphoplasia (82, 83), in the Wiskott-Aldrich syndrome (84), and in children with impaired immunologic response due to reticuloendotheliosis or to immunosuppressive treatment of the nephrotic syndrome (85, 86). Lowered levels of immunoglobulins have been observed in some series (76), while in others the levels of immunoglobulins have been normal.

Hyperlipemia and hyperlipidemia have been reported in association with the hemolytic uremic syndrome (87). The significance of the alterations in lipid metabolism in relation to either etiology or pathogenesis is obscure.

Pathogenesis

A satisfactory hypothesis for the pathogenesis of the hemolytic uremic syndrome must provide an acceptable explanation for the salient clinical features of this disorder, including the abrupt onset in previously healthy children, the variety of etiologic agents thought to be responsible, the pathologic changes in the kidney, the thrombocytopenia, and the hemolytic anemia. Both the thrombocytopenia and the hemolysis may be related to the production or persistence of a renal microangiopathy. What causes the acute onset of a renal microangiopathy? Why should a variety of etiologic agents produce such a uniform pathologic change in the kidney? Although we do not know the answers to these questions, the uniformity of the response strongly suggests that the disorder is mediated via a common mechanism, local or

generalized coagulation being the most likely. However, as will be discussed, the evidence for this is at best indirect, and even if it were to have taken place, the activation of the coagulation mechanism remains to be explained.

It is generally accepted that the hemolytic anemia is microangiopathic. The evidence for intravascular hemolysis and the failure, with rare exceptions, to demonstrate immunoglobulins or complement on the red cells by the Coombs' test or the presence of antibodies in the serum by the indirect Coombs' test preclude an immunologic mechanism for the hemolysis. Furthermore, abnormal red cell morphology with the presence of many fragmented, misshapen, and distorted red cells in the peripheral blood is consistent with microangiopathic hemolysis. The hemolytic anemia is often abrupt in onset and may be transient, but more often it persists. Red cell survival studies, in addition to documenting markedly shortened red cell survival, have demonstrated sequestration of the red cells in the spleen (88). However, it seems likely that this reflects splenic sequestration of the damaged red cells rather than suggesting primary splenic destruction. The hemolytic anemia may subside in the absence of the return of renal function. In other patients, bilateral nephrectomy has been associated with cessation of hemolysis and a concomitant fall in blood pressure (89); more commonly the hemolytic anemia improves concomitantly with improvement in renal function.

The thrombocytopenia probably reflects intravascular platelet damage, and the survival of autologous platelets may be greatly reduced (88). However, as with the red cell, the labeled platelets are sequestered in the spleen rather than in the kidneys, so although it might be postulated that platelet injury may be sustained within the renal circulation, it has not been possible to demonstrate the sequestration of platelets at this site.

The results of both red cell and platelet survival studies are consistent with the persistence of a microangiopathy, and although platelets cannot be shown to be sequestered at the presumed site of the microangiopathy, renal biopsies taken within ten days of the onset of the hemolytic uremic syndrome have shown the accumulation of platelets within the renal glomeruli (90).

Thus both the hemolysis and the thrombocytopenia appear to be related to the presence of a renal microangiopathy.

The pathogenesis of the microangiopathy is obscure. The distribution of the vascular lesions is characteristically focal, both between organs and within organs, but primarily involves the kidney. The not infrequent association of convulsions suggests that focal vascular changes may be present in the brain, and such lesions have been reported in the brain, pancreas, and other organs. In some instances the vascular lesions are sufficiently widespread to justify the classification of such children as examples of thrombotic thrombocytopenic purpura.

In the kidneys the vascular lesions are focally distributed within and between glomeruli. The extent to which the glomeruli are involved is reflected in the degree of renal failure. When serial biopsies have been carried out in children who have recovered, the initial biopsies may show a spectrum of glomerular involvement, some appearing normal, others showing basement membrane thickening and partial glomerular capillary occlusions, while in other areas the whole of the glomerulus may appear occluded or infarcted. In renal biopsies late in the illness, the glomeruli may be either morphologically normal or completely hyalinized. There is rarely, if ever, evidence of a perivascular inflammatory reaction in kidneys or in other organs, and fibrosis is restricted to the glomeruli. Immunofluorescent studies have failed to demonstrate the presence of complement or immunoglobulins, whereas fibrinogen and fibrin have been shown to be present within the capillaries and in subendothelial spaces (91, 92).

The pathologic changes in the kidney appear to be more consistent with the consequences of generalized intravascular coagulation, or a sequel to local platelet and fibrin deposition. However, measurements of the levels of clotting factors have given varied results. The levels of individual coagulation factors may be depressed or increased, and no consistent pattern has emerged. There has been little evidence to suggest the presence of disseminated intravascular coagulation with consumption of coagulation factors at the time at which these coagulation studies have been carried out (93, 94). Measurements of fibrinogen-fibrin–related (FR) antigen have been found to be elevated (95); however, this test is too sensitive to be taken as an indication of disseminated intravascular coagulation, and FR antigen has been shown to be present in the plasma and urine in children with acute glomerulonephritis in the absence of hemolysis. Fibrinogen survival in two infants (in one of whom the study was incomplete) failed to demonstrate increased catabolism or the accumulation of radioactivity in the kidney (88).

The limitation of many of the coagulation studies is that they have been carried out, inevitably, several days or more after the onset of the illness when renal damage as reflected by impaired renal function is already established. So although attempts to detect continuing intravascular coagulation by the rather insensitive indirect measurement of the levels of coagulation factors are frequently negative, platelet survival studies and the tissue obtained at renal biopsy, or at necropsy, strongly suggest that an episode of localized platelet and fibrin deposition has, indeed, taken place. An alternative hypothesis is that the microangiopathy is secondary to the formation of platelet thrombi resulting from the localization of circulating platelet aggregates, such platelet aggregates being brought about by the interaction of platelets with viruses or bacteria. Although fibrin formation would take place locally in such platelet thrombi, it would be unlikely to influence the levels of coagulation factors and might thus account for the discrepancy between the degree of thrombocytopenia and the minimal evidence for intravascular coagulation.

Many workers have drawn an analogy between the hemolytic uremic syndrome and the generalized Shwartzman reaction in experimental animals. The similarity may relate more to the consequences of intravascular coagulation than to the method in its production. The differing response of different mammalian species to endotoxin injection and the circumstances necessary to produce renal cortical necrosis in experimental animals suggest that host variability is an important factor. The same may be true of children with the hemolytic uremic syndrome. It is, perhaps, an idiosyncratic response of particular children in relation to a variety of etiologic stimuli, which can result in the hemolytic uremic syndrome in one child and a mild and clinically undetected episode in another. What might determine this hypothetical variation in the response of children to a variety of virus or other stimuli is currently unknown.

Diagnosis

The diagnosis should be suspected in an infant or young child in whom an episode of gastroenteritis or upper respiratory tract infection is followed by the abrupt onset of pallor. The diagnosis can be confirmed by the recognition of the characteristic red cell morphology accompanying anemia and thrombocytopenia. In the earliest stages of the disease the reticulocyte count may not be elevated, although it often rises to high levels in the ensuing few days. The bone marrow reveals active erythropoiesis and platelet formation, and the plasma and urine may contain free hemoglobin. The urine often contains red cells and hemosiderin casts, in addition to hemoglobin. The white cell count is usually elevated initially, and may show a shift to the left; very rarely leukopenia may be present for a day or so. The impairment of renal function is reflected in the elevation of the blood urea and creatinine, although marked uremia may not develop until a few days after the onset.

Hypertension may be present when the child is first seen and is a fairly common sequel in children with persistent renal damage.

Treatment

The initial treatment should be directed towards management of the renal failure — the provision of adequate nutrition and the avoidance of overhydration. Facilities should be available to carry out peritoneal dialysis or hemodialysis if indicated. The advances in management of renal failure in infants and young children have resulted in an increasing proportion of children recovering from these measures alone (96).

Unfortunately, however, despite improvement in the management of renal failure, a significant proportion of children who recover have impaired renal function and hypertension, and the prognosis of such children would appear to be grave. A small proportion never recover from the anuric or oliguric episode and require regular dialysis; in this group there have been a few reports of dramatic responses to bilateral nephrectomy and renal transplantation, although the long-term prognosis after these procedures is still uncertain (89). Some children make a complete recovery with treatment of the impaired renal function alone.

Ideally, treatment should be directed towards preventing or reversing the underlying renal microvascular damage. For these reasons heparin or fibrinolytic therapy or both have been advocated. The results of such treatment have been varied, good responses being reported by some (77), disappointing results by others (97). At the present time there is insufficient evidence to enable one to either recommend the use of heparin or refute its potential value; nevertheless, the use of heparin has been associated with a reduction in mortality (77). Many would accept that, in view of the probably short period of time in which a postulated episode of intravascular coagulation might have taken place, the introduction of such treatment late in the disease is unlikely to be of value except to lessen the risk of further fibrin deposition through release of thromboplastin from platelets and red cells. If the hemolytic uremic syndrome is detected, early heparin should in theory prove beneficial and justifiable, although the benefits must be considered in relation to the potential risks of inducing hemorrhage.

If it is decided to use heparin, it should be given as a constant intravenous infusion in as small a volume of fluid as is practicable. The initial dose should be 200 U. per kg. body weight, and the dose should be adjusted to keep the partial thromboplastin time (PTT) approximately double the control time. The amount of heparin may initially be considerably greater than anticipated, but once anticoagulation has been achieved, the dose required to produce an adequate prolongation of the PTT may fall. Particular care has to be exercised in the control of heparin in the hemolytic uremic patient owing to the impairment of renal function and reduction in heparin excretion. Heparin treatment should probably be continued for approximately five days and discontinued once adequate urine output has been achieved or the platelet count has returned to normal values.

Fibrinolytic therapy has been used with apparent success, either by the infusion of streptokinase (98, 99) or by the use of phenformin and ethylestrenol, which indirectly activate the fibrinolytic system (100). If streptokinase or urokinase are employed, the euglobulin lysis time should be shortened to approximately one hour. Fibrinolytic agents may be combined with low-dose heparin therapy when particular care should be exercised in monitoring both the fibrinolytic and anticoagulant effects. Furthermore, in view of the risk of delayed hemorrhage from sites of trauma, special care must be taken with venipunctures, and previous arterial punctures or renal biopsies are a contraindication to fibrinolytic therapy.

There is little evidence that corticosteroids influence the outcome of the hemolytic uremic syndrome, and although they have been given frequently, their use is even more empirical than that of heparin therapy and is probably not warranted.

The use of antiplatelet drugs has not been adequately assessed; their use in conjunction with heparin may be hazardous, and it is too early to determine whether they offer a practical alternative to heparin. However, experience with adult patients with vascular-induced platelet damage would suggest that the combination of relatively large doses of aspirin (15 to 20 mg. per kg.) and dipyridamole (7.5 to 10 mg. per kg.) daily would be the most effective treatment.

In patients with persistent severe renal failure and hypertension, bilateral nephrectomy has resulted in dramatic improvement in the hemolysis and hypertension.

Thrombotic Thrombocytopenic Purpura

In many respects this disorder resembles the hemolytic uremic syndrome except for the wider involvement of organs other than the kidney, particularly the nervous system. In many accounts of the hemolytic uremic syndrome, the pathology has been given a descriptive label which overlaps with that described in more classic thrombotic thrombocytopenic purpura (76). Nevertheless, there have been several striking accounts of a relapsing illness in children, associated with episodes of hemolytic anemia, thrombocytopenia, and renal dysfunction, which more closely resembles the disorder thrombotic thrombocytopenic purpura than the hemolytic uremic syndrome (101–103).

Like the hemolytic uremic syndrome, the etiology is obscure, and the relation of the vascular lesions to localized or disseminated coagulation a matter of dispute, although most authorities now regard thrombotic thrombocytopenic purpura as a primary microvascular disease with secondary platelet or fibrin deposition. However, it is equally possible that the microangiopathy is secondary to disseminated platelet aggregation and thrombosis with local fibrin deposition (103a).

The pathogenesis of the hemolysis is probably, as in the hemolytic uremic syndrome, related to the microangiopathy.

Treatment is essentially empirical, and corticosteroids, heparin, antiplatelet drugs, immunosuppression, and splenectomy have their anecdotal advocates. The results of treatment are correspondingly difficult to assess. Perhaps when the etiology of this disorder is better understood, a rational basis for treatment will become better established. A recent review of experience with splenectomy is somewhat encouraging (114).

Malignant Hypertension

The acute arteriolar necrosis which accompanies malignant hypertension may be accompanied by microangiopathic hemolytic anemia and mild to moderate thrombocytopenia. The hemolysis may be corrected by treatment with hypotensive drugs, although others have advocated anticoagulants and antiplatelet drugs (104). Where all else fails, bilateral nephrectomy has corrected both the hypertension and the hemolysis in adults (105, 106).

Cavernous Hemangioma and Malignant Tumors

Microangiopathic hemolytic anemia in association with thrombocytopenia and evidence of intravascular coagulation may complicate massive cutaneous cavernous hemangiomata (107–109).

Smaller hemangioma may regress with growth of the infant; larger hemangioma may respond to treatment with corticosteroids (110, 111), and, should this fail, consideration may have to be given to local radiotherapy.

HEMOLYSIS TO EXTERNAL PHYSICAL AGENTS OR TRAUMA

March Hemoglobinuria

It is now well established that the occurrence of hemoglobinuria after strenuous physical exertion when running on hard surfaces is brought about by the physical injury sustained by the red cells within the soles of the feet (112). Physical trauma to other regions of the body may also result in transient intravascular hemolysis.

Burns

Finally, extensive body burns may induce spherocytosis and hemolysis complicated by intravascular hemolysis (113).

CONCLUSION

This chapter has endeavored to convey how the red cell life span is influenced by the vascular environment, which it enters on release from the bone marrow and from which it is removed after the end of its normal or shortened life span. The normal red cell is remarkably well adapted to survive in the circulation, whether it be in the sluggish circulation of the spleen or in rapid transit through the heart and blood vessels. Nevertheless, in both situations alterations in the environment can lead to hemolysis. Furthermore, the microcirculation in the spleen is such that it effectively removes both the effete normal red cell and the abnormal red cell found in hemolytic anemia.

References

1. Stuart, A. E.: *The Reticuloendothelial System.* Edinburgh, Livingstone, 1970.
2. Weiss, L.: The role of the spleen in the removal of normally aged red cells. Am. J. Anat. *111*: 175, 1962.
3. Ehrenstein, G. V., and Lockner, D.: Sites of the physiological breakdown of the red blood corpuscles. Nature (Lond.) *181*:911, 1958.
4. Ebaugh, F. G., Jr., Emerson, C. P., et al.: Use of radioactive chromium 51 as an erythrocyte tagging agent for the determination of red cell survival in vivo. J. Clin. Invest. 32:1260, 1953.
5. Kaplan, E., and Hsu, K. S.: Determination of erythrocyte survival in newborn infants by means of ^{51}Cr-labelled erythrocytes. Pediatrics 27:354, 1961.
6. Lewis, S. M., Szur, L., et al.: The pattern of erythrocyte destruction in haemolytic anaemia, as studied with radioactive chromium. Br. J. Haematol. 6:122, 1960.
7. Vest, M. F., and Frieder, H. R.: Erythrocyte survival in newborn infants, as measured by chromium 51 and its relation to postnatal bilirubin level. J. Pediatr. 59:194, 1961.
8. Jandl, J. H., Greenberg, M. S., et al.: Clinical determination of the sites of red cell sequestration in hemolytic anemia. J. Clin. Invest. 35:842, 1956.
9. Szur, L., March, G. W., et al.: Studies of splenic function by means of radioisotope-labelled red cells. Br. J. Haematol. 23 (Suppl.):*183*, 1972.
10. Harris, I. M., McAllister, J. M., et al.: Splenomegaly and the circulating red cell. Br. J. Haematol. 4:970, 1958.
11. Toghill, P. J.: Red cell pooling in enlarged spleens. Br. J. Haematol. *10*:347, 1964.
12. Jandl, J. H., and Aster, R. H.: Increased splenic pooling and the pathogenesis of hypersplenism. Am. J. Med. Sci. 253:383, 1967.
13. Song, S. H., and Groom, A. C.: The distribution of red cells in the spleen. Can. J. Physiol. Pharmacol. 49:734, 1971.
14. Dacie, J. V.: Familial haemolytic anaemia (acholuric jaundice), with particular reference to changes in fragility produced by splenectomy. Quart. J. Med. 36:101, 1943.
15. Young, L. E.: Hereditary spherocytosis. Am. J. Med. *18*:486, 1955.
16. Weisman, R., Ham, T. H., et al.: Studies of the role of the spleen in the destruction of erythrocytes. Trans. Assoc. Am. Physicians 58: 181, 1955.
17. Wennberg, E., and Weiss, L.: The structure of the spleen and hemolysis. Annu. Rev. Med. 20:29, 1969.
18. Burke, J. S., and Simon, G. T.: Electron micros-

copy of the spleen. I. Anatomy and micro-circulation. Am. J. Pathol. 58:127, 1970.

19. Hirasawa, Y., and Tokuhiro, H.: Electron micro-scopic studies on the normal human spleen: especially on the red pulp and the reticulo-endothelial cells. Blood 35:201, 1970.

20. Weiss, L., and Tavassoli, M.: Anatomical hazards to the passage of erythrocytes through the spleen. Semin. Hematol. 7:372, 1970.

21. Chen, L-T., and Weiss, L.: Electron microscopy of the red pulp of the human spleen. Am. J. Anat. 134:425, 1972.

22. Rifkind, R. A.: Destruction of injured red cells in vivo. Am. J. Med. 41:721, 1966.

23. Weed, R. I., and Weiss, L.: The relationship be-tween red cell fragmentation occurring with-in the spleen in cell destruction. Trans. Assoc. Am. Physicians 179:426, 1966.

24. Wennberg, E., and Weiss, L.: Splenic erythro-clasia: An electron microscopic study of hemoglobin H disease. Blood 31:778, 1968.

25. Nathan, D. G., and Gunn, R. B.: Thalassemia: consequences of unbalanced hemoglobin synthesis. Am. J. Med. 41:815, 1966.

26. Jacob, H. S., MacDonald, R. A., et al.: Regula-tion of spleen growth and sequestering func-tion. J. Clin. Invest. 42:1476, 1963.

27. Jandl, J. H., Files, N. M., et al.: Proliferative response of the spleen and liver to he-molysis. J. Exp. Med. 122:299, 1965.

28. Ivemark, B. I.: Implication of agenesis of the spleen on the pathogenesis of cono-truncus anomalies in childhood. Acta Pediatr. 44 (Suppl. 104):1, 1955.

29. Putschar, W. G. J., and Namion, W. C.: Congeni-tal absence of the spleen and associated anomalies. Am. J. Clin. Path., 26:429, 1956.

30. Lyons, W. S., Hanlon, D. G., et al.: Congenital cardiac disease and asplenia; report of seven cases. Mayo Clin. Proc. 32:277, 1957.

31. Ruttenberg, H. D., Nuefeld, H. N., et al.: Syn-drome of congenital cardiac disease with asplenia. Am. J. Cardiol. 13:387, 1964.

32. Padmanabhan, J., Risemberg, H. M., et al.: Howell-Jolly bodies in the peripheral blood of full-term and premature neonates. Johns Hopkins Med. J. 132:146, 1973.

33. Holroyde, C. P., Oski, F. A., et al.: The "pocked" erythrocyte. New. Engl. J. Med. 281:516, 1969.

34. Fraser, I. D., McCarthy, C. F., et al.: Howell-Jolly bodies in idiopathic steatorrhea. J. Clin. Pathol. 19:190, 1966.

35. Marsh, G. W., and Stewart, J. S.: Splenic function in adult coeliac disease. Br. J. Haematol. 19:445, 1970.

36. Pearson, H. A., Spencer, R. P., et al.: Functional asplenia in sickle-cell anemia. New Engl. J. Med. 281:923, 1969.

37. Samuels, I. D., and Stewart, C.: Estimation of splenic size in sickle-cell anemia. J. Nucl. Med. 11:12, 1969.

38. Mollison, P. L., Crome, P., et al.: Rate of removal from the circulation of red cells sensitized with different amounts of antibody. Br. J. Haematol. 11:461, 1969.

39. Archer, G. T.: Phagocytosis by human monocytes of red cells coated with Rh antibodies. Vox Sang. 10:590, 1965.

40. Bessis, M., and Boisfleury, A. D.: Étude des différentes étapes de l'érythro-phagocytose par microcinémato-graphie et microscopie électronique à balayage. Nouv. Rev. Fr. Hematol. 10:223, 1970.

41. Gilcher, R., and Conrad, M.: The relationship of RBC surface charge to RBC deformability. Blood 38:807, 1971.

42. Jandl, J. H., Simmons, R. C., et al.: Red cell filtration and the pathogenesis of certain hemolytic anemias. Blood 18:133, 1961.

43. Teitel, P.: Le test de la filtrabilité érythrocytaire (TFE). Une méthode simple d'étude de certaines propriétés microrhéologiques des globules rouges. Nouv. Rev. Fr. 7:195, 1967.

44. Weed, R. I., Lacelle, P. L., et al.: Metabolic de-pendence of red cell deformability. J. Clin. Invest. 45:1137, 1969.

45. Nathan, D. G., and Shohet, S. B.: Erythrocyte ion transport defects and hemolytic anemia. Semin. Hematol. 7:381, 1970.

46. Ham, T. H., Dunn, R. F., et al.: Physical prop-erties of red cells as related to effects in vivo. I. Increased rigidity of erythrocytes as meas-ured by viscosity of cells altered by chemical fixation, sickling and hypertonicity. Blood 32:847, 1968.

47. Charache, S., Conley, C. L., et al.: Pathogene-sis of hemolytic anemia in homozygous hemoglobin C disease. J. Clin. Invest. 46: 1795, 1967.

48. Murphy, J. R.: The influence of pH and tempera-ture in some physical properties of normal erythrocytes and erythrocytes from patients with hereditary spherocytosis. J. Lab. Clin. Med. 69:756, 1967.

49. Jandl, J. H.: Hereditary spherocytosis, In Heredi-tary Disorders of Erythrocyte Metabolism. Beutler, E. (ed.), New York, Grune & Strat-ton, 1968, p 203.

50. Smith, C. H., Erlandson, M. E., et al.: The role of splenectomy in the management of thalas-semia. Blood 15:197, 1960.

51. Weatherall, D. J., and Clegg, J. B.: The Thalas-semia Syndromes. Oxford, Blackwell, 1972, p. 278.

52. Smith, C. H., Erlandson, M. E., et al.: Post-splenectomy infection in Cooley's anemia. An appraisal of the problem in this and other blood disorders. New Engl. J. Med. 266:737, 1962.

53. Eraklis, A. J., Kevy, S. V., et al.: Hazard of over-whelming infection after splenectomy in childhood. New Engl. J. Med. 276:1225, 1967.

54. Eraklis, A. J., and Filler, R. M.: Splenectomy in childhood. A review of 1413 cases. J. Pediatr. Surg. 7:382, 1972.

55. Schumacher, M. J.: Serum immunoglobulin and transferrin levels after childhood splenec-tomy. Arch. Dis. Child. 45:114, 1970.

56. Weiss, L.: Transmural cellular passage in vascu-lar sinuses of rat bone marrow. Blood 36: 189, 1970.

57. Brodeur, M. T. H., Sutherland, D. W., et al.: Red cell survival in patients with aortic valvular disease and ball valve prosthesis. Circulation 32:570, 1965.

58. Westring, D. W.: Aortic valve disease and he-

molytic anemia. Ann. Intern. Med. 65:203, 1966.

59. Ravenel, S. D., Johnson, J. D., et al.: Intravascular hemolysis associated with coarctation of the aorta. J. Pediatr. 75:67, 1969.

60. Westphal, R. G., and Azem, E. A.: Macroangiopathic hemolytic anemia due to congenital cardiac anomalies. J.A.M.A. 216:1477, 1971.

61. Moisey, C. U., Manohitharajah, S. M., et al.: Hemolytic anemia in a child in association with congenital mitral valve disease. J. Thorac. Cardiovasc. Surg. 63:765, 1972.

62. Marsh, G. W., and Lewis, S. M.: Cardiac haemolytic anaemia. Semin. Hematol. 6:133, 1969.

63. Nevaril, C. G., Lynch, E. C., et al.: Erythrocyte destruction and damage induced by shearing stress. J. Lab. Clin. Med. 71:784, 1968.

64. Blackshear, P. L., Jr., Dorman, F. D., et al.: Shear, wall interaction and hemolysis. Trans. Am. Soc. Artif. Intern. Organs 12:113, 1966.

65. Sears, D. A., and Crosby, W. H.: Intravascular hemolysis due to intracardiac prosthetic devices. Diurnal variations related to activity. Am. J. Med. 39:341, 1965.

66. Myhre, E., Rasmussen, K., et al.: Serum lactic dehydrogenase activity in patients with prosthetic heart valves: A parameter of intravascular hemolysis. Am. Heart J. 80:463, 1970.

67. Eysters, E., Mayer, K., et al.: Traumatic hemolysis with iron deficiency anemia in patients with aortic valve lesions. Ann. Intern. Med. 68:995, 1968.

68. Brain, M. C.: Microangiopathic hemolytic anemia. Br. J. Haematol. 23(Suppl.):45, 1972.

69. Brain, M. C., Dacie, J. V., et al.: Microangiopathic haemolytic anaemia: The possible role of vascular lesions in pathogenesis. Br. J. Haematol. 8:358, 1962.

70. Monroe, W. M., and Strauss, A. F.: Intravascular hemolysis: A morphologic study of schizocytes in thrombotic purpura and other diseases. South. Med. J. 46:837, 1953.

71. Rubenberg, M. L., Regoeczi, E., et al.: Microangiopathic haemolytic anaemia: The experimental production of haemolysis and red-cell fragmentation by defibrination in vivo. Br. J. Haematol. 14:627, 1967.

72. Venkatachalam, M. A., Jones, D. B., et al.: Microangiopathic hemolytic anemia in rats with malignant hypertension. Blood 328:276, 1968.

73. Bull, B. S., Rubenberg, M. L., et al.: Microangiopathic haemolytic anaemia: Mechanisms of red-cell fragmentation: in vitro studies. Br. J. Haematol. 14:643, 1968.

74. Bull, B. S., and Kuhn, I. N.: The production of schistocytes by fibrin strands (a scanning electron microscope study). Blood 35:104, 1970.

75. Gasser, C., Gautier, E., et al.: Hämolytisch-urämische syndrome: bilaterale Nierenrindennekrosen bei akuten erworbenen hämolytischen Anämien. Schweiz. Med. Wochenschr. 85:905, 1955.

76. Brain, M. C.: The haemolytic uraemic syndrome. Semin. Hematol. 6:162, 1969.

77. Lieberman, E.: Hemolytic-uremic syndrome. J. Pediatr. 80:1, 1972.

78. Kaplan, B. S., and Koornhof, H. J.: Haemolytic-uraemic syndrome: Failure to demonstrate circulating endotoxin. Lancet 2:1424, 1969.

79. Ray, C. G., Tucker, V. L., et al.: Enteroviruses associated with the hemolytic-uremic syndrome. Pediatrics 46:378, 1970.

80. Gianatonio, C., Vitaccio, M., et al.: The hemolytic-uremic syndrome. J. Pediatr. 64:478, 1964.

81. Kibel, M. A., and Barnard, P. J.: The haemolytic-uraemic syndrome: A survey in South Africa. S. Afr. Med. J. 42:692, 1968.

82. Frick, P. G., and Hitzig, W. H.: Zur klinik und Pathogenese der Thrombotischen Mikroangiopathie. Vorkommen bei Antiköpermangel. Schweiz. Med. Wochenschr. 89:58, 1959.

83. Dubilier, L. D., Chadwick, J. A., et al.: Thymic lymphoplasia associated with the hemolytic-syndrome. J. Pediatr. 73:714, 1968.

84. Krivit, W., and Good, R. A.: Aldrich's syndrome (thrombocytopenia, eczema and infection in infants). Studies of the defense mechanisms. Am. J. Dis. Child. 97:137, 1959.

85. Fluge, G., and Moe, P. J.: Hemolytic uremic (nephropathic syndrome). Acta Pediatr. Scand. 56:665, 1967.

86. Mathieu, H., Lederc, F., et al.: Etude clinique et biologique de 38 observations de syndrome hémolytique et urémique. Arch. Fr. Pediatr. 26:369, 1969.

87. Kaplan, B. S., Gale, D., et al.: Hyperlipidemia in the hemolytic-uremic syndrome. Pediatrics 47:776, 1971.

88. Metz, J.: Observations on the mechanism of the hematological changes in the haemolytic uraemic syndrome of infancy. Br. J. Haematol. 23(Suppl.):53, 1972.

89. Cerilli, G. J., Nelsen, C., et al.: Renal homotransplantation in infants and children with the hemolytic uremic syndrome. Surgery 71:66, 1972.

90. Bartmann, J., Jacques, M., et al.: Anémie hémolytique purpura thrombopénique et néphropathie aiguë chez un nourisson. Etude au microscope électronique des lésions rénales. Rev. Belge Pathol. 30:5, 1964.

91. Habbib, R., Courtecuisse, V., et al.: Etude anatomo-pathologique entre les formes mortelles et curables du syndrome hémolytique et urémique. Arch. Fr. Pediatr. 26:417, 1969.

92. Gervais, M., Richardson, J. B., et al.: Pathology of the hemolytic-uremic syndrome. Pediatrics 47:352, 1971.

93. Gilchrist, G. S., Lieberman, E., et al.: Heparin therapy in the haemolytic-uraemic syndrome. Lancet 1:1123, 1969.

94. Avalos, J. S., Vitacco, M., et al.: Coagulation studies in the hemolytic-uremic syndrome. J. Pediatr. 76:538, 1970.

95. Katz, J., Lurie, A., et al.: Coagulation findings in the hemolytic-uremic syndrome of infancy: Similarities of hyperactive renal transplant rejection. J. Pediatr. 78:426, 1971.

96. Tune, B. M., Leavitt, T. J., et al.: The hemolytic uremic syndrome in California: A review of 28 non-heparinized cases with long-term follow up. J. Pediatr. 82:304, 1973.

97. Kaplan, B. S., Katz, J., et al.: An analysis of the

results of therapy in 67 cases of the hemolytic-uremic syndrome. J. Pediatr. 78:420, 1971.

98. Monnens, L., and Schretlen, E.: Haemolytic-uraemic syndrome. Lancet 2:735, 1968.

99. Bergstein, J. M., Edson, J. R., et al.: Fibrinolytic treatment of the hemolytic uremic syndrome. Lancet 1:448, 1972.

100. Mandal, B. K., and McNulty, M.: Treatment of the haemolytic-uraemic syndrome with phenformin and ethyloestrenol. Lancet 2:1036, 1971.

101. Shumway, C. N., Jr., and Miller, G.: An unusual syndrome of hemolytic anemia, thrombocytopenic purpura, and renal disease. Blood 12:1045, 1957.

102. MacWhinney, J. B., Jr., Packer, J. T., et al.: Thrombotic thrombocytopenic purpura in childhood. Blood 19:181, 1962.

103. Dacie, J. V.: *The Haemolytic Anaemias.* 2nd ed. Part III. *Secondary or Symptomatic Haemolytic Anaemias.* London, Churchill, 1967, p. 863.

103a. Neame, P. B., Lechago, J., et al.: Thrombotic thrombocytopenic purpura: Report of a case with disseminated intravascular platelet aggregation. Blood 42:805, 1973.

104. Kincaid-Smith, P., Laver, M. C., et al.: Dipyridamole and anticoagulants in renal disease due to glomerular and vascular lesions. A new approach to therapy. Med. J. Aust. 1:145, 1970.

105. Giromini, M., and Laperbonza, C.: Prolonged survival after bilateral nephrectomy in an adult with haemolytic uraemic syndrome. Lancet 2:169, 1969.

106. Gavras, H., Brown, W. C. B., et al.: Microangiopathic hemolytic anemia and the development of malignant phase of hypertension. Circ. Res. 28(Suppl. 2):127, 1971.

107. Propp, R. P., and Scharfman, W. B.: Hemangioma-thrombocytopenia syndrome associated with microangiopathic hemolytic anemia. Blood 28:623, 1966.

108. Inceman, S., and Tanguin, Y.: Chronic defibrination syndrome due to giant hemangioma associated with microangiopathic hemolytic anemia. Am. J. Med. 46:997, 1969.

109. Hendricksson, P., Nilsson, I. M., et al.: Giant hemangioma with a disorder of coagulation. Acta Pediatr. Scand. 60:227, 1971.

110. Fost, N. C., and Esterly, N. B.: Successful treatment of juvenile hemangiomas with prednisone. J. Pediatr. 72:351, 1968.

111. Goldberg, S. J., and Fonkalsrod, E.: Successful treatment of hepatic hemangioma with corticosteroids. J.A.M.A. 208:2473, 1969.

112. Davidson, R. J. L.: March or exertional haemoglobinuria. Semin. Hematol. 6:150, 1969.

113. Dacie, J. V.: *The Haemolytic Anaemias.* 2nd ed. Part III. *Secondary or Symptomatic Haemolytic Anaemias.* London, Churchill, 1967, p. 950.

114. Cuttner, J.: Splenectomy, steroids, and dextran 70 in thrombotic thrombocytopenic purpura. J.A.M.A. 227:397, 1974.

Chapter 8

Immunohemolytic Anemia

by Neil Abramson

INTRODUCTION

Jaundice resulting from hemolytic anemia was first described in 1871 when Vanlair and Masius (1) differentiated from liver disease a form of jaundice related to release of "blood cell coloring material" into plasma. In 1904 Donath and Landsteiner (2) described in a patient with syphilis a cold active serum factor, later recognized as an immunoglobulin, which was responsible for destruction of red cells. This constituted the first clinical presentation of what is now termed "paroxysmal cold hemoglobinuria." Several years later other factors were reported which caused agglutination rather than lysis (3, 4). From 1910 to 1913 studies involving heterologous antibody against red cells (5–7) significantly contributed to the understanding of immunohemolytic anemia. Banti's experiments were clear and reproducible, but their interpretation remained uncertain for the next half century. He showed that an antibody produced in a rabbit against dog red cells caused hemolytic anemia, splenomegaly, and spherocytosis in the dog when it was injected. However, when the dog red cells were added to the same antibody in vitro, neither hemolysis nor spherocytosis occurred. This "incomplete" antibody eluded further understanding until Coombs reported the antiglobulin test (Coombs' test) (8). This relatively simple technique allowed the immunologist and hematologist to characterize red cell antibodies and components of serum complement when attached to red cells, to identify red cell antibodies present in the serum, and to delineate some of the red cell antigens. The method further showed the "incomplete" antibody to be an IgG globulin.

Modern understanding of immunohemolytic anemia has required a union of immunology and hematology. As a result pathophysiologic mechanisms have been studied in much more precise terms. Serum factors of past decades referred to descriptively as warm and cold agglutinins, warm and cold hemolysins, and incomplete and complete antibodies have been replaced by immunochemical terminology, such as IgG and IgM antibodies and complement (Table 8–1). Though the precise interrelationships of these proteins with the red cell and the reticuloendothelial system are not fully understood, major advances have been made. The purpose of this chapter is to describe these advances.

TABLE 8–1*

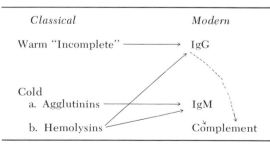

Classical	Modern
Warm "Incomplete"	IgG
Cold	
a. Agglutinins	IgM
b. Hemolysins	Complement

*Equivalent terms are represented. All of the warm antibodies are IgG. With few exceptions, most of the agglutinins are IgM. Hemolysins involve complement and may be either IgG or IgM.

PATHOPHYSIOLOGIC MECHANISMS OF IMMUNE DESTRUCTION

IgG Antibodies

IgG globulins are the most prevalent red cell antibodies clinically and are commonly found in hemolytic anemia associated with lymphoproliferative diseases, connective tissue disorders, infections, malignancies, idiopathic acquired ("autoimmune") hemolytic anemia, drug-induced immunohemolytic anemia, hemolytic disease of the newborn, and transfusion reactions. These antibodies are identical to serum IgG globulins (7S, 160,000 M.W., heat-stable at 56°C, and resistant to 2-mercaptoethanol) (Table 8–2). Since their maximum interaction with red cells is at 37°C, they have been referred to in the past as "warm" antibodies. Many are directed against the Rh antigen. They cause much less fixation of complement than IgM antibodies (8a) and do not cause agglutination, changes in cell metabolism, or morphologic abnormalities in vitro. Their presence on red cells may go unnoticed until the result of the Coombs' test is positive using monospecific antibody against IgG. Although IgG antibodies lack any activity against red cells in vitro, they are usually associated with hemolytic anemia, spherocytosis, and splenomegaly in vivo.

An IgG red cell antibody maximally active at cold temperatures is rarely found. In contrast to the warm IgG antibody, this so-called "cold hemolysin" or Donath-Landsteiner antibody is commonly directed against a particular red cell antigen (P antigen). It is active in the process of complement fixation and complement-mediated lysis. Like the warm IgG antibody, it may also cause spherocytosis.

Much of the information concerning the mechanism of red cell destruction induced by IgG antibodies has come from studies using the anti-Rh (anti-D) antibody (9–11). When infused in vivo, red cells coated with IgG are selectively sequestered by the spleen, undergo spherocytosis, and are destroyed. This occurs in several experimental procedures: (1) when cells are coated with anti-Rh in vitro and are injected in vivo, (2) when cells are coated with anti-Rh in vivo, and (3) when IgG is

nonspecifically and nonimmunologically coupled to red cells and injected in vivo. The final common pathway for the induction of spherocytosis appears to depend on an in vivo environment, usually the spleen.

The first clear demonstration of red cell morphologic abnormalities in vitro associated with attachment of IgG occurred in 1958 (9). Red cells coated with anti-D were observed bound circumferentially about a central white cell into a "rosette." The attached cells appeared spherocytic, whereas those unattached had a normal surface to volume ratio. The white cell was a typical blood monocyte (Fig. 8–1); also some rosette-forming cells appeared as activated monocytes or macrophages, and a few had lymphocytic properties. Polymorphonuclear leukocytes rarely formed rosettes (12, 13). The successor cells of monocytes, the tissue macrophages, isolated from the Rebuck-type skin window or those harvested from spleens at splenectomy formed typical rosettes when tested with IgG-coated red cells (12).

Red cell morphologic abnormalities resulting from rosette formations varied. Osmotic fragility increased, suggesting loss of surface membrane (12). The area of attachment between red cells and mononuclear cells viewed by the electron microscope suggested that hemoglobin-filled deposits or "fragments" were appearing in the intercellular space (13).

Figure 8–2 illustrates the attachment of a red cell to a mononuclear cell. The electron-dense marker on the outer surface

TABLE 8–2.   FEATURES OF CLASSICAL ANTIBODIES

Warm	Cold (EXCEPT FOR COLD HEMOLYSIN)
IgG	IgM
7S	19S
Frequent Rh specificity	Often I specificity clinically or
	A or B specificity naturally
"Incomplete" in vitro	"Complete" in vitro and in vivo
a. No agglutination	a. Agglutination
b. Little or no complement fixation	b. Complement fixation
c. No complement lysis	c. May cause complement lysis
Spherocytic hemolytic anemia in vivo	

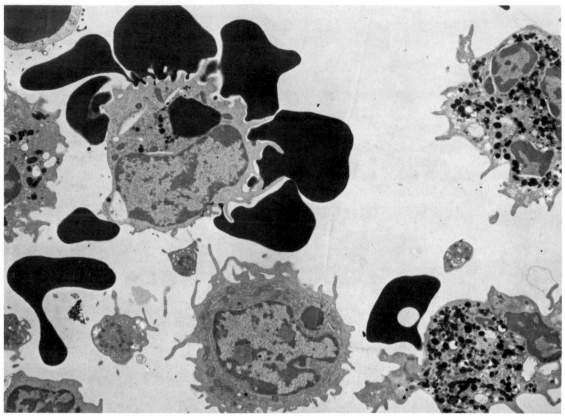

Figure 8–1. Photoelectromicrograph surveying a rosette from a preparation stained for peroxidase. This rosette-forming cell is a monocyte. Note the extreme distortion of the attached red cells and the biconcave shape of the unattached red cell above. The polymorphonuclear leukocytes have no attached red cells (approximately × 3500). (Kindly provided by Dr. R. S. Cotran.)

of the red cell membrane is chromic chloride, a multivalent cation used to couple IgG to the membrane. These markers rim hemoglobin-filled deposits, which appear to be within the cytoplasm of the monocyte. Red cells released from the monocyte frequently remain deformed (Fig. 8–3), and the increased osmotic fragility persists. An actual loss of membrane lipid of attached cells has not been demonstrated; however, studies in man and in rats have shown antibody-related lipid loss (14–15).

Monocytes selectively bind red cells coated with IgG globulins. Other proteins, such as IgM, IgA, transferrin, and albumin, present on red cells in some clinical situations do not produce rosettes (16). A variety of red cell antibodies mediate rosette forma-

TABLE 8–3.   TYPES OF IgG THAT BIND TO MONOCYTES*

1. Drug-induced
   a. α-Methyldopa
   b. L-dopa
   c. Penicillin

2. Blood group antibodies
   a. Anti-D
   b. Anti-A (IgG)
   c. Anti-B (IgG)
   d. Anti-P (Donath-Landsteiner)

3. Idiopathic acquired ("autoimmune") antibodies

4. Nonimmune IgG

*These types of IgG will mediate rosette formation with human mononuclear cells. The antipenicillin antibody was placed on red cells coated with penicillin. The nonimmune IgG was complexed to cells with a coupling agent (chromic chloride).

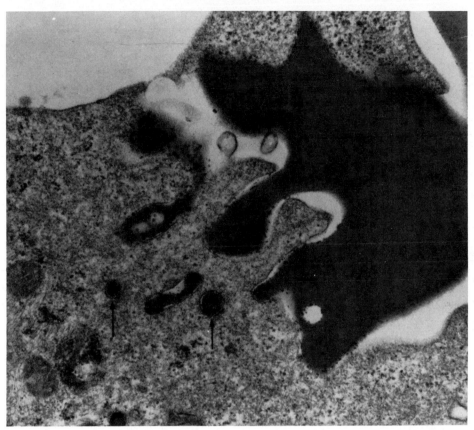

Figure 8–2. A small area of a rosette involving red cells coated with IgG by means of chromic chloride. The chromic chloride–IgG appears as electron-opaque deposits on the surface of the red cell and around the hemoglobin-filled fragments within the cytoplasm of the white cell (arrows) (approximately × 30,000). (From Abramson N., et al.: J. Exp. Med. *132*:1191, 1971.)

tion, and without exception these are IgG globulins (Table 8–3).

The activity of IgG globulins, such as the induction of complement fixation, placental transfer, and immune adherence, resides in certain of the four IgG subclasses. Monocyte binding or rosette formation resides in only two, IgG_1 and IgG_3 (Fig. 8–4). Many isoantibodies (Table 8–4) and red cell antibodies from patients with various diseases may be composed of restricted IgG subclasses (17–19). The quantity (35) and subclass specificity of bound antibody therefore provide some understanding of why certain patients' Coombs'-positive red cells hemolyze and others do not. In addition, the antigen site density on the surface of the erythrocyte influences the binding of antibody (19a, 19b) and hence the severity of hemolysis.

In summary, the "incomplete" IgG red cell antibody is only incompete in vitro.

Presumably red cells coated with this type of antibody circulating in vivo arc detained in tissues such as the spleen by splenic macrophages. Deformity occurs because of loss of membrane, perhaps by the fragmentation mechanism observed in experimental rosettes. Either the more fragile spherocyte is allowed back into the circulation and perhaps destroyed at the next

TABLE 8–4. IgG SUBCLASS SPECIFICITY OF ISOANTIBODIES

	IgG_1	IgG_2	IgG_3	IgG_4
Anti-D	+	0	+	0
Anti-CD	+	±	+	0
Anti-c	+	0	+	0
Anti-s	0	0	+	0
Anti-K	+	0	0	0
Anti-Kp[b]	+	0	+	0
Anti-Jk[a]	0	+	0	0

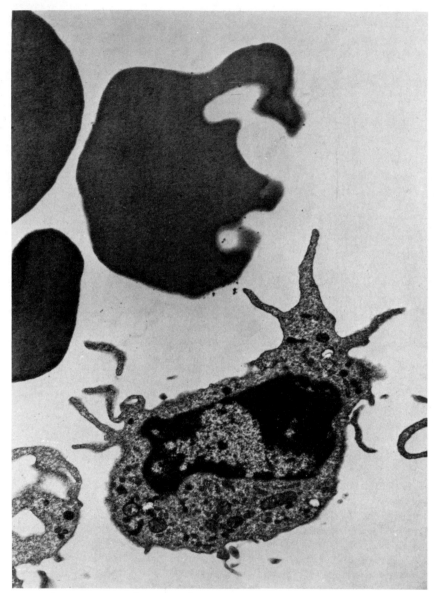

Figure 8–3. View of a preparation of rosettes after incubation with papain. Note the deformed red cell and the monocyte with exposed pseudopodia (approximately × 9000). [From Cotran, R. S.: Immunohemolytic anemias. Advances Immunol. (in press).]

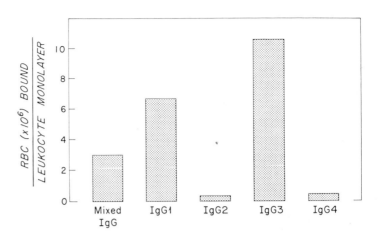

Figure 8–4. Binding of red cells coated with IgG subclasses to white cell monolayers. IgG subclasses were purified from myeloma serum and were coupled to red cells with chromic chloride. Red cells were radiolabeled with $Na_2^{51}CrO_4$. (From Abramson, N., et al.: J. Exp. Med. *132*:1207, 1971.

capillary bed or on its return to the spleen, or the cell may remain in the spleen, where at the low glucose and low pH environment it is highly susceptible to local destruction.

IgM Antibodies

With few exceptions, serum factors referred to as agglutinins are macromolecular substances, 19S, 1,000,000 M.W., IgM globulins (Table 8–2). Frequently the antibody is more active at temperatures less than 37° C. It is referred to as "complete" antibody because it causes macroscopic or microscopic red cell agglutination or both, activates the complement system, and at times causes complement-mediated lysis. The antibody is heat-labile at 56°C for 30 minutes, is destroyed by 2-mercaptoethanol, and possesses multiple antigenic combining sites.

Red cells ordinarily exist as negatively charged units. Hence they repel one another and resist agglutination. Agglutination may occur when the charge is altered, when the suspension medium is altered, or when cell surface properties are modified. Rabbit red cells differ in intracellular charge and are easily agglutinated, whereas the reverse is true of rat red cells. The attachment of proteins such as antibody to the cell surface or alteration of the membrane with proteolytic agents (ficin, trypsin, and papain) alters the surface charge and affects agglutinability. Suspension of cells in solutions containing large anisometric molecules, such as albumin, fibrinogen,

and polyvinylpyrrolidone, also increases potential agglutination. In man the IgM molecule, unlike IgG, is large enough to span the distance between red cells and form the necessary lattice for agglutination.

The mechanism of red cell destruction by IgM antibodies is best studied with anti-A agglutinins as a model (9, 20). Small quantities of radiolabeled ABO incompatible cells infused in man are precipitously removed from the circulation in contrast to the slower removal of anti-D coated cells. The radioactivity appears in the liver rather than in the spleen. The small amount of hemoglobin in plasma indicates overt hemolysis, presumably by complement-mediated lysis. Other IgM antibodies, such as the anti-I agglutinins, destroy human red cells in a similar manner (21).

IgM antibodies fix complement; however, they result in little complement-induced lysis in vitro and in vivo. Most of the C3 fixed to the IgM-coated red cells is in the inactive form (21a). A monocyte-macrophage receptor for IgM has not been described (12, 13, 16, 22), but one for C3 has been noted (26–28). Thus the destruction of red cells by IgM antibodies appears to be primarily the result of agglutination and subsequent sequestration of red cell products in the reticuloendothelial organ of greatest flow, such as the liver. However, rapid fixation of C3 to the red cells by an IgM cold agglutinin during exposure to cold may induce hemolysis (21a).

Recent studies of IgG and IgM antibodies raised against guinea pig erythrocytes have revealed additional information concerning the interaction of these antibodies with mammalian red cells and the reticuloendo-thelial system (8a). At least 60 complement-fixing sites per cell were required for rapid clearance of IgM-coated red cells. The liver initially cleared most of these cells, but the clearance was not irreversible. Many returned to the circulation and survived favorably. However, as few as 1.4 IgG complement-fixing sites per cell caused decreased survival of erythrocytes. The trapping and destruction of IgG-sensitized cells was progressive. Few if any of the cells returned to the circulation. These results may not necessarily reflect the behavior of human red cells and human antibodies, but they do indicate that IgG antibodies are apt to be more deleterious than IgM antibodies.

Complement System

In 1900 a heat-labile serum factor capable of lysis of red cells was described (23). Since that time the factor referred to as complement has been found to be an arcane mixture of proteins characterized by at least 11 different components and many interacting inhibitors, activators, and stabilizers. For a complete discussion, see Chapter 18.

The complement system may be activated by several agents, including antigen-antibody complexes. More commonly the "classical" pathway is triggered through C1, C4, C2, and, less commonly, the "alternate" pathway is activated starting at C3. The system is proteolytic in both pathways; an enzyme cleaves a polypeptide from substrates, thereby activating another enzyme, which in turn acts upon natural substrates in repetitive fashion. When the complement system is activated on the surface of red cells through the ninth component (C9), lysis occurs. At this juncture defects in the membrane, which by osmotic measurements appear to be large enough to permit extravasation of hemoglobin (24), can be observed by electron microscopy. Electron microscopic studies of red cells affected by proteins up to and including C5, without participation of the subsequent components, also show apparent lesions which resemble those induced by C9; however, lysis does not occur (25). When

the third component is attached to red cells, which occurs commonly in vivo, little or no evidence of a decreased life span is observed. However, C3-coated cells may adhere to platelets and phagocytes, predominantly polymorphonuclear leukocytes in vitro (immune adherence), or they may trigger the production of an antibody (immunoconglutinin) against the cell-bound C3. A specific receptor on monocytes for C3 has been reported (26–28), and recent evidence has been presented which suggests that the process of fragmentation induced by macrophage interaction with IgG-coated red cells also occurs when red cells coated with complement interact with macrophages in the spleen (28a). In spite of the potency of the complement system, complement-induced lysis in man in vivo is uncommon; more commonly C3-coated cells are found. Red cell destruction associated with complement activation may also be secondary to coincidental coating with IgG or IgM antibodies. The inability of the complement system to continue through C9 in vivo and cause lysis whenever activation occurs has not been adequately explained. The inactivators, inhibitors, and stabilizers of complement system components may be important in this regard. The C3 inactivator studied in vitro and in vivo (29–33) illustrates some of the pathophysiologic consequences when this potentially lytic system is altered by an interacting protein.

The fixation of complement onto red cells is a function of both antibody class and the antigenic structure on the cell surface. IgM easily fixes complement, and IgG functions poorly. Some IgG antibodies, such as anti-Rh, do not fix complement, but others (anti-P, IgG fraction of anti-A, and anti-B) are active at complement fixation. Serum IgG_1 and IgG_3 are also considered to be active at complement fixation; however, differences among the IgG red cell antibodies are not related to the subclasses solely, since IgG_3 occurs in anti-Rh and anti-P antibodies. Thus the inability of anti-Rh to fix complement suggests that the antigen itself is important in this regard. Ordinarily the activation of complement requires "doublets" of IgG. Rh antigens are infrequent and may be too widely separated to serve as a receptor for IgG "doublets."

On the other hand, A antigens are numerous and perhaps close enough to facilitate formation of IgG doublets.

LABORATORY TESTS FOR DEMONSTRATION OF IMMUNE FACTORS

The hallmark of an immunohemolytic anemia is the demonstration of antibody or complement deposited on red cells or antibody present in the serum which can react with the cell membrane. The antiglobulin test (Coombs' test) identifies these abnormalities. Coombs produced an antibody in rabbits against normal serum proteins which, after absorption with normal red cells, was highly specific in identifying a protein or proteins attached to the red cell membrane. In the "direct" Coombs' test, the patient's red cells are washed free of serum proteins before the antiserum (Coombs' serum) is added. If proteins are attached to the cells, then the antiserum binds to them and agglutinates the cells. Agglutinates are viewed and graded either macroscopically or microscopically. In the "indirect" Coombs' test, normal red cells are added to the serum which is being tested for anti-red cell activity. After incubation the test serum is removed by washing, and the cells are tested with antiserum (Coombs' serum). If proteins are deposited onto cells, the antiserum causes agglutination.

The terms "gamma" and "nongamma" Coombs' test have led to much confusion. For practical purposes the positive gamma test indicates the presence of IgG red cell antibodies, and the positive nongamma test the third component of complement (C3). However, any serum protein attached to red cells other than IgG may also be identified by the nongamma Coombs' reagent. For example, transferrin, which is present naturally on reticulocytes, may be detected by Coombs' serum. In addition, cell-bound albumin or the fourth component of complement (C4) may react with the nongamma Coombs' reagent. To obviate these problems monospecific antisera are available which may permit accurate identification and the replacement of the terms gamma and nongamma Coombs' test by IgG Coombs' test, C3 Coombs' test, and so forth.

Other tests have been used to identify serum factors, but few are clinically useful. Agglutination of red cells with fibrinogen, polyvinylpyrrolidone, albumin, and dextran demonstrates the presence of "incomplete" antibodies by alterations in the electrical charge between cells (zeta potential). Certain proteolytic enzymes alter the surface of red cells and render them hypersusceptible to agglutination by otherwise "incomplete" antibodies. The Coombs' test has replaced these procedures for routine purposes. Immunohemolytic anemia rarely occurs when the Coombs' reaction is negative or very weakly positive. In these rare instances, immune factors can sometimes be demonstrated, utilizing a modified radioactive Coombs' consumption test (34), the Cla transfer test (35), cold Coombs' test (36), or rosette formation (17).

It should be emphasized that the red cell life span is not always diminished when IgG antibodies are adherent to the cells. In fact, treatment of immune hemolytic anemia with steroids may produce a complete remission of hemolysis without marked reduction of the intensity of the direct Coombs' test reaction. Thus the avidity of the reticuloendothelial system for the antibody coated cells may influence clinical severity.

IgM antibodies may be identified by agglutination and complement fixation. Normal red cells incubated in test serum are observed for agglutination (macroscopically and microscopically) or for complement-mediated lysis. Complement coating by IgG or IgM without lysis is tested by a Coombs' test using monospecific antisera against C3. When agglutination occurs with maximum activity at temperatures less than 37°C, a "cold agglutinin" is present. The use of cells with known antigens allows for the identification of anti-I, anti-i, anti-A, and so forth. A rapid screening test has been described which may be used at the bedside (37). An unusual cold active complement-fixing antibody, the Donath-Landsteiner antibody of paroxysmal cold hemoglobinuria, is an IgG antibody directed against the P antigen. Red cells are incubated in test serum in the cold to allow the attachment of the cold antibody. The temperature of the mixture then is brought to 37°C to permit complement activation. Lysis indicates the cold hemolysin. Some cells are not hemolyzed but coated with C3 with or without immunoglobulin and may be Coombs-positive when monospecific antisera are used.

The acid serum lysis test (Ham test) or sucrose lysis test (sugar water test) identifies red cell membrane abnormalities in a rare hemolytic anemia associated with hypersusceptibility to complement, paroxysmal nocturnal hemoglobinuria. Both tests take advantage of complement activation and the lysis of sensitive cells when complement is attached to the membrane. Other cells of bone marrow origin, platelets and white cells, are similarly hypersusceptible in this unusual disease. Tests to demonstrate white cell and platelet abnormalities are not available for routine use. The sucrose lysis or sugar water test is the simplest and most commonly used. In this test the cells are suspended in a sugar solution that is isosmotic but low in ionic concentration. At low ionic strength, serum proteins including complement components aggregate on particulate surfaces (cell membranes) and lysis follows. This test can be performed at the bedside (38). False-negative results may occur because of incorrect anticoagulant (EDTA) (39) or iron deficiency (40). False-positive results which occur infrequently are usually associated with red cell damage due to mishandling in vitro (vigorous defibrination) (39). In hereditary erythrocytic multinuclearity with a positive acidified serum (HEMPAS), the acid serum lysis test is positive, and the sucrose lysis is negative (*vide infra*).

CLINICAL DISORDERS

The immunohemolytic anemias may be classified in two major categories. Cases which occur in the absence of an underlying or associated illness or in the absence of drug ingestion are referred to as idiopathic acquired immunohemolytic anemias. Those associated with drugs, infections, neoplastic diseases, and connective tissue disorders are secondary immunohemolytic anemias. Paroxysmal nocturnal hemoglobinuria must be considered separately,

since this disease represents an abnormality of the cell membrane rather than of the immune system (see also Chapter 6).

Immunohemolytic anemia is an acquired rather than a congenital disease, with the notable exception of hemolytic disease of the newborn period, during which maternal red cell antibodies traverse the placenta (see Chapter 9). In most patients weakness and pallor due to anemia develop, and a variable amount of jaundice without bilirubinuria occurs. History of drug ingestion or infection or physical examination may reveal the etiology of a secondary immunohemolytic anemia. In most immunohemolytic anemias, splenomegaly and mild liver enlargement are common. Laboratory findings include anemia, reticulocytosis, increased indirect bilirubin and serum LDH, a decreased serum haptoglobin, and increased urine urobilinogen and stercobilinogen. These are common in all hemolytic anemias, but, in addition, the demonstration of immune factors in the serum or on the cells indicates that the anemia is immunohemolytic.

Immunohemolytic anemia is most commonly associated with IgG ("incomplete") antibodies; therefore, a positive Coombs' test is of paramount importance in the diagnosis. The frequency of positive tests depends upon the type of patient population, the sensitivity of the test, and the precision of patient evaluation. The diagnosis of idiopathic immunohemolytic anemia was made in as many as 70 per cent of all cases of acquired immunohemolytic anemia in England in 1962 (41). Following discovery of drug-associated positivity, this figure was revised to 50 per cent. More recent data show that the idiopathic form occurs with a frequency of only 10 per cent (42).

Idiopathic Acquired Immunohemolytic Anemia

In idiopathic acquired immunohemolytic anemia, the red cell life span is foreshortened by acquired serum factors with no underlying etiology. A previous history of mild viral infection is common. This disorder affects all races and ages and both sexes. A review of the clinical course of a large group of children with idiopathic acquired immunohemolytic anemia has recently been published (42a). Such patients have been observed in the first months of life (43–45). The signs and symptoms vary, but more commonly it is an acute disorder of mild to severe degree. The peripheral smear may contain many dense-appearing, small red cells (spherocytes) and large polychromatophilic cells, presumably reticulocytes (Fig. 8–5). Red cell indices may not be reliable because of packing abnormalities of spherocytes and the large number of reticulocytes. The Coombs' test usually differentiates this disease from hereditary spherocytosis. The osmotic fragility and autohemolysis test are not helpful. The white cell and platelet counts are usually normal to increased; however; coincident thrombocytopenia and leukopenia may be found rarely (Evans' syndrome) (46).

Treatment begins with a careful search for secondary or associated causes of Coombs' positivity. If none are found, prednisone is administered in a dose of 1 to 2 mg. per kg. per day, resulting in remission in about two-thirds to three-fourths of patients; however, spontaneous remissions occur. Larger doses of prednisone, 6 to 10 mg. per kg., when used at the outset of treatment appear to increase the chances for an earlier response and reduce the need for transfusions. Splenectomy or a trial of immunosuppressive medication or both is sometimes recommended in resistant cases. However, serious attempts to avoid splenectomy should be made in children with this disease. Certainly the operation should be limited to those who have clear-cut splenic sequestration by the [51]chromium scan technique (47). But even in this group, splenectomy is apt to fail and may leave the child vulnerable to overwhelming sepsis. Obviously the operation must be performed on occasion. The risk of splenectomy is worth taking if severe iatrogenic Cushing's disease is the alternative, but it should not be quickly advised.

On the basis of uncontrolled clinical observations, treatment with so-called "immunosuppressive" drugs is of little use

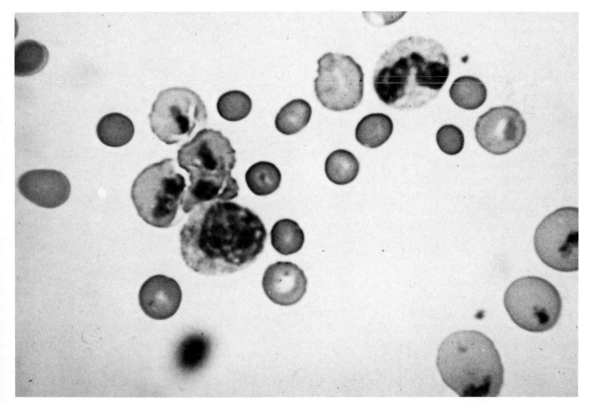

Figure 8–5. Photomicrograph of blood smear (reticulocyte stain) from a patient with IgG Coombs'-positive hemolytic anemia. Note the dense spherocytes, the large red cells, which are reticulocytes, and the nucleated red cell.

in severe immunohemolytic anemia unless the spleen is first removed. Then the addition of drugs, such as azathioprine, may make possible a reduction of the necessary dose of prednisone for maintenance of a reasonable hemoglobin concentration. The use of azathroprine and other immunosuppressive agents has been recently reviewed (47a). The precise mechanism by which steroids and immunosuppressive agents alter red cell survival is unclear, but they may affect reticuloendothelial clearance or even the binding properties of red cell antibodies, as well as diminish the rate of antibody production. Heparin therapy or thymectomy has been proposed, and in isolated case reports remissions have been observed. The latter procedure is obviously one performed in desperation.

Secondary Immunohemolytic Anemia

Drugs

Drug-induced immunohemolytic anemia has been appreciated only recently. Drug-associated hemolysis has become more important as drugs are more commonly used in modern society. Several reviews are available (48, 49). Drugs mediate an immune type of red cell destruction by four general mechanisms: complement fixation, hapten antibody formation, aggregation, and "autoimmunity."

Harris described the complement-fixation mechanism of destruction in 1954 (50). He reported a patient with hemolytic anemia associated with stibophen, an antimonial compound still used in treating schistosomiasis. The patient's plasma transfused into a normal recipient would not cause hemolysis until the recipient was challenged with stibophen. The red cell destruction was related to fixation of complement onto the membrane, a phenomenon initiated by formation of the drug-antidrug antibody complex. It is unclear whether this complex actually attached to the red blood cell or not, but in either case the red cell was an "innocent bystander"

in the reaction. The drugs associated with this reaction include quinidine, quinine, para-aminosalicylic acid, aminopyrine, phenacetin, isoniazid, streptomycin, chlorpromazine, chlorpropamide, and tolbutamide. Antibodies formed against the drugs may be IgG or IgM. A similar pathophysiologic mechanism occurs in drug-induced immunothrombocytopenia.

The laboratory examination clearly identifying this disorder is the Coombs' test (Table 8–5). The patient's red cells (A) may contain C3 (C3 Coombs'-positive). The routine indirect Coombs' test (B), which tests the patient's serum, is negative despite the presence of the antibody. When the antigen (drug) is added to the indirect Coombs' test (C), antigen-antibody complexes occur, some red cells are lysed, others remain coated with C3 and can be detected by monospecific Coombs' sera. That this phenomenon is complement-mediated can be documented by retesting the indirect Coombs' test with the drug, but using heated serum with (E) and without (D) added complement. Treatment consists of discontinuation of the particular drug. Hemolysis abates when the drug is catabolized.

The hapten mechanism of drug-induced hemolytic anemia is illustrated by penicillin. It is an incomplete antigen (hapten), hence unable in itself to induce production

TABLE 8–5. LABORATORY TESTS TO IDENTIFY COMPLEMENT-FIXING DRUG-ASSOCIATED ANTIBODIES

	C3 COOMBS'	LYSIS
A. Patient's red cells	+	
B. Normal red cells plus patient's serum	−	−
C. Normal red cells plus patient's serum plus drug	+	±
D. Same as C, except patient's serum is heated to inactivate complement	−	−
E. Same as D plus fresh serum containing complement factors	+	±

A represents the direct Coombs' test, and *B* the indirect Coombs' test using monospecific antisera against C3. *C, D,* and *E* are indirect Coombs' tests with modifications as shown.

of antibody. Penicillin bound to a macro-molecular substance or tissue protein, how-ever, forms a complete antigen and then has the capability to induce the production of several antibodies – IgM, IgG, and IgE. Penicillin avidly binds to red cells, and the IgG formed is responsible for Coombs' posi-tivity. This antibody does not bind to red cells, but only to cells coated with peni-cillin. Procedures designed to delineate the drug etiology include modifications of the Coombs' test (Table 8–6). The patho-physiologic mechanism of red cell destruc-tion appears similar to, if not identical with, the mechanisms associated with all IgG antibodies. The antibody causes rosette for-mation in vitro. High doses of penicillin or impaired excretion of the drug elevate blood levels and facilitate the binding of penicillin to cells. Antibodies formed react with penicillin-coated cells causing Coombs' positivity. Penicillin induced he-molysis is uncommon but occurs during long-term intravenous administration of the drug, such as in bacterial endocarditis. Anti-penicillin red cell antibodies cross-react with penicillin analogs or with drugs sharing the beta lactam configuration, such as cephalothin. Abatement of hemolysis fol-lows discontinuation of the drug. The hemo-lytic process is eliminated as soon as peni-cillin elutes from the cells or the penicillin-coated red cells are removed.

Aggregation is illustrated by cephalothin. Like penicillin, this drug actively binds to the red cell membrane; however, in so do-ing normal serum proteins are aggregated. Thus the Coombs' test using monospecific antisera against IgG (gamma Coombs' test) is positive, and when the third component of complement is aggregated or fixed by aggregated IgG, the Coombs' test with monospecific antisera against C3 (non-gamma Coombs') is positive. Hemolysis is unusual or mild. It is unclear whether the hemolysis occurs from the nonimmuno-logic coupling of immunoglobulins or com-plement or of both to the cell membrane. Sometimes, anticephalothin or antipeni-cillin antibody reacts with cephalothin-coated red cells. High levels of the drug and Coombs' positivity may occur with renal dysfunction, and the observed he-molysis may be associated with chronic renal disease or infection rather than drugs.

TABLE 8–6. TESTS TO IDENTIFY ANTIPENICILLIN ANTIBODY

	IgG COOMBS'
A. Patient's red cells	+
B. Normal red cells plus patient's serum	–
C. Normal red cells coated with penicillin plus patient's serum	+

A is the direct Coombs' using monospecific antisera against IgG. B is an indirect Coombs'. C is an indirect Coombs' using penicillin-coated red cells.

However, drug-induced Coombs' positivity has been produced in normal subjects and in subhuman primates after the intramuscu-lar injection of cephaloridine (51).

The fourth example of drug-induced Coombs' positivity is illustrated by the ac-tion of α-methyldopa. In 1966 a large num-ber of hypertensive patients in England were reported with Coombs-positive red cells after receiving this drug (52). The in-cidence was proportional to the dose of the drug (10 per cent of patients receiving 1 gm. per day, 20 per cent to 30 per cent of those receiving 2 gm. per day). The anti-body responsible was a typical IgG with specificity directed against the Rh locus. It was similar if not identical to anti-Rh anti-bodies associated with erythroblastosis fetalis, idiopathic acquired immunohemo-lytic anemia, and penicillin. In contrast to the antipenicillin red cell antibody, the antibody associated with α-methyldopa oc-curred after three to four months of adminis-tration of the drug. In addition, it reacted with normal red cells in the absence of the drug. L-dopa causes a similar phenomenon. Apparently the antibodies are induced by the drug, but they cross-react in vitro with normal or patient's red cells in the absence of the drug. Hemolysis is rare but occurs in association with splenomegaly and spherocytosis. Discontinuation of the drug is required only when evidence of hemo-lytic anemia is present. Coombs' positivity without hemolysis is no indication for terminating the drug.

This is an example of allergy rather than "autoimmunity" and is of great signifi-

cance. Clearly the differentiation of idiopathic acquired hemolytic anemia from secondary hemolytic anemia is important in
terms of prognosis and therapy. Corticosteroids, immunosuppressive drugs, and
splenectomy may be used in patients with
immunohemolytic anemia; however, proper
treatment may simply require removing
the antigen from the patient rather than
removing portions of the reticuloendothelial system either surgically or by chemotherapy.

Infections

Immunohemolytic anemia is commonly
associated with infections. Either IgG or
IgM antibodies have been reported in association with acute and chronic infections.
These antibodies include classic "warm
incomplete" cold agglutinins and cold
hemolysins. Best known is the association
between cold agglutinins and *Mycoplasma
pneumoniae* infections.

In the early 1900's Clough and Richter
(53) described microscopic agglutination
of blood associated with pneumonia. The
agglutination was caused by a serum factor
which could affect normal red cells. In
1943 changes in cold agglutinin titers were
reported in association with primary atypical pneumonia (54), later identified as infection due to *Mycoplasma pneumoniae*.
I antigenic specificity is common for most
cold agglutinins. The precise relationship
is unclear; however, some evidence indicates that the microorganism is capable
of altering the I antigen of red cells in
vitro. Cold agglutinins may be produced
experimentally in man by *Mycoplasma* and
in rabbits by *Listeria monocytogenes*. Those

described frequently in patients with infectious mononucleosis have anti-i specificity.

Although most cold agglutinins are IgM
globulins which frequently react with the
I antigen, they have different characteristics
and result in a wide variety of pathophysiologic consequences (Table 8–7). The cold
agglutinins present in normal serum are of
low titer and have no clinical significance.
Those associated with *Mycoplasma pneumoniae* are of higher titer, are frequently
polyclonal (kappa and lambda light chains),
and consist of only a small quantity of the
total serum level of IgM (55). Hemolytic
anemia occurs uncommonly, but when it
does, hemolysis may be severe. Treatment
of the underlying infection with antibiotics
reduces the cold agglutinin titer; however,
with or without therapy the elevated levels
continue only weeks to months. In the adult
population, very high titers may be found
with lymphoproliferative diseases or in the
elderly patient with no underlying disease
(idiopathic cold agglutinin hemolytic anemia). This form of cold agglutinin is often
monoclonal (frequently kappa chains) and
may be visible on serum electrophoresis
as an "M-component" (54). In spite of
these high titers, these patients have only
a mild hemolytic anemia. In fact, infarction
of the ear lobes and the nose, together with
Raynaud's syndrome, is often more troublesome in cold agglutinin disease than is
hemolysis.

Acute hemolytic anemia associated with
viral infections is well recognized (56, 57).
The infections include influenza, Coxsackie
virus, measles, varicella, cytomegalic virus,
and encephalitis. Typical cold agglutinins
or IgG antibody–causing spherocytic hemolytic anemia have been noted. Uncommonly,

TABLE 8–7.   COLD AGGLUTININ CHARACTERISTICS

		TITER	TYPE	HEMOLYSIS
Normal	— Anti-I — Anti-i — Anti-H	<1:50	Polyclonal	None
Postinfection	— Anti-I — Anti-i	$1:10^2 - 1:10^4$	Polyclonal	May be severe
Lymphoproliferative	Anti-I	$1:10^2 - 1:10^6$	Often monoclonal	Mild
Idiopathic	Anti-I	$1:10^2 - 1:10^6$	Often monoclonal	Mild

a cold active complement-fixing IgG antibody causing a syndrome resembling that reported by Donath and Landsteiner is found, and this may result in profound hemolysis and spherocytosis. The Donath-Landsteiner antibody may also occur in syphilis or with no underlying etiology. Laboratory tests demonstrate evidence of hemolysis, spherocytosis, and cold hemolysin. The Coombs' test may be positive with monospecific antibody against IgG or C3. Buffy coat preparations may reveal typical rosettes with monocytes and phagocytosis with polymorphonuclear leukocytes (58). Treatment of hemolytic anemia associated with infections is directed against the inciting agent. The hemolysis is a transient phenomenon and may disappear without specific therapy. Results of steroid therapy vary.

"Connective Tissue" Disease

Coombs' positivity and hemolytic anemia are found associated with diseases such as systemic lupus erythematosus and rheumatoid arthritis, both the adult and juvenile forms. The antigen is obscure but may relate to endogenous nucleic acid liberated from cells, to viral agents, or to others. Usually the red cell antibody is IgG, and cells may contain IgG, a combination of IgG and C3, or C3 alone. Spherocytosis and splenomegaly are common, and the course and prognosis depend upon the successful treatment of the underlying disease. Steroids are frequently beneficial. In some resistant cases, antimetabolites and splenectomy are employed.

Neoplasia

Immunohemolytic anemia is also associated with a variety of neoplasias. These include lymphoproliferative diseases, much less commonly myeloproliferative diseases, and solid tumors (dermoid cysts, teratomas, carcinomas, and so forth). In fact, lymphatic malignancy was observed in 25 per cent of one series of patients (41). Frequently the antibody is an IgG which may fix complement. Agglutinins are also reported. Treatment includes an attack on the neoplasm.

Removal of solid tumors may result in remission. Steroids may be helpful as well. It is unclear whether red cell antibodies are directed against the tumor and cross-react with red cell antigens, whether the tumor alters normal red cell antigens, or whether the immune apparatus is affected by the tumor.

Immune Deficiency States

Immunohemolytic anemia occurs infrequently in association with congenital and acquired defects in the immune defense mechanisms. Defects in humoral immunity, such as congenital agammaglobulinemia and dysgammaglobulinemia, have been associated with unusual antibodies (anti-N, anti-LW) (59, 60). Treatment with steroids is frequently beneficial. In one case known to this writer, immunosuppressive therapy was not helpful. Most reports of hemolysis and defects in cellular immunity are examples of acquired immunohemolytic anemia (such as lymphomas). In these instances therapy is directed toward the malignancy. Steroid therapy which is effective for lymphoma is also helpful for the hemolysis.

It is unknown why antibodies which react with self-antigens are formed in disorders of the immune system. There is no evidence that the antibody produced by the affected individual is abnormal per se; commonly the antibody has normal immunoglobulin structure and function. Foreign antigens may invade the host with impaired defenses and alter certain self-antigens; however, this thesis is unproven. Alternatively, antibodies formed against the foreign antigen may cross-react with self-antigens.

Perinatal Immunohemolytic Anemia

Most of these anemias are examples of "hemolytic disease of the newborn" (see Chapter 9). Rare instances are reported of IgG "incomplete" antibodies present in the mother for unknown reasons (idiopathic acquired immunohemolytic) or in secondary immunohemolytic anemia in which the antibody traverses the placenta and affects the neonate (61). Since IgG is catabolized with a half-life of several weeks, the immunohemolytic anemia exists only until maternal antibody is destroyed by the newborn or is mechanically removed (exchange transfusion). Other therapy includes transfusion of compatible blood and steroids.

Paroxysmal Nocturnal Hemoglobinuria

Paroxysmal nocturnal hemoglobinuria was originally described as a disease in which hemolysis occurred with sleep. This condition is an acquired uncommon disorder which may follow or be accompanied by aplastic or hypoplastic anemia. In some patients, the marrow may be injured by drugs, but in others there is no explanation for the injury. Some of the red cells lyse when the blood is acidified in vitro, a situation which enhances complement activation. It is now known that the PNH lesion is variable in its distribution, so that some populations of the red cells are much more affected than others. In fact, some of the cells may be entirely normal (62). The membrane of the PNH cell is exquisitely sensitive to the effects of complement, but the mechanism is unknown. Furthermore, there is no evidence to indicate that complement is deposited onto red cells in vivo as a result of antigen-antibody activation. These patients may be of both sexes and all ages and races. They manifest pancytopenia and a positive acid serum lysis test (Ham test) and sucrose lysis test (sugar water test). Frequent complications include infection and thrombosis.

The thrombotic manifestations include intrahepatic thrombosis with portal hypertension, mesenteric thrombosis, and deep vein thrombosis of the legs. The basis for the thrombotic tendency is not clearly established but may be related to release of thromboplastic agents present in red cell membranes during intravascular lysis. Treatment with anticoagulants, such as warfarin, is advocated by some, but it should be managed with caution since thrombocytopenia is commonly present in this disease. The thrombocytopenia may be in part due to shortening of platelet life span and decreased production secondary to the hypoplasia which accompanies the disease. Acute leukemia develops in some

patients terminally. Iron deficiency may occur because of chronic hemosiderinuria. Iron therapy may be hazardous because the iron-induced reticulocytosis causes the release of complement-sensitive cells from the bone marrow, which may precipitate a hemolytic crisis. Androgens are of some benefit; however, complications, such as hepatotoxicity, hirsutism, and salt retention, limit their use.

Hereditary Erythroblastic Multinuclearity with a Positive Acidified Serum Test (HEMPAS)

In 1966 Crookston et al. (63) described two unrelated young males with dyserythropoietic anemia with striking hyperplasia and multinuclearity of the marrow erythroblasts. Both had positive acid serum hemolysis, but sucrose lysis was absent. In subsequent studies of other patients, the hereditary nature of the disorder became apparent, and its autosomal recessive character was established. The acronym HEMPAS was assigned. Several additional serologic characteristics were noted. The cells are lysed by a high serum to cell ratio, and lysis is increased by prior cooling of the serum cell mixture. The lytic activity of normal serum is removed by prior absorption with HEMPAS cells but not by PNH cells. Hence the factor in the serum responsible for lysis is a naturally occurring IgM cold isoantibody, the so-called HEMPAS antibody. The cells are highly sensitive to agglutination by anti-i serum, and anti-I serum provides marked cellular uptake of C3. Freeze cleavage of the HEMPAS membrane reveals large pits and plaques on the external surface. There is a marked increase in the activities of certain red cell enzymes (64).

Thorough reviews of the present status of HEMPAS and a comparison of the disorder to PNH, another disorder of the red cell membrane, have been recently published (65, 65a). This specific disorder must be distinguished from the several types of dyserythropoiesis and multinuclearity which are not associated with the serologic characteristics typical of HEMPAS (66, 67).

SUMMARY

Immunohemolytic anemia has been a late development in the history of clinical medicine. In the past century, basic bedside observations have brought together the hematologist and the immunologist, thus providing clinical immunohematology with a theoretical and practical base. The classic terms warm and cold agglutinins, incomplete agglutinins, and warm and cold hemolysins have been replaced by IgG, IgM, and complement. The destructive pathway for IgG-coated red cells is spherocytosis and splenomegaly, perhaps by a model in vivo which resembles rosette formation. The mechanism of destruction of IgM-agglutinated red cells appears to be sequestration in capillary beds of the reticuloendothelial organs of high blood flow, specifically the liver rather than the spleen. Complement may cause frank lysis of red cells or partial injury. Some complement-coated cells may be destroyed in the reticuloendothelial system because of the coexistent presence of IgG or IgM.

These observations have allowed the clinician and the investigator to understand better the pathophysiologic consequences of the immune factors and hopefully will provide the pediatrician, clinician, and hematologist with a more modern and beneficial therapeutic armamentarium for this type of anemia.

References

1. Vanlair, C. F., and Masius, J. R.: De la microcytémia. Bull. Acad. R. Med. Belg. 5:515, 1871.
2. Donath, J., and Landsteiner, K.: Über paroxysmale hemoglobinuria. Munch. Med. Wochenschr. 51:1590, 1904.
3. Chauffard, A., and Troisier, J.: Contribution à l'étude des hémolysines dans leur rapport avec les anémics graves. Bull. Mem. Soc. Med. Hop. Paris 26:94, 1908.
4. Widal, F., Abrami, P., et al.: Auto-agglutination des hématies dans l'ictère hémolytique acquis. C. R. Soc. Biol. (Paris) 64:655, 1908.
5. Banti, G.: Splénomégalie hémolytique anhémopoiétique: le ròle de la rate dans l'hémolyse. Semaine Med. 33:313, 1913.
6. Moss, W. L.: Studies on isoagglutinins and isohemolysins. Bull. Johns Hopkins Hosp. 21:63, 1910.
7. Muir, R., and McNee, J. R.: The anemia produced by a hemolytic serum. J. Pathol. Bact. 16:410, 1911–1912.
8. Coombs, R. R. A., Mourant, A. E., et al.: A new test for the detection of weak and "incomplete" RH agglutinins. Brit. J. Exp. Pathol. 26:255, 1945.
8a. Schreiber, A. D., and Frank, M. M.: Role of antibody and complement in the immune clearance and destruction of erythrocytes I and II. J. Clin. Invest. 51:575, 583, 1972.
9. Jandl, J. H., and Tomlinson, A. S.: The destruction of red cells by antibodies in man. II. Pyrogenic, leukocytic, and dermal responses to immune hemolysis. J. Clin. Invest. 37:1202, 1958.
10. Jandl, J. H., and Kaplan, M. E.: The destruction of red cells by antibodies in man. III. Quantitative factors influencing the patterns of hemolysis in vivo. J. Clin. Invest. 39:1145, 1960.
11. Mollison, P. I.: Blood group antibodies and red-cell destruction. Br. Med. J. 2:1035, 1959.
12. LoBuglio, A. F., Cotran, R. S., et al.: Red cells washed with immunoglobulin G: Binding and sphering by mononuclear cells in man. Science 158:1582, 1967.
13. Abramson, N., LoBuglio, A. F., et al.: The interaction between human monocytes and red cells. Binding characteristics. J. Exp. Med. 132:1191, 1970.
14. Brabec, V., Michalec, C., et al.: Red cell lipids in auto-immune hemolytic anemia. Blood 34:414, 1969.
15. Cooper, R. A.: Loss of membrane components in the pathogenesis of antibody-induced spherocytosis. J. Clin. Invest. 51:16, 1972.
16. Abramson, N., Gelfand, E. W., et al.: Specificity of monocyte receptor in man and monkey. Clin. Res. 18:317, 1970.
17. Gelfand, E. W., Abramson, N., et al.: Buffy coat observations and red cell antibodies in acquired hemolytic anemia. New Engl. J. Med. 284:1250, 1971.
18. Gergely, J., Fudenberg, H. H., et al.: The papain susceptibility of myeloma proteins of heavy chain subclasses. Immunochemistry 7:1, 1970.
19. Abramson, N., and Schur, P. H.: The IgG subclasses of red cell antibodies and relationship to monocyte binding. Blood 40:500, 1972.
19a. Hoyer, L. W., and Trabold, N. C.: The significance of erythrocyte site density. I. Hemagglutination. J. Clin. Invest. 49:87, 1969.
19b. Hoyer, L. W., and Trabold, N. C.: The significance of erythrocyte site density. II. Hemolysis. J. Clin. Invest. 50:1840, 1971.
20. Cutbush, M., and Mollison, P. L.: Relation between characteristics of blood group antibodies in vitro and associated patterns of red cell destruction in vivo. Br. J. Haematol. 4:115, 1958.
21. Evans, R. S., Turner, E., et al.: Chronic hemolytic anemia due to cold agglutinins: The mechanism of resistance of red cells to complement-hemolysis by cold agglutinins. J. Clin. Invest. 46:1461, 1967.
21a. Loque, G. L., Rosse, W. F., et al.: Measurement of the third component of complement bound to red blood cells in patients with the cold agglutinin syndrome. J. Clin. Invest. 52:493, 1973.
22. Huber, H., and Fudenberg, H. H.: Receptor sites of human monocytes for IgG. Int. Arch. Allergy Appl. Immunol. 34:18, 1968.

23. Ehrlich, P., and Morgenroth, J.: Ueber haemoly-sine. *Berl. Klin. Wochenschr.* 37:453, 1900.

24. Rosse, W. F., Dourmashkin, R. R., et al.: Immune lysis of normal human and paroxysmal noctur-nal hemoglobinuria (PNH) red blood cells. III. The membrane defects caused by comple-ment lysis. J. Exp. Med. *123*:969, 1966.

25. Polley, M. J., Muller-Eberhard, H. J., et al.: Pro-duction of ultrastructural membrane lesions by the fifth component of complement. J. Exp. Med. *133*:53, 1971.

26. Huber, H., Polley, M. J., et al.: Human monocytes: Distinct receptor sites for the third component of complement and for immunoglobulin G. Science *162*:1281, 1968.

27. Lay, W. H., and Nussenzweig, V.: Receptors for complement on leukocytes. J. Exp. Med. *128*: 991, 1968.

28. Brown, D. L., Lachman, P. J., et al.: The in vivo behavior of complement-coated red cells: Studies in C6-deficient, C3-deficient and nor-mal rabbits. Clin. Exp. Immunol. 7:401, 1970.

28a. Brown, D. L., and Nelson, D. A.: Surface micro-fragmentation of red cells as a mechanism for complement-mediated immune spherocytosis. Br. J. Haematol. *24*:301, 1973.

29. Nelson, R. A., Jr., Jenson, J., et al.: Methods for the separation, purification and measurement of nine components of hemolytic complement in guinea-pig serum. Immunochemistry 3: 111, 1966.

30. Lachmann, P. J., and Muller-Eberhard, H. J.: The demonstration in human serum of "con-glutinogen-activating factor" and its effects on the third component of complement. J. Immunol. 7:401, 1968.

31. Abramson, N., Alper, C. A., et al.: A normal serum protein that removes C′3 from red cells. Clin. Res. *17*:318, 1969.

32. Abramson, N., Alper, C. A., et al.: Deficiency of C3 inactivator in man. J. Immunol. *107*:19, 1971.

33. Ruddy, S., and Austen, K. F.: C3 inactivator of man. I. Hemolytic measurement by the inac-tivation of cell-bound C3. J. Immunol. *102*: 533, 1969.

34. Gilliland, B. C., Baxter, E., et al.: Red cell anti-bodies in Coombs-negative hemolytic anemia. New Engl. J. Med. 285:252, 1971.

35. Rosse, W. F.: Quantitative immunology of immune hemolytic anemia. II. The relationship of cell-bound antibody to hemolysis and the ef-fect of treatment. J. Clin. Invest. 50:734, 1971.

36. MacKenzie, M. R., and Creevy, N. C.: Hemolytic anemia with cold detectable IgG antibodies. Blood 36:549, 1971.

37. Griffin, J. P.: Rapid screening for cold agglutinins in pneumonia. Ann. Intern. Med. 70:701, 1969.

38. Hartmann, R. C., and Jenkins, D. E.: The sugar water test for paroxysmal nocturnal hemo-globinuria. New Engl. J. Med. 275:155, 1966.

39. Hartmann, R. C., Jenkins, D. E., et al.: Diagnostic specificity of sucrose hemolysis test for par-oxysmal nocturnal hemoglobinuria. Blood 35: 462, 1970.

40. Kann, H. E., Jr., Mengel, C. E., et al.: Increased hemolysis after intramuscular iron adminis-tration in patients with paroxysmal nocturnal hemoglobinuria. Report of six occurrences in four patients and speculations on a possible mechanism. Ann. Intern. Med. 67:593, 1965.

41. Dacie, J. V.: *The Hemolytic Anemias,* Part 2. 2nd ed. New York, Grune & Stratton, 1962.

42. Sawitsky, A., and Ozaeta, P. B., Jr.: Disease-asso-ciated autoimmune hemolytic anemia. Bull. N. Y. Acad. Med. *46*:411, 1970.

42a. Habibi, B., Homberg, J-C., et al.: Autoimmune hemolytic anemia in children. A review of 80 cases. Am. J. Med. *56*:61, 1974.

43. Unger, L. J., Weiner, A. A., et al.: Anémie auto-hémolytique chez un nouveau-né. Rev. Hema-tol. 7:495, 1952.

44. Wirtheimer, C.: Pregnancy and hemolytic anemia. Brux. Med. *37*:539, 1957.

45. Laski, B., Wake, E. J., et al.: Autohemolytic anemia in young infants. J. Pediatr. 59:42, 1961.

46. Evans, R. S., Takahashi, K., et al.: Primary throm-bocytopenic purpura and acquired hemolytic anemia. Arch. Intern. Med. 87:48, 1951.

47. Allgood, J. W., and Chaplin, H., Jr.: Idiopathic acquired autoimmune hemolytic anemia. A review of forty-seven cases treated from 1955 through 1965. Am. J. Med. *43*:254, 1967.

47a. Skinner, M. D., and Schwartz, R. S.: Immuno-suppressive therapy. New Engl. J. Med. *287*: 221, 281, 1972.

48. Croft, J. D., Swisher, S. N., et al.: Coombs'-test positivity induced by drugs. Mechanisms of immunologic reactions and red cell destruc-tion. Ann. Intern. Med. 68:176, 1968.

49. Dacie, J. V., Carstairs, K., et al.: Auto-immune hemolytic anemia. Proc. R. Soc. Med. *61*: 1307, 1968.

50. Harris, J. W.: Studies on the mechanism of a drug-induced hemolytic anemia. J. Lab. Clin. Med. *44*:809, 1954.

51. Perkins, R. L., Mengel, C. E., et al.: Direct Coombs' test reactivity after cephalothin or cephaloridine in man and monkey. Proc. Soc. Exp. Biol. Med. *129*:397, 1968.

52. Carstairs, K. C., Breckenridge, A., et al.: Incidence of a positive direct Coombs test in patients on alpha-1 dopa. Lancet 2:133, 1966.

53. Clough, M. C., and Richter, I. M.: A study of an autoagglutinin occurring in a human serum. Bull. Johns Hopkins Hosp. 29:86, 1918.

54. Peterson, O. L., Ham, T. H., et al.: Cold agglutinins (autohemagglutinins) in primary atypical pneumonias. Science 97:107, 1943.

55. Wollheim, F. A., Williams, R. C., Jr., et al.: Studies on the macroglobulin of human serum. III. Quantitative aspects related to cold agglu-tinins. Blood 29:203, 1967.

56. Zuelzer, W. W., Stulberg, C. S., et al.: The Emily Cooley Lecture—Etiology and pathogenesis of acquired hemolytic anemia. Transfusion 6:438–61, September-October, 1966.

57. Zuelzer, W. W., Mastrangelo, R., et al.: Auto-immune hemolytic anemia. Natural history and viral-immunologic interactions in child-hood. Am. J. Med. *49*:80, 1970.

58. Zinkham, W. H., and Diamond, J. K.: In vitro erythrophagocytosis in acquired hemolytic anemia. Blood 7:592, 1952.

59. Hinz, C. F., and Boyer, J. T.: Dysgammaglobuli-nemia in the adult manifested as autoimmune

hemolytic anemia. Serologic and immunochemical characterization of an antibody of
unusual specificity. New Engl. J. Med. *269*:
1329, 1903.

60. Robbins, J. B., Skinner, R. G., et al.: Autoimmune
hemolytic anemia in a child with congenital
X-linked hypogammaglobulinemia. New
Engl. J. Med. *280*:75, 1969.

61. Vedovini, F., and Benedetti, P. A.: Anemia
emolitica neonatale da auto anticorp materni.
Riv. Clin. Pediatr. *72*:339, 1966.

62. Rosse, W. F.: Variations in the red cells in paroxysmal nocturnal hemoglobinuria. Br. J. Haema-
tol. *24*:317, 1973.

63. Crookston, J. H., Godwin, T. F., et al.: Congenital
dyserythropoietic anemia. *Proceedings 11th
Congr. Int. Soc. Haematol.*, Sydney (abstract),
p. 18.

64. Valentine, W. N., Crookston, J. H., et al.: Erythrocyte enzymatic abnormalities in HEMPAS
(Hereditary erythroblastic multinuclearity
with a positive acidified-serum test). Br. J.
Haematol. *23*:107, 1972.

65. Crookston, J. H., Crookston, M. C., et al.: Red cell
abnormalities in HEMPAS (hereditary erythroblastic multinuclearity with a positive acidified-serum test). Br. J. Haematol. *23*(Suppl.):
83, 1972.

65a. Verwilghen, R. L., Lewis, S. M., et al.: HEMPAS:
Congenital dyserythropoietic anaemia (type
II). Quart. J. Med. *42*:257, 1973.

66. Faille, A., Najean, Y., et al.: Genetique dè l'érythropoiese dans 14 cas "d'érythropoiese in-
efficoce" avec anomolies morphologiques des
érythroblastes et polynucléarite. Nouv. Rev.
Fr. Hematol. *12*:631, 1972.

67. Clauvel, J. P., Cesson, A., et al.: Dysérythropoiese
congénitale. Etude de 6 observations. Nouv.
Rev. Fr. Hematol. *12*:653, 1972.

Chapter 9

Hemolytic Disease of the Newborn

by A. Zipursky

Rh HEMOLYTIC DISEASE

Introduction

The relationship between hemolytic disease in the newborn and sensitization to Rh was established by Levine in 1941 (1). With an increased understanding of the disease, its diagnosis and prognosis, there now exist carefully defined criteria for therapy of the affected newborn or fetus. In the last few years, an approach to the prevention and eradication of this disease has been developed by the technique of preventing immunization in the mother.

Before considering the pathophysiology of the disease, it is well to review the extent of the problem. The incidence of Rh disease in a population will depend in part on the prevalence of the Rh-negative genotype. This differs greatly among races and ethnic groups, as shown in Table 9–1. From these data (2) it will be understood that Rh disease is very rare in many races (e.g., Chinese, Japanese). Among whites, the prevalence is approximately 15 per cent. This varies somewhat; for example, the prevalence is 11 per cent in Greece and Yugoslavia and 20 per cent in Ireland. For every 1000 pregnancies in white women, approximately 90 will be ones in which there is an Rh-positive fetus and an Rh-negative mother. The incidence of hemolytic disease of the newborn in large studies has been found to be six to seven per thousand

births, or one out of every fifteen pregnancies potentially at risk (3). Why is only one out of fifteen pregnancies affected? To begin with, Rh immunization of the mother rarely appears during a first pregnancy (3). Secondly, many of the second infants will be Rh-negative. Finally, as discussed later, only a fraction of women at risk will develop antibodies.

The severity of the disease in the affected infants varies greatly. Thus, of all cases of hemolytic disease of the newborn, approximately 14 per cent result in stillbirth, a figure which has changed surprisingly little in the past fifteen years (3). Forty per cent of the live births will not require therapy, and the remainder have varying degrees of hemolytic disease. The perinatal

TABLE 9–1. PREVALENCE OF Rh-NEGATIVE GENOTYPE (cde/cde; r/r) IN VARIOUS POPULATIONS*

	% OF POPULATION
Caucasians	
Europeans	11–21
Americans (U.S.A.)	14.4
Australians	14.7
Indians (India)	8
American Blacks	5.5
Japanese	0
Chinese	0
North American Indians	0

*From Prokop, O., and Uhlenbruck, G.: *Human Blood and Serum Groups.* New York, Wiley Interscience, 1969, p. 218.

280

mortality per 100 cases of hemolytic disease of the newborn is approximately 17.5, with about 14 due to stillbirth and the remainder due to neonatal death (3). These figures will change as a result of intrauterine transfusions, more accurate antenatal assessment, improved postnatal care, and, of course, a more complete understanding of the physiology of the disease and its treatment.

In the subsequent sections, we will examine the mechanisms by which immunization occurs in the mother, how disease is produced in the fetus, and how the fetus and newborn respond to these disease processes. In this way, we should be able to perceive the logic of the present approach to the diagnosis, prognosis, and therapy of Rh hemolytic disease of the newborn.

Nature of the "Rh-positive" Erythrocyte*

Erythrocytes consist of a membrane enclosing a liquid containing hemoglobin. The erythrocyte blood groups represent antigenic material on the surface of that membrane. That they exist on or in the membrane is evident because of the nature of blood group antibody reactions, all of which depend on the interaction of an antibody with a material on the surface of the erythrocyte. The Rh blood groups represent many different types of antigens. In this section, we shall deal with the most important and clinically significant of those antigens, namely the Rh$_0$ or D antigen. The presence of this antigen on the erythrocyte renders that cell "Rh-positive," and its absence makes it "Rh-negative."

There are two major groups of antigens related to the D antigen, and these are referred to as Cc and Ee. However, to understand them better, let us examine their re-

lation to the D antigen, using three genotypes as examples (Fig. 9–1). Let us assume that the D antigen represents a structural characteristic of a membrane protein or of its product. In this scheme, related antigens represent neighboring configurational and chemical characteristics related to one protein molecule and, therefore, to a single gene product. This would be similar in concept to the many antigenic sites found on other proteins (e.g., hemoglobin) which are determined by a single structural gene.

Thus we can regard the three antigenic sites as the product of a single gene containing structural characteristics which permit them to react with anti-C, anti-c, anti-E, anti-e, or anti-D. There is no anti-d. The frequency of the three genes in a Caucasian population is cDE (R^2) = 0.14, CDe (R^1) = 0.41, and cde (r) = 0.39 (4). These, of course, represent single genes; however, since chromosomes are paired, it means that the antigens of each cell will be determined by two Rh genes. Therefore, one can calculate that the prevalence of rr will be 0.39 × 0.39, or 0.15 (15 per cent). The prevalence of R^1/r will be 0.41 × 0.39 × 2 (because there may be an R^1 or r on either chromosome), which is approximately 32 per cent of the population.

Let us return then to the matter of the "Rh-positive" red cell, which refers to those cells with the D antigen. A cell may be Rh-positive if it contains the gene CDe (R^1) or cDE (R^2), or other genes determining the D antigen. An individual whose erythrocytes contain both the R' and r antigens is referred to as heterozygous Rh-positive. If both genes contain D [e.g., CDe/cDE (R^1/R^2) = 11.4 per cent of the population], that subject is referred to as homozygous Rh-positive. Finally, the formula cde/cde (rr) refers to the "Rh-negative" subject, representing about 15 per cent of the population. The other genes lacking D (Rh$_0$) are infrequent, but it should be understood that a formula such as Cde/cde (r/r) also represents an Rh-negative erythrocyte.

From this discussion, it would appear that D (Rh$_0$) represents one of the antigens in the erythrocyte membrane determined by a specific gene. Furthermore, it can be postulated that in the homozygous state there should be more D sites than in the heterozygous state, not unlike the amount of hemoglobin S in the erythrocytes

---

*The terminology in the Rh system has been the subject of much discussion and, as a result, is the basis of much confusion. In this chapter we shall refer to the D (Rh$_0$) antigen as D; however, we will make reference frequently to the "Rh-positive" or "Rh-negative" erythrocyte, which refers to cells containing or lacking the D (Rh$_0$) antigen, respectively. The Rh-positive subject is one whose erythrocytes are Rh-positive [i.e., contain the D (Rh$_0$) antigen]. A complete survey of the genetics of blood groups is presented in Chapter 26.

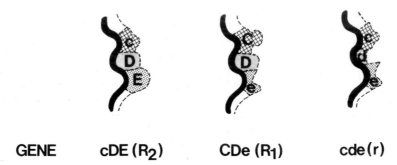

GENE   **cDE (R$_2$)**   **CDe (R$_1$)**   **cde(r)**

Figure 9–1. A schematic representation of the Rh antigens on the red cell membrane (represented as the heavy black line). There are three antigenic sites occupied by the antigens C or c, D or d, and E or e. It is likely that these three sites are products of a single gene, but each of the antigens shown (other than d) can react specifically with the appropriate antibody (anti-C, anti-c, etc.). The genes are named by their content of antigens (cDE, CDe, or cde – Fisher nomenclature) or by a single letter (Rr, R, or r – Wiener classification).

of the sickle cell trait (heterozygote) versus the homozygous case of sickle cell disease. That this is so is shown in Table 9–2, in which the number of D sites are listed in cells of various genotypes (5). D antigenic sites have been determined by the amount of radiolabeled anti-D bound by specific cells. Thus the homozygous *CDe/CDe* contains more D sites than the heterozygous *CDe/cde*, but not twice as many.

If one considers that the D site represents a structural characteristic of a specific membrane material, it is not surprising that its reactivity may differ as a result of other characteristics of that material. This phenomenon is also shown in Table 9–2. Thus, if the number of D sites in the *CDe/cde* cell and in the *cDE/cde* cell are compared, there is a significant difference between them. Although both gene products contain the D antigen, other features of that product have altered its reactivity. It is of interest that the D reactivity is altered not only by a change on the gene of which it is a part

(a cis effect) but also by a change in the second gene, modifying the reactivity of the other gene (a trans effect). For example, it has been reported that the genotype *CDe/Cde* may have a diminished D reactivity (6). This diminished reactivity appears to result from the presence of the Cde gene. When that same CDe gene is associated with another gene, e.g., cde, it expresses as a normal D.

The number of antigenic sites influences the reactivity of the cell with various anti-D antibodies and, accordingly, the interpretation of certain tests. Furthermore, it would appear that the number of antigenic sites bears a close relationship to the immunogenicity of the cell (i.e., the ability to induce anti-D formation in an Rh-negative subject) or to its susceptibility to anti-D antibodies in vivo or both. Thus the severity of hemolytic disease in first-affected infants of genotype R^2/r is more severe than in those infants whose genotype is R^1/r (7). D^u refers to a D antigen of very low reactivity, and this may occur as CD^{u}e or as cD^{u}E, for example. The importance of this group is that these subjects may be grouped as Rh-negative. There is a slight risk if their blood is infused into an Rh-negative subject because it may result in the development of anti-D antibodies in such a recipient (4). There is a very small risk of anti-D development in the D^u recipient following infusion of D cells. A D^u infant can suffer from hemolytic disease of the newborn (4). The diminished reactivity of these cells is supported by quantitative observations suggesting that such cells pick up less anti-D than D cells (8).

TABLE 9–2. THE NUMBER OF D SITES ON ERYTHROCYTES OF DIFFERENT GENOTYPE°

GENOTYPE		D ANTIGEN SITES PER CELL
CDe/cde	*(R^1/r)*	9,900–14,600
CDe/CDe	*(R^1/R^1)*	14,500–19,300
cDE/cDE	*(R^2/R^2)*	15,800–33,300
cDE/cde	*(R^2/r)*	12,000–20,000

°From Rochna, E., and Hughes-Jones, N. C.: Vox Sang. *10*:675, 1965.

The importance of determining D^u in erythrocytes is to distinguish such cells from Rh-negative cells. This will be discussed further in the section on antibody reaction; however, at this point it would be fair to emphasize that, for the detection of D^u, one must test by the use of anti-D antibody in an indirect Coombs' reaction.

Nature of Rh Antibody

In this section, we will consider only anti-D antibodies. Antibodies to other Rh groups will be dealt with in a subsequent section.

Anti-D antibody has been the subject of considerable study over the past 30 years; however, with the clarification of the nature of antibodies, a great deal of the complexity and confusion that existed previously has disappeared. Let us now consider these antibodies on the basis of our present understanding of immunoglobulin structure and function.

The Rh antibodies are primarily IgM or IgG antibodies. There have been a few reported instances of IgA antibodies (9); however, these are of interest only, and are not of significance regarding the pathogenesis of hemolytic disease of the newborn, since IgA antibodies cannot cross the placenta (10).

The appearance of IgM and IgG antibodies in response to antigenic stimulus will be discussed in the section on the pathogenesis of Rh isoimmunization. However, as in other antibody systems, IgM is the first to appear, followed by IgG. It is important to distinguish these two types of antibodies because of their different significance in the pathogenesis of Rh disease and the interpretation of serologic reactions. IgM antibody is of no significance in the pathogenesis of hemolytic disease in the newborn because it cannot cross the placenta to enter the fetal circulation. Only IgG can cross the placenta (10).

Serologic Reactions

In this section we will describe four tests for the detection of anti-D antibodies. To understand these better, in terms of our

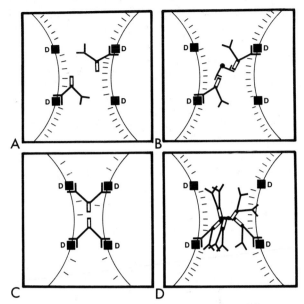

Figure 9–2. A schematic representation of the interaction of anti-D antibodies with D-positive erythrocytes. A, Erythrocytes sensitized with an IgG anti-D are held apart because of their negative charge. Agglutination does not occur. B, Agglutination occurs when the sensitized erythrocytes are treated with an antibody against IgG, which then forms a "bridge" between the two molecules and, therefore, the two cells. C, If the effective charge of the erythrocyte is reduced by either enzyme treatment or suspension of the cells in albumin, the cells can approximate one another, and agglutination will occur. D, Agglutination by the large IgM molecule.

present knowledge of antibody structure and function, their mechanism of action is conceptually represented in Figure 9–2.

Normally, erythrocytes have a negative surface charge at physiologic pH; this will maintain them apart. Thus in Figure 9–2 erythrocytes suspended in saline and sensitized with an IgG anti-D are depicted as being unable to "bridge the gap," and agglutination does not occur (Fig. 9–2,A). The IgG molecule is a bivalent antibody having a molecular weight of 160,000. "Bridging" presumably occurs with the larger IgM molecule (Fig. 9–2,D), which brings about agglutination of the erythrocytes suspended in saline. Such an antibody capable of agglutinating erythrocytes suspended in saline is referred to as a "complete" antibody, whereas the IgG antibody described above would be referred to as "incomplete" (11, 12).

Returning now to the IgG-sensitized cell (Fig. 9–2), agglutination can occur (1) if the sensitized cells are treated with an anti-IgG antibody (i.e., a Coombs' reaction) (Fig. 9–2,B), and (2) if the sensitized cells are brought closer together by suspending them in albumin or by treating them with an enzyme (bromelin, ficin, or papain), which reduces the effective charge and permits agglutination (13) (Fig. 9–2,C).

It will be understood, therefore, that, in interpreting the various serologic tests, the "saline" or complete antibody representing IgM (which cannot cross the placenta) is of no significance in the pathogenesis of the disease, and therefore its level in the serum of an Rh-negative mother is of little value in predicting the severity of hemolytic disease in her fetus. For example, a woman may have a very low "saline" titer in the presence of very high concentrations of IgG anti-D.

Recently, several reports have described another type of IgM antibody, M.W. 1,000,000, which reacts only with enzyme-treated erythrocytes (12, 14). This is of considerable importance in the pathogenesis of Rh immunization (see below), since these antibodies appear to represent the earliest detectable antibodies in the primary immune response. The full explanation of this phenomenon is not yet available; however, it indicates why screening for evidence of Rh immunization must include testing with enzyme-treated erythrocytes.

Complement Fixation

The interaction of anti-D with a D-positive erythrocyte does not result in activation of the complement system [rare exceptions have been noted (4)]. In contrast, anti-A reacting with A cells does activate complement. It is likely that the difference results from the relatively greater number of A sites (about 500,000) than D sites (Table 9–2) on an erythrocyte. Complement activation appears to result from the interaction of several IgG antibodies or from the binding of one IgM molecule to several antigenic sites.

This means that in vivo D erythrocytes are destroyed by anti-D antibody by mechanisms other than that involving complement activation (see subsequent sections). Failure to bind complement also means that serologic tests for anti-D will not be evidenced by free hemolysis (dependent on complement activation) or by binding of complement molecules.

Placental Transfer of Anti-D Antibodies

The transfer of anti-D antibody into the fetal circulation is dependent on the Fc component of the IgG molecule (10). IgM and IgA antibodies lack this component and will not enter the fetal circulation. The rate at which IgG enters the fetal circulation has been reported to be rather slow, with a half-time of entry of approximately three weeks. This is of importance, of course, in the pathogenesis of Rh disease, since the amount of anti-D entering the fetal circulation will determine the severity of the disease. In a pregnancy in which antibodies only begin to appear late in the pregnancy, the slow rate of transplacental passage may protect the Rh-positive fetus. This may be one of the reasons the first affected child is usually not as sick as subsequent children (3). Since the majority of antibodies in a first-affected pregnancy appear after 22 weeks of gestation (15), it would seem reasonable that the severity of disease in such a fetus should not be as marked as in later pregnancies, in which antibodies are present from the beginning.

Although hemolytic disease tends to be more severe in a second than in a first pregnancy, the severity of disease in subsequent pregnancies tends to be more uniform (3).

Pathogenesis of Rh Immunization in Rh-negative Women

If Rh-negative women are transfused with D-positive erythrocytes, they may develop anti-D antibodies. Fortunately, such Rh-incompatible transfusions are now rare and are not a significant cause of Rh immunization. At present, immunization occurs almost exclusively as a result of a pregnancy in which the fetus is Rh-positive. Under these circumstances, the fetal erythrocyte crosses the placenta to enter the maternal circulation, representing thereby an Rh-incompatible transfusion.

TABLE 9–3. THE DEVELOPMENT OF ANTI-D (Rh$_0$) ANTIBODIES IN EXPERIMENTAL SUBJECTS AFTER A SINGLE INJECTION OF D-POSITIVE ERYTHROCYTES

VOLUME OF CELLS (ML.)	SOURCE OF CELLS	NO. DEVELOPING ANTIBODIES PER NO. INJECTED
0.1	Cord (16)	1/16
1.0	Adult (17)	7/13
10	Adult (18)	6/13
20	Adult (19)	5/6
250	Adult (20)	30/60

Antigenicity of Rh-positive Erythrocytes

To understand the process of Rh immunization, let us first consider findings in experimental subjects (Table 9–3). Rh immunization [i.e., the development of anti-D (Rh$_0$) antibodies] can be produced by injection of fetal or adult Rh-positive erythrocytes (16–20). The chance of immunization after a single injection is less when the volume of cells is small (i.e., 0.1 ml.). Repeated injections of small quantities increase the likelihood of immunization; however, not all subjects will develop antibodies, even though many injections are given or the volume of blood is great (Tables 9–3 and 9–4).

Pattern of Rh Isoimmunization

Figure 9–3 demonstrates examples of the various patterns of appearance of anti-D antibodies following an injection of D-positive erythrocytes. There are several characteristic features of Rh immunization depicted. Primary immunization with the appearance of anti-D antibodies may not be evident for several months following the immunogenic stimulus. The first antibody to appear tends to be an IgM ("saline," "complete") anti-D, followed by the IgG ("incomplete") antibody, as demonstrated by testing erythrocytes suspended in albumin. During primary immunization, the first antibody to appear may be demonstrable only by using enzyme-treated cells. This is an IgM antibody, which has been discussed in the section, Nature of Rh Antibody. Following a second injection of cells in an immunized subject, there is a rapid appearance of antibodies in high titer (a secondary response). The titer of antibody may decrease over time, and antibodies may not be demonstrable, even though the subject is immunized, as evidenced by the "secondary response" to another injection of D-positive erythrocytes (Fig. 9–3, *B*).

To these observations, we may now add another feature: primary immunization may first appear as a state in which D-positive erythrocytes have a shortened survival in the immunized subject, but there is no serologic evidence of anti-D antibodies. Such a state is usually followed by the appearance of demonstrable antibodies (17).

Fetal Erythrocytes and the Pathogenesis of Rh Immunization

Since the D antigen is found only on the erythrocyte, it seems reasonable to postulate that its entry into the maternal circula-

TABLE 9–4. THE DEVELOPMENT OF ANTI-D (Rh$_0$) ANTIBODIES IN EXPERIMENTAL SUBJECTS AFTER REPEATED INJECTIONS OF D-POSITIVE ERYTHROCYTES

VOLUME OF CELLS (ML.)	SOURCE OF CELLS AND REFERENCES	NO. OF INJECTIONS	INTERVALS BETWEEN INJECTIONS (WEEKS)	NO. DEVELOPING ANTIBODIES PER NO. INJECTED
0.1	Cord (15, 16)	5	6	5/16
3–5	Adult (21)	4	12–15	27/42
3–5	Adult (22)	5	12–15	15/32
5	Adult (19)	4	4	10/16

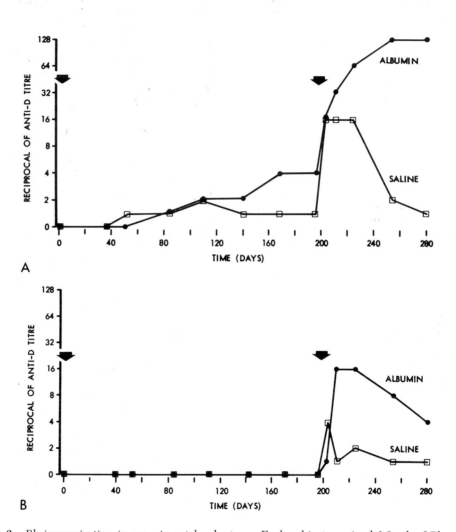

Figure 9–3. Rh immunization in experimental volunteers. Each subject received 2.0 ml. of Rh-positive cord erythrocytes on day 0 and day 196 (indicated by arrows). *A,* An antibody reacting with red cells suspended in saline (i.e., saline antibody) was demonstrable on day 52, and antibody reacting with cells suspended in albuumin (albumin antibody) was demonstrated later. These antibodies persisted and rose within seven days after the second injection (a secondary response). *B,* No saline or albumin antibodies were seen by day 196. A weak reaction was noted with papain-treated cells. Note the profound secondary response achieved and its similarity to that in *A.*

tion is the cause of Rh isoimmunization. The following observations support that hypothesis:

1. Fetal erythrocytes can be found in the maternal circulation as early as the second month of pregnancy and each month thereafter (23). The volume of cells is usually about 0.05 to 0.1 ml., a quantity which can produce primary immunization (see Table 9–3), particularly if given repeatedly (Table 9–4).

2. If pregnant women are studied often enough, most will be found to have fetal cells in their circulation at one time or another during pregnancy (23).

3. Rh immunization tends to occur more frequently when pregnancy has been complicated by toxemia, caesarean section, or manual removal of the placenta. Transplacental hemorrhage occurs more frequently and in greater volume under these circumstances (23–25).

Mechanism of Rh Immunization During Pregnancy

In Figure 9–4 there is a diagrammatic representation of the pathogenesis of Rh immunization. Fetal erythrocytes enter the maternal circulation in most pregnancies; the quantities are small, and, as shown in Tables 9–3 and 9–4, immunization would occur infrequently unless repeated hemor-

TABLE 9–5. THE RISK OF Rh IMMUNIZATION IN RELATION TO THE VOLUME OF FETAL CELLS FOUND IN THE MATERNAL CIRCULATION POST PARTUM*

VOLUME OF FETAL CELLS (ML.)	WOMEN IMMUNIZED PER TOTAL GROUP	%
0–0.1	16/538	3
>0.1	5/35	14.3
TOTAL	21/573	

*From Zipursky, A., and Israels, L. G.: Can. Med. Assoc. J. 97:1245, 1967.

rhages occur. Later in pregnancy, hemorrhages may be larger, particularly if there is interference with, or an abnormality of, the placental site (e.g., toxemia, manual removal of the placenta).

When a relatively large amount of fetal blood is present in the maternal circulation, the likelihood of Rh immunization is much greater (see Table 9–5) (26). Thus women who have received large volumes of fetal Rh-positive erythrocytes are a "high-risk" group in terms of developing Rh immunization. Nevertheless, Table 9–5 reveals that most cases of immunization do not result from a detectable bleed at delivery, but presumably from the smaller (<0.1 ml.) bleeds which occurred during pregnancy.

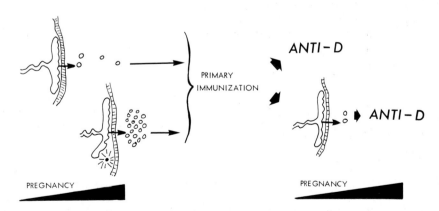

Figure 9–4. Hypothetical representation of the pathogenesis of Rh immunization during pregnancy. Two pregnancies are represented. In the first, primary immunization is shown to occur as a result either of a "large" hemorrhage at delivery or of smaller hemorrhages during pregnancy. Primary immunization can become manifest by the appearance of demonstrable antibodies, or a state of immunization can exist without demonstrable antibodies, which requires the antigenic stimulus of a second pregnancy to evoke the appearance of antibodies. (From Zipursky, A.; Pollock, J.; Chown, B. and Israels, L. G.: Transplacental Isoimmunization by Fetal Red Blood Cells. In *Birth Defects: Orig. Art. Ser.*, ed. D. Bergsma. *Symposium on the Placenta*, The National Foundation, New York, N. Y. Vol. I(1):87, 1965.)

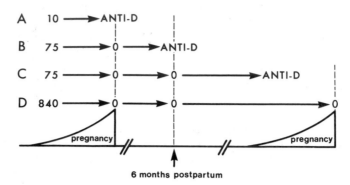

Figure 9–5. This is a hypothetical consideration of the pattern of Rh immunization during two pregnancies of 1000 Rh-negative women. The fetuses are all Rh-positive ABO-compatible.

A, Ten women develop antibodies during their first pregnancies. These are usually very weak, demonstrable only by reaction with enzyme-treated, Rh-positive erythrocytes.

B, Seventy-five women develop anti-D antibodies serologically demonstrable within six months post partum.

C, Seventy-five women have no antibodies at six months (they may have been present as weakly reactive antibodies earlier); antibodies appear during their second pregnancies as a result of the stimulus of fetal erythrocytes.

D, The remaining 840 women are not immunized.

Figure 9–4 also shows that primary immunization may manifest as serologically demonstrable antibodies or as a state of immunization which requires a second stimulus of fetal cells during the next Rh-positive pregnancy.

Let us summarize our present understanding of Rh immunization by considering what would happen to a group of 1000 Rh-negative women pregnant with their first Rh-positive fetuses (Fig. 9–5). Of these, 10 would develop antibodies prior to delivery. Another 75 would develop antibodies during the first six months after delivery. A further 75 would show no evidence of immunization at six months, but they would develop antibodies during their next pregnancy as a result of the stimulus of fetal Rh-positive erythrocytes.

Destruction of Fetal Erythrocytes by Anti-D (Rh₀) Antibody

Erythrocyte Destruction In Vivo

The transfer of anti-D antibody into the fetal circulation and the subsequent destruction of Rh-positive fetal erythrocytes represent the basic pathogenic mechanisms responsible for Rh hemolytic disease of the newborn.

The destruction of these cells can be followed by observing the fate of radio-labeled cells in circulation. Figure 9–6 is taken from the original work of Jandl et al. on the fate of Rh-sensitized cells (27). In this study, erythrocytes were sensitized in vitro with anti-D serum, labeled with chromium-51, and injected into the circulation of a normal subject. Since these cells had been sensitized by an IgG anti-D, they would have had a positive Coombs' reaction. It can be observed that half of the erythrocytes were destroyed within thirty minutes, and that the radioactivity appeared in the spleen, displaying this as the major organ of destruction.

This pattern of splenic destruction of IgG-sensitized erythrocytes is referred to as extravascular hemolysis, in contrast to the intravascular hemolysis which occurs with complement-fixing antibodies (see subsequent section). In the latter instance, red cell destruction occurs in the blood stream, and the radioactivity released from chromium-labeled cells would appear in the liver (27).

In Figure 9–7, it is shown that the rate of destruction of anti-D–sensitized cells is proportional to the amount of anti-D on the cells (28). At the highest levels of sensitization (i.e., more than 32 μg. per ml.), erythrocyte destruction exceeds that which can be accounted for by splenic trapping and radioactivity accumulates in the liver and is found in the plasma hemoglobin fraction. Thus, with extremely high levels

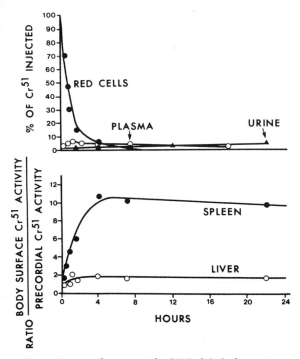

of Rh sensitization, intravascular hemolysis can occur in addition to lysis in the spleen.

The above data therefore tell us that in hemolytic disease of the newborn erythrocyte destruction occurs primarily in the spleen.

Let us now consider the mechanism by which this destruction occurs. If all sensitized erythrocytes are cleared during a single passage through the spleen, the half-life of survival would be approximately thirty minutes, as in Figure 9–6.

How does one explain the observation that the erythrocytes of a newborn with Rh hemolytic disease [which may be sensitized with up to 18 μg. anti-D per ml. (29)] have a survival greater than three days in their own circulation (30), yet last only minutes when infused into a normal recipient (27)?

It would appear that the rate-limiting step for erythrocyte destruction under these circumstances is the capacity of the reticuloendothelial cells of the spleen. When only minute quantities of sensitized erythrocytes are infused into a normal recipient, the spleen can trap and destroy all the cells passing through it. On the other hand, in the subject with hemolytic disease, the "splenic trap" is working fully and can

Figure 9–6. The survival of ^{51}Cr-labeled, anti-D–sensitized erythrocytes after injection into a normal recipient. Note the rapid disappearance of erythrocyte radioactivity ($t_{1/2}$ = 30 minutes), with the appearance of radioactivity over the spleen. Little radioactivity appears in the plasma or urine, compared to the large amounts which would result from intravascular hemolysis. (From Jandl, J. H., Jones, A. R., et al.: J. Clin. Invest. 36:1428, 1957.)

Figure 9–7. The in vivo survival of minute quantities (0.2–1.0 ml.) of Rh-positive erythrocytes, sensitized with varying concentrations of anti-D antibody. The figures represent the amount of antibody on the red cell in μg. of antibody per ml. of red cells. (From Mollison, P. L., Crome, P., et al.: Br. J. Haematol. 11:461, 1965.)

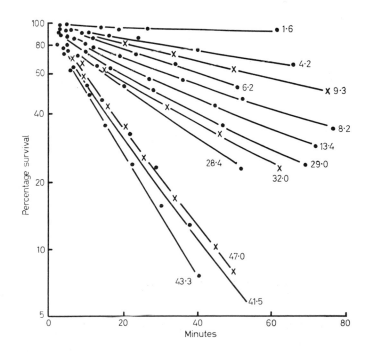

destroy only a small fraction of the large mass of sensitized cells.

It can be concluded, therefore, that the rate of red cell destruction in hemolytic disease of the newborn is related to both the amount of anti-D on the red cells and the capacity of the reticuloendothelial system to destroy these cells.

Destruction of Anti-D–Sensitized Cells in the Spleen

The spleen contains sinusoids through which erythrocytes flow and a system of cords in which erythrocytes are packed at high hematocrit in a plasma of low pH and high protein content (31). These environmental characteristics would enhance agglutination of IgG-sensitized cells (see preceding section). It has been postulated, therefore, that agglutinate formation in the spleen might be the mechanism of splenic trapping and destruction of anti-D–sensitized cells (27). This hypothesis is difficult to support, since minute (< 1 ml.) quantities of D-positive–sensitized cells are readily destroyed by anti-D antibodies in the circulation of an Rh-negative subject (Fig. 9–7). It is difficult to see how these dilute concentrations (less than 1 in 5000) of Rh-positive erythrocytes could be cleared by a single passage through the spleen. Furthermore, a process of agglutination would not explain the "saturation" of the trapping mechanism which occurs during the hemolytic process as described above.

Erythrocytes with membrane abnormalities (e.g., hereditary spherocytosis) are trapped and destroyed in the spleen. It has been suggested that the reduced deformability of such cells results in their trapping (32). Several studies have suggested abnormalities of membrane function of anti-D–sensitized cells (e.g., decreased ATP synthesis (33) and diminished filterability (34), but there is no direct evidence that this is the cause of splenic trapping and destruction. Spherocytosis does not occur in Rh hemolytic disease of the newborn.

Erythrophagocytosis by Monocytes and Macrophages

The destruction of anti-D–sensitized cells within the spleen may occur by macrophage ingestion. Monocytes and macrophages have membrane receptors for the Fc fragment of the IgG molecule (35, 36, 37).

Attachment of the anti-D–sensitized cell results in its almost immediate ingestion (37). It has been suggested that erythrocyte binding to a macrophage may be sufficient to lead to its destruction, possibly through an intermediate step of sphering (36). This postulate was based on in vitro observations in which sensitized erythrocytes were bound to, but not ingested by, macrophages. Our own studies have shown that any interference with macrophage function (e.g., cooling, metabolic inhibitors, centrifugation) will prevent phagocytosis although binding occurs (37). With viable, functioning macrophages, the major process is erythrophagocytosis in vitro and in vivo (Fig. 9–8). It is possible, however, that in vivo, under certain circumstances (see below), binding may occur which leads to erythrocyte destruction on the surface of the monocyte.

There are several reports of monocyte erythrophagocytosis in the peripheral blood of newborns with Rh hemolytic disease (38). However, there is difficulty in accepting the thesis that the major mechanism of destruction of anti-D–sensitized cells occurs by macrophage binding or phagocytosis. These processes are inhibited by as little as two μg. per ml. of nonspecific IgG, presumably by competing for the Fc receptor site on the macrophage surface (36, 37). The normal plasma concentration of IgG is 10,000 μg. per ml. How, then, can erythrophagocytosis occur in the spleen?

Recently it has been shown that this inhibitory effect of IgG can be overcome if the sensitized erythrocytes are brought into contact with the macrophages by centrifugation (37). This also can be demonstrated in vivo by placing the sensitized erythrocytes in a cutaneous exudate (i.e., Rebuck skin window, as shown in Fig. 9–8), where they come into direct contact with the macrophages. Erythrophagocytosis occurs despite the high concentration of IgG present in the exudate.

In the spleen, erythrocytes pass through sinusoids and cords, both of which contain macrophages. In the cords, particularly, the erythrocytes are packed against the macrophages (Fig. 9–9), overcoming the potential inhibition of IgG and resulting

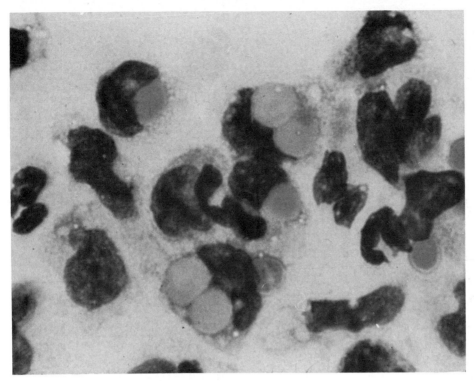

Figure 9–8. A Rebuck skin window preparation, in which anti-D–sensitized erythrocytes have been ingested by macrophages. Note that neutrophil erythrophagocytosis is not seen.

in destruction either on the macrophage surface or more likely by erythrophagocytosis.

The Spleen in Hemolytic Disease of the Newborn

Is there evidence that erythrocyte destruction occurs in the spleen in hemolytic disease of the newborn? The spleen is enlarged in this disease due to engorgement with erythrocytes, to extramedullary hemopoiesis (see below), and to hyperplasia of reticuloendothelial cells (i.e., macrophages). The latter phenomenon has been demonstrated experimentally in animals by producing hemolytic anemia; parenthetically, it should be added that when the rate of red cell destruction is reduced in such animals, splenic size decreases (39). Further evidence of erythrocyte destruction is found in the accumulation of hemosiderin (agglomerates of ferritin) in the macrophages of the spleen of these infants (40). There is little evidence of erythrophagocytosis by light microscopy; however, detailed electron microscopic examinations

would be necessary to establish its presence (41).

Destruction of the Erythrocyte and Disposal of Its Products

Erythrocytes or their products are ingested in the spleen by macrophages which contain the necessary enzymes for hemoglobin digestion. The globin portion of the molecule is digested by lysosomal proteolytic enzymes, presumably releasing the heme.

Heme oxygenase is a microsomal enzyme which digests heme, opening the tetrapyrrole ring by release of a molecule of carbon monoxide from the α-methene bridge (42). This produces the greenish pigment biliverdin, which is reduced to bilirubin by the enzyme, bilirubin reductase. The iron released from heme is taken up by apoferritin to form the storage molecule, ferritin. Thus erythrocyte digestion produces ferritin (which can aggregate to form hemosiderin), bilirubin, and carbon monoxide. The proteolytic enzymes necessary for globin digestion and heme oxygenase increase in concentration as a result of erythrophagocytosis (43).

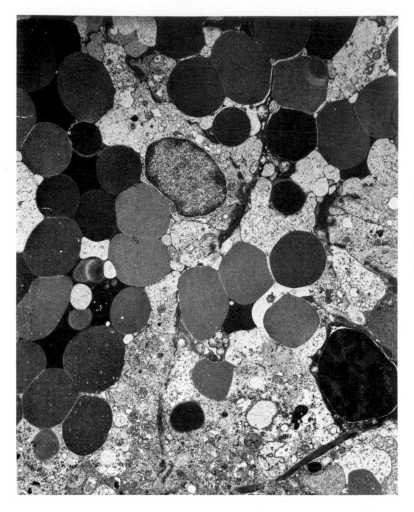

Figure 9–9. An electron photomicrograph of the spleen of a mouse with hereditary spherocytosis, showing the intimate contact between erythrocytes (dark circles) and macrophage cytoplasm (pale, granular background) within the splenic cord. (Prepared by Dr. David Mayman.)

As noted above, one molecule of carbon monoxide is released for each molecule of heme degraded. Hence the production of carbon monoxide should reflect the rate of erythrocyte destruction. Indeed, the blood concentration (44) and production (45) of carbon monoxide are significantly increased in Rh hemolytic disease.

Intravascular Hemolysis in Rh Hemolytic Disease

As noted above, erythrocytes sensitized with high concentrations are destroyed in vivo at rates greater than that which can be accounted for by the spleen. Under these circumstances, free hemoglobin appears in the plasma, presumably because of intravascular hemolysis. In severe hemolytic disease of the newborn, one may find elevated levels of plasma hemoglobin and, as a result, the accumulation of the oxidized product of hemoglobin, methemalbumin (46). The plasma concentrations of haptoglobin (hemoglobin-binding protein) and hemopexin (heme-binding protein) tend to be low as a result of intravascular hemolysis. In the normal newborn, these proteins may be absent or very low and consequently of little value in the diagnosis of intravascular hemolysis (47).

Response of the Fetus to Erythrocyte Destruction

Fetal Erythropoiesis

The fetus is not at risk from hyperbilirubinemia because of the placenta's capacity to clear bilirubin. The risk of Rh hemolytic disease in the fetus is directly related to erythrocyte destruction and the resulting anemia. The fetus responds to erythrocyte destruction by the production of erythropoietin, as do older human beings. Erythropoietin has been found in high levels in the cord blood of newborns with Rh hemolytic disease (48). Red cell production is greatly increased, as evidenced by the high level of normoblasts in the peripheral blood, as well as the high percentage of reticulocytes.

As a result of the sustained demand for red cell production, active erythropoietic tissue is increased in the marrow and appears in other sites throughout the body, particularly in the liver and spleen (49). A major portion of the hepatosplenomegaly of hemolytic disease of the newborn is extramedullary hematopoiesis.

Fetal Anemia

In severe Rh disease, erythrocyte destruction cannot be compensated for by erythropoiesis, and anemia develops. The results of this anemia are many. The body's response to a decrease in circulating red cell mass is an increase in plasma volume; total blood volume is normal. As anemia proceeds, cardiovascular compensation fails, and tissue hypoxia develops, with resultant metabolic acidosis and death (50).

Hydrops Fetalis

There is a characteristic syndrome of massive edema and anasarca associated with very severe hemolytic disease of the newborn referred to as hydrops fetalis. This tends to occur in severely anemic infants, and it has been postulated, therefore, that it is the result of heart failure secondary to anemia. However, infants with hemoglobins as high as 10 g. per 100 ml. have shown evidence of hydrops, and conversely infants with hemoglobins as low as 3 g. per 100 ml. have not developed hydrops (51). It would appear, therefore, that there are additional factors which influence the development of hydrops in severe hemolytic

disease of the fetus. It is known that venous pressure can be very high in afflicted newborns, and this has been related to cardiac failure and expanded blood volume. It is likely, however, that the elevated central venous and arterial pressures are related directly to fetal asphyxia, and when these are corrected, both the above values return to normal (50). Hydrops fetalis has also been associated with depressed levels of serum protein (52), although serum protein values do not bear a direct relationship to the development of hydrops. More recently, the nonprotein oncotic pressure of plasma has been found to be very low in infants with hydrops, and this may contribute to the pathogenesis of this syndrome (52).

Bringing all the above information together, it would appear that hydrops fetalis is associated with severe hemolytic disease of the newborn, usually with profound anemia. The accumulation of fluid may in part be related to heart failure or to the elevated venous pressure associated with fetal asphyxia. The reasons for the fall in oncotic pressure (in part due to a lowering of serum proteins, but in part to other factors) is not clear at this point, but it also seems to play a role in the pathogenesis of this syndrome. Associated with hydrops, there is a characteristic increase in the weight of the placenta with edema of the chorionic villi, which also may play a role in the development of hydrops, possibly by interfering with water transport across the villus.

Other Pathology

There is involvement of other organs in Rh hemolytic disease, the nature of which is not clearly understood. The pancreas shows distinct islet cell hyperplasia, and this has been associated with the development postnatally of hypoglycemia. In the liver, cellular necrosis has been noted, and this is often associated with the presence of high levels of direct bilirubin at birth and subsequently the development of a prolonged obstructive jaundice in the neonate. These phenomena tend to occur particularly in the severe forms of hemolytic disease.

Bilirubin Metabolism in the Fetus and Newborn With Rh Hemolytic Disease
(see also Chapter 3)

Bilirubin Metabolism in the Fetus

Bilirubin produced in the reticuloendothelial cell is lipid-soluble and therefore can traverse the membrane to enter the plasma, where it tends to bind to plasma albumin. The binding of the bilirubin to the albumin molecule is due to the steric configuration of that molecule, which permits certain hydrophobic areas to develop in which the lipid-soluble bilirubin molecule can reside and be held (53). Thus, in circulation, bilirubin is for the most part bound to albumin, but there is a small component in plasma which is free and is in equilibrium with that bound to the albumin. The relative amounts of soluble and bound bilirubin are dependent on the association constants of the bilirubin binding sites, the pH of the blood, the relative quantities of bilirubin and albumin, and the presence of factors which will compete for the bilirubin binding sites (54, 55) (see below and Fig. 9–10).

Under normal circumstances, bilirubin circulating in the plasma is mostly in the bound state, and it is very difficult to dissociate the bilirubin from the albumin. Even prolonged dialysis of plasma does not remove all the bilirubin from albumin (53). We therefore may assume that bilirubin is distributed throughout the body, very much in keeping with the size of the albumin pool, which is approximately twice the size of the plasma volume (4).

In the fetus, bilirubin levels are not high, but they increase rapidly after birth, causing the characteristic jaundice of hemolytic disease. Accordingly, there must be some means for the removal of bilirubin from the fetus in utero. Clearly, this is through the placenta, which has now been shown to freely transport unconjugated bilirubin as a lipid-soluble material (56).

It has been shown clearly that the rate of transport of bilirubin across the placental membrane is far greater than that of albumin (57). Thus the transport of bilirubin into the maternal sinusoids of the placenta

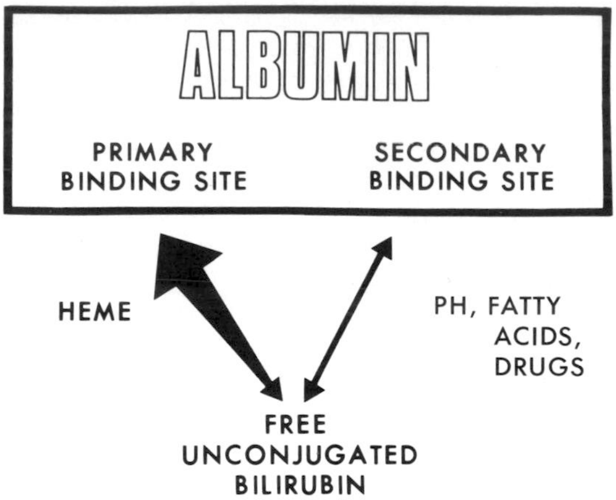

Figure 9–10. A hypothetical presentation of the phenomenon of bilirubin binding to serum albumin (54, 55).

The primary site can bind one molecule of bilirubin with great avidity. Heme also can bind to that site, so that, in the presence of intravascular hemolysis, considerably less bilirubin is bound to the primary site (71).

It should be noted that the primary site is completely saturated at a serum bilirubin/albumin ratio of approximately 25 mg. per 3.0 g.

Therefore, at higher serum bilirubin concentrations (above 20 mg. per 100 ml.), the secondary binding site (or sites) is occupied by bilirubin. The binding affinity of this site is much lower than that of the primary site, and therefore the bilirubin is readily displaced by lowering the pH, by major increases in the fatty acid levels, or by a variety of drugs, such as salicylate, diazepam, sulfisoxazole, caffeine sodium benzoate, tolbutamide, furosemide, sodium oxacillin, hydrocortisone, gentamycin, and sulfadiazine (76).

is, in its free form, then followed by binding to the maternal albumin.

Another path of excretion is into the amniotic fluid. It is clear now that small quantities of bilirubin enter the amniotic fluid (58); in fact, this phenomenon serves as the basis for the antepartum diagnostic tests utilizing amniocentesis to determine bilirubin levels. Heme pigments are also found in the amniotic fluid.

It can be calculated that the total amount of bilirubin in the amniotic fluid which turns over relatively slowly, is seldom more than 2 mg. and therefore constitutes a relatively insignificant excretory mechanism for removing bilirubin from the baby with Rh hemolytic disease (58). In summary, because of the ability of the placenta to transport and remove bilirubin, there is little problem with hyperbilirubinemia in the fetus. Kernicterus does not occur in utero, and there is no other evidence of bilirubin tissue damage.

Bilirubin Metabolism After Birth

After birth, the protective mechanism of the placenta is lost, and the baby must fare for himself in removing bilirubin from the circulation. The major mechanism by which this is done is through the liver. The unconjugated bilirubin, circulating predominantly as albumin-bound, must be taken up by the liver. Bilirubin enters the hepatic cell in the free form, since albumin cannot cross the membrane (53). The free bilirubin within the cell is quickly bound to the binding proteins of the liver cell. The concept of specific bilirubin binding proteins ("Y and Z" or "ligandin") in liver cells has been demonstrated recently (59), and is of considerable importance to the newborn because these particular bilirubin binding proteins are in low concentration in newborn animals (60). Obviously if a deficiency of the binding proteins exists, then it is difficult to maintain a free bilirubin gradient into the cell, and bilirubin clearance from the plasma is reduced. This may be a major cause of hyperbilirubinemia in the newborn infant (60).

The next step in the metabolism of bilirubin is conjugation as a bilirubin glucuronide. The enzyme glucuronyl transferase, which is central to this mechanism, is markedly deficient in the newborn and contributes to the relative inability of the newborn infant to conjugate and remove bilirubin from the body (55).

In adults and older children, severe hemolytic disease almost never results in bilirubin levels greater than 4 mg. per 100 ml. Clearly the excess hyperbilirubinemia that occurs in hemolytic disease of the newborn reflects more than excessive destruction; it represents, in fact, a failure of the liver to handle the bilirubin load. Specifically the areas of deficiency in the newborn may be the binding proteins Y and Z ("ligandin") and the enzyme, glucuronyl transferase. Recently, it has been shown both in humans and in experimental animals that phenobarbital increases both the enzyme system (55) and the binding proteins in the liver of the newborn (56). Accordingly,

phenobarbital administered to newborns or to antepartum mothers results in a more rapid rate of clearance of bilirubin and a lower serum bilirubin level (61, 62).

In the newborn and in experimental animals, there are few other ways in which bilirubin can be cleared. A small amount is lost through the wall of the intestine, and it is likely that a small proportion of bilirubin is broken down into water-soluble products (presumably dipyrroles and tetrapyrroles) (63). Exposure of bilirubin in vitro or in vivo to light results in an increase in these water-soluble products. This, then, is the basis of phototherapy, namely, the production of relatively non-toxic, water-soluble products which are capable of entering both the bile and the urine for excretion (63). The toxicity of these products has been questioned from time to time, but at present there is no evidence, either in vitro or in vivo, to suggest that the soluble photo-oxidation products of bilirubin are in themselves toxic. They do not compete with bilirubin for the bilirubin binding sites of albumin, nor do they enter the brain or cerebrospinal fluid (63).

Bilirubin Toxicity

Hyperbilirubinemia causes brain damage resulting in death or residual neurologic defects (ataxia, deafness, mental retardation). At postmortem examination, the brains show yellow staining of basal ganglia and cerebellum (i.e., kernicterus). Many in vitro studies have been done to determine the nature of bilirubin toxicity. It was once believed that bilirubin interfered specifically with oxidative phosphorylation. This is now considered unlikely (64), and there is evidence that there is an effect of free bilirubin on brain cell mitochondria. Concentrations of free bilirubin of 0.1 mg. per 100 ml. cause mitochondrial swelling (65). Furthermore, brain cell mitochondrial swelling has been demonstrated by electron microscopy in hyperbilirubinemic rats (66). It may be that brain cells are particularly susceptible because they do not contain the bilirubin binding protein, "ligandin," and as a result free bilirubin can accumulate within the cell (67). Certainly it has been shown that, with hyperbilirubinemia, free bilirubin (lipid-soluble) enters many tissues and, in particular, the brain. In experimental systems, it has been shown to enter most parts of the brain (68); however, the pathologic process known as kernicterus refers to staining of specific areas of the brain, particularly the basal ganglia and cerebellum. It may well be that the entry of bilirubin initially into all areas tends to produce toxicity only in certain suceptible tissues, namely, the basal ganglia and the cerebellum. Once injured (e.g., by bilirubin or by anoxia), brain tissue tends to be more susceptible to further bilirubin accumulation (68).

Since most babies are hyperbilirubinemic, and since all babies with clinical Rh hemolytic disease are severely hyperbilirubinemic, what determines whether babies will develop kernicterus or not? It had been suggested that bilirubin accumulates in the brain of the newborn because of "immaturity of the blood-brain barrier." Diamond and Schmid, using ^{14}C-labeled bilirubin, have refuted this hypothesis by showing bilirubin accumulation in the brain of the adult Gunn rat (68); furthermore, proven cases of kernicterus in older children (as old as 15 years) have occurred with the profound hyperbilirubinemia (unconjugated) of the Crigler-Najjar syndrome (68). It would appear now that the level of free unconjugated bilirubin in the plasma is the determining toxicity factor. There is much evidence to suggest that conjugated bilirubin and unconjugated bilirubin bound to albumin do not enter the central nervous system and are not toxic to cells (68). The concentration of free bilirubin in the plasma is dependent, as noted previously (Fig. 9–10), on many factors. As a result, considerable effort has been undertaken to develop suitable means for the estimation of free unconjugated bilirubin in the plasma. Certain specific dyes (HBABA, PSP) bind to albumin; their ability to bind to albumin is reduced if bilirubin is present on the albumin molecule (69). Accordingly, the HBABA or PSP-binding capacity of the plasma should reflect the available bilirubin binding sites on the albumin, hence the risk of free bilirubin accumulation. Since these dyes do not compete specifically with the bilirubin binding site, they have not proven to be an effective means of esti-

mating the bilirubin binding capacity of albumin (69).

Lucey has reported a series of infants who developed kernicterus despite the presence of available dye-binding sites on the plasma albumin (70). Accordingly, at the present time, dye-binding techniques cannot be recommended.

Odell and his group have carried out studies in which they have attempted to measure the amount of bilirubin bound to albumin by observing the amount which could be displaced by salicylate (Fig. 9–10) (71). These studies determine the amount of bilirubin on the secondary binding sites of albumin; when this is great, the risk of free bilirubin accumulation increases. It would appear that infants who have had high indices of displaceable bilirubin, determined in this way, are at greater risk of kernicterus and brain damage (72). More recently, studies using column chromatographic techniques have endeavored to measure the amount of free unconjugated bilirubin present in plasma.

It has been shown that, in hyperbilirubinemic babies, free unconjugated bilirubin levels may be 0.1 to 0.5 mg. per 100 ml. (73); rarely a level as high as 1.0 mg. per 100 ml. has been found. Kernicterus is more likely to develop at the higher levels. Thus there appears to be a relationship between the presence of brain damage and the amount of unconjugated free bilirubin.

At the present time, techniques are available for the determination of free bilirubin levels (74) and potentially, therefore, the risk of brain damage. More recently, it has become possible to determine the bilirubin reserve binding capacity, so that one can predict the level at which albumin becomes saturated and exchange transfusion should be performed (75). Until these methods are definitively coordinated with clinical outcome, we must continue to use the criteria which have evolved from many clinical studies concerning the danger levels of total bilirubin in plasma. These are discussed in a subsequent section. However, in considering hyperbilirubinemia, the clinician must bear in mind the importance of competing molecules, such as free fatty acids or sulfa drugs, the albumin level, and the presence or absence of acidosis (76) (Fig. 9–10).

Prevention and Treatment of Rh Hemolytic Disease of the Newborn

Prevention of Rh Immunization in the Mother at Risk

Approximately 16 per cent of the Rh-negative women who have delivered an Rh-positive, ABO-compatible baby will develop anti-D antibodies as a result of the pregnancy (Fig. 9–5). For most of these women, Rh immunization can be prevented by the administration of anti-D–containing gamma globulin within the first three days following delivery. Accordingly, it can be stated that all Rh-negative women should receive anti-D gamma globulin within 72 hours following the delivery of an Rh-positive, ABO-compatible infant. The recommended dose is 300 μg. of anti-D. The effectiveness of this therapy has been shown by worldwide cooperative studies. In one such study, 15 per cent of the untreated controls developed anti-Rh antibodies, compared to 1 per cent of the treated subjects (Tables 9–6 and 9–7) (77).

It has been described above that fetal cells enter the circulation during most of pregnancy and are found following abortions. Accordingly, it would seem reasonable to conclude that Rh-negative women are also at risk of developing antibodies following an abortion. In fact, this has been described in one study, in which 4 per cent of women developed antibodies following abortion (78). This study requires confirmation, but it is unlikely that such a prospective study would be undertaken now. Therefore, it must be assumed that these women are at risk, and it can be recommended that 300 μg. of anti-Rh immunoglobulin should be administered to all nonimmunized Rh-

negative women after abortion. The correct dosage and effectiveness of such treatment remains to be determined.

In our own studies (77), we have shown that approximately one in 250 Rh-negative women will, at the time of delivery, have a "massive" fetal transplacental hemorrhage. In these women, the volume of blood is such that it demands a greater dosage of the anti-Rh immunoglobulin than commonly recommended. We recommend therefore that all Rh-negative women should be screened for massive transplacental hemorrhage using the Kleihauer acid elution technique. If such hemorrhages are found, anti-Rh immunoglobulin should be given at a dosage of 10 μg. per ml. of fetal blood.

Passive immunization postpartum does not prevent all cases of Rh immunization. As shown in Tables 9–6 and 9–7, for every 15 women protected, one woman will develop Rh antibodies. It is likely that most of these antibodies develop as a result of an immunogenic stimulus well before delivery, so that the immune processes are sufficiently well developed that passive immunization will not stop it. Since fetal red blood cells enter the circulation throughout most of pregnancy, it is possible that the antigenic stimulus can occur very early indeed. Various studies now suggest that 1 to 2 per cent of Rh-negative women will develop antibodies prior to delivery, and, for them, anti-Rh immunoglobulin is of no use (77). The question now remains as to whether this group should have prophylaxis during pregnancy. No definitive information is available, and, at the present time, this procedure cannot be recommended.

I have stated above that anti-Rh immunoglobulin should be used following the delivery of an Rh-positive, ABO-compatible infant. The qualification "ABO-compatible" relates to the fact that Rh immunization is

TABLE 9-6. PREVENTION OF Rh IMMUNIZATION BY TREATING POSTPARTUM WOMEN WITH ANTI-Rh IMMUNOGLOBULIN*

CONTROLS			TREATED		
No.	No. Immunized	% Immunized	No.	No. Immunized	% Immunized
3390	220	6	2920	10	0.34

*From Zipursky, A.: Clin. Obstet. Gynecol. *14*:869, 1971.

TABLE 9–7. THE APPEARANCE OF ANTI-Rh_0 (D) ANTIBODIES IN
SUBSEQUENT Rh-POSITIVE PREGNANCIES OF Rh-NEGATIVE WOMEN
INCLUDED IN THE SERIES IN TABLE 9–6*

CONTROLS			TREATED		
No.	No. Immunized	% Immunized	No.	No. Immunized	% Immunized
533	50	9	297	2	0.7

*From Zipursky, A.: Clin. Obstet. Gynecol. *14*:869, 1971.

very uncommon following an ABO-incompatible pregnancy. It would appear that the risk is approximately 1/10 to 1/25 that of the ABO-compatible pregnancy. Therefore its use is of much lower priority than in compatible pregnancies. Nevertheless, immunization can occur, and although the risk is less, prophylaxis is recommended (77).

*Prevention of Death in the
"Fetus at Risk"*

DIAGNOSIS. The entry of maternal anti-D antibody into the fetal circulation causes the destruction of D-positive erythrocytes, with resulting anemia. Death may result with or without hydrops.

As described earlier, the fetus is not at risk from hyperbilirubinemia. Accordingly, therapy of the fetus is directed towards the prevention of stillbirth. Fifty per cent of stillbirths will occur before 32 weeks of gestation, and, for them, intrauterine trans-

fusion remains the only hope of survival at this stage.

Let us now consider the means by which stillbirths can be predicted in utero, and then we shall discuss the matter of prevention of stillbirths.

History. The severity of Rh hemolytic disease tends to be somewhat consistent in successive pregnancies. Thus the Rh-negative woman who has had a severely affected infant in the past is at high risk of having a stillbirth, as shown in Figure 9–11. However, even in those women who have had a previous stillbirth, approximately 40 per cent of their infants will be born alive. Furthermore, 35 per cent of stillbirths occur in a first-affected pregnancy (i.e., no history of disease). It is clear, therefore, that history alone is of limited predictive value in individual pregnancies.

Maternal Anti-D (Rh_0) Titer. The severity of Rh disease is dependent on the amount of maternal anti-D entering the fetal circulation. Accordingly, the titer of anti-D has been used as a prognostic index

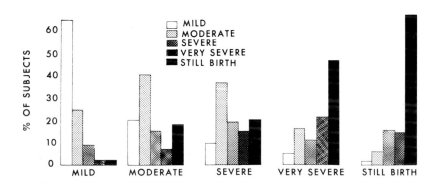

Figure 9–11. The relation between severity in a given case of Rh hemolytic disease and the severity in the previous affected infant.

Mild = no transfusion requirement; moderate = Hb >11.0 g.; severe = cord Hb <11.0 g. and/or bilirubin >5.0 mg. per 100 ml.; very severe = cord Hb <7.5 g. per 100 ml. and/or hydrops. [After Walker, W., In *Recent Advances in Pediatrics.* 4th ed. Gairdner, D., and Hull, D. (eds.), London, J. A. Churchill, 1971, p. 119.]

(Table 9–8). However, as described earlier, the severity of disease is dependent on additional factors other than the amount of antibody bound to the erythrocyte.

Bowman and Pollock state that stillbirths rarely occur in mothers whose anti-D concentration (by albumin technique) does not exceed 1/8 (79). Walker found that a titer (by indirect Coombs') of less than 1/16 seldom was associated with stillbirth (Fig. 9–12) (3). In pregnancies in which the father is heterozygous, the maternal anti-D titer is of limited value, since the fetus may be Rh-negative.

It is evident, therefore, that history and antibody titers are of limited value for prognosis. Their value is to alert the physician to perform a more accurate diagnostic test, namely amniocentesis. If the previous history includes a stillbirth or severe Rh disease, or if the antibody titer (indirect Coombs') is greater than 1/8, amniocentesis should be performed. Since antibody techniques vary, the critical level should be established by each laboratory.

Amniocentesis. Bilirubin accumulates in the amniotic fluid, where it turns over very slowly (58); its concentration reflects the concentration of fetal plasma bilirubin and the severity of hemolytic disease (61). The mechanism of entry of bilirubin into the amniotic fluid is not clearly understood, although it is thought to pass from the fetal plasma possibly through the membranes covering the umbilical cord (61).

The accumulation of bilirubin in amniotic fluid relates to the fetal serum bilirubin level. However, in severe fetal disease, these values no longer correlate in that considerably higher bilirubin levels are found in amniotic fluid than those in the serum. It is likely, therefore, that this accumulation results from the higher con-

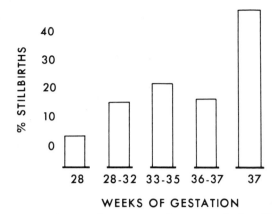

Figure 9–12. The gestational age at which stillbirths result from Rh hemolytic disease of the newborn. [After Walker, W., In *Recent Advances in Pediatrics.* 4th ed. Gairdner, D., and Hull, D. (eds.), London, J. A. Churchill, 1971, p. 119.]

centration of protein found in the amniotic fluid of these patients. Thus the high amniotic fluid bilirubin levels in severe Rh disease result both from excessive bilirubin production and increased bilirubin binding protein in the amniotic fluid (80).

Amniocentesis should be performed at 22 weeks gestation; it is unreasonable to perform it earlier since intrauterine transfusion is not recommended prior to that time (81). The procedure of amniocentesis is well described (82), and care should be taken to avoid striking the placenta, which may result in massive transplacental hemorrhage, possibly increasing the degree of isoimmunization (83) or causing fetal death. Placental localization by ultrasound or radioisotope screening can prevent this complication (77).

The concentration of bilirubin in the amniotic fluid is quite low. For example, normal levels are 0.04 mg. per 100 ml.; values above 0.1 mg. per 100 ml. occur in Rh hemolytic disease, and if the level reaches 0.8 mg. per 100 ml., fetal death is almost certain (84). As a result, it has been difficult to determine amniotic fluid bilirubins accurately. The spectrophotometric technique originally developed by Liley (85) has received the greatest attention and has been used as the basis for many large studies of intrauterine transfusions.

Using this technique, the accuracy of diagnosis of the severity of hemolytic disease is quite good. Bowman and Pollack

TABLE 9–8. RELATION BETWEEN MATERNAL ANTIBODY TITER AND SEVERITY OF DISEASE IN NEWBORN

Titer	Mild (No Treatment)	Treated	Stillbirth
<1/8	53	23	1
1/16–1/64	18	42	9
>1/64	0	16	3

point out that this technique is 100 per cent accurate in determining whether the fetus of a mother who has a significant titer of anti-D (see above) is Rh-positive or -negative (79). They also believe that the technique is 97 per cent accurate in determining the severity of disease, so that appropriate therapy can be given.

As shown in Figure 9–13, amniotic fluid values in zone 3 or high zone 2 are indicative of severe fetal disease. In addition, a rising level is further evidence of severe disease (81). Accordingly it is now recommended that repeat amniocentesis be performed at one- to two-week intervals (depending on initial O.D. values) to determine whether a rising trend is seen. Decision regarding intrauterine transfusion is based on a high zone 2 or zone 3 level associated with a rising trend.

The analysis of amniotic fluid must be done with care, since values can decline because of light exposure or can be misinterpreted because of contamination by meconium, hemoglobin, heme, or cellular debris.

TREATMENT. If it is determined that severe disease exists in the fetus, a decision regarding therapy must be made. As shown in Figure 9–12, the majority of cases of stillbirth occur after 33 weeks of gestation. If gestation is greater than 33 weeks, premature induction is recommended, since survival may be as high as 98 per cent (86). Even in the best of hands, intrauterine transfusion carries a risk of death to the fetus (6.4 per cent) (81). Therefore, it should be reserved for those fetuses in whom chance of survival by premature induction is less than 6 per cent.

A decision regarding premature induction of labor now should include an analysis of the lecithin-sphingomyelin ratio of the amniotic fluid (87). If this ratio is high (> 1.5) the chances of developing the respiratory distress syndrome are low, and it is safer to proceed with premature induction.

For such infants (severe disease at less than 33 weeks gestation), intrauterine transfusion offers the only hope when death appears certain. Intrauterine transfusions have been employed extensively since the first description by Liley in 1963 (88).

Since it is a relatively new and compli-

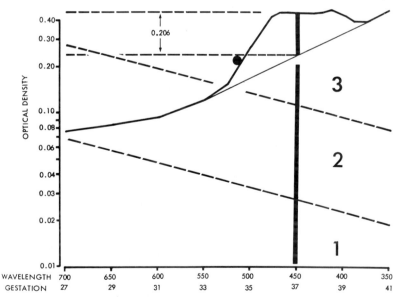

Figure 9–13. The spectrophotometric method of estimating amniotic fluid bilirubin levels. The optical density is measured from wavelength 350 mμ to 700 mμ. The optical density rise at 450 mμ (due to bilirubin) is measured by the rise in optical density at that point above the projected base line. The graph shown is of the amniotic fluid of a woman at 34.5 weeks gestation. The optical density at 450 mμ in this case was 0.206.

The value 0.206 is then plotted on the graph superimposed in this figure and shown in slanted dotted lines, which delineate three zones—1, 2, and 3. In this case, 0.206 lies in zone 3. Zone 3 represents severe disease with impending fetal death; zone 2 = less severe disease; zone 1 = Rh-negative infant or very mild disease.

The calculated optical density must be plotted in this way because the optical density decreases with gestational age. (From Bowman, J. M., and Pollock, J. M.: Pediatrics 35:815, 1965.)

cated technique, its indications, risks, and effectiveness are still being determined. The best results have recently been reported by Bowman et al., who found fetal survival to be 62 per cent, compared to an earlier experience of 28 per cent (81). Maternal morbidity was low and mortality zero.

The data suggest that 62 per cent of fetuses, in whom certain death would have occurred, survived. In the absence of controlled trials, it cannot be considered certain that all these babies would have died; however, it is likely that most would have. Furthermore, overall mortality from intrauterine deaths has fallen as a result of the institution of these programs (86).

The technique of intrauterine transfusion has been well described elsewhere (82). Essentially it consists of localization of the fetal peritoneal cavity and the injection of packed (hematocrit approximately 90 per cent), Rh-negative red cells into the fetal peritoneal cavity. Probably 80 per cent of these cells eventually are absorbed, presumably through lymphatic channels, and survive in the fetal circulation. The amount of fetal blood administered appears to be significant, since excessive quantities are associated with a higher fetal mortality. Accordingly, it is recommended that the volumes used should be increased with gestational age. [50 ml. at 24 weeks to 110 ml. at 30 weeks (89)]. Subsequent transfusions are given at approximately two-week intervals.

The surviving Rh-negative adult erythrocytes now compensate for the profound anemia due to destruction of Rh-positive fetal cells. As a result of continuing destruction and subsequent intrauterine transfusions, these babies can be born with little or no fetal erythrocytes in circulation. In one series, more than 50 per cent of newborns born after intrauterine transfusion had negative Coombs' tests, and 72 per cent had less than 2.0 g. per 100 ml. Hb F in their blood (81). The absence of fetal Rh-positive erythrocytes and the low reticulocyte count may be due to suppression of fetal erythropoiesis by the infused adult blood, or to continuing destruction of mature fetal cells and reticulocytes by anti-D antibody.

Despite the small number of fetal erythrocytes in the circulation of these babies at birth, severe hyperbilirubinemia occurs, requiring multiple exchange transfusions (81). These babies are often very ill, suffering from anemia, heart failure, and potential hemorrhagic disease. Obstructive jaundice is seen very commonly but tends to clear spontaneously (81).

Hydrops fetalis is a very bad sign prognostically; this diagnosis can be made in utero by radiology or by detection of ascitic fluid during intrauterine transfusion (82). Previously it was recommended that there was no point in treating such fetuses; however, survivals of hydropic fetuses following intrauterine transfusion have now been reported (90).

The subsequent development of infants surviving intrauterine transfusion appears to be satisfactory. Developmental failure has been reported but in very low incidence, and generally it would appear that development of survivors has been quite good (81, 91, 92).

It had been speculated that one effect of intrauterine transfusion could be infusion of foreign lymphocytes which could "take" in an immunologically immature or "tolerant" fetus. Naiman et al. described an infant who apparently suffered a graft-versus-host reaction after intrauterine transfusion (93). Bowman et al. (81) in a large series found no evidence of graft-versus-host disease, although there have been other reports of donor lymphocytes persisting 18 months after intrauterine transfusion (94). At present, therefore, the risk of this complication seems minimal.

Prevention of Hyperbilirubinemia and Death in the Newborn at Risk

INTRODUCTION. The preceding sections have described the mechanisms whereby anti-D antibody sensitizes fetal erythrocytes, leading to their destruction both in utero and after delivery. In the severe form of the disease, erythrocyte destruction can be so profound that death occurs in utero or shortly after delivery, with clinical signs of profound anemia with or without gross edema and anasarca (hydrops fetalis). If the infant is less severely affected and is not at risk of death due to anemia, the major problem is hyperbilirubinemia and the resulting risk of brain damage and death.

The key to the treatment of the affected

newborn is exchange transfusion, whereby donor Rh-negative erythrocytes are substituted for the "doomed," sensitized, Rh-positive cells of the infant. This can correct the anemia of the severely affected child, help prevent hyperbilirubinemia (by removing the "doomed" erythrocytes), and wash out bilirubin from the jaundiced child. In the succeeding sections, we shall discuss the physiology of exchange transfusion and its application to the care of the child with Rh hemolytic disease.

PHYSIOLOGY OF EXCHANGE TRANSFUSION. The theory of this procedure is simple. Small volumes of the infant's blood (10 to 20 ml.) are removed and replaced by donor blood. This is usually continued until the volume of donor blood used is approximately 180 ml. per kg. body weight.

Let us now consider these changes:

1. *The exchange of red blood cells:* An exchange transfusion equal to two times the blood volume (i.e., 180 ml. per kg.) effects the exchange of approximately 90 per cent of the circulating red blood cells by donor cells (95). Approximately 75 per cent of the red cells are removed after the first one-volume exchange (95).

2. *The removal of bilirubin:* In the previous sections, the relationship between bilirubin and albumin was described. Clearly most of the intravascular unconjugated bilirubin is in association with albumin. It can be expected, therefore, that bilirubin will also be found throughout the albumin pool. It has been demonstrated that the albumin pool is located in a volume twice the size of the plasma pool (4). Stated in another way, one-half of the body albumin is located outside the plasma. Nevertheless it has been shown that this extravascular albumin is in rapid equilibrium with plasma albumin, so that an exchange transfusion of 180 ml. per kg. will effect approximately a 90 per cent removal of albumin (96). Repeated studies, however, have shown that the bilirubin pool is greatly in excess of that calculated either from the plasma or the albumin pool. Valaes has shown that a two-volume exchange transfusion will remove approximately 150 per cent of the bilirubin calculated to be in the intravascular pool (95). Therefore, bilirubin must be located outside the vascular pool, and presumably much of this is bound to albumin as described above. It should be

added, however, that an exchange transfusion, although removing 90 per cent of the infant's serum albumin, effects a drop of serum bilirubin to only about 55 per cent of the original value (95). This must mean that unconjugated bilirubin exists in three pools: (1) in association with plasma albumin in the blood stream; (2) in association with plasma albumin in an extravascular site; and (3) in a third, slowly equilibrating pool.

These observations explain several phenomena relating to bilirubin and exchange transfusion:

A. *Immediate rebound:* Following an exchange transfusion, there is in the 30 to 60 minutes afterwards an increase in serum bilirubin presumably due to equilibration between the third pool and the plasma.

B. *The limited effectiveness of exchange transfusion in removing serum bilirubin:* In the severely jaundiced infant, large amounts of bilirubin exist in each of the three pools. Exchange transfusion, as noted above, has a limited capacity in removing bilirubin from the third pool. Accordingly, it is advised that when exchange transfusion is certain to be required, it should be done as soon as possible. In this way, "potential bilirubin" (i.e., red blood cells) can be removed more effectively than tissue bilirubin.

In an attempt to increase the amount of bilirubin removed by exchange transfusion, it has been recommended that the bilirubin binding capacity of the infant's blood be increased by the administration of plasma albumin, either before or during the exchange transfusion (97). In some series (97, 98) this has resulted in an approximately 30 per cent increase in bilirubin removed. It has been suggested that the albumin be given before the exchange to permit bilirubin binding, and then be removed during exchange, whereas in other series the albumin has been administered with the blood (97, 98). Some feel that albumin has little role as an adjunct to exchange transfusion (3).

If albumin is to be used, however, it should be used with caution in severely anemic children. These patients are liable to be in congestive heart failure, and any sudden expansion of blood volume, such as that occurring from infusion of serum albumin (99), could have an untoward effect.

3. *Removal of other blood components:* There is a rapid fall in neutrophils during exchange transfusions to levels of 20 to 50 per cent of the original value (100). Recovery is slow, often taking several hours. This rather acute fall suggests that neutrophil reserves are considerably less in newborns than in adults, since rapid removal of leukocytes from adults does not result in a significant fall in neutrophil levels (101).

Exchange transfusion with stored blood may result in a lowering of platelet count to one-half or less of the original value. Recovery may take several days. The fall in platelets is less if fresh (less than 24 hours old) 4° C blood is used (4).

Anti-D antibody is also removed by exchange transfusion, and this may diminish the severity of subsequent hemolysis. However, anti-D is a protein of the IgG class, and therefore is distributed both in the plasma and in an equally large extravascular pool (4). Since exchange transfusion does not remove all of the anti-D, the residual antibody can contribute to subsequent hemolysis of Rh-positive cells and thereby to the "rebound" hyperbilirubinemia (see subsequent section).

INDICATIONS FOR EXCHANGE TRANSFUSION. The infant born with Rh disease may be perfectly normal in appearance and have as the only laboratory evidence of disease a positive direct Coombs' test. Increasing severity of disease is suggested by mild jaundice noted on the cord, anemia, and hepatosplenomegaly. Severe disease will appear as anemia, and there may or may not be gross edema (hydrops fetalis).

For the severely affected child, immediate treatment is required to prevent death. For less severely affected infants, exchange transfusion should be performed as soon as possible to prevent profound hyperbilirubinemia. It is necessary, therefore, that we have criteria by which to select as early as possible those babies who will undoubtedly require exchange transfusion. Experience has taught that relatively accurate predictions can be made by study of cord blood. Thereafter, the need for exchange transfusion is determined by the rate of rise of serum bilirubin. The goal is to keep the bilirubin level below that at which the bilirubin binding capacity is exceeded. Usually the level is considered as 20 mg. per 100 ml.; however, lower levels are used for the hypoxic, acidotic, or hypothermic infant. Clearly an estimate of free (unbound) unconjugated bilirubin is what is required. This problem is discussed in an earlier section.

Cord Hemoglobin and Bilirubin as Predictive Guides for Exchange Transfusion. Walker, after detailed analysis of a large series, has recommended that babies with cord hemoglobin concentrations of less than 13 g. per 100 ml. or a bilirubin of greater than 4 mg. per 100 ml. will (if left untreated) become severely jaundiced (bilirubin more than 20 mg. per 100 ml.) (3). For them, exchange transfusion should be done as soon as possible after birth. An early exchange removes a large source of potential bilirubin (in other words, red cells) before they are destroyed and bilirubin accumulates in body tissue, whence removal is more difficult. Bowman (89), drawing on extensive experience, uses a hemoglobin less than 10.5 g. per 100 ml. or bilirubin of greater than 4 mg. per 100 ml. (3.5 in prematures) as cord blood indications for exchange transfusion.

Rate of Bilirubin Rise as an Indication for Exchange Transfusion. Babies with Rh hemolytic disease must be followed carefully in the first few days of life to be certain that serum bilirubin levels do not exceed either 20 mg. per 100 ml. or the bilirubin binding capacity of the serum. As a guide, Walker suggested that if bilirubin (mg. per 100 ml.) exceeds the baby's age in hours, an exchange transfusion should be performed (3). Graphs are available on which serum bilirubin concentrations can be plotted to determine the need for exchange (102). Whatever method is employed, serum bilirubin levels must be checked frequently until it is certain that the level has reached a plateau or is falling.

Anemia as an Indication for Exchange Transfusion. As described above, anemia at birth is an indication. Recently, however, with the advent of phototherapy, hyperbilirubinemia can be controlled in some cases, even though hemolysis continues. As a result, hemoglobin levels could fall without obvious hyperbilirubinemia, and profound anemia could develop. In fact, cases such as this have been reported (103), and therefore it is recommended that hemoglobin levels must be followed during the first week of life to prevent severe anemia from developing in a minimally jaundiced child.

TECHNIQUE OF EXCHANGE TRANSFUSION. The specific details of the technical procedures involved are contained in other reports (89) and will not be reviewed here.

The blood used should be ABO-compatible and Rh-negative. The erythrocytes should be compatible in a crossmatch with the mother's serum. There has been considerable discussion regarding the relative merits of ACD (acid-citrate-dextrose) blood versus heparinized blood. The vast majority of exchange transfusions have been done using citrated blood (3, 89). There are, however, several objections to the use of this type of blood.

The infusion of large amounts of citrate can result in a fall in ionized calcium, with the potential risk of tetany. Although very few cases of tetany have been reported during exchange transfusion, repeated infusions of calcium gluconate are recommended during exchange transfusion (89). Recently, studies have suggested that calcium gluconate is of little value in improving the low ionized calcium levels that occurred during exchange transfusion (104). Furthermore, it has been shown that during this exchange transfusion there is a total increase in serum calcium, and it can be questioned therefore whether repeated injections of calcium gluconate are in fact necessary. Nevertheless, it has been common practice to employ calcium gluconate during exchange transfusion, and this has been associated with a low mortality rate (89).

A second objection raised to the use of this type of blood is that the blood itself is acidic. As a result, during exchange transfusion, the pH of an infant's blood will drop, particularly in small prematures (105). For these infants, it has been recommended that an additional quantity of sodium bicarbonate be added to the donor blood (106). The recommended volume would be 1.8 mEq. of sodium bicarbonate per 100 ml. during the first half of the exchange, and 0.9 mEq. during the second half. Using this, the pH of the infant does not change during exchange transfusion.

It should be noted that, following exchange transfusion, citrate is metabolized, and there occurs a postexchange alkalosis (105). This, however, has not proved to be detrimental to the child.

In order to circumvent the problems occasioned by citrated blood, it has been recommended that heparinized blood be employed. Certainly there is no fall in the blood pH, there is no risk of hypocalcemia, and success has been reported utilizing heparinized blood (107). It should be recalled, however, that in severely affected cases of Rh hemolytic disease there is a risk of hemorrhagic complications. Pulmonary hemorrhage and intraventricular hemorrhage are recognized complications in association with the respiratory distress syndrome seen most commonly in fatal cases of erythroblastosis (108). It could be questioned, therefore, whether heparinization for one hour or a longer period (in other words, during exchange transfusion) is an entirely innocuous procedure. Furthermore, the neutralization recommendations utilizing protamine are arbitrary indeed, and usually are not based on heparin assays. Accordingly, it could be recommended that, if heparinized blood is to be utilized for exchange transfusion, protamine neutralization subsequently should be complete and should be checked thereafter by appropriate heparin assays.

Fresh blood, whenever possible, should be utilized for exchange transfusion. As noted above, if blood is 24 hours of age or less, the fall in platelets will be minimized. Furthermore, erythrocytes stored longer than 24 hours will commence to lose potassium, and the serum potassium may rise, constituting the hazard of hyperkalemia. Finally, stored blood gradually loses 2,3-diphosphoglycerate concentration, as a result of which the oxygen dissociation curve shifts so that the blood is less able to deliver oxygen to the tissues, a theoretical but possible hazard (102). Accordingly, it is recommended that fresh blood (less than 24 hours of age) be utilized for exchange transfusion.

Many experienced groups remove plasma from ACD blood in order to concentrate the cells. ACD blood is diluted by the anticoagulant solution, and as a result the hemoglobin concentration is considerably less than that of the donor blood. It is recommended, therefore, that a volume of plasma equal to the amount of anticoagulant solution initially present should be removed (3, 89). The removal of plasma will lower the citrate and potassium load on the baby, presumably a beneficial effect. In addition, it will leave the baby with a higher postexchange hemoglobin than unconcentrated blood (109). There is reason to believe (see below) that this is of value in terms of preventing rebound hyperbilirubinemia and subsequent development of "late" anemia (109).

In summary, it can be recommended that for the majority of exchange transfusions ACD blood is satisfactory. The blood should be collected in bags, stored at 4° C, and used within 24 hours. Immediately prior to use, a volume of plasma equivalent to the volume of anticoagulant should be removed. In the severely affected infant, sodium bicarbonate can be added to the blood, as described above.

COMPLICATIONS OF EXCHANGE TRANSFUSION. There are many complications, some of which are common to any transfusion. The metabolic and hemorrhagic complications have been discussed above. Vascular problems, such as thrombosis of the portal vein with subsequent portal hypertension and hemorrhagic infarction of the bowel (102), are rare, but must be suspected if the infant suddenly becomes ill.

TREATMENT OF SPECIFIC PROBLEMS ASSOCIATED WITH HEMOLYTIC DISEASE OF THE NEWBORN

Severe Anemia With or Without Hydrops Fetalis. Until recently, hydrops fetalis was considered to be lethal, either in utero or after birth. As noted in an earlier section, salvage of these cases can be achieved by intrauterine transfusion. Furthermore, recently it has been shown that these severely affected children can be salvaged by sophisticated and careful pediatric care (89, 108).

Death in the first few hours of life of the severely affected newborn infant is due to anemia. It has been pointed out that anemia in utero and particularly during labor results in tissue hypoxia and the signs of asphyxia at birth (in other words, low apgar score and low pH). Characteristically, these in-

fants have an elevated peripheral venous pressure originally thought to be a manifestation of heart failure but more likely due to asphyxia and acidosis (110). Accordingly, therapy of these infants should be directed towards immediate handling of the problems of asphyxia and acidosis and early exchange transfusion (108). This approach and that of others (89) have resulted in survival of hydropic infants.

"Rebound" Hyperbilirubinemia. In the minutes after exchange transfusion, serum bilirubin rises as tissue bilirubin reaches equilibrium with the plasma pool. This takes about 30 minutes (95), as described in an earlier section.

In severe cases, bilirubin levels continue to rise, often necessitating more than one exchange transfusion. One possible source of bilirubin is the residual Rh-positive cells left after an exchange transfusion. These amount to 5 to 10 per cent of the original cells (95, 96). Let us recall (as noted in an earlier section) that the limiting factor in red cell destruction in this disease is the capacity of the reticuloendothelial system to destroy sensitized cells. It seems reasonable, therefore, that the residual cells after one exchange may be a sufficient source of bilirubin. But what about severe hyperbilirubinemia after three or more exchanges? Certainly few of the baby's original cells will be left. Here it would seem that continued production of Rh-positive cells may be an explanation. Red cell production often continues for many days after birth, and these cells, even at the reticulocyte stage, will be destroyed rapidly, serving as a source of bilirubin. That red cell destruction occurs after exchange transfusion is attested to by increased carbon monoxide production in these infants (111) (carbon monoxide is released when the heme ring opens) and by rapidly falling haptoglobin levels after exchange transfusion (112).

Hemorrhagic Diathesis. A bleeding disorder can complicate the severe case of hemolytic disease. Most commonly there is thrombocytopenia with or without other laboratory evidence of intravascular coagulation (i.e., hypofibrinogenemia, fibrin split products, and so forth). Post mortem one frequently finds small vessel thrombi along with intracranial and pulmonary hemorrhage (113). It is possible that intravascular coagulation results directly from intravascular hemolysis (113); in my opinion it is more likely that it is related, at least in part, to the hypoxia which occurs in these babies. There is evidence now in experimental animals (114) and in newborn infants (115) that hypoxia can induce intravascular coagulation.

There is no evidence to support an immunologic basis to the thrombocytopenia, although several studies have shown depressed platelet counts as a frequent finding in less severe cases in which there is no evidence of intravascular coagulation (116). The Rh antigen is not present on platelets, and therefore thrombocytopenia could not be due directly to the anti-D antibodies. Platelets are known to bind antigen-antibody complexes, and in vivo this has resulted in thrombocytopenia, in which the platelet has suffered as an "innocent bystander." We considered this possibility and found that, unlike other antigen-antibody complexes, anti-D–sensitized erythrocytes do not adhere to platelets (37).

Practically these observations mean that the severely affected patient with hemorrhagic disease of the newborn is at risk of developing a hemorrhagic diathesis. If thrombocytopenia is a major problem, and it may be, especially after an exchange transfusion, a platelet infusion should be given. If, however, there is evidence of profound intravascular coagulation, consideration should be given to heparin therapy. The latter should be approached very cautiously and must be monitored continually by either heparin levels or degree of anticoagulation (e.g., prolongation of partial thromboplastin time). Heparin therapy in the newborn is difficult, the indications are vague, and the effectiveness unproven. We rarely use it.

Obstructive Jaundice. This occurs in approximately 8 per cent of cases of hemolytic disease of the newborn. Most of these are severe cases of hemolytic disease; the obstructive jaundice is evident in the cord blood, where the direct bilirubin is elevated. Conjugated bilirubinemia may be very profound, with levels exceeding 20 mg. per 100 ml. There is no explanation for this phenomenon; liver function tests are otherwise not abnormal, and we must conclude that the picture is most like a cholestatic jaundice, in some way related to the severe hemolytic disease. No specific therapy appears necessary, although corticosteroids have been recommended (117).

Hypoglycemia. Hypertrophy and hyperplasia of the islets of Langerhans have been found in infants who have died of hemolytic disease of the newborn. In addition, the level of insulin in the pancreas is increased (118).

It is not surprising, therefore, that hypoglycemia is found in newborns suffering from hemolytic disease more often than in normals. Price (119) found it in 4 per cent of cases, and usually these were the sickest infants. Hypoglycemia appeared as early as four hours and usually within the first 24 hours.

Schiff et al. (120) pointed out that hyperglycemia exists during an exchange transfusion and hyperinsulinemia is found at the end of the transfusion. In the subsequent two hours, there occurs a rapid drop in blood glucose, and symptoms of hypoglycemia may appear.

"Late" Anemia. Anemia developing during the first weeks of life may occur in affected babies. This may occur following exchange transfusion or in those babies who have not been treated. The latter group may be seen more frequently now because of phototherapy which may control hyperbilirubinemia, even though hemolysis continues (103). Continued low-grade hemolysis may result in anemia in babies who have not received an exchange transfusion.

Anemia following exchange transfusions is not infrequent and must be anticipated. Following one or more exchange transfusions, more than 90 per cent of the baby's erythrocytes are Rh-negative. Why should anemia occur? There would appear to be several reasons.

First, postexchange hemoglobin concentrations are frequently much lower than those in normal infants. At five days of age, the mean hemoglobin concentration of normal babies is 19 g. per 100 ml. in our experience. Following an exchange with ACD blood, the hemoglobin may be 15 g. per 100 ml. if the blood has been concentrated (see above), or 13 g. per 100 ml. if unconcentrated.

As babies grow during the first weeks of life, there is a rapid expansion of blood volume, as a result of which hemoglobin concentration may fall; the fall will be more apparent if the baby starts at a lower level (i.e., after exchange transfusion). Another factor contributing to the rapid fall in hemoglobin concentration may be the reduced survival of donor Rh-negative cells, which has been found in some cases (4). This nonspecific destruction may relate to hypersplenism and although mild, would contribute to the "late" anemia.

Does the baby respond to this evolving anemia? There have been several reports of severe "late anemia" in these babies, in whom reticulocyte counts were close to zero (121). This suggested that bone marrow failure was contributing to the late anemia. However, Dillon and Krivit (122) showed that bone marrow normoblast activity did appear to respond to the anemia. The lower the hemoglobin concentration, the greater the marrow erythroid activity. Thus, in the affected infant, marrow activity is normal for that age of life. [Note: erythroid activity in the first month of life normally is reduced unless there are profound hypoxic or anemic stimuli (102)].

The paradox of active marrow erythropoiesis and low peripheral reticulocyte count presumably results from the destruction of reticulocytes by anti-D antibody. The D antigen is present on reticulocytes, as evidenced by the ingestion of anti-D-sensitized reticulocytes by macrophages in vitro (37).

OTHER THERAPY. Recently there have been two major approaches to the care of infants with hyperbilirubinemia—namely, light therapy and phenobarbital therapy (see also Chapter 3). Several well-controlled clinical trials have demonstrated that phototherapy is effective in lowering serum bilirubin levels. These studies have recently been well summarized (138, 139).

Light converts unconjugated bilirubin, in the presence of oxygen, to more polar, diazonegative, water-soluble products, which are excreted in both the bile and the urine (see p. 92). Bilirubin absorbs light maximally at 450 to 460 nm., and therefore light sources whose spectra include peak emission in this range should be employed. The principal peak of the blue light is 425 to 475 nm., and for special blue 420 to 480 nm.

The use of phototherapy has enjoyed its greatest success in the treatment of idiopathic hyperbilirubinemia in premature infants. It can reduce the incidence of bilirubin values in excess of 15 mg. per 100 ml. from 20 to 2 per cent in a premature nursery unit (140). It has also been demonstrated to reduce the need for exchange transfusion in infants with ABO incompatibility and to reduce the need for repeat exchange transfusions in infants with Rh incompatibility.

No recognizable undesirable long-term consequences of phototherapy have been observed. Minor complications associated with its use include the occurrence of green, loose stools, transient skin rashes, and transient bronze discoloration of the skin, particularly in those infants with associated liver disease.

More serious problems may occur when phototherapy is improperly employed. Infants receiving phototherapy must have frequent bilirubin and hemoglobin determinations performed. As bilirubin is broken down in the skin, the appearance of jaundice disappears, and the physician can no longer estimate the bilirubin level on the basis of physical examination of the infant. When phototherapy is utilized to treat hemolytic disease and exchange transfusion is avoided, severe anemia may develop during the first weeks of life if attention is not paid to the infant's hemoglobin level.

The greatest potential danger of phototherapy lies in its substitution for diagnostic precision in the evaluation of the cause of jaundice. Jaundice appearing during the first week of life is a valuable sign of many illnesses (see Table 9–9). The liberal use of phototherapy, particularly on a prophylactic basis, may remove this valuable diagnostic sign unless the decision to employ phototherapy in the treatment of jaundice is always coupled with efforts to determine its etiology.

Phenobarbital is one of a group of agents that will induce proliferation of the endoplasmic reticulum of liver cells and increase enzymatic activity. It can enhance both bilirubin conjugation and excretion. When phenobarbital is given in a sufficient dose to the mother, to the baby, or to both, it is effective in lowering serum bilirubin levels (139). When phenobarbital is given to infants, an effect on bilirubin reduction may be observed within 48

TABLE 9-9. PATHOLOGIC CAUSES OF NEONATAL JAUNDICE

Hemolytic Diseases
   Erythroblastosis fetalis, Rh or ABO incompatibility, and so forth
   Inherited red cell defects: hereditary spherocytosis, enzyme deficiencies (± drugs): glucose-6-phosphate
      dehydrogenase, pyruvate kinase, and so forth
   Drugs and toxins: vitamin K_3 (excessive doses), naphthalene (moth balls)

Infections
   Bacterial: sepsis, congenital syphilis
   Viral: cytomegalic inclusion disease, disseminated herpes simplex, congenital rubella syndrome
   Protozoal: congenital toxoplasmosis

Enclosed Hemorrhage

Metabolic Disorders
   Galactosemia
   Crigler-Najjar syndrome
   Breast milk jaundice
   Transient familial neonatal hyperbilirubinemia
   Cretinism

Neonatal (Giant-Cell) Hepatitis

hours, although really significant reduction in bilirubin values requires three to five days.

The indications for its use in the newborn period are not well defined. Its slow onset of action, its effect on other enzyme systems, and the recognition that, when given in large doses to mothers prior to delivery, it may produce severe depression of the infant's vitamin K–dependent factors (141) have all served to limit its usefulness.

ABO HEMOLYTIC DISEASE

Introduction

Twenty per cent of pregnancies are ABO-incompatible, meaning that the serum of the mother contains anti-A or anti-B antibodies, while the fetal erythrocytes contain the respective antigen. Hyperbilirubinemia occurs more frequently in this group of infants and would appear to result from the destruction of the baby's red cells by the maternal isoantibody.

The disease is limited to mothers of blood group O and affects babies of blood group A or B. This association occurs in 15 per cent of pregnancies, yet evidence of ABO incompatibility disease (see below) is found only in 3 per cent of pregnancies, and is a cause of exchange transfusion in only 1 in 1000 to 1 in 4000 pregnancies (4).

Why is severe ABO hemolytic disease so rare when 15 per cent of pregnancies are

potentially at risk? The answer is in the maternal antibody and the ability of these antibodies to interact with and destroy fetal erythrocytes.

Maternal Antibody

Anti-A and anti-B antibodies develop early in life and are found in all subjects whose erythrocytes lack the related antigen (i.e., all group O subjects have anti-A and anti-B antibodies). These "naturally" occurring antibodies result from immune stimulation by the A or B substance contained in food and bacteria. It is not known why some women develop unusually high levels of anti-A or -B, but this may arise from continued antigenic stimulus, as, for example, by repeated bacterial infections. ABO hemolytic disease tends to occur in newborns whose mothers have high levels of antibody (4, 123, 124).

Anti-A and anti-B antibodies are found in the IgA, IgM, and IgG fractions of plasma. Only IgG crosses the placenta and is responsible for the occurrence of ABO hemolytic disease in the newborn. Therefore, the occurrence and severity of disease relates, in part, to the level of IgG anti-A (or -B) in the mother (4, 123, 124, 125). The direct determination of this type of antibody is difficult, and most studies have relied on indirect methods of detecting the IgG antibody (often referred to as the "immune antibody"). These methods can be summarized as follows:

1. Antibody activity after neutralization with A or B blood group substance (126, 127).

2. Thermostable antibody.

3. Indirect Coombs' technique (127).

4. Antibody against pig A erythrocytes (128).

5. Hemolytic activity (4).

6. Antibody in purified IgG fractions (125).

7. Mercaptoethanol-resistant antibody (126).

These techniques singly or in combination provide an assay of IgG anti-A or -B which correlates well with the occurrence of ABO incompatibility disease. Unfortunately none of these tests can predict with certainty the presence of ABO hemolytic disease in the newborn. However, failure to demonstrate them in the maternal serum of an infant with suspected ABO hemolytic disease makes that diagnosis most unlikely.

The diagnosis of ABO hemolytic disease depends largely on the hematologic findings in the newborn.

Erythrocytes of the Newborn

The red blood cell of the newborn differs in many respects from that of the adult. Among these differences is a much lower content of reactive A or B sites. The number of reactive A sites in various red cells is shown in Table 9-10 (129).

Fewer A (or B) sites on the newborn's erythrocytes explains the weakly reactive Coombs' test in ABO hemolytic disease, presumably related to the large distance between each A site. As a result, fewer anti-A molecules are firmly bound to the cell, and the reaction with anti-globulin serum [i.e., Coombs' test (Fig. 9-2)] is less marked (4, 130). Antibody eluted from these cells reacts strongly with adult Group A erythrocytes, in which the A sites are close to one another (131).

The sparse distribution of A sites on the newborn erythrocytes explains also the observation that erythrocyte life span in ABO hemolytic disease is only slightly shortened. If, however, adult Group A erythrocytes are infused into such subjects, they are destroyed very quickly, often with evidence of intravascular lysis (4).

It has been suggested that the infant affected with ABO hemolytic disease may have inherited an unusually reactive A antigen. The available evidence would not support this thesis (132).

Erythrocyte Destruction in ABO Hemolytic Disease

As described above, the disease appears to be due to the entrance of maternal IgG anti-A (or -B) into the fetal circulation and to the reaction there with fetal erythrocytes. The degree of interaction is determined by the A-antigen strength of the erythrocyte, as noted above. It is probably modified by the presence of soluble A or B substance in the plasma of these infants, since it has been shown that the reaction of a weak anti-A with A cells is depressed by the presence of such substances (133). The ubiquitous nature of A substance may further modulate the activity of the anti-A antibodies. This is supported by the observation that anti-A and anti-B antibodies rapidly disappear from the circulation of the newborn in the first three days of life (134). This results presumably from uptake of antibody by A or B substance in the body's tissues.

Red blood cell destruction can occur either by intravascular or extravascular hemolysis. In ABO-incompatible disease, destruction would appear to result primarily from extravascular hemolysis, since hyperbilirubinemia predominates and there is

TABLE 9-10. THE NUMBER OF A SITES ON VARIOUS TYPES OF RED CELLS*

CELL TYPE†	AVERAGE NO. OF A SITES PER CELL
Adult A¹	26,000
Adult A²	6,000
Newborn A¹	7,500

*From Voak, D., and Williams, M. A.: Br. J. Haematol. 20:9, 1971.

†These values for A sites are relative only; A² refers to a subgroup of A (about 20 per cent of Group A subjects), whose erythrocytes are considerably less reactive than the major subgroup of A (i.e., A¹).

little if any evidence of intravascular lysis (i.e., hemoglobinemia or hemoglobinuria). In severe forms of the disease, splenomegaly occurs, presumably in response to the splenic destruction of erythrocytes (39).

It has been demonstrated in adults, both experimentally and in disease, that A or B erythrocytes are destroyed by intravascular lysis (27, 28). Why, then, does this not occur in ABO hemolytic disease? In the adult, anti-A (or -B) causes destruction either by gross agglutination (due to IgM or IgA antibodies), with subsequent trapping, or by complement-induced lysis by IgM or IgG antibodies.

In the newborn, only maternal IgG antibody is of significance. There is no evidence of complement-induced red cell destruction in ABO hemolytic disease; serum complement levels are normal, and complement components are not found on the sensitized erythrocytes (135). That the newborn is capable of lysing A (or B) cells can be shown by injecting A or B adult erythrocytes into the circulation of a newborn with ABO hemolytic disease; intravascular lysis occurs (4).

It is likely that intravascular lysis of the erythrocytes of the newborn does not occur because relatively few antibody molecules bind to the cell (for the reasons cited above), and, as a result, the critical IgG aggregation necessary to activate complement does not occur.

A prominent feature of ABO hemolytic disease is the presence of microspherocytosis. This can be observed on blood smears and has been documented by demonstration of their increased osmotic fragility (4). Why do spherocytes occur? It has been suggested that erythrocytes trapped in contact with cells of the reticuloendothelial system (e.g., splenic histiocytes, Kupffer cells in the liver) lose part of their membranes, and the resulting cells have a lower membrane/volume ratio and therefore assume a spherocytic shape. This mechanism has been invoked to explain the development of sphering in hereditary spherocytosis and in experimental complement-deficient animals in which erythrocytes had been sensitized by antibody and $C'3$ component of complement (136, 137). Spherocytes are much less common in Rh hemolytic disease; the basis for this difference is obscure.

Clinical Features of ABO Hemolytic Disease

Hyperbilirubinemia, commencing usually within 24 hours of birth, is the hallmark of this disorder (hence the name "icterus praecox"). There may be little or no evidence of a hemolytic process; the hemoglobin, reticulocyte count, and normoblast count may be normal or only moderately abnormal. A severe hemolytic process is extremely rare.

As a result, there is no risk of anemia in the fetus and hence no need for antenatal diagnosis or therapy.

The diagnosis of ABO-incompatible hemolytic disease is often difficult, since there are no absolutely definitive diagnostic criteria. The following guidelines can be used:

1. The presence of unexplained hyperbilirubinemia in an A or B newborn of an O mother.

2. The presence of mild anemia, reticulocytosis, and normoblastemia supports the diagnosis; however, their absence does not rule it out.

3. In most laboratories, a weakly positive direct Coombs' test (on the infant's erythrocytes) can be detected. In all laboratories anti-A (or -B) can be eluted from the erythrocytes of the affected newborn; these antibodies will react strongly with the respective A (or B) adult cells.

4. The presence of free anti-A (or -B) in the serum of the newborn is strong confirmatory evidence (134).

5. The mother's serum should contain relatively high levels of anti-A (or -B); these should be of the IgG type, as determined by the indirect or direct tests described above.

HEMOLYTIC DISEASE OF THE NEWBORN DUE TO "MINOR GROUP" ANTIBODIES

Less than 1 per cent of cases of hemolytic disease of the newborn are due to minor group antibodies (in other words, antibodies other than anti-A, anti-B, or anti-D). The vast majority of these are either anti-c, anti-E, or anti-Kell.

The infrequency of "minor group" hemolytic disease is due to the relatively low potency of these antigens. Thus K, E, and c are 1 to 5 per cent as potent in inducing antibodies as D. All other antigens have potencies less than 0.1 per cent that of D (4).

The diagnosis and therapy of these diseases are identical to those of Rh hemolytic disease of the newborn.

References

1. Levine, P., Katzin, E. M., et al.: Isoimmunization in pregnancy, its possible bearing on the etiology of erythroblastosis fetalis. J.A.M.A. *116*:825, 1941.
2. Prokop, O., and Uhlenbruck, G.: *Human Blood and Serum Groups.* New York, Wiley Interscience, 1969.
3. Walker, W.: Hemolytic disease of the newborn, In *Recent Advances in Pediatrics*, 4th ed. Gairdner, D., and Hull, D. (eds.), London, J. A. Churchill, 1971, p. 119.
4. Mollison, P. L.: Blood transfusion, In *Clinical Medicine.* Oxford, Blackwell Scientific Publications, Ltd., 1967.
5. Rochna, E., and Hughes-Jones, N. C.: The use of purified ^{125}I-labelled anti-γ globulin in the determination of the number of D antigen sites on red cells of different phenotypes. Vox Sang. *10*:675, 1965.
6. Race, R. R., and Sanger, R.: *Blood Groups in Man*, 2nd ed. Oxford, Blackwell Scientific Publications, Ltd., 1954.
7. Murray, S., Knox, G., et al.: Haemolytic disease and the rhesus genotypes. Vox Sang. *10*:257, 1965.
8. Masouridis, S. P.: Reaction of I^{131} trace labelled human anti-Rh$_o$ (D) with red cells. J. Clin. Invest. *38*:279, 1959.
9. Adinolfi, A., Mollison, P. L., et al.: γA blood group antibodies. J. Exp. Med. *123*:951, 1966.
10. Brambell, F. W. R.: *The Transmission of Passive Immunity from Mother to Young.* Amsterdam, North-Holland Publishing Co., 1970.
11. Van der Giessen, M., Van der Hart, M., et al.: Fractionation of sera containing antibodies against red cells or platelets with special reference to anti-D sera. Vox Sang. *9*:25, 1964.
12. Dodd, B. E., and Wilkinson, P. C.: A study of the distribution of incomplete rhesus antibodies among the serum immunoglobulin fractions. J. Exp. Med. *120*:45, 1964.
13. Pollack, W., Hager, H. J., et al.: A study of the forces involved in the second stage of hemagglutination. Transfusion *5*:158, 1965.
14. Murray, S.: Early "Enzyme" Rh antibodies and second pregnancies. Vox Sang. *21*:217, 1971.
15. Zipursky, A., Pollock, J., et al.: Transplacental isoimmunization by foetal red blood cells. Birth Defects *1*:84, 1965.
16. Zipursky, A., Pollock, J., et al.: The pathogenesis and prevention of Rh immunization in pregnancy. Bibl. Haematol. *29*:280, 1968.
17. Mollison, P. L., Frame, M., et al.: Differences between Rh(D)-negative subjects in response to Rh(D) antigen. Br. J. Haematol. *19*:257, 1970.
18. Freda, V. J., Gorman, J. G., et al.: Rh factor: Prevention of immunization and clinical trials on mothers. Science *151*:828, 1966.
19. Cook, I. A.: Primary rhesus immunization in male volunteers. Br. J. Haematol. *21*:369, 1971.
20. Pickles, M. M., quoted in Mollison, P. L.: Blood transfusion, In *Clinical Medicine.* Oxford, Blackwell Scientific Publications, Ltd., 1967, p. 303.
21. Wiener, A. S.: Further observations on isosensitization to the Rh factor. Proc. Soc. Exp. Biol. Med. *70*:576, 1949.
22. Clarke, C. A., Donohoe, W. T. A., et al.: Further experimental studies on the prevention of Rh haemolytic disease. Br. Med. J. *1*:979, 1963.
23. Zipursky, A., Pollock, J., et al.: The transplacental passage of foetal red blood-cells and the pathogenesis of Rh immunisation during pregnancy. Lancet *2*:489, 1963.
24. Finn, R., Harper, D. T., et al.: Transplacental hemorrhage. Transfusion *3*:114, 1963.
25. Wimhöfer, H., Schneider, J., et al.: Untersuchungen über die einschwemmung fetaler erythrozyten in den mütterlichen Kreislauf bei spontangeburten und geburtshilflichen eingriffen. Geburtshilfe Frauenheilkd. *22*:589, 1962.
26. Zipursky, A., and Israels, L. G.: The pathogenesis and prevention of Rh immunization. Can. Med. Assoc. J. *97*:1245, 1967.
27. Jandl. J. H., Jones, A. R., et al.: The destruction of red cells by antibodies in man. I. Observations on the sequestration and lysis of red cells altered by immune mechanisms. J. Clin. Invest. *36*:1428, 1957.
28. Mollison, P. L., Crome, P., et al.: Rate of removal from the circulation of red cells sensitized with different amounts of antibody. Br. J. Haematol. *11*:461, 1965.
29. Hughes-Jones, N. C., Hughes, M. I. J., et al.: The amount of anti-D on red cells in haemolytic disease of the newborn. Vox Sang. *12*:279, 1967.
30. Mollison, P. L.: The survival of transfused cells in haemolytic disease of the newborn. Arch. Dis. Child. *18*:161, 1943.
31. Weiss, L.: The structure of fine splenic arterial vessels in relation to hemoconcentration and red cell destruction. Am. J. Anat. *111*:131, 1962.
32. LaCelle, P. L.: Alteration of membrane deformability in hemolytic anemias. Semin. Hematol. *7*:355, 1970.
33. Schrier, S. L., Moore, L. D., et al.: Inhibition of human erythrocyte membrane-mediated ATP synthesis by anti-D antibody. Am. J. Med. Sci. *256*:340, 1968.
34. Teitel, P.: Le test de la filtrabilité erythrocytaire (TFE). Nouv. Rev. Fr. Hematol. *7*:195, 1967.
35. Huber, H., and Fudenberg, H. H.: Receptor sites of human monocytes for IgG. Int. Arch. Allergy Appl. Immunol. *34*:18, 1968.

36. LoBuglio, A. F., Cotran, R. S., et al.: Red cells coated with immunoglobulin G.: Binding and sphering by mononuclear cells in man. Science 158:1582, 1967.

37. Brown, E. J., and Zipursky, A.: Unpublished observations.

38. Cooper, M. B.: Erythrophagocytosis in hemolytic disease of the newborn. Blood 5:678, 1950.

39. Jandl, J. H., Files, N. M., et al.: Proliferative response of the spleen and liver to hemolysis. J. Exp. Med. 122:299, 1965.

40. Lindsay, S.: Hemolytic disease of the newborn infant (erythroblastosis fetalis). J. Pediatr. 37, 582, 1950.

41. Simon, G. T., and Burke, J. S.: Electron microscopy of the spleen. III. Erythroleukophagocytosis. Am. J. Pathol. 58:451, 1970.

42. Pimstone, N. R., Tenhunen, R., et al.: The enzymatic degradation to bile pigments by macrophages. J. Exp. Med. 133:1264, 1971.

43. Pimstone, N. R., Engel, P., et al.: Inducible heme oxygenase in the kidney: A model for the homeostatic control of hemoglobin catabolism. J. Clin. Invest. 50:2042, 1971.

44. Fallstrom, S. P.: On the endogenous formation of carbon monoxide in full-term infants. Acta Paediatr. Scand. Suppl. 189, 1969.

45. Maisels, M. J., Pathak, A., et al.: Endogenous production of carbon monoxide in normal and erythroblastic infants. J. Clin. Invest. 50: 1, 1971.

46. Zetterstrom, R., Stempful, R., et al.: Methemalbuminemia in the neonatal period with special reference to hemolytic disease of the newborn. Acta Paediatr. 45:241, 1956.

47. Lundh, B., Oski, F. A., et al.: Plasma hemopexin and haptoglobin in hemolytic diseases of the newborn. Acta Paediatr. Scand. 59:121, 1970.

48. Halvorsen, S.: Plasma erythropoietic levels in cord blood and in blood during the first week of life. Acta Paediatr. 52:425, 1963.

49. Gilmour, J. R.: Erythroblastosis fetalis. Arch. Dis. Child. 19:1, 1944.

50. Phibbs. R. H., Johnson, P., et al.: Circulatory changes in newborns with erythroblastosis fetalis. Pediatr. Res. 1:321, 1967.

51. Parkin, J., and Walker, W.: Peritoneal dialysis in severe hydrops fetalis. Lancet 2:283, 1968.

52. Baum, J. D., and Harris, D.: Colloid osmotic pressure in erythroblastosis fetalis. Br. Med. J. 1:601, 1972.

53. Ostrow, J. D., and Schmid, R.: The protein-binding of C^{14}-bilirubin in human and murine serum. J. Clin. Invest. 42:1286, 1963.

54. Schmid, R.: Bilirubin metabolism in man. New Engl. J. Med. 287:703, 1972.

55. Thaler, M. M.: Perinatal bilirubin metabolism. Adv. Pediatr. 19:215, 1972.

56. Schier, R. W., Dilts, P. V., Jr., et al.: Bilirubin transfer across the human placenta. Am. J. Obstet. Gynecol. 111:677, 1971.

57. Bashore, R. A., Smith, F., et al.: Placental transfer and disposition of bilirubin in the pregnant monkey. Am. J. Obstet. Gynecol. 103: 950, 1969.

58. Cherry, S. H., Rosenfield, R. E., et al.: Mechanism of accumulation of amniotic fluid pigment in erythroblastosis fetalis. Am. J. Obstet. Gynecol. 106:297, 1970.

59. Litwack, G., Ketterer, B., et al.: Ligandin: a hepatic protein which binds steroids, bilirubin, carcinogens and a number of exogenous organic amines. Nature (Lond.) 234: 466, 1971.

60. Levi, A. J., Gatmaitan, Z., et al.: Deficiency of hepatic organic anion-binding protein, impaired organic anion uptake by liver and "physiologic" jaundice in newborn monkeys. New Engl. J. Med. 283:1136, 1970.

61. Maisels, M. J.: Bilirubin. On understanding and influencing its metabolism in the newborn infant. Pediatr. Clin. North Am. 19:447, 1972.

62. Yeung, C. Y., Tam, L. S., et al.: Phenobarbitone prophylaxis for neonatal hyperbilirubinemia. Pediatrics 48:372, 1971.

63. Diamond, I., and Schmid, R.: Neonatal hyperbilirubinemia and kernicterus. Arch. Neurol. 18:699, 1968.

64. Diamond, I., and Schmid, R.: Oxidative phosphorylation in experimental bilirubin encephalopathy. Science 155:1288, 1967.

65. Mustafa, M. G., Cowger, M. L., et al.: Effects of bilirubin on mitochondrial reactions. J. Biol. Chem. 244:6403, 1969.

66. Schutta, H. S., Johnson, L., et al.: Mitochondrial abnormalities in bilirubin encephalopathy. J. Neuropathol. Exp. Neurol. 29:296, 1970.

67. Fleischner, G., Robbins, J., et al.: A major cytoplasmic organic anion-binding protein in rat liver. J. Clin. Invest. 51:677, 1972.

68. Diamond, I., and Schmid, R.: Experimental bilirubin encephalopathy. The mode of entry of bilirubin-C^{14} into the central nervous system. J. Clin. Invest. 45:678, 1966.

69. Chan, G., Schiff, D., et al.: Competitive binding of free fatty acids and bilirubin to albumin: differences in HBABA dye versus Sephadex G-25. Interpretation of results. Clin. Biochem. 4:208, 1971.

70. Lucey, J. F., Valaes, T., et al.: Serum albumin reserve PSP dye-binding capacity in infants with kernicterus. Pediatrics 39:876, 1967.

71. Odell, G. B., Cohen, S. M., et al.: Studies in kernicterus. II. The determination of the saturation of serum albumin with bilirubin. J. Pediatr. 74:214, 1969.

72. Odell, G. B., Storey, G. N. B., et al.: Studies in kernicterus. III. The saturation of serum protein with bilirubin during neonatal life and its relationship to brain damage at five years. J. Pediatr. 76:12, 1970.

73. Zamet, P., and Chunga, F.: Separation by gel filtration and microdetermination of unbound bilirubin. Acta Paediatr. Scand. 60:33, 1971.

74. Chunga, F., and Lardinois, R.: Separation by gel filtration and microdetermination of unbound bilirubin. 1. In vitro albumin and acidosis effects on albumin-bilirubin binding. Acta Paediatr. Scand. 60:27, 1971.

75. Schiff, D., Chan, G., et al.: Sephadex G-25 quantitative estimation of free bilirubin potential in jaundiced newborn infants' sera: A guide to the prevention of kernicterus. J. Lab. Clin. Med. 80:455, 1972.

76. Stern, L.: Drugs, the newborn infant, and the binding of bilirubin to albumin. Pediatrics 49:916, 1972.

77. Zipursky, A.: The universal prevention of Rh

immunization. Clin. Obstet. Gynecol. *14*: 869, 1971.

78. Freda, V. J., Gorman, J. G., et al.: The threat of Rh immunization from abortion. Lancet 2: 147, 1970.

79. Bowman, J. M., and Pollock, J. M.: Amniotic fluid spectrophotometry and early delivery in the management of erythroblastosis fetalis. Pediatrics 35:815, 1965.

80. Polacek, K., and Zwinger, A.: Factors influencing the accumulation of bilirubin in amniotic fluid in Rh hemolytic disease. Biol. Neonate 19:253, 1971.

81. Bowman, J. M., Friesen, R. F., et al.: Fetal transfusion in severe Rh isoimmunization. J.A.M.A. 207:1101, 1969.

82. Queenan, J. T.: *Modern Management of the Rh Problem.* New York, Hoeber Medical Division, Harper and Row, 1967.

83. Zipursky, A., Pollock, J., et al.: Transplacental foetal hemorrhage after placental injury during delivery or amniocentesis. Lancet 2: 493, 1963.

84. Watson, D., Mackay, E. V., et al.: Amniotic fluid analysis and foetal erythroblastosis. Clin. Chim. Acta 12:500, 1965.

85. Liley, A. W.: The use of amniocentesis and fetal transfusion in erythroblastosis fetalis. Pediatrics 35:836, 1965.

86. Boggs, T. R., Jr.: Proper place of intrauterine transfusions in management of fetuses with Rh hemolytic disease. Clin. Pediatr. 9:636, 1970.

87. Gluck, L., Kulovich, M., et al.: Diagnosis of the respiratory distress syndrome by amniocentesis. Am. J. Obstet. Gynecol. 109:440, 1971.

88. Liley, A. W.: Intrauterine transfusion of foetus in haemolytic disease. Br. Med. J. 2:1107, 1963.

89. Bowman, J. M., and Friesen, R. F.: Homolytic disease of the newborn, In *Current Pediatric Therapy.* Gellis, S. S., and Kagan, B. M. (eds.), Philadelphia, W. B. Saunders Company, 1968.

90. Friesen, R. F.: Complications of intrauterine transfusion. Clin. Obstet. Gynecol. 14:572, 1971.

91. Phibbs, R. H., Harvin, D., et al.: Development of children who had received intrauterine transfusions. Pediatrics 47:689, 1971.

92. Gregg, G. S., and Hutchinson, D. L.: Developmental characteristics of infants surviving fetal transfusions. J.A.M.A. 209:1059, 1969.

93. Naiman, J. L., Punnett, H. H., et al.: Possible graft-versus-host reaction after erythroblastosis fetalis. New Engl. J. Med. 281: 697, 1969.

94. Hutchinson, D. L., Maxwell, N. D., et al.: Advantages of use of maternal erythrocytes for fetal transfusion. Am. J. Obstet. Gynecol. 99:702, 1967.

95. Valaes, T.: Bilirubin distribution and dynamics of bilirubin removal by exchange transfusion. Acta Paediatr. Suppl. 149, 1963.

96. Sproul, A., and Smith, L.: Bilirubin equilibration during exchange transfusion in hemolytic disease of the newborn. J. Pediatr. 65:12, 1964.

97. Odell, G. B., Cohen, S. N., et al.: Administration of albumin in the management of hyperbilirubinemia by exchange transfusions. Pediatrics 30:613, 1962.

98. Comley, A., and Wood, B.: Albumin administration in exchange transfusion for hyperbilirubinemia. Arch. Dis. Child. 43:151, 1968.

99. Ruys, J. H., and van Gelderen, H. H.: Administration of albumin in exchange transfusion. J. Pediatr. 61:413, 1962.

100. Phibbs, R. H.: Response of newborn infants to leukocyte depletion during exchange transfusion. Biol. Neonate 15:112, 1970.

101. Bierman, H. R., Kelley, K. H., et al.: Leucapheresis in man. I. Haematological observations following leucocyte withdrawal in patients with non-haematological disorders. Br. J. Haematol. 7:51, 1961.

102. Oski, F. A., and Naiman, J. L.: *Hematologic Problems in the Newborn.* Philadelphia, W. B. Saunders Company, 1972.

103. Lanzkowsky, P., Salemi, M., et al.: Phototherapy —a note of caution. Pediatrics 48:914, 1970.

104. Radde, I. C., Parkinson, D. K., et al.: Ionized calcium in infants treated with exchange transfusions. Abstract, Soc. Pediatr. Res. Atlantic City, May, 1970, p. 235.

105. Calladine, M., Gairdner, D., et al.: Acid-base changes following exchange transfusion with citrated blood. Arch. Dis. Child. 40:626, 1965.

106. Gaudy, G., Partridge, J. W., et al.: Control of acidosis during exchange transfusion with citrated blood. Arch. Dis. Child. 43:147, 1968.

107. Bentley, H. P., Jr., Ziegler, N. R., et al.: The use of heparinized blood for exchange transfusion in infants. A.M.A. J. Dis. Child. 99:8, 1960.

108. Phibbs, R. H., Johnson, P., et al.: Cardiorespiratory status of erythroblastotic infants. 1. Relationship of gestational age, severity of hemolytic disease and birth asphyxia to idiopathic respiratory distress syndrome and survival. Pediatrics 49:5, 1972.

109. Sisson, T. R. C., Whalen, L. E., et al.: A comparison of the effects of whole blood and sedimented erythrocytes in exchange transfusion. Pediatrics 21:81, 1958.

110. Phibbs, R. H., Johnson, P., et al.: Circulatory changes in newborns with erythroblastosis fetalis with or without hydrops. Pediatr. Res. 1:321, 1971.

111. Maisels, M. J., Pathak, A., et al.: The effect of exchange transfusion on endogenous carbon monoxide production in erythroblastotic infants. J. Pediatr. 81:705, 1972.

112. Kauder, E., and Mauer, A. M.: Hemolysis as a contributing factor in the bilirubin rebound after exchange transfusion. J. Pediatr. 60: 163, 1962.

113. Chessels, J. M., and Wigglesworth, J. S.: Hemostatic failure in babies with Rhesus isoimmunization. Arch. Dis. Child. 46:38, 1971.

114. Latour, J. G., McKay, D. G., et al.: Activation of Hageman factor by cardiac arrest. Thromb. Diath. Haemorrh. 27:543, 1972.

115. Chessels, J. M., and Wigglesworth, J. S.: Coagulation studies in severe birth asphyxia. Arch. Dis. Child. 46:253, 1971.

116. Ekert, H., and Mathew, R. Y.: Platelet counts and plasma fibrinogen levels in erythroblastosis foetalis. Med. J. Aust. 2:844, 1967.

117. Dunn, P. M.: Obstructive jaundice and hemolytic disease of the newborn. Arch. Dis. Child. 38: 54, 1963.

118. Driscoll, S. C., and Steinke, J.: Pancreatic insulin content in severe erythroblastosis fetalis. Pediatrics. 39:448, 1967.

119. Price, H. V.: Hypoglycemia complicating hemolytic disease of the newborn. Arch. Dis. Child. 44:248, 1969.

120. Schiff, D., Aranda, J. V., et al.: Metabolic effects of exchange transfusion. II. Delayed hypoglycemia following exchange transfusion with citrated blood. J. Pediatr. 79:589, 1971.

121. Giblett, E. R., Varela, J. E., et al.: Damage of the bone marrow due to Rh antibody. Pediatrics 17:37, 1956.

122. Dillon, H. C., and Krivit, W.: Serial study of bone marrow in hemolytic disease of the newborn (erythroblastosis fetalis). Pediatrics 23:314, 1959.

123. Voak, D.: The serological specificity of the sensitizing antibodies in ABO heterospecific pregnancy of the Group O mother. Vox Sang. 14:271, 1968.

124. Denborough, M. H., and Downing, H. J.: The incidence of anti-A and anti-B isoagglutinins in cord blood and maternal saliva. Br. J. Haematol. 16:111, 1969.

125. Kochwa, S., Rosenfeld, R. E., et al.: Isoagglutinins associated with erythroblastosis. J. Clin. Invest. 40:874, 1961.

126. Moores, P., Grobbelaar, B. G., et al.: Hemolytic disease of the newborn due to ABO incompatibility. Acta Haematol. 44:47, 1970.

127. Polley, M. J., Mollison, P. L., et al.: A simple serological test for antibodies causing ABO-haemolytic disease of the newborn. Lancet 1:291, 1965.

128. Winstanley, D. P., Konugres, A. A., et al.: Studies on human anti-A sera with special reference to so-called immune anti-A. I. The A^p antigen and the specificity of the haemolysin in anti-A sera. Br. J. Haematol. 3:341, 1957.

129. Voak, D., and Williams, M. A.: An explanation of the failure of the direct antiglobulin test to detect erythrocyte sensitization in ABO

haemolytic disease of the newborn and observations on pinocytosis of IgG anti-A antibodies by input (cord) red cells. Br. J. Haematol. 20:9, 1971.

130. Rosenfeld, R. E., and Ohno, G.: A-B hemolytic disease of the newborn. Rev. Hematol. 10: 231, 1955.

131. Yunis, E., and Bridges, R.: The serological diagnosis of ABO hemolytic disease of the newborn. Am. J. Clin. Pathol. 41:1, 1964.

132. Grundbacher, F. J.: ABO hemolytic disease of the newborn: A family study with emphasis on the strength of A antigen. Pediatrics 35: 916, 1965.

133. Denborough, M. A., Downing, H. J., et al.: Serum blood group substances and ABO haemolytic disease. Br. J. Haematol. 16:103, 1969.

134. Gunson, H. H.: An evaluation of the immunological tests used in the diagnosis of AB hemolytic disease. Am. J. Dis. Child. 94: 123, 1957.

135. Wang, M. Y. F. W., and Desfarges, J. F.: Complement in ABO-hemolytic disease of the newborn. Pediatrics 48:650, 1971.

136. Weed, R. I., and Weiss, L.: The relationship of red cell fragmentation occurring within the spleen to cell destruction. Trans. Assoc. Am. Physicians 79:426, 1966.

137. Brown, D. L., Lachmann, P. J., et al.: The in vivo behaviour of complement-coated red cells: Studies in C6-deficient, C3-depleted and normal rabbits. Clin. Exp. Immunol. 7:401, 1970.

138. Lucey, J. F.: Neonatal jaundice and phototherapy. Pediatr. Clin. North Am. 19:827, 1972.

139. Maisels, M. J.: Bilirubin: On understanding and influencing its metabolism in the newborn infant. Pediatr. Clin. North Am. 19:447, 1972.

140. Lucey, J. F.: Phototherapy jaundice 1969. Bilirubin Metabolism. Birth Defects Orig. Art. Ser. 6:63, 1970.

141. Mountain, K. R., Hirsh, J., et al.: Neonatal coagulation defect due to anticonvulsant treatment in pregnancy. Lancet 1:265, 1970.

Chapter 10

Pyruvate Kinase Deficiency and Disorders of Glycolysis

By William C. Mentzer, Jr.

INTRODUCTION

The mature erythrocyte, devoid of nucleus, mitochondria, ribosomes, and other organelles, has no capacity for cell replication, protein synthesis, or oxidative phosphorylation. The glycolytic production of ATP, the sole known energy source of such erythrocytes, is sufficient to meet their limited metabolic requirements. The discovery during the past decade that hemolytic anemia may result from any of several glycolytic enzymopathies has underscored the dependence of erythrocytes upon glycolysis. More recently, acquired abnormalities of the chemical milieu within the erythrocyte have also been shown to influence glycolysis, leading to altered hemoglobin function and sometimes to premature hemolysis. Acquired deficiencies of certain glycolytic enzymes have also been found in erythrocytes from a few individuals harboring malignancies of the hemopoietic system. In the following paragraphs, the clinical, biochemical, and genetic features associated with abnormalities of erythrocyte glycolysis will be described in detail. Because they have been more thoroughly studied, the congenital hemolytic anemias will be discussed at length, while the various acquired disorders will be briefly described.

Hereditary anemias resulting from altered erythrocyte metabolism are distinguished from hereditary spherocytosis by the absence of spherocytes on the peripheral blood smear, by normal osmotic fragility of fresh erythrocytes, by a partial rather than complete therapeutic response to splenectomy, and by a recessive rather than dominant mode of inheritance. Hemoglobin structure and synthesis are normal. Because no specific morphologic abnormality is associated with these disorders, they have become known as the congenital nonspherocytic hemolytic anemias (CNSHA) (1). Initial attempts at classification were based on the autohemolysis test, in which saline-washed erythrocytes were incubated in vitro at 37°C under sterile conditions and the percentage hemolysis determined after 48 hours (2). Autohemolysis was greater than normal in almost all cases of CNSHA. If glucose was added prior to incubation, hemolysis was reduced in controls and in some cases of CNSHA (Type I), but was unchanged or actually increased in others (Type II). Robinson, Loder, and DeGruchy (3) found that Type II erythrocytes contained subnormal amounts of ATP but markedly increased amounts of 2,3-DPG. These observations, coupled with the demonstrable inability of such cells to metabolize glucose (2) led Robinson and her co-workers to suggest the existence of a specific glycolytic enzyme defect below the site of 2,3-DPG synthesis. In 1961, Valentine, Tanaka, and Miwa provided dramatic confirmation of the suggested glycolytic defect by reporting a deficiency of erythrocyte pyruvate kinase in three patients with CNSHA (4). Subsequently, abnormalities

315

of other glycolytic enzymes have been associated with CNSHA, as indicated in Figure 10–1.

The presence of a glycolytic enzymopathy should be suspected when chronic hemolysis occurs in the absence of marked abnormalities of erythrocyte morphology or osmotic fragility. Hemoglobin electrophoresis, stains for inclusion bodies, hemoglobin heat stability, acid hemolysis, and appropriate studies for immune hemolysis are normal. The autohemolysis test is usually abnormal but lacks specificity. Inheritance is customarily autosomal recessive, with the exception of phosphoglycerate kinase, which is X-linked. Dominant inheritance favors an abnormality of hemoglobin or membrane. Although appropriate clinical and laboratory findings may suggest its presence, definitive diagnosis depends upon quantitative assay of the activity of the suspect enzyme. The availability of such assays is somewhat limited, but screening tests for deficiencies of pyruvate kinase, triose phosphate isomerase, and phosphoglucose isomerase can be carried out in any well-equipped clinical laboratory (5–7). Mutant enzyme proteins vary in their in vitro properties (Table 10–1), and characterization of such properties has improved understanding of the genetics and pathogenesis of anemias associated with defective glycolytic enzymes. Measurement of glycolytic intermediates extracted from freshly obtained erythrocytes has provided confirmation of the in vivo significance of such in vitro abnormalities of enzyme function. The usual finding is an accumulation of proximal, and a depletion of distal,

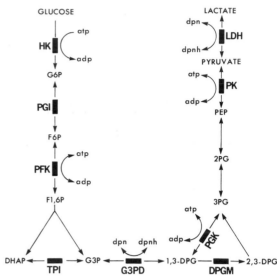

Figure 10–1. The Embden-Meyerhof pathway. Recognized enzyme defects are indicated by solid bars. HK = hexokinase; PGI = phosphoglucose isomerase; PFK = phosphofructokinase; TPI = triosephosphate isomerase; G3PD = glucose-3-phosphate dehydrogenase; PGK = phosphoglycerate kinase; DPGM = 2,3-diphosphoglycerate mutase; PK = pyruvate kinase; LDH = lactate dehydrogenase.

intermediates, giving rise to a characteristic transition or cross-over pattern at the locus of an abnormal enzyme. Secondary cross-overs are sometimes observed, reflecting the influence of altered concentrations of metabolites upon key regulatory enzymes, such as hexokinase, phosphofructokinase, and pyruvate kinase.

As will be seen later, a certain amount of caution is necessary in interpreting results, even when quantitative assays are employed. First, only surviving cells are available for sampling in the circulating blood, and the metabolic circumstances of these favored cells cannot be extrapolated to indicate the status of cells either already hemolyzed or sequestered under conditions such as hypoxia, acidosis, and hypoglycemia in the spleen. Second, assay in vitro under optimal conditions of pH, cofactor availability, and substrate concentration may not adequately reflect the performance of an enzyme under less favorable circumstances in vivo. Third, the high specific activity of certain enzymes in leukocytes may result in spurious normal values for erythrocyte enzyme activity unless such leukocytes are either removed prior to

TABLE 10–1. PARAMETERS COMMONLY USED IN VITRO TO CHARACTERIZE MUTANT ENZYME PROTEIN

Vmax	Maximal enzyme velocity obtainable with saturating substrate concentrations.
Km	The substrate concentration yielding half maximal activity. An index of catalytic efficiency.
pH optimum	That pH at which maximal enzyme activity is present.
Heat stability	Resistance of enzyme protein to heat denaturation.
Electrophoretic mobility	Migration of enzyme protein in an electric field.

assay or their contribution to total activity is compensated for by appropriate calculations. Fourth, transfusion therapy with normal erythrocytes within several months prior to assay may obscure the presence of an enzyme defect. Finally, the mean enzyme activity determined fails to portray distribution of activity within individual erythrocytes. The endowment of intracellular enzymes is fixed with the disappearance of protein synthetic ability at the reticulocyte stage; thereafter the inevitable denaturation of enzyme protein which accompanies cell aging reduces enzymatic activity at a rate characteristic of each enzyme. Transient accentuation of reticulocytosis, therefore, is often accompanied by rising mean enzyme activity. At such a time the true magnitude of an enzyme deficiency may not be apparent unless comparison is made to equally reticulocyte-rich blood.

HEXOKINASE DEFICIENCY

Enzyme

$$\text{Glucose} \xrightarrow[\text{ATP} \, \diagdown \text{Mg}^{2+} \, \diagup \text{ADP}]{\text{Hexokinase}} \text{Glucose-6-phosphate}$$

Clinical Manifestations

Fewer than ten cases of congenital nonspherocytic hemolytic anemia have thus far been attributed to deficient erythrocyte hexokinase (HK). Severely affected individuals may exhibit neonatal hyperbilirubinemia and thereafter require transfusion at regular intervals for intractable anemia, but in mild cases, hemolysis is fully compensated for by increased erythropoiesis, and anemia is absent. However, jaundice, reticulocytosis, and splenomegaly are usually present in such patients. Transient bone marrow aplasia, induced by certain infections, may lead to anemia, even in mild cases, as well as to exacerbations of anemia in severely affected patients. In contrast to G6PD deficiency, hyperhemolytic episodes are not a feature of the disorder. Macrocytosis and polychromatophilia are found on examination of the peripheral blood smear, in keeping with the reticulocytosis present, but red cell morphology is

usually otherwise unremarkable. After splenectomy, occasional burr cells, target cells, stippled cells, and densely stained spiculated cells may be observed. The osmotic fragility of fresh erythrocytes is normal, but after incubation at 37°C, a fragile population of cells may be produced in some cases. The autohemolysis test may be normal or exhibit varying degrees of increased hemolysis in saline with partial correction by glucose.

Deficient erythrocyte hexokinase activity has also been found in four young males who exhibited the renal, skeletal, dermatologic, endocrinologic, and chromosomal abnormalities characteristic of Fanconi's aplastic anemia (8), and who thus differed from patients with isolated congenital hemolytic anemia. Thrombocytopenia and leukopenia were present, and both platelet and white cell hexokinase activity was reduced. Macrocytic hemolytic anemia without reticulocytosis was observed in all cases. Other patients with Fanconi's anemia have not been hexokinase-deficient, complicating interpretation of the role of hexokinase in the pathogenesis of this disorder.

Biochemistry

The maximal activity (Vmax) of erythrocyte hexokinase from deficient patients has varied from 35 to 90 per cent of normal. Although it might seem unlikely that such modest reduction in enzyme activity would result in hemolysis, it should be recalled that hexokinase activity declines rapidly as erythrocytes age. Comparisons of enzyme activity must, therefore, be made between red cell populations of equivalent age. In the case described by Valentine, for example (Fig. 10–2), although hexokinase activity was 62 per cent of the normal for mature erythrocytes, it was only 14 per cent of the activity found in high reticulocyte blood. A separation of young and old red cell populations by centrifugation revealed only the expected moderate diminution (to 0.11 μM. per min. per 10^{10} RBC) of hexokinase activity in older cells from this patient (12). Hexokinase activity was even lower (0.075 μM. per min. per 10^{10} RBC) in an asymptomatic brother, yet no evidence of undue hemolysis was present. However, reference to Figure 10–2 will

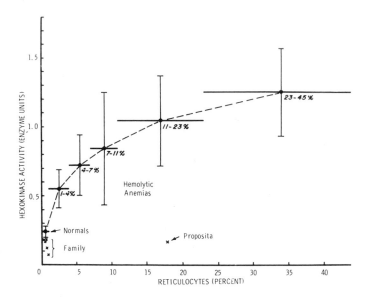

Figure 10–2. Hexokinase (HK) activity observed in 54 cases of hemolytic anemia of various etiologies plotted against reticulocyte percentages in cells assayed. Cases are grouped according to reticulocyte levels. Mean HK activity for each group is plotted against mean reticulocyte percentage in cells of that group. Standard deviations are indicated by vertical bars. Values for a single HK-deficient patient (proposita) and her family are designated separately. [Reproduced by permission from Valentine, W. N., et al., In *Hereditary Disorders of Erythrocyte Metabolism.* Beutler, E. (ed.), New York, Grune & Stratton, 1968, p. 294.]

establish that the brother's cells are actually far less deficient with respect to cell age than are the immature cells of the proposita. In fact, diminished hexokinase activity should impose a greater limitation on energetic young cells with increased metabolic needs than on aged, metabolically indolent cells. A defect present in youth then might curtail survival, while the same defect emerging later in the life of the cell would not (12). As the erythrocyte ages, in vivo changes in stability or kinetics peculiar to mutant hexokinase may also render older cells liable to premature hemolysis. In rats and rabbits, hexokinase from immature erythrocytes exhibits a higher Km glucose than is seen in mature cells, but such is not the case in normal human erythrocytes (14). No evidence is yet available on possible age-associated changes in mutant hexokinase, and the relationship of such changes to hemolysis is at present undefined.

In keeping with their enzymatic defect, hexokinase deficient erythrocytes have invariably demonstrated subnormal glucose consumption and lactate production in vitro. Such cells also metabolize fructose poorly, but utilize mannose or galactose normally (12). Apparently the latter two substrates enter the glycolytic sequence through the action of kinases other than hexokinase. Some hexokinase-deficient erythrocytes are capable of normal glucose consumption at the glucose concentrations

(5 mM.) customarily found in plasma. However, such cells utilize glucose poorly or not at all at lower glucose concentrations, either because of an abnormally low affinity for glucose (11) or because of enzyme instability under conditions of low substrate availability (10). Such erythrocytes may encounter a particularly unfavorable metabolic environment within the spleen. The concentration of glucose in normal splenic homogenates has been found by Necheles to be only 5 to 11 μM. per gram of tissue, and in a hexokinase-deficient patient the concentration was even lower (1.1 μM. per gram of tissue) (11). Furthermore, because splenic tissue metabolizes glucose rapidly (15), prolonged vascular pooling in the spleen is probably accompanied by profound local hypoglycemia. Erythrocytes containing high Km hexokinase are clearly at a disadvantage competing with reticuloendothelial cells for such a reduced glucose supply. Another disadvantage of the splenic environment is its relative acidity. The pH optimum of erythrocyte hexokinase is approximately 8; at lower pH values diminished enzyme activity may be expected. Possibly of greater importance at low pH, glucose-6-phosphate, a potent inhibitor of hexokinase, accumulates because of phosphofructokinase inhibition (16). An erythrocyte whose hexokinase activity is diminished, even under optimal pH conditions, will be further compromised in the acidic environment of the spleen. The clinical

improvement which attends splenectomy attests to the importance of this organ in the pathogenesis of hemolysis; the fact that hemolysis persists after splenectomy indicates that other factors are also involved. Detailed isotopic studies to define red cell kinetics and sites of hemolysis have yet to be reported. While in one patient no splenic sequestration of chromated autologous erythrocytes was noted (13), in another patient such sequestration was present (8).

Significant alterations in intracellular metabolites are associated with defective hexokinase function. With a single exception (11), erythrocyte ATP concentration has been subnormal in all reported cases. Glucose-6-phosphate is reduced to approximately half normal concentrations, and other more distal intermediates, most notably 2,3-DPG, are also reduced in concentration. These metabolites may exert a significant regulatory influence upon glycolysis. For example, Brewer has shown that concentrations of 2,3-DPG in the physiologic range inhibit hexokinase (17). The partial relief of 2,3-DPG inhibition afforded by the reduced concentration of this metabolite in hexokinase-deficient red cells may facilitate utilization of available hexokinase by deficient cells. The increased hemoglobin-oxygen affinity customarily associated with subnormal 2,3-DPG levels has been investigated in one anemic hexokinase-deficient patient by Delivoria-Papadopoulos and her co-workers (18) and by Oski et al. (19). This patient, whose whole blood oxygen affinity (P_{50}) was 19 mm. Hg (normal = 27 ± 1.2), was capable of only minimal exercise on a bicycle ergometer despite only moderate anemia (hemoglobin = 9.8 gm. per 100 ml.). On exercise, her central venous pO_2 promptly fell to minimal levels as oxygen consumption rose. Increased oxygen delivery was achieved largely by an increase in cardiac output since the unfavorable oxygen affinity curve precluded any substantial further desaturation of hemoglobin (19). Thus the altered concentration of intracellular metabolites induced by hexokinase deficiency may, as in this patient, accentuate the usual clinical manifestations of anemia.

Because of its reactive sulfhydryl group, hexokinase is susceptible to oxidant inactivation in the absence of sufficient glutathione (20). Both normal (8, 21) and low (13) glutathione levels have been reported in hexokinase deficiency, and while Heinz bodies were discovered in Löhr's patients with Fanconi's anemia (8), they have not been observed in other enzymopenic individuals. Resting hexose monophosphate shunt activity, measured with glucose-1-^{14}C, was quantitatively normal in one case despite subnormal glucose consumption, but stimulation with methylene blue produced only a meager 6-fold rise in activity, compared to a 22-fold rise in control blood (22). Failure of the shunt at low glucose concentrations has also been noted in a high Km glucose hexokinase mutant (11). These studies, while not indicating a central role for defective shunt activity in the pathogenesis of hemolysis, do suggest that in certain circumstances hexokinase-deficient cells might be compromised by a limited shunt. Such circumstances, for example, might arise upon exposure to a potent oxidant in the low glucose environment of the spleen. Episodic hemolysis has not been a feature of the cases reported to date.

Genetics

An autosomal recessive mode of inheritance has been proposed, with hematologically normal heterozygotes exhibiting enzyme activity approximately half that of normals. Biochemical identification of such asymptomatic carriers is not always possible, as enzyme activity often falls within the low-normal range. Thus in none of the cases of hemolytic anemia thus far described have there been unequivocal deficiencies of enzyme activity in both parents. Furthermore, in the normal parent no qualitative enzyme abnormalities have appeared on electrophoresis or kinetic studies. It remains possible that anemic patients rather than being homozygotes are double heterozygotes for two separate traits, only one of which has thus far been biochemically defined. Such a patient who appeared to be doubly heterozygous for hexokinase and G6PD deficiency has recently been reported (21).

The qualitative abnormalities characteristic of variant hexokinase (Table 10–2) may reflect either a structural or regulatory gene mutation. The electrophoretic pattern of normal erythrocyte hexokinase is charac-

TABLE 10–2. HEXOKINASE VARIANTS

AUTHOR (REFERENCE)	NUMBER OF CASES	CLINICAL STATUS	ERYTHROCYTE HEXOKINASE				
			$Vmax°$	Km Glucose	Km ATP	Stability In Vitro	Electrophoresis Bands Present
Altay (9)	1	Asymptomatic	100	Normal	---	---	—, II, III
Keitt (10)	2	Hemolytic anemia	89–93	---†	Normal	Unstable	I, II, III
Necheles (11)	2	Hemolytic anemia	75	Increased	---	Normal	I, II, —
Valentine (12)	1	Hemolytic anemia	62	Normal	Normal	---	I, —, —
Moser (13)	1	Hemolytic anemia	50	Increased	Increased	---	---
Löhr (8)	4	Fanconi's pancytopenia	35–60	Increased	Increased	---	---

°Vmax = maximal enzyme activity expressed as percentage of the mean normal activity.
†High concentrations of glucose, required for stability in vitro, precluded determination of Km glucose.
— = Absent band; --- = not examined.

terized by different bands of varying intensity (I, II, and III). On electrophoresis, mutant hexokinase lacks one or more of the normal bands of activity, but no bands migrating in an abnormal position have been observed. The various bands represent the presence of several isozymes of hexokinase, each with different kinetic properties. Therefore, diminished synthesis of one or more isozymes with predominance of the remaining isozyme(s) could account for apparent qualitative changes in enzyme protein. The normal glucose kinetics found by Altay (9) in mutant hexokinase which lacked band I on electrophoresis indicate that unbalanced representation of isozymes need not result in kinetic abnormalities. Furthermore, although normal on electrophoresis, the mutant described by Keitt (10) exhibited qualitative abnormalities in enzyme stability and kinetics. It is probable, therefore, that many of the abnormalities noted in Table 10–2 do, in fact, reflect structural abnormalities of enzyme protein, although a definite answer must await isolation and characterization of the mutant enzymes.

Studies of the distribution of hexokinase deficiency have been limited to blood cells, although the widespread abnormalities seen in Fanconi's pancytopenia suggest involvement of nonhematologic tissues in these patients. Electrophoresis of leukocyte or platelet hexokinase reveals three isozymes (IV, V, VI) distinct from those of the erythrocyte as well as a shared isozyme (I) (9). Abnormalities in leukocyte hexokinase were not observed in the patients reported by Valentine (12) and Keitt (10), emphasizing the separate nature of erythrocyte and leukocyte hexokinase. However, the deficient leukocyte and platelet hexokinase found in the patients of Löhr (8), as well as the qualitative abnormality of leukocyte hexokinase described by Necheles (11), indicates that to some extent the enzyme is under common genetic control in different tissues.

Therapy

The supportive care customarily employed in chronic hemolytic anemia—blood transfusion as indicated, supplemental folic acid, and close observation for cholelithiasis—is appropriate in hexokinase deficiency as well. Experience with splenectomy has been limited to three cases; none were cured but all benefited. Preexisting transfusion requirements were abolished in two severe cases (11, 12), while in the third case (10), which was milder and did not require transfusion, evidence of diminished hemolysis was obtained. Treatment by circumventing the aberrant enzyme with alternate substrates such as inosine, although theoretically of possible benefit, has not been explored.

PHOSPHOGLUCOSE ISOMERASE

Enzyme

Phosphoglucose isomerase
Glucose-6-phosphate ↔ Fructose-6-phosphate

Clinical Manifestations

Deficient phosphoglucose isomerase (PGI) has been found in the erythrocytes of 13 anemic patients from 10 different pedigrees (23–30). In most cases, hemolytic anemia has first appeared in infancy and has been severe enough to warrant blood transfusion therapy. Aplastic marrow crises with reticulocytopenia and accentuation of anemia have occurred following infections. Two patients have experienced hyperhemolytic crises; in one, G6PD as well as phosphoglucose isomerase was deficient (30), while in the other no single precipitating cause was identified (23). The blood smear, in general, resembles that seen in other types of congenital nonspherocytic hemolytic anemia. In several severely anemic patients, dense, spiculated, or "whiskered" microspherocytes have been noted after splenectomy. In one instance, sufficient numbers of such cells were present before splenectomy to suggest the diagnosis of hereditary spherocytosis (28). Reticulocytosis may be profound; levels as high as 81 per cent have been observed. The mean corpuscular volume is elevated (97 to 139 μ^3). When incubated at 37°C, a variable fraction of erythrocytes exhibits abnormally increased osmotic fragility, whereas fresh cells are indistinguishable from normal. Autohemolysis is increased in saline, partly corrected by glucose, and further corrected by nucleotides (ATP, adenosine, or inosine). The survival of chromated autologous red cells is reduced ($t_{1/2}$ = 2.5 to 12 days), with evidence of splenic sequestration (23–25, 30).

Biochemistry

The metabolic events which precede hemolysis of PGI-deficient erythrocytes are poorly understood. There is good evidence that erythrocyte glycolysis is impaired in vivo, since accumulation of glucose-6-phosphate has been a consistent finding in freshly obtained enzymopenic cells. Paradoxically, such cells are fully capable of glycolysis in vitro, even at the maximal rate imposed by a high-phosphate medium (18 mM) (23). In contrast to hexokinase deficiency, in which 2,3-DPG levels are low, sufficient glycolysis occurs in PGI defi-

ciency to maintain the 2,3-DPG concentration at or above the normal level. Although in most cases intracellular ATP concentrations have been normal, two exceptions with diminished ATP and reduced in vitro glycolysis for cell age have been reported (28, 30). One such exception (30) was G6PD- as well as PGI-deficient, and exhibited unusually high glucose-6-phosphate levels. It was thought that inhibition of hexokinase by the increased concentration of glucose-6-phosphate present might have contributed importantly to the reduced glycolytic rate observed. On the other hand, increased glucose-6-phosphate availability might have favorably influenced the PGI reaction by bringing the enzyme closer to saturation with its substrate.

Although in vitro the mainstream of glycolysis is relatively uninfluenced by PGI deficiency, a profound defect in recycling of fructose-6-phosphate through the pentose phosphate shunt has been repeatedly observed (24, 28, 29). Shunt activity in vivo appears to be uncompromised, however, since Heinz bodies are absent, glutathione concentration is normal, and glutathione stability is unimpaired in PGI-deficient erythrocytes.

Genetics

Like most other glycolytic enzymopathies, PGI deficiency is inherited as an autosomal recessive. Obligate heterozygotes are hematologically normal but exhibit reduced erythrocyte PGI activity. At least 12 variants of the erythrocyte enzyme have been revealed by electrophoretic studies in humans, many with decreased activity and hemolysis. The properties of several mutant forms of erythrocyte PGI are presented in Table 10–3. The frequency of the wild (type 1) PGI phenotype exceeds 99 per cent in all human populations surveyed; most variants reflect the heterozygous inheritance of type 1 plus another rare type (31). The resultant electrophoretic pattern usually demonstrates three bands, which represent the association into dimers of like subunits of type 1 or of the variant as well as a third hybrid dimer with unlike subunits. In one pedigree (29), a single band of PGI activity with decreased cathodal migration was present in anemic mem-

TABLE 10–3.   PHOSPHOGLUCOSEISOMERASE VARIANTS

REFERENCE	VMAX°	KM F6P	pH OPTIMUM	THERMAL STABILITY	ELECTROPHORESIS
Baughan (24)	19	Normal	– – –	– – –	Abnormal‡
Paglia (29)	16	Normal	– – –	– – –	Abnormal
Cartier (26)	40	– – –	– – –	– – –	Normal
Nakashima (26a)	57	Normal	Normal	Unstable	Abnormal
Arnold (23, 23a)	32.4	Normal	Normal	Unstable†	Abnormal
Nakashima (26a)	53	Normal	Abnormal	Unstable	Normal
Blume (25)	14	Normal	Normal	Unstable	Abnormal
Blume (25)	29	Normal	Normal	Unstable	Abnormal

°Vmax expressed as per cent of normal.

†PGI activity was unusually low in the older erythrocytes of this patient, suggesting that the mutant may be unstable in vivo as well as in vitro.

‡The electrophoretic patterns described here as abnormal differed from each other, as well as from the wild type. – – – = not examined.

bers, while their parents' enzyme migrated normally but exhibited reduced activity. Such results are puzzling since, if the abnormal band seen in these anemic patients represents a dimer composed solely of mutant subunits, such a dimer should also have been evident in the parents.

Leukocytes also exhibit reduced PGI activity (5 to 73 per cent of normal), but are capable of normal phagocytosis and chemotaxis despite their enzyme defect (28). Similarly, platelet PGI is reduced (23), but clot formation, platelet aggregation, and other clotting studies are normal. Since the electrophoretic pattern of PGI from other human tissues resembles that of erythrocytes (31), many of these tissues are probably also deficient in PGI. Cultured skin fibroblasts exhibited only half-normal PGI activity in one patient (32), and plasma PGI activity was absent in another (24). The absence of clinical abnormalities outside the hemopoietic system, however, suggests that PGI deficiency is not critically important to such tissues.

Therapy

Transfusion requirements are usually eliminated by removal of the spleen, but anemia persists. The postsplenectomy hemoglobin levels of 6.7 to 10.3 g. per 100

ml. and reticulocyte counts of 36 to 73 per cent observed in three siblings by Paglia and his co-workers (29) reflect the magnitude of continued hemolysis which may be present. Arnold and his colleagues (23) have attempted to reduce the elevated erythrocyte glucose-6-phosphate concentration characteristic of PGI deficiency and thereby relieve hexokinase inhibition. Intravenous methylene blue (100 mg.) was given daily for four days in an effort to increase utilization of glucose-6-phosphate by the stimulated hexose monophosphate shunt. A moderate decrease in erythrocyte glucose-6-phosphate was observed 2 hours after methylene blue administration both in two normal controls and in one anemic patient, but 24 hours later baseline concentrations of glucose-6-phosphate had reappeared. No change in either hemoglobin concentration or reticulocyte count was noted. Because previous in vitro studies had demonstrated a 230 per cent increase in glycolysis when PGI deficient erythrocytes were incubated in a high-phosphate medium, the same patient then received 500 ml. of 0.22 M sodium phosphate (pH 7.4) solution by intravenous infusion daily for ten days. The reticulocyte count fell from 10 per cent to 7 per cent, and the hemoglobin rose 2 g. per 100 ml. A second trial of phosphate therapy for four days, however, failed to reproduce the therapeutic effect.

PHOSPHOFRUCTOKINASE

Enzyme

$$\text{Fructose-6-phosphate} \xleftrightarrow{\text{Phosphofructokinase}} \text{Fructose-1,6-diphosphate}$$

$$\text{ATP} \quad \text{Mg}^{2+} \quad \text{ADP}$$

Clinical Manifestations

Several individuals with a myopathy clinically indistinguishable from McArdle's disease have been found to lack muscle phosphofructokinase (PFK) (33, 34). Red cell PFK activity was reduced to about 50 per cent of normal, and mild hemolysis was present. Physical activity was limited not by anemia but by severe muscular cramps associated with the myopathy. A single example of hemolysis without evidence of myopathy has been described in an asymptomatic 23-year-old physician who was not anemic but exhibited mild icterus, splenomegaly, reticulocytosis, and shortened survival of chromated autologous erythrocytes (35). Hematologic findings were those typical of congenital nonspherocytic hemolytic anemia: normal osmotic fragility, increased autohemolysis (Type I), and no striking abnormalities of erythrocyte morphology.

Biochemistry

Studies of inactivation of human erythrocyte PFK by rabbit anti-human muscle PFK antibody have indicated that about 50 per cent of the erythrocyte enzyme is identical to muscle PFK (36). Antibody inactivation studies have further shown that the muscle component of the erythrocyte enzyme is lacking both in patients with myopathy and muscle PFK deficiency, and in the single individual with isolated hemolysis. Characterization of the mutant enzyme in the latter patient revealed an abnormal sensitivity to ATP inhibition and unusual fructose-6-phosphate kinetics. Mutant enzyme was unstable on storage at 4°C, but assay of PFK in young and old red cells separated by centrifugation disclosed no evidence for age-associated enzyme instability in vivo. Leukocytes did not share the enzyme defect either in this patient or in those with myopathy.

A variety of studies have established the central role of PFK in the regulation of erythrocyte metabolism (see Chapter 1). It is not surprising to find a deficiency of this important enzyme associated with hemolysis. However, little information is thus far available on the mechanism of hemolysis of PFK-deficient red cells. Erythrocyte sodium and potassium concentration, sodium influx, and lactate production were normal in one patient (35). Despite their normal glycolytic capabilities in vitro, deficient cells were incapable of maintaining normal ATP concentrations in vivo. The reduced (73 per cent of normal) intracellular ATP concentration in these cells, while indicative of an abnormality of cellular metabolism, might also be of benefit by partially relieving the inhibitory influence of ATP on the unduly sensitive mutant PFK. It is of interest that erythrocytes from newborn infants have PFK activity about 50 to 60 per cent that of normal adult cells (37). Although proof is thus far lacking, the demonstration that PFK deficiency may be associated with hemolytic anemia suggests that such a deficiency may contribute to the shortened mean survival of newborn red cells.

Genetics

Inheritance is probably autosomal recessive, although sometimes only one parent has exhibited biochemical evidence of PFK deficiency. For unknown reasons, the biochemical defect as measured in vitro may be more severe in asymptomatic relatives than in patients with anemia or myopathy.

The erythrocytes but not the leukocytes and platelets of individuals with trisomy 22 consistently contain increased PFK activity (38–40). Localization of a gene governing erythrocyte PFK synthesis on the 21 chromosome is suggested but by no means established by this observation. Although a third gene for PFK synthesis should lead to a 50 per cent increase in enzyme activity, the measured increase has often fallen short of this mark, ranging from 48 per cent (39) to 29 per cent (38). Since evidence suggests that PFK in erythrocytes is composed of at least two subunits, one identical to that found in muscle and the other unique to erythrocytes, genetic control of enzyme synthesis is likely to be complex. For this reason, an increase of less than 50 per cent in PFK activity remains consistent with a gene dosage effect, although other explanations now appear more likely (40).

TRIOSEPHOSPHATE ISOMERASE

Enzyme

Triosephosphate isomerase
$$\text{Dihydroxyacetone phosphate} \longleftrightarrow \text{Glyceraldehyde-3-phosphate}$$

Clinical Manifestations

An association with triosephosphate isomerase (TPI) deficiency has been proven or suspected on clinical and genetic grounds in nine cases of congenital hemolytic anemia (41–47). In addition to the familiar signs and symptoms of chronic hemolysis — pallor, jaundice, and splenomegaly — a severe neurologic disorder characterized initially by spasticity and motor retardation, often progressing to weakness and hypotonia, has been a feature of all cases surviving beyond the neonatal period. Such neurologic abnormalities, which are usually not manifest before 6 months of age, are almost certainly not related to kernicterus, since most patients have not exhibited neonatal hyperbilirubinemia. The neurologic abnormality stabilized during adolescence in the only adult patient thus far discovered (43, 44). Other affected individuals have died before the age of 5, often suddenly and without obvious explanation. Increased susceptibility to bacterial infection has been noted in both splenectomized and unsplenectomized patients.

Anemia has ranged from severe to moderate, with most patients requiring at least occasional blood transfusions. Macrocytosis and polychromatophilia are evident on the blood smear, reflecting the presence of reticulocytosis, which may reach 50 per cent on occasion. Aside from occasional small, dense, spiculated cells, no striking changes in erythrocyte morphology are present. Unincubated erythrocyte osmotic fragility is normal, while incubation produces both fragile and resistant subpopulations. The autohemolysis test is abnormal (Type 1).

Biochemistry

When measured in vitro, erythrocyte TPI activity is approximately 1000 times that of hexokinase, the least active glycolytic enzyme. Even deficient erythrocytes with only 5 to 35 per cent of normal TPI activity possess far more TPI than hexokinase activity. No qualitative abnormalities of enzyme protein have been reported. In view of the foregoing, it should not be surprising to learn that TPI-deficient erythrocytes are capable of normal glycolysis in vitro, even when compared to reticulocyte-rich control blood (42). Nonetheless, a striking accumulation of dihydroxyacetone phosphate (DHAP) is present in freshly obtained enzymopenic erythrocytes, and this intermediate accumulates further on incubation. In addition, erythrocyte ATP is low for cell age. Such results indicate the presence of a substantial impairment of glycolysis in vivo.

The enzymatic defect can be partially by-passed via the hexose monophosphate shunt, which generates glyceraldehyde-3-phosphate from glucose without the participation of TPI. Methylene blue stimulation of the shunt in TPI-deficient erythrocytes produces a lesser increase in glycolysis, relative to the rate found without additives, than is found in reticulocyte-rich control blood (42). This has been interpreted as indicating a markedly greater "resting" shunt rate in the deficient cells, consistent with the proposed reliance of such cells on the shunt. If the shunt is as active as has been suggested, it is difficult to explain the marked susceptibility of one patient's erythrocytes to Heinz body formation following incubation with acetylphenylhydrazine (46). Glutathione and glutathione stability were normal, however, in this patient.

The enzyme deficiency is manifest not only in red cells but also in leukocytes, muscle, serum, and cerebral spinal fluid. Tissues other than the above have not yet been analyzed, but the cerebral spinal fluid deficiency suggests the possibility that deficient TPI activity in neural tissue may be responsible for the neurologic abnormalities observed in enzymopenic patients. Although increased susceptibility to infection might be the consequence of defective function by TPI-deficient leukocytes, the limited studies thus far carried out on such cells indicate that they phagocytose normally (47).

Genetics

Studies of several large pedigrees are consistent with an autosomal recessive mode of inheritance. Obligate heterozygotes have been clinically normal, but their erythrocytes contain approximately half the TPI activity of control erythrocytes. As is often the case in other glycolytic enzymopathies, there is no clear boundary between heterozygous-deficient and low-normal enzyme activity. Partial deletion of the short arm of the fifth chromosome has been associated with a reduction of erythrocyte TPI to half the normal activity in two children with the cri-du-chat syndrome (48). In at least one case, both parents had normal erythrocyte TPI activity, raising the possibility of localization on the fifth chromosome of a gene associated with TPI. However, 13 additional cases of cri-du-chat syndrome, some with karyotypes indistinguishable from the two cases already mentioned, have had normal erythrocyte TPI (49). Simultaneous heterozygous inheritance of TPI deficiency and either G6PD deficiency or sickle cell trait has not altered the typical clinical pattern of the disorders when present alone (46). Of two female patients who inherited all three traits, one was hematologically normal, while the other exhibited evidence of chronic hemolytic anemia. The contribution, if any, of heterozygous TPI deficiency to the latter condition is unknown.

Therapy

Aside from transfusions and folic acid supplement, no other means of therapy are currently at hand. Splenectomy in one pa-

tient did not alter the intensity of hemolysis (47).

GLYCERALDEHYDE-3-PHOSPHATE DEHYDROGENASE

Enzyme

$$
\text{Glyceraldehyde-3-phosphate} \underset{NAD \quad P_i}{\overset{\text{Glyceraldehyde-3-phosphate dehydrogenase}}{\longleftrightarrow}} \text{1.3-Diphosphoglycerate} \quad NADH
$$

Clinical Manifestations, Biochemistry, and Genetics

Three males in whom hemolytic anemia was associated with reduced erythrocyte glyceraldehyde-3-phosphate dehydrogenase (G3PD) have been briefly described (50, 51). Differences in erythrocyte osmotic fragility and in G3PD activity indicate that the disorder in one patient may not be identical to that in the other two. In the former, infection and an antimalarial drug, dapsone, accelerated hemolysis, yet in all three, glutathione and glutathione stability were normal. Changes in the pattern of glycolytic intermediates similar to those induced by iodoacetic acid, a known inhibitor of G3PD, were found in the erythrocytes of one patient. Iodoacetic acid inhibited glycolysis more in affected erythrocytes than in control erythrocytes. The disorder is probably hereditary, since both father and son were affected in one pedigree, but the mode of inheritance has not yet been defined. In one patient enzyme activity was normal in platelets and reduced in leukocytes.

PHOSPHOGLYCERATE KINASE

Enzyme

$$
\text{1,3-Diphosphoglycerate} \underset{ADP \quad Mg^{2+}}{\overset{\text{Phosphoglycerate kinase}}{\longleftrightarrow}} \text{3-Phosphoglycerate} \quad ATP
$$

Clinical Manifestations

A severe form of congenital hemolytic anemia (Hb 6 to 10 g. per 100 ml.) has been reported in a 12-year-old Chinese boy whose erythrocyte phosphoglycerate kinase (PGK) activity was only 6 per cent of normal (52). This patient first presented with seizures, motor retardation, and anemia at 2½ years of age. A male maternal cousin, aged 4, with similar evidence of hemolytic anemia, motor retardation, and emotional instability, but without a history of seizures, was found to have no measurable erythrocyte PGK activity. Erythrocyte morphology was not remarkable aside from changes attributed to splenectomy; the osmotic fragility test was normal, and the autohemolysis test revealed moderately increased hemolysis not correctable by glucose (Type II). The mother and grandmother of the first case had higher erythrocyte PGK activity (42 to 77 per cent of normal), milder hemolytic anemia, and no neurologic abnormalities. The hematologic and neurologic abnormalities seen in males from this pedigree have also been noted in other PGK-deficient males (52a, 52b).

Biochemistry

PKG-deficient cells are capable of normal glycolysis in vitro (52). Nevertheless, intracellular ATP concentration is low when compared to normal cells of equivalent age (52). These results presumably indicate increased flow through the 2,3-DPG cycle (Fig. 10–1) at the expense of the ATP-generating PGK reaction. The 2,3-DPG concentration in deficient cells is elevated to twice the normal in affected males and to a lesser degree in females (52). The pattern of glycolytic intermediates in one female demonstrated a crossover between 3-phosphoglycerate and phosphoenolpyruvate, suggesting that the activity of other enzymes may sometimes be compromised in PGK deficiency (53).

Substantial PGK activity is membrane associated (54). ADP derived from membrane ATPase exerts an important regulatory influence on glycolysis by its participation in the PGK reaction (55); the ATP thus generated is then available for ATPase-mediated cation transport. Despite this relationship, the cation pump operates normally in PGK-deficient erythrocytes, probably because sufficient substrate flows through the residual enzyme (56). Sodium accumulation has been implicated in the hemolysis of other congenitally abnormal erythrocytes (57). It is not yet known, however, whether PGK-deficient erythrocytes accumulate sodium in vivo.

Several rare, clinically asymptomatic, electrophoretic variants of erythrocyte PGK have been discovered (58, 59). Yoshida has succeeded in purifying both normal erythrocyte PGK and that of the "New Guinea" variant (59). The two enzymes, clearly distinct on electrophoresis or isoelectric focusing but with identical molecular weights of approximately 50,000, differ from one another by the substitution of a single amino acid. Threonine has been replaced by arginine in the variant enzyme. The properties of purified normal PGK are known (60), but those of the variant enzymes have not yet been reported. In crude hemolysate from a 63-year-old female with mild hemolytic anemia whose PGK activity was approximately 80 per cent of normal, the Km for an unspecified substrate as well as enzyme stability at 4 and 37°C were normal (61). No evidence for more than a single isozyme of PGK has been obtained by studies of human nonhematopoietic tissues obtained at autopsy (62). It is therefore possible that the neurologic disorder found in PGK-deficient males results from an abnormality of this enzyme in neural tissue.

PGK activity in leukocytes from one anemic male was reduced to 5.6 per cent of normal, while in contrast, 50 to 100 per cent of normal PGK activity has been found in the leukocytes of affected females. Although ingestion of bacteria is normal, deficient leukocytes are unable to effectively kill or iodinate ingested *Staphylococcus aureus* in vitro. PGK-deficient leukocytes exhibit increased Krebs cycle activity both at rest and during phagocytosis. Abolition of Krebs cycle metabolism with cyanide severely impairs the ingestion of bacteria by such cells but has little or no effect on normal leukocytes (63). Thus the PGK-deficient leukocyte appears to compensate for its glycolytic defect, at least in part, by increased Krebs cycle activity. Leukocyte function in vivo is probably not compromised, since an increased incidence of infection has not been a feature of PGK deficiency.

Genetics

The structural gene for PGK in man is X-linked (58, 64). As in G6PD deficiency, deficient male hemizygotes have little or no active enzyme and are more symptomatic than heterozygous females with intermediate levels of activity. Curiously, although the mothers of the two anemic PGK-deficient boys mentioned previously are sisters, one has mild anemia and a partial enzyme deficiency, while the other is both hematologically and biochemically normal. Despite these differences, both have given birth to similarly afflicted male offspring. The fathers of both boys are normal by clinical and biochemical criteria.

When young and old erythrocytes from a female heterozygote are separated by centrifugation, greater PGK activity is noted in old cells than in young cells (Fig. 10–3) (52). In contrast, pyruvate kinase activity is lower in old cells than in young cells, conforming to the normal decline in enzyme activity associated with aging of the red cell. These results have been interpreted as resulting from random inactivation of the X chromosome. Cells possessing an active chromosome dictating the synthesis of normal PGK have normal enzyme activity, while those in whom the X chromosome for mutant PGK is activated should be markedly enzymopenic. The selective survival of enzyme replete cells would then result in higher enzyme activity in the population of older erythrocytes. Similar study of another anemic female, however, has yielded contradictory results, with higher enzyme activity in young cells (61).

Therapy

Splenectomy in one patient failed to influence the chronic anemia, but did abolish episodes of more severe anemia which had required transfusion on several previous occasions (52).

2,3-DIPHOSPHOGLYCERATE MUTASE

Enzyme

Diphosphoglycerate mutase

1,3-Diphosphoglycerate $\longrightarrow$ 2,3-Diphosphoglycerate

3PG   3PG

Clinical Manifestations

A 50 per cent reduction in erythrocyte DPGM was found in a young woman, her father, and her infant daughter by Cartier and his co-workers (65). The infant was jaundiced and anemic at birth but, in contrast, both affected adults were clinically normal. Although hemoglobin and bilirubin levels were not abnormal, the possibility of compensated hemolysis was suggested in one adult patient by a modestly elevated reticulocyte count.

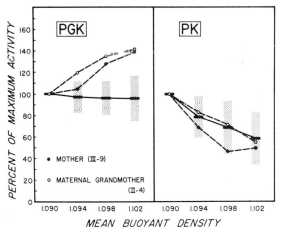

Figure 10–3. Erythrocytes fractionated on the basis of buoyant density. PGK indicates phosphoglycerate kinase activity, and PK pyruvate kinase activity. The solid line represents the mean activity, and the shaded bars the range of activity in four normal controls and 14 unaffected paternal and maternal relatives in the kindred. Comparison is made with the same activities in the affected mother and maternal grandmother. In each, enzyme activity in each fraction is compared with the activity of the least dense red cell fraction taken as 100 per cent. (From Valentine, W. N., et al.: New Engl. J. Med. 280:532, 1969.)

Schröter (66) described an infant who developed anemia and hepatosplenomegaly in the newborn period, required blood transfusion at increasingly frequent intervals, and died at 3 months of overwhelming infection. Erythrocyte DPGM activity and 2,3-DPG concentration were reduced to approximately 50 per cent of normal in both parents, a sister, and a grandmother. These presumed heterozygotes were hematologically normal despite their enzyme deficiency. In vitro, their erythrocytes exhibited normal glycolysis. Biochemical studies of the anemic infant's erythrocytes were precluded by the necessity for frequent transfusion. It was inferred that he was severely DPGM-deficient and probably represented the homozygous form of the enzymopathy. His minimal reticulocytosis and lack of jaundice, as well as the severe foreshortening of the survival of normal erythrocytes when transfused into the patient, however, were findings at variance with previous experience in other glycolytic enzymopathies.

Biochemistry

In the pedigree described by Cartier et al. (65), the most striking biochemical abnormality in affected erythrocytes was a reduction to 30 to 42 per cent of normal in 2,3-DPG concentration, resulting in a pronounced left shift in the hemoglobin oxygen dissociation curve. The pattern of glycolytic intermediates indicated increased activity at the HK, PFK, and PGK loci, consistent with relief of the inhibitory influence of 2,3-DPG upon these enzymes (65). Erythrocyte AMP and ADP were normal, while ATP was somewhat increased in one individual but normal in the second. Increased ATP would be compatible with diversion of 1,3-DPG into the PGK reaction as a consequence of reduced flow through DPGM. Erythrocyte glycolysis and pentose shunt activity were normal in vitro.

Genetics

The findings in both pedigrees were consistent with an autosomal recessive mode of inheritance.

PYRUVATE KINASE

Enzyme

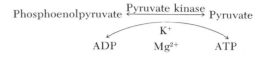

$$\text{Phosphoenolpyruvate} \underset{ADP}{\overset{\text{Pyruvate kinase}}{\rightleftarrows}} \underset{Mg^{2+}}{\overset{K^+}{}} \underset{ATP}{\text{Pyruvate}}$$

Clinical Manifestations (67–96)

Pyruvate kinase (PK) deficiency is the most frequently encountered glycolytic enzymopathy associated with anemia. Of the approximately 150 cases thus far reported, the majority have been of Northern European extraction, although sporadic cases have also been encountered in Blacks, Japanese, Chinese, Mexicans, Southern Europeans, and Syrians. The clinical abnormalities customarily associated with chronic hemolysis—anemia, jaundice, and splenomegaly—are regularly present in PK deficiency. Anemia may be profound, presenting in early infancy and requiring frequent blood transfusions for survival or, conversely, be so mild as to evade discovery until later childhood or even adulthood. In a few cases, anemia is absent, hemolysis is fully compensated, and jaundice may be the sole clinical abnormality. When present, anemia is lifelong and usually varies little in intensity. Exacerbations of anemia are uncommon and usually result from transient erythroid hypoplasia following infections or, rarely, from increased hemolysis of unknown cause.

Hyperbilirubinemia is frequently encountered in PK-deficient newborns and may require exchange transfusion. Serum unconjugated bilirubin levels remain elevated in later life. Gallstones may appear as early as 8 years of age and eventually occur in at least 10 per cent of patients. Unconjugated bilirubin levels in excess of 6 mg. per 100 ml. are occasionally seen; one brother and sister regularly had levels greater than 20 mg. per 100 ml. These patients have abnormal hepatic function in addition to hemolysis. Whether abnormalities of liver PK contribute to such hyperbilirubinemia is unknown.

Routine laboratory studies reveal no distinctive abnormalities. Leukocytes and platelets are normal in number and appearance. Macrocytosis, occasional shrunken, spiculated erythrocytes and, rarely, acanthocytes may be observed on examination of the blood smear; these changes may be accentuated by splenectomy. More extreme alterations in erythrocyte morphology are sometimes encountered (Fig. 10–4). Such abnormalities in shape may result from the inadequate ATP synthesis characteristic of PK-deficient erythrocytes (68). Plasma lipid abnormalities, although associated with similar morphologic changes, have not been found in PK deficiency. A paradoxical rise in the reticulocyte count often follows splenectomy, despite evidence of a beneficial reduction in the rate of hemolysis. Reticulocyte counts may exceed 90 per cent, and many patients maintain counts of 40 to 70 per cent for years. Conversely, other patients exhibit the expected reduction in reticulocyte count after splenectomy. The osmotic fragility of fresh and incubated erythrocytes is most often normal, although in occasional patients minor populations of fragile or resistant cells may be encountered after incubation. The autohemolysis test is usually but not invariably abnormal, with hemolysis of as many as 50 per cent of erythrocytes after 48 hours' incubation in saline. Prior addition of glucose may reduce hemolysis in some instances, but more frequently glucose has little or no effect. In fact, if the reticulocyte count exceeds 25 per cent, incubation with glucose regularly accentuates hemolysis. This phenomenon has been attributed to inhibition of oxidative phosphorylation by glucose (Crabtree effect), with unfavorable consequences in PK-deficient reticulocytes due to their reliance upon oxidative phosphorylation for ATP synthesis (69). Phosphorylated adenine nucleotides almost always reduce autohemolysis of PK-deficient cells to less than 2 per cent, while adenosine has a less predictable effect, sometimes accentuating and other times ameliorating hemolysis. Ethacrynic acid, ouabain, NAD, NADP, coenzyme A, and reduced glutathione have also been shown to have a beneficial influence on autohemolysis. If a common mechanism of action underlies the similar effect of these diverse agents on incubated PK-deficient cells, it has thus far escaped detection.

Biochemistry

The molecular weight of purified human erythrocyte PK has been variously reported to be 150,000 (97), 195,000 (98), 205,000 (99), 237,000 (100), or 235,000 to 245,000 (101). By analogy with rabbit muscle PK, the erythrocyte enzyme is probably a

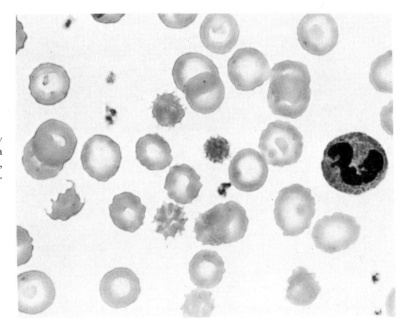

Figure 10–4. Postsplenectomy blood smear from a patient with severe PK deficiency. (From Oski, F. A., et al.: New Engl. J. Med. 270:1024, 1964.)

tetramer composed of four subunits whose nature is as yet undefined. The enzyme may exist in either of two physical conformations, analogous to the R and T forms proposed by Monod, Wyman, and Changeaux for allosteric proteins (102).

Partially purified enzyme preparations usually exhibit sigmoid kinetics in the presence of increasing concentrations of phosphoenolpyruvate (PEP) (Fig. 10–5). Small amounts of PEP appear to facilitate further binding of substrate by the enzyme in a manner analogous to heme-heme interactions. Fructose diphosphate (FDP) induces a transition from sigmoid to hyperbolic kinetics, probably by acting directly at the PEP binding site (103).

Transition between an FDP-sensitive conformation with sigmoid kinetics and an insensitive form with hyperbolic kinetics has been achieved by varying pH (104), temperature (104, 105), and conditions of storage (100, 105, 106, 106a). Aging of the enzyme in vivo appears to favor the FDP-sensitive conformation (107). Such transitions may in part reflect interconversions between polymeric species of the enzyme composed of two, three, or more subunits (100) or alternatively represent conformational changes in the tetramer thought to be the natural form of the enzyme. In either case, these transitions may play a significant role in modulation of PK activity in vivo.

The enzyme is subject to numerous other regulatory influences. ATP is a competitive inhibitor ($K_i = 3.5 \times 10^{-4}M$) (97); at physiologic ATP concentrations (approximately 1 mM), erythrocyte PK activity should be significantly constrained by ATP. Both potassium (103) and magnesium (108) activate PK; Rb^+ or NH_4^+ may substitute for K^+, while Mn^{2+} or Co^{2+} can replace Mg^{2+} (109). The enzyme is inhibited by sulfhydryl reagents, such as PCMB (109), indicating the presence of exposed sulfhydryl groups on the surface of the molecule. Activation of purified PK by FDP has been demonstrated at concentrations normally found within the erythrocyte (98). At higher concentration (0.5 mM) another glycolytic intermediate, glucose-6-phosphate, activates PK, while yet other intermediates have no apparent influence on the enzyme (99). 2,3-DPG, of particular interest because of its high concentration in PK-deficient erythrocytes, has no influence upon PK in hemolysates (110), but has variously been reported to inhibit (111) or activate (99) purified PK. It is clear that intracellular PK activity will be determined by the complex interplay of a number of regulatory factors and may bear little relation to meas-

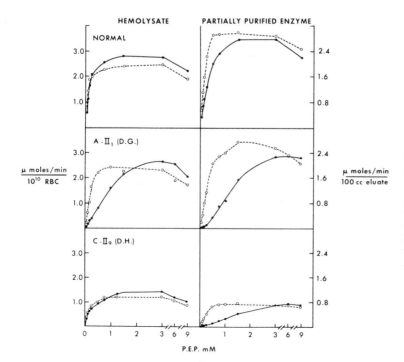

Figure 10–5. PK activity at varying PEP concentrations. Results for crude hemolysate are compared with those for partially purified enzyme in the presence of FDP, 10 μM (O————O), and without FDP (●————●). Top, normal; middle and bottom, two mutant forms of PK associated with hemolysis. The partially purified enzymes exhibit sigmoid kinetics, while in crude hemolysate hyperbolic kinetics are obtained. (From Mentzer, W. C., and Alpers, J. A.: Clin. Res. 29:209, 1971.)

ures of activity determined in vitro under optimal condition.

Human tissues contain one or more of three PK isoenzymes separable on the basis of their differing kinetic, antigenic, and physicochemical properties. Type I is found in erythrocytes and liver, type II in kidney, and type III in leukocytes, platelets, kidney, muscle, liver, and brain (112). As the different isoenzymes are presumably under separate genetic control, it is not surprising that leukocyte and platelet PK are normal in patients with abnormalities of the erythrocyte enzyme. On the other hand, when erythrocyte PK is abnormal, hepatic PK may also be affected. In two anemic PK-deficient individuals, liver PK was reduced to 59 per cent (70) and 46 per cent (71) of normal. Residual liver PK, measured in the latter case, was largely type III. No disorders of hepatic function appear to result from such partial deficiency of PK.

PK-deficient erythrocytes vary considerably in their metabolic capabilities in vitro. Although resting hexose monophosphate shunt activity is slightly to moderately low for cell age (113), no significant effect on either oxidized or reduced glutathione levels has been observed (72–75), even following incubation with acetylphenylhydrazine (69, 74–77). In many instances, glycolysis, as measured by the glucose consumption or lactate production of incubated erythrocytes, is markedly subnormal (69, 78, 113). Such diminished glycolysis is relative rather than absolute, since the glycolytic rate of enzymopenic cells can be increased substantially by incubation in a high–inorganic phosphate medium (69, 114, 115). A reduction of residual PK activity within the erythrocyte to 10 per cent of normal will still leave sufficient enzyme to support normal glycolysis if full enzyme activity is utilized. Such considerations indicate that intracellular regulators of PK function must play an important role in the reduced glycolysis characteristic of enzymopenic cells. Frequently, particularly in the case of kinetic variants of PK, glycolytic rates characteristic of mature normal erythrocytes are achieved (75, 79–81, 114, 116). However, such rates are clearly subnormal when compared to those obtained by reticulocyte-rich control blood of an equivalent mean cell age (79). Furthermore, the glucose consumption of incubated normal hemolysate is unchanged when supplemental purified PK is added, whereas addition of supplemental PK to hemolysate from PK-deficient erythrocytes produces a substantial rise in glucose consumption (79).

Accumulation of glycolytic intermediates proximal to the enzyme defect has customarily (72, 75, 79, 105, 116), although not invariably (79, 81), been observed. The pattern of intermediates obtained in a mildly anemic patient with a high Km PEP mutant enzyme (D.G.) is contrasted in Figure 10–6 with that found in a severely anemic child (C.D.) with a low activity PK mutant and a marked reticulocytosis of 50 per cent. Intermediates have accumulated just proximal to PK in both instances, and in C.D. a striking accumulation of more distant intermediates is noted as well, extending as far proximal as the triose phosphates, F6P, and G6P. Alterations in the normal ratio of NADH to NAD, as well as complex changes in the substrates governing the rate of PK and DPGM, ap-

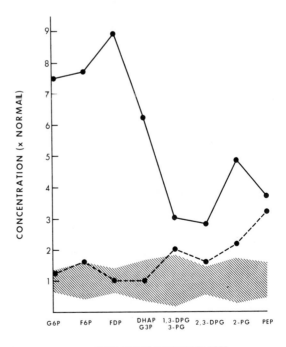

Figure 10–6. Changes in erythrocyte glycolytic intermediates in PK deficiency. Results, expressed as multiples of normal values, are shown for D. G., a patient with mild anemia (●------●), and for C. D. (●——●), whose anemia was severe. (From Mentzer, W.: Unpublished data.)

pear to be responsible for triose phosphate accumulation when glycolysis is accelerated by P_i in normal red cells (117). Such striking elevations in triose phosphate intermediates can be returned to normal both in red cells of controls and in PK-deficient red cells by addition of exogenous pyruvate or other oxidant (115). The concentration of both NAD and NADH is reduced in PK-deficient erythrocytes (105, 113), or, if normal in fresh cells, the level of NAD falls with undue rapidity on incubation in vitro (77).

The concentration of 2,3-DPG in PK-deficient erythrocytes may exceed three times normal values. The expected rightward shift of the hemoglobin-oxygen dissociation curve associated with such high 2,3-DPG levels is found in PK-deficient blood (18, 19). The ability to extract a greater percentage of available oxygen from hemoglobin at any given pO_2 associated with such a right-shifted curve increases the exercise tolerance of PK-deficient patients (19). Such patients, although anemic, may exhibit none of the expected symptoms of fatigue and exercise intolerance.

Erythrocyte ATP is often abnormally low in PK deficiency, although patients with reticulocyte counts greater than 25 per cent usually have normal ATP levels. In such high reticulocyte blood, ATP is unstable on incubation with glucose in contrast to normal reticulocyte-rich blood. When incubated without glucose, however, the PK-deficient reticulocyte conserves ATP more successfully than does the normal (69). The reticulocyte, able to generate ATP from sources other than glucose via oxidative phosphorylation, can circumvent its glycolytic defect. When forced to utilize glucose, however (i.e., in a high-glucose environment), the PK-deficient reticulocyte fares poorly, and ATP levels plummet. The PK-deficient reticulocyte is thus exquisitely dependent upon oxidative phosphorylation for maintenance of ATP, as was first shown by Keitt (69). Incubation of PK-deficient blood with cyanide, which inhibits oxidative phosphorylation, produces a striking and rapid decrease in cell ATP content, whereas control reticulocytes are immune to this effect of cyanide. However, fluoride, which inhibits enolase and thus simulates the lesion of PK deficiency, renders normal reticulocytes equally susceptible to the

effect of inhibitors of oxidative phosphorylation. The increased oxygen consumption of PK-deficient reticulocytes compared to normal (3.75 ± 1.55 vs. 0.56 ± 0.5 μL. O_2 per 10^9 reticulocytes per hour) (78) further demonstrates the reliance of such cells upon oxidative phosphorylation. Oxygen consumption is abolished by hypoxia in vitro at approximately venous pO_2 levels (Fig. 10–7). When exposed to prolonged periods of hypoxia in vivo, therefore, or upon maturation with consequent loss of mitochondria, the PK-deficient immature erythrocyte will become reliant upon its demonstrably inadequate glycolytic apparatus, with loss of cell ATP the inevitable consequence. In contrast, the reduced ATP needs of the mature erythrocyte may be marginally but adequately served for a time by the diminished glycolytic activity of the PK-deficient cell.

ATP depletion greatly increases the cation permeability of PK-deficient erythrocytes (78). In part, this is the consequence of failure of the ouabain inhibitable ATPase cation pump, which transports approximately 1 to 2 mEq. K^+ per hour per liter

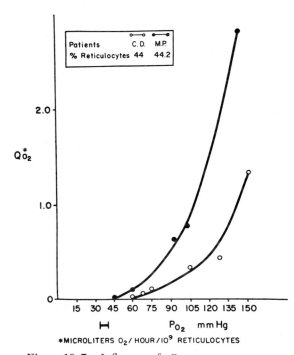

Figure 10–7. Influence of pO_2 on oxygen consumption by PK-deficient reticulocytes. The normal range for venous pO_2 is indicated by the solid bar between 30 and 45 mm. Hg. (From Mentzer, W., et al.: J. Clin. Invest. 50:688, 1971.)

of erythrocytes (118). Even in freshly obtained PK-deficient blood, such a pump rate is insufficient, although adequate membrane ATPase is present (79, 119), and a net loss of from 0.2 to 6.3 mEq. K$^+$ per hour per liter of cells occurs (68, 79, 118). Following ATP depletion, net K$^+$ loss may exceed 20 mEq. per hour per liter of cells (78). Failure of the cation pump cannot explain such large losses of K$^+$. The effect is thought to be related to altered binding of membrane-associated Ca^{2+} and can be partially prevented by EDTA, even though EDTA has no direct influence on the rate or extent of ATP depletion (78).

Initially in the ATP-depleted cell, potassium loss exceeds sodium gain. The resultant net loss of cations is accompanied by an obligate osmotic loss of water and a reduction in cell volume. The shrunken, crenated cells produced by ATP depletion in PK-deficient reticulocytes are shown in Figure 10–8. These spiculated cells pass with difficulty through 8-μ millipore filters, and cell suspensions demonstrate increased viscosity in the Wells-Brookfield viscometer (78). The destiny of such ATP-depleted erythrocytes then is to become dehydrated, rigid "dessicytes," whose unfavorable characteristics may well prematurely terminate their existence (57).

As enzyme-deficient erythrocytes age, a progressive reduction in glycolysis should accompany the inevitable gradual degrada-

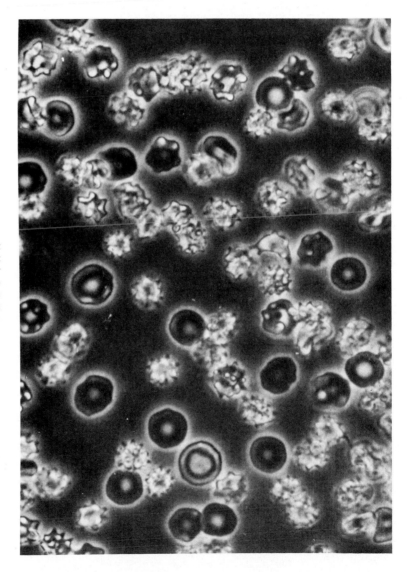

Figure 10–8. Phase contrast photomicrograph of PK-deficient blood (patient C.D.) after 2-hour exposure to 5 mM cyanide to deplete ATP. The spiculated cells are, for the most part, reticulocytes ($\times$ 6600). (From Mentzer, W., et al.: J. Clin. Invest. 50:688, 1971.)

tion of enzyme protein. Such deteriorating glycolysis will eventually result in ATP depletion and subsequently in hemolysis. However, centrifuge studies have not revealed dramatic differences in the PK activity of enzymopenic young and old cells (71), with the exception of one unstable PK variant (82), in which accelerated denaturation of enzyme protein was present in vivo as well as in vitro. Deterioration in catalytic efficiency, reported to occur in both normal (107) and variant (120) enzyme on aging in vivo, may also hasten the demise of enzymopenic cells.

Erythrokinetics

The normal or near-normal survival of labeled, severely PK-deficient erythrocytes reported by several investigators (78, 80, 81, 83, 105) indicates that diminished PK activity need not significantly curtail the life span of affected erythrocytes. Biphasic erythrocyte survival curves are sometimes obtained (121, 122) and suggest that two populations of cells are present, one destined for almost immediate destruction, and the other with a considerably better outlook for survival.

Ferrokinetic studies in ten patients (78, 84, 122) indicate that destruction of newly made erythrocytes in the bone marrow, spleen, or liver may indeed be the major source of hemolysis in this disorder. Organ monitoring has shown that, as reticulocytes are released from the marrow, some are almost immediately sequestered in the spleen. The paradoxical reticulocytosis which follows splenectomy is probably the consequence of improved survival of this population of reticulocytes.

Spleens removed from anemic PK-deficient patients contain an unduly large number of reticulocytes (76, 123). Splenic histology contrasts with that seen in hereditary spherocytosis in that the pulp spaces are empty rather than packed with erythrocytes. Erythrophagocytosis by RE histiocytes is prominent in PK deficiency but rare in spherocytosis; and many more crenated, deformed cells are seen in PK deficiency (123). The hypoxic, acidic environment of the spleen would be expected to produce just such crenation in reticulocytes through the sequence of events out-

lined earlier: inhibition of oxidative phosphorylation, ATP depletion, selective K^+ leakage, loss of cell water, and resultant loss of cell volume. These rigid dessicytes should negotiate only with difficulty the $3\text{-}\mu$ fenestrations between the splenic cords and sinuses. Thus doomed to a stay of uncertain duration in the metabolically unfavorable splenic environment, further deterioration in cell capabilities would seem inevitable. Isotope studies show that the final *coup de grâce* is often administered in the liver (121, 122).

Splenic destruction of reticulocytes is a variable feature of PK deficiency; in some instances, either bone marrow or liver destruction predominates. Why some reticulocytes are destroyed while others survive to reach maturity and thereafter enjoy a near-normal existence despite their enzyme defect is unclear. It is possible that chance determines which reticulocytes will be detained in unfavorable metabolic circumstances. On the other hand, there is some evidence for actual variation in PK activity amongst reticulocytes (78). Those most adequately endowed would be more likely to survive. The genetic and molecular basis for such variability requires clarification.

Genetics

Autosomal recessive transmission of the enzyme defect has been encountered in all pedigrees adequately studied in this regard. Homozygotes exhibit hemolytic anemia, but heterozygotes remain clinically normal despite a 50 per cent reduction in erythrocyte PK activity. In a recent population survey in Germany, the incidence of apparent heterozygosity for PK deficiency was 1.4 per cent in healthy young adults (124). Using the fluorescent screening method of Beutler, PK deficiency was found in 3.4 per cent of 700 consecutive newborn Chinese infants in Hong Kong (125). Some of the deficient infants, thought to be heterozygotes on the basis of family studies, developed neonatal hyperbilirubinemia in the absence of other known causes of jaundice. A transient further reduction in PK activity during the neonatal period was associated with hemolysis in one apparent heterozygote (85). Such hemolysis in neonates is an exception to the benign nature of the carrier state in later life. The simple measures of enzyme activity employed to ascertain heterozygosity in these studies do not exclude the possibility that affected neonates may have been doubly heterozygous for two different mutant forms of PK, only one of which was detected.

There is little correlation between severity of anemia in homozygotes and the level of erythrocyte PK activity as measured by the conventional in vitro assay system. This seeming inconsistency is explained, at least in part, by the existence of numerous mutant forms of the enzyme whose differing properties result in variable degrees of hemolysis. Such mutants when studied in vitro either in crude hemolysates or in partially purified form are distinguishable from one another on the basis of maximal activity, electrophoretic mobility, substrate kinetics, thermal stability, and response to the activator FDP, as shown in Table 10-4. The true number of PK mutants will remain unknown until standardized means of preparation and methods of biochemical characterization of variant enzymes are agreed upon. Some high Km PEP enzymes

have had normal or increased activity in vitro but have, nevertheless, been associated with hemolysis. Such enzymes may appear to be at little disadvantage when studied in vitro at saturating substrate concentrations, but are nearly inactive at the low PEP concentrations found within the erythrocyte. Low Km PEP enzymes, conversely, should be catalytically more efficient than normal at the usual intracellular concentrations of PEP. Instability in vivo rather than catalytic inefficiency may explain the deleterious effect of the latter enzymes on erythrocyte survival.

If erythrocyte PK is a polymer composed of multiples of a single subunit, its inheritance may well be governed by a single gene locus. Although definitive studies of the peptide gene product are not yet available, pedigree analysis of families in which mutant PK has appeared have been consistent with such a mode of inheritance. Since nothing is known of the factors governing PK synthesis in normal and enzymopenic erythroid precursors, structural or regulatory gene mutations may conceivably lead to deficient enzyme

TABLE 10-4. VARIANTS OF ERYTHROCYTE PK

REFERENCE	V_{MAX}^H % NORMAL	KM PEP × NORMAL	SIGMOID PEP KINETICS	FDP ACTIVATION	THERMAL STABILITY	ELECTRO-PHORESIS	pH OPTIMUM
Normal Km PEP							
Staal (82)	50	Normal[P]	Present[P]	Present[P]	Dec.	Normal	
Staal (120, 126)		Normal[P]	Absent[P]	Present[P]	Dec.	Abnormal	
Low Km PEP							
Staal (120)		0.25 − 0.33[P]	Absent[P]		Dec.		
Boivin (127, 127a)	10–50	0.2[H], 0.5[P]					
Oski (79)							
Gilman (86)	36–150	0.1[H]			Dec.		Normal
Brandt (87)	1000	0.1[H]			Dec.	Abnormal	Abnormal
High Km PEP							
Gulbis (84)	33	3[H]					Abnormal
Paglia (88)	40	4[H]5[H]	Absent[H]	Reduced[H]			
Mentzer (89)	41–71	2[H] − 4[P]	Absent[H] Present[P]	Reduced[HP]	Dec.		
Boivin (90, 127a)	88	6[H] − 9[P]		Reduced[H] Normal[P]	Dec.	Normal	
Miwa (116)	100	4[H]			Dec.		Normal
Paglia (80)	66–145	10[H] − 13[H]	Present[H]	Normal[H]	Dec.		Abnormal
Munro (108)	160	10[H]	Present[HP]	Abnormal[P]	Normal		Abnormal
Ohyama (91)	138	5[P]			Normal		Abnormal

H = Hemolysate.
P = Partially purified enzyme.
Dec. = Decreased.

activity in mature erythrocytes. When kinetic abnormalities have been discovered in anemic patients, at least one parent has exhibited similar abnormalities. The other parent may also have kinetically aberrant PK (89, 92), or may be found to have a low activity variant with normal kinetics (88); the anemic child is considered to be a homozygote in the former instance and a double heterozygote in the latter. Occasionally, it has not been possible to demonstrate an abnormality of erythrocyte PK in one (89, 93) or both (82) parents of patients with PK activity in the homozygous deficient range. Staal (82) has speculated that in some heterozygotes a compensatory increase in synthesis of enzyme protein by the normal allele may result in enzyme activity indistinguishable from normal. More complete characterization of PK in these heterozygotes may reveal the presence of mutant enzyme. In at least one instance increased thermolability was the only abnormality discovered in PK from an obligate heterozygote (89).

To date, no evidence suggests interaction between PK deficiency and other disorders of the erythrocyte. The clinical and hematologic presentation of beta thalassemia minor is not altered by the concomitant presence of heterozygous PK deficiency (94). Although autologous erythrocyte survival was reduced in one woman doubly heterozygous for PK and G6PD deficiency, similarly reduced erythrocyte survival was present in a female relative heterozygous only for G6PD deficiency (67). Reports of spherocytosis or paroxysmal nocturnal hemoglobinuria in PK heterozygotes have not mentioned unusual features of either disease in such heterozygotes. Markedly increased involvement of the kidneys was noted at autopsy in a patient with Gaucher's disease who also exhibited hemolytic anemia and deficiency of erythrocyte PK. It was suggested that cerebroside production was enhanced as a result of hemolysis (95).

Therapy

Unlike hereditary spherocytosis, a complete cure is not achieved by splenectomy, but elimination or amelioration of transfusion requirements, a fall in bilirubin, and a rise in hemoglobin are quite often obtained. While in severely anemic individuals splenectomy may be life saving (76, 81), anemia in mild cases may be uninfluenced by the procedure. Where significant morbidity exists, it would seem reasonable to recommend splenectomy, bearing in mind that the degree of benefit cannot be predicted with certainty. Standard studies of erythrocyte survival and sequestration using ^{51}Cr-labeled cells are often not useful in selecting patients for surgery, particularly where hemolysis of newly made cells predominates. Such cells are unavailable for tagging in the circulating blood, and their presence and fate is not reflected in the results obtained. Ferrokinetics with appropriate organ monitoring allows a better assessment of the role of the spleen in such circumstances, but the value of such studies in predicting the results of splenectomy has yet to be determined.

Therapeutic intervention with agents which either circumvent the metabolic aberrations induced by the defective enzyme or which directly modify enzyme activity is theoretically possible. For example, a redox agent, such as methylene blue or ascorbic acid, might alleviate secondary inhibition of glyceraldehyde-3-phosphate dehydrogenase by increasing the amount of available NAD. Preliminary trial of these agents in one PK-deficient patient produced no change in reticulocyte count or hemoglobin concentration (128). Activation of a relatively FDP-insensitive mutant form of PK was apparently achieved in a single patient by intravenous infusion of 20 mM inosine and 1 mM adenine over a period of three hours. Although the induced change in erythrocyte FDP concentration was modest (9×10^{-6} M to 5×10^{-5} M), a threefold increase in the survival of labeled red cells, a rise in hemoglobin concentration, and a fall in bilirubin level and reticulocyte count ensued (96). Whether the effect is reproducible in the same or in other patients has yet to be established; in one other individual with a different PK mutant, nucleotide therapy was ineffective. Such agents are potentially hazardous, and their use remains experimental and controversial at the present time. In another attempt to increase erythrocyte FDP, mannose, galactose, and fructose were given orally to one PK-deficient patient, but no increase in PK activity was noted (82).

LACTATE DEHYDROGENASE

Enzyme

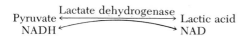

$$\text{Pyruvate} \underset{\text{NADH}}{\overset{\text{Lactate dehydrogenase}}{\rightleftharpoons}} \overset{\text{Lactic acid}}{\underset{\text{NAD}}{}}$$

Clinical Manifestations, Biochemistry, and Genetics

A severe deficiency of erythrocyte lactate dehydrogenase (LDH) was recently discovered in a 64-year-old Japanese male with mild diabetes, but there was no evidence of anemia or hemolysis (129). Activity of the deficient enzyme was reduced to 6 per cent of normal in erythrocytes and was also low in serum. Electrophoresis demonstrated a complete absence of the H subunit of LDH in erythrocytes, leukocytes, platelets, and serum. All five children of this suspected homozygote for deficiency of the H subunit of LDH exhibited approximately a 50 per cent reduction in erythrocyte LDH activity, as well as corresponding changes on electrophoresis, and were presumed to be heterozygotes. Blood lactate levels were subnormal in all affected family members. Measurement of glycolytic intermediates in freshly obtained red cells revealed accumulation of trioses, suggesting insufficient cycling of NADH to NAD via LDH to support adequate glyceraldehyde-3-phosphate dehydrogenase activity. It is of interest that such low LDH activity can result in impairment of glycolysis without apparent shortening of the red cell life span.

ABNORMALITIES OF ATP METABOLISM

It is apparent from the foregoing discussion that reduced erythrocyte ATP often plays a central role in the pathogenesis of hemolysis. A number of individuals with

unusually high erythrocyte ATP levels have also been discovered (130–133), but the relationship of the nucleotide abnormality to hemolysis is not clear. Twice normal erythrocyte PK activity has been found in one high-ATP pedigree but not in another; in neither pedigree was hemolysis present (130, 131). In a third family, two infants with hemolytic anemia, high erythrocyte ATP, and low 2,3-DPG had reduced DPG phosphatase activity (132). The relationship of these enzyme abnormalities to the unusual elevation of erythrocyte ATP or to hemolysis is uncertain. The same may be said of a recently reported case of chronic nonspherocytic hemolytic anemia, in which affected erythrocytes had only 20 to 30 per cent of the ribosephosphate pyrophosphokinase (RPK) activity of equally reticulocyte-rich control blood (133). The patient's erythrocytes exhibited pronounced basophilic stippling, Type II autohemolysis, and an adenine nucleotide concentration twice normal, with balanced elevation of ATP, ADP, and AMP. No abnormalities of PK or other glycolytic enzymes were discovered. In fact, adequate lactate was produced from either glucose or adenosine, confirming that glycolysis and the enzymatic sequence from nucleoside phosphorylase to G3PD were normal. It is possible to account for increased nucleotide content on the basis of RPK deficiency, but the link between these biochemical observations and premature hemolysis needs clarification.

Mild to moderate hemolytic anemia was present in two unrelated individuals whose erythrocyte adenylate kinase activity was less than 13 per cent of normal (134, 135). Autosomal recessive inheritance and Type I autohemolysis were features of the disorder. Although an alteration in the amount or relative proportion of the adenine nucleotides might be expected, ATP was normal, ADP was slightly increased, and AMP was normal or increased in the erythrocytes of both patients. Similar results were obtained in the brother of one patient, in whom concomitant deficiency of both adenylate kinase and G6PD were associated with severe hemolysis. Although the hemolytic anemia in these patients suggests an indispensable function for adenylate kinase in erythrocyte metabolism, the nature of this function is obscure since only minimal derangements in adenine nucleotide content characterized the deficient cells.

ACQUIRED DISORDERS OF ERYTHROCYTE GLYCOLYSIS

Alterations in the external chemical milieu may profoundly influence erythrocyte metabolism. The rate of glycolysis, for example, is in part governed by the availability of inorganic phosphate. High concentrations of inorganic phosphate augment the glycolytic synthesis of ATP and 2,3-DPG, while low concentrations impede synthesis of these important organic phosphates. Erythrocytes from uremic patients with hyperphosphatemia contain an average of 70 per cent more ATP than do normal erythrocytes, and a lesser but significant increase in 2,3-DPG concentration is also found in the hyperphosphatemic cells (136). Equivalent changes in organic phosphates can be induced in normal erythrocytes by incubation either in hyperphosphatemic uremic plasma or in autologous normal plasma supplemented with inorganic phosphate (136). Conversely, hypophosphatemia induced by hyperalimentation with low phosphate nutrients (137) or by anion resin therapy of hyperphosphatemia (138) is associated with a reduction in erythrocyte organic phosphates. The magnitude of such changes is shown in Table 10–5. Organic phosphate depletion consequent to hypophosphatemia may be sufficient to displace the oxyhemoglobin dissociation curve to the left, unfavorably influencing tissue oxygenation. In one patient (139) whose serum inorganic phosphate was unmeasurably low, a transient hemolytic anemia associated with the appearance of spherocytes on the peripheral blood smear and an increase in the osmotic fragility of unincubated erythrocytes was attributed to a profound fall in erythrocyte ATP concentration to 11 per cent of normal. Normal erythrocytes become rigid when ATP falls below 15 per cent of the normal concentration (140), and such changes in erythrocyte deformability also characterized the short-lived hypophosphatemic cells. With correction of hypophosphatemia, the erythrocyte abnormalities disappeared, and red cell survival improved. Klock and his co-workers (141) have also observed transient hemolytic anemia and spherocytosis in a hypophosphatemic patient. Red cell membrane phospholipid composition was altered in this patient during the hypophosphatemic interval. Correction of the membrane lipid abnormalities accompanied the return of the serum phosphorus to normal. The effects of phosphate on normal erythrocyte glycolysis are discussed in Chapter 1. In hypophosphatemic erythrocytes, a remarkable accumulation of triose phosphate intermediates occurs when the serum phosphorus falls below 2 mg. per 100 ml. This may be attributed to inhibition of glyceraldehyde-3-phosphate dehydrogenase by lack of inorganic phosphorus, a cofactor in the reaction (137). In addition, the low concentration of ATP and 2,3-DPG which accompanies hypophosphatemia partly relieves inhibition of phosphofructokinase by these metabolites, accelerating the production of triose phos-

TABLE 10–5. MEAN ATP, 2,3-DPG, and P_{50} IN FIVE PATIENTS WITH SERUM Pi OF LESS THAN 1 MG. PER 100 ML. AND IN 20 NORMAL SUBJECTS

GROUP	Pi (MG/100 ML.)	ATP (μMOLES/ML. OF RED CELLS)	2,3-DPG (μMOLES/ML. OF RED CELLS)	P_{50}(MM. HG)
Patients				
Mean	0.50	0.41	2.6	19.5
Range	0.40 − 0.70	0.20 − 0.65	2.2 − 3.2	16.5 − 23.3
Normal°	3.4 ± 1.0	1.1 ± 0.2	5.1 ± 0.8	27.0 ± 2.2

°Mean ± 2 SD.
Reprinted by permission from Travis, S. F., et al.: New Engl. J. Med. 285:763, 1971.

phate. Overall, in hypophosphatemia inhibitory influences on glycolysis predominate, and there is a measurable reduction in erythrocyte glucose consumption and lactate production (142). The opposite effect, acceleration of glycolysis, is observed in hyperphosphatemia. The clinically significant abnormalities of oxygen transport or of erythrocyte shape, rigidity, and life span which attend alterations in the normal level of plasma phosphate are ultimately the consequence of such changes in erythrocyte glycolysis.

The lower hemoblobin levels characteristic of childhood may be the result of phosphate-mediated changes in red cell metabolism (142a). The high serum inorganic phosphate levels found in normal children are associated with increased red cell organic phosphate concentrations and with a rightward shift in the whole blood oxygen affinity curve. During maturation serum phosphate levels fall, the oxygen affinity curve shifts to the left, and hemoglobin levels then presumably rise to maintain normal oxygen transport. These same changes in serum phosphate and oxygen affinity accompany maturation in sickle cell anemia and may explain the reduced frequency of painful crises noted by many adults and adolescents with this disorder (142b). Increased oxygen affinity allows red cells to remain more saturated with oxygen and thus less susceptible to sickling at physiologic oxygen tensions.

Less is known about the influence of other components of the chemical environment upon erythrocyte glycolysis. Experimental magnesium deficiency in the rat resembles hypophosphatemia in that erythrocyte glycolysis is inhibited, ATP and 2,3-DPG levels are subnormal, and red cell rigidity is increased. Spherocytes are evident on the blood smear, and red cell survival is reduced (143). Magnesium is essential for the normal function of a variety of glycolytic and nonglycolytic enzymes. The relative contribution of these various enzymes to the observed inhibition of energy metabolism in magnesium-deficient red cells has not yet been defined, nor is it known whether hematologic changes similar to those seen in the rat occur in human magnesium deficiency.

Iron deficiency not only decreases the production of red cells but also accelerates their destruction (144). Studies of the metabolic properties of iron-deficient red cells have revealed several abnormalities that might reduce cell viability. The activity of both catalase and glutathione peroxidase is reduced in deficient cells (145); in vitro hydrogen peroxide hemolysis is increased, and increased susceptibility to peroxidation of membrane lipids can be inferred from these findings. Although erythrocyte glycolysis in vitro is normal for cell age (146), cell ATP is unstable on incubation. ATP concentration in freshly obtained red cells may either be normal (147) or low (148, 149). The spontaneous autohemolysis of iron-deficient red cells incubated at 37°C is increased (150). The increased rigidity characteristic of the ATP-depleted cell is present in iron-deficient cells as well (150). These findings suggest that a defect in energy metabolism may contribute to the shortened survival of iron-deficient red cells, but the nature of this hypothetical defect has not yet been defined.

Little is known about the possible influence of hormones upon erythrocyte glycolytic enzymes. The activity of hexokinase, phosphofructokinase, pyruvate kinase, and glucose-6-phosphate dehydrogenase is often reduced in the erythrocytes of diabetics (151). The same enzymes were remarkably increased in activity in one patient with an insulinoma prior to removal of the tumor. The activity of several erythrocyte enzymes is reduced in hypothyroidism and becomes normal after therapy (152), probably reflecting changes in the mean erythrocyte cell age rather than a direct influence of the hormone on the enzymes. However, Snyder (153) has shown that 2,3-DPG synthesis in vitro by hemoglobin− and membrane-free extracts of erythrocytes is enchanced by thyroid hormone. The site of action of this effect is unknown, but may well involve one of several glycolytic enzymes.

Alterations in erythrocyte enzyme activity are often found during the course of either acute or chronic leukemia, but no consistent pattern has emerged (154–158). Enzyme abnormalities have also been observed in nonmalignant pancytopenias (155, 159–161), congenital dyserythropoietic anemia (162), acquired dyserythropoietic anemia (155, 163), myeloid metaplasia (155), and polycythemia vera (155). One, a few, or many enzymes may be involved. For example, the activity of enolase may be increased as much as three- to fourfold in erythroleukemia or in monomyelogenous leukemia. Conversely, in these types of leukemia, pyruvate kinase activity has sometimes, but not invariably, been reduced to approximately half normal. These changes do not merely reflect alterations in the mean red cell life span, since enolase activity is normally little different in young and old erythrocytes, and since appropriate changes on other enzymes whose activity is clearly related to red cell age do not occur. It is thought that the enzymatic abnormalities reflect fundamental alterations in the chromosomal composition of the erythroid cell line induced by the malignant state. No evidence for structural alteration of enzyme protein or for the presence of activators or inhibitors has yet been obtained (155). The possibility that these enzyme abnormalities may be familial and antedate the onset of leukemia has not been explored.

References

1. Dacie, J. V., Mollison, P. L., et al.: Atypical congenital hemolytic anemia. Quart. J. Med. 22: 79, 1953.
2. Selwyn, J. G., and Dacie J. V.: Autohemolysis and other changes resulting from the incubation in vitro of red cells from patients with congenital hemolytic anemia. Blood 9:414, 1954.
3. Robinson, M. A., Loder, P. B., et al.: Red cell metabolism in non-spherocytic congenital haemolytic anemia. Br. J. Haematol. 7:327, 1961.
4. Valentine, W. N., Tanaka, K. R., et al.: A specific erythrocyte enzyme defect (pyruvate kinase) in three subjects with congenital non-spherocytic hemolytic anemia. Trans. Assoc. Am. Physicians 74:100, 1961.
5. Beutler, E.: A series of new screening procedures for pyruvate kinase deficiency, glucose-6-phosphate dehydrogenase deficiency, and glutathione reductase deficiency. Blood 28: 553, 1966.
6. Kaplan, J. C., Shore, N., et al.: The rapid detection of triose phosphate isomerase deficiency. Am. J. Clin. Pathol. 50:656, 1968.
7. Blume, K. G., and Beutler, E.: Detection of glucose-phosphate isomerase deficiency by a screening procedure. Blood 39:685, 1972.
8. Löhr, G. W., Waller, H. D., et al.: Hexokinasemangel in Blutzellen bei einer Sippe mit familiärer Panmyelopathie (Typ Fanconi). Klin. Wochenschr. 43:870, 1965.
9. Altay, C., Alper, C. A., et al.: Normal and variant isoenzymes of human blood cell hexokinase and the isoenzyme patterns in hemolytic anemia. Blood 36:219, 1970.
10. Keitt, A. S.: Hemolytic anemia with impaired hexokinase activity. J. Clin. Invest. 48:1997, 1969.
11. Necheles, T. F., Rai, U. S., et al.: Congenital non-spherocytic hemolytic anemia associated with an unusual erythrocyte hexokinase abnormality. J. Lab. Clin. Med. 76:593, 1970.
12. Valentine, W. N., Oski, F. A., et al.: Erythrocyte hexokinase and hereditary hemolytic anemia, In Hereditary Disorders of Erythrocyte Metabolism. Beutler, E. (ed.), New York, Grune & Stratton, 1968. p. 288.
13. Moser, K., Ciresa, M., et al.: Hexokinasemangel bei hämolytischer Anämie. Med. Welt 21: 1977, 1970.
14. Gerber, G. K., Schultze, M., et al.: Occurrence and function of a high Km hexokinase in immature red blood cells. Eur. J. Biochem. 17:445, 1970.
15. Jandl, J. H., and Aster, R. H.: Increased splenic pooling and the pathogenesis of hypersplenism. Am. J. Med. Sci. 253:282, 1967.
16. Rakitzis, E. T., and Mills, G. C.: Relation of red-cell hexokinase activity to extracellular pH. Biochem. Biophys. Acta 141:439, 1967.
17. Brewer, G. J.: Erythrocyte metabolism and function: Hexokinase inhibition by 2,3-diphosphoglycerate and interaction with ATP and Mg^{2+}. Biochim. Biophys. Acta 192:157, 1969.
18. Delivoria-Papadopoulos, M., Oski, F. A., et al.: Oxygen-hemoglobin dissociation curves: Effect of inherited enzyme defects of the red cell. Science 165:601, 1969.
19. Oski, F. A., Marshall, B. E., et al.: Exercise with anemia. The role of the left-shifted or right-shifted oxygen-hemoglobin equilibrium curve. Ann. Intern. Med. 74:44, 1971.
20. Kosower, N. S., Vanderhoff, G. A., et al.: Hexokinase activity in normal and glucose-6-phosphate dehydrogenase deficient erythrocytes. Nature (Lond.) 201:684, 1964.
21. Bethenod, M., Kissin, C., et al.: Déficit en hexokinase intra-erythrocytaire. Ann. Pediatr. (Paris) 50:825, 1967.
22. Valentine, W. N., Oski, F. A., et al.: Hereditary hemolytic anemia with hexokinase deficiency. New Engl. J. Med. 276:1, 1967.
23. Arnold, H., Blume, K-G., et al.: Klinische und biochemische Untersuchungen zur Glucosephosphatisomerase normaler menschlicher Erythrocyten und bei Glucosephosphatisomerase Mangel. Klin. Wochenschr. 21:1299, 1970.
23a. Arnold, H., Blume, K-G., et al.: Glucosephosphate isomerase deficiency: Evidence for in vivo instability of an enzyme variant with hemolysis. Blood 41:691, 1973.
24. Baughan, M., Valentine, W. N., et al.: Hereditary hemolytic anemia associated with glucosephosphate isomerase (GPI) deficiency — A new enzyme defect of human erythrocytes. Blood 32:236, 1968.
25. Blume, K. G., Hryniuk, W., et al.: Characterization of two new variants of glucose-phosphate-isomerase deficiency with hereditary non-spherocytic hemolytic anemia. J. Lab. Clin. Med. 79:942, 1972.

26. Cartier, P., Temkine, H., et al.: Étude biochemique d'une anémie hémolytique avec déficit familial en phosphohexo-isomerase. 7th Int. Congr. Clin. Chem., Geneva/Evian, 1969. Vol. 2: *Clinical Enzymology*. Basel, S. Karger, 1970, p. 139.

26a. Nakashima, K., Miwa, S., et al.: Electrophoretic and kinetic studies of glucosephosphate isomerase (GPI) in two different Japanese families with GPI deficiency. Am. J. Hum. Genet. 25:294, 1973.

27. Leger, J., Bost, M., et al.: Anémie hémolytique congénitale et familiale avec déficit en phospho-hexose-isomerase (PHI) et elliptocytose. *Proceedings 13th Int. Congr. Hematol.*, Munich, 1970.

28. Oski, F., and Fuller, E.: Glucose-phosphate isomerase (GPI) deficiency associated with abnormal osmotic fragility and spherocytes. Clin. Res. 19:427, 1971.

29. Paglia, D. E., Holland, P., et al.: Occurrence of defective hexosephosphate isomerization in human erythrocytes and leukocytes. New Engl. J. Med. 280:66, 1969.

30. Schroter, W., Brittinger, G., et al.: Combined glucosephosphate isomerase and glucose-6-phosphate dehydrogenase deficiency of the erythrocytes: A new hemolytic syndrome. Br. J. Haematol. 20:249, 1971.

31. Detter, J. C., Ways, P. O., et al.: Inherited variations in human phosphohexose isomerase. Ann. Hum. Genet. 31:329, 1968.

32. Krone, W., Schneider, G., et al.: Detection of phosphohexose isomerase deficiency in human fibroblast cultures. Humangenetik 10:224, 1970.

33. Layzer, R. B., Rowland, L. P., et al.: Muscle phosphofructokinase deficiency. Arch. Neurol. 17:512, 1967.

34. Tarui, S., Okuno, G., et al.: Phosphofructokinase deficiency in skeletal muscle. A new type of glycogenolysis. Biochem. Biophys. Res. Commun. 19:517, 1965.

35. Waterbury, L., and Frenkel, E. P.: Hereditary nonspherocytic hemolysis with erythrocyte phosphofructokinase deficiency. Blood 39:415, 1972.

36. Tarui, S., Kono, N., et al.: Enzymatic basis for the coexistence of myopathy and hemolytic disease in inherited muscle phosphofructokinase deficiency. Biochem. Biophys. Res. Commun. 34:77, 1969.

37. Oski, F. A.: Red cell metabolism in the newborn infant. V. Glycolytic intermediates and glycolytic enzymes. Pediatrics 44:84, 1969.

38. Conway, M. M., and Layzer, R. B.: Blood cell phosphofructokinase in Down's syndrome. Humangenetik 9:135, 1970.

39. Bartels, S., and Kruse, K.: Enzymbestimmungen in Erythrocyten bei Kindern mit Down-Syndrom. Humangenetik 5:305, 1968.

40. Layzer, R. B., and Epstein, C. J.: Phosphofructokinase and chromosome 21. Am. J. Hum. Genet. 24:533, 1972.

41. Schneider, A. S., Valentine, W. N., et al.: Triosephosphate isomerase deficiency. A multisystem inherited enzyme disorder. Clinical and genetic aspects, In *Hereditary Disorders of Erythrocyte Metabolism*. Beutler, E. (ed.), New York, Grune & Stratton. 1968, p. 265.

42. Schneider, A. S., Dunn, I., et al.: Triosephosphate isomerase deficiency. B. Inherited triosephosphate isomerase deficiency. Erythrocyte carbohydrate metabolism and preliminary studies of the erythrocyte enzyme, In *Hereditary Disorders of Erythrocyte Metabolism*. Buetler, E. (ed.), New York, Grune & Stratton, 1968, p. 273.

43. Harris, S. R., Paglia, D. E., et al.: Triosephosphate isomerase deficiency in an adult. Clin. Res. 18:529, 1970.

44. Jaffé, E. R., Paglia, D. E., et al.: Triosephosphate isomerase deficiency and hemolytic anemia in an adult. *Proceedings 13th Int. Congr. Hematol.*, Munich, 1970, p. 122.

45. Kleihauer, E., Kleeberg, U. R., et al.: Methylene blue induced hemolytic Heinz body anemia in a newborn infant with glutathione reductase and triosephosphate isomerase deficiency. *Proceedings 13th Int. Congr. Hematol.*, Munich, 1970.

46. Valentine, W. N., Schneider, A. S., et al.: Hereditary hemolytic anemia with triosephosphate isomerase deficiency. Am. J. Med. 41:27, 1966.

47. Schneider, A. S., Valentine, W. N., et al.: Hereditary hemolytic anemia with triosephosphate isomerase deficiency. New Engl. J. Med. 272:229, 1965.

48. Sparkes, R. S., Carrel, R. E., et al.: Probable localization of a triosephosphate isomerase gene to the short arm of the number 5 human chromosome. Nature (Lond.) 224:367, 1969.

49. Brock, D. J., and Singer, J. D.: Red cell triosephosphate isomerase and chromosome 5. Lancet 2:1136, 1970.

50. Harkness, D. R.: A new erythrocytic enzyme defect with hemolytic anemia: Glyceraldehyde 3-phosphate dehydrogenase deficiency. J. Lab. Clin. Med. 68:879, 1966.

51. Oski, F. A., and Whaun, J.: Hemolytic anemia and red cell glyceraldehyde-3-phosphate dehydrogenase. *Proceedings Soc. Pediatr. Res.* 39th Annual Meeting, Atlantic City, 1969, p. 151.

52. Valentine, W. N., Hsieh, H. S., et al.: Hereditary hemolytic anemia associated with phosphoglycerate kinase deficiency in erythrocytes and leukocytes. New Engl. J. Med. 280:528, 1969.

52a. Cartier, P., Habibi, B., et al.: Anémie hémolytique congénitale associée à un déficit en phosphoglycerate-kinase dans les globules rouges, les polynucleaires et les lymphocytes. Nouv. Rev. Fr. Hematol. 11:565, 1971.

52b. Konrad, P., McCarthy, D. J., et al.: Erythrocyte and leukocyte phosphoglycerate kinase deficiency with neurologic disease. J. Pediatr. 82:456, 1973.

53. Mazza, U., Arese, P., et al.: Red cell metabolism in a case of 3-phosphoglycerate kinase deficiency. *Proceedings 13th Int. Congr. Hematol.* Munich, 1970.

54. Schrier, S. L.: Organization of enzymes in human erythrocyte membranes. Am. J. Physiol. 210:139, 1966.

55. Parker, J. C., and Hoffman, J. F.: The role of mem-

brane phosphoglycerate kinase in the control of glycolytic rate by active cation transport in human red blood cells. J. Gen. Physiol. *50*: 893, 1967.

56. Segel, G. B., Feig, S. A., et al.: An essential role for phosphoglycerate kinase–dependent red cell cation transport. Blood *42*:982, 1973.

57. Nathan, D. G., and Shohet, S. B.: Erythrocyte ion transport defects and hemolytic anemia: "Hydrocytosis" and "dessicocytosis." Semin. Hematol. 7:381, 1970.

58. Chen, S. H., Malcolm, L. A., et al.: Phosphoglycerate kinase: An X-linked polymorphism in man. Am. J. Hum. Genet. *23*:87, 1971.

59. Yoshida, A., Watanabe, S., et al.: Human phosphoglycerate kinase. II. Structure of a variant enzyme. J. Biol. Chem. *247*:446, 1972.

60. Yoshida, A., and Watanabe, S.: Human phosphoglycerate kinase. I. Crystallization and characterization of normal enzyme. J. Biol. Chem. *247*:440, 1972.

61. Kraus, A. P., Langston, M. F., Jr., et al.: Red cell phosphoglycerate kinase deficiency. Biochem. Biophys. Res. Commun. *30*:173, 1968.

62. Beutler, E.: Electrophoresis of phosphoglycerate kinase. Biochem. Genet. *3*:189, 1969.

63. Baehner, R. L., Feig, S. A., et al.: Metabolic, phagocytic, and bacteriocidal properties of phosphoglycerate kinase deficient polymorphonuclear leukocytes. Blood *38*:833, 1971.

64. Peys, B. F., Grzeschick, K. H., et al.: Human phosphoglycerate kinase and inactivation of the X chromosome. Science *175*:1002, 1972.

65. Cartier, P., Labie, P., et al.: Déficit familial en diphosphoglycerate mutase: Étude hématologique et biochemique. Nouv. Rev. Fr. Hematol. *12*:269, 1972.

66. Schröter, W.: Kongenitale nichtsphärocytäre hämolytische Anämie bei 2,3-Diphosphoglyceratemutase-Mangel der Erythrocyten im frühen Sauglingsalter. Klin. Wochenschr. *43*: 1147, 1965.

67. Oski, F. A., Nathan, D. G., et al.: Extreme hemolysis and red-cell distortion in erythrocyte pyruvate kinase deficiency. I. Morphology, erythrokinetics, and family enzyme studies. New Engl. J. Med. *270*:1023, 1964.

68. Nathan, D. G., Oski, F. A., et al.: Studies of erythrocyte spicule formation in haemolytic anaemia. Br. J. Haematol. *12*:385, 1966.

69. Keitt, A. S.: Pyruvate kinase deficiency and related disorders of red cell glycolysis. Am. J. Med. *41*:762, 1966.

70. Brunetti, P., Puxeddu, A., et al.: Anemia emolitica congenita non sferocitica de carenza di piruvico-chinase (PK). Haematol. Arch. *47*: 505, 1962.

71. Bigley, R. H., and Koler, R. D.: Liver pyruvate kinase (PK) isoenzymes in a PK-deficient patient. Ann. Hum. Genet. *31*:383, 1968.

72. Waller, H. D., and Löhr, G. W.: Hereditary nonspherocytic enzymopenic hemolytic anemia with pyruvate kinase deficiency. *Proceedings 9th Congr. Int. Soc. Hematol.*, Mexico City, 1962. Mexico, D. F., Universidad Nacional Autonoma de Mexico, Vol. I., 1964, p. 257.

73. Miwa, S., and Nagate M.: Pyruvate kinase deficiency hereditary nonspherocytic hemolytic anemia. Report of two cases in a Japanese family and review of literature. Acta Haematol. Jap. *28*:1, 1965.

74. Necheles, T. F., Finkel, H. E., et al.: Red cell pyruvate kinase deficiency. The effect of splenectomy. Arch. Intern. Med. *118*:75, 1966.

75. Busch, D.: Erythrocyte metabolism in three persons with hereditary nonspherocytic hemolytic anemia, deficient in pyruvate-kinase, In *Proceedings 9th Congr. Eur. Soc. Hematol.*, Lisbon, Vol II. Basel, S. Karger, 1963, p. 783.

76. Bowman, H. S., and Procopio, F.: Hereditary nonspherocytic hemolytic anemia of the pyruvate-kinase deficient type. Ann. Intern. Med. *58*: 567, 1963.

77. Oski, F. A., and Diamond, L. K.: Erythrocyte pyruvate kinase deficiency resulting in congenital nonspherocytic hemolytic anemia. New Engl. J. Med. *269*:269, 1963.

78. Mentzer, W. C., Baehner, R. L., et al.: Selective reticulocyte destruction in erythrocyte pyruvate kinase deficiency. J. Clin. Invest. *50*:688, 1971.

79. Oski, F. A., and Bowman, H.: A low K_m phosphoenolpyruvate mutant in the Amish with red cell pyruvate kinase deficiency. Br. J. Haematol. *17*:289, 1969.

80. Paglia, D. E., Valentine, W. N., et al.: An inherited molecular lesion of erythrocyte pyruvate kinase. Identification of a kinetically aberrant isoenzyme associated with premature hemolysis. J. Clin. Invest. *47*:1929, 1968.

81. Zuelzer, W. W., Robinson, A. R., et al.: Erythrocyte pyruvate kinase deficiency in nonspherocytic hemolytic anemia: A system of multiple genetic markers? Blood *32*:33, 1968.

82. Staal, G. E. J., Sybesma, H. B., et al.: Familial hemolytic anaemia due to pyruvate kinase deficiency. Folia Med. Neerl. *14*:72, 1971.

83. Mallarmé, J., Boivin, P., et al.: L'anémie hémolytique congénitale non sphérocytaire par déficit en pyruvate-kinase. Bull. Soc. Med. Hop. Paris *115*:483, 1964.

84. Gulbis, E., Weber, A., et al.: Contribution à l'étude de l'anémie hémolytique congénitale avec déficit en pyruvate kinase. Arch. Fr. Pediatr. 27:31, 1970.

85. Bossu, M., Dacha, M., et al.: Neonatal hemolysis due to a transient severity of inherited pyruvate kinase deficiency. Acta Haematol. (Basel) *40*:166, 1968.

86. Gilman, P. A.: An unusual form of pyruvate kinase in congenital nonspherocytic hemolytic anemia. *Proceedings 39th Ann. Meeting Soc. Pediatr. Res.*, Atlantic City. 1969, p. 158.

87. Brandt, N. J., and Hanel, H. K.: Atypical pyruvate kinase in a patient with haemolytic anemia. Scand. J. Haematol. 8:126, 1971.

88. Paglia, D. E., Valentine, W. N., et al.: Defective erythrocyte pyruvate kinase with impaired kinetics and reduced optimal activity. Br. J. Haematol. 22:651, 1972.

89. Mentzer, W., and Alpers, J.: Mild anemia with abnormal RBC pyruvate kinase. Clin. Res. 29: 209, 1971.

90. Boivin, P., Galand, C., et al.: Mise en évidence d'un enzyme a cinétique anormale dans deux nouveaux cas de déficit en pyruvate-

kinase érythrocytaire. Pathol. Biol. (Paris) 17: 597, 1969.

91. Ohyama, H., Kumatori, T., et al.: Functionally abnormal pyruvate kinase in congenital hemolytic anemia. Acta Haematol. Jap. 32: 330, 1969.

92. Sachs, J. R., Wicker, D. J., et al.: Familial hemolytic anemia resulting from an abnormal red blood cell pyruvate kinase. J. Lab. Clin. Med. 72:359, 1968.

93. Busch, D., Witt, I., et al.: Deficiency of pyruvate kinase in the erythrocytes of a child with hereditary non-spherocytic hemolytic anemia. Acta Paediatr. Scand. 55:177, 1966.

94. Baughan, M. A., Paglia, D. E., et al.: An unusual hematological syndrome with pyruvate kinase deficiency and thalassemia minor in the kindreds. Acta Haematol. (Basel) 39:345, 1968.

95. Eudlerink, F., and Cleton, F. S.: Gaucher's disease with severe renal involvement combined with pyruvate-kinase deficiency. Pathol. Eur. 5:409, 1970.

96. Blume, K. G., Busch, D., et al.: The polymorphism of nucleoside effect in pyruvate kinase deficiency. Humangenetik 9:257, 1970.

97. Koler, R. D., Bigley, R. H., et al.: Pyruvate kinase: molecular differences between human red cell and leukocyte enzyme. Symp. Quant. Biol. 29:213, 1964.

98. Blume, K. G., Hoffbauer, R. W., et al.: Purification and properties of pyruvate kinase in normal and in pyruvate kinase deficient human red blood cells. Biochim. Biophys. Acta 227:364, 1971.

99. Staal, G. E. J., Koster, J. F., et al.: Human erythrocyte pyruvate kinase. Its purification and some properties. Biochim. Biophys. Acta 227:86, 1971

100. Ibsen, K. H., Schiller, K. W., et al.: Interconvertible kinetic and physical forms of human erythrocyte pyruvate kinase. J. Biol. Chem. 246:1233, 1971.

101. Calbreath, D. F.: PhD dissertation, The Ohio State University, 1968, University Microfilm 69-11, 618, Ann Arbor, Michigan, 1970.

102. Monod, J., Wyman, J., et al.: On the nature of allosteric transitions: A plausible model. J. Mol. Biol. 12:88, 1964.

103. Koler, R. D., and Vanbellinghen, P.: The mechanism of precursor modulation of human pyruvate kinase I by fructose diphosphate. Adv. Enzyme Regul. 6:127, 1968.

104. Koster, J. F., Staal, G. E. J., et al.: The effect of urea and temperature on red blood cell pyruvate kinase. Biochim. Biophys. Acta 236:362, 1971.

105. Cartier, P., Najman, A., et al.: Les anomalies de la glycolyse au cours l'anémie hémolytique par déficit du globule rouge en pyruvate kinase. Clin. Chim. Acta 22:165, 1968.

106. Boivin, P., Galand, C., et al.: Coexistence de deux types de pyruvate-kinase cinétiquement différents dans les globules rouges humains normaux. Nouv. Rev. Fr. Hematol. 12:159, 1972.

106a. Boivin, P., Galand, C., et al.: Études sur la pyruvate-kinase érythrocytaire. I. Propriétés de l'enzyme normale. Pathol. Biol. 30:383, 1972.

107. Paglia, D. E., and Valentine, W. N.: Evidence for molecular alteration of pyruvate kinase as a consequence of erythrocyte aging. J. Lab. Clin. Med. 76:202, 1970.

108. Munro, G. F., and Miller, D. R.: Mechanism of fructose diphosphate activation of a mutant pyruvate kinase from human red cells. Biochim. Biophys. Acta 206:87, 1970.

109. Solovonuk, P. F., and Collier, H. B.: The pyruvic phosphoferase of erythrocytes. I. Properties of the enzyme and its activity in erythrocytes of various species. Can. J. Biochem. Physiol. 33: 38, 1955.

110. Srivastava, S. K., and Beutler, E.: The effect of normal red cell constituents on the activities of red cell enzymes. Arch. Biochem. Biophys. 148:249, 1972.

111. Ponce, J., Roth, S., et al.: Kinetic studies on the inhibition of glycolytic kinases of human erythrocytes by 2,3-diphosphoglycerate acid. Biochim. Biophys. Acta 250:63, 1971.

112. Bigley, R. H., Stenzel, P., et al.: Tissue distribution of human pyruvate kinase isoenzymes. Enzymol. Biol. Clin. (Basel) 9:10, 1968.

113. Grimes, A. J., Meisler, A., et al.: Hereditary non-spherocytic haemolytic anaemia. A study of red-cell carbohydrate metabolism in twelve cases of pyruvate-kinase deficiency. Br. J. Haematol. 10:403, 1964.

114. Jacobasch, G., and Boese, C.: Regulation des Kohlenhydratstoff-wechsels roter Blutzellen bei Pyruvatkinasemangel. Folia Haematol. (Leipz.) 91:70, 1969.

115. Rose, I. A., and Warms, J. V. B.: Control of glycolysis in the human red blood cell. J. Biol. Chem. 241:4848, 1966.

116. Miwa, S., Nishina, T., et al.: Studies on erythrocyte metabolism in various hemolytic anemias: With special reference to pyruvate kinase deficiency. Acta Haematol. Jap. 33: 501, 1970.

117. Rose, I. W., and Warms, J. V. B.: Control of red cell glycolysis. The cause of triose phosphate accumulation. J. Biol. Chem. 245:4009, 1970.

118. Nathan, D. G., Oski, F. A., et al.: Extreme hemolysis and red cell distortion in erythrocyte pyruvate kinase deficiency. II. Measurements of erythrocyte glucose consumption, potassium flux, and adenosine triphosphate stability. New Engl. J. Med. 272:118, 1965.

119. Twomey, J. J., O'Neal, F. B., et al.: ATP metabolism in pyruvate kinase deficient erythrocytes. Blood 30:576, 1967.

120. Staal, G. E. J., Koster, J. F., et al.: A new variant of red blood cell pyruvate kinase deficiency. Biochim. Biophys. Acta 258:685, 1972.

121. Nathan, D. G., Oski, F. A., et al.: Life-span and organ sequestration of the red cells in pyruvate kinase deficiency. New Engl. J. Med. 278:73, 1968.

122. Najean, Y., Dresch, C., et al.: Étude de l'érythrocinétique dans 8 cas de déficit homozygote en pyruvate kinase. Nouv. Rev. Fr. Hematol. 9:850, 1969.

123. Bowman, H. S., and Oski, F. A.: Splenic macrophage interaction with red cells in pyruvate kinase deficiency and hereditary spherocytosis. Vox Sang. 19:168, 1970.

124. Blume, K. G., Löhr, G. W., et al.: Beitrag zur

Populationsgenetik der Pyruvat-kinase menschlicher Erythrocyten. Humangenetik 6: 261, 1968.

125. Fung, R. H. P., Keung, Y. K., et al.: Screening of pyruvate kinase deficiency and G6PD deficiency in Chinese newborn in Hong Kong. Arch. Dis. Child. 44:373, 1969.

126. Staal, G. E. J., Koster, J. F., et al.: Some properties of abnormal red blood cell pyruvate kinase. Biochem. Biophys. Acta 220:613, 1970.

127. Boivin, P., and Galand, C.: Recherche d'une anomalie moleculaire lors des déficits en pyruvate kinase éythrocytaire. Nouv. Rev. Fr. Hematol. 8:201, 1968.

127a. Boivin, P., Galand, C., et al.: Études sur la pyruvate-kinase éythrocytaire. II. Hétérogénéité enzymologique des déficits. Études à propos de 28 cas avec anémie hémolytique congénitale. Nouv. Rev. Fr. Hématol. 12: 569, 1972.

128. Mentzer, W. C.; unpublished data.

129. Miwa, S., Nishina, T., et al.: Studies on erythrocyte metabolism in a case with hereditary deficiency of H-subunit of lactate dehydrogenase. Acta Haematol. Jap. 34:228, 1971.

130. Loos, J. A., Prins, H. K., et al.: Elevated ATP levels in human erythrocytes, In Hereditary Disorders of Erythrocyte Metabolism. Beutler, E. (ed.), New York, Grune & Stratton, 1968, p. 280.

131. Brewer, G. J.: A new inherited abnormality of human erythrocytes: Elevated erythrocyte adenosine triphosphate. Biochem. Biophys. Res. Commun. 18:430, 1965.

132. Jacobasch, G., Syllm-Rapoport, I., et al.: 2,3-PGase-mangel als mögliche Ursache erhohten ATP-Gehaltes. Clin. Chim. Acta 10:477, 1964.

133. Valentine, W. N., Anderson, H. M., et al.: Studies on human erythrocyte nucleotide metabolism. II. Nonspherocytic hemolytic anemia, high red cell ATP, and ribosephosphate pyrophosphokinase deficiency. Blood 39: 674, 1972.

134. Szeinberg, A., Kahana, D., et al.: Hereditary deficiency of adenylate kinase in red blood cells. Acta Haematol. 42:111, 1969.

135. Boivin, P., Galand, C., et al.: Anémie hémolytique congénitale non sphérocytaire et déficit héréditaire en adenylate-kinase érythrocytaire. Presse Med. 79:215, 1971.

136. Lichtman, M. A., and Miller, D. R.: Erythrocyte glycolysis, 2,3-diphosphoglycerate and adenosine triphosphate concentration in uremic subjects: Relationship to extracellular phosphate concentration. J. Lab. Clin. Med. 76: 267, 1970.

137. Travis, S. F., Sugerman, H. J., et al.: Red cell metabolic alterations induced by intravenous hyperalimentation. New Engl. J. Med. 285: 763, 1971.

138. Lichtman, M. A., Miller, D. R., et al.: Energy metabolism in uremic red cells: Relationship of red cell adenosine triphosphate concentration to extracellular phosphate. Trans. Assoc. Am. Physicians 82:331, 1969.

139. Jacob, H. S., and Amsden, T.: Acute hemolytic anemia with rigid red cells in hypophosphatemia. New Engl. J. Med. 285:1446, 1971.

140. Weed, R. I., LaCelle, P. L., et al.: Metabolic dependence of red cell deformability. J. Clin. Invest. 48:795, 1969.

141. Klock, J. C., Williams, H. E., et al.: Glycolysis, glycogenolysis, and erythrocyte phospholipids in severe hypophosphatemia. Arch. Intern. Med., 1974.

142. Lichtman, M. A., Miller, D. R., et al.: Reduced red cell glycolysis, 2,3-diphosphoglycerate, and adenosine triphosphate concentration, and increased hemoglobin oxygen affinity caused by hypophosphatemia. Ann. Intern. Med. 74:562, 1971.

142a. Card, R. T., and Brain, M. C.: The anemia of childhood: Physiologic response to hyperphosphatemia. New Engl. J. Med. 288:388, 1973.

142b. Mentzer, W. C., Addiego, J., et al.: Modulation of oxygen affinity by phosphate in sickle cell anemia. Clin. Res. 22:225a, 1974.

143. Oken, M. M., Lichtman, M. A., et al.: Spherocytic hemolytic disease during magnesium deprivation in the rat. Blood 38:468, 1971.

144. Macdougall, L. G., Judisch, J. M., et al.: Red cell metabolism in iron deficiency anemia. II. The relationship between red cell survival and alterations in red cell metabolism. J. Pediatr. 76:660, 1970.

145. Macdougall, L. G.: Red cell metabolism in iron deficiency anemia. III. The relationship between glutathione peroxide, catalase, serum vitamin E, and susceptibility of iron-deficient red cells to oxidative hemolysis. J. Pediatr. 80:775, 1972.

146. Macdougall, L. G.: Red cell metabolism in iron-deficiency anemia. J. Pediatr. 72:303, 1968.

147. Slawsky, P., and Desforges, J. F.: Erythrocyte 2,3-diphosphoglycerate in iron deficiency. Arch. Intern. Med. 129:914, 1972.

148. Brewer, G. J.: Metabolism of ATP in thalassemic and iron-deficient erythrocytes. J. Lab. Clin. Med. 70:1016, 1967.

149. Ramot, B., Brok-Simoni, F., et al.: Glucose 6-phosphate dehydrogenase, hexokinase activities and ATP levels as a function of cell density in thalassemia and iron deficiency anemia. Ann. N.Y. Acad. Sci. 165:400, 1968.

150. Card, R. T., and Weintraub, L. R.: Metabolic abnormalities of erythrocytes in severe iron deficiency. Blood 37:725, 1971.

151. Kimura, H., Horiuchi, N., et al.: Hormonal response of glycolytic key enzymes of erythrocytes in insulinoma. Metabolism 20:1119, 1971.

152. Butenandt, O.: Erythrocytic enzyme activities in hypothyroid children. Acta Haematol. 47: 335, 1972.

153. Snyder, L. M., and Reddy, W. J.: Thyroid hormone control of erythrocyte 2,3-diphosphoglyceric acid. Science 169:879, 1970.

154. Najman, A., Leroux, J. P., et al.: Déficit en pyruvate kinase érythrocytaire au cours des leucémies aigues. Rev. Fr. Etud. Clin. Biol. 14:795, 1969.

155. Boivin, P., Galand, C., et al.: Érythroenzymop-

athies acquises. 1. Anomalies quantitatives observées dans 100 cas d'hemopathies diverses. Pathol. Biol. (Paris) *18*:175, 1970.

156. Emerson, P. M., and Ganow, D. H.: Differences in the two red-cell populations in erythroleukemia. Lancet 2:1150, 1971.

157. Kahn, A., Vroclans, M., et al.: Differences in the two red-cell populations in erythroleukemia. Lancet 2:933, 1971.

158. Pagnier, J., Labie, D., et al.: Étude biochemique d'un cas d'erythroleucémie. Nouv. Rev. Fr. Hematol. *12*:317, 1972.

159. Moser, K., Fischer, M., et al.: Glutathionreductase—und Triosephosphatisomerasemangel in Erythrocyten und Thrombocyten bei Pancytopenie (Typ Estren-Damastrek) Klin. Wochenschr. *46*:995, 1968.

160. Schroter, W.: Chronische idiopathische infantile Panzytopenie. Ein neues Syndrom mit rela- tivem Pyruvatkinase und Glutathionreduktasemangel der Erythrozyten und Hyperplasie des erythropoetischen Gewebes. Schweiz. Med. Wochenschr. *100*:1101, 1970.

161. Kleeberg, U. R., Heimpel, H., et al.: Relativer Glutathion und/oder Pyruvatkinasemangel in den Erythrocyten bei Panmyelopathien und akuten Leukamien. Klin. Wochenschr. *49*:557, 1971.

162. Valentine, W. N., Crookston, J. H., et al.: Erythrocyte enzymatic abnormalities in HEMPAS (hereditary erythroblastic mulitnuclearity with a positive acidified-serum test). Br. J. Haematol. *23*:107, 1972.

163. Dreyfus, B., Sultan, C., et al.: Anomalies of blood group antigens and erythrocyte enzymes in two types of chronic refractory anaemia. Br. J. Haematol. *16*:303, 1969.

Chapter 11

G6PD Deficiency and Related Disorders of the Pentose Pathway

by Sergio Piomelli

INTRODUCTION

The discovery of G6PD deficiency made it possible for the first time to identify a specific metabolic defect responsible for hemolysis. Thus a sound scientific basis could be proposed to explain the abnormal response of some individuals to drugs harmless to the majority of people. This phenomenon ("the individual variability") had been observed empirically by physicians since the beginning of medicine.

The discovery and understanding of this enzyme deficiency has been an exciting scientific endeavour. The combined observations of investigators from various parts of the world have contributed in less than two decades to the present coherent picture of this inherited abnormality.

The deficiency of G6PD in the red cells of certain individuals was discovered by a group at the University of Chicago. These investigators, studying the hemolytic effect of antimalarial drugs, first postulated a defect intrinsic to the red cell (39). In less than two years they demonstrated the relationship between hemolysis and reduced glutathione levels and finally localized the specific lesion to a defect in the enzyme G6PD (29). One of the participants in the original studies has given a detailed historical account (8).

It soon became apparent that G6PD deficiency was a widespread, worldwide genetic defect. The same deficiency was also responsible for favism, the acute hemolysis following ingestion of fava beans, known for centuries in semitropical areas (123). Shortly thereafter, the sex-linkage of the gene for G6PD was demonstrated by Childs et al. in Baltimore (31) and conclusively confirmed by Siniscalco et al. in Sardinia (132), who demonstrated its close linkage with color blindness. In view of the great frequency of G6PD deficiency among individuals from tropical areas, a protective effect on malaria was postulated by Allison in England (3) and by Motulsky in the United States (85). The elegant cytologic and epidemiologic studies of Luzzatto et al. in Nigeria have confirmed this hypothesis (16, 77).

G6PD deficiency represents one of the best examples of human genetic polymorphism. The discovery of G6PD deficiency and its genetic inheritance provided both the tools and the knowledge required to expand some basic genetic theories. The X-inactivation hypothesis was elaborated by Lyon on the basis of X-linked color coat genes in mice (78), and by Beutler in his observations on human females deficient in G6PD (15). Using G6PD as a marker, Davidson et al. demonstrated the cellular mosaicism of the human female (35).

G6PD has been a unique tool in the study of clonal origin of tumors (70) and in somatic cell genetics. A map of the human

346

X chromosome has been recently drawn for the first time (122). This could not have been possible without the availability of G6PD as a marker. The enzyme has been used to obtain critical information in experiments employing entirely different techniques, such as human pedigree analysis and studies of interspecies somatic cell hybrids in tissue culture (90).

Marks and Gross demonstrated that the enzyme deficiency was due to a different mutation in Africans than in Caucasians (80). Several dozen different mutants at the G6PD locus have since been demonstrated (146). This was made possible by the development of electrophoretic techniques (22) and the demonstration of heterogeneity in certain kinetic characteristics (62). The differences between mutant enzymes are not limited to their physical properties. Different variants may produce widely different clinical conditions. These range from the asymptomatic state to the extreme debilitation of individuals with chronic hemolysis (CNSHA).

The enzyme has been extensively purified (33), crystallized (149), and viewed under the electron microscope (148). Yoshida has demonstrated in at least two mutants a single amino acid substitution (150, 151). The enzyme defect has been shown in at least two mutants to be due to the synthesis of an unstable enzyme (105). Cytologic techniques have been developed for the visualization of enzyme activity in single cells (43, 125).

Thus, in less than two decades, the discovery of G6PD deficiency has greatly contributed not only to the clarification of the mechanism of hemolysis but also to the advancement of human genetics. Several excellent reviews in recent years have covered some of these aspects (10, 11, 55, 59, 60, 154).

THE ENZYME AND ITS FUNCTION

G6PD and the Pentose Pathway

Glucose-6-phosphate dehydrogenase is the enzyme that catalyzes the conversion of glucose-6-P to 6-phosphogluconate, and at the same time reduces NADP to NADPH (Fig. 11–1). Glucose-6-P can be utilized either through the main Embden-Meyerhof pathway or through the pentose pathway. Under ordinary conditions in the red cell only a small fraction of the glucose-6-P is utilized through the pentose pathway; most of the metabolic flow is directed through glycolysis to the generation of ATP, 2,3-DPG, and lactate (88). Glucose-6-P occupies a key position in the regulation of glycolysis, since its level controls the activity of hexokinase (117). Thus a decrease in intracellular G6P concentration (consequent to accelerated utilization) derepresses the hexokinase, which phosphorylates more glucose to G6P. Through this equilibrium a constant G6P level is maintained, and accelerated glucose utilization can be directed through the pentose pathway, if so required.

G6PD controls the first step in a chain of reactions that comprise the pentose pathway. This is schematically represented in Figure 11–2. Glucose-6-P is converted through 6-phosphogluconate into ribulose-5-P. In this process, the two main by-products of the pathway, NADPH and CO_2, are generated. The fact that the carbon atom in position 1 is converted to CO_2 in this step can be conveniently utilized in the laboratory to follow the course of the reaction with glucose-1-^{14}C. Every molecule of radioactive CO_2 formed is, in fact, representative of the utilization of one molecule of G6P. The subsequent reactions of the pentose pathway result in the molecular rearrangement of the sugars formed through transaldolation and transketolation. For every three moles of glucose-6-P utilized, two moles of fructose-6-P and one of glyceraldehyde-3-P are formed. Fructose-6-P can be either metabolized through glycolysis to lactate or converted back to glucose-6-P by hexose isomerase to restart the cycle. For every two cycles of the pentose pathway, six moles of glucose-6-P are utilized, and four moles of fructose-6-P and two moles of glyceraldehyde-3-P are produced. The two moles of glyceraldehyde-3-P could, in turn, be converted into another molecule of fructose-6-P. Thus the sum of these series of reactions shows that one of every six moles of glucose metabolized through this pathway is totally converted to CO_2.

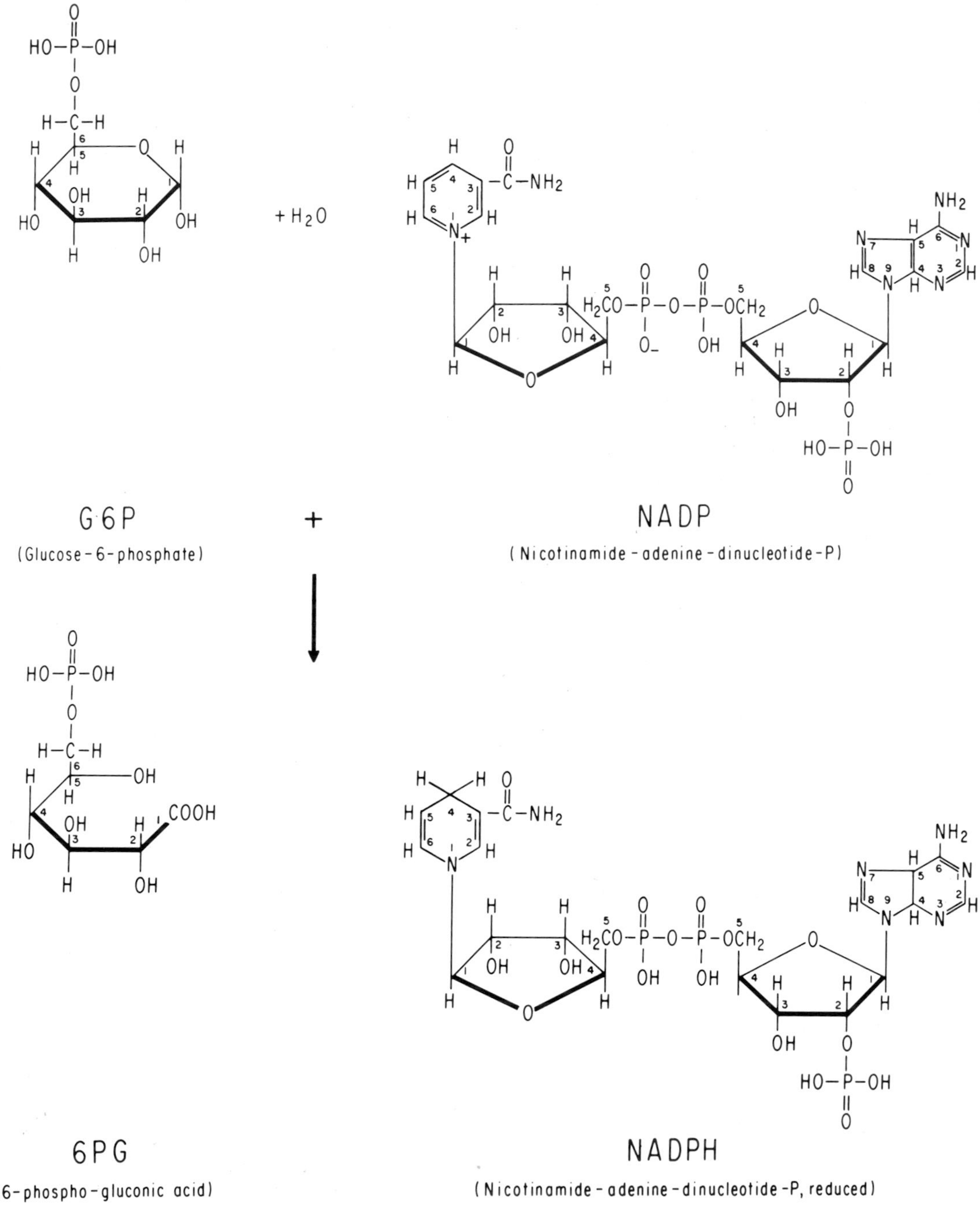

G·6·P

(Glucose-6-phosphate)

NADP

(Nicotinamide-adenine-dinucleotide-P)

6PG

(6-phospho-gluconic acid)

NADPH

(Nicotinamide-adenine-dinucleotide-P, reduced)

Figure 11-1. The reaction catalyzed by glucose-6-phosphate dehydrogenase.

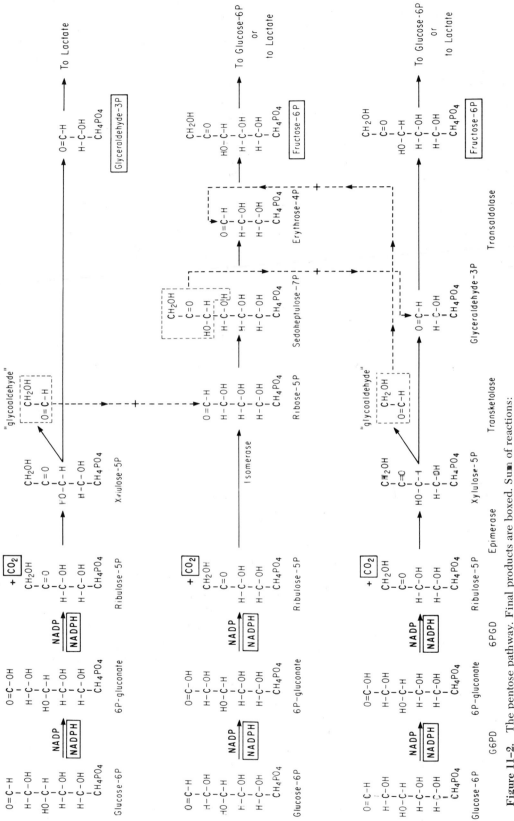

Figure 11–2. The pentose pathway. Final products are boxed. Sum of reactions:

1 cycle: $3 \, G6P + 6 \, NADP = 2 \, F6F + 1 \, G3P + 6 \, NADPH + 3 \, CO_2$
2 cycles: $6 \, G6P + 12 \, NADP = 4 \, F6P + 2 \, G3P + 12 \, NADPH + 6 \, CO_2$

Since F6P can be reconverted to G6P, and 3PGa is converted to lactate, the final result is that, of the six G6P that enter the cycle, one is converted to lactate, one is converted to CO_2, and four are recycled.

For this reason, the pentose pathway is also called the oxidative pathway. In the process, 12 molecules of NADP are reduced to NADPH.

In human red cells, recycling is mostly channeled through the production of fructose-6-P (79). In fact, only negligible amounts of $^{14}CO_2$ are produced using glucose-6-^{14}C as a substrate. This suggests that very little recycling occurs through the formation of glyceraldehyde-3-P. The glyceraldehyde-3-P formed is probably mostly converted to lactate. The net balance of the reaction remains unchanged. For each six moles of glucose entering the cycle, one mole of glucose disappears, one is converted to lactate, and only four are re-utilized; still six moles of CO_2 and 12 of NADPH are formed.

The product of the pentose pathway which is of great physiologic significance is NADPH. The importance of G6PD in the overall cell metabolism resides in its role in the maintenance of an adequate supply of NADPH, which, in turn, plays a key role in maintaining several cellular systems in the reduced state. G6PD is therefore of greatest importance in tissue like the red cell, which has no other source of NADPH.

It has been suggested that the NADP/NADPH system represents a more recent evolutionary development from the NAD/NADH system. In the primitive earth when oxygen appeared in the atmosphere, hydrogen, NH_3, and CH_4 became scarcer. Hence the need for a different coenzyme which was not in rapid equilibrium with oxygen. NADPH is in fact less prone to direct oxidation by O_2 than NADH, and it is therefore more valuable in maintaining reduced intracellular components (51).

The Trigger of the Pentose Pathway

G6PD has been the object of extensive purification and characterization (20, 33, 58, 82, 149). The techniques for its purification have been standardized for purposes of interlaboratory comparison (146). With some of the most recently developed methods, considerable purification of the enzyme can be achieved, even from small quantities of normal blood (112). Several physical characteristics have been eluci-

dated by the study of the purified enzyme. This knowledge permits a better understanding of its intracellular function.

The enzyme is a protein composed of two apparently equal monomers, each with a molecular weight of approximately 52,000 (33, 111, 153). The monomers are almost completely inactive. Thus the active enzyme is a dimer with a molecular weight of about 104,000, consisting of two monomers joined by one mole of NADP (1, 19, 76, 153). The monomers viewed under the electron microscope appear cylindrical, with an axial ratio of 2 and dimensions of 68 Å. × 34 Å. Dimers are formed at 90° angles, and their formation is accompanied by a reduction of the axial ratio to 1.4. Tetramers can also be formed under experimental conditions; these have a tetrahedral structure (148). Evidence for the dimeric structure and for the presence of structural NADP in the active form of the enzyme has also been gathered from hybridization experiments (13). If two enzymes of different electrophoretic mobility (such as human and rat G6PD) are first incubated together at low concentration of NADP, and then the concentration of NADP is raised, a third "hybrid" band of intermediate mobility appears (116). These experiments confirm that the active form is composed of an even number of subunits, and NADP is necessary for its polymerization and function. In this system, in fact, the enzyme is detected only if it is in active form.

The enzyme has different affinities for glucose-6-P and NADP. The Km for glucose-6-P is of the order of 60 to 90 μM. The affinity for NADP is much greater, since the Km for this substrate is of the order of only 1 to 3 μM. Recent data suggest that the curve of the NADP affinity is not hyperbolic but rather sigmoid, and therefore it does not fit the Michaelis-Menten equation (1, 20, 76). These observations, together with the evidence for dimeric structure and for the inhibitory effect of NADPH, have led to the formulation of the hypothesis that G6PD is another regulator enzymatic system with allosteric kinetics. At low concentration of NADP, the enzyme is in a sub-active form; at higher concentration the enzyme is activated. Since the concentration of NADP inside the red cell is of the order of magnitude of only 1 μM (96), the enzyme is probably in normal conditions in the subactive form. Any increase in oxidative level that converts NADPH to NADP at the same time (a) increases the concentration of NADP, (b) removes the inhibitory effect of NADPH, (c) results in the activation of the enzyme, (d) suddenly increases the enzyme Vmax, (e) triggers the pentose pathway cycle, (f) decreases the concentration of G6P, (g) derepresses the hexokinase, and (h) induces the utilization of additional glucose.

This sequence of events leads to a rapid increase of glucose metabolism through the pentose pathway and ultimately to rapid regeneration of NADPH. As soon as the level of NADPH is restored, G6PD activity is again inhibited, and the pentose pathway returns to its nearly inactive state.

Through these mechanisms G6PD plays a regulatory role in the flow of glucose metabolism through the pentose pathway. Any "redox stress" that produces oxidation of NADPH is counterbalanced by a burst of activity from the pentose pathway: G6PD acts as the trigger of the pentose shunt, since it is extremely sensitive to any change in the NADPH/NADP ratio. The flux of glucose via hexokinase may be increased several times by these mechanisms. Normal cells in which G6PD potential activity is present in great excess can easily cope with the greater metabolic flux. In enzyme-deficient cells, G6PD activity becomes rate-limiting, and little or no acceleration of glucose flow through the pentose pathway (and NADPH regeneration) can occur.

GENETICS OF G6PD DEFICIENCY

Sex Linkage

The gene for G6PD in man as well as in other mammals is located on the X chromosome (31, 132). Studies of populations with a high incidence of enzyme deficiency have shown that the distribution of the enzyme activity is different in the two sexes (31). Among males only two categories are observed—normal and deficient; among females, there is also a third group with intermediate values. Similar observations are made in populations in which two electro-phoretically different enzymes are present. Males have either one or the other type of enzyme, but females may have both.

These differences can be easily explained in terms of X chromosome–linked inheritance. Since males only have one X chromosome, they may belong exclusively to one or the other category. (The term "hemizygotes" is applied to males when describing the inheritance of X-linked genes.) By contrast, females may be homozygous for either gene (the same gene on both X chromosomes) or heterozygous for both (one different gene on each X chromosome) (Table 11–1).

Sex-linked inheritance had been known for years in the case of hemophilia (110). Typically, a sex-linked deficiency is detected in the males and is transmitted from grandfather to grandson, apparently skipping one generation (crisscross heredity). In the case of G6PD deficiency, however, the heterozygous female can be identified, and homozygous-deficient females may be observed. In certain areas of the world where G6PD deficiency is a common mutation, homozygous deficient females are found at relatively high frequency (146). The percentage of homozygous females may be predicted from the Hardy-Weinberg equilibrium ($1 = p^2 + 2\ pq + q^2$, where p is the frequency of normal males and q is the frequency of enzyme-deficient males). For instance, in a population in whom the frequency of G6PD deficiency among males is 11 per cent (q = 0.11), the frequency of heterozygous females is 19.5 per cent, and that of deficient homozygous females is 1.2 per cent ($1 = 0.7921 + 2\ (0.0979) + 0.0121$). These values closely approximate the frequencies of G6PD deficiency ob-

TABLE 11–1. POSSIBLE GENOTYPES IN G6PD DEFICIENCY

MALES	
XY	X⁻Y
Hemizygous normal	Hemizygous deficient

FEMALES		
XX	X⁻X	X⁻X⁻
Homozygous normal	Heterozygote	Homozygous deficient

X = Chromosome for normal gene; X⁻ = chromosome for deficient gene.

served, for instance, among Afro-Americans in New York City (107).

Inactivation of the X Chromosome

Since the human female has two X chromosomes, she also has two of each X-linked gene. A double dose of a gene that controls the quantitative production of enzyme proteins (such as the gene for G6PD) should produce in the cells of females twice the level of activity that is found in those of males. Instead, in both sexes the level is nearly the same. The mechanism responsible for this phenomenon is also called the "dosage compensation" effect. Even in the cells of individuals with more than two X chromosomes, the G6PD activity (and presumably the amount of protein produced) is always of the same order of magnitude as in males (47). Careful quantitative studies have shown a slightly higher enzyme activity in the red cells of normal females; the activity per unit volume of blood is, however, the same as in males, since females have a lower hematocrit (108).

The mechanism by which dosage compensation occurs in the normal female has been greatly clarified by the study of females heterozygous for G6PD. Certain women are known to be "obligatory heterozygotes" by family study. For instance, a woman who has both normal and deficient sons cannot be anything except heterozygous. When the G6PD level is measured in obligatory heterozygotes, an average value of 50 per cent of the normal activity is found (46). Some individuals in this group, however, appear to have either normal or totally deficient enzyme activity. Thus certain females exhibit a discrepancy between the phenotypic expression and the known genotype.

This phenomenon can be explained by the X-inactivation hypothesis (78). The three postulates of this hypothesis are as follows:

1. In every cell of the female, only one of the two X chromosomes is active, and the other is dormant.

2. The relative proportion of cells in which one of the two X chromosomes is inactive is randomly determined in an early developmental stage.

3. In the progeny of each cell, the same X chromosome thereafter remains inactive.

Thus a female heterozygous for G6PD deficiency does not have uniformly decreased enzyme activity in every cell. Instead, two different populations of cells coexist in the same individual—one "normal," the other "deficient." Since the relative proportion of normal and enzyme-deficient cells in each individual is determined at random, the level of enzyme activity that may be found in the red cells of heterozygous females varies according to a normal type of distribution. On the average, 50 per cent of the cells will appear normal and 50 per cent enzyme-deficient, but some individuals will have an excess of normal cells, some an excess of deficient cells. At the extreme of the distribution, a few individuals will have such a large excess of cells of one type or another as to appear normal or enzyme-deficient, respectively. In reality, however, all heterozygous females still carry in their mature germ cells both the normal and the deficient X chromosome; therefore, they may transmit either one and may have both normal and deficient sons.

The ultimate percentage of red cells of one type or the other observed in an individual heterozygous female can also be influenced by postinactivation selection. The concomitant presence on one X chromosome of other genes with selective value may result in an advantage for the cells in which that chromosome remains active (95). This effect could modify the percentage of cells with one X chromosome and explain some of the deviations from the expected 50 per cent value.

All of the postulates of the X-inactivation hypothesis have been verified in the human female heterozygous for G6PD by the histochemical demonstration in the same individuals of two populations of red cells (and fibroblasts) (36)—one deficient, one normal (43, 125) (Fig. 11–3). More definitive evidence was given by the demonstration of two different types of fibroblasts in female heterozygotes for two electrophoretically different enzymes. In cell clones, in fact, either one or the other enzyme was found, but never both (35). In artificial in vitro mixtures of two different enzymes, a third hybrid band is easily formed. Hybrid bands are also formed when both X chromo-

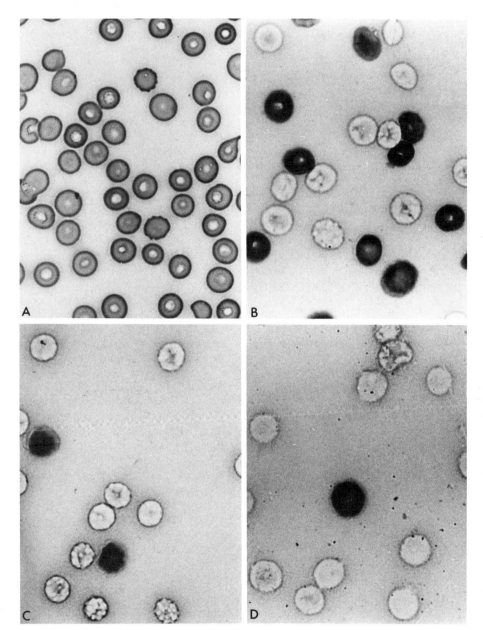

Figure 11–3. Methemoglobin elution test (according to Gall et al., 43). *A*, Normal (Gd^B+) blood; *B*, heterozygous Gd^Mediterranean female: mosaicism; *C*, hemizygous Gd^A− male: pseudomosaicism; *D*, hemizygous Gd^Mediterranean male: occasional stained cell (reticulocyte).

somes are active in the same cell, as, for instance, in hybrid cells formed in vitro by Sendai virus–mediated fusion (48). There are no hybrid bands in freshly prepared extracts of tissues from human females heterozygous for different enzymes. Their absence further confirms that only one molecular species is present in any single cell.

Genetic Heterogeneity

Several different mutants of G6PD have been described, all apparently allelic and under the control of genes located on the X chromosome. The genetic heterogeneity results from qualitative as well as quantitative differences.

Several dozen mutants have been described and characterized sufficiently well to be considered unique (154). The list is continuously expanded by the description of new mutants and by the further subdivision of mutants originally considered homogenous with the use of finer biochemical techniques (137). An exhaustive listing would be outside the scope of this book and would become rapidly outdated. Identification of new mutants has, at present, descriptive value. When more detailed structural analysis of mutants becomes possible, this will permit correlation of the nature of the mutation and the functional change. The recent development of techniques for purification of the enzyme from small amounts of blood makes this goal more realistic (112).

The different mutants have been classified according to their degree of deficiency and clinical behavior into five groups (11, 154):

1. Increased enzyme activity.
2. Very mild or no enzyme deficiency.
3. Moderate to mild enzyme deficiency.
4. Severe enzyme deficiency.
5. Severe enzyme deficiency associated with congenital nonspherocytic hemolytic anemia (CNSHA).

This classification can be further refined if other characteristics, such as electrophoretic mobility, are used to further subdivide each group. The characteristic that best correlates with clinical expression is the enzyme level of the red cell. Increased (group 1) or nearly normal (group 2) enzyme activity has no clinical consequence. In the

group with moderate enzyme deficiency (group 3), overt clinical hemolysis is not present, but it may be acutely induced by several drugs and other agents. In the group with severe enzyme deficiency (group 4), the sensitivity to hemolysis-inducing agents and the severity of the individual episodes are more marked. In the group in which the deficiency is associated with congenital nonspherocytic anemia (group 5), clinically overt hemolysis is, by definition, constantly present; the degree of severity varies in different types.

The level of the enzyme activity is not the only characteristic that influences the clinical manifestations. In fact, certain mutants associated with congenital nonspherocytic hemolytic anemia have, at least in vitro, much higher activity in the red cells than other mutants in which hemolysis only occurs after exposure to drugs.

The individuality of each of the several dozen distinct mutants of G6PD has been established on the basis of unique physical characteristics. In the two mutants studied to date, the amino acid analysis has led to the conclusion that a single substitution is involved. In the case of Gd^{A+}, aspartic acid replaces asparagine (150); in the case of $Gd^{Hektoen}$, tyrosine replaces histidine (151). It appears from these observations that G6PD is similar to human hemoglobin in that the substitution of a single amino acid may result in profound differences in physical properties, biological activity, and ultimately in clinical expression.

The genetic heterogeneity of G6PD is expressed through several dozen distinct isozymes. Most of these are either unique to certain individuals or families or limited to small ethnic groups (146). However, certain enzyme mutants are very frequent in some populations and can be called "common types." The normal enzyme, also called Gd^B, is the most common type and represents the standard of normal activity. $Gd^{Mediterranean}$ (an enzyme with nearly absent activity, normal electrophoretic mobility, and increased affinity for both NADP and G6P) is commonly observed among populations in the southern Mediterranean area, where it was originally described. This enzyme is, however, also found frequently among Indians and Southeast Asians (10, 60, 146).

Two different mutant enzymes are frequently observed in Western and Central Africa. Both enzymes have fast electrophoretic mobility and normal kinetic characteristics. One, Gd^{A-}, is associated with decreased activity (5 to 15 per cent of normal) in the red cells; the other, Gd^{A+}, has nearly normal activity, although in one series it was found to average only 80 per cent of normal (72).

These four enzymes are the most common and widespread. Other enzymes with decreased activity observed with relatively high frequency are $Gd^{Debrousse}$ (63) in North Africa and Gd^{Canton} (89) in southern Asia.

Racial Distribution of G6PD Deficiency: The Malarial Hypothesis

G6PD deficiency is among the most common of the inborn errors of metabolism. Several million males throughout the world are enzyme-deficient. There are also between approximately one and a half and twice as many heterozygous females. In many individuals the defect is only partial, because they are carriers of a gene responsible for mild deficiency.

The frequency of G6PD deficiency is clearly different among various ethnic groups. It is extremely rare among Northern Europeans, but it is quite common among populations from subtropical and tropical areas. This distribution suggests that in tropical areas some environmental selective pressure maintains the high incidence of a possibly deleterious gene (3). The geographic distribution of G6PD deficiency is strikingly superimposable on that of the endemicity of *Plasmodium falciparum* malaria (85). The hypothesis was therefore put forward that the higher incidence of G6PD deficiency in certain populations was being maintained by a protective effect against malaria for individual carriers of the defect.

Indirect evidence for this hypothesis was obtained by population studies in small villages in Sardinia. These communities had been isolated for centuries and resembled closely true mendelian isolates. The enzyme deficiency was found to be more common in the villages at sea level than in those at higher elevation (131). An extremely good correlation was observed between previous malarial endemicity and the present-day distribution of enzyme deficiency.

Direct evidence supporting the protective effect of G6PD deficiency against malaria has been provided by the elegant cytologic studies of Luzzatto et al. (77) in Nigerian heterozygous G6PD-deficient females affected with malaria. These authors demonstrated a greater incidence of parasites in the normal cells than in the G6PD-deficient red cells. The two categories of cells were distinguished by cytochemical staining on the same slide on which the malarial parasites were demonstrated. In normal individuals, *Plasmodium falciparum* does not preferentially parasitize young red cells. This was the first clear demonstration that absence of G6PD activity in a red cell may modify its relationship with the malarial parasite. A biochemical hypothesis has been advanced by Kosower and Kosower to explain this mechanism (67). These authors proposed that, since oxidized glutathione (GSSG) inhibits protein synthesis, its higher level in the deficient cell might inhibit parasite growth. G6PD-deficient cells do, indeed, have an increased level of GSSG (135).

Several studies, on the other hand, have failed to show in hemizygous deficient males a clear decrease in either parasitemia or mortality rates from malaria (71). Recently, the parasitemia has been measured in children of both sexes by Bienzle et al. (16) in Nigeria. These studies have clearly shown a much lower parasite count in the Gd^B/Gd^{A-} heterozygous female. These data suggest that the high frequency of the enzyme deficiency is maintained primarily, and perhaps exclusively, by the advantage of the heterozygous females against malaria (71).

The biological disadvantage of the hemizygous and homozygous G6PD-deficient individual is certainly smaller than that of the individual with sickle cell anemia. The advantage required to maintain a high frequency of G6PD deficiency must accordingly also be smaller. In most populations, the average frequency of the enzyme deficiency is fixed at a value of about 20 per cent (71). This is compatible with the hypothesis of maximum fitness of the heterozygote and decreased fitness of hemizygote and homozygote deficient. There are populations, however, where the frequency of the G6PD deficiency among males exceeds 50 per cent (146). These unusually high frequencies require a greater fitness of the hemizygous deficient individual himself; it is possible that in these rare situations some other factor besides malaria could contribute further selective pressure.

In Western Africa, both the Gd^{A-} and the Gd^{A+} mutants are found with equally increased frequency. To explain this finding it is necessary to postulate a similar net advantage *vis-à-vis* malaria. Since the Gd^{A+} mutation is not intrinsically deleterious, its high frequency could result from a minimal selective advantage. Data supporting a very mild selective advantage of the Gd^{A+} hemizygote himself have been reported by Bienzle et al. (16). In their survey in Nigeria, a decreased frequency of "very severe" parasitemia was observed in the Gd^{A+} hemizygotes.

G6PD and the Map of the Human X Chromosome

The discovery of the genetic heterogeneity of G6PD has greatly contributed to the studies that led to a preliminary map of the human X chromosome (122). Linkage between two genes on the same chromosome may be estimated by the classical genetic approach of counting the percentage of recombinant children in a series of families. With this technique, the X-linkage of G6PD itself was definitively established (132). The frequency of recombination of G6PD with the deutan type of color blindness (a well-known X-linked gene) was in fact found to be extremely low. Population studies have provided evidence for the close linkage between the locus for G6PD and those for both deutan and protan types of color blindness, as well as the locus for Factor VIII (122). From pedigree analysis it has also been shown that the locus for G6PD is at a nonmeasurable distance from the locus for the blood group Xg (the latter is probably located at the extreme end of the short arm) and from the loci for Factor IX and Duchenne muscular dystrophy. Frequent recombination has been demonstrated in two separate kindreds between G6PD and the X-linked gene for hypoxan-

thine-guanine-phosphoribosyl transferase (HGPRT) (a defect of this enzyme is responsible for the Lesch-Nyhan syndrome) (34, 95).

Mapping of human chromosomes has been greatly facilitated by the recent progress in the field of somatic cell genetics (90). It has become possible to detect the recombination of human genes in vitro, utilizing somatic hybrid cells prepared by Sendai virus–mediated fusion. With this technique it is possible to study the recombination frequency of those genes, such as G6PD, which are known to be X-linked and which express themselves in cultured fibroblasts. Briefly, human cells are fused with mouse or hamster cells which are deficient in HGPRT activity. These hybrid cells rapidly lose human chromosomes; by adding hypoxanthine-aminopterin-thymidine (HAT) to the medium, only those cells which have retained the human X chromosome (and thus the HGPRT enzyme) are permitted to grow. With this technique, it has been possible, for instance, to definitely demonstrate the sex linkage of the gene for phosphoglycerate kinase (PGK) (48), which had been suspected by study of one family with PGK deficiency hemolytic anemia (141).

The technique of cell hybridization combined with cytogenetics provides even more precise localizations. Utilizing cells from a woman with an X-autosomal translocation, for instance, the PGK gene was located on the long arm of the X chromosome (48). Since PGK has been shown to undergo X-inactivation, these studies also suggest that the long arm of the X chromosome undergoes X-inactivation (40).

The X chromosome is probably fairly long, approximately 250 centiMorgans [1 centiMorgan = cross-over frequency of 1 per cent] (115). From the data presently accumulated a preliminary map of the X chromosome can be drawn. The gene for G6PD appears located near the centromere in a cluster of genes, including those for Factor VIII, deuteranopia, and protanopia. Another cluster of genes is located on the short arm. This includes Xg, retinitis pigmentosa, ichthyosis, ocular albinism, and Fabry's disease. The gene for HGPRT is most likely located in between the two clusters closer to Xg. The basis for the location of PGK on the long arm has been discussed. The positions of other X-linked genes outside these clusters is not established yet with certainty.

THE BIOCHEMICAL DEFECT OF THE G6PD-DEFICIENT CELL

Relationship Between G6PD Activity and Red Cell Age

It was originally observed that the G6PD activity of the red cell increases during reticulocytosis (81). This suggested that the younger red cells have higher enzyme activity, which then decreases as the red cell ages. These observations introduced in red cell biochemistry the concept of "age-dependent" enzymes.

Recently, techniques have become available to measure in the erythrocytes the in vivo life span of individual enzymes. It has been found that the activity of the normal G6PD enzyme declines exponentially with a $t_{1/2}$ of 62 days (105). Thus the youngest red cells have twice the G6PD activity of the average red cells, and the oldest ones have only one half of it. The enzyme activity, therefore, shows a fourfold decline during the life span of the cell. In certain situations, such as hemolysis, there is an increased number of young red cells in the circulation. These have proportionally more enzyme activity, and result in an increased enzyme level in the peripheral blood.

The in vivo instability of G6PD plays an important role in the development of enzyme deficiency and in the clinical course of drug-induced hemolysis. Genotypically G6PD-deficient individuals of the Gd^{A-} type may exhibit normal levels of enzyme activity during a hemolytic crisis (87). In these individuals if the administration of the hemolytic drug is continued, anemia and reticulocytosis level off (37). These observations suggest that the only red cells susceptible to hemolysis are the oldest and that their selective destruction leaves in the circulation only the younger cells with a greater level of activity (9).

With techniques of red cell ultracentrifugation on albumin gradients, it has been possible to demonstrate in Gd^{A-} individuals that their newly formed red cells have the same enzymatic activity as newly formed cells from normal Gd^{B+} individuals. Their activity rapidly declines, since the life span in vivo of the Gd^{A-} enzyme is only 13 days (105). The enzyme deficiency in these individuals is due to neither a homogenously decreased level of activity of all their red cells nor the existence of a double population, as in the heterozygous female. Rather, in the circulation of the Gd^{A-} male there is a mixture of cells of continuously decreasing level of activity. The reticulocytes have a higher than average enzyme level, but most mature red cells have grossly deficient activity.

In individual cells enzyme activity may be demonstrated cytologically with the methemoglobin elution test (43). This technique has a threshold, and it gives the impression that even in deficient males two distinct populations of cells are present. This histochemical artifact has been called "pseudomosaicism" to distinguish it from the true genetic mosaicism of the heterozygous female (12, 101). It has, in fact, no genetic basis, since it is due to the difference in age between circulating red cells (Fig. 11–3).

The difference between the age dependency of the normal and the Gd^{A-} enzyme is clearly visible in Figure 11–4. In normal blood a fourfold reduction in mean red cell age (from 60 to 15 days) increases the enzyme activity from 5 to 8.3 units. In the blood of Gd^{A-} individuals a comparable fourfold reduction in mean cell age (from 50 to 12 days) would raise the enzyme level from 0.6 to 5 units (an almost tenfold increase) and would bring it into the normal range. Thus, in Gd^{A-} individuals with acute or chronic hemolysis, the enzyme deficiency might not be apparent. In these circumstances, the oldest enzyme-deficient cells are destroyed, and, at the same time, bone marrow compensatory activity results in a large number of reticulocytes. The net result is a drastic reduction in mean cell age. If the mean cell age becomes less than 12 days, the enzyme activity of the circulating red cells may appear even higher than normal. For these reasons in the Gd^{A-} individuals the diagnosis of G6PD deficiency may become extremely difficult at the time of acute hemolysis [when it is most important] (87). A correct diagnosis still may be obtained in the presence of reticulo-

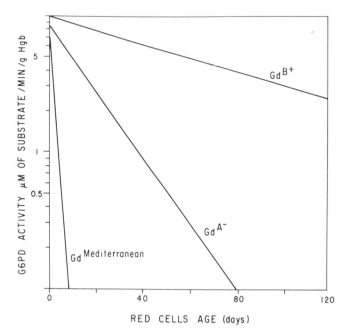

Figure 11–4. Rate of decline of G6PD in vivo in different mutants.

cytosis by either separation of cells on the basis of age (50) or cytochemical demonstration of enzyme deficiency in individual cells or, whenever this is feasible, by a combination of electrophoretic and family studies (107).

The decreased level of enzyme in the red cells of Gd^{A-} individuals does not result from a defect in synthesis but rather from the in vivo instability of the enzyme. A similar mechanism underlies the other common type of deficiency, Gd^{Mediterranean}. In this mutant, the instability is so pronounced that the enzyme activity disappears from the red cells in just a few hours (104). The reticulocytes are released into the circulation of these individuals with an already greatly reduced level of activity, and mature erythrocytes have no detectable enzyme level.

The level of enzyme activity in the red cell is a function of the amount synthesized in the bone marrow and of its rate of decline. In tissues other than the red cell, the level is also determined by a balance between rate of synthesis and decay. A clear example of this effect is observed in the leukocytes of Gd^{A-} individuals. These cells have a normal G6PD activity. The life span of the leukocytes is much shorter than the $t_{1/2}$ of the enzyme, and possibly an increased synthesis compensates for the accelerated decay. In the leukocytes from Gd^{Mediterranean}, the enzyme level is only approximately 20 per cent of normal. Since the rate of decay of this type of enzyme is even shorter than the life span of the leukocyte itself, increased synthesis can only in part compensate for such a rapid disappearance. Hence the enzyme activity is greatly decreased, but to a lesser degree than in the red cells.

The balance between rates of synthesis and decay in different G6PD mutants results in tissue levels of enzyme which are sometimes normal and sometimes decreased, but they are never as low as in the red cells (30). In certain mutants, such as Gd^{A-}, the defect is indeed exclusively limited to the red cells and possibly to the lens of the eye. In other mutants, such as Gd^{Mediterranean}, with almost negligible levels of enzyme activity in the peripheral blood, it is surprising to detect nearly normal levels of activity in the bone marrow normoblasts (104).

A biochemical basis has recently been suggested for the instability in vivo of at least one deficient mutant. Babalola et al. have shown that the purified Gd^{A-} enzyme can be readily converted in vitro into another form (Fraction II) (4). This transformation appears to be due to the formation of a disulfide bond. The oxidized form tends to become inactive, and has clearly abnormal kinetics. This conversion appears to be peculiar to Gd[A−], since the normal enzyme in similar conditions remains unmodified. If the oxidized form of the enzyme is also labile in vivo, such change could represent the molecular lesion leading to enzyme instability and ultimately to the deficiency in the peripheral blood.

The Hemolytic Crisis

A nearly normal hemoglobin level in the G6PD-deficient individual is maintained by a delicate balance. This can be abruptly offset by what has been called a "redox stress." This usually results from the administration of a drug or from infections (such as hepatitis) (121). Diabetic acidosis may also induce a hemolytic crisis. The sequence of events seems to be triggered by the production of H_2O_2 by the hemolytic agent (or one of its metabolites) (32). Other free radicals or even peroxyhemoglobin can be produced. These compounds in turn convert the reduced glutathione (GSH) to oxidized glutathione. Mixed disulfides (hemoglobin-S-SG) may be formed (2). The system glutathione peroxidase–glutathione reductase is used in these situations to return the glutathione to the reduced state and to remove the dangerous peroxides (53) (Fig. 11–5). In the G6PD-deficient cells this pathway is inadequate, since NADPH cannot be regenerated at a fast enough rate. Hemoglobin then precipitates in the form of Heinz bodies; these are "pitted" in the microcirculation of the spleen, with consequent fragmentation of the cell and intravascular hemolysis. It has been pointed

out that this coherent sequence of events is not necessarily the only mechanism by which red cells can be damaged (56). The "redox stress" might cause direct, or H_2O_2-mediated, peroxidation of lipids, with membrane destruction and hemolysis. These effects, in turn, could not be reversed in the absence of an adequate level of NADPH (and GSH) in the cell (28). Whatever its exact mechanism, it is certain that the abrupt hemolysis results from inability of the enzyme-deficient red cells to produce the necessary sudden metabolic surge through the pentose pathway cycle.

The Biochemical Defect in Chronic Hemolysis: CNSHA-Associated Mutants

Unless acute hemolysis is induced by a "redox stress," G6PD-deficient red cells have a survival time which is only slightly shorter than normal (7). These observations may suggest that G6PD and the pentose pathway are mainly potential mechanisms, rather than indispensable for the daily survival of the red cell. In other words, G6PD deficiency and the consequent inadequate function of the pentose pathway would be responsible for the susceptibility to oxidant stress, but in the absence of stress the defect could be largely tolerated by the cell.

However, shortly after the discovery of G6PD, in 1958 Newton and Frajola first described a new category of patients in whom an apparently similar defect in G6PD activity was accompanied by severe extra-

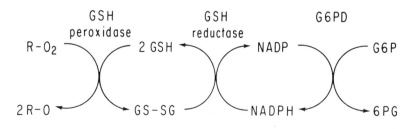

Figure 11–5. The relationship between G6PD, glutathione, and intracellular peroxides.

R = H₂   = Hydrogen peroxide

Hgb = Peroxyhemoglobin

Lipid = Lipid peroxidation

vascular chronic hemolysis (CNSHA) (94). This report demonstrated that G6PD deficiency may produce a completely different syndrome in certain individuals. The reason for this difference remains largely unexplained. It is now clear, however, that the mutants responsible for CNSHA are different from the common types and also from all other types associated with drug sensitivity only.

It has as yet been impossible to find for all the CNSHA-associated mutants a common biochemical denominator that could explain their more severe and continuous effect. Most CNSHA-associated mutants have very low activity, but some of them actually have only moderate deficiencies. In the standard biochemical assay some mutants appear to have higher activity than the clinically silent $Gd^{Mediterranean}$ and Gd^{A-}. These observations suggest that a qualitative rather than a quantitative difference of these mutant enzymes is responsible for the severity and chronicity of the clinical syndrome.

Since the majority of CNSHA-associated G6PD mutant enzymes exhibit an abnormal thermal stability in vitro, it was suggested that this physical characteristic might be responsible for the clinical severity. However, some clinically severe CNSHA-associated mutants appear stable in vitro under similar conditions (114). On the other hand, in vivo instability is a prominent feature of G6PD mutants (such as Gd^{A-} and $Gd^{Mediterranean}$) not associated with CNSHA (105); $Gd^{Mediterranean}$ is also very unstable in vitro (146).

Kirkman first suggested that the intracellular efficiency of the enzyme rather than its apparent activity in the artificially optimal conditions of the in vitro assay may be of true physiologic significance (59). His original hypothesis was based on the observation of abnormally decreased affinity for glucose-6-P in at least one CNSHA-associated G6PD mutant ($Gd^{Oklahoma}$) (62). This feature, however, is not observed in many other CNSHA-associated G6PD mutants (114). Thus, although it may represent the basis for the clinical severity of $Gd^{Oklahoma}$ and a few other similar mutants, it is certainly not the common biochemical denominator for all these syndromes.

In line with the general hypothesis of Kirkman, attention has been directed recently to the affinity of the enzyme for its other substrate (NADP) and to the inhibitory effect of one of its products (NADPH).

One current hypothesis (114) emphasizes that, within the cell, G6PD functions at totally different rates, depending on the absolute concentration of NADP and on the NADP/NADPH ratio (76, 114). In the steady state, the intracellular concentration of NADP is of the order of 1 μM. At this concentration of NADP (and very low NADP/NADPH ratio), the prevalent molecular form of enzyme within the cell is probably the subactive monomer. The extremely low rate of activity of the enzyme in this state is still sufficient to support the minimal activity (0.1 per cent of the maximum potential) required to maintain a slow flow of glucose metabolism through the pentose pathway (23, 24) and thus a level of NADPH compatible with normal cell survival. When a "redox stress" occurs, NADPH is rapidly oxidized to NADP. In these conditions of increased intracellular concentration of NADP (= increased NADP/NADPH ratio), the prevalent molecular form of G6PD within the cell becomes the active dimer. The rate of activity of G6PD is thus greatly increased and becomes adequate to cope with most "redox stress." According to this hypothesis of enzyme function, a mutant G6PD may be defective (a) in the activity of the monomer, (b) in the activity or formation of the dimer, or (c) in the activity of both.

Mutants in which the catalytic activity of the monomer is impaired result in chronic hemolysis, since the enzyme function is inadequate, even in the steady state. In some of these mutants the activity of the dimer is present, although reduced; hence significant activity is shown in the assay, which is always performed in conditions favoring dimer formation. In other mutants, the activity of the dimer is also impaired: hence, the virtual absence of activity in the assay. Mutants in which the low level of activity of the monomer is maintained but the activity (or formation) of the dimer is impaired are not associated with chronic hemolysis, but only with acute hemolysis during "redox stress" (e.g., $Gd^{Mediterranean}$). These mutants appear less efficient than they actually are within the cell. This complex hypothesis rests on the assumption that the minimal activity associated with the enzyme in the monomeric form is responsible for the maintenance of intracellular NADPH level. Direct verification requires measurement of affinity curves for NADP at the very low levels present in the cell. However, since NADP even at low concentration produces the dimerization of the enzyme, these measurements are technically extremely difficult.

Recently, attention has been directed also to the inhibitory effect of NADPH (152). At least some CNSHA-associated G6PD mutants exhibit in vitro an abnormal sensitivity to NADPH inhibition. On the other hand, some very low-activity G6PD mutants not associated with CNSHA (such as Gd^{Mediterranean}) have normal sensitivity to NADPH inhibition but greater affinity for NADP.

The different emphasis placed by these two hypotheses on the respective importance of NADP and NADPH concentration is not contradictory. In fact, dimer dissociation into monomer can be induced by low NADP as well as by high NADPH concentration. In other words, the ratio NADP/NADPH controls the molecular form of and the activity state of the enzyme within the cell.

It appears at present that CNSHA is the result of functional failure of G6PD within the red cell, even in the steady state. This might result from one of several kinetic abnormalities: decreased affinity for NADP or G6P or both, increased sensitivity to inhibition by NADPH, total inactivity of the monomeric form, extreme instability, or any combination of these factors.

CLINICAL EFFECTS ASSOCIATED WITH G6PD DEFICIENCY

The deficiency of G6PD is always associated with a reduction in the life span of the red cells. This effect, however, can be of a different order of magnitude, depending on the particular gene mutation. Chronic hemolysis is extremely mild and only subclinical in the common types, Gd^{A-} and Gd^{Mediterranean}. In certain types of CNSHA, on the contrary, the chronic hemolysis results in severe physical impairment. Most types of G6PD deficiency are associated with acute exacerbation of the hemolysis coinciding with drug administration or infections or both.

The Steady State

In normal conditions, the common types of G6PD deficiency are clinically silent. Several millions of individuals carry one or the other of these defects, unaware of it. Careful clinical and hematologic examinations would not detect any anomaly in the majority of these individuals. Thus the diagnosis can only be performed by specific screening tests.

Several observations have made it apparent that a very mild, subclinical state of chronic hemolysis is invariably present in both Gd^{A-}- and Gd^{Mediterranean}-deficient males. The red cell life span was found to be decreased in both Gd^{A-} and Gd^{Mediterranean} males in two independent studies (7, 27). Although the techniques used were quite different, the estimates of life span were very similar (96 days for Gd^{A-} and 100 days for Gd^{Mediterranean}). A slight but significant increase in reticulocytes has been reported (1.7 per cent for Gd^{A-} and 1.5 per cent for Gd^{Mediterranean}, compared with 0.8 per cent for normal males) (105). Hexokinase levels were found to be elevated in Gd^{A-} males (25). Since hexokinase is one of the most age-dependent red cell enzymes, its increased level is a very sensitive indicator of decreased mean cell age. These data indicate that although not clinically obvious, a small degree of subclinical hemolysis always occurs in G6PD-deficient males. In the only controlled study available, Gd^{Mediterranean} males had a slight but significantly lower mean hemoglobin (14.1 g. per 100 ml.) than control males (15.7 g. per 100 ml.) simultaneously examined (108), indicating less than perfect bone marrow compensation. In the females, it is presumable that this mild degree of hemolysis would be even less prominent, since only a fraction of their red cells is enzyme-deficient. The life span of the deficient red cells in heterozygous females for either Gd^{A-} or Gd^{Mediterranean} cannot be greatly decreased in comparison with that of the normal red cells. If this were the case, in fact, there would be in their peripheral blood a much smaller percentage of detectable enzyme-deficient cells than is actually found.

Except for subclinical chronic hemolysis, the enzyme-deficient individuals lead an apparently normal life. It was, therefore, greatly surprising that in 1970 Petrakis et al. suggested that the enzyme deficiency might result in a reduction in the individual's life span (103). This hypothesis resulted from the observation of a decrease in incidence of G6PD deficiency with increasing age in a large group of Afro-Americans. The incidence in the group up to 20 years was 12 per cent, but was only 5.6 per cent in the group between 21 and 49 years and 3.8 per cent in the oldest group. In the same study the frequency of sickle cell trait (another African gene) did not decline with age; a bias of ascertainment could thus be reasonably excluded. A later study from the same group suggested higher mean blood pressure, pulse rate, and serum creatinine levels among individuals with G6PD deficiency (145). On the other hand a previous study had suggested a decreased frequency of coronary artery disease among individuals with Gd^A and Gd^{A-} (72). An initial suggestion of increased incidence of schizophrenia among Gd^{A-} individuals (38) could not be confirmed by detailed analysis of a larger group of patients (21).

The Hemolytic Crisis

The sequence of biochemical events that leads to intravascular hemolysis of the G6PD-deficient red cell under "redox stress" has been discussed in the previous section.

This biochemical tempest inside the circulating red cells becomes clinically apparent as one of the most severe and dramatic forms of hemolysis. Depending on the nature of the offending agent and the severity of the individual's enzyme deficiency, hemolysis may be severe to the point of being fatal. The difference between the extreme deficiency of the $Gd^{Mediterranean}$ and the milder deficiency of the Gd^{A-} plays an important role in the severity of the hemolytic episode. In the Gd^{A-}, hemolysis may be severe, but it is always self-limited. In the $Gd^{Mediterranean}$, hemolysis is often abrupt and very severe and, if not promptly treated with transfusion, may be fatal.

Moreover, the incidence of hemolysis with certain drugs is less in Gd^{A-} than in $Gd^{Mediterranean}$ (146). Agents reported to trigger acute hemolysis in $Gd^{Mediterranean}$ may be well tolerated by Gd^{A-}-deficient (10).

The hemolytic episode occurs from within a few hours to two to three days after the administration of the responsible agent. The length of this interval is also a function of the nature of the "redox stress" and of the type of enzyme deficiency. The episode is characterized by intravascular hemolysis: anemia with Heinz bodies (Fig. 11–6) and reticulocytosis is accompanied by hemoglobinemia and hemoglobinuria and followed by jaundice. The peripheral smear may reveal numerous "pincer cells." These probably represent cells from which oxidized hemoglobin and membrane have been removed by phagocytes in the spleen and elsewhere (Fig. 11–7). The intravascular nature of the hemolysis may not always be apparent at times of observation, since Heinz bodies, hemoglobinuria, and hemoglobinemia may have subsided. In these situations it is often possible to establish the nature of the hemolysis by demonstration of methemalbumin spectroscopically or visually (dark brown serum).

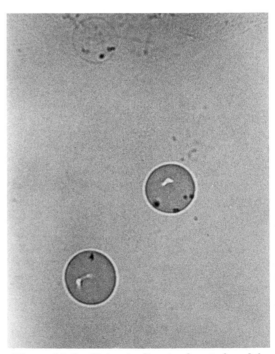

Figure 11–6. Heinz bodies in drug-induced hemolysis.

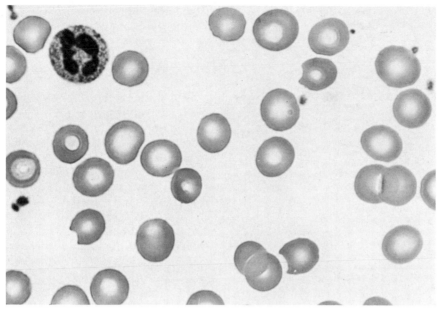

Figure 11–7. Peripheral blood of a 1-year-old Caucasian male with severe G6PD deficiency one day following aspirin treatment of a flulike illness. The infant was brought to our attention because of sudden pallor and pink diapers. Note numerous "pincer cells." Three weeks later the smear was entirely normal.

In Gd^{A-} males and females (37), as well as in heterozygous $Gd^{Mediterranean}$ females (120), hemolysis is self-limited. Even if the administration of the offending drug is continued, the patient survives the episode and anemia and reticulocytosis decrease (37). Both genetic mosaicism (in the female) and age-dependent pseudo-mosaicism (in the Gd^{A-} male) may produce refractoriness to hemolysis. In both instances, in fact, there is only selective destruction of the enzyme-deficient cells; the residual cells have normal activity and are not susceptible to hemolysis. In $Gd^{Mediterranean}$ males, on the other hand, the life span of the defective enzyme is so short that the newly formed cells become susceptible to hemolysis within a few hours of entering the circulation. Most of these patients' red cells are hemolysis prone, and, if the hemolytic agent is not removed, transfusion with normal cells is necessary to prevent death from acute anemia (57, 124).

The major clinical differences between the Gd^{A-} and the $Gd^{Mediterranean}$ variant are summarized in Table 11–2. The types of drugs and other agents capable of inducing hemolysis in G6PD-deficient individuals are listed in Table 11–3. An important corollary to the racial distribution of G6PD de-

TABLE 11–2. CLINICAL DIFFERENCES BETWEEN Gd^{A-} AND $Gd^{Mediterranean}$ MALES

	Gd^{A-}	$Gd^{Mediterranean}$
Steady State		
Activity of RBC's	5–15%	0–5%
Activity of WBC's	100%	20%
RBC's life span	100 days	100 days
Hemolytic Crisis		
Interval after exposure to hemolytic agent	24–36 hrs.	3–24 hrs.
Hemoglobinuria	Common	Constant
Jaundice	Common	Constant
Anemia	Moderate	Severe
	(rarely < 6 g. Hgb.)	(often < 6 g. Hgb.)
Duration of hemolysis	Self-limited	May be fatal

Drugs*
  Sulfonamides (diaphenylsulfone, sulfanilamide, sul-
    fapyridine, sulfisoxazole)
  Antibacterial (chloramphenicol, nalidixic acid, nitro-
    furantoin)
  Antimalarials (chloroquine, pamaquine, primaquine,
    quinacrine)
  Miscellaneous (acetylsalicylic acid, ascorbic acid,
    methylene blue)

Chemicals
  Benzene, naphthalene

Infections
  Hepatitis

Diabetic acidosis

*For a more complete list of drugs, see Beutler, E.:
Drug-induced hemolytic anemia. Pharmacol. Rev. *21*:
73, 1969.

ficiency is that the patient who is undergoing acute hemolysis should be transfused
with non–G6PD-deficient blood. This necessitates screening of the donors for G6PD
deficiency in areas where the enzyme deficiency is common (139). For instance, in
Sardinia, the chances of receiving a transfusion of G6PD-deficient blood are more
than 1 in 3 without donor screening (131).

Special Situations

Favism

This is the acute hemolysis that follows
the ingestion of fava beans (*Vicia faba*).
The syndrome seems to be restricted to the
Mediterranean countries, and it appears
exclusively in G6PD-deficient individuals
of the Gd^Mediterranean type (124).

The syndrome is more frequent, as expected, among males than females. There
is an increased incidence between the
ages of 2 and 6. Favism can occur in breast-
fed infants, whose mother has ingested
fava beans (usually without any ill effects
to her) (57). Favism may occur after eating
dry beans, but it is most common after ingestion of fresh beans. Acute hemolysis has
also been reported occasionally after inhalation of pollen from the fava plant, but
these observations are difficult to substan-

tiate. The hemolytic crisis of favism is in
all respects similar to that triggered by
drugs or other agents. The clinical severity
is often extreme (with hemoglobin dropping
below 3 g. per 100 ml.) and may be fatal
(57).

Ingestion of fava beans does not always
necessarily produce hemolysis in G6PD-
deficient individuals. Many patients have
eaten fava beans on several occasions without apparent ill effects before developing
the hemolytic crisis. These observations
suggest that, in the same individual, there
might also be a variable susceptibility to
the effect of fava beans on different days.
In a controlled study, ⁵¹Cr-labeled G6PD-
deficient cells from individuals with a
clinical history of favism were transfused
to 24 normal volunteers. Primaquine always induced disappearance of the ⁵¹Cr-
labeled red cells, but ingestion of fava
beans resulted in hemolysis only in 1 out
of 12 such experiments. These results suggest a variability in the absorption of the
hemolytic principle between individuals
(106). Besides G6PD deficiency and fava
bean ingestion, a third factor not genetically
determined is required for the hemolytic
crisis.

*G6PD Deficiency and Neonatal Jaundice
(see also Chapter 9)*

The equilibrium between hemolysis and
the ability of the liver to convert heme by-
products into bilirubin is precarious in the
newborn. Any factor that either increases
hemolysis or decreases bilirubin conjugation may easily shift the delicate balance
and result in hyperbilirubinemia. Newborn
red cells are particularly defective in the
enzymatic machinery required to maintain
hemoglobin in the reduced state; NADH-
dependent diaphorase (118), as well as
glutathione peroxidase (45), is less active
than in adult red cells. It is conceivable that
the additional deficiency of G6PD might
make the red cells of the newborn even
more prone to hemolysis and, consequently,
the infant more prone to hyperbilirubinemia.

G6PD deficiency per se does not result
in obligatory hyperbilirubinemia. Several
studies suggest that jaundice might be
more easily induced, more frequent, and

more severe in G6PD-deficient newborns. Increased incidence of neonatal hyperbilirubinemia associated with G6PD deficiency has been reported from Greece, Turkey, Sardinia, and China (73, 100, 128). These are all geographic areas where the more severe deficiency, Gd^{Mediterranean}, is observed. On the other hand, no increased hyperbilirubinemia was observed in Gd^{Mediterranean}-deficient newborns from Israel (138). No detectable increase in the incidence of neonatal hyperbilirubinemia was observed among full-term Afro-American newborns with G6PD deficiency (147), but both prematurity and perinatal hypoxia were shown to increase the incidence of neonatal jaundice (42).

In a survey of newborns from three different locations in Greece, an increased incidence of neonatal jaundice was observed in G6PD-deficient newborns, but there were striking local differences (140). In one of the locations (Lesbos), severe jaundice without blood group incompatibility or low birth weight was much more frequent among both G6PD-deficient and normal newborn males.

These findings support the view that G6PD deficiency further aggravates the predisposition of the newborn to hyperbilirubinemia. Some additional factors responsible for an increased incidence of hyperbilirubinemia in G6PD-deficient newborns may occur with different frequency in different locations. Additional causes, such as alpha thalassemia or the herbs used in traditional Chinese medicine, have been suspected but not proven. A reduction in the activity of red cell acid phosphomonoesterase was observed in Caucasian G6PD-deficient individuals (99), but not in Chinese newborns (74).

G6PD deficiency is only a predisposing factor in the pathogenesis of neonatal jaundice. Thus, once this diagnosis is established in a jaundiced newborn, the search must continue for other factors (such as hypoxia, infection, or acidosis) that could be corrected. On the other hand, in a jaundiced G6PD-deficient newborn, the exchange transfusion could be more effective than in a non–G6PD-deficient jaundiced newborn. The procedure in this case replaces the bulk of the hemolysis-prone G6PD-deficient red cells, while in other forms of unexplained neonatal jaundice, only removal of bilirubin is achieved.

A mechanism by which G6PD deficiency might result in neonatal jaundice is often overlooked. Hemolysis-inducing drugs administered to a heterozygous female during the latter part of gestation may result in little or no maternal hemolysis. Transplacental passage of these agents may, however, induce acute neonatal hemolysis (and jaundice) if the male offspring is enzyme-deficient (52).

The rare types of G6PD deficiencies associated with CNSHA frequently produce extreme hyperbilirubinemia in the newborn (114). These infants have severe hemolysis with extreme reticulocytosis and require exchange transfusion in the first hours of life.

G6PD Deficiency and Sickle Cell Anemia

Sickle cell anemia is associated with chronic hemolysis. The young red cell population in this disorder always results in increased G6PD activity of the red cells. Gd^{A-}, the type of deficient enzyme common among Africans, is more age-dependent than the enzymes with normal activity (Gd^{B+} or Gd^{A+}). In the individual with sickle cell anemia who also inherits the Gd^{A-} gene, the G6PD activity of the red cells might increase to a normal or supernormal level. In these individuals the diagnosis of G6PD deficiency may be extremely difficult. If the G6PD assay shows low or normal activity, the diagnosis of G6PD deficiency is established. If the assay shows high activity, it still remains possible that the patient is genotypically G6PD-deficient. The situation is analogous to that observed in Gd^{A-} nonsicklers during a hemolytic crisis. A correct diagnosis, at least in the male, can be established by a combination of electrophoresis and either pedigree analysis or cytochemical demonstration of individual enzyme-deficient cells (107).

The correct diagnosis of G6PD deficiency in patients with sickle cell anemia is not just a matter of academic interest. The average red cell enzyme activity may be elevated owing to a preponderance of very young cells, but still many deficient cells remain in the circulation of these individuals. Sudden reduction of bone marrow output in sickle cell anemia during infections may increase the percentage of old deficient cells susceptible to hemolysis. Thus, at the very moment that he is most liable to hemolysis, the Gd^{A-} sickle cell anemia patient is also more likely to be exposed to a hemolytic insult (through the administration of drugs or the infection itself). Hemolytic crises have in fact been described in patients with sickle cell anemia and G6PD deficiency in such situations (133).

Another aspect of the interactions between sickle cell anemia and G6PD deficiency is at the moment still controversial. The incidence of G6PD deficiency in male patients with sickle cell anemia has been found greatly increased in three studies, one in New York (107), one in Ghana (69), and one in California (155). In an earlier survey in Chicago, however, the increased incidence had not been observed (91). In this report only individuals with a clearly decreased enzyme level were classified "deficient." Thus many sicklers were misclassified as nondeficient on the basis of a normal level. The mechanism underlying the greater frequency of G6PD deficiency among males with sickle cell anemia is still unclear. Since the two genes are independently inherited and are even on different chromosomes, an increased frequency of individuals with both conditions cannot be explained by a genetic mechanism. Thus it must result from either a protective effect or sampling bias. Konotey-Ahulu has suggested that the increased frequency observed might result from the greater morbidity of patients with Gd^{A-} and sickle cell anemia. In his experience, these individuals are more frequently ill and attend clinics more often (65). However, this hypothesis implies that sickle cell anemia may be subclinical in the absence of G6PD deficiency. All available studies, including those from Ghana of Konotey-Ahulu himself (64), indicate that sickle cell anemia is a severe illness, and more than 50 per cent of the patients die before age 20 (129). In a recent study of the prevalence of G6PD deficiency in sickle cell disease (156), the incidence of Gd^{A-} was also increased (as expected) in the brothers of SS patients.

G6PD Deficiency and Thalassemia Trait

Since G6PD deficiency and thalassemia appear to exert a protective effect against malaria (71), both traits are often observed at elevated incidence in the same population (131). Gd^{Mediterranean} is the type of G6PD mutant most commonly involved. Several individuals who have simultaneously inherited both traits have been studied (108). The hematologic effects seem to be additive. The average hemoglobin in males with the combined defect was 12.5 g., compared with 15.7 g. in normal male controls, 14.1 g. in males with only Gd^{Mediterranean}, and 13.6 g. in males with only thalassemia trait. The ^{51}Cr red cell survival in individuals with both defects was identical to that in individuals with only Gd^{Mediterranean} (7). The combined defect does not aggravate the clinical expression of either conditions. Individuals with both defects, therefore, are clinically asymptomatic, as are those with only one defect.

The Rare Mutants Associated With Chronic Hemolysis (CNSHA)

In contrast to the widespread occurrence of the common types of G6PD deficiency, G6PD mutants associated with CNSHA are extremely rare. In a recent review 70 patients from almost as many families have been analyzed (114). The severity of the hemolysis in this syndrome is quite variable. Hemoglobin may be as low as 6 g. per 100 ml. and as high as (in one case) 14 g. per 100 ml. Most patients have 8 to 9 g. Reticulocytosis is always present (by definition), and this can range between 4 and 35 per cent; most patients have 10 to 15 per cent. The red cell life span has been measured in 16 patients with ^{51}Cr; the $t_{1/2}$ ranged between 2 and 17 days. Neonatal jaundice was noticed in at least 26 cases; hyperbilirubinemia was frequently observed. At variance with other congenital hemolytic anemias, the spleen is rarely enlarged and splenectomy generally ineffective. There appears to be a positive correlation between age and hemoglobin level; it has been suggested that this is the result of increased red cell production with puberty (130).

It is apparent that CNSHA associated with G6PD deficiency can be a syndrome of varying severity. A separate category should probably include some patients with G6PD deficiency with a normal or slightly elevated reticulocyte count and questionable clinical history of chronic hemolysis (5, 6). Some of these individuals were found to have a reduction in the $t_{1/2}$ of ^{51}Cr-labeled red cells disproportionate to the level of reticulocytosis (109). It is not clear whether this discrepancy results from an artifact, from the selective destruction of reticulocytes, or from some extraneous factor contributing to the increased hemolysis.

In the CNSHA-associated G6PD mutants, in contrast to the common types, the patients' mothers have normal levels of G6PD in the periphcral blood (94). This apparent exception is due to postinactivation selection. These women manufacture, as do all other heterozygotes, a double population of red cells, one normal and one deficient. However, the deficient red cells are extremely short-lived and disappear from the circulation extremely rapidly. This hypothesis is proved by the demonstration of a double population of cells, either in the reticulocytes separated from the peripheral blood (104) or in the fibroblasts in those mutants in which the G6PD deficiency is demonstrable in the fibroblasts (36) (Fig. 11–8).

TESTING FOR G6PD DEFICIENCY

Methods

Methods for measurement of G6PD activity are all based on the detection of NADPH. NADPH can be demonstrated directly either spectrophotometrically by its absorbance at 340 nm. or by its fluorescence under long-wave ultraviolet light. The spectrophotometric (or spectrofluorometric) methods are very accurate and are the basis of the biochemical assay. The techniques for measurement of G6PD activity have been standardized by a WHO appointed committee for the purpose of interlaboratory comparison (146).

Several simple screening tests have been proposed for use either in the field or in the routine hospital laboratory. One technique utilizes the direct fluorescence of NADPH (14), but most other methods utilize some hydrogen (electron) acceptor linked to NADPH [methylene blue (98, 126), nile blue, and brilliant cresyl bluc (86)], which form colorless compounds when reduced. Tetrazolium salts, such as

nitroblue tetrazolium and methyl tetrazolium (MTT), form insoluble dark blue granules in the reduced form. The latter compounds are particularly suited for the demonstration of enzyme activity in situ. They have been used for cytochemical demonstration of the enzyme (119), as well as for staining of the enzyme after electrophoresis (61). Compounds such as phenazine methosulfate or methylene blue are often used as electron carriers to facilitate the transfer of H^+ from NADPH in the reduction of methemoglobin to diagnose G6PD deficiency. The methemoglobin reduction test is based on this principle (26). A modification of this test (43), combined with a cytochemical technique for elution of methemoglobin, permits the detection of enzyme activity in individual cells. The conversion of methemoglobin to oxyhemoglobin is also at the basis of the ascorbic acid cyanide test (54). This test is nonspecific, which in fact enhances its value as a screening test for all of the conditions in which glutathione stability is compromised. In experienced hands it is also useful in the diagnosis of female heterozygotes, since a small proportion of G6PD-deficient red cells can be detected by this technique.

Several methods are therefore available for the laboratory diagnosis of G6PD (75). The proliferation of methodology for screening testifies that none of the techniques available is simple enough to be readily adaptable to mass screening, although most techniques are both rapid and accurate.

Two tcchniques which had been used in the past for the diagnosis of G6PD still retain an interest. These techniques are the glutathione stability test and the Heinz body formation test (8). In both tests the red cells are incubated with acetylphenylhydrazine in controlled conditions in the presence of glucose. Normal cells maintain their level of reduced glutathione and form only very few Heinz bodies. Enzyme-deficient cells drop their reduced glutathione level to very low values and form much more numerous Heinz bodies. Both tests have now been superseded, but they provide a model of the sequence of events that takes place in the deficient red cell exposed to "redox stress."

Besides measurements of quantitative variations of the enzyme, several methods are directed to the study of qualitative aspects and are employed to characterize

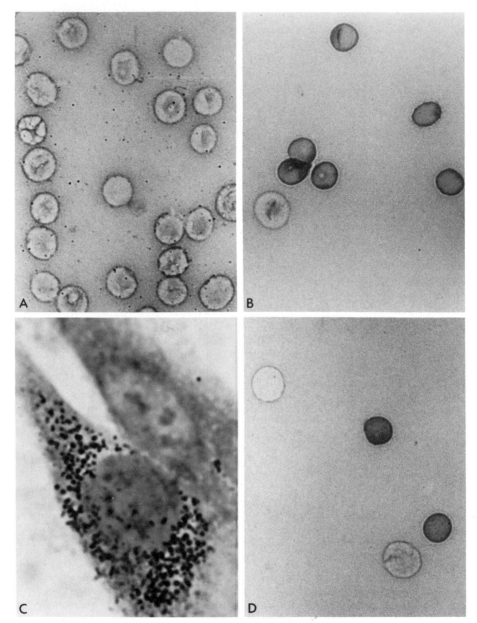

Figure 11–8. Gd^New York (114) associated with CNSHA: demonstration of mosaicism in the patient's mother. *A*, Blood smear from patient: total absence of activity; *B*, mother's blood smear: only occasional (0.4 per cent) unstained cell; *C*, mother's fibroblasts showing mosaicism; *D*, mother's isolated reticulocytes: 46 per cent unstained cells. Blood smears stained according to Gall (43); fibroblasts stained by a modification of the technique of Rozenszajn (119) (dark granules indicate enzyme activity).

mutant enzymes. Electrophoretic mobility can be studied on various media, including starch (61), agar (49), cellulose acetate gel (113), and cellulose acetate itself (134). On this basis, the enzymes can be classified as slow, normal, and fast. Thermal stability and pH optima can be studied by classic biochemical techniques (146). The enzymes can also be distinguished by their capability for utilizing substrate analogs, such as galactose-6-P, and by their affinity (Km) for deoxyglucose-6-P and acetyl–NADP (137).

The Detection of the Heterozygote

Since G6PD is an X-linked gene, some female heterozygote deficients may appear either normal or deficient on assay or screening. This is not a failure of the technique, but rather is the result of random X-inactivation. It must be emphasized that in the vast majority of cases the heterozygous females have clearly intermediate values. However, in females it is not possible to exclude heterozygosity just because the assay is either normal or markedly deficient. The correct recognition of all heterozygotes is necessary in population genetics. An exact diagnosis may also be necessary clinically.

The methemoglobin elution test, as modified by Gall and Brewer, allows the analysis of individual cells for enzyme activity (43). In normal individuals less than 5 per cent of the cells appear unstained. A percentage of unstained cells higher than 5 per cent permits establishment of the diagnosis of heterozygosity. Thus, with this technique, only those hypothetical heterozygous females in whom the X chromosome carrying the gene for G6PD deficiency has been inactivated in more than 95 per cent of the cells would be missed. On the other hand, the methemoglobin slide elution test cannot clearly distinguish heterozygous and homozygous deficient females since, as in hemizygous males, a certain amount of age-dependent pseudomosaicism is present in homozygous females. From these considerations it appears clear that heterozygosity can be diagnosed if either an intermediate value in the assay, the results of the methemoglobin elution test, or family studies provide direct evidence. If none of these is conclusive, it is impossible to ascertain with absolute certainty the correct genotype, since heterozygosity cannot be ruled out definitively.

The difficulties inherent in the detection of female heterozygotes for G6PD deficiency are illustrated by the results of a study of the red cells of family members of the Caucasian male infant whose blood smear is illustrated in Figure 11–7. G6PD activity was barely detectable in the red cells of the propositus and his mother. The propositus' father was normal. The mother had two female siblings and one male sibling. All of them and the maternal grandfather exhibited severe red cell G6PD deficiency. The maternal grandmother, however, had normal red cell G6PD activity. Suspecting that the affected X chromosome in the maternal grandmother was largely inactivated, a test for mosaicism was performed on her red cells. This revealed that the percentage of G6PD-deficient red cells in her blood was twice as high as that observed in normal female controls. Thus we concluded that the affected X chromosome had indeed been largely inactivated in the precursors of the maternal grandmother's red cell population. The abnormal gene had been inherited by all of her children, the females having also inherited the abnormal gene of their father. The parental source of the abnormal gene in the propositus was not determined by analysis of other potential X markers.

The complexity of X-inactivation is illustrated by the fact that females heterozygous for CNSHA-associated mutants do not have a double population in the red cells (94). Similarly, females heterozygous for HGPRT deficiency only have normal cells in their peripheral blood (95). The presence on one X chromosome of the abnormal HGPRT gene apparently results in selection against the cell population in which that chromosome remains active. If a gene for a G6PD mutant is present on the same X chromosome, it will not be expressed in the peripheral blood. This phenomenon has been clearly demonstrated by Nyhan et al. in two families in which Gd^{A-} and HGPRT deficiency coexisted (95).

The Value of Screening

Progress in our knowledge of genetic disorders becomes particularly useful when new information is applied either in preventive medicine or in genetic counseling.

Genetic counseling in the case of G6PD deficiency would be indicated only for those mutants associated with CNSHA. It would be practically impossible to screen women for this trait, since it is not expressed in the peripheral blood (94). The diagnosis may be established on fibroblasts, with a demonstration of a double population. [This may require, in certain mutants with a higher level of activity, the analysis of the cell culture after heat inactivation (36).] The double population can also be demonstrated in isolated reticulocytes (Fig. 11–8). Although these techniques could be applied to prenatal diagnosis in families in which the disease has already occurred, CNSHA is usually not severe enough to warrant interruption of pregnancy when an affected fetus is detected.

The screening of large numbers of individuals in susceptible populations, on the other hand, is obviously of great value in preventive medicine. Individuals deficient in G6PD are indeed susceptible to a variety of hemolytic agents. Knowledge of their susceptibility is important for the prevention of hemolytic episodes. Individuals found deficient by screening should be given a clear explanation of the risk of being exposed to certain drugs and agents; their physician should be notified.

Screening for G6PD deficiency requires a great amount of education not only of the public at large but also of the medical profession. In the author's experience, many physicians are not aware of the exact implications of G6PD deficiency and tend to ignore it or overestimate its importance when detected. Both of these attitudes could be corrected by more precise knowledge of the problem.

Editor's Note: The value of widespread screening for G6PD deficiency is not accepted by all experts in the field. It has been cogently argued that screening should be restricted to newborns, hospitalized patients, pregnant women, and donors to blood banks supplying blood to small children. Screening of entire Black populations may not be useful, since the drugs to which Gd^{A-} cells may be sensitive [i.e., sulfa compounds, dapsone, nitrofurantoin, and antimalarials] are not available without prescription and usually cause mild hemolysis (33a). The over-the-counter mild oxidants, such as aspirin and phenacetin derivatives, are virtually harmless in the Black population. Sporadic reports of hemolysis due to acetanilide are available (43a).

It is true that Caucasians with severe G6PD deficiency may develop hemolytic reactions due to mild oxidants such as aspirin (Fig. 11–7), but widespread screening of all individuals with Mediterranean ancestry would be financially prohibitive. The funds would be better spent in the education of physicians, many of whom are still unaware of the complexity of the problem.

TREATMENT OF G6PD DEFICIENCY

No form of treatment is available. Indeed, except in the case of a mutant associated with CNSHA, none is required in the steady state. Treatment of the hemolytic episode is supportive. The hemolytic episode is often self-limited. It will always subside upon removal of the causative agent and sometimes, in Gd^{A-} males, even when this persists. Transfusions are often required in the severe hemolytic crisis of $Gd^{Mediterranean}$, but they are rarely required by Gd^{A-} individuals.

The causative agent of the hemolysis should be removed whenever possible. In pediatrics, it is important to keep in mind that the responsible agent may also be acquired by transplacental passage or breastfeeding or both. The investigation of the possible cause should always be extended to the mother.

An intriguing new avenue of treatment could be offered by the recent report that human red cells can produce NADPH through the xylulose pathway independently from G6PD (144). This possibility appears particularly important to individuals with CNSHA-associated mutants. However, the activity of the xylulose pathway is only one thousandth that of the pentose pathway, and the Km for xylulose is extremely high (0.1 M) (143). The practical value of this observation thus appears very limited. Moreover, severe side reactions have been reported in individuals receiving xylulose infusions, although it appears possible that these were not secondary to xylulose itself but to impurities in the preparation.

OTHER DEFECTS OF THE PENTOSE PATHWAY

6PGD Deficiency

6PGD is the enzyme that catalyzes the conversion of 6-phosphogluconate to ribulose-5-phosphate, with production of both NADPH and CO_2 (Fig. 11–2). Numerous electrophoretic variants of 6PGD are known, but they are not associated with either biochemical defects or clinical significance.

Lack of this enzyme does not completely curtail NADPH production, since G6PD activity persists. Both partial and total enzyme deficiencies have been reported (11, 68, 102).

The clinical expression is quite variable, ranging from absence of hemolysis in one case to severe anemia in another. The deficiency is extremely rare, and only a handful of cases has been described.

Abnormalities of Glutathione Metabolism

Glutathione plays a key role in the maintenance of intracellular constituents in the reduced state. The conversion of reduced glutathione to disulfide via glutathione peroxidase and its subsequent reduction by glutathione reductase provides an efficient system for removal of peroxides from the red cells (53). The red cell synthesizes glutathione de novo (83); the half-life of glutathione in the red cells is only four days (41).

Defects in reduced glutathione may be secondary either to defects of glutathione synthesis or to lack of the enzymes connected with glutathione metabolism.

Glutathione Deficiency

Five families have been described with total or near-total absence of glutathione in the red cells (17, 66, 84, 97).

Glutathione can be synthesized directly in the red cells in two consecutive steps (Figure 11-9).

In the first step glutamic acid and cysteine form glutamyl cysteine; in the second, glycine is attached to form glutathione.

Of the five families described, four have been shown to have a defect in the second step; only recently Konrad et al. have described a family with a defect in the enzyme that catalyzes the initial step: glutamyl cysteine synthetase (66). Glutathione deficiency of both types is transmitted as an autosomal recessive.

The clinical syndrome associated with a defect in glutathione is one of mild chronic hemolysis. Hemoglobin is only slightly reduced, but the reticulocyte count is constantly increased.

Glutathione Peroxidase Deficiency

An autosomal recessive gene is also responsible for the transmission of the defect in glutathione peroxidase. The homozygous state is associated with chronic hemolysis and is probably extremely rare; only three cases have been described to date (18, 93). Partial deficiency, however, could be more common. The enzyme level is also generally reduced in the newborn, but the decrease is not related to the susceptibility to oxidative damage observed in newborn cells (43b). Four newborn infants have been described with a further

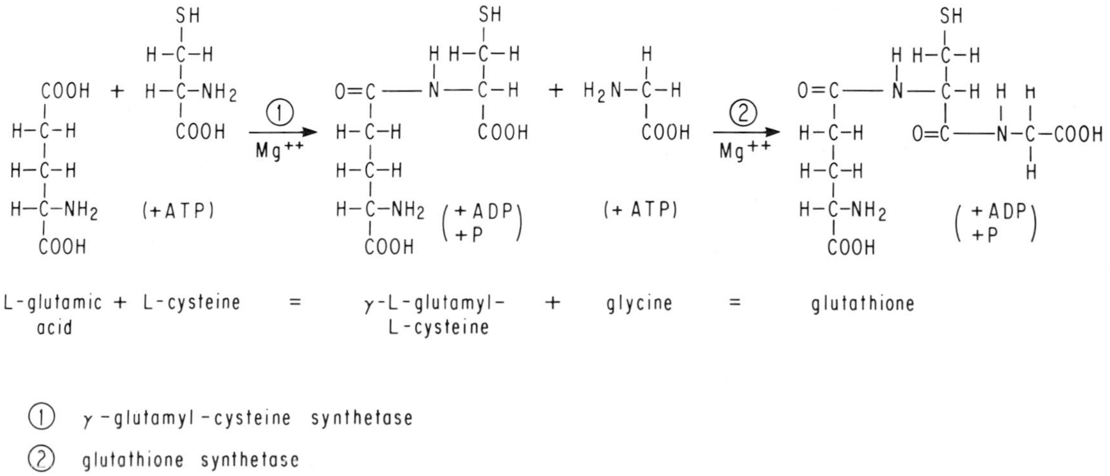

① γ-glutamyl-cysteine synthetase

② glutathione synthetase

Figure 11-9. Biosynthesis of glutathione.

reduced enzyme level (92). In these, the enzyme level was still decreased at 3 months of age, when normal infants have a higher value approaching the adult range. Since moderate hyperbilirubinemia was observed in these infants, it is possible that heterozygous deficiency for glutathione peroxidase may be related to perinatal jaundice. The partial deficiency is probably clinically silent in later life.

Glutathione Reductase Deficiency

A partial defect seems to be a relatively common disorder. This is, however, not associated with any hematologic manifestation. The defect has been demonstrated in disorders as diverse as hemoglobin C disease, thrombocytopenia, and chronic disease (142). These peculiar frequencies cast serious doubts on the genetic nature of this defect.

Further doubts have been raised by the demonstration that flavine adenine dinucleotide (FAD) stimulates the enzyme in vitro (44), and administration of riboflavin can correct the defect in vivo (136). These observations suggest that many described instances of glutathione reductase deficiency could be in reality cases of suboptimal riboflavin intake or storage. In a few cases a truly genetically determined defect persists, even after riboflavin treatment. The data presently available, however, suggest that reductions in glutathione reductase, at least in the moderate degree reported, do not result in hematologic side effects. Probably, glutathione reductase is not a limiting step in the chain of reactions necessary for the maintenance of glutathione in the reduced state. Electrophoretic variants of the enzyme without impaired activity have also been described.

Deficiency in NADPH Diaphorase

A single individual has been described with this deficiency. This was a chance finding, since the defect was detected because of an abnormal methylene blue screening test for G6PD. No clinical or hematologic manifestations were evident (127).

ACKNOWLEDGMENTS

The author is indebted to Drs. M. Rattazzi, L. Corash, and M. Siniscalco for helpful revisions of the manuscript and to Mrs. Leonora LaForte for careful and patient secretarial assistance.

The author is a Career Investigator of the Health Research Council of the City of New York (under contract I-383).

The studies of the author referred to in this manuscript have been sponsored by Grant No. AM 09274-08 from the National Institutes of Health.

References

1. Afolayan, A., and Luzzatto, L.: Genetic variants of human erythrocyte glucose-6-phosphate dehydrogenase. I. Regulation of activity by oxidized and reduced nicotinamide-adenine dinucleotide phosphate. Biochemistry 10: 415, 1971.

2. Allen, D. W., and Jandl, J. H.: Oxidative hemolysis and precipitation of hemoglobin. II. Role of thiols in oxidant drug action. J. Clin. Invest. 40:454, 1961.

3. Allison, A. C.: Glucose-6-phosphate dehydrogenase in red blood cells of East Africans. Nature (Lond.) 186:531, 1960.

4. Babalola, O., Cancedda, R., et al.: Genetic variants of glucose-6-phosphate dehydrogenase from human erythrocytes: Unique properties of the A⁻ variant isolated from "deficient" cells. Proc. Natl. Acad. Sci. USA 69:946, 1972.

5. Benbassat, J., and Ben-Ishay, D.: Hereditary hemolytic anemia associated with glucose-6-phosphate dehydrogenase deficiency (Mediterranean type). Is. J. Med. Sci. 5:1053, 1969.

6. Ben-Ishay, D., and Izak, G.: Chronic hemolysis associated with glucose-6-phosphate dehydrogenase deficiency. J. Lab. Clin. Med. 63:1002, 1964.

7. Bernini, L., Latte, B., et al.: Survival of ^{51}Cr-labelled red cells in subjects with thalassemia-trait or G6PD deficiency or both abnormalities. Br. J. Haematol. 10:171, 1964.

8. Beutler, E.: The hemolytic effect of primaquine and related compounds: A review. Blood 14: 103, 1959.

9. Beutler, E.: Glucose-6-phosphate-dehydrogenase deficiency: Diagnosis, clinical and genetic implications. Am. J. Clin. Pathol. 47:303, 1967.

10. Beutler, E.: Drug-induced hemolytic anemia. Pharmacol. Rev. 21:73, 1969.

11. Beutler, E.: Abnormalities of the hexose monophosphate shunt. Semin. Hematol. 8:311, 1971.

12. Beutler, E., and Collins, Z.: Pseudo-mosaicism in males with mild glucose-6-phosphate dehydrogenase deficiency. Lancet 1:552, 1965.

13. Beutler, E., and Collins, Z.: Hybridization of

glucose-6-phosphate dehydrogenase from rat and human erythrocytes. Science *150*: 1306, 1965.

14. Beutler, E., and Mitchell, M.: Special modifications of the fluorescent screening method for glucose-6-phosphate dehydrogenase deficiency. Blood *32*:816, 1968.

15. Beutler, E., Yeh, M., et al.: The normal human female as a mosaic of X-chromosome activity: Studies using the gene for G6PD deficiency as a marker. Proc. Natl. Acad. Sci. USA *48*: 9, 1962.

16. Bienzle, U., Ayeni, O., et al.: Glucose-6-phosphate dehydrogenase and malaria. Greater resistance of females heterozygous for enzyme deficiency and of males with nondeficient variant. Lancet *1*:107, 1972.

17. Boivin, P., Galand, C., et al.: Anémies hémolytiques congénitales avec déficit isolé en glutathion réduit par déficit en glutathion synthétase. Nouv. Rev. Fr. Hematol. 6:859, 1966.

18. Boivin, P., Galand, C., et al.: Déficit en glutathion-peroxydase érythrocytaire et anémie hémolytique médicamenteuse. Presse Méd. 78:171, 1970.

19. Bonsignore, A., Lorenzoni, I., et al.: Distinctive patterns of NADP binding to dimeric and tetrameric glucose-6-phosphate dehydrogenase from human red cells. Biochem. Biophys. Res. Commun. 39:142, 1970.

20. Bonsignore, A., Lorenzoni, I., et al.: Purification of glucose-6-phosphate dehydrogenase from human erythrocytes. Ital. J. Biochem. *19*: 165, 1970.

21. Bowman, J. E., Brewer, G. J., et al.: A re-evaluation of the relationship between glucose-6-phosphate dehydrogenase deficiency and the behavioral manifestations of schizophrenia. J. Lab. Clin. Med. 65:222, 1965.

22. Boyer, S. H., Porter, I. H., et al.: Electrophoretic heterogeneity of glucose-6-phosphate dehydrogenase and its relationship to enzyme deficiency in man. Proc. Natl. Acad. Sci. USA 48:1868, 1962.

23. Brand, K., Arese, P., et al.: Bedeutung und regulation des pentosephosphatweges in menschlichen erythrozyten, I. Hoppe Seyler Z. Physiol. Chem. *351*:501, 1970.

24. Brand, K., Arese, P., et al.: Bedeutung und regulation des pentosephosphatweges in menschlichen erythrozyten, II. Hoppe Seyler Z. Physiol. Chem. *351*:509, 1970.

25. Brewer, G. J., Powell, R. D., et al.: Hemolytic effect of primaquine. XVII. Hexokinase activity of glucose-6-phosphate dehydrogenase deficient and normal erythrocytes. J. Lab. Clin. Med. *64*:601, 1964.

26. Brewer, G. J., Tarlov, A. R., et al.: The methemoglobin reduction test for primaquine-type sensitivity of erythrocytes: A simplified procedure for detecting a specific hypersusceptibility to drug hemolysis. J.A.M.A. *180*: 386, 1962.

27. Brewer, G. J., Tarlov, A. R., et al.: The hemolytic effect of primaquine. XII. Shortened erythrocyte life span in primaquine-sensitive male Negroes in the absence of drug administration. J. Lab. Clin. Med. 58:217, 1961.

28. Bunn, H. F.: Erythrocyte destruction and hemoglobin catabolism. Semin. Hematol. 9:3, 1972.

29. Carson, P. E., Flanagan, C. L., et al.: Enzymatic deficiency in primaquine-sensitive erythrocytes. Science *124*:484, 1956.

30. Chan, T. K., Todd, D., et al.: Tissue enzyme levels in erythrocyte glucose-6-phosphate dehydrogenase deficiency. J. Lab. Clin. Med. 66:937, 1965.

31. Childs, B., Zinkham, W., et al.: A genetic study of a defect in glutathione metabolism of the erythrocyte. Bull. Johns Hopkins Hosp. *102*: 21, 1958.

32. Cohen, G., and Hocstein, P.: Glutathione peroxidase: The primary agent for the elimination of hydrogen peroxide in erythrocytes. Biochemistry 2:1420, 1963.

33. Cohen, P., and Rosenmeyer, M. A.: Human glucose-6-phosphate dehydrogenase: Purification of the erythrocyte enzyme and the influence of ions on its activity. Eur. J. Biochem. 8:1, 1969.

33a. Conrad, M. E.: Military ethics and G-6-PD deficiency. New Engl. J. Med. *286*:1418, 1972.

34. Dancis, J., Yip, L. C., et al.: Disparate enzyme activity in erythrocytes and leucocytes: A variant of hypoxanthine phosphoribosyl transferase deficiency with an unstable enzyme. J. Clin. Invest. *52*:2068, 1973.

35. Davidson, R. G., Nitowsky, H. M., et al.: Demonstration of two populations of cells in the human female heterozygous for glucose-6-phosphate dehydrogenase variants. Proc. Natl. Acad. Sci. USA *50*:481, 1963.

36. Demars, R.: A temperature-sensitive glucose-6-phosphate dehydrogenase in mutant cultured human cells. Proc. Natl. Acad. Sci. USA *61*: 562, 1968.

37. Dern, R. J., Beutler, E., et al.: The hemolytic effect of primaquine. II. The natural course of the hemolytic anemia and the mechanism of its self-limited character. J. Lab. Clin. Med. *44*:171, 1954.

38. Dern, R. J., Glynn, M. F., et al.: Studies on the correlation of the genetically determined trait, glucose-6-phosphate dehydrogenase deficiency, with behavioral manifestations in schizophrenia. J. Lab. Clin. Med. 62:319, 1963.

39. Dern, R. J., Weinstein, I. M., et al.: The hemolytic effect of primaquine. I. The localization of the drug-induced hemolytic defect in primaquine sensitive individuals. J. Lab. Clin. Med. 43:303, 1954.

40. Deys, B. F., Grzeschik, K. M., et al.: Human phosphoglycerate kinase and inactivation of the X-chromosome. Science *175*:1002, 1972.

41. Dimant, E., Landsberg, E., et al.: The metabolic behavior of reduced glutathione in human and avian erythrocytes. J. Biol. Chem. *213*: 769, 1955.

42. Eshaghpour, E., Oski, F. A., et al.: The relationship of erythrocyte glucose-6-phosphate dehydrogenase deficiency to hyperbilirubinemia in Negro premature infants. J. Pediatr. 70:595, 1967.

43. Gall, J. C., Jr., Brewer, G. J., et al.: Studies of glucose-6-phosphate dehydrogenase activity

of individual erythrocytes: The methemo-globin-elution test for identification of females heterozygous for G-6-PD deficiency. Am. J. Hum. Genet. 17:359, 1965.

43a. Gilles, H. M., and Ikeme, A. C.: Haemoglobin-nuria among adult Nigerians due to glucose-6-phosphate dehydrogenase deficiency with drug sensitivity. Lancet 1:889, 1960.

43b. Glader, B. E., and Conrad, M. E.: Decreased glutathione peroxidase in neonatal erythrocytes: Lack of relation to hydrogen peroxide metabolism. Pediatr. Res. 6:900, 1972.

44. Glatzle, D., Weber, F., et al.: Enzymatic test for the detection of a riboflavin deficiency. NADPH-dependent glutathione reductase of red blood cells and its activation by FAD in vitro. Experientia 24:1122, 1968.

45. Gross, R. T., Bracci, R., et al.: Hydrogen peroxide toxicity and detoxification in erythrocytes of newborn infants. Blood 29:481, 1967.

46. Gross, R. T., Hurwitz, R. E., et al.: An hereditary enzymatic defect in erythrocyte metabolism: Glucose-6-phosphate dehydrogenase deficiency. J. Clin. Invest. 37:1176, 1958.

47. Grumbach, M. N., Marks, P. A., et al.: Erythrocyte glucose-6-phosphate dehydrogenase activity and X-chromosome polysomy. Lancet 1:1330, 1962.

48. Grzeschik, K. M., Allerdice, P. W., et al.: Cytological mapping of human X-linked genes by use of somatic cell hybrids involving an X-autosome translocation. Proc. Natl. Acad. Sci. USA 69:69, 1972.

49. Haywood, B. J., Storkweather, W. H., et al.: Electrophoretic separation of glucose-6-phosphate dehydrogenase from human erythrocytes with agar gels. J. Lab. Clin. Med. 324:327, 1963.

50. Herz, F., Kaplan, E., et al.: Diagnosis of erythrocyte glucose-6-phosphate dehydrogenase deficiency in the Negro male despite hemolytic crisis. Blood 35:90, 1970.

51. Horecker, B. L.: Glucose-6-phosphate dehydrogenase: The pentose phosphate cycle and its place in carbohydrate metabolism. Am. J. Clin. Pathol. 47:271, 1967.

52. Ifekwunigwe, A. E., and Luzzatto, L.: Kernicterus in G.-6-P.D.-deficiency. Lancet 1:667, 1966.

53. Jacob, H. S., and Jandl, J. M.: Effects of sulfhydryl inhibition on red blood cells. I. Mechanism of hemolysis. J. Clin. Invest. 41:779, 1962.

54. Jacob, H. S., and Jandl, J. H.: A simple visual screening test for G-6-PD deficiency employing ascorbate and cyanide. New Engl. J. Med. 274:1162, 1966.

55. Jaffé, E. R.: Hereditary hemolytic disorders and enzymatic deficiencies of human erythrocytes. Blood 35:116, 1970.

56. Jaffé, E. R.: Oxidative hemolysis, or "what made the red cell break?" New Engl. J. Med. 286:156, 1972.

57. Kattamis, C. S., Kariazakous, M., et al.: Favism: Clinical and biochemical data. J. Med. Genet. 6:34, 1969.

58. Kirkman, H. N.: Glucose-6-phosphate dehydrogenase from human erythrocytes. I. Further purification and characterization. J. Biol. Chem. 237:2364, 1962.

59. Kirkman, H. N.: Glucose-6-phosphate variants and drug-induced hemolysis. Ann. N.Y. Acad. Sci. 151:753, 1968.

60. Kirkman, H. N.: Glucose-6-phosphate dehydrogenase. Adv. Hum. Genet. 2:1, 1971.

61. Kirkman, H. N., and Hendrickson, E. M.: Sex-linked electrophoretic difference in glucose-6-phosphate dehydrogenase. Am. J. Hum. Genet. 15:241, 1963.

62. Kirkman, H. N., Riley, H. D., et al.: Different enzymic expressions of mutants of human glucose-6-phosphate dehydrogenase. Proc. Natl. Acad. Sci. USA 46:938, 1960.

63. Kissin, C., Dorche, C., et al.: Le glucose 6-phosphate deshydrogenase type debrousse: Problème d'un type enzymatique propre aux algerien de race arabe. Bull. Soc. Chim. Biol. (Paris) 52:1233, 1972.

64. Konotey-Ahulu, F. I. D.: Computer assisted analysis of data on 1,697 patients attending the sickle-cell haemoglobinopathy clinic of Korle Bu Teaching Hospital, Accra, Ghana. Clinical Features: I. Sex, genotype, age, rheumatism and dactylitis frequencies. Ghana Med. J. 10:241, 1971.

65. Konotey-Ahulu, F. I. D.: Glucose-6-phosphate dehydrogenase deficiency and sickle cell anemia. New Engl. J. Med. 287:887, 1972.

66. Konrad, P. N., Richards, F. R., II, et al.: γ-Glutamyl-cysteine-synthetase deficiency. A cause of hereditary hemolytic anemia. New Engl. J. Med. 286:557, 1972.

67. Kosower, N. S., and Kosower, E. M.: Molecular basis for selective advantage of glucose-6-phosphate dehydrogenase deficient subjects. Lancet 2:23, 1970.

68. Lausecker, C., Heidt, P., et al.: Anémie hémolytique constitutionnelle avec déficit en 6-phospho-gluconate-dehydrogenase. Arch. Fr. Pediatr. 22:789, 1965.

69. Lewis, R. A., and Hathorn, M.: Glucose-6-phosphate dehydrogenase deficiency correlated with S hemoglobin. Ghana Med. J. 2:131, 1969.

70. Linder, D., and Gartler, S. M.: Glucose-6-phosphate dehydrogenase mosaicism: Utilization as a cell marker in the study of leiomyomas. Science 150:67, 1965.

71. Livingstone, F. B.: Malaria and human polymorphism. Ann. Rev. Genet. 5:33, 1971.

72. Long, W. K., Wilson, S. W., et al.: Associations between red cell glucose-6-phosphate dehydrogenase variants and vascular diseases. Am. J. Hum. Genet. 19:35, 1967.

73. Lu, T. C., Wei, H., et al.: Increased incidence of severe hyperbilirubinemia among newborn Chinese infants with G6PD deficiency. Pediatrics 37:994, 1966.

74. Lu, T. C., Wei, H., et al.: Erythrocyte acid phosphomonoesterase activity in newly born Chinese deficient in glucose-6-phosphate dehydrogenase. Nature (Lond.) 213:707, 1967.

75. Lubin, B. M., and Oski, F. A.: An evaluation of screening procedures for red cell glucose-6-phosphate dehydrogenase deficiency in the newborn infant. J. Pediatr. 70:788, 1967.

76. Luzzatto, L.: Regulation of the activity of glucose-6-phosphate dehydrogenase by NADP+

and NADPH. Biochim. Biophys. Acta *146*: 18, 1967.

77. Luzzatto, L., Usanga, E. A., et al.: Glucose-6-phosphate dehydrogenase deficient red cells: Resistance to infection by malarial parasites. Science *164*:839, 1969.

78. Lyon, M. F.: Gene action in the X-chromosome of the mouse (*Mus musculus* L.). Nature (Lond.) *190*:372, 1961.

79. Marks, P. A.: Glucose-6-phosphate dehydrogenase in mature erythrocytes. Am. J. Clin. Path. *47*:287, 1967.

80. Marks, P. A., and Gross, R. T.: Erythrocyte glucose-6-phosphate dehydrogenase deficiency: Evidence of differences between Negroes and Caucasians with respect to this genetically determined trait. J. Clin. Invest. *38*: 2253, 1959.

81. Marks, P. A., and Johnson, A. B.: Relationship between the age of human erythrocytes and their osmotic resistance: A basis for separating young and old erythrocytes. J. Clin. Invest. *37*:1542, 1958.

82. Marks, P. A., Szeinberg, A., et al.: Erythrocyte glucose-6-phosphate dehydrogenase of normal and mutant human subjects. Properties of the purified enzymes. J. Biol. Chem. *236*: 10, 1961.

83. Minnich, V., Smith, M. B., et al.: Glutathione biosynthesis in human erythrocyte. I. Identification of the enzyme of glutathione synthesis in hemolysates. J. Clin. Invest. *50*:507, 1971.

84. Mohler, D. N., Majerus, P. W., et al.: Glutathione synthetase deficiency as a cause of hereditary hemolytic disease. New Engl. J. Med. *283*: 1253, 1970.

85. Motulsky, A. G.: Metabolic polymorphisms and the role of infectious diseases in human evolution. Hum. Biol. *32*:28, 1960.

86. Motulsky, A. G., and Campbell-Kraut, J. M.: Population genetics of glucose-6-phosphate dehydrogenase deficiency of the red cell, In *Proceedings of Conference on Genetic Polymorphisms and Geographic Variations in Disease*. Blumberg, B. S. (ed.), New York, Grune & Stratton, 1961, p. 159.

87. Motulsky, A. G., and Stamatoyannopoulos, G.: Clinical implications of glucose-6-phosphate dehydrogenase deficiency. Ann. Intern. Med. *70*:222, 1969.

88. Murphy, J. R.: Erythrocyte metabolism. II. Glucose metabolism and pathways. J. Lab. Clin. Med. *55*:28, 1960.

89. McCurdy, P. R., Kirkman, H. N., et al.: A Chinese variant of glucose-6-phosphate dehydrogenase. J. Lab. Clin. Med. *67*:374, 1966.

90. McKusick, V. A.: The mapping of human chromosomes. Sci. Am. *224*:104, 1971.

91. Naylor, J., Rosenthal, I., et al.: Activity of glucose-6-phosphate dehydrogenase in erythrocytes of patients with various abnormal hemoglobins. Pediatrics *26*:285, 1960.

92. Necheles, T. F., Boles, T. A., et al.: Erythrocyte glutathione-peroxidase deficiency and hemolytic disease of the newborn infant. J. Pediatr. *72*:319, 1968.

93. Necheles, T. F., Maldonado, N., et al.: Homozygous, erythrocyte glutathione-peroxidase deficiency: Clinical and biochemical studies. Blood *33*:164, 1969.

94. Newton, W. A., and Frajola, W. J.: Drug-sensitive chronic hemolytic anemia: Family studies. Clin. Res. *6*:392, 1958.

95. Nyhan, W. L., Bakay, B., et al.: Hemizygous expression of glucose-6-phosphate dehydrogenase in erythrocytes of heterozygotes for the Lesch-Nyhan syndrome. Proc. Natl. Acad. Sci. USA *65*:214, 1970.

96. Omachi, A., Scott, C. B., et al.: Pyridine nucleotides in human erythrocytes in different metabolic states. Biochim. Biophys. Acta *184*:139, 1969.

97. Oort, M., Loos, J. A., et al.: Hereditary absence of reduced glutathione in the erythrocytes—a new clinical and biochemical entity? Vox Sang. *6*:370, 1961.

98. Oski, F. A., and Growney, M. P.: A simple micromethod for the detection of erythrocyte glucose-6-phosphate dehydrogenase deficiency. J. Pediatr. *66*:90, 1965.

99. Oski, F. A., Shahidi, N. T., et al.: Erythrocyte acid phosphomonoesterase and glucose-6-phosphate dehydrogenase deficiency in Caucasians. Science *139*:409, 1963.

100. Panizon, F.: Erythrocyte enzyme deficiency in unexplained kernicterus. Lancet *2*:1093, 1960.

101. Papayannopoulou, T., and Stamatoyannopoulos, G.: Pseudo-mosaicism in males with mild glucose-6-phosphate dehydrogenase deficiency. Lancet *2*:1215, 1964.

102. Parr, C. W., and Fitch, L. I.: Hereditary partial deficiency of human erythrocyte phosphogluconate dehydrogenase. Biochem. J. *93*: 28c, 1964.

103. Petrakis, N. L., Wiesenfeld, S. L., et al.: Prevalence of sickle cell trait and glucose-6-phosphate dehydrogenase deficiency. New Engl. J. Med. *282*:767, 1970.

104. Piomelli, S., Amorosi, E. L., et al.: In vivo life span of different variants of G6PD in the RBCs. Proceedings 12th Meeting *Int. Soc. Hematol.*, 110, 1968.

105. Piomelli, S., Corash, L. M., et al.: In vivo lability of glucose-6-phosphate dehydrogenase in Gd^{A-} and Gd^{Mediterranean} deficiency. J. Clin. Invest. *47*:940, 1968.

106. Piomelli, S., Puca, F., et al.: Possibili variazioni individuali nell'assorbimento del principio attivo delle fave in rapporto al favismo clinico. Atti Assoc. Genet. Ital. *8*:99, 1963.

107. Piomelli, S., Reindorf, C. A., et al.: Clinical and biochemical interactions of glucose-6-phosphate dehydrogenase deficiency and sickle cell anemia. New Engl. J. Med. *287*:213, 1972.

108. Piomelli, S., and Siniscalco, M.: The haematological effects of glucose-6-phosphate dehydrogenase deficiency and thalassemia trait: Interaction between the two genes at the phenotype level. Br. J. Haematol. *16*:537, 1969.

109. Ramot, B., Ben-Bassat, I., et al.: New glucose-6-phosphate dehydrogenase variants observed in Israel and their association with congenital nonspherocytic hemolytic disease. J. Lab. Clin. Med. *74*:895, 1969.

110. Ratnoff, O. D., and Bennett, B.: The genetics of hereditary disorders of blood coagulation. Science 179:1291, 1973.

111. Rattazzi, M. C.: Glucose-6-phosphate dehydrogenase from human erythrocytes: Molecular weight determination by gel filtration. Biochem. Biophys. Res. Commun. 31:16, 1968.

112. Rattazzi, M. C.: Isolation and purification of human erythrocyte glucose-6-phosphate dehydrogenase from small amounts of blood. Biochim. Biophys. Acta 181:1, 1969.

113. Rattazzi, M. C., Bernini, L. F., et al.: Electrophoresis of glucose-6-phosphate dehydrogenase: A new technique. Nature (Lond.) 213:79, 1967.

114. Rattazzi, M. C., Corash, L. M., et al.: G6PD deficiency and chronic hemolysis: Four new mutants. Relationship between clinical syndrome and enzyme kinetics. Blood 38:205, 1971.

115. Renwick, J. H.: The mapping of human chromosomes. Ann. Rev. Genet. 5:81, 1971.

116. Rosa, R., and Dreyfus, J. C.: Hybridation de la glucose-6-phosphate deshydrogenase des globules rouges et des globules blancs humains avec l'enzyme de différents tissus de rat. Clin. Chim. Acta 24:199, 1969.

117. Rose, I. A., and O'Connell, E. L.: The role of glucose-6-phosphate in the regulation of glucose metabolism in human erythrocytes. J. Biol. Chem. 239:12, 1964.

118. Ross, J. P.: Deficient activity of DPNH-dependent methemoglobin diaphorase in Gd blood erythrocytes. Blood 21:51, 1963.

119. Rozenszajn, L., and Shoham, D.: Demonstration of dehydrogenases and diaphorases in cells of peripheral blood and bone marrow. Blood 29:737, 1967.

120. Russo, G., Mollica, F., et al.: Hemolytic crises of favism in Sicilian females heterozygous for G6PD deficiency. Pediatrics 49:854, 1972.

121. Salen, G., Goldstein, F., et al.: Acute hemolytic anemia complicating viral hepatitis in patients with glucose-6-phosphate dehydrogenase deficiency. Ann. Intern. Med. 65:1210, 1966.

122. Sanger, R., and Race, R. R.: Towards mapping the X-chromosome, In Modern Trends in Human Genetics. Emery, A. E. M. (ed.), London, Butterworth, 1972.

123. Sansone, G., and Segni, G.: Prime determinazioni del glutatione (GSH) ematico nel favismo. Boll. Soc. Ital. Biol. Sper. 32:456, 1956.

124. Sansone, G., Piga, A. M., et al.: Favism. Turin, Italy, Minerva Medica, 1958.

125. Sansone, G., Rasore-Quartino, A., et al.: Demonstration of blood smears of a double erythrocytic population in females heterozygous for glucose-6-phosphate dehydrogenase deficiency. Pathologica 55:371, 1963.

126. Sass, M. D., Caruso, C. J., et al.: Rapid screening for D-glucose-6-phosphate: NADP oxidoreductase deficiency with methylene blue. J. Lab. Clin. Med. 68:156, 1966.

127. Sass, M. D., Caruso, C. J., et al.: TPNH-methemoglobin reductase deficiency: A new red-cell enzyme defect. J. Lab. Clin. Med. 70:760, 1967.

128. Say, B., Ozand, P., et al.: Erythrocyte glucose-6-phosphate dehydrogenase deficiency in Turkey. Acta Paediatr. Scand. 54:319, 1965.

129. Scott, R. B.: Health care priority and sickle cell anemia. J.A.M.A. 214:731, 1970.

130. Shahidi, N. T., and Clatanoff, D. V.: The role of puberty in red-cell production in hereditary hemolytic anaemias. Br. J. Haematol. 17:335, 1969.

131. Siniscalco, M., Bernini, L., et al.: Population genetics of haemoglobin variants, thalassaemia and G-6-PD deficiency, with particular reference to the malaria hypothesis. Bull. WHO 34:379, 1966.

132. Siniscalco, M., Motulsky, A. G., et al.: Indagini genetiche sulla predisposizione al favismo. II. Dati familiari. Associazione genica con il daltonismo. Accad. Nazionale dei Lincei 28:1, 1960.

133. Smits, H. L., Oski, F. A., et al.: The hemolytic crisis of sickle cell disease: The role of glucose-6-phosphate dehydrogenase deficiency. J. Pediatr. 74:544, 1969.

134. Sparks, R. S., Baluda, M. C., et al.: Cellulose acetate electrophoresis of human glucose-6-phosphate dehydrogenase. J. Lab. Clin. Med. 73:531, 1969.

135. Srivastava, S. K., and Beutler, E.: Oxidized glutathione levels in erythrocytes of glucose-6-phosphate-dehydrogenase−deficient subjects. Lancet 2:23, 1968.

136. Staal, G. E. J., Visser, J., et al.: Purification and properties of glutathione reductase of human erythrocytes. Biochim. Biophys. Acta 185:39, 1969.

137. Stamatoyannopoulos, G., Voitglander, V., et al.: Genetic diversity of the "Mediterranean" glucose-6-phosphate dehydrogenase deficiency phenotype. J. Clin. Invest. 50:1253, 1971.

138. Szeinberg, A., Oliver, M., et al.: Glucose-6-phosphate dehydrogenase deficiency and hemolytic disease of the newborn in Israel. Arch. Dis. Child. 38:23, 1963.

139. Tizianello, A., Panaeeiulli, I., et al.: Erythrocyte glucose-6-phosphate dehydrogenase deficiency as a problem in the selection of blood donors. Vox Sang. 8:47, 1963.

140. Valaes, T., Karaklis, A., et al.: Incidence and mechanism of neonatal jaundice related to glucose-6-phosphate dehydrogenase deficiency. Pediatr. Res. 3:448, 1969.

141. Valentine, W. N., Hsieh, H. S., et al.: Hereditary hemolytic anemia associated with phosphoglycerate kinase deficiency in erythrocytes and leukocytes: A probable X-chromosome linked syndrome. New Engl. J. Med. 280:528, 1969.

142. Waller, H. D., Benohr, H. C., et al.: Die glutathionreduktion in erythrocyten von gesunden und enzymdefektragern. Klin. Wochenschr. 48:79, 1970.

143. Wang, Y. M., and van Eys, J.: The enzymatic defect in essential pentosuria. New Engl. J. Med. 282:892, 1970.

144. Wang, Y. M., Patterson, J. H., et al.: The potential use of xylitol in glucose-6-phosphate dehydrogenase deficiency anemia. J. Clin. Invest. 50:1421, 1971.

145. Wiesenfeld, S. L., Petrakis, N. L., et al.: Elevated

blood pressure, pulse rate and serum creatinine in Negro males deficient in glucose-6-phosphate dehydrogenase. New Engl. J. Med. 282:1001, 1970.

146. WHO Scientific Group: Standardization of procedures for the study of glucose-6-phosphate dehydrogenase. WHO Tech. Rep. Ser. No. 366, Geneva, 1967.

147. Wolff, J. A., Grossman, B. H., et al.: Neonatal serum bilirubin and glucose-6-phosphate dehydrogenase. Am. J. Dis. Child. 113:251, 1967.

148. Wrigley, N. G., Heather, J. V., et al.: Human erythrocyte glucose-6-phosphate dehydrogenase. Electron microscope studies on structure and interconversion of tetramers, dimers and monomers. J. Mol. Biol. 68:483, 1972.

149. Yoshida, A.: Glucose-6-phosphate dehydrogenase of human erythrocytes. I. Purification and characterization of normal (B+) enzyme. J. Biol. Chem. 241:4966, 1966.

150. Yoshida, A.: A single amino acid substitution (asparagine to aspartic acid) between normal (B+) and the common Negro variant (A+)

of human glucose-6-phosphate dehydrogenase. Proc. Natl. Acad. Sci. USA 57:835, 1967.

151. Yoshida, A.: Amino acid substitution (histidine to tyrosine) in a glucose-6-phosphate dehydrogenase variant (G6PD Hektoen) associated with overproduction. J. Mol. Biol. 52:483, 1970.

152. Yoshida, A.: Hemolytic anemia and G6PD deficiency. Science 179:532, 1973.

153. Yoshida, A., and Hoagland, V. D.: Active molecular unit and NADP content of human glucose-6-phosphate dehydrogenase. Biochim. Biophys. Acta 40:1167, 1970.

154. Yoshida, A., Stamatoyannopoulos, G., et al.: Biochemical genetics of glucose-6-phosphate dehydrogenase variation. Ann. N.Y. Acad. Sci. 155:868, 1968.

155. Johnson, C., Beutler, E., et al.: The relationship between G-6-P-D genotype and SS disease (abstract). Clin. Res. 22:178A, 1974.

156. Beutler, E., Johnson, C., et al.: Prevalence of glucose-6-phosphate dehydrogenase deficiency in sickle-cell disease. New Engl. J. Med. 290:826, 1974.

Section IV

Red Cell Destruction: Disorders of Hemoglobin

Chapter 12

Methemoglobinemia

by Stephen A. Feig

INTRODUCTION

The valence of heme iron is a critical determinant of the capacity of hemoglobin to interact reversibly with oxygen. In the various forms of methemoglobinemia, heme iron is oxidized to the ferri form, rendering the hemoglobin incapable of oxygen binding at physiologic partial pressures. Although usually mild, methemoglobinemia can pose a serious threat of tissue anoxia, and fatalities under this circumstance have been reported.

The heme of normal hemoglobin is gradually oxidized to the met or ferri hemoglobin form in vivo (1). Several metabolic pathways are present in erythrocytes to counteract this phenomenon and restore oxygen-carrying capacity (2). These pathways mediate the transfer of electrons via reduced pyridine nucleotides to methemoglobin. One enzyme, in particular, links NADH and glycolysis to methemoglobin reduction. Genetic variation or specific deficiency of this NADH-methemoglobin reductase (MHR) is responsible for methemoglobi-

378

nemia in most patients with the congenital form of the disease (2, 3).

Less common forms of congenital methemoglobinemia are due to alteration of the amino acid sequence of hemoglobin, which renders the molecule more susceptible to the assumption of the met or ferri configuration (4). These hemoglobinopathic forms of congenital methemoglobinemia are discussed in detail in Chapter 13.

Acquired methemoglobinemia is the commonest form of the disorder (3), a condition which prevails when the normal tendency to heme oxidation is increased by exposure to an oxidant chemical or drug which stimulates the rate of ferri heme formation to exceed the rate of heme iron reduction. In extreme cases, the concentration of methemoglobin may suddenly increase to lethal levels.

This chapter is designed to develop an understanding of how specific genetic abnormalities and environmental factors affect the metabolism of the erythrocyte, alter the chemistry of hemoglobin, and interfere with its essential function. Regardless of its etiology, the clinical result of methemoglobinemia is the same. The need for and urgency of therapy are dictated by the degree of hypoxia, i.e., the absolute capacity of methemoglobinemic blood to carry and release oxygen.

HISTORICAL REVIEW

The concept of methemoglobinemia dates from 1845, when François described a cyanotic patient who did not have apparent cardiopulmonary disease (5). Subsequently, several authors recognized that certain drugs could cause methemoglobinemia, and in 1891 Dittrich demonstrated that red cells possess the capacity to reverse this toxic pigment change (6). Forty years later Hitzenberger recognized the familial form of methemoglobinemia (7), but it remained for Gibson to link the familial form of methemoglobinemia to a deficiency of red cell diaphorase (8). This condition was associated with a classic autosomal recessive mode of inheritance. Hörlein and Weber observed a family with methemoglobinemia in which the genetic pattern was autosomal, but dominant (9), and established that this occurrence was indicative of a hemoglobinopathy. In recent years, structural variants of methemoglobin reductase have been identified. These have been associated with methemoglobinemia due to decreased function rather than reduced amount of enzyme protein (10–14).

BIOCHEMICAL ASPECTS

The biochemical pathophysiology of methemoglobinemia encompasses nearly the entire range of red cell metabolism. An understanding of the relationship of this syndrome to normal and pathologic metabolism is essential to the formulation of rational therapy.

The Role of Iron

The heme iron of deoxy-hemoglobin must be in the ferrous state to allow reversible binding with oxygen (15). In erythrocytes there is a constant tendency to oxidize heme iron to the ferric state. The rate at which heme iron is normally oxidized in vivo has been estimated to be approximately 3 per cent per day (1).

Recent observations have clarified the role of iron in the binding of oxygen and the disruption of this function in methemoglobinemia (16–18). As oxygen is bound, one of the electrons of the ferrous iron is partially transferred to the oxygen. Effectively, then, the iron of oxyhemoglobin is in the ferric state, and the oxygen exists as the superoxide (O_2^-) anion (Fig. 12–1). As the oxygen is released, the electron is returned to the iron. This sharing of an electron places the iron in a low-spin ferric state; the loss is partial and reversible. This condition must be distinguished from the complete loss of an electron which places the iron in a high-spin ferric state (Fig. 12–1). In this state, it cannot combine with oxygen. This form of iron has five unpaired electrons; the sixth coordinate position is usually taken by water or an anion. These ligands are not easily dislodged from methemoglobin, nor can the electron be returned easily to the iron. Reduction of methemoglobin therefore requires activity of one of the reductive pathways and one or more cofactors.

In an aqueous environment, the superoxide anion is a highly reactive species. Both the iron and the globin are protected from it by the tertiary structure of hemo-

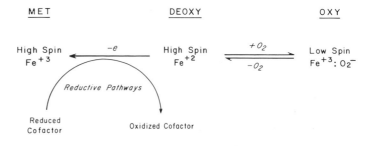

Figure 12–1. The oxidative states of hemoglobin iron.

globin, which results in an extremely hydrophobic heme pocket and renders the superoxide anion stable (19).

Reductive Pathways

Several pathways exist in red cells to provide reducing capacity. Each involves one or more cofactors, and, through these, is linked to red cell metabolism. Although a wide variety of substrates may support methemoglobin reduction, this effect is always mediated through the production of reduced pyridine nucleotides (Figs. 12–2 and 12–3).

Scott and his associates have isolated two NADH-linked methemoglobin reductases from normal erythrocytes (20). One of these is deficient in the enzymopenic form of methemoglobinemia. These enzymes account for nearly 70 per cent of methemoglobin reduction in normal cells.

In mature adult erythrocytes, NADH may be produced at two steps in glycolysis, the oxidations of glyceraldehyde-3-phosphate and lactate (Fig. 12–2). Physiologic conditions in the erythrocyte, however, favor the reduction of pyruvate over the oxidation of lactate. Thus, lactate oxidation is not usually considered a source of NADH in vivo. In fact, pyruvate may be considered in competition with methemoglobin for available NADH. Under ordinary circumstances pyruvate is produced more than 100 times faster than methemoglobin. Hence the requirement of the red cell for NADH for the reduction of methemoglobin is only a small part of its total needs for that cofactor. Another reductive system, the polyol pathway, may also contribute NADH for methemoglobin formation under certain circumstances (20a).

In vitro, however, with either glucose or lactate as metabolic substrate, the reduction of methemoglobin is matched by equimolar accumulation of pyruvate (8). In cells deficient in MHR, the lactate:pyruvate production ratio is greater than it is in normal RBC's. When purine nucleoside is the metabolic substrate for normal red cells, pyruvate does not accumulate as readily as it does in the presence of glucose (21). Inosine, for instance, is a source of ribose-5-phosphate, which is an intermediate in the hexose monophosphate shunt, and is metabolized to provide glyceraldehyde-3-phosphate. In contrast to the first steps of glycolysis, the production of glyceraldehyde-3-phosphate from inosine occurs without the expenditure of ATP. In the presence of adequate concentrations of phosphate and a hydrogen acceptor such as methemoglobin, the concentration of 2,3-DPG increases when inosine is the substrate. This expansion of the 2,3-DPG pool provides a subsequent metabolic source of ATP, but limits pyruvate build-up which would compete with methemoglobin for the NADH made available by glyceraldehyde-phosphate dehydrogenase (22).

Inhibitors of glycolysis have variable effects on methemoglobin reduction. Iodoacetate, which inhibits glyceraldehyde-phosphate dehydrogenase, blocks the syn-

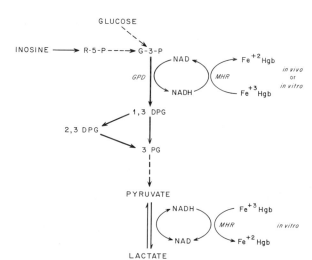

Figure 12–2. Glycolysis and methemoglobin reduction. R-5-P, ribose-5-phosphate; G-3-P, glyceraldehyde-3-phosphate; GPD, glyceraldehyde-phosphate dehydrogenase; DPG, diphosphoglycerate; 3-PG, 3-phosphoglycerate; NADH, nicotinamide adenine dinucleotide, reduced; NAD, nicotinamide adenine dinucleotide; MHR, methemoglobin reductase; Fe^{+3} Hgb, ferri(met)hemoglobin; Fe^{+2} Hgb, ferrohemoglobin.

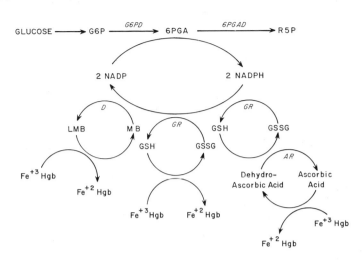

Figure 12–3. Hexose monophosphate shunt and methemoglobin reduction. G6P(D), glucose-6-phosphate (dehydrogenase); 6PGA(D), 6-phosphogluconic acid (dehydrogenase); R5P, ribose-5-phosphate; NADP, nicotinamide adenine dinucleotide phosphate, oxidized; NADPH, nicotinamide adenine dinucleotide phosphate, reduced; MB, methylene blue, oxidized; LMB, leukomethylene blue, reduced; D, diaphorase; GR, glutathione reductase; GSH, reduced glutathione; GSSG, oxidized glutathione; AR, ascorbate reductase; Fe^{+3}Hgb, ferri(met)-hemoglobin; Fe^{+2}Hgb, ferrohemoglobin.

thesis of NADH from glucose and thus interferes with methemoglobin reduction. This interference is prevented when lactate is used as a metabolic substrate (2). Fluoride is an inhibitor of enolase and causes secondary accumulation of trioses, because of lack of NAD produced at lactate dehydrogenase (23). The presence of a hydrogen acceptor such as methemoglobin provides an alternate path of NAD production. This may, in turn, permit triose oxidation and maintenance of ATP levels. Even the competitive inhibition of enolase by fluoride may be overcome when methemoglobin is present (23a).

Several NADPH-linked methemoglobin reductases have been identified (20, 24). These enzymes account for less than 10 per cent of normal methemoglobin reduction (20), although they are of significance in the treatment of methemoglobinemia. The ordinary clinical insignificance of this pathway was demonstrated by observation of a patient whose red cells were deficient in this enzyme but did not accumulate methemoglobin (25). Furthermore, although the sources of erythrocyte NADPH are glucose-6-phosphate dehydrogenase (G6PD) and 6-phosphogluconic dehydrogenase, patients with deficiencies of either of these enzymes do not have chronic methemoglobinemia (26, 27). In fact, the red cells of such patients reduce methemoglobin normally in vitro (28), unless the globin moiety of hemoglobin is irreversibly oxidized. Finally, even severe methemoglobin accumulation is not associated with in-

creased hexose monophosphate shunt activity in vitro (29).

Despite the lack of importance of the NADPH-methemoglobin reductases in the ordinary maintenance of ferro hemoglobin, the NADPH-dependent diaphorases are vitally important in the therapy of methemoglobinemia which results from congenital deficiency of the NADH-dependent enzymes. It is currently believed that therapy with methylene blue depends upon reduction of the dye to leukomethylene blue by NADPH diaphorase (Fig. 12–3). The reduced (leuko) methylene blue then directly reduces ferri to ferro hemoglobin (30, 31). When methemoglobinemia occurs in a patient with G6PD deficiency, NADPH is not produced in sufficient amount to support the reduction of methylene blue, and treatment failures have been reported (32).

Reduced glutathione (GSH) and ascorbic acid may directly reduce methemoglobin (Fig. 12–3). GSH reacts slowly with methemoglobin, and Scott has estimated that less than 15 per cent of methemoglobin could be reduced by this cofactor in normal cells (20). This estimate was made by measuring the kinetics of the NADPH-diaphorases and estimating the reducing capacity of the enzyme at physiologic concentrations of the reactants. Since methemoglobinemia does not occur in the presence of low reduced glutathione (as in G6PD deficiency) (26, 27) or low total glutathione (33), this pathway must be relatively insignificant.

Ascorbic acid may reduce methemoglobin in vivo and in vitro (34), and has been used successfully in the therapy of methemoglobinemia (35). Dehydroascorbic acid is reduced by GSH in the presence of a specific reductase, and the reduced ascorbic acid probably reacts nonenzymatically with methemoglobin (Fig. 12–3) (36). Kinetic estimates by Scott suggest that perhaps 15 per cent of methemoglobin reduction is accomplished by this mechanism in normal erythrocytes (20). The absence of methemoglobinemia in scurvy also suggests that this is not a major pathway of methemoglobin reduction (2). Ascorbic acid levels in methemoglobinemia are variable (3).

Methemoglobin Reductases

Considerable effort has been devoted to the characterization of the enzymes which mediate the reduction of methemoglobin (20, 24, 37–45). The literature is complicated by the fact that methemoglobin is reduced very slowly by the direct mediation of these enzymes. A wide variety of other electron acceptors react more quickly with this enzyme and have been used to study patients with methemoglobinemia. In general, the results obtained with one acceptor are comparable to those obtained with another, and vary primarily with the ease with which the oxidoreductase will transfer electrons to the final acceptor (3). All the reactions require reduced pyridine nucleotide as an electron and hydrogen donor.

Scott first observed the presence of a species of NADH-diaphorase (20). One enzyme (NADH-dehydrogenase I) is responsible for the majority of methemoglobin reduction in normal red cells. Decrease or absence of activity of this enzyme is observed in homozygous enzymopenic methemoglobinemia and in obligatory heterozygotes. This enzyme was differentiated from NADH-diaphorase II by chromatography, kinetic behavior, and the effects of pH and temperature. The type II enzyme is responsible for residual diaphorase activity in patients with homozygous enzyme deficiency; however, its kinetic properties and the substrate concentrations present in the red cell make it an inadequate alternative when type I is deficient.

Hegesh and co-workers have amplified this work with the technique of polyacrylamide gel electrophoresis (38). They have observed four or five different bands of enzyme activity. The more anodal bands are less prominent in patients with enzyme deficiency (homozygotes, heterozygotes, and neonates) and do not cross-react with NADPH (38). The two cathodal bands have cross-reactivity with NADPH, are present in the hemolysates of deficient individuals, and presumably correspond to Scott's NADH-diaphorase II. The rate at which the enzymes utilize NADH is proportional to the concentration of inorganic phosphate (39).

Scott also observed two species of NADPH-diaphorase (20), and Hegesh has detected two or more bands which correspond to each (38). The appearance of multiple bands for each diaphorase may be due to the presence or absence of bound pyridine nucleotide (40).

NADH-diaphorase I has a molecular weight of approximately 30,000 (38, 41, 42), and can be separated by gel filtration from NADPH-diaphorase, which has a molecular weight of approximately 20,000 (38, 40). It is generally agreed that there is no prosthetic heme compound associated with these enzymes (41–43); however, some groups have detected an associated flavin moiety (FAD) (41, 44), which has not been confirmed by others (42, 43).

Functional differences between purified NADH- and NADPH-dependent enzymes are most clearly demonstrated using ferrocyanide and dichlorophenolindophenol (DCIP) as the final electron acceptor (38). The direct reduction of methemoglobin with either pyridine nucleotide occurs too slowly to be of significance (38, 46). In the presence of ferrocyanide, however, the NADH-associated enzyme reduces methemoglobin rapidly (38). NADPH does not act as a cofactor in the reduction of the methemoglobin ferrocyanide complex with either purified enzyme (14, 38).

Recently Hultquist and Passon have detected the presence of cytochrome b_5 in human erythrocytes (46). These workers have purified and characterized an erythrocyte cytochrome b_5 reductase which appeared identical to NADH-diaphorase I (46). This enzyme is incapable of mediating the transfer of electrons from NADPH. In low concentrations, it is minimally capable of transferring electrons directly from NADH to methemoglobin, but this activity is markedly enhanced in the presence of cytochrome b_5. Indeed, Sugita et al. have found cytochrome b_5 to be the most effective known acceptor of electrons from NADH (42). Both groups suggest that the physiologic pathway of methemoglobin reduction in human erythrocytes may be initiated through the reduction of cytochrome b_5. Since the rate of methemoglobin reduction occurs at the same rate as the production of reduced cytochrome b_5 and this is achieved in the presence of minute amounts of the cytochrome, it has been proposed that the transfer of electrons from cytochrome b_5 to methemoglobin occurs directly and nonenzymatically in a manner analogous to the transfer of electrons from leukomethylene blue to methemoglobin (Fig. 12–4) (42).

Clinical Correlations

Normal red cells maintain methemoglobin at a concentration below 1 per cent by the mechanisms outlined above. Methemoglobinemia occurs when the oxidative tendency is sufficiently increased or the reducing capacity is markedly impaired.

Scott has estimated that in normal red cells the mean capacity to reduce methemoglobin is 250 times greater than the rate at which hemoglobin is oxidized (47). Individuals heterozygous for enzyme deficiency have 125 times the heme-reducing capacity compared with the normal rate of heme oxidation, and this reducing potential is sufficient to maintain the methemoglobin concentration in heterozygote cells below 1 per cent. Similar estimates reveal that the reducing capacity of homozygous deficient cells must be only four times greater than the normal oxidizing rate. These estimates indicate the abundance of reducing capac-

ity in normal cells. Oxidant stress or impairment of reducing capacity must be severe to produce methemoglobinemia. The majority of patients with methemoglobin reductase deficiency appear to have suppressed production of the enzyme (2). Whether this represents a true lack of enzyme protein or the synthesis of an inactive variant is not known. Several electrophoretic variants of methemoglobin reductase have been described (10–13a, 48, 49). One individual has been reported who has inherited two electrophoretic variants (14), although most patients have the normal isozyme in addition to a variant (3).

The presence of an enzyme with abnormal electrophoretic mobility does not necessarily indicate functional impairment (48). The primary structure of the normal enzyme has not been elucidated, nor have any of the amino acid substitutions which presumably cause the electrophoretic heterogeneity been defined.

In addition to simple decrease in enzyme activity, two functional abnormalities have been observed. Schwartz has documented the presence of a kinetic variant of NADH-diaphorase in three patients with methemoglobinemia who carry the "Puerto Rican" isoenzyme. The enzyme migrates more rapidly than normal. Schwartz and his co-workers have reported a decreased Km DCIP, and an increased Km NADH for this partially purified enzyme, which also was relatively heat labile (13).

In 1966, Keitt, Smith, and Jandl reported a patient with congenital methemoglobinemia in whose red cells they observed an uneven distribution of methemoglobin (50). They noted that the concentration of methemoglobin was greater in the older, denser erythrocytes, although in contrast to the studies of Rigas and Koler (51) the activity of NADH-diaphorase did not decrease with

Figure 12–4. Proposed physiologic pathway of methemoglobin reduction. G3P, glyceraldehyde-3-phosphate; GPD, glyceraldehyde phosphate dehydrogenase; DPG, diphosphoglycerate; NAD, nicotinamide adenine dinucleotide, oxidized; NADH, nicotinamide adenine dinucleotide, reduced; Cb5R, cytochrome b_5 reductase; Fe^{+2}Hgb, ferrohemoglobin; Fe^{+3}Hgb, ferri(met)hemoglobin.

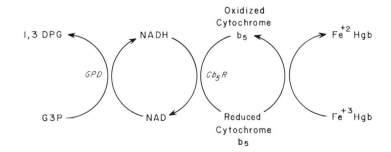

cell aging either in normal cells or in the patient's cells. This patient was subsequently shown to have the "Boston-slow" variant of NADH-diaphorase (48, 49). In a later study, using the methemoglobin-ferrocyanide assay, Feig and co-workers observed that the older cells of this patient retained only 10 per cent of the methemoglobin-reducing capacity of her younger cells, while in normal red cells the loss of activity with aging was negligible (14). Two other patients with mild methemoglobinemia and a different isoenzyme variant demonstrated age lability of approximately 40 per cent. Thus, these patients appeared to lose most of the enzyme activity associated with the labile variant during the life span of their red cells. In all three patients, the concentration of methemoglobin in the older cells was consistent with the enzyme activity of those cells.

GENETIC ASPECTS

Congenital methemoglobinemia is a rare entity. Although it is encountered throughout the world, several inbred populations have been reported to demonstrate an exceptionally high incidence of this disorder (52, 53). The pattern of inheritance of the enzyme deficiency is considered to be autosomal recessive (2). This concept has been strengthened by the inheritance of the isoenzyme variants (Fig. 12–5). Under normal circumstances, heterozygous subjects encounter no clinical difficulty, consistent with the calculations of Scott (47). These individuals are easily recognized by tests of enzyme activity (54), and are more susceptible to oxidant stress than are normals (55). Heterozygous neonates may appear as severely affected as homozygotes (14, 56) because of the transient diaphorase deficiency which occurs in the newborn (57, 58). Recent studies of fetal red cells document even more severe diaphorase deficiency in early gestation (59). In view of the increased incidence of mental retardation among patients with enzymopenic methemoglobinemia, it is recommended that oxidant drugs be avoided in pregnant women in order to reduce potential intra-uterine cerebral anoxia on the basis of fetal methemoglobinemia. The alleged association of mental retardation with intrauterine cerebral hypoxia on the basis of fetal methemoglobinemia is not supported, however, by the fact that intrauterine methemoglobinemia must occur in subjects with alpha chain hemoglobin M variants, in whom no retardation is reported. No consistent general or unifying feature distinguishes those families in which methemoglobinemia is associated with retardation from those in which it is not (3, 60, 61).

The autosomal dominant inheritance pattern of the hemoglobinopathic form of methemoglobinemia clearly distinguishes it from the enzyme deficiency (9).

CLINICAL ASPECTS

Methemoglobinemia is classically characterized by slate-gray cyanosis. Quite naturally, these patients are initially evaluated for cardiac or pulmonary disease. Indeed, it is frequently the failure to uncover such an etiology for cyanosis which raises the possibility of methemoglobinemia. An early clue to the correct diagnosis is usually derived from the fact that cyanosis in methemoglobinemia is entirely out of propor-

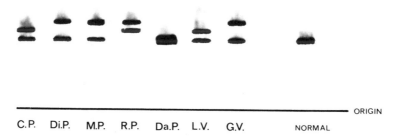

C.P.   Di.P.   M.P.   R.P.   Da.P.   L.V.   G.V.   NORMAL

——————————————————————————————— ORIGIN

Figure 12–5. Diagrammatic representation of electrophoresis of NADH-methemoglobin reductase of P family. The method used was that of Bloom and Zarkowsky (49). C. P. and Di.P. are siblings of the propositus, M.P. R.P. and Da.P. are the mother and father of the propositus. L.V. and G.V. are the maternal grandparents. The figure demonstrates the allelic nature of these isoenzymes and their autosomal inheritance.

tion to the severity of hypoxic symptomatology. Finch has observed clinical cyanosis at methemoglobin concentrations below 2 g. per 100 ml., while recognizable cyanosis due to deoxyhemoglobin does not occur until the concentration is greater than 5 g. per 100 ml (62).

The clinical sequelae of methemoglobinemia are the result of reduced oxygen-carrying capacity and tissue hypoxia. Methemoglobin concentrations of 25 to 30 per cent are often well tolerated (2), but as the concentration rises further, progressive symptoms of hypoxia are observed. Early symptoms, such as headache and exercise intolerance, are usually observed when methemoglobin concentrations approach 35 to 40 per cent (62), and depression of consciousness may be observed at levels of 50 to 60 per cent (63). Fatalities, usually the result of toxic drug ingestion, have been reported (64).

Since the symptoms reflect tissue oxygen deprivation, other conditions which affect tissue oxygenation would be expected to interact with methemoglobinemia. Thus, earlier and more severe symptoms occur in anemic patients. This situation would be more likely to arise in acquired methemoglobinemia, when toxicity is superimposed upon an unrelated anemia. In fact, patients with moderate or severe congenital methemoglobinemia frequently manifest a compensatory erythrocytosis (1, 35, 52, 61). Another condition which may interact to increase the severity of methemoglobinemia is occlusive vascular disease, an infrequent pediatric problem.

Quite obviously, acquired or toxic methemoglobinemia is of variable severity and, in general, proportional to the severity of the oxidant stress. This is determined by several factors: the dose of oxidant absorbed, its redox potential, and the rate at which it is metabolized or excreted. In addition, the capacity of red cells to reduce methemoglobin may vary among patients. Although heterozygous deficiency of methemoglobin reductase (MHR) is relatively rare and asymptomatic, these individuals are exceptionally susceptible to methemoglobinemia after the administration of certain oxidant drugs (55). Similarly, some patients with abnormal hemoglobins, especially some of the unstable variants, are

also more susceptible to the effects of oxidants (65).

Premature and newborn infants have an increased incidence of methemoglobinemia (66, 67). Several studies have correlated this observation with decreased MHR levels or reducing capacity (57, 58). Thus, normal neonates are more susceptible to oxidants, and several nursery epidemics due to disinfectants (68, 69), formulas containing nitrites (made from water with high concentrations of nitrates) (67), and absorption of aniline marker dyes (70, 71) have been reported. Several authors have observed apparently spontaneous methemoglobinemia in neonates who had extremely low MHR activity and who were later shown to be heterozygous for MHR deficiency (14, 56). An additional factor rendering newborns more susceptible is the relative ease with which Hb F can be oxidized compared with Hb A (72).

Hereditary methemoglobinemia is entirely compatible with a normal life expectancy (64). Pregnancies are uncomplicated (64), but oxidant drugs (especially local anesthetics) have been reported to cause methemoglobinemia in both the mother and the neonate (73). Methemoglobinemia of the toxic or enzymopenic varieties is not associated with shortened erythrocyte survival (74), and the induction of methemoglobinemia in vitro is likewise not associated with increased hemolysis (39, 75).

Rapid differentiation of methemoglobinemia from other forms of cyanosis is usually possible at the bedside because deoxyhemoglobin will oxygenate at ambient oxygen tensions. This can be easily seen as a change in the color of the blood from brownish red to bright red in the test tube. Harley and Celermajer have reported a modification of this simple test using a drop of blood on a piece of filter paper (76). They report that gentle waving in air for 30 seconds is sufficient to oxygenate normal hemoglobin. Failure to turn color is suggestive of methemoglobinemia, and more quantitative assessment should then be performed. The most widely used of these assays was described by Evelyn and Malloy (77). It depends upon the characteristic absorption maximum of methemoglobin at 634 nm., which is lost upon the addition of cyanide.

Once the diagnosis of methemoglobinemia has been documented, it is essential to determine whether the cause is genetic, toxic, or a combination of the two. A careful history to exclude or confirm exposure to toxic chemicals or drugs is essential. A list of some of the offending oxidants is presented in Table 12–1. The diagnosis of hemoglobin M is best made by hemoglobin electrophoresis, but a positive heat stability test may be observed. In the neonatal period, only an alpha chain abnormality would be present in sufficient quantity to produce symptomatic hemoglobinopathic methemoglobinemia.

Two simple enzyme assays are available to document enzyme deficiency. The diaphorase assay measures the ability of a hemolysate to reduce (and decolorize) a blue dye, 2,6-dichlorophenolindophenol (DCIP) (54). The MHR assay measures the ability of a hemolysate to reduce a methemoglobin-ferrocyanide complex (78). Although neither assay measures directly the reduction of methemoglobin, reduced activity by either assay (using NADH as an electron donor) correlates well with enzymopenic methemoglobinemia or the heterozygous state (48, 54, 78).

Treatment of methemoglobinemia, regardless of etiology, is dictated by the severity of hypoxia. The majority of patients with hereditary disease require no therapy. Severe methemoglobinemia, whether toxic or hereditary, should be treated initially with 1 to 2 mg. per kg. of methylene blue administered intravenously as a 1 per cent solution in saline. This is usually sufficient to reduce the concentration of methemoglobin to less than 1 per cent in less than an hour (2). In the event of oxidant exposure, the agent should be identified and eliminated immediately. Further treatment, if necessary, can usually be accomplished with oral methylene blue. The necessary dose is determined empirically but adult chronic doses usually range from 100 to 300 mg. per day.

A universal side effect of methylene blue administration is the production of blue urine, which though frequently distressing, is totally harmless. It should be recognized that methylene blue is, itself, an oxidant. In overdose, it may cause methemoglobinemia or hemolytic anemia in susceptible individuals (32, 79). The utility of methylene blue is based upon the presence of an NADPH-linked diaphorase in red cells. Thus, methylene blue is reduced to leukomethylene blue, which, in turn, is capable of the nonenzymatic reduction of methemoglobin (30, 31). In the presence of a defect in the hexose monophosphate shunt, low availability of NADPH has been shown to limit the effectiveness of methylene blue therapy in methemoglobinemia and to result in hemolytic anemia (32). The failure of methylene blue treatment of methemoglobinemia should suggest the presence of G6PD deficiency. An alternate oxidant which may be used in chronic therapy is ascorbic acid (300 to 400 mg. per day, orally), but it is, in general, less effective than methylene blue and also requires an intact hexose monophosphate shunt. Severe acquired methemoglobinemia in the patient with G6PD deficiency may require exchange transfusion to eliminate the offending oxidant and to improve the patient's oxygen carrying capacity. Hyperbaric oxygen has also been recommended in the therapy of toxic methemoglobinemia (80).

TABLE 12–1. OXIDANTS REPORTED TO CAUSE METHEMOGLOBINEMIA

1. Analgesics
   Acetophenetidin
2. Anesthetics
   Benzocaine (topical, rectal)
   Prilocaine (obstetrical)
3. Aniline Derivatives
   Marking dyes (topical)
   Disinfectants (topical)
   Crayons
4. Antimalarials
5. Nitrites
   Nitrate contamination of well water
   Bismuth subnitrate
   Nitroglycerin
   Nitrate food additives
6. Pyridium
7. Sulfonamides
8. Vitamin K Analogs

References

1. Eder, H. A., Finch, C., et al.: Congenital methemoglobinemia. A clinical and biochemical study of a case. J. Clin. Invest. 28:265, 1949.
2. Jaffé, E. R.: Hereditary methemoglobinemias associated with abnormalities of erythrocytes. Am. J. Med. 41:786, 1966.
3. Jaffé, E. R., and Hsieh, H. S.: DPNH-methemoglobin reductase deficiency and heredtiary

methemoglobinemia. Semin. Hematol. 8:417, 1971.

4. Gerald, P. S., and Efron, M. L.: Chemical studies of several varieties of Hb M. Proc. Natl. Acad. Sci. USA 47:1758, 1961.

5. François: Cas de cyanose congénitale sans cause apparente. Bull. Acad. R. Med. Belg. 4:698, 1845.

6. Dittrich, P.: Ueber methämoglobinbildende gifte. Naunyn-Schmiedebergs. Arch. Exper. Path. U. Pharmacol. 29:247, 1891.

7. Hitzenberger, K.: Autotoxische zyanose (intraglobuläre methämoglobinämie). Wien. Arch. Inn. Med. 23:85, 1933.

8. Gibson, Q. H.: The reduction of methaemoglobin in red blood cells and studies on the cause of idiopathic methaemoglobinaemia. Biochem. J. 42:13, 1948.

9. Hörlein, H., and Weber, G.: Über chronische familiäre methämoglobinämie und eine neue modifikation des methämoglobins. Dsch. Med. Wochenschr. 73:476, 1948.

10. West, C. A., Gomperts, B. D., et al.: Demonstration of an enzyme variant in a case of congenital methaemoglobinaemia. Br. Med. J. 4:212, 1967.

11. Brewer, G. J., Eaton, J. W., et al.: A starch-gel electrophoretic method for the study of diaphorase isozymes and preliminary results with sheep and human erythrocytes. Biochem. Biophys. Res. Commun. 29:198, 1967.

12. Kaplan, J. C., and Beutler, E.: Electrophoresis of red cell NADH- and NADPH-diaphorases in normal subjects and patients with congenital methemoglobinemia. Biochem. Biophys Res. Commun. 29:605, 1967.

13. Schwartz, J. M., Ross, J. M., et al.: Electrophoretic and kinetic characterization of a DPNH-diaphorase variant in a methemoglobinemic subject, In Red Cell Structure and Metabolism. Ramot, B. (ed.), New York, Academic Press, 1971, p. 135.

13a. Schwartz, J. M., Paress, P. S., et al.: Unstable variant of NADH methemoglobin reductase in Puerto Ricans with hereditary methemoglobinemia. J. Clin. Invest. 51:1594, 1972.

14. Feig, S. A., Nathan, D. G., et al.: Congenital methemoglobinemia: The result of age-dependent decay of methemoglobin reductase. Blood 39:407, 1972.

15. Pauling, L.: The electronic structure of hemoglobin, In Haemoglobin. Roughton, F. J. W., and Kendrew, J. C. (eds.), London, Butterworth & Company, 1949, p. 57.

16. Weiss, J. J.: Nature of the iron-oxygen bond in oxyhaemoglobin. Nature (Lond.) 202:83, 1964.

17. Peisach, J., Blumberg, W. E., et al.: The electronic structure of protoheme proteins. III. Configuration of the heme and its ligands. J. Biol. Chem. 243:1871, 1968.

18. Wittenberg, J. B., Wittenberg, B. A., et al.: On the state of the iron and the nature of the ligand in oxyhemoglobin. Proc. Natl. Acad. Sci. USA 67:1846, 1970.

19. Perutz, M. F., and Lehmann, H.: Molecular pathology of human hemoglobin. Nature (Lond.) 219:902, 1968.

20. Scott, E. M., Duncan, I. W., et al.: The reduced pyridine nucleotide dehydrogenases of human erythrocytes. J. Biol. Chem. 240:481, 1965.

20a. Travis, S. F., Oski, F. A., et al.: Polyol pathway and methemoglobin reduction in human RBC's (abstract). Blood 38:831, 1971.

21. Reinauer, H., and Bruns, F. H.: Limitierende Faktoren der Glykolyse in roten Blutzellen des Menschen. Biochem. Z. 340:503, 1964.

22. Schröter, W., and Heyden, H. V.: Kinetik des 2,3-Diphosphoglyceratumsatzes in menschlichen Erythrocyten. Biochem. Z. 341:387, 1965.

23. Feig, S. A., Shohct, S. B., et al.: Energy metabolism in human erythrocytes. I. Effects of sodium fluoride. J. Clin. Invest. 50:1731, 1971.

23a. Keitt, A. S.: Asynchronous glycolysis induced by fluoride. Clin. Res. 15:282, 1967.

24. Kajita, A., Kerwar, G. K., et al.: Multiple forms of methemoglobin reductase. Arch. Biochem. Biophys. 130:662, 1969.

25. Sass, M. D., Caruso, C. J., et al.: TPNH-methemoglobin reductase deficiency: A new red-cell enzyme defect. J. Lab. Clin. Med. 70:760, 1967.

26. Beutler, E., Dern, R. J., et al.: The hemolytic effect of primaquine. III. A study of primaquine-sensitive erythrocytes. J. Lab. Clin. Med. 44:177, 1954.

27. Dawson, J. P., Thayer, W. W., et al.: Acute hemolytic anemia in the newborn infant due to naphthalene poisoning: Report of two cases with investigations into the mechanism of the disease. Blood 13:1113, 1958.

28. Jaffé, E. R.: The reduction of methemoglobin in erythrocytes of a patient with congenital methemoglobinemia, subjects with erythrocyte glucose-6-phosphate dehydrogenase deficiency, and normal individuals. Blood 21:561, 1963.

29. Keitt, A. S.: Hereditary methemoglobinemia with deficiency of NADH methemoglobin reductase, In The Metabolic Basis of Inherited Disease. 3rd ed., Stanbury, J. B., Wyngaarden, J. B., and Fredrickson, D. S. (eds.), New York, McGraw-Hill, 1972, p. 1389.

30. Beutler, E., and Baluda, M.: Methemoglobin reduction. Studies of the interaction between cell populations and of the role of methylene blue. Blood 22:323, 1963.

31. Sass, M. D., Caruso, C. J., et al.: Mechanisms of the TPNH-linked reduction of methemoglobin by methylene blue. Clin. Chim. Acta 24:77, 1969.

32. Rosen, P. J., Johnson, C., et al.: Failure of methylene blue treatment in toxic methemoglobinemia. Association with glucose-6-phosphate dehydrogenase deficiency. Ann. Intern. Med. 75:83, 1971.

33. Prins, H. K., Oort, M., et al.: Congenital nonspherocytic hemolytic anemia, associated with glutathione deficiency of the erythrocytes. Hematologic, biochemical, and genetic studies. Blood 27:145, 1966.

34. Jaffé, E. R.: Metabolic processes involved in the formation and reduction of methemoglobin in human erythrocytes, In The Red Blood Cell. Bishop, C., and Surgenor, D. M. (eds.), New York, Academic Press, 1964, p. 397.

35. Barcroft, H., Gibson, Q. H., et al.: Familial idio-

pathic methaemoglobinaemia and its treatment with ascorbic acid. Clin. Sci. 5:145, 1945.

36. Cristine, L., Thomson, G., et al.: The reduction of dehydroascorbic acid by human erythrocytes. Clin. Chim. Acta. 1:557, 1956.

37. Kiese, M., Schneider, C., et al.: Hämiglobinreduktase. Arch. Exp. Path. Pharmak. 231:158, 1957.

38. Hegesh, E., Calmanovici, N., et al.: The diaphorase bands of human erythrocytes. J. Lab. Clin. Med. 77:859, 1971.

39. Kuma, F., Ishizawa, S., et al.: Studies on methemoglobin reductase. I. Comparative studies of diaphorases from normal and methemoglobinemic erythrocytes. J. Biol. Chem. 247:550, 1972.

40. Niethammer, D., and Huennekens, F. M.: Bound TPN as the determinant of polymorphism in methemoglobin reductase. Biochem. Biophys. Res. Commun. 45:345, 1971.

41. Kuma, F., and Inomata, H.: Studies on methemoglobin reductase. II. The purification and molecular properties of reduced nicotinamide adenine dinucleotide–dependent methemoglobin reductase. J. Biol. Chem. 247:556, 1972.

42. Sugita, Y., Nomura, S., et al.: Purification of reduced pyridine nucleotide dehydrogenase from human erythrocytes and methemoglobin reduction by the enzyme. J. Biol. Chem. 246:6072, 1971.

43. Hegesh, E., and Avron, M.: The enzymatic reduction of ferrihemoglobin. II. Purification of a ferrihemoglobin reductase from human erythrocytes. Biochim. Biophys. Acta. 146:397, 1967.

44. Scott, E. M., and McGraw, J. C.: Purification and properties of diphosphopyridine nucleotide diaphorase of human erythrocytes. J. Biol. Chem. 237:249, 1962.

45. Huennekens, F. M., Caffrey, R. W., et al.: Erythrocyte metabolism. IV. Isolation and properties of methemoglobin reductase. J. Biol. Chem. 227:261, 1957.

46. Hultquist, D. E., and Passon, P. G.: Catalysis of methaemoglobin reduction by erythrocyte cytochrome b_5 and cytochrome b_5 reductase. Nature [New Biol.] 229:252, 1971.

47. Scott, E. M.: Congenital methemoglobinemia due to DPNH-diaphorase deficiency, In *Hereditary Disorders of Erythrocyte Metabolism*. Beutler, E. (ed.), New York, Grune & Stratton, 1968, p. 102.

48. Hsieh, H. S., and Jaffé, E. R.: Electrophoretic and functional variants of NADH-methemoglobin reductase in hereditary methemoglobinemia. J. Clin. Invest. 50:196, 1971.

49. Bloom, G. E., and Zarkowsky, H. S.: Heterogeneity of the enzymatic defect in congenital methemoglobinemia. New Engl. J. Med. 281:919, 1969.

50. Keitt, A. S., Smith, T. W., et al.: Red-cell "pseudomosaicism" in congenital methemoglobinemia. New Engl. J. Med. 275:398, 1966.

51. Rigas, D. A., and Koler, R. D.: Erythrocyte enzymes and reduced glutathione (GSH) in hemoglobin H disease: Relation to cell age and denaturation of hemoglobin H. J. Lab. Clin. Med. 58:417, 1961.

52. Scott, E. M., and Hoskins, D. D.: Hereditary

methemoglobinemia in Alaskan Eskimos and Indians. Blood 13:795, 1968.

53. Balsamo, P., Hardy, W. R., et al.: Hereditary methemoglobinemia due to diaphorase deficiency in Navajo Indians. J. Pediatr. 65:928, 1964.

54. Scott, E. M.: The relation of diaphorase of human erythrocytes to inheritance of methemoglobinemia. J. Clin. Invest. 39:1176, 1960.

55. Cohen, R. J., Sachs, J. R., et al.: Methemoglobinemia provoked by malarial chemoprophylaxis in Vietnam. New Engl. J. Med. 279:1127, 1968.

56. Harper, M. A., Robin, H., et al.: Transient infantile cyanosis in a diaphorase-deficient male. Aust. Paediatr. J. 4:144, 1968.

57. Bartos, H. R., and Desforges, J. F.: Erythrocyte DPNH-dependent diaphorase levels in infants. Pediatrics 37:991, 1966.

58. Ross, J. D.: Deficient activity of DPNH-dependent methemoglobin diaphorase in cord blood erythrocytes. Blood 21:51, 1963.

59. Vetrella, M., Åstedt, B., et al.: Activity of NADH- and NADPH-dependent methemoglobin reductases in erythrocytes from fetal to adult age. Klin. Wochenschr. 49:972, 1971.

60. Fialkow, P. J., Browder, J. A., et al.: Mental retardation in methemoglobinemia due to diaphorase deficiency. New Engl. J. Med. 273:840, 1965.

61. Jaffé, E. R., Neumann, G., et al.: Hereditary methemoglobinemia with and without mental retardation. A study of three families. Am. J. Med. 41:42, 1966.

62. Finch, C. A.: Methemoglobinemia and sulfhemoglobinemia. New Engl. J. Med. 239:470, 1948.

63. Bodansky, O.: Methemoglobinemia and methemoglobin-producing compounds. Pharmacol. Rev. 3:144, 1951.

64. Jaffé, E. R., and Heller, P.: Methemoglobinemia in man. Progr. Hematol. 4:48, 1964.

65. Carrell, R. W., and Lehmann, H.: The unstable hemoglobin hemolytic anemias. Semin. Hematol. 6:116, 1969.

66. Kravitz, H., Elegant, L. D., et al.: Methemoglobin values in premature and mature infants and children. Am. J. Dis. Child. 91:1, 1956.

67. Knotek, Z., and Schmidt, P.: Pathogenesis, incidence and possibilities of preventing alimentary nitrate methemoglobinemia in infants. Pediatrics 34:78, 1964.

68. Johnson, R. R., Navone, R., et al.: An unusual epidemic of methemoglobinemia. Pediatrics 31:222, 1963.

69. Fisch, R. O., Berglund, E. B., et al.: Methemoglobinemia in a hospital nursery. J.A.M.A. 185:760, 1963.

70. Graubarth, J., Bloom, C. J., et al.: Dye poisoning in the nursery. J.A.M.A. 128:1155, 1945.

71. Scott, E. P., Prince, G. E., et al.: Dye poisoning in infancy. J. Pediatr. 28:713, 1946.

72. Martin, H., and Huisman, T. H. J.: Formation of ferrihaemoglobin of isolated human hemoglobin types by sodium nitrite. Nature (Lond.) 200:898, 1963.

73. Climie, C. R., McLean, S., et al.: Methaemoglobinaemia in mother and foetus following continuous epidermal analysis with prilocaine. Br. J. Anaesth. 39:155, 1967.

74. Harris, J. W., and Kellermeyer, R. W.: *The Red Cell*. Cambridge, Harvard University Press, 1970, p. 495.

75. Jaffé, E. R.: The reduction of methemoglobin in human erythrocytes incubated with purine nucleosides. J. Clin. Invest. 38:1555, 1959.

76. Harley, J. D., and Celermajer, J. M.: Neonatal methaemoglobinaemia and the "red-brown" screening-test. Lancet 2:1223, 1970.

77. Evelyn, K. A., and Malloy, H. T.: Microdetermination of oxyhemoglobin, methemoglobin, and sulfhemoglobin in a single sample of blood. J. Biol. Chem. 126:655, 1938.

78. Hegesh, E., Calmanovici, N., et al.: New method for determining ferrihemoglobin reductase (NADH-methemoglobin reductase) in erythrocytes. J. Lab. Clin. Med. 72:339, 1968.

79. Goluboff, N., and Wheaton, R.: Methylene blue–induced cyanosis and acute hemolytic anemia complicating the treatment of methemoglobinemia. J. Pediatr. 58:86, 1961.

80. Goldstein, G., and Doull, J.: Treatment of nitrite-induced methemoglobinemia with hyperbaric oxygen. Proc. Soc. Exp. Biol. Med. 138:137, 1971.

Chapter 13

The Structure and Function of Normal and Abnormal Human Hemoglobins

by H. Franklin Bunn

The determination of the structure of hemoglobin is one of the milestones of molecular biology. This information has provided an intimate understanding of the way in which the molecule functions physiologically. Study of hemoglobin has proved relevant to a number of biomedical disciplines. This protein is a suitable prototype of a general class of enzymes whose function depends on allosteric transition. Recently, attention has been focused on environmental factors, including 2,3-DPG, hydrogen ion concentration, and CO_2, which can modify and perhaps regulate the behavior of hemoglobin within the red cell. Comparisons of primary amino acid sequences of animal hemoglobins have provided new and independent phylogenetic insights. Furthermore, surveys of human hemoglobin phenotypes have been of considerable utility in the study of population genetics. Finally, certain variants are responsible for specific clinical syndromes. As we shall discuss in detail, in most cases the clinical features can be directly attributed to lesions at a submolecular level. This chapter will first present a detailed account of interrelationships between hemoglobin structure and function. Secondly, we will consider the various factors in health and disease which can modify hemoglobin's physiologic role. This background information will be useful in the consideration of inherited and acquired disorders of hemoglobin structure and function.

HEMOGLOBIN STRUCTURE

Hemoglobin is a tetramer approximately $50 \times 55 \times 64$ Å, with a molecular weight of 64,400. It consists of two pairs of unlike polypeptide chains. A heme group, ferroprotoporphyrin IX, is linked covalently at a specific site to each globin polypeptide chain. When heme iron is in the reduced (ferrous) state, it can bind reversibly with gaseous ligands, such as oxygen or carbon monoxide. The ferrihemes of methemoglobin are incapable of oxygenation but can bind tightly to anionic ligands, such as cyanide. Such modifications of hemoglobin cause specific alterations in its color and absorption spectrum.

Human Hemoglobin Phenotypes

There are at least five genes which govern globin synthesis in developing human erythroblasts, resulting in the formation of structurally different globin polypeptide chains, designated as α, β, γ, δ, and ϵ. There is indirect evidence in man (1) and primates (2) that the α chain gene is duplicated. Furthermore, structural heterogeneity in the γ chain can be best explained by the presence of more than one gene (3). The β, γ, and δ genes are probably closely linked. Chapter 15 contains a detailed description of hemoglobin synthesis. This subject is directly relevant to an understanding of the thalassemia syndromes in which there is a defect in the synthesis of one (or rarely two) globin subunit(s).

The various normal human hemoglobins are listed in Table 13-1. In adult red cells, Hb A ($\alpha_2\beta_2$) comprises over 90 per cent of the total. The structure and function of this molecule will be described in detail below.

About 2.5 per cent of the hemoglobin is A$_2$ ($\alpha_2\delta_2$). This minor component is evenly distributed among red cells (4). Its functional behavior is probably the same as that of Hb A (5). The amino acid sequence of the δ chain differs from that of the β chain in 10 out of 146 residues (6). The increased percentage of Hb A$_2$ in beta thalassemia is a useful diagnostic aid (see Chapter 15). In addition, Hb A$_2$ may be increased in megaloblastic anemia (7). In contrast, Hb A$_2$ is decreased in iron deficiency (8) and sideroblastic anemias (9). The marked differences in the amount of Hb A$_2$ in these disorders of red cell maturation may be related to the fact that the relative rate of synthesis of this minor component is markedly curtailed in the final stages of erythoid development (10).

The main component during fetal development is Hb F ($\alpha_2\gamma_2$). Most other mammalian species which have been tested appear to have structurally different fetal hemoglobin(s). Exceptions include the horse and perhaps the dog (11). The γ chain differs from the β chain in 39 of 146 residues (6). The oxygen equilibrium of purified Hb F is nearly identical to that of Hb A. However, fetal red cells have a considerably higher oxygen affinity than do adult red cells. This phenomenon has been observed in a number of mammalian species (12) and may facilitate the transport of oxygen across the placenta. In the human, this discrepancy in relative oxygen affinities is due to the diminished interaction of Hb F with red cell organic phosphates (13) (see below). Hemoglobin F has the special property of being remarkably resistant to denaturation at extremes of pH. This may be owing to increased bonding energy between α and γ chains. The measurement of alkali-resistant hemoglobin (14, 15) has proved to be a very useful, although indirect, way of estimating the content of Hb F within a hemolysate. However, this approach tends to underestimate Hb F (16).

The red cells of the newborn contain about 80 per cent Hb F, 20 per cent Hb A, and less than 0.5 per cent Hb A$_2$. Occasionally, Hb Bart's (γ_4) may be detected in trace amounts in a normal neonate. Shortly before birth there is a switch from γ chain to β chain synthesis. Hemoglobin F falls steadily following birth, approaching a nadir at about age four months. However, the rate of fall of fetal hemoglobin is quite variable. Fetal hemoglobin persists longer

TABLE 13-1.

HEMOGLOBIN	STRUCTURE	% OF NORMAL ADULT HEMOLYSATE	INCREASED IN	DECREASED IN
A	$\alpha_2\beta_2$	92		
A$_2$	$\alpha_2\delta_2$	2.5	β thalassemia Megaloblastic anemia Malaria	Iron deficiency Sideroachrestic anemia
A$_{IA}$	Not known	<1		
A$_{IB}$	Not known	2		
A$_{IC}$	α_2 (β-N-Hexose)$_2$	6	Diabetes mellitus	
F	$\alpha_2\gamma_2$	<1	Fetal red cells β thalassemia Marrow "stress" (sickle cell anemia, pernicious anemia, and so forth)	
H	β_4	0	α thalassemias	
Bart's	γ_4	0	α thalassemias	
Gower I	ϵ_4	0	Early embryo	
Gower II	$\alpha_2\epsilon_2$	0	Early embryo	

in infants born prematurely (17). Conversely, there is a more rapid decline of Hb F in neonates having increased red cell turnover, such as in erythroblastosis fetalis. Although alkali denaturation is not sensitive enough to detect Hb F in normal adults, recent fluorescent labeling has demonstrated this hemoglobin distributed rather unevenly among red cells (18). Hemoglobin F is increased to a variable extent in several hereditary disorders, including beta thalassemia, hereditary persistence of fetal hemoglobin, and sickle cell anemia. In addition, increased levels of fetal hemoglobin may be seen in a variety of acquired hematologic disorders, including megaloblastic anemia, aplastic anemia, and leukemias. The mechanism underlying this return to γ chain synthesis is unknown.

Hemoglobin H and Hb Bart's are tetramers of β chains and γ chains, respectively. In order for hemoglobin to function physiologically, a tetramer must consist of pairs of α and non-α chains. In contrast, Hb H and Hb Bart's have very high oxygen affinity and absent heme-heme interaction and Bohr effect. These hemoglobins are found to a variable extent in patients with the different types of alpha thalassemia (see Chapter 15).

The Gower hemoglobins ($\alpha_2\epsilon_2$ and ϵ_4) are detectable only in the first three months of fetal development. Epsilon chains are probably synthesized in the yolk sac. Only minute amounts of these hemoglobins can be obtained. For this reason their structure and function have not been determined.

When the hemoglobin from normal adult red cells is carefully analyzed by column chromatography (19, 20), several minor components can be detected which have a lower isoelectric point than the main Hb A. These are designated A_{IA}, A_{IB}, and A_{IC}. On zone electrophoresis at alkaline pH, these components appear as a smear (sometimes designated as Hb A_3) running anodal to the main component. Hemoglobin A_{IC} comprises about 6 per cent of the hemoglobin in normal adult red cells. Its structure differs from Hb A only at the N-terminal amino group of each β chain which is covalently linked to a hexose by a Schiff base (21). It is not known how this structural modification takes place. This glycoprotein is increased in patients with diabetes

mellitus (22, 23). About 20 per cent of Hb F in the developing fetus has a similar structural modification: the N-terminus of each γ chain is acetylated (Hb F_1).

Primary and Secondary Structure

Alpha chains contain 141 amino acids in linear sequence, while β, δ, and γ chains have 146 residues. The amino acid sequence for each of these polypeptide chains has been established by chemical methods, including enzymatic digestion followed by amino acid analysis of the resultant peptides. More recently, Edman degradation has also proved useful for determining primary amino acid sequence. Such techniques are used for the structural analysis of human hemoglobin variants. Furthermore, at this time the primary structure has been worked out for some 12 mammalian hemoglobins and for a few avian and amphibian hemoglobins. This information has been useful in analyzing phylogenetic development. There is strong structural homology among the α chains and β chains of various species. Certain segments of these proteins have specific amino acids in common. Such invariant residues have been shown to be crucial to the molecule's function.

Approximately 80 per cent of hemoglobin in its native state is in the form of an α helix. X-ray analysis has shown that each chain consists of eight helical segments. Figure 13–1 shows the amino acid residues of the α and β chains of human hemoglobin that are oriented in an α helix. Thus, individual residues can be assigned to a specific helix. This has been very useful in establishing homology between globin subunits. Thus, the heme iron is linked covalently to histidines at F8, the eighth residue of the F helix. This is residue number 87 of the α chain and 92 of the β chain (Fig. 13–1). All hemoglobins whose primary structures are known have a histidine residue at F8.[*] Residues which have charged

---

[*]Two of the variant M hemoglobins are exceptions. These will be discussed in detail at the end of this chapter.

side groups, such as lysine, arginine, and glutamic acid, lie on the surface of the molecule in contact with the surrounding water solvent. Uncharged residues are commonly oriented toward the hydrophobic interior of the molecule.

Tertiary and Quaternary Structure

From x-ray analyses of crystals of horse and human hemoglobins, Perutz and his associates in Cambridge, England, have determined the conformation of human hemoglobin in three-dimensional space. This remarkable achievement has allowed considerable progress in relating structure to function (24). The hemoglobin tetramer was shown to be a spheroid with a diameter of about 55 Å and a single (dyad) axis of symmetry. The polypeptide chains are themselves folded in such a way that the four heme groups lie in clefts on the surface of the molecule equidistant from one another. The x-ray analysis is of sufficiently high resolution that the coordinates of all atoms in the molecule are known to within 2.5 Å. As shown in Figure 13–2, the molecule undergoes a marked change in quaternary conformation upon deoxygenation. The β chains rotate apart by about 7 Å. In contrast, liganded forms, including oxyhemoglobin, carboxyhemoglobin, and cyanmethemoglobin, all appear to be isomorphous. This conformational change which occurs upon removal and addition of ligand accounts for the many known differences in physical and chemical properties of oxy- and deoxyhemoglobins. Perutz has shown that deoxyhemoglobin is stabilized in a constrained or taut (T) configuration by the presence of inter- and intra-subunit salt bonds (Fig. 13–3) (24). These include residues responsible for the Bohr effect and for the binding of 2,3-diphosphoglycerate (see below). Upon the addition of ligand, such as oxygen, these salt bonds are sequentially broken. The fully liganded hemoglobin is in the so-called relaxed (R) configuration. In this state, there is considerably less bonding energy between subunits, and the liganded molecule is able to dissociate reversibly according to the

following reaction: $\alpha_2\beta_2 \rightleftharpoons 2\,\alpha\beta$. The formation of $\alpha\beta$ dimers is apparently required for hemoglobin to bind to haptoglobin (25, 26) and to traverse renal glomeruli (27). As shown in Figure 13–2, each subunit in the tetramer is oriented toward the two unlike subunits in different ways (i.e., α_1-β_1 and α_1-β_2). The dissociation of the liganded tetramer into dimers occurs at the $\alpha_1\beta_2$ interface. Thus, there is stronger binding energy between α_1 and β_1 subunits than between α_1 and β_2 subunits. Furthermore, during oxygenation and deoxygenation (T $\rightleftharpoons$ R), there is considerable movement along the $\alpha_1\beta_2$ interface. As we shall discuss at the end of this chapter, hemoglobin variants having an amino acid substitution in this region may have markedly abnormal functional properties.

HEMOGLOBIN FUNCTION

The oxygenation of hemoglobin, as depicted by the classic sigmoid oxyhemoglobin dissociation curve shown in Figure 13–4, can be characterized by two important properties: oxygen affinity and heme-heme interaction.[*] A convenient index of oxygen affinity is P_{50} or partial pressure of oxygen at which hemoglobin is half saturated. If the oxyhemoglobin dissociation curve is shifted to the right, P_{50} is increased and oxygen affinity is decreased. Thus, P_{50} varies inversely with oxygen affinity. As discussed in detail in this section, P_{50} is dependent on temperature, pH, organic phosphates, and pCO_2. Under physiologic conditions (37° C, pH 7.40, 2,3-DPG = 5 mM, pCO_2-40 mm. Hg), the P_{50} of normal adult blood is 26 mm. Hg.

---

[*]Data obtained from measurement of oxygen equilibria can be satisfactorily fitted by the empirical Hill equation: $\left(\dfrac{Y}{1-Y}\right) = \left(\dfrac{pO_2}{P_{50}}\right)^n$, where Y is the fractional saturation of hemoglobin with oxygen and n is an index of heme-heme interaction. If such interaction were absent, n would be 1.0. (This is true for myoglobin and isolated hemoglobin subunits.) If heme-heme interaction were maximal, n would be 4.0. In pure solutions of phosphate-free hemoglobin A, n is about 3.0, while in whole blood n is somewhat less (2.6 to 2.8). At the extremes of oxygen saturation (Y < 0.1, > 0.9), the experimentally derived points deviate from the Hill equation.

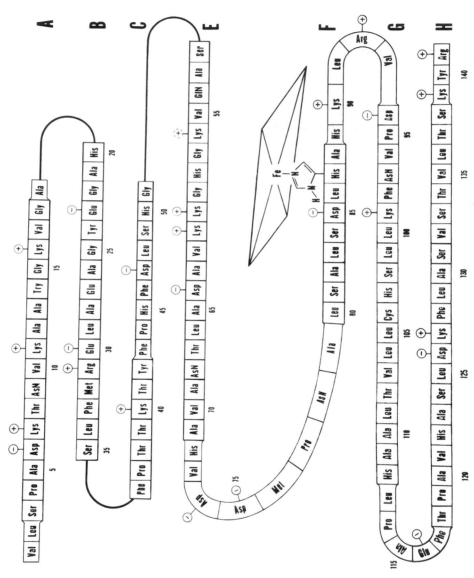

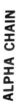

ALPHA CHAIN

Figure 13–1. The primary structure of the α chain (A) and β chain (B) of human hemoglobin A. Those residues which are oriented in the form of an α helix are depicted by squares, and nonhelical residues by rectangles. The site for heme attachment is shown. [From Murayama, M., In *Molecular Aspects of Sickle Cell Hemoglobin*. Nalbandian, R. M. (ed.), 1971. Courtesy of Charles C Thomas, Publisher, Springfield, Illinois.]

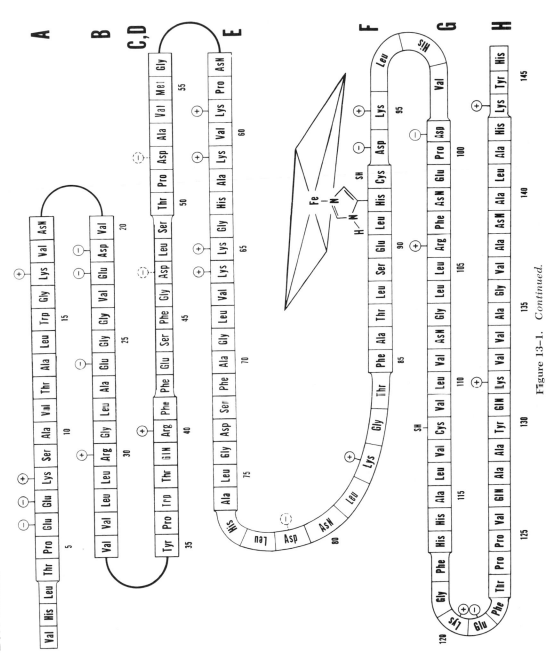

Figure 13–1. *Continued.*

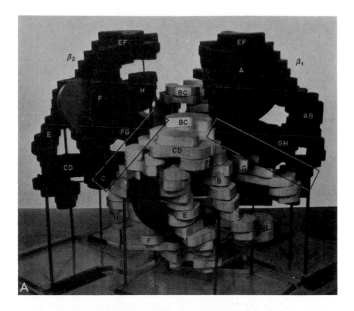

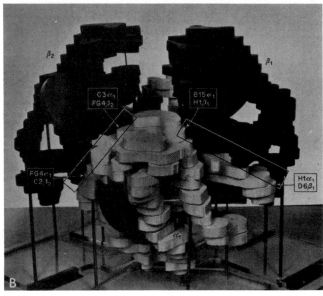

Figure 13–2. A three dimensional model of hemoglobin, based on x-ray crystallographic analysis (*A*, deoxy; *B*, oxy). The α chains are shown in white, the β chains in black. The heme groups are depicted as disks inserted into each subunit. There is an axis of symmetry which is parallel to the plane of the paper. Note the difference in conformation between oxy- and deoxyhemoglobin. (From Muirhead, H., Cox, J. M., et al.: J. Mol. Biol. 28:117, 1967.)

Heme-heme Interaction (Subunit Cooperativity)

When hemoglobin is partially saturated with oxygen, the affinity of the remaining hemes on the tetramer for oxygen increases markedly. This phenomenon can be considered in terms of the two hemoglobin conformations: deoxy (or T) and oxy (or R). The T form has a lower affinity for ligands such as O_2 or CO than has the R form. At some point during the sequential addition of oxygen to the four hemes of the molecule, a transition from the T to R configura-

tion occurs. At this point the oxygen affinity of the partially liganded molecule increases markedly. In this way, hemoglobin can be considered a prototype of a more general class of allosteric enzymes, in which the interaction of protein and ligand alters binding affinity for another ligand at a different site on the same macromolecule. How can the oxygenation of one heme cause sufficient alteration in the environment of other heme groups to affect their oxygen affinity? In deoxyhemoglobin, the iron atoms lie outside the plane of the porphyrin ring by about 0.75 Å (24). The

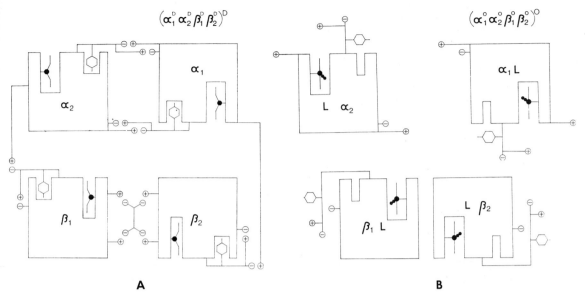

Figure 13–3. Diagrammatic representation of the quaternary configurations of deoxy-(A) and oxyhemoglobin (B). The salt bonds which stabilize the deoxy conformation are broken when the molecule is oxygenated. [From Perutz, M. F.: Nature (Lond.) 228:726, 1970.]

trigger which effects this allosteric transition appears to be the decrease in the atomic radius of heme iron upon the addition of ligand. The smaller iron atom is now able to snap into the plane of the porphyrin ring. The resulting alteration in heme configuration is amplified by a series of intra- and inter-subunit interactions, so that the environments of other hemes within the molecule are perturbed, resulting in increased ligand affinity. From a comparison of the immediate environment around the α and β chain hemes, Perutz (24) has suggested that the first molecule of oxygen is more likely to bind to an α chain. However, there is no information as to which of the remaining three hemes would be oxygenated next. In general, the structural conformation of partially liganded hemoglobin is not well understood.

Heme-heme interaction (or subunit cooperativity) has considerable physiologic importance. This phenomenon dictates the familiar sigmoid shape of the oxyhemoglobin dissociation curve (Fig. 13–4). The S-shaped curve allows a considerable amount of oxygen to be released over a relatively small drop in oxygen tension. In contrast, heme proteins, such as myoglobin and hemoglobins H and Bart's, which lack subunit cooperativity, have a hyperbolic curve, which allows much less oxygen unloading.

The Bohr Effect

In 1904, Bohr, Hasselbalch, and Krogh found that the oxygen affinity of hemoglobin decreased with increasing CO_2 tension (28). It was later shown that this phenomenon was largely pH-dependent. Thus,

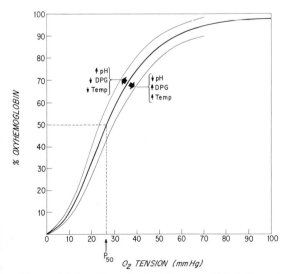

Figure 13–4. The principal factors which influence the position of the oxyhemoglobin dissociation curve.

over a pH range of 6.0 to 8.5, oxygen affinity varies directly with pH (Fig. 13–4). A thermodynamic corollary of this statement is that oxyhemoglobin is a stronger acid than deoxyhemoglobin. Under physiologic conditions, a molecule of hemoglobin releases about 2.8 protons upon oxygenation:

$$Hb \cdot H + 4 \ O_2 \rightleftharpoons Hb \ (O_2)_4 + 2.8 \ H^+$$

The recent high-resolution x-ray data in conjunction with experiments of Kilmartin and Rossi-Bernardi (29) on chemically modified hemoglobins have permitted the identification of specific acid groups on hemoglobin which yield Bohr protons. In deoxyhemoglobin, the N-terminus of each α chain is linked by a salt bridge to the C-terminus of the other α chain. This can be shown schematically as follows:[*]

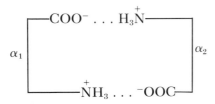

As part of the conformational isomerization that occurs upon oxygenation, these salt bonds are broken with the release of protons. These residues contribute about 25 per cent to the (physiologic or "alkaline") Bohr effect. About 50 per cent of the Bohr effect is due to intra-subunit salt bonds between the positively charged imidazole of β146-histidine and negatively charged carboxyl of β94-aspartate. These salt bridges are among the important bonds which stabilize the deoxy conformation (see Fig. 13–3).

The Bohr effect offers a physiologic advantage in facilitating oxygen unloading. At the tissue level, the drop in pH due to CO_2 influx lowers oxygen affinity, thereby enhancing oxygen release. In contrast, at the pulmonary level the increase in pH due to the efflux of CO_2 increases oxygen affinity and uptake. As further testimony to its adaptational advantage, the Bohr effect is present to a varying degree in virtually all mammalian species which have been tested and also in many types of lower animals.

---

[*]Also depicted diagrammatically in Figure 13–3.

Carbamino Formation

CO_2 affects hemoglobin function in two ways. It readily diffuses into red cells where, in the presence of a generous supply of carbonic anhydrase, carbonic acid is rapidly formed. The resulting decrease in pH lowers oxygen affinity (the Bohr effect). In addition, CO_2 can bind free amino groups on hemoglobin to form carbamino complexes according to the following reaction:

$$RNH_2 + CO_2 \rightleftharpoons RNHCOO^- + H^+$$

Only nonprotonated amino groups can react with CO_2. The only amino groups in globin whose pK's are low enough to be partially nonprotonated at physiologic pH are at the N-termini. It has been recently demonstrated that hemoglobin whose N-terminal amino groups are blocked by cyanate are no longer able to bind CO_2 (29). Deoxyhemoglobin forms carbamino complexes more readily than oxyhemoglobin. From this, it follows that, at a given pH, CO_2 lowers oxygen affinity. This effect becomes more marked as carbamino formation is favored at increasing pH. It is likely that, under physiologic conditions, the relatively low pH of the red cell precludes extensive carbamino formation. It is estimated only about 10 per cent of the CO_2 produced by tissue metabolism is transported to the lungs in the form of carbamino hemoglobin (30). Garby et al. (31) have estimated that under physiologic conditions approximately 0.03 mole of CO_2 becomes bound per mole of oxygen released at oxyhemoglobin saturation between 50 per cent and 100 per cent.

The Interaction of 2,3-Diphosphoglycerate with Hemoglobin

The red cell differs metabolically from other tissues in two important ways: (1) it derives its chemical energy almost solely through anaerobic glycolysis; and (2) it contains an unusually high concentration of 2,3-diphosphoglycerate (2,3-DPG). Normal human erythrocytes contain about 5 mM 2,3-DPG per liter (of packed cells), a concentration about threefold that of the next most abundant organic phosphate, ATP. The *raison d'être* for such large amounts of 2,3-DPG in red cells remained elusive until the recent discovery that this compound is a potent modifier of hemoglobin function (32, 33). The addition of increasing amounts of 2,3-DPG to a solution of purified A hemoglobin results in a progressive lowering of oxygen affinity. This helps to explain the long-known fact that whole blood has a lower oxygen affinity than a solution of dialysed hemoglobin, studied under comparable conditions. The mechanism by which 2,3-DPG lowers oxygen affinity was clarified when Benesch and his associates (34) measured its binding to hemoglobin by a modified form of equilibrium dialysis. They showed that, at physiologic pH and ionic strength, 2,3-DPG bound to human deoxyhemoglobin rather avidly ($K = 2 \times 10^{-5}$ M) in a 1:1 molar ratio (1 molecule 2,3-DPG per hemoglobin tetramer). Furthermore, under these conditions, 2,3-DPG did not bind to liganded forms of hemoglobin such as oxy, carboxy, and cyanmet hemoglobin. Furthermore, 2,3-DPG bound to hemoglobin H (β_4) but not to isolated α chains (34). As shown in Figure 13–5, 2,3-DPG is a strongly anionic compound. At physiologic pH, a molecule of 2,3-DPG has about three and one-half negative charges (Fig. 13–5). From their binding data, the Benesches concluded that 2,3-DPG binds electrostatically with the β chains of deoxyhemoglobin, probably in the central cavity along the dyad axis of symmetry.

A comparison of the reactivities of a number of human and animal hemoglobins of known structure with 2,3-DPG

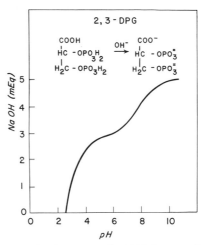

Figure 13–5. Structure of 2,3-DPG. From this titration curve, it is apparent that, at physiologic pH, 2,3-DPG has about 3.5 negative charges per molecule.

has suggested that the N-terminal amino groups of the β chains and the imidazoles of β143-histidine are specific residues responsible for 2,3-DPG binding (5). Model fitting and, more recently, x-ray diffraction measurements have confirmed these as the likely binding sites (24, 35). Figure 13–6 shows a cross section of deoxyhemoglobin, with a plane perpendicular to that of Figure 13–2. The A and H helices of the β chains are shown (compare with Fig. 13–2). 2,3-DPG is situated in the central cavity between the two β chains. Its negative charges are neutralized by positively charged groups mentioned above. In addition, β82-lysine and β2-histidine are also thought to be involved in 2,3-DPG binding (35). In light of this information on the binding of 2,3-DPG to hemoglobin, the fol-

Figure 13–6. The site at which 2,3-DPG binds to deoxyhemoglobin. This diagram shows a cross section of the molecule, the plane of which is perpendicular to the dyad axis of symmetry, at the level of the A and H helices of the β chains (compare with Fig. 13–2). This diagram shows salt bonds between the phosphates of 2,3-DPG and positively charged groups at βNA1-valine and βH21-histidine.

HUMAN DEOXYHEMOGLOBIN

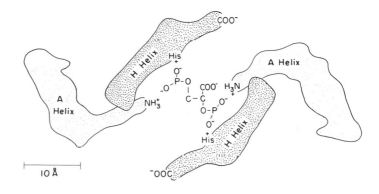

lowing simple reaction can be written:

$$Hb \cdot DPG + 4\ O_2 \rightleftharpoons Hb\ (O_2)_4 + DPG$$

[Note the similarity of this equation and that for the Bohr effect (see above).] This equilibrium expresses both the preferential binding of 2,3-DPG for deoxyhemoglobin and the 1:1 stoichiometry. Furthermore, changing concentrations of 2,3-DPG shift the oxygen binding equilibrium in accord with the experimental results cited above.

Other red cell phosphates are also able to lower the oxygen affinity of hemoglobin. In their degree of interaction with hemoglobin, these compounds can be ranked as follows: 2,3-DPG > ATP > ADP > AMP > pyrophosphate > inorganic phosphate. Although there is almost one-third as much ATP as 2,3-DPG in normal red cells, ATP probably plays an insignificant role in mediating intracellular hemoglobin function. First, it binds to deoxyhemoglobin less avidly than does 2,3-DPG. Second, an appreciable portion of red cell ATP is bound to magnesium ion. This complex does not interact with hemoglobin (36).

Alterations in Blood O₂ Affinity

The position of the oxyhemoglobin dissociation curve may be influenced by a number of factors. As depicted in Figure 13–4, the three most important are temperature, pH, and red cell 2,3-DPG. Oxygen affinity varies inversely with temperature. This phenomenon is physiologically appropriate since, during a period of relative hyperthermia, oxygen requirement is likely to be increased. The decrease in oxygen affinity at elevated body temperature would facilitate unloading of oxygen to tissues. The effects of pH and 2,3-DPG on hemoglobin function have already been discussed. Conventionally, whole blood oxygen saturation curves are corrected to pH 7.40, 37°C. Thus, the main variable leading to fluctuation in the position of the standardized oxygen dissociation curve is red cell 2,3-DPG.

Other factors which can also contribute include red cell ATP, pCO₂, alteration in cell hemoglobin concentration (MCHC),

and extracellular-intracellular pH gradient. Red cell ATP and pCO₂ are probably of limited importance for reasons mentioned above. Changes in MCHC can affect oxygen affinity in several ways (37). Whether the range of MCHC encountered clinically is sufficiently large to influence hemoglobin function is not yet clear. Finally, because of the Bohr effect, any factor which changes the pH of the red cell relative to the plasma will be reflected in altered oxygen affinity. For example, any increase within the cell of an impermeant anion, such as hemoglobin or 2,3-DPG, will lower intracellular pH as a manifestation of the Gibbs-Donnan equilibrium.

How does the oxygen affinity of the blood affect the delivery of oxygen to tissues? Lucid discussions of this topic have appeared in recent reviews by Oski and Gottlieb (38) and Finch and Lenfant (39). At a given blood flow and hemoglobin concentration, the amount of oxygen that is unloaded is dependent upon the position of the oxyhemoglobin dissociation curve. As shown in Figure 13–7, a shift to the right increases oxygen release at a given mixed venous oxygen tension (40 mm. Hg). This is owing to the fact that at this Δ pO₂, a steeper portion of the oxygen dissociation curve is encompassed. In contrast, if the oxyhemoglobin dissociation curve is shifted to the left, less oxygen is unloaded at a given Δ pO₂. From another viewpoint, it is apparent that if the oxygen affinity of the blood is increased, a given amount of oxygen will be extracted at a lower oxygen tension. This phenomenon bears on several clinical states to be discussed in detail, including hemoglobin variants associated with polycythemia, and blood transfusion therapy.

Decreased Oxygen Affinity: Adaptation to Hypoxia

The uptake of oxygen [vO₂ (ml. per min.)] by a given tissue or the whole organism can be expressed in the following equation (40):

$$vO_2 = 1.39 \cdot Hb \cdot Q(Sat_A - Sat_V)$$

where 1.39 = number of ml. of O₂ which can bind to 1 g. hemoglobin; Hb = the hemoglobin concentration of the blood

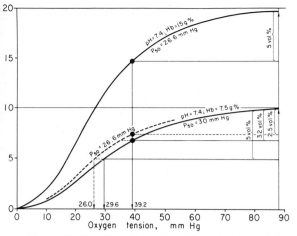

Figure 13–7. The effect of a shift to the right of the oxyhemoglobin dissociation curve of an anemic individual on oxygen unloading. In this figure, the ordinate is oxygen content in vol. %, rather than % oxyhemoglobin (as in Fig. 13–4). As shown in the upper curve, a normal individual with a normal red cell mass carries 19.5 ml. oxygen per 100 ml. of arterial blood. At a mixed venous pO_2 of 39.2 mm. Hg, 5 vol. % oxygen has been unloaded. In contrast, the anemic patient shown here has an arterial oxygen content of only 10 vol. %. At the same mixed venous pO_2 of 39.2 mm. Hg, 2.5% vol. % O_2 would be unloaded if the red cells had normal oxygen affinity (dotted line). However, because of decreased oxygen affinity, the anemic patient unloads 3.2 vol. % at this ΔpO_2. In order for this patient to unload 5 vol. %, the mixed venous pO_2 would have to fall to 29.6 mm. Hg. Without the compensation of a right-shifted oxyhemoglobin dissociation curve, the mixed venous pO_2 would be even lower (26.0 mm. Hg). (From Torrance, J., Jacobs, P., et al.: New Engl. J. Med. 283.165, 1970.)

(g. per 100 ml.); Q = blood flow (ml. per min.); and Sat_A, Sat_V are the per cent saturation of arterial and venous blood, respectively. During hypoxic stress, the organism may increase vO_2 by altering one or more of these three variables:

1. Increase in cardiac output ($\uparrow Q$).
2. Increase in red cell mass ($\uparrow Hb$).
3. Decrease in whole blood oxygen affinity [$\uparrow (Sat_A - Sat_V)$].

A shift to the right (decreased whole blood oxygen affinity) is encountered in various types of hypoxic states (Table 13–2). In each case, the decreased oxygen affinity can be explained by increased levels of red cell 2,3-DPG. In fact, Oski and his associates have shown a close correlation between P_{50} (an index of oxygen affinity) and 2,3-DPG in a number of diverse dis-

orders (38, 39) (Fig. 13–8). It is apparent from such data that a decreased whole blood oxygen affinity, mediated through increased red cell 2,3-DPG, is a rather general phenomenon in a variety of hypoxic states.

2,3-DPG levels are quite variable in patients with chronic lung disease. It is difficult to assess the physiologic significance of the oxygen-binding curve in these individuals, since there may be concomitant respiratory acidosis (see below).

The regulation of the intracellular concentration of 2,3-DPG is poorly understood. (This subject is discussed in detail in references 38 and 41.) In particular, it is not clear how red cell 2,3-DPG can increase as much as twofold in various hypoxic states. One contributing factor may be an increase in intracellular pH. Patients with hypoxia of varying sorts commonly have respiratory alkalosis. Secondly, if there is an increase in the amount of oxygen extracted per red cell, intracellular pH will increase slightly because of the Bohr effect. Alkalosis not only stimulates glycolysis in general but may also affect the relative degree of 2,3-DPG formation and catabolism via the Rapoport-Luebering cycle (see

TABLE 13–2. DISPLACEMENT OF THE OXYHEMOGLOBIN DISSOCIATION CURVE IN VARIOUS CLINICAL DISORDERS

I. Shift to the right
  A. Increase in red cell 2,3-DPG
    1. High altitude adaptation
    2. Pulmonary hypoxemia
    3. Cardiac right to left shunt
    4. Severe anemia; decrease in red cell mass
    5. Congestive heart failure
    6. Decompensated hepatic cirrhosis
    7. Thyrotoxicosis
    8. Hyperphosphatemia (ATP also increased)
  B. Functionally abnormal hemoglobin variants (see Table 13–7)
II. Shift to the left
  A. Decrease in red cell 2,3-DPG
    1. Septic shock
    2. Severe acidosis
    3. Following transfusion of stored blood
    4. Hypophosphatemia
    5. Panhypopituitarism
    6. Neonatal respiratory distress syndrome
  B. Functionally abnormal hemoglobin variants (see Table 13–7)
  C. Methemoglobinemia
  D. Carbon monoxide intoxication

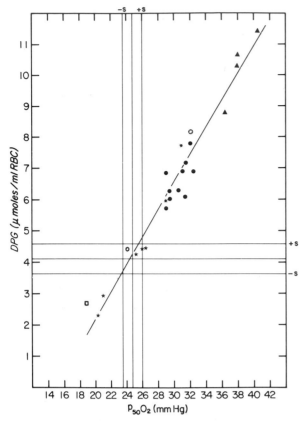

Figure 13-8. Correlation between alterations in red cell 2,3-DPG and P_{50} in a variety of clinical disorders: cyanotic congenital heart disease ●, pyruvate kinase deficiency ▲, hexokinase deficiency □, septic shock ★, postseptic shock ✪, thyrotoxicosis ☉, glucose-6-phosphate dehydrogenase deficiency ○. (From Oski, F. A., Gottlieb, A. J., et al.: Med. Clin. North Am. 54:731, 1970.)

the membrane and therefore not available for interaction with hemoglobin (45). Certain drugs such as propranolol and perhaps endogenous humoral substances may release 2,3-DPG from the membrane, thereby effecting a significant increase in P_{50}.

3. Hormones may influence the absolute level of 2,3-DPG within the red cell. The thyroid hormones, T_3 and T_4, can increase 2,3-DPG in vitro by stimulation of diphosphoglycerate mutase (46). This probably explains increased red cell 2,3-DPG found in a patient with thyrotoxicosis (38). Low levels are found in patients with panhypopituitarism (47) but not in those with myxedema (unpublished observation). The administration of androgens to patients with chronic renal failure can cause a 60 per cent increase in red cell 2,3-DPG (48).

Although decreased oxygen affinity of

Fig. 13-9). A decreased oxygen saturation may also enhance red cell 2,3-DPG because of the specific binding of this organic phosphate to deoxyhemoglobin. The resulting fall in the intracellular concentration of free 2,3-DPG would relieve product inhibition of diphosphoglycerate mutase, thereby stimulating its own synthesis (42). There are several additional factors which may influence the level of 2,3-DPG within red cells.

1. 2,3-DPG falls during in vivo cell aging (43). This may explain why patients with hypoplastic anemia and a relatively old population of red cells have considerably lower 2,3-DPG than those with hemolysis and a comparable degree of anemia (44).

2. It is possible that a significant portion of the total red cell 2,3-DPG is bound to

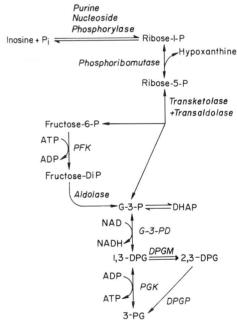

Figure 13-9. The pathway of red cell inosine metabolism to 2,3-DPG. Also shown in this figure is the Rapoport-Luebering cycle, wherein 1,3-DPG can be converted to 3-PG either directly or via 2,3-DPG. PFK, phosphofructokinase; G-3-PD, glyceraldehyde-3-phosphate dehydrogenase; PGK, phosphoglycerate kinase; DPGM, diphosphoglycerate mutase; DPGP, diphosphoglycerate phosphatase; P_i, inorganic phosphate; G-3-P, glyceraldehyde-3-phosphate; DHAP, dihydroxyacetone phosphate; 3-PG, 3-phosphoglycerate. (From Oski, F. A., Travis, S. E., et al.: The in vitro restoration of red cell 2,3-diphosphoglycerate levels in banked blood. Blood 37:52–58, 1971, by permission of Grune & Stratton.)

blood containing normal hemoglobin is generally due to increased 2,3-DPG, some exceptions have been reported. Zimmon (49) has found that the marked right shift (6 to 10 mm. Hg) that develops in patients with hepatic encephalopathy is due to a plasma factor rather than to an increase in red cell 2,3-DPG. A smaller shift to the right (1 to 3 mm. Hg) has also been observed in coronary sinus blood of patients with angina pectoris during atrial pacing (50). This phenomenon also could not be explained by any measurable increase in 2,3-DPG. It is possible that in these instances some humoral factor effects release of organic phosphates from the red cell membrane or perhaps increases the hydrogen ion gradient between the inside and outside of the red cell. Finally, patients with hereditary spherocytosis who have undergone splenectomy have normal red cell 2,3-DPG but reduced whole blood oxygen affinity (shift to the right of 2.6 mm. Hg) (51).

The fact that decreased red cell oxygen affinity is so commonly found in hypoxic states does not constitute proof that the phenomenon is adaptive or beneficial to the organism. Is the position of the oxyhemoglobin dissociation curve an important determinant of tissue oxygenation? This question defies an easy answer. It is a technical challenge to monitor oxygen uptake at the cellular level. Clearly, there is a marked pO_2 gradient between the red cell and various intracellular organelles, such as mitochondria. Therefore, it is difficult to say what constitutes a critical pO_2 for various tissues. Recently, Oski and his associates (52) have addressed themselves to this problem by comparing the hemodynamics of two teen-agers whose oxygen dissociation curves were abnormally fixed because of congenital red cell enzyme defects. Patient 1, with hexokinase deficiency, had a low red cell 2,3-DPG and consequently a left-shifted curve. In contrast, patient 2, with pyruvate kinase deficiency, had elevated red cell 2,3-DPG and a right-shifted curve. Both individuals were equally anemic. However, patient 1 was a semi-invalid, while patient 2 had no appreciable limitations. During graded exercise, the patient with the left-shifted curve had a prompter fall in mixed venous pO_2 and a more marked increase in cardiac output.

The position of the oxygen dissociation curve appears to be one important determinant of red cell mass, presumably via erythropoietin control. From a comparison of various hemolytic disorders, Bellingham and Huehns (53) showed a strong correlation between hemoglobin level and oxygen affinity. The polycythemia secondary to high affinity hemoglobin variants also attests to this relationship (see below).

Increased Oxygen Affinity

From considerations developed here, it appears that increased whole blood oxygen affinity may lead to relative tissue hypoxia. In addition to the congenital disorders discussed above, a "shift to the left" may be encountered in a number of acquired conditions (Table 13–2). As previously noted, the concentration of 2,3-DPG in the red cell is markedly pH-dependent. Accordingly, patients with severe acidosis generally have low 2,3-DPG. The pH "corrected" oxygen dissociation curves of patients with acidosis are left shifted. However, their in vivo curve may be normally placed because the Bohr effect counterbalances the reduction in red cell 2,3-DPG. If metabolic acidosis is rapidly corrected by the infusion of bicarbonate, the prompt rise in blood pH is reflected in a proportional increase in oxygen affinity (the Bohr effect). However, there is a lag of several hours before the red cell 2,3-DPG increases to normal (54). During this time there is a "shift to the left" in both the in vivo and the in vitro oxygen dissociation curves. This phenomenon may compromise tissue oxygenation in patients who have diminished cardiovascular reserves. Low red cell 2,3-DPG has been documented in patients with septic shock (38, 55). This may be in part because of concomitant metabolic acidosis. The resulting left shift in the oxyhemoglobin dissociation curve probably accounts for the increased mixed venous oxygen content often encountered in this condition. Again, an increase in blood oxygen affinity may have untoward effects in patients who already have severe circulatory dysfunction. Low red cell 2,3-DPG may be a grave prognostic sign in patients with sepsis.

In addition to metabolic acidosis, acquired deficiency of red cell 2,3-DPG (and ATP) may also be encountered in patients who have hypophosphatemia, due either to diarrhea (56, 57) or to inadequate phosphate supplements during hyperalimentation (58). In both instances, the expected shift to the left has been observed (56–58).[*] In addition hemolysis may occur in association with rigid red cells (57). Finally, as mentioned above, low red cell 2,3-DPG has been found in patients with pituitary insufficiency (47).

During the first week of storage of blood in acid-citrate-dextrose (ACD), red cells become depleted of 2,3-DPG and, as a result, have increased oxygen affinity (60, 61, 43). Thus, patients who are transfused with large amounts of such blood will have a "left-shifted" oxyhemoglobin dissociation curve (60). The clinical significance of this phenomenon has not been established. At the least, it is safe to say that the recipient does not derive the full physiologic benefit from blood depleted in 2,3-DPG. Following infusion of such donor cells into normal volunteers, their content of 2,3-DPG returns to normal within 6 to 24 hours (62, 63). Considerable attention is now being focused on ways of modifying storage media in order to preserve red cell 2,3-DPG and normal hemoglobin function. 2,3-DPG and P_{50} are better maintained in citrate-phosphate-dextrose (CPD), because of the higher pH of this medium (64). The addition of inosine to the storage medium provides ribose 1-phosphate, a substrate which feeds directly into the glycolytic pathway (Fig. 13–9). The resulting increase in 2,3-DPG is potentiated by the adding of pyruvate or methylene blue, both of which oxidize NADH to NAD, thereby providing cofactor for the glyceraldehyde-3-phosphate dehydrogenase reaction (65). The transfusion of large amounts of blood stored in inosine may be limited by hyperuricemia resulting from the catabolism of this purine.

The oxygen affinity of fetal blood is substantially higher than that of maternal blood (P_{50}: 19 mm. Hg compared with 26 mm. Hg for normal maternal blood). This difference may be of physiologic importance in facili-

---

*In contrast, the slight but significant shift to the right encountered in normal children may be due to physiologically increased levels of plasma phosphate, resulting in a marked increase in red cell ATP and a modest increase in red cell 2,3-DPG (59).

tating the transport of oxygen across the placenta. The content of 2,3-DPG in the red cells of the newborn is at least as high as that of maternal red cells. Furthermore, phosphate-free hemoglobins A and F have nearly the same oxyhemoglobin dissociation curves. The higher oxygen affinity of fetal blood is due to the fact that 2,3-DPG interacts less strongly with Hb F than with Hb A (13). This can be explained by a comparison of the primary structure of the β and γ chains. β143-Histidine of Hb A has been shown to be an important binding site for 2,3-DPG (see above). In Hb F, γ143 is serine. This uncharged residue would not participate in electrostatic binding with 2,3-DPG.

The increased oxygen affinity of fetal blood may become a handicap to the infant following birth. Oski and his associates have found that the mortality of premature newborns (weighing between 750 and 1250 g. at birth) is markedly reduced if these infants are given an exchange transfusion of fresh adult blood, having near normal oxygen affinity (66). These investigators are also studying this therapy in newborns with respiratory distress syndrome (RDS). Infants with this disorder have even more left-shifted curves and lower red cell 2,3-DPG than do normal infants of comparable age and weight. Recent mortality statistics for premature infants with and without RDS are shown in Table 13–3.

HUMAN HEMOGLOBIN VARIANTS

There are several different molecular and genetic mechanisms which are thought to be responsible for the various types of hemoglobinopathies found in man (Table 13–4). A detailed discussion of hemoglobin synthesis in general and the thalassemias in particular appears in Chapter 15. Furthermore, certain types of mutations, such as nonhomologous crossing-over and errors in globin chain termination, will also be covered in that chapter.

Over 160 structurally different human hemoglobin variants have been discovered to date. Each of these constitutes a single amino acid substitution in one of the globin polypeptide chains. In each case the substitution of one residue for another can be

TABLE 13–3. PROPHYLACTIC EXCHANGE TRANSFUSION STUDIES ON NEWBORN INFANTS WEIGHING 1250 GRAMS OR LESS AT BIRTH

	TOTAL	LIVED	DIED
A. Without Severe Respiratory Distress			
Weight Group (750–1000 g.)			
Exchange tx.	6	5 (80%)	1 (20%)
Control	8	3 (38%)	5 (62%)
Weight Group (1001–1250 g.)			
Exchange tx.	16	15 (94%)	1 (6%)
Control	14	8 (57%)	6 (43%)
All Weights (750–1250 g.)			
Exchange tx.	21	19 (90%)	2 (10%)
Control	22	11 (50%)	11 (50%)
B. With Severe Respiratory Distress			
Severe RDS (750–1200 g.)			
Exchange tx.	9	0	9 (100%)
Control	12	0	12 (100%)
Severe RDS (>1250 g.)			
Exchange tx.	16	13 (81%)	3 (19%)
Control	17	8 (47%)	9 (53%)

accounted for by a substitution of a single nucleotide base in the DNA or mRNA codon according to the widely accepted genetic code. In addition, two variants have been encountered thus far in which two amino acid substitutions have been encountered at separate sites on a given globin subunit (Table 13–4). There are about 50 per cent more known β chain mutants than α chain mutants. This is somewhat surprising since there is circumstantial evidence that there are two structural genes for the α chain, one for the β chain (1). In addition, six δ chain and eight γ chain mutants have been described. The vast majority of these hemoglobin variants are unassociated with any clinical manifestations. Many were discovered during the course of large population surveys. The most useful diagnostic tool for the detection of new hemoglobin variants is zone electrophoresis. This technique separates hemoglobins which differ in charge.

Those abnormal hemoglobins which are of clinical importance can be conveniently classified into one of four groups outlined

TABLE 13–4. MOLECULAR BASES OF HUMAN HEMOGLOBIN ABNORMALITIES

	EXAMPLES
I. Unbalanced subunit synthesis (deficient mRNA)	β thalassemia, α thalassemia, and so forth
II. Single amino acid substitution in subunit (single nucleotide base substitution in codon)	β chain—S, C, D, E, etc. (101 variants) α chain—(55 variants) γ chain—(8 variants) δ chain—(6 variants)
Two amino acid substitutions in subunit (two separate nucleotide base substitutions)	C—Harlem (104) J—Singapore (105)
III. Amino acid deletions [deletion of corresponding codon(s)]	Freiburg (106) Gun Hill (107) Leiden (108) Niteroi (109) Tochigi (110) St. Antoine (122) Tours (123)
IV. Error in termination of subunit (nucleotide base substitution in termination codon)	α chain : Constant Spring (111) β chain : ? Tak (112)
V. Fusion hemoglobins (nonhomologous crossover)	The Lepores : $\delta\beta$ (113–115) Miyada : $\beta\delta$ (116) Kenya : $\gamma\beta$ (117)
VI. Frame shift mutation [deletion of one (or two) nucleotide bases in codon]	Wayne (118)

TABLE 13–5. CLINICALLY IMPORTANT HUMAN HEMOGLOBIN VARIANTS

I. Hemolysis due to decreased hemoglobin solubility
    A. Hemoglobin S disease
    B. Hemoglobin C disease
II. Unstable hemoglobins: congenital Heinz body hemolytic anemia
III. Hemoglobins having abnormal oxygen binding
    A. High oxygen affinity
       1. Familial erythrocytosis
    B. Low oxygen affinity
       1. Familial cyanosis (hemoglobin Kansas)
       2. "Anemia" (hemoglobin Seattle)
IV. The M hemoglobins
       1. Familial cyanosis

in Table 13–5. Sickle hemoglobin (Hb S, $\alpha_2\beta_2^{6\ \text{Val}}$) is by far the most frequently encountered variant worldwide. Furthermore, sickle cell anemia has the most severe clinical manifestations of any of the hemoglobinopathies. The sickle syndromes and Hb C disease will be covered in detail in Chapter 14.

The Unstable Hemoglobins (Congenital Heinz Body Hemolytic Anemia)

In 1952, Cathie described a patient with congenital nonspherocytic hemolytic anemia associated with jaundice, splenomegaly, and pigmenturia (67). Subsequently, other patients with similar clinical findings were suspected of having a structurally abnormal hemoglobin by the fact that their hemolysates formed a precipitate readily upon heating. In most cases, structural analyses have demonstrated mutant hemoglobins. So-called congenital Heinz body hemolytic anemia (CHBA) constitutes an important type of congenital hemolytic disease.

CHBA has an autosomal dominant pattern of inheritance. Thus, affected individuals are heterozygotes. Because the spleen selectively removes the Heinz bodies, the unstable hemoglobin comprises only a minority (10 to 30 per cent) of the total. As expected in the heterozygous state, the remainder is predominantly normal Hb A. Because of the low gene frequency, the homozygous state would be a very rare event and almost certainly in-

compatible with life. Such genetic considerations also apply to erythrocytosis due to a hemoglobin variant having abnormally high oxygen affinity (see below). A sizable minority of cases of CHBA appear to have arisen because of a spontaneous mutation, both parents being unaffected. Viewed another way, of the 19 instances of apparent spontaneous mutations among hemoglobin variants reported to date, 16 involved patients with CHBA (68). This is not surprising, since most cases are sufficiently severe that medical attention and evaluation are sought. In contrast, the chances are very remote of finding an asymptomatic individual with a hemoglobin variant due to a spontaneous mutation. Furthermore, the potential of patients with severe CHBA to have fit offspring may be markedly decreased.

Thus far, at least 39 structurally different unstable hemoglobin variants have been documented (Table 13–6). [A very thorough review of this subject has appeared recently (69).] About three-fourths of these are β chain mutants. Many of them are amino acid substitutions in the vicinity of the heme pocket (Fig. 13–10). The majority are neutral substitutions, such as Hb Köln ($\beta^{98\ \text{Val}\rightarrow\text{Met}}$). Such an alteration in primary structure may cause considerable perturbations in the hydrophobic interior of the molecule. Considering the nature of such amino acid substitutions, it is not surprising that many of these variants have electrophoretic mobility identical to that of Hb A. Others may appear as single or multiple bands having isoelectric points higher than that of Hb A. If these bands are no longer visible following the addition of hemin to the hemolysate, it is likely that the abnormal electrophoretic mobility was due to heme loss (or heme displacement) rather than to an alteration in the charge of a globin subunit. Five of the unstable hemoglobins* are leucine to proline substitutions. Proline residues are unable to participate in the formation of an α helix. Thus, instability may result from disruption of the secondary structure of the subunit.

The mechanism by which CHBA red cells hemolyze is still uncertain. There is

---

*Hemoglobins Genova ($\alpha_2\beta_2^{28\ \text{Pro}}$), Santa Ana ($\alpha_2\beta_2^{88\ \text{Pro}}$), Sabine ($\alpha_2\beta_2^{91\ \text{Pro}}$), Caspar ($\alpha_2\beta_2^{106\ \text{Pro}}$), Bibba ($\alpha_2^{136\ \text{Pro}}\beta_2$).

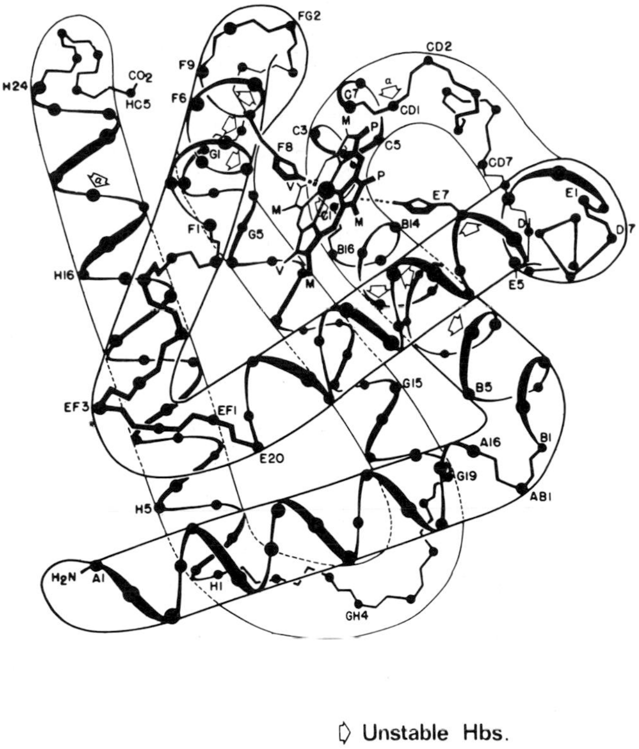

Figure 13-10. Three dimensional representation of β chain. Arrows indicate sites of substitutions in a number of unstable hemoglobins. Note their proximity to the heme group. [This figure was constructed by Dr. Helen Ranney, using a three dimensional diagram of myoglobin which was published by Dickerson, R. E., In *The Proteins: Composition, Structure and Function*. Vol. II. 2nd ed. Neurath, H. (ed.), New York, Academic Press, 1964, pp. 603-778.]

◊ Unstable Hbs.

convincing evidence that normally placed hemes confer considerable stability to their globin subunits. In many of the hemoglobin variants associated with CHBA, the amino acid substitution prevents a stable hemoglobin linkage. Once the heme becomes detached from its normal position in the cleft on the surface of the involved subunit (70), it probably binds nonspecifically on another site on the globin (71). Both spectrophotometric and electron spin resonance measurements indicate that hemichrome may be an intermediate step in the denaturation of unstable hemoglobins (72). Following heme displacement, the globin subunits probably dissociate from their parent tetramer and aggregate to form a coccoid precipitate, having the morphologic characteristics of a Heinz body. Winterbourne and Carrell have recently shown that both the Heinz bodies and the heat-induced precipitate in CHBA contain equal amounts of α and β chains and probably a normal complement of heme (73). Red cells containing Heinz bodies have reduced filterability (74) and are likely to be entrapped in the microcirculation. There is convincing morphologic evidence that

these Heinz bodies become selectively removed or "pitted" during circulation through the sinusoids of the spleen (75). Therefore, it is not surprising that patients who have undergone splenectomy have an increased number of Heinz bodies and, in most cases, a greater percentage of the hemoglobin variant relative to normal Hb A.

The degree of instability of these hemoglobin variants and, therefore, the extent of hemolysis vary considerably. In some, such as Hb Zürich, an additional oxidant stress, such as the ingestion of certain drugs, is required for significant hemolysis. In contrast, patients with Hb Hammersmith have continuous and marked red cell breakdown. The degree of anemia is influenced not only by the severity of the hemolysis but also by the ability of the blood to unload oxygen (53). Thus, patients having unstable variants of high oxygen affinity, such as Hb Köln (71), may have a near normal hemoglobin level, i.e., compensated hemolysis. In contrast, the hemoglobin level is apt to be much lower in patients having variants with decreased oxygen affinity, such as Hb Hammersmith.

These pathophysiologic considerations

TABLE 13–6. UNSTABLE HEMOGLOBIN VARIANTS

NAME	STRUCTURE	HELICAL SITE	INCLUSION BODIES	HEAT LABILE	DARK URINE
I. β Chain Variants					
Leiden	$\alpha_2\beta_2^{6\text{ or }7\ \text{Glu}\rightarrow\text{O}}$	A3 or A4	?		
Sogn	$\alpha_2\beta_2^{14\ \text{Leu}\rightarrow\text{Arg}}$	A11			
Lyon	$\alpha_2\beta_2^{17,\ 18\ \text{Lys, Val}\rightarrow\text{O}}$	A14,15	+		
Freiburg	$\alpha_2\beta_2^{23\ \text{Val}\rightarrow\text{O}}$	B5		+	
Riverdale-Bronx	$\alpha_2\beta_2^{24\ \text{Gly}\rightarrow\text{Arg}}$	B6		+	0
Savannah	$\alpha_2\beta_2^{24\ \text{Gly}\rightarrow\text{Val}}$	B6	+	+	
St. Louis, SaoPaulo	$\alpha_2\beta_2^{28\ \text{Leu}\rightarrow\text{Gln}}$	B10	+		
Genova	$\alpha_2\beta_2^{28\ \text{Leu}\rightarrow\text{Pro}}$	B10	+	+	±
Tacoma	$\alpha_2\beta_2^{30\ \text{Arg}\rightarrow\text{Ser}}$	B12	0	+	0
Philly	$\alpha_2\beta_2^{35\ \text{Tyr}\rightarrow\text{Phe}}$	C1	+	+	?
Hammersmith	$\alpha_2\beta_2^{42\ \text{Phe}-\text{Ser}}$	CD1	+	+	+
Louisville; Bucuresti	$\alpha_2\beta_2^{42\ \text{Phe}\rightarrow\text{Leu}}$	CD1	+	+	
Zürich	$\alpha_2\beta_2^{63\ \text{His}\rightarrow\text{Arg}}$	E7	+	+	+
Toulouse	$\alpha_2\beta_2^{66\ \text{Lys}\rightarrow\text{Glu}}$	E10	0	+	0
Sidney	$\alpha_2\beta_2^{67\ \text{Val}\rightarrow\text{Ala}}$	E11	+	+	+
Bristol	$\alpha_2\beta_2^{67\ \text{Val}\rightarrow\text{Asp}}$	E11	+	+	
Shepherds Bush	$\alpha_2\beta_2^{74\ \text{Gly}\rightarrow\text{Asp}}$	E18			
St. Antoine	$\alpha_2\beta_2^{74,\ 75\ \text{Gly, Leu}\rightarrow\text{O}}$	E18,19	+	+	0
Seattle	$\alpha_2\beta_2^{76\ \text{Ala}\rightarrow\text{Glu}}$	E20	+	+	+
Bryn Mawr	$\alpha_2\beta_2^{85\ \text{Phe}\rightarrow\text{Ser}}$	F1	+	0	0
Tours	$\alpha_2\beta_2^{88\ \text{Leu}\rightarrow\text{O}}$	F4	+	+	0
Boras	$\alpha_2\beta_2^{88\ \text{Leu}\rightarrow\text{Arg}}$	F4	+	+	
Santa Ana	$\alpha_2\beta_2^{88\ \text{Leu}\rightarrow\text{Pro}}$	F4	+	+	+
Gun Hill	$\alpha_2\beta_2^{\sim 91-97\rightarrow\text{O}}$	F + FG	0	+	0
Sabine	$\alpha_2\beta_2^{91\ \text{Leu}\rightarrow\text{Pro}}$	F7	+	+	
Istanbul; St. Etienne	$\alpha_2\beta_2^{92\ \text{His}\rightarrow\text{Gln}}$	F8	+	+	
Köln	$\alpha_2\beta_2^{98\ \text{Val}\rightarrow\text{Met}}$	FG5	+	+	+
Rush	$\alpha_2\beta_2^{101\ \text{Glu}\rightarrow\text{Gln}}$	G3			
Casper	$\alpha_2\beta_2^{106\ \text{Leu}\rightarrow\text{Pro}}$	G8	+	+	
Peterborough	$\alpha_2\beta_2^{111\ \text{Val}\rightarrow\text{Phe}}$	G13	0	+	
Wien	$\alpha_2\beta_2^{130\ \text{Tyr}\rightarrow\text{Asp}}$	H8		+	
Olmstead	$\alpha_2\beta_2^{141\ \text{Leu}\rightarrow\text{Arg}}$	H19			
II. α Chain Variants					
Torino	$\alpha^{43\ \text{Phe}\rightarrow\text{Val}}\beta_2$	CD1	+	+	?
L-Ferrara	$\alpha_2^{47\ \text{Asp}\rightarrow\text{Gly}}\beta_2$	CD5			
Hasharon	$\alpha_2^{47\ \text{Asp}\rightarrow\text{His}}\beta_2$	CD5	0	±	0
Russ	$\alpha_2^{51\ \text{Gly}\rightarrow\text{Arg}}\beta_2$	CD9			
Ann Arbor	$\alpha_2^{80\ \text{Leu}\rightarrow\text{Arg}}\beta_2$	F1			
Etobicoke	$\alpha_2^{84\ \text{Ser}\rightarrow\text{Arg}}\beta_2$	F5		+	
Setif	$\alpha_2^{94\ \text{Asp}\rightarrow\text{Tyr}}\beta_2$	G1		+	0
Dakar	$\alpha_2^{112\ \text{His}\rightarrow\text{Gln}}\beta_2$	G19			
Bibba	$\alpha_2^{136\ \text{Leu}\rightarrow\text{Pro}}\beta_2$	H19	+	+	

°After splenectomy.

†The remainder of the references are cited in the review by White and Dacie (69). Dr. D. Labie and Prof. H. Lehmann kindly provided additional information.

TABLE 13–6.   UNSTABLE HEMOGLOBIN VARIANTS (*Continued*)

HB (G./100 ML.)	RETICULOCYTES (%)	% ABNORMAL HB	OXYGEN AFFINITY	COMMENTS	REFERENCE†
I. β Chain Variants					
11–13	3–6	30	Decreased	Mild; one residue deletion	
12–13	0.4	30		No clinical manifestations	
14.5	4	37	Increased		(146)
13	9	30	Increased	Cyanosis; ↑ methemoglobin, one residue deletion	
11–12	10	30			
4→6°	50	15–30		Severe	(119)
12	10	29	Increased	15% methemoglobin	(120)
8→14°	10–50	10–25	Increased		(122)
13	4		Increased	No clinical manifestations	
12–14	2–8				
6→7°	20–50	30	Decreased		
11–13	7–9	30–35	Decreased		(121)
11–12	5–6	25	Increased	Mild; drug-sensitive	
12–15	1–4	40	Normal	No clinical manifestations	
12	8	30			
7→7°	37	36	Decreased	Severe hemolysis	
12–13	5–8		Increased	Impaired reactivity of hb with 2,3-DPG	
11	8	25	Normal		(122)
9–10	3	40	Decreased		
12–14	8–15		Increased	Compensated hemolysis	(76)
13–14°	9	20	Increased		(122)
8→12°		10			
8→13°	6–28	10		Two hemes per molecule	
13.5	4–10	30	Increased	5 residue deletion; two hemes per molecule	
8–10°	35–65	8		Two hemes per molecule	(123)
9→13°	4	12–15	Increased		(124, 125)
11–13	5–16	10		Commonest of unstable hbs; mild to moderate	
					(126)
4–7→13°	20–90		Increased		(127)
12	3.5		Decreased	Mild	(128)
10°	43				
5→6°	3–8				
II. α Chain Variants					
8→12°	6–16	8	Decreased	Moderately severe; aggravated by drugs	
13–14	9	14–20	Normal	Mild	
Normal	1–5	14–19	Normal	Mild	
					(129)
12	10	2–12		Mild	
11–14	1–3	15	Increased	Mild	
		15	Slightly low		(130)
Normal		10		Mild	
6–7.5	6–16	5–11		Severe	

explain a number of the clinical features of this disorder. Patients usually present in early childhood with a hemolytic anemia, accompanied by jaundice and splenomegaly. The red cell morphology is somewhat variable. Often, patients with a functioning spleen have normal-looking red cells. Slight hypochromia and basophilic stippling are not uncommon. The blood may have to be incubated in order to bring out Heinz bodies (69). In some cases, red cells appear as if a bite had been taken from a margin. It is tempting to speculate that at this site a Heinz body had been pitted. Following splenectomy, red cells appear much more abnormal. Heinz bodies are larger and more numerous. The extent of clinical symptomatology varies markedly with the degree of anemia. As mentioned above, one of the two parents is involved in about two-thirds of cases. Some patients with CHBA give a history of passing dark urine. Although this pigment has not been completely characterized, it appears to be a dipyrrole (mesobilifuscin). This may be the consequence of aberrant (perhaps nonenzymatic) heme catabolism.

The following studies are valuable in establishing the diagnosis of CHBA:

1. *Demonstration of Heinz bodies.* Fresh blood is treated with a supravital stain, such as 1 per cent methyl violet. If the patient's spleen is intact, it may be necessary to incubate (either 60 minutes with acetylphenylhydrazine or with no additive for 24 to 48 hours). A positive test reveals the presence of purple-stained red cell inclusions, often several per cell and up to 1 μ in diameter.

2. *Heat instability.* Freshly prepared hemolysates of the patient and a normal control are diluted in 0.1 M phosphate buffer, pH 7.4. (Final hemoglobin concentration: 0.5 to 1 g. per 100 ml.) After incubating one hour at 50° C, a precipitate will appear in the solution containing an unstable hemoglobin variant. Recently Carrell and Kay (147) have shown that hemolysates containing an unstable hemoglobin will form a flocculent precipitate when incubated in 17 per cent isopropanol, pH 7.4.

3. *Hemoglobin electrophoresis.* Abnormal patterns have been observed in most cases of CHBA (see above discussion on molecular pathogenesis). In some instances, a high resolution method, such as isoelec-tric focusing, may be required to demonstrate an abnormal hemoglobin.

4. *Oxyhemoglobin dissociation curve.* The unstable hemoglobins frequently have abnormal oxygen affinity. A patient presented recently with compensated hemolysis, negative heat instability test, and normal hemoglobin electrophoresis (starch gel, pH 8.6), but a positive incubated Heinz body preparation and increased oxygen affinity of both whole blood and a phosphate-free hemoglobin solution (76). She was found to have a new unstable variant, Hb Bryn Mawr ($\alpha_2\beta_2^{85\ Phe\rightarrow Ser}$).

If these tests are negative in a patient with congenital nonspherocytic hemolytic anemia, a defect of one of the red cell glycolytic enzymes is likely.

The treatment of CHBA is primarily supportive. Anemia is rarely severe enough to warrant blood transfusion. Oxidant drugs should be avoided. Like others with chronic hemolysis, these patients have an increased requirement for folic acid. Those with severe hemolysis should benefit from prophylactic folate therapy. The red cell mass may fall precipitously during a period of bone marrow suppression, such as that resulting from folate deficiency or acute infection. Although patients with severe hemolysis may benefit by splenectomy, this operation is not curative. Because of the risk of bacterial sepsis in infants and young children who have been splenectomized, this treatment should be postponed until the child is over 5 years old. The diagnostic tests cited above become more abnormal following splenectomy. For this reason, in some cases the diagnosis may not be definitely established until after the operation.

Hemoglobin Variants Having Abnormal Oxygen Binding

In 1966, Charache, Weatherall, and Clegg (77) described a family with erythrocytosis due to the presence of a hemoglobin variant, Hb Chesapeake ($\alpha_2^{92\ Leu}\beta_2$). Oxygen equilibria done on both whole blood and the isolated abnormal hemoglobin revealed a marked increase in oxygen affinity and a reduction in subunit cooperativity. Because of the "shift to the left" and consequent reduction in oxygen unloading, these individuals have compensatory erythrocytosis via increased production of erythropoietin (78). To date, twelve other variants with abnormally high oxygen affinity have been discovered (Table 13–7). In each case, affected family members have erythrocytosis. Unlike the unstable hemoglobins, which also may have abnormal oxygen affinity, these variants are unassociated with any hemolysis or abnormal red cell morphology.

The location and nature of the amino acid substitutions in these variants have been utilized to earmark specific sites on the hemoglobin molecule that are critical to its function. A number of these variants have substitutions at the $\alpha_1\beta_2$ interface. Such a structural perturbation may affect the conformational isomerization that exists between the oxy (R) and deoxy (T) forms. For example, there is good experimental evidence that the high oxygen affinity of Hb Bethesda is due to a decreased stability of the T form (79). In contrast, the low oxygen affinity of Hb Kansas can be related to decreased stability of the R form (80).

Other than erythrocytosis, affected individuals have minimal clinical manifestations. An exception may be one family with Hb Malmö, in which there is an increase in coronary artery disease in young members (81). In most cases, the increase in red cell mass is probably appropriate to ensure tissue oxygenation. Hemodynamic studies on individuals with Hb Yakima showed normal cardiac output and mixed venous oxygen tension (82).* Packed cell volumes seldom reach high enough levels so that increased blood viscosity necessitates therapeutic phlebotomy. Affected mothers have carried unaffected offspring to term. In this case, the oxygen affinity of the maternal blood was probably greater than that of the fetus. The lack of any untoward complications may be an argument against the physiologic importance of the normal differential oxygen affinity of fetal and maternal blood.

The possibility of a functionally abnormal hemoglobin should be considered in any case of unexplained erythrocytosis. A positive family history and an abnormal hemoglobin electrophoresis are very helpful. However, we have seen one child in whom neither of these findings was present (68). She was found to have Hb Bethesda, which apparently arose as a spontaneous mutation.

---

*In contrast, hemodynamic studies done on a patient with compensated hemolysis due to an unstable hemoglobin (San Francisco) having high oxygen affinity revealed a normal cardiac output but a decrease in mixed venous pO$_2$ (83). This individual is probably more hypoxic than one with Hb Yakima because of inability to develop supranormal red cell mass.

TABLE 13–7.　STABLE HEMOGLOBIN VARIANTS HAVING ABNORMAL O$_2$ AFFINITY

HEMOGLOBIN	STRUCTURE	BOHR EFFECT	CLINICAL FEATURES	REFERENCE
I. High Oxygen Affinity				
Chesapeake	$\alpha_2^{92\ Arg\to Leu}\beta_2$	Normal	Familial erythrocytosis	(131)
J-Capetown	$\alpha_2^{92\ Arg\to Gln}\beta_2$	Normal	? Mild erythrocytosis	(132)
Olympia	$\alpha_2\beta_2^{20\ Val\to Met}$	Not reported	Familial erythrocytosis	(133)
Malmö	$\alpha_2\beta_2^{97\ His\to Gln}$	Normal	Familial erythrocytosis	(134)
Yakima	$\alpha_2\beta_2^{99\ Asp\to His}$	Present	Familial erythrocytosis	(135)
Kempsey	$\alpha_2\beta_2^{99\ Asp\to Asn}$	Decreased	Familial erythrocytosis	(136)
Ypsilanti	$\alpha_2\beta_2^{99\ Asp\to Tyr}$	Not reported	Familial erythrocytosis	(137)
Brigham	$\alpha_2\beta_2^{100\ Pro\to Leu}$	Normal	Familial erythrocytosis	(138)
Little Rock	$\alpha_2\beta_2^{143\ His\to Gln}$	Normal	Familial erythrocytosis	(140)
Andrew-Minneapolis	$\alpha_2\beta_2^{144\ Lys\to Asn}$	Decreased	Familial erythrocytosis	(148)
Rainier	$\alpha_2\beta_2^{145\to Tyr\to Cys}$	Decreased	Familial erythrocytosis	(139)
Bethesda	$\alpha_2\beta_2^{145\ Tyr\to His}$	Decreased	Familial erythrocytosis	(141)
Hiroshima	$\alpha_2\beta_2^{146\ His\to Asp}$	Decreased	Familial erythrocytosis	(142)
II. Low Oxygen Affinity				
Kansas	$\alpha_2\beta_2^{102\ Asn\to Thr}$	Normal	Cyanosis	(143)
Seattle	$\alpha_2\beta_2^{76\ Ala\to Glu}$	Normal	"Anemia"	(144)
Yoshizuka	$\alpha_2\beta_2^{108\ Asn\to Asp}$	Decreased	None	(145)

M Hemoglobins

Cyanosis is due to an excess of either deoxyhemoglobin or methemoglobin in the blood. Congenital methemoglobinemia may be due to a deficiency of the enzyme diaphorase I (or NADH-dependent methemoglobin reductase), which enables red cell hemoglobin to be maintained in the reduced form. This disorder is discussed thoroughly in Chapter 12. A much more uncommon cause of congenital methemoglobinemia is the presence of one of the M hemoglobins. Like the other two classes of functionally abnormal hemoglobins discussed in detail in this chapter, the M hemoglobins are inherited according to an autosomal dominant pattern. Affected individuals present with cyanosis. They are otherwise asymptomatic. Generally, there is no evidence of anemia. The blood has a peculiar mahogany color. Spectral examination of the hemoglobin shows an abnormal pattern similar to but not identical to that of methemoglobin. Hemoglobin electrophoresis reveals the presence of an abnormal band with a slightly anodal mobility. The normal A and abnormal M hemoglobins may be separated more readily if the entire hemolysate is converted to methemoglobin prior to the electrophoresis (84).

Five M hemoglobins have been described (Table 13–8). The same variants have been detected in unrelated families all over the world. Four represent substitution of either the proximal (F8) or distal (E7) histidine by tyrosine. It is likely that the side group of the substituted tyrosine can serve as an internal ligand, stabilizing the heme iron in the ferric form. As anticipated, the M hemoglobins are functionally abnormal. The two α chain variants have both decreased oxygen affinity and decreased Bohr effect (85). The whole blood oxygen affinity of individuals with Hb M may be markedly decreased owing in part to the intrinsic functional abnormality of the hemoglobin variant and in part to increased 2,3-DPG in the red cell (86). Furthermore, individuals who have one of the β M hemoglobins may have mild hemolysis (87, 88).

In this disorder, no treatment is either indicated or possible. The M hemoglobins are perhaps of more interest and concern to the molecular biologist than to the individuals affected.

ACQUIRED ABNORMALITIES OF HEMOGLOBIN STRUCTURE AND FUNCTION

Hemoglobinopathies are generally classified among the "inborn errors of metabolism." Indeed, the genetic bases for these disorders are well understood. However, a number of acquired abnormalities of hemoglobin structure and function also deserve consideration. Some, such as methemoglobinemia and carbon monoxide poisoning, involve specific alterations of heme, the prosthetic group of the molecule.

TABLE 13–8.   PROPERTIES OF THE M HEMOGLOBINS (102)

M Hemoglobin	Synonyms	Structure	Helical Residue	Oxygen Affinity at P_{50}	Bohr Effect
M$_{Boston}$	Osaka Gothenburg	$\alpha_2^{58\ His\rightarrow Tyr}\beta_2$	E7	Decreased	Decreased
M$_{Iwate}$	Kankakee Oldenburg	$\alpha_2^{87\ His\rightarrow Tyr}\beta_2$	F8	Decreased	Decreased
M$_{Saskatoon}$	Chicago, Radom, Emory, Kurume	$\alpha_2\beta_2^{63\ His\rightarrow Tyr}$	E7	Normal	Present
M$_{Hyde\ Park}$		$\alpha_2\beta_2^{95\ His\rightarrow Tyr}$	F8	Normal	Present
M$_{Milwaukee-1}$		$\alpha_2\beta_2^{67\ Glu\rightarrow Val}$	E11	Decreased	Present

In contrast, modifications of globin structure may accompany such diverse entities as myeloproliferative disorders, diabetes mellitus, and lead poisoning.

Methemoglobinemia

Acquired methemoglobinemia is generally due to exposure to an agent capable of oxidizing heme iron to the ferric state. It has been demonstrated recently that individuals heterozygous for diaphorase I deficiency (NADH-dependent methemoglobin reductase) are much more likely than normals to develop clinically apparent methemoglobinemia following exposure to an oxidant stress (89). Chapter 12 contains a detailed treatment of the interrelationship between red cell metabolism and the reduction of methemoglobin.

The extent of methemoglobinemia depends not only on the dose of the toxic agent but also on the susceptibility of the exposed individual (see Chapter 12). If methemoglobin exceeds 1.5 g. per 100 ml. (10 per cent of the total hemoglobin), cyanosis is readily apparent. At a methemoglobin level of about 35 per cent, the affected individual becomes symptomatic, experiencing headache, weakness, and breathlessness. Levels in excess of 70 per cent are incompatible with life.

The toxicity of methemoglobinemia can be readily explained in terms of our current understanding of hemoglobin function, as outlined in the beginning of this chapter. The fact that a certain proportion of hemes is no longer able to bind oxygen is not a serious physiologic handicap per se. Thirty per cent methemoglobinemia is much more deleterious than a 30 per cent decrement in red cell mass, because the oxidized hemes have a profound effect on the remaining functional hemes in the hemoglobin tetramer. The conformation of methemoglobin (as well as carboxyhemoglobin and cyanmethemoglobin) is very close to that of oxyhemoglobin. Thus, a partially oxidized hemoglobin tetramer has the same tertiary and quaternary structure as a molecule which is comparably oxygenated. In each case, the affinity of the remaining hemes for oxygen is increased. For this reason, methemoglobinemia [as well as carbon monoxide (see below and Table 13–2)] causes a "shift to the left" of the oxyhemoglobin dissociation curve and, consequently, impaired unloading of oxygen to tissues. Recent high-resolution electrophoretic analysis has indicated that in hereditary methemoglobinemia both the α and β chain hemes are oxidized to approximately equal extent (90). However, there appears to be a heterogeneous distribution of methemoglobin among red cells in individuals with this disorder, the older red cells containing more methemoglobin (91–93). The treatment of methemoglobinemia is discussed in Chapter 12.

Carbon Monoxide Intoxication

Carbon monoxide (CO) has received belated recognition as an important and widespread industrial pollutant and toxin. This gas may be engendered from the combustion of any organic material but, in particular, that of hydrocarbons such as petroleum and tobacco tar. In addition, one mole of CO is formed endogenously in the breakdown of heme into bile pigment (see Chapter 3). Accordingly, individuals with significant hemolysis or ineffective erythropoiesis have a measurably increased amount of circulating carboxyhemoglobin.

Like oxygen, CO is a ligand which binds reversibly to hemoglobin when heme iron is in the reduced (ferrous) state. The toxicity of CO is due to its very high affinity for heme, approximately 210 times that of oxygen. Following an acute exposure, CO remains so tightly bound to hemoglobin that about four hours are required for an individual with normal ventilation to expel half of it. Because of its slow disappearance time, a toxic level of carboxyhemoglobin may accumulate from continued exposure to a relatively low dose of CO. CO also binds to other heme proteins, such as cytochrome P-450. Whether this contributes significantly to the toxicity of CO is not yet known.

As expected, the clinical manifestations of CO intoxication are directly related to the duration and extent of exposure. Impaired visual and time discrimination have been documented in individuals with carboxyhemoglobin levels of 5 per cent (94). Above approximately 20 per cent carboxyhemoglobin, more overt and subjective symptoms develop, such as headache, weakness, and so forth (94). At levels of

40 to 60 per cent, unconsciousness is followed by death. Like methemoglobinemia, the toxic effect of CO is primarily due to increased oxygen affinity of the blood.

The mechanism by which CO shifts the oxyhemoglobin dissociation curve to the left is identical to that of methemoglobin (see above). However, a given per cent carboxyhemoglobin appears to be more deleterious than a comparable level of methemoglobin. This may be because of a more even distribution of CO among red cells of all ages.

The treatment of carbon monoxide intoxication is directed primarily at removing the source of toxic exposure and facilitating the expulsion of the gas by the lungs. Thus, it is very important to maintain adequate ventilation. If the patient is transferred from room air to 100 per cent oxygen, the disappearance half-time for CO is reduced from four hours to one hour. Other therapeutic approaches, such as hyperbaric oxygen or exchange transfusion, may have theoretical merit but are not readily available.

Acquired Alterations of Globin Structure

Minor hemoglobin components may increase in certain hematologic disorders. As mentioned previously, Hb A_2 may be elevated in megaloblastic anemia and perhaps in malaria (95). Hemoglobin F may reach levels of about 5 per cent in such diverse diseases as aplastic anemia and pernicious anemia. Much higher levels of hemoglobin F have been encountered in children with chronic myelogenous leukemia. Finally, there are now several case reports of myeloproliferative disease, in which up to 10 per cent Hb H (β_4) has been documented (96).

Hemoglobin A_{IC}, the "main" minor component of normal adults, is significantly increased in diabetics (22, 23). This association is of considerable interest, since this hemoglobin is a glycoprotein. The exact nature of the hexose moiety in Hb A_{IC} is not yet known.

In some children with plumbism, an abnormal hemoglobin of rapid (anodal) electrophoretic mobility has been documented (97). This component was more frequently observed in those children with hypochromic red cells. The hemoglobin did not contain any measurable lead. It is possible that the lead exposure in some way mediated oxidation of globin sulfhydryl groups. However, the abnormal component differed electrophoretically from the mixed disulfide which can be formed in vitro from hemoglobin and glutathione (97). Thus, the structure of this acquired hemoglobinopathy is not yet known.

References

1. Lehmann, H., and Carrell, R. W.: Differences between α- and β-thalassemia: Possible duplication of the α-chain gene. Br. Med. J. 4:748, 1968.
2. Barnicot, N. A., Wade, P. T., et al.: Evidence for a second haemoglobin α-locus duplication in Macca-irus. Nature (Lond.) 228:379, 1970.
3. Schroeder, W. A., Huisman, T. H. J., et al.: Evidence for multiple structural genes for γ chain of human fetal hemoglobin. Proc. Natl. Acad. Sci. USA 60:537, 1968.
4. Heller, P., and Yakulis, V.: The distribution of hemoglobin A_2. Ann. N.Y. Acad. Sci. 165:54, 1969.
5. Bunn, H. F., and Briehl, R. W.: The interaction of 2,3-diphosphoglycerate with various human hemoglobins. J. Clin. Invest. 49:1088, 1970.
6. Dayhoff, M. O.: *Atlas of Protein Sequence and Structure.* Silver Spring, Maryland, National Biomedical Research Foundation, 1969.
7. Josephson, A. M., Masri, M. S., et al.: Starch block electrophoretic studies of human hemoglobin solutions. II. Results in cord blood, thalassemia and other hematologic disorders: Comparison with Tiselius electrophoresis. Blood 13:543, 1958.
8. Chernoff, A. I.: A method for the quantitative determination of hemoglobin A_2. Ann. N.Y. Acad. Sci. 119:557, 1964.
9. Reed, L. J., and Mollin, D. W.: Personal communication.
10. Rieder, R. F., and Weatherall, D. J.: Studies on hemoglobin biosynthesis: Asynchronous synthesis of hemoglobin A and hemoglobin A_2 by erythrocyte precursors. J. Clin. Invest. 44:42, 1965.
11. Bunn, H. F., and Kitchen, H.: Hemoglobin function in the horse: The role of 2,3-diphosphoglycerate in modifying the oxygen affinity of maternal and fetal blood. Blood 42:471, 1973.
12. Novy, M. J., and Parer, J. T.: Absence of high blood oxygen affinity in the fetal cat. Resp. Physiol. 6:144, 1969.
13. Bauer, C. I., Ludwig, I., et al.: Different effects of 2,3-diphosphoglycerate and adenosine triphosphate on the oxygen affinity of adult and fetal human hemoglobin. Life Sci. 7:1339, 1968.
14. Singer, K., Chernoff, A. I., et al.: Studies on abnormal hemoglobins. I. Their demonstration in sickle cell anemia and other hema-

tologic disorders by means of alkali denaturation. Blood 6:413, 1951.

15. Jonxis, J. H. P., and Visser, H. K. A.: Determination of low percentages of fetal hemoglobin in blood of normal children. Am. J. Dis. Child. 92:588, 1956.

16. Schroeder, W. A., Huisman, T. H. J., et al.: An improved method for quantitative determination of human fetal hemoglobin. Anal. Biochem. 35:235, 1970.

17. Garby, L., Sjölin, S., et al.: Studies on erythrokinetics in infancy. II. The relative rate of synthesis of haemoglobin F and haemoglobin A during the first months of life. Acta Paediatr. (Stockholm) 51:245, 1962.

18. Hosoi, T.: Studies on hemoglobin F within a single erythrocyte by fluorescent antibody technique. Exp. Cell Res. 37:680, 1965.

19. Allen, D. W., Schroeder, W. A., et al.: Observations on the chromatographic heterogeneity of normal adult and fetal human hemoglobins. J. Am. Chem. Soc. 80:1628, 1958.

20. Huisman, T. H. J., and Meyering, C. A.: Studies on the heterogeneity of hemoglobin. I. The heterogeneity of different human hemoglobin types in carboxymethylcellulose and in Amberlite IRC-50 chromatography: Qualitative aspects. Clin. Chim. Acta 5.103, 1960.

21. Bookchin, R. M., and Gallop, P. M.: Structure of hemoglobin A_{IC}: Nature of the N-terminal β chain blocking group. Biochem. Biophys. Res. Commun. 32:86, 1968.

22. Rahbar, S.: An abnormal hemoglobin in red cells of diabetics. Clin. Chim. Acta 22:296, 1968.

23. Trivelli, L. A., Ranney, H. M., et al.: Hemoglobin components in patients with diabetes mellitus. New Engl. J. Med. 284:353, 1971.

24. Perutz, M. F.: Stereochemistry of cooperative effects in haemoglobin. Nature (Lond.) 228:728, 1970.

25. Nagel, R. L., and Gibson, Q. H.: Kinetics and mechanism of the complex formation between hemoglobin and haptoglobin. J. Biol. Chem. 242:3428, 1967.

26. Bunn, H. F.: Effect of sulfhydryl reagents on the binding of human hemoglobin to haptoglobin. J. Lab. Clin. Med. 70:606, 1967.

27. Bunn, H. F., Esham, W. T., et al.: The renal handling of hemoglobin. I. Glomerular filtration. J. Exp. Med. 129:909, 1969.

28. Bohr, C., Hasselbalch, K., et al.: Ueber einen in biologischer Beziehung wichtigen Einfluss, den die Kohlensäuerespannung des Blutes auf dessen Sauerstoffbinding übt. Skand. Arch. Physiol. 16:402, 1904.

29. Kilmartin, J. V., and Rossi-Bernardi, L.: Inhibition of CO_2 combination and reduction of the Bohr effect in hemoglobin chemically modified at the α-amino groups. Nature (Lond.) 222:1243, 1969.

30. Rossi-Bernardi, L., Roughton, F. J. W., et al.: The effect of organic phosphates on the binding of CO_2 to human hemoglobin and CO_2 transport in the circulating blood, In Oxygen Affinity of Hemoglobin and Red Cell Acid-Base Status. Rorth, M., and Astrup, P. (eds.), Copenhagen, Munksgaard, 1972, p. 225.

31. Garby, L., Robert, M., et al.: Proton and car-

bamino-linked oxygen affinity of normal human blood. Acta Physiol. Scand. 84:482, 1972.

32. Chanutin, A., and Curnish, R. R.: Effect of organic and inorganic phosphates on the oxygen equilibrium of human erythrocytes. Arch. Biochem. Biophys. 121:96, 1967.

33. Benesch, R., and Benesch, R. E.: The effect of organic phosphates from the human erythrocyte on the allosteric properties of hemoglobin. Biochem. Biophys. Res. Commun. 26:162, 1967.

34. Benesch, R., and Benesch, R. E.: Intracellular organic phosphates as regulators of oxygen release by haemoglobin. Nature (Lond.) 221:618, 1969.

35. Arnone, A.: X-ray diffraction study of binding of 2,3-diphosphoglycerate to human deoxyhaemoglobin. Nature (Lond.) 237:146, 1972.

36. Bunn, H. F., Ransil, B. J., et al.: The interaction between erythrocyte organic phosphates, magnesium ion and hemoglobin. J. Biol. Chem. 246:5273, 1971.

37. Bellingham, A. J., Detter, J. C., et al.: Regulatory mechanisms of hemoglobin oxygen affinity in acidosis and alkalosis. J. Clin. Invest. 50:700, 1971.

38. Oski, F. A., and Gottlieb, A. J.: The interrelationship between red cell metabolites, hemoglobin and the oxygen equilibrium curve. Progr. Hematol. 7:33, 1971.

39. Finch, C. A., and Lenfant, C.: Oxygen transport in man. New Engl. J. Med. 286:407, 1972.

40. deVerdier, C. H., Garby, L., et al.: The role of 2,3-diphosphoglycerate in the erythrocyte as a regulator of tissue oxygen tension. Försvarsmedicin 5:258, 1969.

41. Rorth, M., Nygaard, S. F., et al. Oxygen affinity of hemoglobin and red cell metabolism during exposure to simulated high altitude, In Second International Conference on Red Cell Metabolism and Function. Brewer, G. (ed.), New York, Plenum Press, 1972, p. 361.

42. Oski, F. A., Gottlieb, A. J., et al.: The effects of deoxygenation of adult and fetal hemoglobin on the synthesis of red cell 2,3-diphosphoglycerate and its in vivo consequences. J. Clin. Invest. 49:400, 1970.

43. Bunn, H. F., May, M. H., et al.: Hemoglobin function in stored blood. J. Clin. Invest. 48:311, 1969.

44. Opalinski, A., and Beutler, E.: Creatine, 2,3-diphosphoglycerate and anemia. New Engl. J. Med. 285:483, 1971.

45. Oski, F. A., Miller, L. D., et al.: Oxygen affinity in red cells—changes induced in vivo by propranolol. Science 175:1372, 1972.

46. Synder, L. M., and Reddy, W. J.: Mechanism of action of thyroid hormones on erythrocyte 2,3-diphosphoglyceric acid synthesis. J. Clin. Invest. 49:1993, 1970.

47. Rodriguez, J. M., and Shahidi, N. T.: Erythrocyte 2,3-diphosphoglycerate in adaptive red cell volume deficiency. New Engl. J. Med. 285:479, 1971.

48. Parker, J. P., Beirne, G. J., et al.: Androgen-induced increase in red cell 2,3-diphosphoglycerate. New Engl. J. Med. 287:381, 1972.

49. Zimmon, D. S.: Changing oxyhemoglobin dissociation curve in hepatic encephalopathy. Clin. Res. 20:489, 1972.

50. Shappell, S. H., Murray, J. A., et al.: Acute change in hemoglobin affinity for oxygen during angina pectoris. New Engl. J. Med. 282:1219, 1970.

51. Fernandez, L. A., and Erslev, A. J.: Oxygen affinity and compensated hemolysis in hereditary spherocytosis. J. Lab. Clin. Med. 80: 780, 1972.

52. Oski, F. A., Marshall, B. E., et al.: Exercise with anemia. The role of the left-shifted or right-shifted oxygen hemoglobin equilibrium curve. Ann. Intern. Med. 74:44, 1971.

53. Bellingham, A. J., and Huehns, E. R.: Compensation in haemolytic anemias caused by abnormal haemoglobins. Nature (Lond.) 218: 924, 1968.

54. Bellingham, A. J., Detter, J. C., et al.: The role of hemoglobin oxygen affinity and red cell 2,3-diphosphoglycerate in the management of diabetic ketoacidosis. Trans. Assoc. Am. Phys. 83:113, 1970.

55. Chillar, R. K., Slawsky, P., et al.: Red cell 2,3-diphosphoglycerate and adenosine triphosphate in patients with shock. Br. J. Haematol. 21:183, 1971.

56. Lichtman, M. A., Miller, D. R., et al.: Reduced red cell glycolysis, 2,3-diphosphoglycerate and adenosine triphosphate and increased hemoglobin oxygen affinity caused by hypophosphatemia. Ann. Intern. Med. 74:562, 1971.

57. Jacob, H. S., and Amsden, T.: Acute hemolytic anemia with rigid red cells in hypophosphatemia. New Engl. J. Med. 285:1446, 1971.

58. Travis, S. F., Sugerman, H. J., et al.: Alterations of red cell glycolytic intermediates and oxygen transport as a consequence of hypophosphatemia in patients receiving intravenous hyperalimentation. New Engl. J. Med. 285:763, 1971.

59. Card, R. B., and Brain, M.: The "anemia" of childhood. New Engl. J. Med. 288:388, 1973.

60. Valtis, D. J., and Kennedy, A. C.: Defective gas transport function of stored red blood cells. Lancet 1:119, 1954.

61. Akerblom, O., deVerdier, C. H., et al.: Restoration of defective oxygen transport function of stored red blood cells by addition of inosine. Scand. J. Clin. Lab. Invest. 21:245, 1968.

62. Valeri, C. R., and Hirsch, N. M.: Restoration in vivo of erythrocyte adenosine triphosphate, 2,3-diphosphoglycerate, potassium ion and sodium concentrations following the transfusion of acid-citrate-dextrose stored human red blood cells. J. Lab. Clin. Med. 73:722, 1969.

63. Beutler, E., and Wood, L. A.: The in vivo regeneration of red cell 2,3-diphosphoglyceric acid after transfusion of stored blood. J. Lab. Clin. Med. 74:300, 1969.

64. Huisman, T. H. J., Boyd, E. M., et al.: Oxygen equilibria and chemical changes of whole blood stored in different preservatives. Transfusion 9:180, 1969.

65. Oski, F. A., Travis, S. F., et al.: The in vitro restoration of red cell 2,3-diphosphoglycerate levels in banked blood. Blood 37:52, 1971.

66. Delivoria-Papadopoulos, M., Miller, L. D., et al.: The effect of exchange transfusion on altering mortality in infants weighing less than 1300 grams at birth and its role in the management of severe respiratory distress syndrome (RDS). Pediatr. Res. 6:408, 1972.

67. Cathie, I. A. B.: Apparent idiopathic Heinz body anemia. Great Ormond St. J. 3:43, 1952.

68. Bunn, H. F., Bradley, T. B., et al.: Structural and functional studies on hemoglobin Bethesda $(\alpha_2\beta_2^{145 \text{ his}})$, a variant associated with compensatory erythrocytosis. J. Clin. Invest. 51:2299, 1972.

69. White, J. M., and Dacie, J. V.: The unstable hemoglobins—molecular and clinical features. Progr. Hematol. 7:69, 1971.

70. Jacob, H. S., and Winterhalter, K. H.: The role of hemoglobin heme loss in Heinz body formation: Studies with a partially heme-deficient hemoglobin and with genetically unstable hemoglobins. J. Clin. Invest. 49: 2008, 1970.

71. DeFuria, F. G., and Miller, D. R.: Oxygen affinity in hemoglobin Köln disease. Blood 38:398, 1972.

72. Rachmilewitz, E. A., Peisach, J., et al.: Role of haemichromes in the formation of inclusion bodies in haemoglobin H disease. Nature (Lond.) 222:248, 1969.

73. Winterbourne, C. C., and Carrell, R. W.: Characterization of Heinz bodies in unstable hemoglobin. Nature (Lond.) 240:150, 1972.

74. Jandl, J. H., Simmons, R. L., et al.: Red cell filtration and the pathogenesis of certain hemolytic anemias. Blood 18:133, 1961.

75. Rivkind, R. A.: Heinz body anemia: An ultrastructural study. II. Red cell sequestration and destruction. Blood 26:433, 1965.

76. Bradley, T. B., Wohl, R. C., et al.: Properties of hemoglobin Bryn Mawr $\beta^{85 \text{ Phe} \rightarrow \text{Ser}}$, a new spontaneous mutation producing an unstable hemoglobin with high oxygen affinity (abstract). Blood 40:947, 1972.

77. Charache, S., Weatherall, D. J., et al.: Polycythemia associated with a hemoglobinopathy. J. Clin. Invest. 45:813, 1966.

78. Adamson, J. W., Parer, J. T., et al.: Erythrocytosis associated with hemoglobin Rainier: Oxygen equilibria and marrow regulation. J. Clin. Invest. 48:1376, 1969.

79. Olson, J. S., and Gibson, Q. N.: The functional properties of hemoglobin Bethesda. J. Biol. Chem. 247:3662, 1972.

80. Bonaventura, J., and Riggs, A.: Hemoglobin Kansas, a human hemoglobin with a neutral amino acid substitution and an abnormal oxygen equilibrium. J. Biol. Chem. 243:980, 1968.

81. Fairbanks, V. F., Maldonado, J. E., et al.: Familial erythrocytosis due to a hemoglobin with impaired oxygen dissociation (hemoglobin Malmö, $\alpha_2\beta_2^{97 \text{ Gln}}$). Mayo Clin. Proc. 46:723, 1961.

82. Novy, M. J., Edwards, M. J., et al.: Hemoglobin Yakima II. High blood oxygen affinity associated with compensating erythrocytosis and

hemodynamics. J. Clin. Invest. *46*:1848, 1967.

83. Woodson, R. D., Heywood, J. D., et al.: Oxygen transport in hemoglobin San Francisco. Clin. Res. *18*:134, 1970.

84. Gerald, P. S.: The electrophoretic and spectroscopic characterization of Hgb M. Blood *13*:936, 1958.

85. Ranney, H. M., Nagel, R. L., et al.: Oxygen equilibrium of hemoglobin M$_{Hyde Park}$. Biochim. Biophys. Acta *160*:112, 1968.

86. Byckova, V., Wajcman, H., et al.: Hemoglobin M Saskatoon: Further data on biophysics and oxygen equilibrium. Biochim. Biophys. Acta *243*:117, 1971.

87. Josephson, A. M., Weinstein, H. G., et al.: A new variant of hemoglobin M disease. Hemoglobin M Chicago. J. Lab. Clin. Med. *59*:918, 1962.

88. Stavem, P., Strömme, J., et al.: Hemoglobin M Saskatoon with slight constant hemolysis increased by sulfonamides. Scand. J. Haematol. *9*:566, 1972.

89. Cohen, R. J., Sachs, J. R., et al.: Methemoglobinemia provoked by malarial chemoprophylaxis in Vietnam. New Engl. J. Med. *279*:1127, 1968.

90. Bunn, H. F.: The use of gel electrofocusing in the study of human hemoglobins. Ann. N.Y. Acad. Sci. *209*:345, 1973.

91. Keitt, A. S., Smith, T. W., et al.: Red cell "pseudomosaicism" in congenital methemoglobinemia. New Engl. J. Med. *275*:397, 1966.

92. Feig, S. A., Nathan, D. G., et al.: Congenital methemoglobinemia: The result of age-dependent decay of methemoglobin reductase. Blood *39*:407, 1972.

93. Schwartz, J. M., Paress, P. S., et al.: Unstable variant of NADH methemoglobin reductase in Puerto Ricans with hereditary methemoglobinemia. J. Clin. Invest. *51*:1594, 1972.

94. Coburn, R. F.: Biological effects of carbon monoxide. Ann. N.Y. Acad. Sci. Vol. 174, 1970.

95. Arends, T.: High concentration of haemoglobin A$_2$ in malaria patients. Nature (Lond.) *215*:1517, 1967.

96. Hamilton, R. W., Schwartz, E., et al.: Acquired hemoglobin H disease. New Engl. J. Med. *285*:1217, 1971.

97. Charache, S., and Weatherall, D. J.: Fast hemoglobin in lead poisoning. Blood *28*:377, 1966.

98. Murayama, M.: Molecular mechanism of human red cell (with Hb S) sickling, In *Molecular Aspects of Sickle Cell Hemoglobin*. Nalbandian, R. M. (ed.), Springfield, Ill., Charles C Thomas, 1971.

99. Muirhead, H., Cox, J. M., et al.: Structure and function of haemoglobin III. A three dimensional Fourier synthesis of human haemoglobin at 5.5 Å resolution. J. Mol. Biol. *28*:117, 1967.

100. Torrance, J., Jacobs, P., et al.: Intraerythrocytic adaptation to anemia. New Engl. J. Med. *283*:165, 1970.

101. Oski, F. A., Gottlieb, A. J., et al.: The influences of heredity and environment on the red cells' function of oxygen transport. Med. Clin. North Am. *54*:731, 1970.

102. Ranney, H. M.: Clinically important variants of human hemoglobin. New Engl. J. Med. *282*:144, 1970.

103. Dickerson, R. E.: X-ray analysis and protein structure, In *The Proteins: Composition, Structure and Function*. Vol. 2. 2nd ed. Neurath, H. (ed.), New York, Academic Press, 1964, pp. 603–778.

104. Bookchin, R. M., Nagel, R. L., et al.: Hemoglobin C-Harlem: A sickling variant containing amino acid substitutions in two residues of the β-polypeptide chain. Biochem. Biophys. Res. Commun. *23*:122, 1966.

105. Blackwell, R. Q., Boon, W. H., et al.: Hemoglobin J Singapore: α78 Asn→Asp; α79 Ala→Gly. Biochim. Biophys. Acta *278*:482, 1972.

106. Jones, R. T., Brimhall, B., et al.: Hemoglobin Freiburg: Abnormal hemoglobin due to deletion of a single amino acid residue. Science *134*:1024, 1966.

107. Bradley, T. B., Wohl, R. C., et al.: Hemoglobin Gun Hill: deletion of five amino acid residues and impaired heme-globin binding. Science *157*:1581, 1967.

108. deJong, W. W. W., Went, L. N., et al.: Hemoglobin Leiden. Deletion of β6 or 7 glutamic acid. Nature (Lond.) *220*:788, 1968.

109. Praxedes, H., Wiltshire, B. G., et al.: Submitted for publication.

110. Shibata, S., Miyaji, T., et al.: Hemoglobin Tochigi (β56–59 deleted). A new unstable hemoglobin discovered in a Japanese family. Proc. Jap. Acad. *46*:440, 1970.

111. Clegg, J. B., and Weatherall, D. J.: Hemoglobin H disease due to a unique haemoglobin variant with an elongated α chain. Lancet *1*:729, 1971.

112. Kinderlerer, J. L., Kilmartin, J. V., et al.: Hemoglobin Tak: A variant with additional residues at the end of the β-chains. Lancet *1*:722, 1971.

113. Barnabas, J., and Muller, C. J.: Haemoglobin Lepore Hollandia. Nature (Lond.) *194*:931, 1962.

114. Ostertag, W., and Smith, E. W.: Haemoglobin Lepore Baltimore. A third type of $\delta\beta$ crossover ($\delta^{50}\beta^{86}$). Eur. J. Biochem. *10*:371, 1969.

115. Baglioni, C.: The fusion of two polypeptide chains in hemoglobin Lepore and its interpretation as a genetic deletion. Proc. Natl. Acad. Sci. USA *48*:1880, 1962.

116. Yanese, T., Hanada, M., et al.: Molecular basis of morbidity from a series of studies of hemoglobinopathies in Western Japan. Jap. J. Hum. Gen. *13*:40, 1968.

117. Huisman, T. H. J., Schroeder, W. A., et al.: Hemoglobin Kenya, the product of non-homologous crossover of γ and β genes (abstract). Blood *40*:947, 1972.

118. Seid-Akhaven, M., Winter, W. P., et al.: Hemoglobin Wayne: a frameshift variant occurring in two distinct forms (abstract). Blood *40*:927, 1972.

119. Huisman, T. H. J., Brown, A. K., et al.: Hemoglobin Savannah (B6 (24)β-glycine→valine): An unstable variant causing anemia with inclusion bodies. J. Clin. Invest. *50*:650, 1971.

120. Cohen Solal, M., Seligmann, M., et al.: A new unstable hemoglobin: Hemoglobin St. Louis $\alpha_2^A\beta_2^{B10}$ glutamine. Abstract No. 408, 14th Int. Congr. Hematol., 1972.

121. Keeling, M. M., Ogden, L. L., et al.: Hemoglobin Louisville (β42(CD1) Phe→Leu): An unstable variant causing mild hemolytic anemia. J. Clin. Invest. 50:2395, 1971.

122. Labie, D.: Personal communication.

123. Schneider, R. G., Satoshi, U., et al.: Hemoglobin Sabine Beta 91(F7) Leu→Pro. An unstable variant causing severe anemia with inclusion bodies. New Engl. J. Med. 280: 739, 1969.

124. Aksoy, M., Erdem, S., et al.: Hemoglobin Istanbul: substitution of glutamine for histidine in a proximal histidine (F8(92)β). J. Clin. Invest. 51:2380, 1972.

125. Beuzard, Y., Courvalin, J. C., et al.: Structural studies on hemoglobin St. Etienne β92(F8)-His→Glu: A new abnormal hemoglobin with loss of β proximal histidine and absence of heme on the β chains. FEBS Letters 27: 76, 1972.

126. Adams, J. G., Winter, W. P., et al.: Hemoglobin Rush (β-101(G-3) glu→gln): A new unstable hemoglobin (abstract). Blood 40:941, 1972.

127. Koler, R. D., Jones, R. T., et al.: Hemoglobin Casper β106(G8) Leu→Pro. A contemporary mutation. Am. J. Med. 55:549, 1973.

128. Kung, H. A. R., Wiltshire, B. G., et al.: An unstable haemoglobin with reduced oxygen affinity: Haemoglobin Peterborough, β111 (G13) valine-phenylalanine, its interaction with normal haemoglobin and with haemoglobin Lepore. Br. J. Haematol. 22:125, 1972.

129. Reynolds, C. A., and Huisman, T. H. J.: Hemoglobin Russ or $\alpha_2^{51\ arg}\beta_2$. Biochim. Biophys. Acta 130:541, 1966.

130. Wajcman, H., Belkhodja, O., et al.: Hemoglobin Setif:G1(94) α Asp→Tyr. A new α chain hemoglobin variant with substitution of a residue involved in a hydrogen bond between unlike subunits. FEBS Letters 27: 298, 1972.

131. Charache, S., Weatherall, D. J., et al.: Polycythemia associated with a hemoglobinopathy. J. Clin. Invest. 45:813, 1966.

132. Lines, J. G., and McIntosh, R.: Oxygen binding by hemoglobin J—Capetown. Nature (Lond.) 215:297, 1967.

133. Nute, P. E., Stamatoyannopoulos, G., et al.: Hemoglobin Olympia (β20 val→met): An electrophoretically silent variant associated with high oxygen affinity and erythrocytosis. J. Clin. Invest. 51:70a, 1972.

134. Berglund, S., Lehmann, H., et al.: Familial polycythemia connected with a new abnormal hemoglobin. Proceedings Int. Soc. Hematol. 1970, p. 280.

135. Jones, R. T., Osgood, E. E., et al.: Hemoglobin Yakima: I. Clinical and biochemical studies. J. Clin. Invest. 46:1840, 1967.

136. Reed, C. S., Hampson, R., et al.: Erythrocytosis secondary to increased oxygen affinity of a mutant hemoglobin, Hemoglobin Kempsey. Blood 31:623, 1968.

137. Glynn, K. P., Penner, J. A., et al.: Familial erythrocytosis: Description of three families with Hemoglobin Ypsilanti. Ann. Intern. Med. 69:769, 1968.

138. Lokich, J. J., Moloney, W. C., et al.: Hemoglobin Brigham ($\alpha_2^A\beta^{100\ Pro→leu}$): Hemoglobin variant associated with familial erythrocytosis. J. Clin. Invest. 52:2060, 1973.

139. Adamson, J. W., Parer, J. T., et al.: Erythrocytosis associated with hemoglobin Rainier: Oxygen equilibria and marrow regulation. J. Clin. Invest. 48:1376, 1969.

140. Bromberg, P. A., Alben, J. O., et al.: High oxygen affinity of haemoglobin Little Rock with unique properties. Nature [New Biol.] 243: 177, 1973.

141. Hayashi, A., Stamatoyannopoulos, G., et al.: Hemoglobin Rainier: β^{145} (HC2) Tyrosine→Cysteine and Hemoglobin Bethesda: β^{145} (HC2) Tyrosine→Histidine. Nature (Lond.) 230:265, 1971.

142. Hamilton, H. G., Iuchi, I., et al.: Hemoglobin Hiroshima (β^{143} Histidine→Aspartic acid): A newly identified fast-moving beta chain variant associated with increased oxygen affinity and compensatory erythremia. J. Clin. Invest. 48:525, 1969.

143. Reissmann, K. R., Ruth, W. E., et al.: A human hemoglobin with lowered oxygen affinity and impaired heme-heme interactions. J. Clin. Invest. 40:1826, 1961.

144. Stamatoyannopoulos, G., Parer, J. T., et al.: Physiologic implications of a hemoglobin with decreased oxygen affinity (hemoglobin Seattle). New Engl. J. Med. 281:915, 1969.

145. Imamura, T., Fujita, S., et al.: Hemoglobin Yoshizuka (G10(108) β asparagine→aspartic acid): A new variant with a reduced oxygen affinity from a Japanese family. J. Clin. Invest. 48:2341, 1969.

146. Cohen Solal, M., Blouquit, Y., et al.: Hemoglobin Lyon (submitted for publication).

147. Carrell, R. W., and Kay, R.: A simple method for the detection of unstable haemoglobins. Br. J. Haematol. 23:615, 1972.

148. Zak, S. J., Brunhall, B., et al.: Hemoglobin Andrew Minneapolis β 144 Lys→Asparagine: A new high affinity mutant. J. Clin. Invest. 52:92a, 1973.

Chapter 14

Sickle Cell Syndromes and Hemoglobin C Disease

by David G. Nathan
and Howard A. Pearson

INTRODUCTION

In Chapter 13, Bunn has reviewed the anatomy and synthesis of hemoglobin, the interaction of hemoglobin with organic phosphates, and the molecular basis of the hemoglobinopathies that are associated with premature precipitation of hemoglobin or abnormal oxygen affinity. In this chapter, we will consider the pathophysiology and the clinical manifestations of the sickle hemoglobin syndromes and hemoglobin C disease. No attempt will be made to define all the abnormal hemoglobins or their manifestations, since they either are described in Chapters 13 and 15, are uncommon, or are clinically less consequential.

THE SICKLE SYNDROMES

Sickle Cell Anemia

Incidence

The sickle gene is a common mutant, being prevalent in Central Africa, the Near East, the Mediterranean, and parts of India. The gene frequency usually varies directly with the incidence of falciparum malaria (1–4). Whereas the average incidence among American Blacks, whose roots are largely in Central Africa, is approximately 8 per cent (5), the frequency is much higher in certain areas of Africa where falciparum malaria has been rampant.

The physiologic basis for the influence of falciparum malaria on the sickle gene (so-called "balanced polymorphism") has been studied but without clear-cut results (6). For reasons that are not established, the gene appears to provide some protection to children who might otherwise succumb to cerebral falciparum malaria. Hence the gene has persisted in zones in which falciparum malaria is endemic.

History

Sickle cell anemia was first described in a West Indian student by Herrick in 1910 (7). The pathologic basis of the disorder and its relation to the hemoglobin molecule was defined in 1927 by Hahn and Gillespie (8). Shortly after the application of moving-boundary electrophoresis to the separation of sickle from normal hemoglobin by Pauling and Itano (9), Beet (10), Neel (11), and their co-workers defined the genetics of the disorder and clearly distinguished sickle trait, the heterozygous condition (AS), from sickle cell anemia, the homozygous state (SS). Further understanding of the molecular basis of the disorder was made possible by the finding that normal human hemoglobin is composed of two pairs of globin subunits, one pair of which

419

is invariant, the alpha chain, and the other variable, the epsilon (12, 13), zeta (14), gamma, beta, or delta chain. The relative ease by which sickle hemoglobin could be isolated by chromatography or zone-electrophoresis techniques led to Ingram's application of tryptic digestion, high-voltage electrophoresis, and paper chromatography to the isolated sickle hemoglobin, with the result that the amino acid substitution in sickle hemoglobin is now known to be a valine instead of a glutamic acid in the number 6 position of the beta chain. The alpha chain is normal (15, 16). The proper chemical nomenclature for sickle hemoglobin is therefore $\alpha_2^A\beta_2^{6\ \text{Glu}\to\text{Val}}$.

Pathophysiology of Sickling

MOLECULAR BASIS OF SICKLING. Hahn and Gillespie (8) showed that deoxygenation was responsible for the change of morphology of sickle cells from the biconcave to the sickle shape, and Harris (17) clearly demonstrated that this effect resides in the unusual solubility characteristics of Hb S, which undergoes nematic liquid crystal or "tactoid" formation as it becomes deoxygenated.

The precise structure of sickled hemoglobin molecules in pure S gels and in mixtures is not yet known. The elongation of the sickle cells during sickling and their birefringence suggested to Harris that the nematic crystals or tactoids must be composed of parallel bundles of molecules (17). Electron microscopic studies of sickled cells and of gels of deoxy S by Murayama (18, 19), Stetson (20), White (21), Döbler (22), Lessin (23, 24), and their co-workers showed that aggregates of sickled hemoglobin molecules are arranged in parallel rodlike structures. The diameter of the rod is approximately 150 to 170 angstroms. The rod may actually be a tube with a central hollow core of about 50 angstroms. Murayama has proposed that the β^6-valine–induced alteration of the deoxygenated β^s chain fits into a complementary position in the alpha chain of an accompanying hemoglobin molecule and that the molecules are then stacked on top of each other. He further proposes that six stacks of molecules are twisted around each other in a helix of high pitch to form the rods (18). Finch, Perutz, Bertles, and Döbler also

have shown that "each fiber is a tube made up of six thin filaments that are wound around the tubular surface with a helical pitch of about 3000 Å. Each filament in turn is a strand of single hemoglobin molecules" (42). Although interaction of β^s chains with α chains is probably quite important in the sickling phenomenon (42a), the stacking of molecules in each filament is unlikely to conform to the model proposed by Murayama. This model would not account for the orientation of the mean plane of the heme groups which are perpendicular to the long axis of the gelled filament as described by Micheson and Perutz (25). Bookchin and Nagel have suggested that the molecules in each of the filaments are actually arranged in a single stranded helix of low pitch, six molecules occupying the space necessary for one complete turn (26). Recent x-ray diffraction studies of Magdoff-Fairchild and her co-workers are consistent with the latter view (27), but the exact relationship between the molecules is not established.

Precise understanding of the primary structural alteration induced in deoxy S by the β^6-valine substitution remains to be acquired, and the nature of the complementary site(s) on participating molecules is unknown. That multiple residues provide important complementary sites seems very likely.

The substitution of valine for glutamic acid in the beta chain (the primary binding site) bestows a particular conformation on the surface of the deoxygenated β^s chain which encourages gelation owing to specific interaction of the primary binding site with a complementary site on a neighboring or participating chain (28). Tight apposition of the primary binding sites to the complementary site results in helix formation, the helix being stabilized by many different secondary binding sites. The availability of the latter is dependent upon the primary structure of the participating hemoglobin molecule. In fact the neighboring hemoglobin does not necessarily have to be in the deoxy configuration to participate, i.e., to provide the complementary or $2°$ binding site(s). The different human hemoglobins vary in their capacity to participate in sickling with deoxy S. This variation among the hemoglobins with regard to their participation in sickling has been extensively studied by Bookchin and Nagel (26), and by Milner and his colleagues (29) using the minimum gelling concentration measurements developed by Singer and Singer (30) and by Allison (31). In this technique, known proportions of purified Hb S and an accompanying purified hemoglobin are mixed together in 0.15 M phosphate buffer. The mixture is first completely deoxygenated by exposure to hydrated nitrogen and then concentrated by exposure to dry nitrogen. The concentration at which gelling occurs is the minimum gelling concentration of the mixture.

Some of these measurements are listed in Table 14-1, where it is shown that a mixture of 60 per cent deoxy Korle Bu with 40 per cent deoxy S, or 30 per cent deoxy F with 70 per cent deoxy S requires a much higher hemoglobin concentration for gelation than does a mixture of 60 per cent deoxy D or O_{Arab} with 40 per cent deoxy S. Thus hemoglobins D and O_{Arab} participate much more readily in sickling with deoxy S. Presumably they contain easily accessible complementary or secondary binding site(s) on their surfaces for interaction with the primary binding site. Mixtures of deoxy hemoglobins A and C with deoxy hemoglobin S have intermediate minimum gelling concentrations. Deoxy A participates less readily than deoxy C but more readily than deoxy F or deoxy Korle Bu. It seems likely that participation of other hemoglobins with hemoglobin S in a helix is actually due in part to the formation of molecular hybrids (32), in which two different beta chains, one β^s and one β^{non-s}, are combined with two normal alpha chains.

Certain amino acid substitutions in α and β chains of accompanying hemoglobin molecules may radically alter the firmness of the attachment of the complementary site to the β^6-valine–induced primary binding site in deoxy S, since the tertiary structural changes induced by amino acid substitutions may influence the availability of secondary binding sites. If sickled molecules are arranged in a single stranded helix, it seems likely that such secondary interactions must be established between the molecules to hold them in the helical arrangement. These molecular interactions appear to be strengthened when hemoglobins S, O, or D are present, either as tetramers or more likely as hybrids in the helix, and are weakened if hemoglobins F or Korle Bu are present. In fact, deoxy Hb F appears to be excluded from gels if it is present at equal concentrations with deoxy S (32). The exclusion of F from the gels is all the more striking in light of the paradoxical fact that liganded F tends to participate in sickling much more readily than deoxy F (26). Thus the surface topography of F appears to afford little or no stability to a helix of deoxy S, and, by dilution, its presence may inhibit the ability of deoxy S molecules to make contact with each other. Nonhemoglobin proteins such as albumin might participate more readily in sickling than does F by providing

TABLE 14-1. THE SICKLE SYNDROMES

Syndrome	% S	% Non-S		Minimum Gelling Concentration (g. per 100 ml.)	Clinical Severity
SS	85–95	5–15 (F)		24	4+
S-thalassemia	60–90	10–40 (A+F)		Variable	2–3+
SD	45	55	D	20	3+
SO_{Arab}	50	50	O_{Arab}	22	3+
SC	50	50	C	27	2+
AS	40	60	A	30	±
S–high F	70	30	F	37	±
S Korle Bu	40	60	Korle Bu	37	±

stabilizing surfaces for the helix. In fact, Singer and Singer found in early gelation studies that albumin can participate in sickling (30). Its precise position in the hierarchy from Korle Bu and F to O_{Arab} and D would be of interest.

The structural studies currently available, though incomplete, do suggest that pharmacologic approaches to sickling should be oriented toward development of agents which either favor the oxyconfiguration of S or selectively inhibit either the stability of the putative helix by reduction of available secondary binding sites or the "fit" between the β^6-valine site and the complementary site.

CELLULAR SICKLING. The rate and extent of sickling of cells within a sample of sickle hemoglobin–containing red cells are responsible for the characteristic deoxygenation-induced change in viscosity of sickle whole blood (17). This change in viscosity is intimately related to the clinical severity of any of the so-called S syndromes, the more severe syndromes being those in which significant viscosity increments occur rapidly at physiologic oxygen tensions (33, 34). It must be emphasized that the viscosity of the whole blood of patients with homozygous sickle cell anemia is higher than normal, even at physiologic arterial oxygen tensions (34, 35). The plasma of patients with SS disease is itself somewhat more viscous than normal (35), probably because of the increased level of gamma globulin which occurs in most cases, particularly in patients over 4 years of age (36). The presence of irreversibly sickled cells, to be described below, alters whole blood viscosity perhaps by interfering with the normal apposition and flow of more flexible, disklike cells. Indeed, irreversibly sickled cells, if present in sufficient numbers, delay the passage of oxygenated sickled blood through filters and viscometers (34) and increase the viscosity of sickle blood at any shear rate (35).

Though viscosity is increased in oxygenated SS blood, alterations in viscosity become much more profound when the blood is deoxygenated and SS cells in the biconcave disk form begin to sickle. The clinical results of heightened viscosity in the sickle syndromes are vaso-occlusive phenomena and anemia. The occlusive episodes are heightened by a vicious cycle

of sickling[*] in the microvasculature. The cycle begins when cells containing Hb S enter a deoxygenated area. If they remain for a sufficient time, the Hb S is deoxygenated and some of the cells sickle. The time factor is critical. As Harris and Kellermeyer have emphasized,[*] the entire venous circulation of an individual with homozygous S disease would be occluded with sickle forms, were the red cells to become stagnant in that environment. Most, however, escape from the venous to the arterial circulation before sufficient cell deformity to cause entrapment occurs. If sickling does begin, viscosity of the blood is heightened. Flow slows so that other cells deoxygenate for progressively lengthening periods of time. As flow slows to a critical level and tissue deoxygenation proceeds, acidosis occurs, and the hemoglobin-oxygen saturation curve is shifted further toward decreased oxygen affinity. Deoxygenation then proceeds to completion, and an entire area of tissue is then obstructed by a mass of sickle cells. Since viscosity is strongly influenced by hematocrit, the patient with sickle cell disease is partially protected from occlusive episodes by anemia, and, conversely, occlusive phenomena are apt to occur more severely in areas of hemoconcentration, such as in the spleen.

Hemolytic anemia in sickle cell disease is related to the development of the sickle shape and further shape change during circulation. These elongated cells exhibit increased mechanical fragility (37, 38, 39). Repeated sickling and unsickling by alternating exposure to variable oxygen tensions produces fragmentation of sickle cells with the appearance of platelet-sized "blood dust" in the plasma (40). These "dust" particles contain both the protein and lipid moieties of red cell membranes. As loss of membrane approaches a critical quantity and the membrane surface area to cell volume ratio attains a minimum, the sickle cells become spheroidal during the unsickling process (41). The induction of spheroidicity can be rapidly achieved in sickle cells by laser-induced microsurgical

---

[*]For an excellent review of the pathophysiology of sickling the reader is referred to Harris, J., and Kellermeyer, R.: *The Red Cell.* Cambridge, Mass., Harvard University Press, 1970.

excision of one of the several membrane excrescences which occur when sickle cells are deoxygenated (42). Indeed, a small number of spherocytes are usually present in the peripheral blood of patients with sickle cell disease. Although patients with sickle cell anemia exhibit certain laboratory findings consistent with intravascular hemolysis, such as decreased haptoglobin (43) and hemopexin (44) and increased serum hemoglobin concentration (45), the anemia is largely due to the rapid destruction of erythrocytes (46) by a process of sequestration and erythrophagocytosis (47). This process occurs within the spleen until it is infarcted and shrunken by the sickling process, and then largely in the liver and throughout the reticuloendothelial system (48). Within the sites of sequestration, the stagnant cells probably develop irreversible abnormalities of the membrane, which lead to membrane stiffness and phagocytosis by tissue macrophages. These metabolic alterations are described more fully in the following section.

The Formation of Irreversibly Sickled Cells

The red cells in the peripheral blood of patients with homozygous sickle cell ane-

mia are markedly heterogeneous. The smear reveals target cells, rare spherocytes, biconcave disks, nucleated red cells, Howell-Jolly bodies, and irreversibly sickled cells (ISC) (Fig. 14-1). The latter are defined as sickle-shaped cells that do not resume the biconcave form, even after vigorous oxygenation. They contain less fetal hemoglobin than do non-ISC (49, 50). In some patients, as many as 50 per cent of the peripheral red cells are ISC, the percentage being usually considerably lower in children than in adults. The ISC percentage is not necessarily related to the severity of clinical symptoms, such as painful crises, but does appear to be related to the hemolytic rate (51). Abolition of ISC formation, even if possible, would not be expected to relieve the vaso-occlusive phenomena, since the latter are probably caused by what might be called the "Trojan horse performance" of disk-shaped Hb S cells that slip into the microvasculature because of their normal rheologic properties and then sickle within the vessels. ISC are probably not as readily admitted into the microvessels because they are rigid as well as malformed and cannot adapt to the shape requirements necessary for entrance into very small vessels. The survival of ISC in the circulation is very brief; they

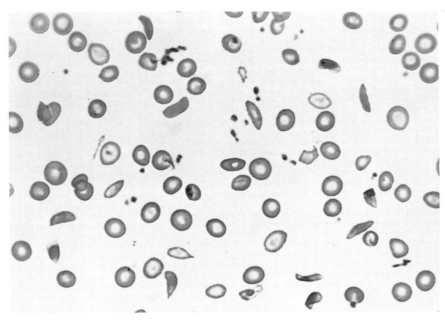

Figure 14-1. Peripheral smear of a patient with sickle cell anemia. Note normal cells, irreversibly sickled cells, and red cell fragments.

are destroyed rapidly throughout the reticuloendothelial system (50).

Despite the sickled appearance of oxygenated ISC, the hemoglobin in the cells is usually not in the gelled state (Fig. 14–2). This has been demonstrated both by lack of birefringence (52) and by electron micrograph sections which fail to demonstrate typical bundles of sickle hemoglobin in these cells (53). Thus it has been concluded that ISC remain in the sickled form because of the development of increased membrane rigidity during some stage of the sickling process (54, 55). Evidence for membrane damage during sickling is relatively easy to acquire. As mentioned above, red cell fragments are formed during sickling and unsickling. Spherocytes develop after mechanical trauma, and they are present in the blood smear. Studies of membrane constituents of ISC compared with unsickled cells from patients with SS disease reveal marked losses of phospholipids (56). The phospholipid loss observed in ISC isolated from the blood of patients with SS disease may be due to fragmentation during the circulation of the ISC after they are formed. When disk-shaped sickle cells undergo sickling, they develop a reversible increase in cation permeability (57, 58). The permeability of ISC membranes to sodium and potassium is increased, with potassium loss exceeding sodium gain (59). Water loss accompanies this cation loss, and therefore the concentration of hemoglobin is relatively increased in these cells, partially accounting for their decreased oxygen affinity (60). For this reason, ISC are dehydrated cells or "desiccytes," according to the classification of hyperpermeable red cells described in Chapter 6.

Production of ISC in vitro can be accomplished by prolonged incubation of sickle cells under nitrogen in a calcium-containing buffer or in plasma under conditions in which cellular ATP, but not membrane phospholipid, is lost. If ATP is maintained or if calcium is removed from the incubation system, the ISC formation is markedly reduced (55). This provides some evidence that ISC formation is not caused primarily by membrane loss, but may instead be due to the irreversible development of membrane rigidity secondary to heightened calcium entrance into the membrane while the cell is in the sickled form (55a, 55b). Indeed, prolonged storage of nonsickled SS cells inhibits the induction of sickling by sodium metabisulfite or by deoxygenation (54), presumably because of the decreased membrane deformability which accompanies ATP depletion in the presence of calcium ions (61). Membrane stiffness is irreversible in ISC (55), whereas in normal cells it is not. Normal flexibility and plasticity cannot be recovered, even when ATP stores are regained.

Clinical Manifestations (62, 63)

Since substantial amounts of beta chain are not present at birth, and deoxy fetal hemoglobin participates poorly with deoxy S in the gelation process, SS disease does not usually become apparent in the first six months of life, although documented symptomatic disease as early as one to three months has been described (63a, 63b). Progressive hemolytic anemia and splenomegaly, with appearance of sickle forms in the blood smear, then occur. The marrow compensation for hemolysis leads to characteristic boney changes with expansion of medullary cavities, such as widening of the diploë which is responsible for the "hair-on-end" appearance of the skull x-ray that is observed in children with sufficient erythroid marrow expansion of any cause. The degree of marrow expansion and thinning of the boney cortex is not usually severe enough to lead to pathologic fractures, as is the case in beta thalassemia. Increased ineffective erythropoiesis is probably present to a certain extent in SS disease (64), but not to the degree which characterizes the severe forms of thalassemia. Although anemia can be a serious problem in sickle cell disease, this is not usually the case except in the first few years of life when intrasplenic "sequestration crisis" may be life threatening (63b). On the contrary, it is the onset of septic complications and vaso-occlusive phenomena during the first or second years of life that constitutes the gravest threat to the patient and causes the most serious symptoms. For example, bacterial meningitis may be 600 times more frequent in these patients than in normal children (75).

THE PAINFUL CRISIS. Vaso-occlusive

episodes are responsible for the commonest symptom in sickle cell disease—the painful crisis. Such crises occur at variable frequencies during the course of the illness and are due to infarction of the various organ systems, the numerous consequences of which are described below. Most commonly the painful crises involve the periosteum, the bones, and the joints and usually begin abruptly with burning or "deep pain" in the bones. The pain may then become excruciating. Occasionally boney infarction may be localized to one or two areas. For example, in infants the small bones of the hands and feet are the most frequent sites of infarction and may become swollen and tender (hand-foot syndrome). A week or so later, characteristic x-ray changes are evident (Fig. 14–3).

The crises may follow any episode of dehydration. This may occur more frequently in hot, dry weather, following vigorous exercise, or during an infection with fever, but in many patients there is no regular or seasonal pattern (63). The course of the painful crisis is variable. The pain may be fleeting and can sometimes be aborted if the patient drinks copious amounts of fluid. However, it may last for days, particularly in adults. When the joints are involved, the pain, tenderness, and bogginess of the synovia (63a) may be mistaken for rheumatic fever with severe joint manifestations, septic arthritis, or, in adults, acute secondary gout. The latter two possibilities must in fact be seriously considered. The pain may also be located in the chest, and a pleuritic component suggesting pulmonary embolism or acute pneumococcal pneumonia may create a difficult differential diagnosis.

Abdominal painful crisis is also common. When the abdominal pain is accompanied by increased icterus, acute cholecystitis or common duct stone must be considered, but these are relatively infrequent. Splenic or bowel infarction or acute appendicitis must also be ruled out. Although many patients with SS disease have had needless abdominal surgery, some have suffered abdominal catastrophes because of overconfidence in the diagnosis of painful abdominal crisis. The presence of bowel sounds usually supports the diagnosis of abdominal painful crisis rather than an acute abdomen. Unfortunately, the white count and differential are usually not helpful, since granulocytes are nearly always increased in patients with SS disease with functional asplenia. Many patients tend to establish a repeated pattern of symptoms in the painful crisis. Deviation from that pattern should suggest a more serious problem.

THE SKIN. Leg ulcers usually do not occur in childhood, but later in life when venous circulation is less competent, they may constitute a crippling symptom. They are more common in tropical areas, perhaps because shoes are infrequently worn and because of the presence of insect bites (65). Usually present over the medial surface of the lower tibia or just posterior to the medial malleolus, they begin as a small depression with central necrosis and then widen, if unattended, to encircle the entire lower leg. Debridement, scrupulous hygiene, topical antibiotics, rest, and elevation are the mainstays of therapy. In some patients protection of the ulcer by the application of a soft sponge-rubber doughnut and low-pressure elastic bandage seems to be beneficial. Prevention of ulcers may result from close attention to improved venous circulation by the use of above-the-knee elastic stockings. If ulcers persist despite optimal care, transfusion therapy should be utilized and consideration given to split-thickness skin grafts. Transfusion therapy is sometimes effective, but in many patients the ulcers recur following discontinuation of this therapy.

THE EYES. Tortuosity and sacculation of conjunctival vessels is commonly observed, but retinal manifestations of SS disease are frequently underdiagnosed, since the lesions, called "black sunbursts" or "sea fans" (66–68), may be so peripheral as to require mydriatics for proper visualization. These proliferative lesions are of importance since they may lead to premature separation of the retina, which can be prevented by laser beam therapy (68). They appear to be particularly common in SC disease and, as is true of skin ulcers, tend to occur much more commonly in adults than in children, at least in this country.

THE LUNGS AND HEART. The lungs are damaged in SS disease not only by extensive occlusion of the pulmonary arterioles but also by repeated infection and occasionally by marrow emboli which occur during episodes of bone infarction (69–71,

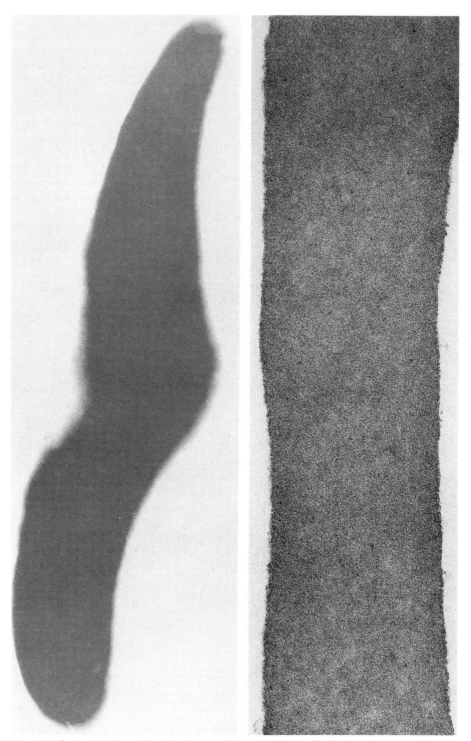

Figure 14–2.   *A,* Electron micrograph of oxygenated, irreversibly sickled cells. The hemoglobin is homogeneously distributed. There is no evidence of sickled hemoglobin in the cells.

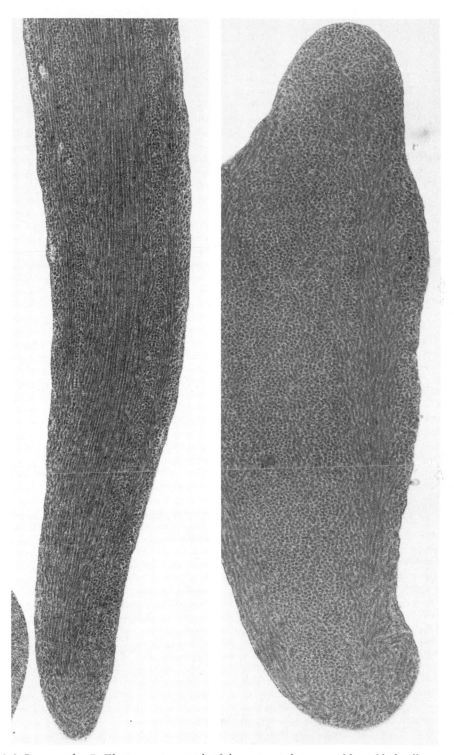

Figure 14–2 *Continued.* *B,* Electron micrograph of deoxygenated, irreversibly sickled cells revealing typical sickled hemoglobin. (From Bertles, J. F., and Döbler, J.: Reversible and irreversible sickling: A distinction by electron microscopy. Blood *33*:884–898, 1969, by permission of Grune & Stratton.)

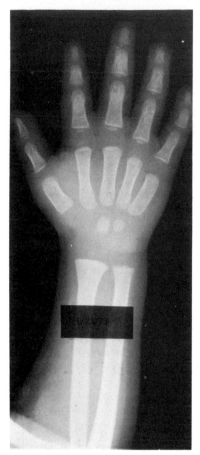 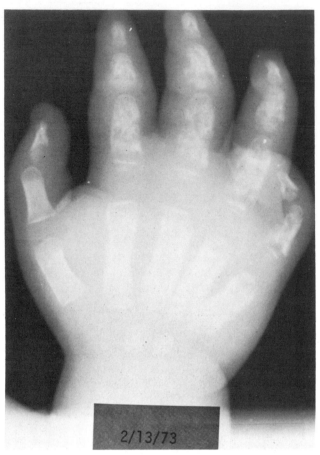

Figure 14–3.   X-rays of the hand of a child with sickle cell anemia. The x-ray on the left was taken on admission during an episode of hand-foot syndrome. There is edema but no evidence of boney destruction. Two weeks later destructive boney lesions are evident, as shown on the right.

160). The result is abnormal gas exchange (72, 73). Pneumonia is a frequent and serious complication of SS disease (74, 75), not only because of the peculiar susceptibility of these patients to infection, as described below, but also because the vascular damage to the lungs creates a fertile soil for further and repeated infection. Prompt and vigorous treatment with antibiotics, pulmonary toilet, and intermittent oxygen therapy by mask in adults and by nasal catheter or a tent in children is necessary to combat interpulmonary sickling which may retard the movement of phagocytes and the diffusion of antibiotics into the infected area. It is in the setting of severe pneumonia and secondary hypoxia that fatal cerebral or diffuse organ sickling may occur (76). Pneumococci and staphylococci are the usual offenders, but Mycoplasma also seem to attack these patients with a high degree of frequency (77).

The cardiomegaly, increased pulmonic second heart sound, and the murmurs which are invariably present in SS patients are usually due to anemia, but rheumatic heart disease provides an important differential diagnosis, and occasionally congenital heart disease may be seen (77a). Repeated episodes of pulmonary vascular obstruction and infection may lead to cor pulmonale and right-sided congestive failure (71, 78, 79). Digitalis and diuretics are then indicated. The symptoms may also require chronic transfusion therapy to maintain adequate oxygen delivery. Transfusion also decreases the incidence of further pulmonary vascular occlusive episodes by reducing the number of sickle cells in the circulation. Cardiomegaly may also result from hypertension of renal origin, the latter due to sickling within the kidney and renal vascular occlusion.

The red cells in coronary radicals should

be particularly susceptible to sickling since oxygen extraction by the heart from the blood is highly efficient. However, the number of sickled forms in coronary sinus blood is no higher than in the general circulation (80), perhaps because of the brief time spent by sickle cells in the coronary circulation. Thus under ordinary circumstances the heart is not particularly involved in vaso-occlusive episodes. However, when these patients undergo slowing of the circulation, such as during hypotensive general anesthesia or as a result of septic or hemorrhagic shock, coronary vascular sickling and myocardial infarction might be expected to occur.

ABDOMEN. The role of the spleen in SS disease has been repeatedly emphasized. In most hemolytic anemias (including S-thalassemia discussed below), the spleen removes the abnormal cells and becomes hyperplastic in the process (81). In young patients with SS disease, the spleen is enlarged but the abnormal cells gradually infarct the spleen and it becomes atrophic. In addition, the spleen is functionally inactive, even when the organ is considerably enlarged. For awhile, loss of splenic reticuloendothelial function is reversible since it may reappear after a short transfusion program (Fig. 14–4). (82, 83). The absence of splenic function contributes to the risk of infection in SS disease (see below), and the loss of the filtration function increases the number of circulating ISC (49), as well as target cells, cells with Howell-Jolly bodies, and siderocytes. In most children splenomegaly persists for at least the first four years of life and sometimes longer (84). Then the spleen begins to decrease in size and is usually no longer palpable by the age of 5 or 6. In some children splenomegaly progressively increases. In such patients severe hemolytic anemia may be alleviated by splenectomy (85–88). The gain from this procedure must be balanced against the increased risk of occlusive phenomena, which would seem likely to occur if the sickle hemoglobin concentration is significantly increased. This is a decision which must be carefully weighed in individual cases. Young children with persistent splenomegaly may undergo life-threatening sequestration crises in which massive numbers of red

cells accumulate in the spleen with a resulting anemic shock. This potentially fatal syndrome provides, in our opinion, an absolute indication for splenectomy.

The liver and biliary system is nearly always affected in sickle cell anemia (89, 90). Pigment stones are nearly always present. They may cause cholecystitis and common duct obstruction for which surgery may be required, even before the age of 10 (91). The stones should not be removed electively. Chronic vascular obstruction may lead to hepatic abscess (92) and fibrosis (93), but portal hypertension is uncommon since the fibrosis is not usually localized around portal vessels (89). The extensive fibrosis caused by infarction and by infection secondary to biliary tract obstruction may lead to liver failure (94) and death. Sequestration crises can also occur in the liver. They do not usually lead to fatal anemic shock, but rather to severe jaundice and hepatomegaly with total bilirubin concentrations, including both direct and indirect fractions, as high as 50 or 60 mg. per 100 ml. The presence of severe hyperbilirubinemia in a patient with sickle cell anemia confronts the physician with a difficult differential diagnosis. The possibilities usually include sequestration crisis, viral hepatitis (95), and biliary obstruction (96, 97).

GENITOURINARY SYSTEM Hyposthenuria (98–100), hematuria, infection, and necrosis are the major renal complications of sickle cell disease. Hyposthenuria probably occurs because of chronic sickling and slow flow in proximity to the loop of Henle, at which point the countercurrent-dependent renal concentration mechanism is particularly sensitive to the rate of blood flow (101, 102). The concentration defect is improved by transfusion with normal red cells during the first five to six years of life (103, 104). The resulting obligatory water loss creates an increased liability to dehydration and resultant painful crisis. Hyposthenuria also forces the physician to judge the adequacy of fluid intake during the treatment of painful crisis without being unduly influenced by the urine output. Hematuria is usually inconsequential, but it may be massive (105–107) and require treatment with blood transfusion or partial exchange transfusion. Epsilon aminocaproic

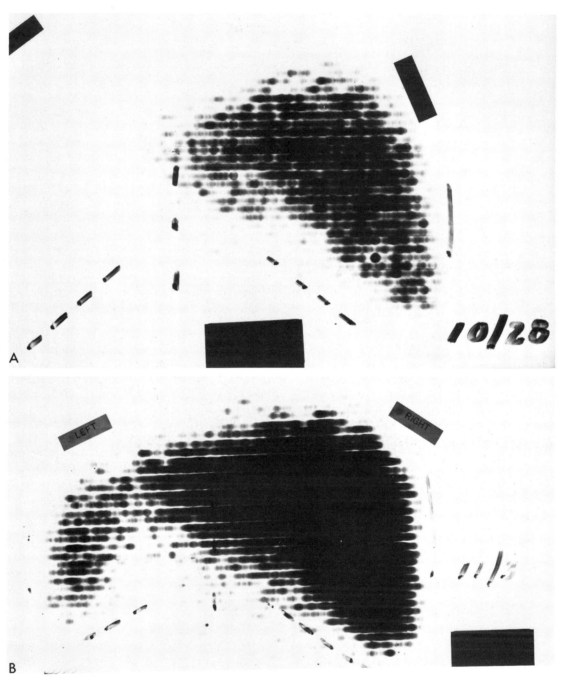

Figure 14–4. *A,* ^{99m}Technetium gelatin sulfur colloid scan of the reticuloendothelial system in a child with sickle cell anemia. Note absence of splenic localization of radioactivity. *B,* After transfusion with normal red cells, splenic reticuloendothelial function is restored, as shown by splenic localization of radioactivity. (From Pearson, H. A., Cornelius, E. A., et al.: New Engl. J. Med. *283:*334, 1970.)

acid has been used successfully to decrease the bleeding (108), but the risk of intra-pelvic or ureteral clotting is considerable. Renal failure due to renal vascular obstruc-tion does occur in some patients (109, 110), and papillary necrosis with or without pyelonephritis is also observed (111, 112). Nephrotic syndrome has also been docu-mented.

Priapism rarely occurs in young children (113), but it may begin as a notable problem during adolescence (114). Though often self-limited or easily treated (115), it can be severe enough to warrant surgical intervention, such as venous bypass (116) and removal of clots from the corpus cavernosum. Early surgical treatment is sometimes advised to prevent impotence, (117), and transfusion therapy is also indi-cated.

Development of secondary sexual char-acteristics and onset of puberty and me-narche are usually delayed in sickle cell anemia (119) and, at least in Africa, may be corrected by administration of folic acid (119).

Amenorrhea and infertility are common, but some patients may be fertile (120). During pregnancy these patients require special attention (121–126a). The incidence of vaso-occlusive and urinary tract com-plications is then often increased. We favor transfusion therapy during the last trimester of the pregnancy in order to protect the placenta as much as possible from infarction and resulting abortion or premature labor.

HEMOPOIETIC SYSTEM. The hemopoi-etic system is itself affected by sickle cell disease. Red cell production may be inter-rupted by viral or bacterial infection lead-ing to severe aplastic crises. The aplastic crisis affords physiologic insight into the heterogeneity of hemoglobin distribution in sickle cell disease. Of the total hemo-globin in SS patients, from 3 to 30 per cent is fetal, with 8 per cent being the average value in one series (127). In contrast to the homogeneous distribution of hemoglobin observed in the S–high F syndrome (128, 129) (to be discussed below), a group of fetal-rich cells is produced in SS disease (130, 131). This heterogeneous distribution of F is present in many of the diseases in which increased fetal hemoglobin synthesis oc-curs as a stress response, e.g., aplastic

anemia (132), juvenile chronic myelogenous leukemia (133–135), various forms of hemolytic anemia, and myelofibrosis. For this reason, fetal hemoglobin in SS dis-ease affords little protection to the patient since it is not equally mixed in the cells in which S-hemoglobin is present. For ex-ample, ISC develop more readily in fetal-poor cells (50). During the aplastic crisis the ratio of circulating hemoglobins S to F decreases because the life span of F-rich cells is considerably longer than that of F-poor cells (136), and the ratios of the rates of synthesis of F and S in the bone marrow are unaltered by changes in the total rate of erythropoiesis (137).

The aplastic crises are rarely severe enough to warrant transfusion therapy, but patients must be observed carefully to be sure that reticulocytosis does in fact re-sume within the usual four to five days following the crisis. Routine transfusion therapy is to be avoided in sickle cell dis-ease for the usual degrees of anemia. Carefully crossmatched blood should be used. Blacks frequently lack certain blood group antigens, such as Duffy and Kell, which a higher percentage of whites possess (138). Immunization could render subse-quent and more necessary transfusions difficult to accomplish.

Hemolytic crises are said to occur regu-larly in sickle cell disease, but they are difficult to document and usually represent reticulocyte responses to preceding aplastic crises. They may occur more frequently in patients who have G6PD deficiency in as-sociation with SS disease, particularly during an infection (139). The coincidence of G6PD deficiency and SS disease appears to be higher than might be explained by chance alone (140, 141). Its genetic signifi-cance and the difficulty of diagnosis of G6PD deficiency in SS disease are dis-cussed in Chapter 11.

Megaloblastic crisis occurs in sickle cell disease as a result of folic acid insufficiency (119, 142–144). In Africa this complication may cause extraordinarily severe anemia in pregnant females with sickle cell disease (145). Cardiopulmonary compensation in such patients may be so limited that ordi-nary packed cell administration may cause pulmonary edema. Partial exchange trans-fusion is recommended as safer therapy. An extraordinary syndrome of sexual retardation associated with sickle cell disease has been described in certain West African patients. Remarkable rates of sexual development are achieved when folic acid therapy is instituted (146). Folic acid deficiency or iron deficiency may alter the rate of S hemoglobin production, since the ratio of S to A has been observed to change during episodes of megaloblastic and iron deficiency anemia in patients with S-trait (147, 148). Patients with sickle cell disease should ingest a 1-mg. daily supplemental dose of folic acid increased to 2 mg. per day during pregnancy, although there is not controlled evidence that this is of significant value in the United States (148a).

The high turnover of erythroid precursors predisposes patients with sickle cell disease to episodes of secondary gout (149, 150). Those with high levels of uric acid and suspicious joint symptoms should receive allopurinol at a dose of 1.5 to 3 mg. per kg. per day.

THE IMMUNE SYSTEM. Peculiar susceptibility to infection in some patients with sickle cell disease has been well documented (75). The infections are pyogenic and include *Salmonella* osteomyelitis as well as the pulmonary infections cited above. The response to immunizations with *Salmonella* vaccines is normal (150a). Infection may be associated with overwhelming septicemia, meningitis (151), and intravascular coagulation (152). The susceptibility is more evident in the first four years of life and tends to occur frequently in certain families. In some patients a defect in serum opsonic factors has been observed (153). Recent preliminary evidence indicates that the opsonic defect resides in the "bypass pathway" of C-3 activation (154). In such patients, fresh plasma infusions are indicated during episodes of severe infection. Impaired splenic reticuloendothelial function despite splenomegaly also predisposes to infection (83); moreover, it has been noted that antibody formation following intravenous antigenic administration is retarded in these patients (155). Despite reduced capacity to clear collodial suspensions and to produce antibodies, the spleens of these patients may retain their capacity to sequester red cells and platelets (156).

THE SKELETON. Skeleton abnormalities occur with a high degree of frequency in sickle cell disease (157, 158). During painful crisis reversible elevations of the periosteum may be apparent (159). As infarctions accumulate in extent and frequency, aseptic necrosis of the femoral head (160, 161) and osteosclerosis (162) may become evident (Fig. 14–5). The latter is usually not evident in childhood. The joint spaces themselves rarely fill with fluid, but the periarticular tissues become thickened and fibrotic (63a). In childhood, polydactylitis is a frequent manifestation of bony crisis (see Fig. 14–3). This complication rarely occurs in adults. Growth during childhood is retarded in sickle cell disease, but continues throughout adolescence (162a). In fact, the habitus of adult patients is characteristically tall and thin (163). The fingers and toes may be excessively long after the adolescent growth spurt. *Salmonella* osteomyelitis is observed with relatively high frequency (164) and creates a difficult diagnostic dilemma between infarction and infection. Marrow infarction may also occur (165) and result in marrow embolism (166).

NEUROLOGIC. The central nervous system may be seriously affected in sickle cell disease, with disastrous results (76). Cerebral sickling or subarachnoid hemorrhage (167) may be fatal or cause severe hemiplegia, diplegia, and speech defects (168). The cerebral vessels may become occluded, perhaps because of sickling of the vasa vasorum and injury to the intima. The high platelet count observed in patients who are autosplenectomized may also contribute to the vascular disorder. Unfortunately the vascular lesions are rarely found within the range of a neurosurgical approach, but patients with newly acquired cerebral symptoms should be studied with angiography after careful preparation by hypertransfusion (169).

PSYCHOLOGICAL. Patients with sickle cell disease may be completely cheerful and well adjusted, but some may be withdrawn and frightened owing to lifelong episodes of pain, inability to keep up with peers, and retardation of sexual development. Parental pressure due to a combination of guilt and misunderstanding may be severe. These patients and families usually

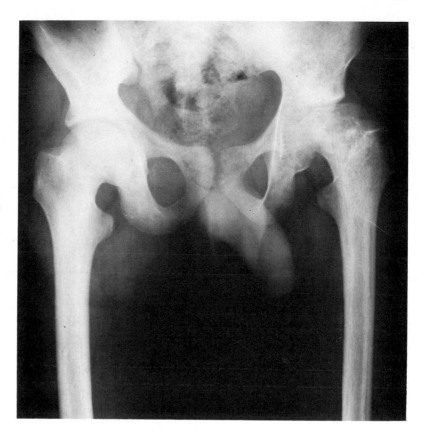

Figure 14–5. Pelvic and upper femur x-ray of a young adult male with sickle cell anemia. Note numerous areas of osteosclerosis.

require more than ordinary support and encouragement from medical facilities (170, 171).

Diagnosis

Although the diagnosis of sickle cell anemia can be made at birth by adaptations of agar gel electrophoresis at pH 6.2, or zonal or iso-focusing electrophoretic methods (Fig. 14–6), it is usually not made until anemia is observed during subsequent observations or when a painful crisis or severe infection occurs. Anemia, abnormal morphology, a positive sickling test with sodium metabisulfite (172) (Fig. 14–7), or a precipitation test with dithionite and phosphate (173), and the presence of hemoglobins S and F in a hemoglobin electrophoresis confirm the diagnosis (Fig. 14–8). The acid elution test (174) confirms the heterogeneous distribution of the Hb F, and the heterozygous state is confirmed in the parents by the sickling test and hemoglobin electrophoresis. All other siblings should be screened at this time.

Treatment

The patient with sickle cell disease needs a physician or a team of physicians, nurses, and social workers which knows him well (170, 171). If "care" is delivered only through sporadic emergency service visits for acute crisis, required attention to details rarely occurs. These details include prompt treatment of infection and attention to nutrition, with particular reference to folic acid and iron requirements. The adage that patients with hemolytic anemia do not develop iron deficiency is a generalization which is incorrect in some infants with sickle cell disease. Hypochromia and microcytosis together with a low serum iron may appear during early childhood or at the onset of menses. However, sickle thalassemia may also be associated with hypochromia and microcytosis and should be differentiated by appropriate studies. Since reduction of the MCHC may be beneficial in sickle cell anemia (26), treatment with oral iron supplements should only be offered if symptoms of iron deficiency are

S   A   F

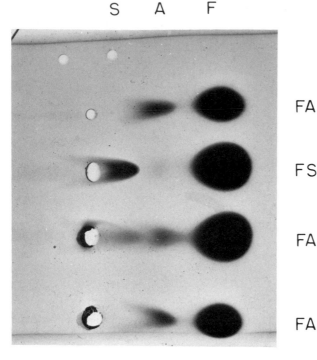

FA

FS

FAS

FA

pH 6.2   ⟶

Figure 14–6. Citrate agar gel electrophoresis of cord blood specimens of normal infants and infants with sickle cell trait or sickle cell anemia. Note that sickle cell anemia can be discriminated from normal or sickle cell trait.

obvious. School and social maladjustments and family conflicts must be approached. The patient and his family must be taught to increase water intake at the earliest sign of a painful crisis. We believe that prompt hydration and mild analgesic therapy can prevent the worsening of the crisis that leads to the requirement for emergency service or prolonged treatment on an inpatient service. Prevention of crisis by

prompt treatment of infections is also important (175).

If the patient does require intravenous fluid for treatment of crises at the hospital, our practice is to treat with 3 ml. per kg. per hour of 5 per cent dextrose to which is added 25 mEq. sodium chloride and 10 mEq. of sodium bicarbonate/1. Potassium at 10 mEq./1 is not added unless therapy is required for more than one day and the

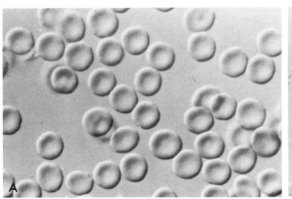
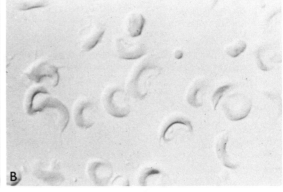

Figure 14–7. Phase photomicrograph of the sodium metabisulfite test in sickle cell trait.
A, *Left:* Cells incubated with 0.9 per cent saline and 0.5 per cent albumin.
B, *Right:* Cells 24 hours after incubation in sodium metabisulfite.

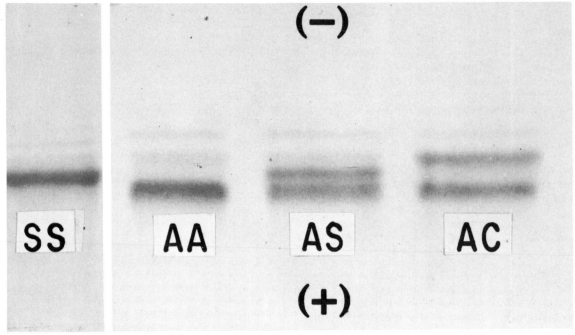

Figure 14–8. Electrophoresis in cellulose acetate at pH 8.6 of normal and various examples of abnormal hemoglobins. The direction of electrophoresis is toward the anode.

patient is unable to take solid foods by mouth. The addition of bicarbonate or citrate, as suggested by Greenberg and Kass (176) and by Barreras and Diggs (177), seems reasonable, although we have not evaluated alkali therapy critically ourselves. If the patient has chronic cor pulmonale, the rate of fluid replacement is slower and sodium administration restricted. Electrolyte therapy must be handled with caution. Inadequate water retention may be accompanied by a renal sodium-losing syndrome in these patients. Large doses of electrolyte-free water may cause a sudden and severe low-sodium syndrome. On the other hand, vigorous sodium and fluid replacement can cause pulmonary edema.

In adolescents and young adults an attempt is made to use non-narcotic analgesics and to utilize phenothiazines as sedatives [not as antisickling compounds (178)] when necessary, since repeated exposure to narcotics or barbiturates might expose the patient to increased risk of drug addiction or habituation.

If the crisis is not terminated in a reasonable period of time, partial exchange transfusion, as advocated by Brody and his co-workers (179), may be used with benefit, although we rarely utilize this approach. It is probably just as effective to use multiple small transfusions with packed red cells to reduce the patient's cells to less than 40 per cent of the total. A chronic hypertransfusion program is used only in patients with severe and frequent crises, in those with neurologic involvement, during the last trimester of pregnancy, and when major surgery is contemplated.

If visceral sickling appears life-threatening, exchange transfusion is indicated. We have not used hyperbaric oxygenation; its efficacy is not clearly established, although reports of its use are available (180, 181).

Adrenal and androgen steroid therapy have been examined in the treatment of sickle cell anemia with conflicting results and conclusions. Kass and co-workers' experiences with ACTH in a patient with sickle cell anemia were most remarkable in that improvement in viscosity as well as hemoglobin concentration did occur (182). Isaacs and Hayhoe noted decreased sickling with sodium metabisulfite after exposure to androgenic steroids in vitro (183), and Isaacs and co-workers claimed a reduction in painful crises in androgen treated patients (184). Lundh and Gardner achieved increases in hemoglobin in several patients after treatment with androgens (185). However, priapism was a significant complication. In one patient, Mentzer, August, and Nathan noted decreased ISC formation following androgen administration (186). At this time it appears that androgen or corticosteroid therapy does not provide enough benefit to warrant its risk, and the treatment is considered entirely experimental. Indeed, there are cogent theoretical reasons to avoid high-dose androgen in sickle cell disease, since the hormone increases erythrocyte 2,3-DPG and would thereby tend to increase erythrocyte sickling (187).

Splenectomy has a limited role in the management of sickle cell anemia. In addition to sequestration crisis, some patients with SS disease have persistent splenic enlargement rather than infarctions and splenic shrinkage. Anemia or thrombocytopenia or both may be particularly severe and limiting in these patients, and these may be alleviated by splenectomy (185–189). The rise in sickle hemoglobin concentration after the procedure might induce a higher incidence of vaso-occlusive manifestations. The indications for the procedure must therefore be unambiguous.

Recently, both urea and cyanate have been suggested as possible modes of therapy and are currently under experimental investigation. Urea has been proposed because at high concentrations (1 molar) it breaks hydrophobic bonds. Nalbandian and Murayama, who are advocates of urea therapy (190, 191), believe that the gelation of sickle hemoglobin involves the formation of hydrophobic bonds. Despite preliminary clinical studies which supported the efficacy of urea therapy (192, 193), there is now considerable doubt about its value at the concentrations which can be achieved in normal human blood (194–196). Indeed, at the "therapeutic range" that has been established by Nalbandian, no effects of urea on sickling in vitro were detected by Segel and his co-workers (195). In addition, urea treatment does cause severe osmotic diuresis, and the fluid losses caused by the drug can achieve major proportions (197).

Cyanate inhibits sickling in vitro and prolongs the life span of sickle cells in vivo (198–201). This compound carbamylates the N-terminal amino group of hemoglobin, and to a much lesser extent, the E amino groups of lysine residues. It alters the oxygen saturation curve and shifts it to a higher affinity (202, 203). Hence sickling is decreased at any given pO_2 (204). At high concentrations cyanate directly inhibits sickling (204). Clinical trials with cyanate are now in progress. Oral cyanate does decrease the rate of destruction of sickle red cells (205) and also leads to somewhat higher hemoglobin levels in the treated patients (206). Whether the drug will decrease vaso-occlusive manifestations is not known. The long-term toxicity is also not well established (273). The drug does depress protein synthesis in reticulocytes in vitro (207), but does not significantly depress erythropoiesis in rats (208). However, rats do develop severe wasting disease and hind limb paralysis when very high doses of cyanate are administered. In addition, alterations of tissue isozymes (209) and hepatic enzyme function (210) occur. Whether much lower doses of cyanate can be safely tolerated for longer periods of time by humans remains to be seen. Careful clinical trials are now being organized by the National Institutes of Health.

Interactions With Sickle Hemoglobin

As described above, the minimum gelling concentration of a mixture of hemoglobin S with other hemoglobins varies markedly. Certain hemoglobins interact with S to reduce the minimum gelling concentration toward that determined when S constitutes 100 per cent of the mixture. Others, such as F or Korle Bu, raise the minimum gelling concentration far above that observed when A is the accompanying hemoglobin. Clinical characteristics of heterozygous states correlate well with these physical qualities, as shown in Table 14–1 and references 26 and 274.

SICKLE CELL TRAIT:
$\alpha_2\beta_2$, $\alpha_2\beta_2^{6\ \text{Val}}$, $\alpha_2\beta^A$, $\beta^{6\ \text{Val}*}$

Individuals who are heterozygous for the beta S gene (AS) are generally free of

---

*This chemical notation is presented to remind the reader that hybrid hemoglobins probably exist in the cell.

symptoms and demonstrate neither selective mortality nor morbidity because of the sickle gene (211–213). The blood counts, red cell morphology, and red cell survival are entirely normal. The red cells contain 20 to 40 per cent Hb S, the mean level being 35 per cent. The remainder are hemoglobins A and A_2. In contrast, the red cells of individuals heterozygous for most structural abnormalities of the alpha chain contain approximately 25 per cent of the abnormal hemoglobin and 75 per cent of Hb A (214). (See Chapter 15.)

The experimentally determined minimum gelling concentration of a mixture of 40 per cent deoxyhemoglobin S and 60 per cent deoxyhemoglobin A is approximately equal to the mean corpuscular hemoglobin concentration of normal red cells (30 g. per 100 ml.) (26). It is not surprising, therefore, that under certain extreme circumstances, symptoms due to sickling occur in sickle cell trait. In fact, bony and visceral sickling crises have been reported in this condition (215–220). The clinical circumstances in which sickling occurs in sickle trait must be sufficient to produce marked deoxygenation of the cells, since the minimum gelling concentration of an AS hemoglobin mixture must be considerably higher than 32 g. per 100 ml. at higher levels of oxygen saturation.

Among the circumstances which are thought to produce organ infarction or even cerebral sickling (221) in sickle cell trait are severe pneumonia, flying, vigorous exercise in a hot, dry climate at a high altitude (222–224), underwater swimming, anesthesia (225), and labor and delivery (226). It must be emphasized that severe sickling is extremely rare in these circumstances and that the reports of fatality are those *associated* with sickle trait and not necessarily *due* to sickle trait. Postmortem sickling is no evidence that sickling occurred ante mortem.

The spleen and kidneys are quite regularly involved in sickle trait. Splenic infarction may occur during flight in aircraft that are not pressurized to less than 7000 feet (227) and has even been reported in a mountain climber at 3000 feet (228). This is not a serious clinical problem, but ordinary safety considerations should eliminate individuals with sickle trait from aviation jobs requiring solo flight status.

The milieu of the loop of Henle appears to encourage sickling, perhaps due to a combination of decreased pH and deoxygenation secondary to efficient oxygen extraction by renal cells. In any case, blood flow to those areas responsible for water extraction from tubular urine is apparently deficient in some individuals with sickle trait as it is in sickle cell anemia, and hyposthenuria results (95, 229). In addition, microinfarction of the renal pelves together with prolonged bouts of hematuria may occur. The hematuria may be extraordinarily persistent. Hypertransfusion or epsilon aminocaproic acid treatment or both may be useful (108), but the latter agent must be used with caution. Chronic pyelonephritis may be a significant problem in women with sickle trait (111), and bacteriuria is common (212). Particularly careful attention should be paid to the elimination of urinary tract infection in such individuals.

Screening for Sickle Trait

As national programs for the detection of sickle trait and suitable educational systems which might lead to a decrease in the birth rate of homozygotes are developed, controversy about their utility and wisdom has mounted (230–232). It is certainly not established that a national screening program including all age groups will be useful. More selective screening and education of hospital or clinic patients, military recruits, blood donors, pregnant women, and couples contemplating marriage would seem both practical and desirable. Screening in the newborn nursery may reveal patients with SS disease for whom close attention can then be provided (232a).

SC DISEASE:
$$\alpha_2\beta_2^{6\ Val}, \alpha_2\beta_2^{6\ Lys}, \alpha_2\beta^{6\ Val}\beta^{6\ Lys}$$

Hemoglobin SC disease is characterized by mild chronic hemolytic anemia (hemoglobin 8 to 11 g. per 100 ml.) with splenomegaly. The smear reveals many target cells and a few irreversibly sickled cells. There is a high incidence of vaso-occlusive disorders (233–236), including painful crisis, retinal thrombosis and detachment

(66–68), pulmonary thrombosis with cor pulmonale (237), aseptic necrosis of the femoral head (238), renal papillary necrosis (239), and, above all, placental infarction with multiple complications in pregnancy (240). Hemolysis is less severe in SC disease than it is in SS disease (64). Hence the hematocrit is usually higher. Although the minimum gelling concentration of a mixture of S and C is higher than that of pure S (26), any sickling in SC blood might be expected to induce a higher increment of viscosity than a similar amount of sickling in SS, since the hematocrit so strongly influences viscosity. For this reason, the vaso-occlusive complications mentioned above, rather than anemia, characterize the clinical manifestations of SC disease (239a).

Patients with SC disease appear to be particularly susceptible to infections with *Salmonella*. Osteomyelitis due to *Salmonella* is a frequent problem (238).

SO_{Arab}:
$$\alpha_2\beta_2^{6\ Val}, \alpha_2\beta_2^{121\ Lys}, \alpha_2\beta^{6\ Val}\beta^{121\ Lys}$$

SO_{Arab} double heterozygotes usually have more severe anemia and painful crises than do patients with SC disease, and the increase in severity correlates with the lower minimum gelling concentrations of mixtures of S and O_{Arab} (29). O_{Arab} migrates with hemoglobin C during filter paper electrophoresis. Investigation of putative SC double heterozygotes with unusually severe symptoms has sometimes revealed that such individuals actually have hemoglobins S and O_{Arab}.

SD:
$$\alpha_2\beta_2^{6\ Val}, \alpha_2\beta_2^{121\ Gln}, \alpha_2\beta^{6\ Val}\beta^{121\ Gln}$$

Individuals heterozygous for hemoglobins S and D of the Punjab variety also have moderately severe symptoms, comparable to those of patients with SO_{Arab} (240a, 240b), and this result is predictable from the minimum gelling concentrations of mixtures of S and D (26). The presence of hemoglobin D, which migrates electrophoretically with hemoglobin S, is detected by its solubility characteristics and by its characteristic migration pattern during electrophoresis on agar gels at pH 6.5 (241).

SD is suspected when only one parent has a positive sickling test but both have Hb A and another hemoglobin which migrates electrophoretically like S.

S KORLE BU:
$$\alpha_2\beta_2^{6\ Val}, \alpha_2\beta_2^{73\ Asn}, \alpha_2\beta^{6\ Val}\beta^{73\ Asn}$$

Hemoglobin Korle Bu is a rare hemoglobin mutant (242). It is mentioned here only because it illustrates an important pathophysiologic point. Korle Bu participates poorly in sickling, as illustrated by the high minimum gelling concentration of mixtures of S and Korle Bu (26). The S Korle Bu double heterozygotes who have been reported are entirely symptom free, and one would surmise that even the rare sickling manifestations reported in AS heterozygotes would not be observed in S Korle Bu individuals.

HEMOGLOBIN C_{Harlem}:
$$\alpha_2\beta_2^{6\ Val,\ 73\ Asn}$$

This hemoglobin is now known to be identical to hemoglobin $C_{Georgetown}$ and represents two mutations in the beta chain. One is the sickle mutation $\beta^{6\ Glu\rightarrow Val}$ and the other the Korle Bu mutation $\beta^{73\ Asp\rightarrow Asn}$ (243). As might be expected, this double mutant causes few, if any, symptoms of sickling, since the minimum gelling concentration of the hemoglobin is about 40 g. per 100 ml., a value higher than that observed with mixtures of S and A (26).

HEMOGLOBIN S MEMPHIS:
$$\alpha_2\beta_2^{6\ Val}, \alpha_2^{23\ Gln}\beta_2^{6\ Val}, \alpha\alpha^{23\ Gln}\beta_2^{6\ Val}$$

Individuals homozygous for sickle hemoglobin have extremely mild clinical disease if they are also heterozygotes for the alpha chain mutant, hemoglobin Memphis $\alpha^{23\ Glu\rightarrow Gln}$ (244). This mutation in the alpha chain must reduce the available complementary or secondary binding sites for interaction with the $\beta^{6\ Val}$-induced primary binding site. The mild disease observed in an elderly patient with homozygous S and the Memphis alpha chain variant is of considerable importance. Such alpha chain variants may explain mild sickling in other individuals with homozygous S. The syndrome also provides a clinical basis for the development of drugs which might be specifically designed to interact with particular residues of alpha and beta chains and thereby reduce available complementary or secondary binding sites. This would lead to decreased stability of the deoxy S helix.

HEMOGLOBIN S AND FETAL HEMOGLOBIN

As mentioned above, fetal hemoglobin participates poorly, if at all, in sickling. It is heterogeneously distributed among red cells in SS disease, and those cells with the highest propensity to sickle during deoxygenation or to develop into irreversibly sickled forms contain the least amount of Hb F (50). Indeed, clinical severity of SS disease is mitigated by the capacity of the marrow to synthesize fetal hemoglobin in a broad cellular distribution and in relatively high amounts. This is not to say that all mildly affected patients with SS disease have increased amounts of fetal hemoglobin in their cells (245, 246), but increased F (in the absence of an aplastic crisis in which S is preferentially destroyed) is usually associated with mild clinical symptoms (247, 248).

S-High F

The mutation which produces hereditary persistence of fetal hemoglobin is associated with absence of beta-A production, and substantial γ production by the F gene on the same chromosome (128, 249–251). When present with a β^A or a β^S gene in trans, the hemoglobin mixture is approximately 70 per cent A or S and 30 per cent F. The F is equally distributed in the cells (128, 251), and the minimum gelling concentration of this mixture approximates that of 40 per cent S and 60 per cent A (26). Hence, symptoms of sickling in the S–high F syndrome are minimal (128, 252), even though the S concentration in the cells is

double that which is observed in the AS heterozygote.

S-Thalassemia

Individuals who are doubly heterozygous for a beta thalassemia gene and a β^S gene usually have clinical manifestations similar to those of patients with mild to moderate SS disease or SC disease (253–256a). Painful crises and visceral vaso-occlusive phenomena do occur, but they are infrequent in most patients. Since the hemoglobin electrophoresis in many S-thalassemia patients may reveal between 70 and 90 per cent Hb S and the remainder Hb F, the differential diagnosis between S-thalassemia and SS disease may be somewhat difficult. Certain criteria are helpful. First, most patients with S-thalassemia have splenomegaly rather than splenic atrophy, indicating splenic erythroclasia rather than infarction. This implies that erythrocytes in S-thalassemia are less prone to sickle than are the cells in SS disease, but are sufficiently misshapen to render them liable to splenic destruction. In some cases the decreased tendency to sickle may be due to relatively high concentrations of Hb F distributed widely among the cells. In others with substantial Hb A production, the percentage of S is lower than is usually observed in SS disease. Of additional protective importance is the low MCHC due to the thalassemia gene in S-thalassemia. A reduction of total hemoglobin concentration reduces the capacity of the cell to sickle at any given oxygen tension, because the minimum gelling concentration is less readily achieved. Indeed, irreversibly sickled cells are considerably less evident in the peripheral smears of patients with S-thalassemia than in those of patients with SS disease, and it is believed that intravascular blockade is also less severe because the S-thalassemia cells do not sickle as readily. The cells are hypochromic and deformed, however, and they are readily phagocytosed by the splenic littoral cells. It may be stated, therefore, that in S-thalassemia the spleen destroys the cells, whereas in SS disease the cells destroy the spleen.

Another important diagnostic feature of S-thalassemia is the presence of variable amounts of Hb A. In some patients with a so-called β^0 thalassemia gene in trans, no Hb A is present. In patients with a β^+ thalassemia gene, some Hb A is present. Finally, Hb A_2 is often increased in S-thalassemia patients.

None of the above features, except the presence of small amounts of Hb A, are diagnostic of S-thalassemia. Splenomegaly may persist in some patients with mild SS disease and even lead to a requirement for splenectomy. Electrophoretic quantitation of Hb A_2 may be difficult in the presence of S (it is impossible in the presence of Hb C). Small amounts of Hb A may be difficult to define when Hb F is present, unless very reliable separation procedures, such as isoelectric focusing, are available. If the parents of the patient are unambiguously identified, the detection of sickle trait in one and hypochromic microcytosis without sickling in the other is extremely useful. If the MCV and MCHC are reduced in the absence of iron deficiency, the diagnosis of S-thalassemia should be seriously considered.

Splenomegaly in S-thalassemia may be extensive enough to produce severe thrombocytopenia or hemolytic anemia, which may necessitate splenectomy. This procedure should be attempted only in highly selected cases, since an elevation of the hematocrit in any sickle syndrome enhances the risk of vaso-occlusive disease.

When the Hb S gene is present with an alpha thalassemia gene, the percentage of Hb S in the hemoglobin mixture is often somewhat lower than it is in ordinary sickle cell trait (255). There are hypochromia and microcytosis. The clinical sequelae of S–alpha thalassemia are minimal.

HEMOGLOBIN C DISEASE:
$\alpha_2 \beta_2^{6\ Lys}$

Homozygous Hb C disease is a mild disorder characterized by hemolytic anemia and splenomegaly (257–259). The tendency of Hb C to aggregate into precipitates (260, 261) is probably responsible for the characteristic target morphology of the dried red cell in homozygous C disease and in Hb C trait, and for the rapid removal of homozygous C cells by splenic littoral cells. Vaso-occlusive phenomena are rare, but do occur (262, 263). Bone infarction is extremely uncommon. In Hb C trait, the target cell is the only manifestation of the anomaly. Approximately 35 to 45 per cent of the hemoglobin is Hb C. Hemolytic anemia is not present. The morphology of the red cells in Hb C disease and in Hb C trait is an interesting exception to the general rule concerning the formation of target cells. These cells usually occur under circumstances in which the ratio of the cell surface area to the cell volume is increased, such as in obstructive liver disease, when excess lipid accumulates on the cell (264), or in volume depletion syndromes, such as iron deficiency or thalassemia. In Hb C trait, the area:volume ratio is normal, but the target shape occurs, probably because the Hb C tends to aggregate into a puddle in the middle of the cell when the cell dries on a glass slide. Wet preparations of Hb C trait cells do not reveal large numbers in the target shape.

The basis of the aggregation and crystal formation of Hb C cells during drying is not precisely understood. It is thought that the substantial charge difference between Hb C and Hb A is in some way responsible for the tendency toward aggregation of C molecules, which leads to local increments of hemoglobin concentration in excess of its solubility (260).

HEMOGLOBIN SYNTHESIS IN THE SICKLE SYNDROMES

The beta-S gene is capable of a wide range of synthetic rates, depending upon the nature of the non-alpha gene in trans. In ordinary AS trait, S is synthesized at approximately 40 per cent of the rate of beta-A. In S-high F, S is synthesized at almost twice the rate observed when the trans beta gene synthesizes beta-A. In S–beta thalassemia, S synthesis from the beta-S gene is not as high as it is in S–high F, but it is higher than that observed in AS. The nature of the control of S production, whether by transcriptional modification or by some feedback control of translation, is not known. This is an important area of research for which the tools are beginning to become available.

FUTURE THERAPY OF SICKLE CELL DISEASE

Modification of Hemoglobin Function

The clinical and experimental experience with cyanate has demonstrated the potential utility of drug-induced alteration of the hemoglobin-oxygen saturation curve in sickle cell anemia. Cyanate, which predominantly carbamylates the N-terminus of hemoglobin, increases the affinity of Hb S or Hb A for oxygen, and therefore reduces the likelihood of sickling at any given partial pressure of oxygen. This effect of cyanate may be seen at levels of carbamylation of between 0.5 and 1 mole of cyanate per mole of hemoglobin tetramer. At higher levels of carbamylation, a direct inhibition by cyanate, which is independent of the drug effect on the oxygen saturation curve, is also observed (204).

2,3-diphosphoglycerate also affects sickling in an interesting fashion (265). At low levels of intracellular 2,3-DPG, the oxygen saturation curve is shifted to a higher affinity state, which decreases the tendency to sickle at any given pO_2. At high levels of 2,3-DPG, the affinity curve is shifted toward lower affinity, and sickling is enhanced. As is true of cyanate, 2,3-DPG also exerts an oxygen affinity–independent effect on sickling. High levels of 2,3-DPG enhance sickling at any pO_2 or oxygen saturation (204, 266).

These results indicate that a class of drugs which could be transported across the red cell membrane and "fit" into a critical position within the hemoglobin molecule might develop as potent antisickling compounds. Such a drug might be designed to interfere with the interrelationship of 2,3-DPG with the hemoglobin molecule, or it might by another mechanism shift the configuration of the oxygen saturation curve in such a way as to increase the affinity of hemoglobin for oxygen.

It may well be that cyanate itself will serve this purpose in sickle cell anemia. If studies of its toxicity and efficacy prove promising, its development as a potential antisickling compound will be pursued with vigor. Recently a technique for mea-surement of the life span of SS red cells in a rodent model has been developed. This may aid in the determination of the utility of potential therapeutic agents (266a).

Genetic Control

Control of the synthesis of Hb S with substitution of fetal globin synthesis for S globin synthesis is the long-term objective of many studies of the molecular biology of hemoglobin synthesis, in man and in animals. As yet, no therapeutic advantages have been generated by this approach, but it is hoped that future efforts will reveal methods by which genetic messages can be influenced by the administration of genetic material or drugs or both which influence the translation of preformed message.

Prevention of Sickle Cell Anemia

Genetic Counseling

It is clear that persuasive efforts to eliminate reproduction by partners with sickle cell trait would decrease the incidence of sickle cell anemia. This is one of the goals of screening and educational programs which have achieved high national priority for the past several years. The record of accomplishment of many other educational and screening programs devoted to the understanding of inherited diseases and their elimination by out-breeding has not been particularly encouraging (267). In addition, the charge of "genocide" has understandably arisen as a result of such programs (232).

Efforts are in progress to establish methods of prenatal diagnosis of sickle cell disease and thalassemia in order to apply what might be termed "focused genetic counseling" on a particular pregnancy at risk. It has been shown that the beta chain of human hemoglobin is synthesized in the first trimester (268, 269), and it has been further demonstrated that heterozygotes for the sickle cell gene can be detected in 6- to 8-cm. fetuses (270, 271). Further studies are now in progress to determine whether suitable samples of fetal or mixed placental blood can be acquired safely and reliably and if homozygous sickle disease and thalassemia can be detected in them (272). If this is accomplished, the methods can be applied in highly selected cases. If such techniques could be established, partners with sickle trait could plan to have children without the fear of producing a child with sickle cell anemia.

CONCLUSION

Sickle cell disease has been the object of many years of intensive investigation, and its study has provided vital information of critical value in human biology. Practical clinical application of this information has lagged behind, as would be expected from the complexity of the problem. However, significant strides have been made. It is important for the clinician to understand that relatively simple principles of care can offer reasonably rapid relief from painful crises and, in many cases, a prolonged and useful life span. While we await further progress in molecular therapy and prevention by prenatal diagnosis, the patient with sickle cell anemia will depend upon an optimistic and skilled medical and social service team and an understanding family.

References

1. Allison, A. C.: Recent developments in the study of inherited anemias. Eugen. Quart. 6:155, 1959.
2. Rucknagel, D. L., and Neel, J. V.: The hemoglobinopathies, In *Medical Genetics*. New York, Steinberg, A. G. (ed.), Grune and Stratton, 1961, p. 1.
3. Wiesenfeld, S. L.: Sickle-cell trait in human biological and cultural evolution. Science 157:1134, 1967.
4. Konotey-Ahulu, F. I. D., and Kuma, E.: Maintenance of high sickling rate in Africa. Role of polygamy. J. Trop. Med. Hyg. 73:19, 1970.
5. Motulsky, A. G.: Frequency of sickling disorders in U.S. Blacks. New Engl. J. Med. 288:31, 1973.
6. Luzzatto, L., Nwachuku-Jarrett, E. S., et al.: Increased sickling of parasitised erythrocytes as mechanism of resistance against malaria in the sickle-cell trait. Lancet 1:319, 1970.
7. Herrick, J. B.: Peculiar elongated and sickle-shaped red corpuscles in a case of severe anemia. Arch. Intern. Med. 6:517, 1910.
8. Hahn, E. V., and Gillespie, E. B.: Sickle-cell

anemia: Report of a case greatly improved by splenectomy. Arch. Intern. Med. 39:233, 1927.
9. Pauling, L., Itano, H. A., et al.: Sickle cell anemia: A molecular disease. Science 110:543, 1949.
10. Beet, E. A.: Genetics of the sickle-cell trait in a Bantu tribe. Ann. Eugen. (Lond.) 14:279, 1949.
11. Neel, J. V.: Inheritance of the sickling phenomenon with particular reference to sickle-cell disease. Blood 6:389, 1951.
12. Huehns, E. R., and Shooter, E. M.: Human hemoglobins. J. Med. Genet. 2:1, 1965.
13. Huehns, E. R., Dance, N., et al.: Human embryonic haemoglobins. Nature (Lond.) 201:1095, 1964.
14. Capp, G. L., Rigas, D. A., et al.: Evidence for a new haemoglobin chain (ζ chain). Nature (Lond.) 228:278, 1970.
15. Ingram, V. M.: *Hemoglobin and Its Abnormalities*. Monograph in American Lecture Series. Springfield, Illinois, Charles C Thomas, 1961.
16. Ingram, V. M.: Gene mutations in human haemoglobin: The chemical difference between normal and sickle cell haemoglobin. Nature (Lond.) 180:326, 1957.
17. Harris, J. W.: Studies on the destruction of red blood cells. VIII. Molecular orientation in sickle-cell hemoglobin solutions. Proc. Soc. Exp. Biol. Med. 75:197, 1950.
18. Murayama, M.: A molecular mechanism of sickle erythrocyte formation. Nature (Lond.) 202:258, 1964.
19. Murayama, M.: Structure of sickle cell hemoglobin and molecular mechanisms of the sickling phenomenon. Clin. Chem. 13:578, 1967.
20. Stetson, C. A., Jr.: The state of hemoglobin in sickled erythrocytes. J. Exp. Med. 123:341, 1966.
21. White, J. G.: The fine structure of sickled hemoglobin in situ. Blood 31:561, 1968.
22. Döbler, J., and Bertles, J. F.: The physical state of hemoglobin in sickle cell anemia erythrocytes in vivo. J. Exp. Med. 127:711, 1968.
23. Lessin, L. S.: Helical polymerization of hemoglobin molecules in falciform erythrocytes. A study using unmasking by cold. C. R. Acad. Sci. (Paris) 266:1806, 1968.
24. Lessin, L. S., Jensen, W. N., et al.: Molecular rearrangement in intraerythrocyte crystallization in hemoglobin C disease. Clin. Res. 16:307, 1968.
25. Perutz, M. F., and Mitcheson, J. M.: State of haemoglobin in sickle-cell anaemia. Nature (Lond.) 166:677, 1950.
26. Bookchin, R. M., and Nagel, R. L.: Ligand-induced conformational dependence of hemoglobin in sickling interactions. J. Mol. Biol. 60:262, 1971.
27. Magdoff-Fairchild, B., Swerdlow, P. H., et al.: Intermolecular organization of deoxygenated sickle hemoglobin determined by X-ray diffraction. Nature (Lond.) 239:217, 1972.
28. Perutz, M., and Lehmann, H.: Molecular pathology of human haemoglobins. Nature (Lond.) 219:902, 1968.

29. Milner, P. F., Miller, C., et al.: Hemoglobin O Arab in 4 Negro families and its interaction with hemoglobin S and hemoglobin C. New Engl. J. Med. 283:1417, 1970.

30. Singer, K., and Singer, L.: Studies on abnormal hemoglobins. VIII. The gelling phenomenon of sickle cell hemoglobin: Its biologic and diagnostic significance. Blood 8:1008, 1953.

31. Allison, A. C.: Properties of sickle cell haemoglobin. Biochem. J. 65:212, 1957.

32. Bertles, J. F., Rabinowitz, R., et al.: Hemoglobin interaction: Modification of solid phase composition in the sickling phenomenon. Science 169:375, 1970.

33. Dintenfaas, L.: Rheology of packed red blood cells containing hemoglobins A-A, S-A and S-S. J. Lab. Clin. Med. 64:594, 1964.

34. Jandl, J. H., Simmons, R. L., et al.: Red cell filtration and the pathogenesis of certain hemolytic anemias. Blood 18:133, 1961.

35. Chien, S., Usami, S., et al.: Abnormal rheology of oxygenated blood in sickle cell anemia. J. Clin. Invest. 49:623, 1970.

36. Evans, H. E., and Reindorf, C.: Serum immunoglobulin levels in sickle cell disease and thalassemia major. Am. J. Dis. Child. 116:586, 1968.

37. Lange, R. D., Minnich, V., et al.: Effect of oxygen tension and of pH on the sickling and mechanical fragility of erythrocytes from patients with sickle cell anemia and the sickle cell trait. J. Lab. Clin. Med. 37:789, 1951.

38. Harris, J. W., Brewster, H. A., et al.: Studies on the destruction of red blood cells. X. The biophysics and biology of sickle-cell disease. A.M.A. Arch. Intern. Med. 97:145, 1956.

39. Jensen, W. N., Bromberg, P. A., et al.: Microincision of sickled erythrocytes by a laser beam. Science 155:704, 1967.

40. Holroyde, C. P., Lundh, B., et al.: Erythrocyte fragmentation; A mechanism of red cell destruction in sickle cell anemia. J. Clin. Invest. 48:39a, 1969.

41. Jensen, W. N.: Fragmentation and the freakish poikilocyte (editorial). Am. J. Med. Sci. 257:355, 1969.

42. Finch, J. T., Perutz, M. F., et al.: Structure of sickled erythrocytes and of sickle-cell hemoglobin fibers. Proc. Natl. Acad. Sci. USA 70:718, 1973.

42a. Benesch, R., Benesch, R. E., et al.: The solubility of hemoglobin β_4^S, the mutant subunits of sickle cell hemoglobin. Biochem. Biophys. Res. Commun. 55:261, 1973.

43. Herman, E. C., Jr.: Serum haptoglobins in hemolytic disorders. J. Lab. Clin. Med. 57:834, 1961.

44. Muller-Eberhardt, H. J., and Miescher, P. A.: Textbook of Immunopathology. New York, Grune & Stratton, 1968.

45. Crosby, W. H.: Metabolism of hemoglobin and bile pigment in hemolytic disease. Am. J. Med. 18:112, 1955.

46. Erlandson, M. E., Schulman, I., et al.: Studies on congenital hemolytic syndromes. III. Rate of destruction and production of erythrocytes in sickle cell anemia. Pediatrics 25:629, 1960.

47. Weisman, R., Jr., Hurley, T. H., et al.: Studies of the function of the spleen in the hemolysis of red cells in hereditary spherocytosis and sickle-cell disorders. J. Lab. Clin. Med. 42:965, 1954.

48. Jandl, J. H., Greenberg, M. S., et al.: Clinical determination of the sites of red cell sequestration in hemolytic anemias. J. Clin. Invest. 35:842, 1956.

49. Serjeant, G. R.: Irreversibly sickled cells and splenomegaly in sickle cell-anemia. Br. J. Haematol. 19:635, 1970.

50. Bertles, J. F., and Milner, P. F.: Irreversibly sickled erythrocytes: A consequence of the heterogeneous distribution of hemoglobin types in sickle cell anemia. J. Clin. Invest. 47:1731, 1968.

51. Serjeant, G. R., Serjeant, B. E., et al.: The irreversibly sickled cell; a determinant of haemolysis in sickle cell anemia. Br. J. Haematol. 17:527, 1969.

52. Sherman, I. J.: The sickling phenomenon, with special reference to differentiation of sickle cell anemia from the sickle cell trait. Bull. Johns Hopkins Hosp. 67:309, 1940.

53. Bertles, J. F., and Döbler, J.: Reversible and irreversible sickling: A distinction by electron microscopy. Blood 33:884, 1969.

54. Shen, S. C., Fleming, E. M., et al.: Studies on the destruction of red blood cells. V. Irreversibly sickled erythrocytes: Their experimental production in vitro. Blood 4:498, 1949.

55. Jensen, M., Shohet, S. B., et al.: The role of red cell energy metabolism in the generation of irreversibly sickled cells in vitro. Blood 42:835, 1973.

55a. Palek, J.: Calcium accumulation during sickling of hemoglobin S[Hb SS] red cells (abstract). Blood 42:988, 1973.

55b. Eaton, J. W., Skelton, T. O., et al.: Elevated erythrocyte calcium in sickle cell disease. Nature (Lond.) 246:105, 1973.

56. Shohet, S. B.: Personal communication.

57. Tosteson, D. C., Carlsen, E., et al.: The effects of sickling on ion transport. I. Effects of sickling on potassium transport. J. Gen. Physiol. 39:31, 1956.

58. Tosteson, D. C.: The effects of sickling on ion transport. II. The effect of sickling on sodium and cesium transport. J. Gen. Physiol. 39:55, 1956.

59. Mentzer, W. C.: Personal communication.

60. Seakins, M., Gibbs, W. N., et al.: Erythrocyte Hb-S concentration, an important factor in the low oxygen affinity of blood in sickle cell anemia. J. Clin. Invest. 52:422, 1973.

61. Weed, R. I., LaCelle, P. L., et al.: Metabolic dependence of red cell deformability. J. Clin. Invest. 48:795, 1969.

62. Margolies, S. I., and Minkin, S. D.: Sickle cell disease. The roentgenologic manifestations of urinary tract abnormalities in adults. Am. J. Roentgenol. Radium Ther. Nucl. Med. 107:702, 1969.

63. Diggs, L. W.: Sickle cell crises. Am. J. Clin. Pathol. 44:1, 1965.

63a. Porter, F. S., and Thurman, W. G.: Studies of sickle cell disease: Diagnosis in childhood. Am. J. Dis. Child. 106:35, 1963.

63b. Jenkins, M. E., Scott, R. B., et al.: Studies in sickle cell anemia. XVI. Sudden death during SCA crises in young children. J. Pediatr. 56: 30, 1960.

64. McCurdy, P. R.: Erythrokinetics in abnormal hemoglobin syndromes. Blood 20:686, 1962.

65. Wolfort, F. G., and Krizek, T. J.: Skin ulceration in sickle cell anemia. Plast. Reconstr. Surg. 43:71, 1969.

66. Goldberg, M. F.: Natural history of untreated proliferative sickle retinopathy. Arch. Ophthalmol. 85:428, 1971.

67. Ryan, S. J., and Goldberg, M. F.: Anterior segment ischemia following scleral buckling in sickle cell hemoglobinopathy. Am. J. Ophthalmol. 72:35, 1971.

68. Goldberg, M. F.: Treatment of proliferative sickle retinopathy. Trans. Am. Acad. Ophthalmol. Otolaryngol. 75:532, 1971.

69. Diggs, L. W.: Pulmonary lesions in sickle cell anemia. Blood 34:734, 1969.

70. Diggs, L. W., and Berraras, L.: Pulmonary emboli versus pneumonia in patients with sickle cell anemia. Memphis Med. J. 42:375, 1967.

71. Moser, K. M., and Shea, J. C.: The relationship between pulmonary infarction, cor pulmonale and the sickle states. Am. J. Med. 22:561, 1957.

72. Miller, G. J., and Serjeant, G. R.: An assessment of lung volumes and gas transfer in sickle cell anaemia. Thorax 26:309, 1971.

73. Sproule, B. J., Halden, E. R., et al.: A study of cardiopulmonary alterations in patients with sickle cell disease and its variants. J. Clin. Invest. 37:486, 1957.

74. Kabins, S. A., and Lerner, C.: Fulminant pneumococcemia and sickle cell anemia. J.A.M.A. 211:467, 1970.

75. Barrett-Connor, E.: Bacterial infection and sickle cell anemia. An analysis of 250 infections in 166 patients and a review of the literature. Medicine 50:97, 1971.

76. Baird, R. L., Weiss, D. L., et al.: Studies in sickle cell anemia. XXI. Clinicopathological aspects of neurological manifestations. Pediatrics 34:92, 1964.

77. Shulman, S., Bartlett, J., et al.: Unusual severity of Mycoplasma pneumonia in children with sickle cell disease. New Engl. J. Med. 287: 164, 1972.

77a. Pearson, H. A.: Sickle-cell anemia associated with tetralogy of Fallot. New Engl. J. Med. 273:1079, 1965.

78. Beeson, C. W., 2nd: Sickle cell heart disease. J. Med. Assoc. Georgia 57:438, 1968.

79. Shubin, H., Kaufman, R., et al.: Cardiovascular findings in children with sickle cell anemia. Am. J. Cardiol. 6:875, 1960.

80. Jensen, W. N., Rucknagel, D. L., et al.: In vivo study of the sickle cell phenomenon. J. Lab. Clin. Med. 56:854, 1960.

81. Jacob, H. S., MacDonald, R. A., et al.: Regulation of spleen growth and sequestering function. J. Clin. Invest. 42:1476, 1963.

82. Pearson, H. A., Spencer, R. P., et al.: Functional asplenia in sickle-cell anemia. New Engl. J. Med. 281:923, 1969.

83. Pearson, H. A., Cornelius, E. A., et al.: Transfusion-reversible functional asplenia in young children with sickle-cell anemia. New Engl. J. Med. 283:334, 1970.

84. Haggard, M. E., and Schneider, R. G.: Sickle cell anemia in the first two years of life. J. Pediatr. 58:785, 1961.

85. Ham, T. H., and Battle, J. D.: Viscosity of sickle cells: A thirty-four-year study of an Italian family with sickle-cell and thalassemia traits: Splenectomy in two members. Trans. Am. Clin. Climatol. Assoc. 68:146, 1957.

86. Lam, R. C.: Splenectomy for treatment of sickle cell anemia. Am. J. Surg. 95:150, 1958.

87. Lichtman, H., Shapiro, H., et al.: Splenic hyperfunction in sickle cell anemia. Am. J. Med. 14:516, 1952.

88. Rossi, E. C., Westring, D. W., et al.: Hypersplenism in sickle cell anemia. A.M.A. Arch. Intern. Med. 114:408, 1964.

89. Alli, A. F., and Lewis, E. A.: The liver in sickle cell disease—pathological aspects based on a report on the pathological study of 77 necropsy and 5 biopsy specimens of liver. Ghana Med. J. 8:119, 1969.

90. Bogoch, A., Casselman, W. G. B., et al.: Liver disease in sickle cell anemia: A correlation of clinical, biochemical and histochemical observations. Am. J. Med. 19:583, 1955.

91. Barrett-Connor, E.: Cholelithiasis in sickle cell anemia. Am. J. Med. 45:889, 1968.

92. Brittain, H. P., DeLa Torre, A., et al.: A case of sickle cell disease with an abscess arising in an infarct of the liver. Ann. Intern. Med. 65:560, 1966.

93. Green, T. W., Conley, C. L., et al.: Liver in sickle cell anemia. Bull. Johns Hopkins Hosp. 92: 99, 1953.

94. Ferguson, A. D., and Scott, R. B.: Studies in sickle-cell anemia. XII. Further studies on hepatic function in sickle-cell anemia. A.M.A. Am. J. Dis. Child. 97:418, 1959.

95. Barrett-Connor, E.: Sickle cell disease and viral hepatitis. Ann. Intern. Med. 69:517, 1968a.

96. Flye, M. W., and Silver, D.: Biliary tract disorders and sickle cell disease. Surgery 72: 361, 1972.

97. Cameron, J. L., Maddrey, W. C., et al.: Biliary tract disease in sickle cell anemia: Surgical considerations. Ann. Surg. 174:702, 1971.

98. Whitten, C. F., Younes, A. A., et al.: Comparative study of renal concentrating ability in children with sickle cell anemia and in normal children. J. Lab. Clin. Med. 55:400, 1960.

99. Hatch, F. E., Culbertson, J. W., et al.: Nature of the renal concentrating defect in sickle cell disease. J. Clin. Invest. 46:336, 1967.

100. Schlitt, L. E., and Keital, H. G.: Renal manifestations of sickle cell disease. A review. Am. J. Med. Sci. 239:773, 1960.

101. Perillie, P. E., and Epstein, F. H.: Sickling phenomenon produced by hypertonic solutions: A possible explanation for the hyposthenuria of sicklemia. J. Clin. Invest. 42:570, 1963.

102. Whitten, C. F.: Effect of dietary protein on the renal concentrating process in sickle cell anemia. Am. J. Dis. Child. 115:262, 1968.

103. Statius van Eps, L. W., Schouten, H., et al.: The influence of red blood cell transfusions

on the hyposthenuria and renal hemodynamics of sickle cell anemia. Clin. Chem.
Acta 17:449, 1967.

104. Statius van Eps, L. W., Pinedo-Veels, C., et al.:
Nature of concentrating defect in sickle-cell
nephropathy. Lancet 1:450, 1970.

105. Mostofi, F. K., Bruegge, C. F. V., et al.: Lesions
in kidneys removed for unilateral hematuria
in sickle cell disease. Arch. Pathol. 63:336,
1957.

106. Lucas, W. M., and Bullock, W.: Hematuria in
sickle cell disease. J. Urol. 83:733, 1960.

107. Allen, T. D.: Sickle cell disease and hematuria:
A report of 29 cases. J. Urol. 91:177, 1964.

108. Bilinsky, R. T., Kandel, G. L., et al.: Epsilon
aminocaproic acid therapy of hematuria due
to heterozygous sickle cell diseases. J. Urol.
102:93, 1969.

109. Bernstein, J., and Whitten, C. F.: Histologic
appraisal of the kidney in sickle cell anemia.
A.M.A. Arch. Pathol. 70:407, 1960.

110. Femi-Pearse, D., and Odunjo, E. O.: Renal cortical infarcts in sickle-cell trait. Br. Med. J.
3:34, 1968.

111. Akinkugbe, O. O.: Renal papillary necrosis in
sickle-cell hemoglobinopathy. Br. Med. J.
3:283, 1967.

112. Plunket, D. C., Leiken, S. L., et al.: Renal radiologic changes in sickle cell anemia. Pediatrics 35:955, 1965.

113. Sccler, R. A.: Priapism in children with sickle
cell anemia. Clin. Pediatr. 10:418, 1971.

114. Campbell, J. H., and Cummings, S. D.: Priapism
in sickle cell anemia. J. Urol. 66:697, 1951.

115. Harrow, B. R.: Simple technique for treating
priapism. J. Urol. 101:71, 1969.

116. Grayhack, J. T., McCullough, W., et al.: Venous
bypass to control priapism. Invest. Urol. 1:
509, 1964.

117. Grace, D. A., and Winter, C. C.: Priapism: An
appraisal of management of twenty-three
patients. J. Urol. 99:301, 1968.

118. Jimenez, C. T., Scott, R. B., et al.: Studies in
sickle cell anemia. Am. J. Dis. Child. 111:
497, 1966.

119. Watson-Williams, E. J.: The role of folic acid in
the treatment of sickle cell disease. East
Afr. Med. J. 39:213, 1962.

120. Pearson, H. A., and Vaughan, E. O.: Lack of influence of sickle cell trait on fertility and
successful pregnancy. Am. J. Obstet. Gynecol.
105:203, 1969.

121. Curtis, E. M.: Pregnancy in sickle cell anemia,
sickle cell-hemoglobin C disease, and the
variants thereof. Am. J. Obstet. Gynecol.
77:1312, 1959.

122. Anderson, M., Went, L. N., et al.: Sickle-cell
disease in pregnancy. Lancet 2:516, 1960.

123. Henderson, A. B., Prince, A. E., et al.: Sickle-
cell disease variants and pregnancy. New
Engl. J. Med. 264:1279, 1961.

124. Whalley, P. J., Martin, F. G., et al.: Sickle cell
trait and urinary tract infection during pregnancy. J.A.M.A. 189:903, 1964.

125. Apthorp, G. H., Measday, B., et al.: Pregnancy in
sickle cell anemia. Lancet 1:1344, 1966.

126. Laros, R. K.: Sickle cell disease and pregnancy.
Penn. Med. J. 70:73, 1967.

126a. Pritchard, J. A.: The effects of maternal sickle

cell hemoglobinopathies and sickle cell
trait on reproductive performance. Am. J.
Obstet. Gynecol. 117:662, 1973.

127. Beaven, G. H., Ellis, M. J., et al.: Studies on
human foetal hemoglobin. III. The hereditary haemoglobinopathies and thalassemias.
Br. J. Haematol. 7:196, 1961.

128. Charache, S., and Conley, C. L.: Hereditary
persistence of fetal hemoglobin. Ann. N.Y.
Acad. Sci. 165:37, 1969.

129. Shepard, M. K., Weatherall, D. J., et al.: Semi-
quantitative estimation of the distribution
of fetal hemoglobin in red cell populations.
Bull. Johns Hopkins Hosp. 110:293, 1962.

130. Singer, K., and Chernoff, A. I.: Studies on abnormal hemoglobins. III. The interrelationship
of Type S (sickle cell) hemoglobin and
Type F (alkali-resistant) hemoglobin in
sickle cell anemia. Blood 7:47, 1952.

131. Singer, K., and Fisher, B.: Studies on abnormal
hemoglobins. V. The distribution of Type S
(sickle cell) hemoglobin and Type F (alkali-
resistant) hemoglobin within the red cell
population in sickle cell anemia. Blood 7:
1216, 1952.

132. Bloom, G. E., and Diamond, L. K.: Prognostic
value of fetal hemoglobin levels in acquired
aplastic anemia. New Engl. J. Med. 278:304,
1971.

133. Miller, D. R.: Raised foetal haemoglobin in chil-
hood leukemia. Br. J. Haematol. 17:103, 1969.

134. Weatherall, D. J., Edwards, J. A., et al.: Haemoglobin and red cell enzyme changes in juvenile myeloid leukemia. Br. Med. J. 1:679,
1968.

135. Maurer, H. S., Vida, L. N., et al.: Similarities of
the erythrocytes in juvenile chronic myelogenous leukemia to fetal erythrocytes. Blood
39:778, 1972.

136. MacIver, J. E., and Parker-Williams, E. I.:
Aplastic crisis in sickle-cell anemia. Lancet
1:1086, 1961.

137. Gabuzda, T. G., and Gardner, F. H.: Regulation
of fetal and adult hemoglobin formation in
patients with sickle cell disease transfused
to normal hematocrits. Blood 29:126, 1967.

138. Race, R. R., and Sanger, R.: Blood Groups in
Man. 5th ed. Oxford, Blackwell Scientific
Publications, 1968.

139. Smits, H. L., Oski, F. A., et al.: The hemolytic
crisis of sickle cell disease; the role of glu-
cose-6-phosphate dehydrogenase deficiency.
J. Pediatr. 74:544, 1969.

140. Lewis, R. A., Kay, R. W., et al.: Sickle cell disease
and glucose-6-phosphate dehydrogenase.
Acta Haematol. 36:399, 1966.

141. Piomelli, S., Reindorf, C. A., et al.: Interactions
of G6PD deficiency and sickle cell anemia.
New Engl. J. Med. 287:213, 1972.

142. Jonsson, U., Roath, O. S., et al.: Nutritional
megaloblastic anemia associated with sickle
cell states. Blood 14:535, 1959.

143. Lindenbaum, J., and Klipstein, F. A.: Folic acid
deficiency in sickle cell anemia. New Engl.
J. Med. 269:875, 1963.

144. Pierce, L. E., and Rath, C. E.: Evidence for folic
acid deficiency in the genesis of anemic
sickle cell crisis. Blood 20:19, 1962.

145. Watson-Williams, E. J.: Folic acid deficiency in

sickle-cell anaemia. East Afr. Med. J. *39*: 213, 1962.

146. Watson-Williams, E. J.: Folic acid, sickle cell anemia and growth, In *Abnormal Haemoglobins in Africa.* Jonxis, J. H. P. (ed.), C.I.O.M.S. Symposium, Philadelphia, F. A. Davis Co., 1965.

147. Grode, H. E., and Laszlo, J.: Sickle cell trait, refractory anemia, and nutritional anemia with variable expression of A and S hemoglobin. Arch. Intern. Med. *65*:321, 1966.

148. Heller, P., Yakulis, V., et al.: Variation in the amount of hemoglobin S in a patient with sickle cell trait and megaloblastic anemia. Blood *21*:479, 1963.

148a. Schiebler, G. L., Krovetz, L. T., et al.: Folic acid studies in sickle-cell anemia. J. Lab. Clin. Med. *64*:913, 1964.

149. Gold, M. S., Williams, J. C., et al.: Sickle cell anemia and hyperuricemia. J.A.M.A. *206*: 1572, 1968.

150. Walker, B. R., and Alexander, F.: Uric acid excretion in sickle cell anemia. J.A.M.A. *215*: 255, 1971.

150a. Robbins, J. B., and Pearson, H. A.: Normal response of sickle cell anemia patients to immunization with salmonella vaccines. J. Pediatr. *66*:877, 1965.

151. Robinson, M., and Watson, R. J.: Pneumococcal meningitis in sickle cell anemia. New Engl. J. Med. *274*:1006, 1966.

152. Whitaker, A. N.: Infection and the spleen: Association between hyposplenism, pneumococcal sepsis and disseminated intravascular coagulation. Med. J. Aust. *1*:1213, 1969.

153. Winkelstein, J. A., and Drachman, R. H.: Deficiency of pneumococcal serum opsonizing activity in sickle-cell disease. New Engl. J. Med. *279*:459, 1968.

154. Johnston, R. B., Jr., Newman, S. L., et al.: Serum opsonins and the alternate pathway in sickle cell disease. New Engl. J. Med. *288*:803, 1973.

155. Schwartz, A. D., and Pearson, H. A.: Impaired antibody response to immunization in sickle cell anemia. Pediatr. Res. *6*:145, 1972.

156. Schwartz, A. D.: The splenic platelet reservoir in sickle cell anemia. Blood *40*:678, 1972.

157. Golding, J. S. R., MacIver, J. E., et al.: Bone changes in sickle-cell anemia and its genetic variants. J. Bone Joint Surg. (Am.) *41B*:711, 1959.

158. Diggs, L. W.: Bone and joint lesions in sickle-cell disease. Clin. Orthop. *51*:119, 1967.

159. Johnson, A., Davis, T. W., et al.: Studies in sickle cell anemia. XXXII. Roentgenographic aspects of osseous changes. Med. Ann. D.C. *36*:651, 1967.

160. Konotey-Ahulu, F. I. D., and Kuma, E.: Skeletal crumbling in sickle cell anemia complicated by *Salmonella typhi* infection. Br. J. Clin. Pract. *19*:575, 1965.

161. Chung, S. M. K., and Ralston, E. L.: Necrosis of the femoral head associated with sickle-cell anemia and its genetic variants. A review of the literature and study of thirteen cases. J. Bone Joint Surg. *51A*:33, 1969.

162. Rowe, C. W., and Haggard, M. E.: Bone infarcts in sickle cell anemia. Radiology *68*:661, 1957.

162a. Serjeant, G. R., and Ashcroft, M. T.: Delayed skeletal maturation in sickle cell anemia in Jamaica. Johns Hopkins Med. J. *132*:95, 1973.

163. Whitten, C. F.: Growth status of children with sickle cell anemia. A.M.A. J. Dis. Child. *102*:101, 1961.

164. deTorregrosa, M. V., Dapena, R. B., et al.: Association of salmonella-caused osteomyelitis and sickle-cell disease. J.A.M.A. *174*:354, 1960.

165. Charache, S., and Page, D. L.: Infarction of bone marrow in the sickle cell disorders. Ann. Intern. Med. *67*:1195, 1967.

166. Shelley, W. M., and Curtis, E. M.: Bone marrow and fat embolism in sickle cell anemia and sickle cell-hemoglobin C disease. Bull. Johns Hopkins Hosp. *103*:8, 1958.

167. Ballard, H. S., and Bondar, H.: Spontaneous subarachnoid hemorrhage in sickle cell anemia. Neurology *7*:443, 1957.

168. Portnoy, B., and Herion, J. C.: Neurological manifestations in sickle cell disease. Ann. Intern. Med. *76*:643, 1972.

169. Stockman, J. A., Nigro, M. A., et al.: Occlusion of large cerebral vessels in sickle cell anemia. New Engl. J. Med. *287*:846, 1972.

170. Scott, R. B., and Ferguson, A. D.: Studies in sickle-cell anemia. XIV. Management of the child with sickle-cell anemia. A.M.A. J. Dis. Child. *100*:85, 1960.

171. Scott, R. B., and Kessler, A. D.: Sickle cell anemia and your child: Questions and answers on sickle cell anemia for parents (13-page booklet). Howard University College of Medicine, Washington, D.C., 1960.

172. Daland, G. A., and Castle, W. B.: A simple and rapid method for demonstrating sickling of the red blood cells: The use of reducing agents. J. Lab. Clin. Med. *33*:1082, 1948.

173. Greenberg, M. S., Harvey, H. A., et al.: A simple and inexpensive screening test for sickle hemoglobin. New Engl. J. Med. *286*:1143, 1972.

174. Betke, K.: Cytological differentiation of haemoglobin. Bibl. Haematol. *29*:1085, 1968.

175. Konotey-Ahulu, F. I. D.: Treatment and prevention of sickle cell crisis. Lancet *2*:1255, 1971.

176. Greenberg, M. S., and Kass, E. H.: Studies on the destruction of red blood cells. XIII. Observations on the role of pH in the pathogenesis and treatment of painful crisis in sickle-cell disease. A.M.A. Arch. Intern. Med. *101*:355, 1958.

177. Barreras, L., and Diggs, L. W.: Sodium citrate orally for painful sickle cell crisis. J.A.M.A. *215*:762, 1971.

178. Pearson, H. A., and Noyes, W. D.: Failure of phenothiazines in sickle cell anemia. J.A.M.A. *199*:33, 1967.

179. Brody, J. I., Goldsmith, M. H., et al.: Symptomatic crisis of sickle cell anemia treated by limited exchange transfusion. Ann. Intern. Med. *72*:327, 1970.

180. Laszlo, J., Obenous, W., et al.: Effects of hyper-

baric oxygenation on sickle syndromes. South. Med. J. *62*:453, 1969.

181. Reynolds, J. D. H.: Painful sickle cell crisis. Successful treatment with hyperbaric oxygen therapy. J.A.M.A. *216*:1977, 1971.

182. Kass, E. H., Geiman, Q. M., et al.: Some diseases which may be activated by ACTH: Observations on sickle cell anemia and malaria. *Proc. 2nd Clinical ACTH Conference on Therapeutics.* Vol. 2. Philadelphia, Blakiston, 1951, p. 376.

183. Isaacs, W. A., and Hayhoe, F. G. J.: Steroid hormones in sickle-cell disease. Nature (Lond.) *215*:1139, 1967.

184. Isaacs, W. A., Effiong, C. E., et al.: Steroid treatment in the prevention of painful episodes in sickle-cell disease. Lancet *1*:570, 1972.

185. Lundh, B., and Gardner, F. H.: The hematologic response to androgens in sickle cell anemia. Scand. J. Haematol. 7:389, 1970.

186. Mentzer, W. C., August, C. S., et al.: The irreversibly sickled cell (abstract). Blood *34*:733, 1969.

187. Feig, S. A., and Segel, G. B.: Androgens, 2,3-DPG and sickling. New Engl. J. Med. *287*:1097, 1972.

188. Eraklis, A. J., Kevy, S. V., et al.: Hazard of overwhelming infection after splenectomy in childhood. New Engl. J. Med. *276*:1125, 1967.

189. Diamond, L. K.: Splenectomy in childhood and the hazard of overwhelming infection. Pediatrics *43*:886, 1969.

190. Nalbandian, R. M., Henry, R. L., et al.: Sickling crisis treated successfully by urea in invert sugar. Ann. Intern. Med. 74:827, 1971.

191. Nalbandian, R. M.: *Molecular Aspects of Sickle Cell Hemoglobin: Clinical Applications.* Springfield, Illinois, Charles C Thomas, 1971.

192. McCurdy, P. R., and Mahmood, L.: Intravenous urea treatment of the painful crisis of sickle cell disease: A preliminary report. New Engl. J. Med. *285*:992, 1971.

193. Lusher, J. M., and Barnhart, M. I.: Evaluation of oral urea in the management of sickle cell anemia, In *Hemoglobin and Red Cell Structure and Function. Advances in Experimental Medicine and Biology.* Vol. 28. Brewer, G. L. (ed.), New York, Plenum Press, 1972, p. 303.

194. Opio, E., and Barnes, P. M.: Intravenous urea in treatment of bone pain crises of sickle cell disease — a double blind trial. Lancet 2:160, 1972.

195. Segel, G. B., Feig, S. A., et al.: Effects of urea and cyanate on sickling *in vitro.* New Engl. J. Med. *287*:59, 1972.

196. Lubin, B., and Oski, F. A.: An evaluation of oral urea therapy for sickle cell anemia (abstract). American Society of Hematology. Fifteenth Annual Meeting, Hollywood, Florida, Dec. 3-6, 1972, p. 38.

197. Brodie, J. I.: Treatment of sickle cell crises. New Engl. J. Med. *287*:616, 1972.

198. Cerami, A., and Manning, J. M.: Potassium cyanate as an inhibitor of the sickling of erythrocytes in vitro. Proc. Natl. Acad. Sci. USA 68:1180, 1971.

199. Gillette, P. N., Manning, J. M., et al.: Increased survival of sickle-cell erythrocytes after treatment *in vitro* with sodium cyanate. Proc. Natl. Acad. Sci. USA 68:2791, 1971.

200. May, A., Bellingham, A. J., et al.: Effect of cyanate on sickling. Lancet *1*:658, 1972.

201. Alter, B. P., Kan, Y. W., et al.: Reticulocyte survival in sickle cell anemia: Effect of cyanate. Blood *40*:733, 1972.

202. Diederich, D.: Relationship between the oxygen affinity and in vitro sickling propensity of carbamylated sickle erythrocytes. Biochem. Biophys. Res. Commun. *46*:1255, 1972.

203. Diederich, D., Carreras, J., et al.: Carbamylation-induced alterations in red cell function. Blood *38*:795, 1971.

204. Jensen, M., Bunn, H. F., et al.: Effects of cyanate and 2,3-diphosphoglycerate on sickling. Relationship to oxygenation. J. Clin. Invest. *52*:2542, 1973.

205. Gillette, P. N., Manning, J. M., et al.: Increased survival of sickle-cell erythrocytes after treatment *in vitro.* Proc. Natl. Acad. Sci. USA 68:2791, 1971.

206. Gillette, P. N., Peterson, C. M., et al.: Preliminary clinical trials with cyanate, In *Hemoglobin and Red Cell Structure and Function. Advances in Experimental Medicine and Biology.* Vol. 28. Brewer, G. L. (ed.), New York, Plenum Press, 1972, p. 261.

207. Alter, B. P., Kan, Y. W., et al.: Inhibition of hemoglobin synthesis by cyanate *in vitro.* Blood *43*:57, 1974.

208. Alter, B. P., Kan, Y. W., et al.: Toxic effects of high-dose cyanate administration in rodents. Blood *43*:69, 1974.

209. Papayannopoulou, T., Stamatoyannopoulos, G., et al.: Tissue isozyme alterations in cyanate treated animals. Life Sci. *12*:127, 1973.

210. Toskes, P., Hildebrandt, P., et al.: In vivo toxicity of cyanate in rats (abstract). J. Clin. Invest. *52*:85a, 1973.

211. Boyle, E., Jr., Thompson, C., et al.: Prevalence of sickle cell trait in adults of Charleston County. Arch. Environ. Health *17*:891, 1968.

212. Ashcroft, M. T., Miall, W. E., et al.: Comparison between characteristics of Jamaican adults with normal hemoglobin and those with sickle cell trait. Amer. J. Epidemiol. *90*:236, 1969.

213. Drew, F. L., Brereton, H., et al.: Prevalence of abnormal hemoglobins in a Negro population over 50 years of age. Personal communication, 1969.

214. Koler, R. D., Jones, R. T., et al.: Genetics of haemoglobin H and α-thalassemia. Ann. Hum. Genet. *34*:371, 1971.

215. Levin, W. C., Baird, W. D., et al.: Experimental production of splenic sequestration of erythrocytes in patients with sickle cell trait. J. Lab. Clin. Med. *50*:926, 1957.

216. Levin, W. C., Thurm, R. H., et al.: Chronic hypoxia and heterozygous S hemoglobinopathies. J. Lab. Clin. Med. *59*:792, 1962.

217. Green, T. W., and Conley, C. L.: Occurrence of symptoms of sickle cell disease in the absence of persistent anemia. Ann. Intern. Med. *34*:849, 1951.

218. Rashamtolla, S., Good, C. J., et al.: Pulmonary infarction in disorders associated with sickle cell trait. Thorax 15:320, 1960.

219. Mengel, C. E., Schauble, J. F., et al.: Infarct necrosis of the liver in a patient with SA hemoglobin. A.M.A. Arch. Intern. Med. 111: 93, 1963.

220. Ratcliff, R. G., and Wolf, M. D.: Avascular necrosis of the femoral head associated with sickle cell trait (AS hemoglobin). Ann. Intern. Med. 57:299, 1962.

221. Schenk, E. A.: Sickle cell trait and superior longitudinal sinus thrombosis. Ann. Intern. Med. 60:465, 1964.

222. Ober, W. B., Bruno, M. S., et al.: Fatal intravascular sickling in a patient with sickle cell trait. New Engl. J. Med. 263:947, 1960.

223. McCormick, W. F.: Abnormal hemoglobins. II. The pathology of sickle cell trait. Am. J. Med. Sci. 241:329, 1961.

224. Jones, S. R., Binder, R. A., et al.: Sudden death in sickle-cell trait. New Engl. J. Med. 282: 323, 1970.

225. Konotey-Ahulu, F. I. D.: Anesthetic deaths and the sickle cell. Lancet 1:267, 1969.

226. Platt, H. S.: Effect of maternal sickle cell trait on perinatal mortality. Br. Med. J. 6:334, 1971.

227. Smith, E. W., and Conley, C. L.: Clinical features of the genetic variants of sickle cell disease. Bull. Johns Hopkins Hosp. 94:289, 1954.

228. O'Brien, R. T., Pearson, H. A., et al.: Splenic infarct and sickle-(cell) trait. New Engl. J. Med. 287:720, 1972.

229. Welt, L. G., and Lyle, C. B.: The kidney in sickle cell anemia, In Diseases of the kidney. 2nd ed. Strauss, M., and Welt, L. G. (eds.), Boston, Little, Brown and Co., 1971.

230. Mentzer, W. C., Jr., Lubin, B. H., et al.: Screening for sickle cell trait and G6PD deficiency (editorial). New Engl. J. Med. 282:1155, 1970.

231. Beutler, E., Boggs, D. R., et al.: Hazards of indiscriminate screening for sickling. New Engl. J. Med. 285:1485, 1971.

232. Whitton, C.: Sickle cell programming—An imperiled promise. New Engl. J. Med. 288: 318, 1973.

232a. Pearson, H. A., and O'Brien, R. T.: Sickle cell anemia testing programs. J. Pediatr. 81: 1201, 1972.

233. Tuttle, A. H., and Koch, B.: Clinical and hematological manifestations of hemoglobin C-S disease in children. J. Pediatr. 56:331, 1960.

234. River, G. L., Robbins, A. B., et al.: S-C hemoglobin: A clinical study. Blood 18:385, 1961.

235. Lecocq, F. R., and Harper, J. Y., Jr.: Sickle cell-hemoglobin C crisis precipitation by fever therapy. A.M.A. Arch. Intern. Med. 111:149, 1963.

236. Smith, E. W., and Conley, C. L.: Clinical features of the genetic variants of sickle cell disease. Bull. Johns Hopkins Hosp. 94:289, 1954.

237. Rowley, P. T., and Enlander, D.: Hemoglobin S-C disease presenting as acute cor pulmonale. Am. Rev. Resp. Dis. 98:494, 1968.

238. Barton, C. J., and Cockshott, W. P.: Bone changes in hemoglobin SC disease. Am. J. Roentgenol. 88:523, 1962.

239. Kay, C. J.: Renal papillary necrosis in hemoglobin SC disease. Radiology 90:897, 1968.

239a. Serjeant, G. R., Ashcroft, M. T., et al.: The clinical features of haemoglobin SC disease in Jamaica. Br. J. Haematol. 24:491, 1973.

240. Fullerton, W. T., de V. Hendrickse, J. P., et al.: Haemoglobin SC disease in pregnancy, In Abnormal Haemoglobins in Africa. Jonxis, J. H. P. (ed.), Philadelphia, F. A. Davis Co., 1965.

240a. Sturgeon, P., Itano, H. A., et al.: Clinical manifestations of inherited abnormal hemoglobins. I. The interaction of hemoglobin S with hemoglobin D. Blood 10:389, 1955.

240b. Schneider, R. G., Veda, S., et al.: Hemoglobin D Los Angeles in two Caucasian families: Hemoglobin SD disease and hemoglobin D thalassemia. Blood 32:250, 1968.

241. Robinson, A. R., Robson, M., et al.: A new technique for differentiation of hemoglobin. J. Lab. Clin. Med. 50:745, 1957.

242. Konotey-Ahulu, F. I. D., Gallo, E., et al.: Haemoglobin Korle-Bu (β^{73} aspartic acid → asparagine) showing one of the two amino acid substitutions of haemoglobin C Harlem. J. Med. Genet. 5:107, 1968.

243. Bookchin, R. M., Nagel, R. L., et al.: Structure and properties of hemoglobin C Harlem, a human hemoglobin variant with amino acid substitutions in 2 residues of the beta polypeptide chain. J. Biol. Chem. 242:248, 1967.

244. Kraus, L. M., Miyaji, T., et al.: Characterization of $\alpha^{23\ GluNH_2}$ in hemoglobin Memphis. Hemoglobin Memphis /S, a new variant of molecular disease. Biochemistry 5:3701, 1966.

245. Charache, S., and Richardson, S. N.: Prolonged survival of a patient with sickle cell anemia. Arch. Intern. Med. 113:844, 1964.

246. Serjeant, G. R., Richards, R., et al.: Relatively benign sickle-cell anemia in 60 patients over 30 in the West Indies. Br. Med. J. 3:86, 1968.

247. Weatherall, D. J., Clegg, J. B., et al.: A new sickling disorder resulting from interaction of the genes for haemoglobin S and alpha-thalassaemia. Br. J. Haematol. 17:517, 1969.

248. Perrine, R. P., Brown, M. J., et al.: Benign sickle cell anaemia. Lancet 1:1163, 1972.

249. Bradley, T. B., Jr., Brawner, J. N., III, et al.: Further observations on an inherited anomaly characterized by persistence of fetal hemoglobin. Bull. Johns Hopkins Hosp. 108:242, 1961.

250. Jacob, G. F., and Raper, A. B.: Hereditary persistence of foetal hemoglobin production and its interaction with the sickle cell trait. Br. J. Haematol. 4:138, 1958.

251. Weatherall, D. J., and Clegg, J. B.: The Thalassemia Syndromes. 2nd ed. Oxford, Blackwell Scientific Publications, 1972, p. 195.

252. Charache, S., and Conley, C. L.: Rate of sickling of red cells during deoxygenation of blood from persons with various sickling disorders. Blood 24:25, 1964.

253. Silvestroni, E., and Bianco, I., La Molattra Microchepanocitica. II Pensiero Scintifico, Editore, Roma, 1955.

254. Weatherall, D. J.: Biochemical phenotypes of thalassemia in the American Negro population. Ann. N. Y. Acad. Sci. 119:450, 1964.

255. Pearson, H. A.: Hemoglobin S-thalassemia syndrome in Negro children. Ann. N. Y. Acad. Sci. *165*:83, 1969.

256. Weatherall, D. J., and Clegg, J. B.: *The Thalassemia Syndromes.* 2nd ed. Oxford, Blackwell Scientific Publications, 1972, p. 252.

256a. Serjeant, G. R., Ashcroft, M. T., et al.: The clinical features of sickle cell/β thalassemia in Jamaica, Br. J. Haematol. *24*:19, 1973.

257. Itano, H. A.: A third abnormal hemoglobin associated with hereditary hemolytic anemia. Proc. Natl. Acad. Sci. USA *37*:775, 1951.

258. Thomas, E. D., Motulsky, A. G., et al.: Homozygous hemoglobin C disease. Am. J. Med. *18*:832, 1955.

259. Jensen, W. N., Schoefield, R. A., et al.: Clinical and necropsy findings in hemoglobin C disease. Blood *12*:74, 1957.

260. Charache, S., Conley, C. L., et al.: Pathogenesis of hemolytic anemia in homozygous hemoglobin C disease. J. Clin. Invest. *46*:1795, 1967.

261. Kraus, A. P., and Diggs, L. W.: In vitro crystallization of hemoglobin occurring in citrated blood from patients with hemoglobin C. J. Lab. Clin. Med. *47*:700, 1956.

262. Smith, E. W., and Krevans, J. R.: Clinical manifestations of hemoglobin C disorders. Bull. Johns Hopkins Hosp. *104*:17, 1959.

263. Redetzki, J. E., Bickers, J. N., et al.: Homozygous hemoglobin C disease. Clinical review of fifteen patients. South. Med. J. *61*:238, 1968.

264. Cooper, R. A.: Anemia with spur cells. A red cell defect acquired in serum and modified in the incubation. J. Clin. Invest. *48*:1820, 1969.

265. Paniker, N. V., Ben-Bassat, I., et al.: Evaluation of sickle hemoglobin and desickling agents by falling ball viscometry. J. Lab. Clin. Med. *80*:282, 1972.

266. Briehl, R. W., and Evert, S.: Effects of pH, 2,3-diphosphoglycerate and salts on gelation of sickle cell deoxyhemoglobin. J. Mol. Biol. *80*:445, 1973.

266a. Castro, O., Orlin, J., et al.: Survival of human sickle-cell erythrocytes in heterologous species. Response to variations in oxygen tension. Proc. Natl. Acad. Sci. USA *70*: 2356, 1973.

267. Stevenson, A. C., and Davison, B. C. C.: *Genetic Counseling.* Philadelphia, J. B. Lippincott Company, 1970.

268. Hollenberg, M. D., Kaback, M. M., et al.: Adult hemoglobin synthesis by reticulocytes from human fetus at mid trimester. Science *174*: 698, 1971.

269. Basch, R. S.: Hemoglobin synthesis in short term cultures of human fetal hematopoietic tissue. Blood *39*:530, 1972.

270. Kan, Y. W., Dozy, A. M., et al.: Detection of the sickle gene in the human fetus. Potential for intrauterine diagnosis of sickle-cell anemia. New Engl. J. Med. *287*:1, 1972.

271. Kazazian, H. H., Jr., and Woodhead, A. P.: Hemoglobin A synthesis in the developing fetus. New Engl. J. Med. *289*:58, 1973.

272. Cividalli, G., Nathan, D., et al.: Relationship of β to γ synthesis during the first trimester: An approach to prenatal diagnosis of thalassemia. Pediatr. Res., May, 1974.

273. Gillette, P. N., Peterson, C. M., et al.: Sodium cyanate as a potential treatment for sickle-cell disease. New Engl. J. Med. *290*:654, 1974.

274. Moffat, K.: Gelation of sickle cell hemoglobin: Effects of hybrid tetramer formation in hemoglobin mixtures. Science, *185*:274, 1974.

Chapter 15

Thalassemia and the Genetics of Hemoglobin

by Bernard G. Forget and Yuet Wai Kan

DEFINITION

The thalassemia syndromes are a group of hereditary disorders in which there is a defect in the synthesis of one or more of the normal polypeptide chains of hemoglobin. This defect causes absent or decreased synthesis of the affected chain and therefore results in a low hemoglobin content of the red blood cells, which are characterized by microcytosis and hypochromia. In addition, the continued normal synthesis of the unaffected chain leads to the accumulation of unstable aggregates of these chains, which precipitate and cause the premature destruction of red blood cells in the peripheral circulation and of their precursors in the bone marrow. The anemia of thalassemia is therefore hemolytic as well as hypochromic.

HISTORY AND INCIDENCE

The historical development of thalassemia has recently been summarized (1, 2). The disease has been known for some time to affect primarily people of Mediterranean and African origin. However, thalassemia has also been recently recognized as an important disease in the Middle East and the Far East (3–5), and therefore it is probably the commonest hemoglobinopathy to affect man. Sporadic cases have been described in many varied ethnic groups (4).

It is believed that malaria has exerted a selective pressure for the propagation of the thalassemia genes (2, 4), although the scientific basis for the supposed protection of the thalassemia heterozygote against malaria is unknown.

GENETICS OF HUMAN HEMOGLOBIN

The structure of the different normal hemoglobin types is discussed in Chapter 13. In summary, the protein portion of all normal hemoglobin molecules is made up of two alpha and two non-alpha polypeptide chains which, in normal adult hemoglobin (Hb A), are the beta chains; in fetal hemoglobin (Hb F), the gamma chains; in the minor hemoglobin, Hb A_2, the delta chains; and in early embryonic hemoglobin (Gower 2), the epsilon chains (6, 6a). Another embryonic hemoglobin (Gower 1) consists of four epsilon chains (6, 6a). Normal cord blood also contains trace elements of Hb Portland, which is made up of two gamma chains and two new globin chains called zeta chains (7). Beta 4 tetramers (Hb H) and gamma 4 tetramers (Hb Bart's) occur only in pathologic situations and have very high oxygen affinity. They will be discussed in relation to alpha thalassemia. Alpha chain aggregates are unstable and precipitate to form the inclusion bodies found in beta thalassemia.

There exists at least one pair of allelic

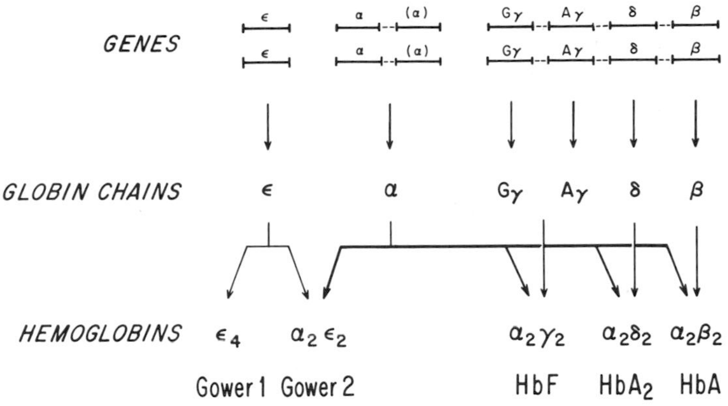

Figure 15–1. Schematic representation of the genes for the different human globin chains, and their gene products.

genes for each globin chain (Fig. 15–1). Although many animal species have duplicated alpha chain genes, controversy still exists over the possibility of duplication of the human alpha chain structural gene (8). The evidence in favor of duplication is the report of a Hungarian family (8a), in which three siblings were heterozygous for two different alpha chain variants and still had approximately 50 per cent Hb A. In addition, another individual has been described in which two different alpha chain variants have been present in addition to normal Hb A (9). The finding of two abnormal alpha chains in addition to the normal alpha chain in heterozygotes for the alpha chain variant, Hopkins-2, has been used as further evidence of duplication of the human alpha gene (9a). Also in favor of alpha chain duplication, without providing conclusive evidence for it, is the genetic basis for Hb H disease (10–12), and its association with Hb Constant Spring (8), which will be discussed in detail later. Finally, alpha chain duplication is suggested by the fact that heterozygotes for most (but not all) alpha chain variants have a lower percentage of the abnormal hemoglobin than do heterozygotes for beta chain structural variants (10, 13, 14). The evidence against duplication is the finding, in a Melanesian family, of absent Hb A in two homozygotes for Hb J Tongariki (15). Three other individuals homozygous for Hb J Tongariki have been found in New Guinea, and they all lack Hb A (16). Absence of Hb A in a Hb G Philadelphia homozygote and in Hb Q alpha thalassemia also favors the theory of a single alpha chain locus (8). The possibility exists, therefore, that alpha

gene duplication may occur in some, but not necessarily all, human populations.

The presence of at least two structural genes for the gamma chain has been established by the finding, in individuals from a number of different populations, of two forms of γ chain which have either glycine or alanine in position 136 of their amino acid sequence (17, 18); these chains are referred to as $^G\gamma$ and $^A\gamma$, respectively. The ratio of $^G\gamma$ to $^A\gamma$ in the cord blood of neonates is 3:1, whereas in the blood of adults it is 2:3. When increased fetal hemoglobin is present in the course of various hematologic conditions in the adult, either the 3:1 or the 2:3 ratio may be found (18). The reason for this variable ratio is not known; it may be related to the presence of more than one copy of either or both of the γ genes, or due to other unknown regulatory mechanisms.

Huisman, Schroeder, and their colleagues have proposed an interesting model for the number of γ-chain genes, based on the study of the occurrence and relative proportions (per cent of total Hb F) of various fetal hemoglobin structural variants (18a, 18b). According to this model there would be four nonallelic structural genes for the γ chain: two $^A\gamma$ and two $^G\gamma$ genes, each with a different quantitative output of gene product. These genes have been labeled $^G_m\gamma$, $^G_1\gamma$, $^A_m\gamma$, $^A_1\gamma$, or $^G\gamma$, $^g\gamma$, $^A\gamma$, $^a\gamma$, respectively; [the lower case letters (or the subscript 1) indicate genes with a relative decrease in output of gene product]. They would be arranged in the following order on the chromosome (going from N-terminus to C-terminus, or from left to right, as in Figure 15–1): $^G\gamma$, $^g\gamma$, $^A\gamma$, $^a\gamma$. If the production rate by $^a\gamma$ (the lowest output of the four genes) is arbitrarily given a value of one, the proportion of $^G\gamma$ and $^A\gamma$ in fetal and adult red cells may be explained by the following scheme:

	Gene			
or	$^G_m\gamma$	$^G_1\gamma$	$^A_m\gamma$	$^A_1\gamma$
	$^G\gamma$	$^g\gamma$	$^A\gamma$	$^a\gamma$
production in fetal cells	4	2	2	1
production in adult cells	0	2	2	1

This model is a totally arbitrary one, but it does explain the fact that fetal cells have a $^G\gamma{:}^A\gamma$ ratio of approximately 3:1 (70:30), whereas adult cells have a ratio of 2:3. This model, if it is correct, may prove quite useful in furthering our understanding of the fetal to adult hemoglobin "switch" and the distribution of fetal hemoglobin subtypes in hereditary persistence of fetal hemoglobin (HPFH) and thalassemia.

There is no evidence for multiple beta, delta, or epsilon genes.

The location of the hemoglobin genes on the human chromosomes is not known. There is a report of presumptive identification of the chromosomes bearing the human globin genes by means of in situ hybridization of ^{32}P-labeled rabbit globin mRNA to metaphase chromosomes of human lymphocytes (19). However, there are serious criticisms of the data (20, 21). There is slight evidence favoring linkage of the beta (and delta) locus with the Duffy blood group locus (22), and it is known that the Duffy locus is located on chromosome no. 1 (23). Although there is increased fetal hemoglobin associated with the D_1 trisomy (trisomy 13), this is thought to result from a defect in normal fetal maturation rather than being an indication of localization of the gamma genes on chromosome 13 (24, 25).

Linkage studies show clearly that the alpha and beta genes are not closely linked to each other and may even be on different chromosomes (26, 27). However, the beta and delta genes are closely linked to one another, as evidenced by the study of a number of families in which both a delta and beta chain variant are present: there was no recombination, in 41 opportunities, between the two loci (28). The occurrence of a delta-beta hybrid globin chain (Hb Lepore) (29), presumably the result of nonhomologous crossover between delta and

beta structural genes (30), also supports the close proximity of these two genes. The location of the gamma genes is not certain, but there is evidence to indicate close proximity of the gamma genes to the beta and delta genes: (a) in families in which a beta chain structural variant (or beta thalassemia) occurs in association with hereditary persistence of Hb F (HPFH), beta chain and HPFH genes behave as alleles, indicating close linkage between the two loci (2); (b) in individuals homozygous for HPFH or doubly heterozygous for HPFH and a beta or delta chain structural variant, there is no synthesis of normal beta or delta chain associated with the HPFH gene (2); this is the so-called "cis effect," i.e., the beta and delta chain genes in the cis position of the HPFH gene are totally inactive; (c) finally, a gamma-beta hybrid globin chain (Hb Kenya) has been described (31a, 31b), which presumably resulted from nonhomologous crossing-over of the gamma and beta structural genes.

The location of the epsilon chain gene is unknown.

GENETICS OF THE THALASSEMIA SYNDROMES

The location of the alpha and beta thalassemia genes is not known with certainty, but there is good evidence that they are closely linked, respectively, to the structural genes for the alpha and beta globin chains. This conclusion is based on the study of interaction of alpha and beta thalassemia with alpha and beta globin chain structural variants: the genes for beta chain structural variants and beta thalassemia behave as alleles, as do the genes for alpha chain structural variants and alpha thalassemia (2).

There has been no convincing evidence of crossing-over between the beta thalassemia and beta structural genes (2). The study of families in which genes for both beta thalassemia and a delta chain variant coexist makes it possible to evaluate the proximity of these two genes: in four such families, providing 31 opportunities for crossing-over between beta thalassemia and delta structural genes, there is indeed evidence of two likely instances of such a crossover (32, 33). On the other hand there has been no evidence of recombination, in 50 opportunities, between beta structural and delta structural genes (2). These findings suggest that the beta thalassemia gene is located further away from the delta structural gene than is the beta structural gene. Further family studies are necessary to confirm this somewhat surprising conclusion.

The genetics of alpha thalassemia are quite confusing (see review in reference 2), and much of the confusion centers on whether or not the alpha chain locus is duplicated in man and, if it is duplicated, whether the two genes are linked or independent. Study of various alpha thalassemia syndromes and the interaction of alpha thalassemia with alpha globin chain structural variants has not clearly ruled out either the one- or the two-alpha chain gene theory. In most instances it is possible to construct models consistent with either theory (2). There is only one family which provides genetic evidence for the linkage of the alpha thalassemia and alpha chain structural loci: in three offspring of an individual doubly heterozygous for alpha thalassemia and the alpha chain structural variant, Hb I, no crossing-over occurred, indicating close linkage of the alpha thalassemia gene to the alpha structural gene(s) (34).

The genetics of the alpha and beta thalassemia syndromes will be discussed again, later in this chapter, in relation to the clinical description of the different specific syndromes.

DEVELOPMENT OF HEMOGLOBIN

The time of appearance and relative proportions of the various globin chains during fetal and neonatal development are schematically represented in Figure 15–2. Alpha chains appear early and persist throughout development. From an early age, epsilon chains can be detected in the fetus, and they disappear by the tenth to twelfth week of gestation (6, 6a), when gamma chains begin to appear in large quantity. Alpha and gamma chain syntheses predominate during the rest of fetal development. A small amount of beta chain synthesis can be detected in fetuses as early as six to eight weeks of gestation (35–39). However, beta chain only becomes a major component near term. Studies of globin synthesis of cord blood (40, 41) show that there is approximately half as much beta as gamma chain synthesis at term. The mechanism of the switch from gamma to beta chain synthesis is unknown (2, 42). The finding of increased maternal synthesis of fetal hemoglobin during pregnancy (6a, 42, 43) suggests the role of a humoral factor. There is no evidence, however, that erythropoietin is involved. The switch seems to be regulated more by gestational age than by extrauterine environment, since prematurity seems to have little effect on the process (44). However, various forms of anoxia (42), intrauterine growth retardation, maternal anoxia (40), and the D₁ trisomy syndrome

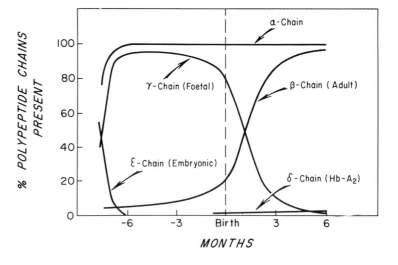

Figure 15–2. Diagrammatic representation of the changes in human globin synthesis during prenatal and neonatal development. (Modified from Huehns, E. R., Dance, N., et al.: Cold Spring Harbor Symp. Quant. Biol. *19*:327, 1964.)

(24, 25) seem to delay the switch. The cord blood of infants with erythroblastosis fetalis contains increased amounts of Hb A compared to normal cord blood (42, 45). However, this finding is not universal (46), and it is not related to the actual levels of synthesis of gamma and beta chains by the reticulocytes of the infants: the relative amounts of Hb A and Hb F synthesized are not different from those of normal neonates of the same gestational age (40, 41). The preponderance of Hb A probably results from the destruction of the older Hb F-containing cells and the presence, in the circulation, of predominantly young red blood cells. Previous intrauterine transfusion (40) or exchange transfusion at birth (45) does not seem to affect the relative synthesis of Hb A to Hb F at birth or during neonatal development. In hereditary persistence of fetal hemoglobin (HPFH), to be discussed later, the gamma to beta chain switch fails completely, and, in the homozygous state, no Hb A is synthesized. Once the switch has occurred it is not reversible, although in certain conditions (6a, 42) usually associated with some hematologic stress, an increase in fetal hemoglobin is observed. In such instances, only a small proportion of the red cells contain Hb F (so-called clonal distribution of Hb F), in contrast to the equal distribution of Hb F seen in all the red cells in HPFH.

Delta chain synthesis appears in the third trimester and never achieves significant proportions.

This sequence of appearance of globin chains is important for the understanding of the development of clinical manifestations in the thalassemia syndromes. A deficiency in alpha chain or gamma chain synthesis should be recognizable at birth, while beta chain deficiency will not become manifest until several months of age. Knowledge of the different types of Hb F distribution in red blood cells is also important in the differential diagnosis of thalassemia and other hemoglobinopathies. Finally, further knowledge of the control of the gamma to beta globin chain "switch" is of great theoretical and practical interest, because the ability to preserve gamma chain synthesis might provide an effective means of treatment of beta thalassemia, as will be discussed later.

MOLECULAR PATHOLOGY OF THE THALASSEMIA SYNDROMES

As stated in the introduction to this chapter, the thalassemia syndromes are all characterized by absent or decreased synthesis of one or more of the globin chains of human hemoglobin. In those cases in which some of the affected globin chain is synthesized, the resulting globin chain is structurally normal (47–49). In this respect, the thalassemia syndromes differ from the other hemoglobinopathies, such as sickle cell anemia, in which a structurally abnormal globin chain with one or more amino acid substitutions is synthesized.

There are two rare thalassemia-like disorders, however, in which an abnormal globin chain is, in fact, synthesized. The first is hemoglobin Lepore syndrome (29), in which the abnormal globin chain appears to be a hybrid chain, having the N-terminal amino acid sequence of the normal delta chain, and the carboxy-terminal amino acid sequence of the normal beta chain. (30). This defect appears to have resulted from nonhomologous crossing-over of the chromosomes at meiosis in the region of the adjacent delta and beta loci (30). As illustrated in Figure 15–3, this phenomenon would yield a fused delta-beta locus only, on one chromosome, and on the other chromosome, a hybrid locus containing the N-terminal amino acid sequence of the beta chain and the carboxy-terminal sequence of the delta chain, between the normal delta chain and beta chain loci. The Hb Lepore gene resembles beta thalassemia because there is a marked decrease in the synthesis of the gene product and presumably absence of the normal beta chain locus on the affected chromosome. This latter assumption is confirmed by the findings in patients homozygous for Hb Lepore, in whom there is total absence of normal Hb A and Hb A_2 (2).

The condition in which the delta, beta-delta, and beta loci all occur on one chromosome is called the anti-Lepore syndrome, and its demonstration is important in confirming the Lepore crossover hypothesis. Two instances of such an abnormal hybrid

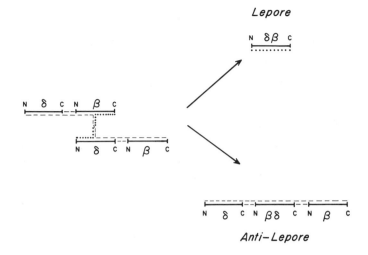

Figure 15–3. Schematic representation of the phenomenon of "unequal crossing-over" between delta and beta globin genes to explain origin of Lepore and anti-Lepore globin chains. N and C refer to amino-terminal (N) and carboxy-terminal (C) ends of the globin chains.

N beta–C delta chain have recently been demonstrated, in Hb P Congo (Hb P Nilotic) (50, 50a) and Hb Miyada (51). The anti-Lepore syndrome does not resemble thalassemia because the affected chromosome carries, in addition to the mutant gene, normal beta and delta genes with normal output.

The second thalassemia-like condition in which a structurally abnormal globin chain is synthesized is the hemoglobin Constant Spring syndrome (Hb CS) (52, 53), which has been described in association with Hb H disease. In the heterozygous state, it resembles the silent carrier state of alpha thalassemia (or α-thal 2 gene), which will be described below. In Hb CS an abnormally long alpha globin chain is synthesized, which is elongated at its carboxy-terminal end by an additional 31 amino acids. This globin chain is present in only small amounts, and therefore the gene resembles an alpha thalassemic gene. The possible molecular mechanism for this disorder will be discussed later.

Studies of Globin Synthesis in Intact Thalassemic Erythroid Cells

The thalassemia defect, the imbalance of globin chain synthesis, was first directly demonstrated in thalassemic cells by three different laboratories between 1964 and 1966 (54–57). The technique which was used consists of incubating peripheral blood reticulocytes for one to two hours in the presence of a radioactive amino acid precursor, usually leucine or valine. Globin is then prepared from the total cell lysate or from the Hb A purified from the lysate by column chromatography. The globin is fractionated by carboxymethyl cellulose column chromatography in the presence of 8 molar urea, which separates the gamma, beta, and alpha globin chains. The chromatogram obtained from normal nonthalassemic peripheral reticulocytes is shown in Figure 15–4, A. It can be seen that there is an equal amount of radioactive, newly synthesized, alpha and beta globin chains under the alpha and beta globin chain peaks. One can thus obtain a quantitative ratio of beta to alpha globin chain synthesis which, in a normal cell, will be equal to 1.0. When applied to the study of thalassemic reticulocytes, the initial studies (54–57) all demonstrated a decrease in incorporation of radioactivity into the beta chain of Hb A in beta thalassemic reticulocytes. Similar studies have since been repeated in a number of laboratories, and the results of these studies all indicate marked decrease of beta chain synthesis relative to alpha chain synthesis in beta thalassemia (58–61).

In the usual heterozygotes for beta thalassemia, approximately half as much radioactivity is incorporated into beta chains as into alpha chains, but in American Blacks with beta thalassemia trait, the beta/alpha ratio can be normal (61a, 61b, 68). In homozygotes for beta thalassemia, there is either absent beta chain radioactivity or marked

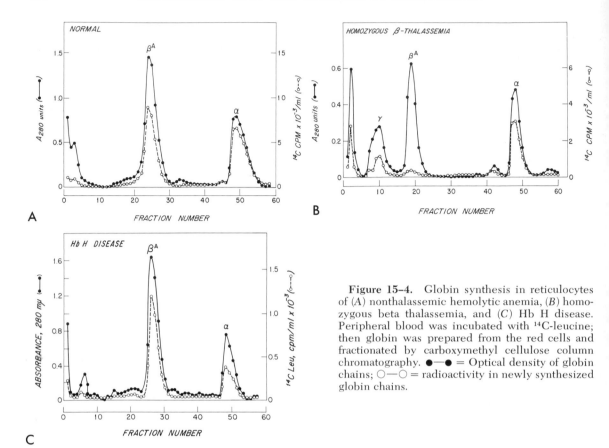

Figure 15–4. Globin synthesis in reticulocytes of (A) nonthalassemic hemolytic anemia, (B) homozygous beta thalassemia, and (C) Hb H disease. Peripheral blood was incubated with ^{14}C-leucine; then globin was prepared from the red cells and fractionated by carboxymethyl cellulose column chromatography. ●—● = Optical density of globin chains; ○—○ = radioactivity in newly synthesized globin chains.

decrease in beta chain radioactivity with a beta to alpha ratio of 0.1 to 0.3 (Fig. 15–4, B). It should be pointed out that this technique does not measure absolute rates of alpha and beta chains but only expresses a ratio of one to the other. An attempt has been made to express the data in terms of absolute rates (62), and the findings are consistent with a normal rate of alpha chain synthesis in beta thalassemia.

The same techniques were applied to the study of alpha thalassemia (56, 63, 64). In Hb H disease or mild homozygous alpha thalassemia, the globin synthesis profile reveals decreased incorporation of radioactivity into alpha chains when compared to beta chain synthesis. The alpha to beta ratio in this instance is 0.3 to 0.6, with a mean of 0.4 (Fig. 15–4, C). Recently, a hydropic infant with severe homozygous alpha thalassemia (Hb Bart's syndrome) was studied by this technique, and total absence of alpha chain synthesis was demonstrated (65). When alpha thalassemia heterozygotes are studied by this technique, less striking imbalance in globin synthesis is observed

than in the beta thalassemia heterozygotes (64). In the obvious alpha thalassemia heterozygotes (α-thal 1 trait), the alpha/beta ratio is 0.7 to 0.8, and in the "silent carrier" or α-thal 2 trait, it is 0.8 to 0.95 (64). Alpha thalassemia in the American Black does not demonstrate as marked or as consistent an imbalance in globin chain synthesis (66).

When the technique was applied to the study of globin synthesis in marrow from patients with homozygous beta thalassemia, interesting observations were noted. In this condition the beta to alpha synthetic ratio was still abnormal in the marrow, but the value was closer to 1 than in the peripheral blood (67, 68). Other workers have not been able to demonstrate such a striking difference between marrow and peripheral blood globin synthesis in homozygous beta thalassemia (58, 69, 70).

In heterozygous beta thalassemia, an even more interesting observation has been made by Dr. E. Schwartz. In the marrow of such persons, the beta to alpha synthetic ratio is very close to 1.0 (71). This observation has been confirmed in a number of different laboratories in simple β-thalassemia trait (69, 70, 72, 73) and in Hb Lepore trait (74, 75). The findings are difficult to interpret. It is unlikely that there is simple instability of beta chain synthesis between marrow and reticulocytes, because over 90 per cent of globin synthesis occurs in the marrow, and if decreased beta chain synthesis occurred only at the reticulocyte stage, then the beta thalassemic heterozygotes should not be anemic and the red cells should not be hypochromic. Another possible explanation for hypochromia despite relatively equal amounts of alpha and beta chain synthesis is that the alpha chain synthesis is decreased as well as beta chain synthesis in marrow cells of patients with heterozygous beta thalassemia, whereas in the reticulocytes, the imbalance becomes obvious. There is as yet no experimental evidence to support this type of presumed feedback inhibition of synthesis of the non-affected globin chain in thalassemia. Studies by Clegg and Weatherall on globin synthesis in heterozygous beta thalassemic marrow (73) indicate that, despite the synthetic ratio of 1, there is indeed imbalance between beta and alpha globin synthesis, as evidenced by the finding of a free pool of alpha globin chains in such marrow cells.

The authors postulate two explanations for the equal ratio: first, in marrow, non-globin peptides may co-chromatograph with the beta chain, thereby falsely increasing the radioactivity in the beta chain region; second, there is evidence provided by the authors that, in vitro, alpha chains are more unstable in marrow, as compared to peripheral blood, and may undergo proteolysis in time, thereby falsely lowering the radioactivity found in the alpha chain peak. The question is still the subject of intense debate. More recently, cases of heterozygous beta thalassemia of unusual severity have been described in which the marrow beta to alpha synthetic ratio ranges between 0.7 and 0.8, whereas the peripheral blood ratio is 0.5 (75a, 75b).

Molecular Biology of Protein Synthesis

As outlined in the previous section, studies of protein synthesis in intact thalas-semic erythroid cells demonstrate that the major biosynthetic defect in the thalassemia syndromes is absent or decreased synthesis of one or another globin chain of adult hemoglobin. To understand how this process could arise, we will review, very schematically, the major steps involved in protein synthesis, as illustrated in Figure 15–5 (see review in reference 76).

The genetic information for the amount and structure of a given protein is encoded in the nucleotide sequence of the DNA, which makes up the gene located on the chromosome within the cell nucleus. Each amino acid is specified by a sequence of three nucleotide bases, called a codon. There are many different codons possible for the same amino acid, but each codon is specific for only one amino acid and the unique transfer RNA (tRNA) molecule necessary for transporting that amino acid. The genetic information is relayed to the cytoplasm of the cell (where protein synthesis occurs) by the synthesis of a strand of RNA, which is complementary to, or the mirror image of, the DNA. According to Watson-Crick base pairing, C in DNA gives G, A gives U, G gives C, and T gives A. This RNA is called messenger RNA (mRNA), and its synthesis from DNA is called transcription. The messenger RNA then leaves the nucleus for the cytoplasm, where it binds to ribosomes, which are the subcellular organelles on which protein synthesis occurs. The initial step in which messenger RNA binds to the ribosomes is a complex enzymatic reaction which brings together the messenger RNA, the smaller ribosomal subunit, the initiator transfer RNA (which carries the amino acid methionine), and the larger ribosomal subunit. The reaction requires many separate protein factors (or initiation factors), and the entire process is called initiation. In mammalian systems, just as in bacterial systems, the first amino acid incorporated into a protein chain is methionine, but contrary to the bacterial systems, this amino acid is later cleaved from the protein chain, and is not present in the completed polypeptide chain. Once initiated, the synthesis of a protein chain continues by the process of elongation, which involves the sequential addition of amino acids to the initial amino acid by peptide bond formation, resulting in gradual growth of a polypeptide chain. Each

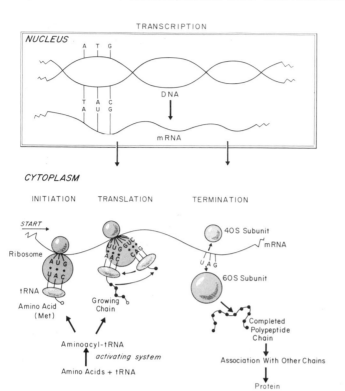

Figure 15–5. Schematic representation of the molecular biology of protein synthesis.

amino acid is brought to its specific position by a specific tRNA to which it is attached (the complex is called amino acyl-tRNA). The amino acyl-tRNA binds to the ribosome and to the specific codon sequence of the messenger RNA by a complementary nucleotide sequence of its own, located in a specific site of the tRNA. This sequence is called the anticodon. The nascent chain which is attached to the previous tRNA is transferred to the new tRNA, and a peptide bond is formed with the new amino acid. This new peptidyl-tRNA complex then moves to the position of the previous tRNA, which is then released as the ribosome moves along to the next codons. A new amino acyl-tRNA binds to this codon, and the process is repeated. Chain elongation is also a complex enzymatic reaction which involves many cofactors. This process continues until the ribosome, traveling down the messenger RNA in a ticker tape fashion, reaches a specific nucleotide codon which signifies chain termination. At this time the polypeptide chain is released from the ribosome, which in turn dissociates into two subunits and separates from the mRNA. The polypeptide chain then assumes its secondary and tertiary structure, and may bind to

other polypeptide subunits to form a functional protein.

Molecular Pathology of Protein Synthesis in Thalassemia

It is easy to see that, in the complex process of protein synthesis, a number of regulatory events could occur which would affect the rate of synthesis of a given protein and result in the presence of decreased amounts of this protein in the cells. If chain termination were slowed, completed protein would accumulate in the cell more slowly. In thalassemia, however, there is no evidence for slow release of chains from ribosomes to cytoplasm (77). At the level of elongation, decreased output of a structurally normal protein chain could result from a nucleotide sequence change in the messenger RNA, which results in its coding, not for a different amino acid, but for a different transfer RNA of the same amino acid. If this specific tRNA were in short supply in the cell, an overall slowing of the rate of synthesis of the affected chain would result. This is the so-called modulation hypothesis to explain thalassemia (77a, 77b). However, there is good evidence that this does not occur in thalassemia, since pulse-labeling experiments and peptide analysis of the nascent globin chains in beta thalassemia have revealed normal rates of elongation and termination of the beta globin chain (77, 78). Decreased synthesis could occur if there is decreased initiation of the messenger RNA due either to an abnormality in the messenger RNA, to an abnormality of the ribosome, or to abnormalities in the various initiation factors. The following areas of study have revealed no abnormalities or differences in thalassemic cells compared to nonthalassemic cells: ribosome quantity (79); radioactive profile of polysomes (79); effect of added nonthalassemic ribosomal subunits to thalassemic ribosomes (80); translation of synthetic mRNA (poly U) (81) and natural mRNA (rabbit globin mRNA) (82) by thalassemic ribosomes; effect of added human or rabbit initiation factors or both to thalassemic ribosomes (83); distribution of nascent alpha and beta chains on thalassemic reticulocyte and marrow polysomes, as an index of specific chain initiation (and elongation) (84, 85). The specific mechanism of globin chain initiation (use of initiator tRNA and initial dipeptide formation) (85a) is also normal in beta thalassemia.

All the evidence, therefore, indicates the presence of a defect in the messenger RNA for the affected globin chain as the basis for the imbalanced globin chain synthesis which occurs in the thalassemia syndromes. The messenger RNA may be either quantitatively deficient or qualitatively (structurally) abnormal in its nontranslated portions. Such a structural defect might lead to more rapid degradation and, subsequently, to quantitative deficiency of the mRNA; or it might lead to abnormal function of the mRNA, such as absent or decreased binding to ribosomes. In fact, a number of laboratories have now shown that messenger RNA isolated from thalassemic reticulocytes will duplicate the imbalance of globin chain synthesis characteristic of the intact thalassemic reticulocyte, when it is translated in a heterologous, cell-free, protein-synthesizing system (86–90b). Similar findings were observed with cell-free translation of globin mRNA isolated from thalassemic marrow cells (69, 90b). However, these observations still do not differentiate between overall quantitative deficiency of mRNA and simple deficiency of functional mRNA. On the other hand, RNA-DNA hybridization studies (91, 91a) and primary structure studies (90a, 92) of the messenger RNA isolated from thalassemic reticulocytes indicate that the messenger RNA present in these reticulocytes is indeed quantitatively deficient for the affected globin chain. These observations, however, leave open the question of whether the messenger RNA is initially transcribed in abnormally low amounts from the DNA, or whether it is transcribed initially in normal amounts, but with some structural defect which renders it unstable and rapidly destroyed.

A different set of hypotheses and molecular mechanisms may have to be proposed for the cases of thalassemia in which there is totally absent synthesis of the affected globin chain (beta^0 and alpha^0 thalassemia). A gene deletion and therefore total absence of mRNA could explain the findings, but other mechanisms must be ruled out. A nonsense mutation is one in which there is a nucleotide base substitution in the mRNA which converts an amino acid codon into a chain termination codon: only a short portion of the globin chain would be synthesized, then prematurely released (93). In such an instance, one should find within the cells alpha or beta peptides corresponding to these fragments, assuming there is no proteolytic destruction of the abnormally short chains (93). Such peptides have been sought but not found both in beta^0 thalassemia of the Ferrara type (94) and in the alpha^0 thalassemia syndrome of Hb Bart's hydrops fetalis (65). In the beta^0 thalassemia of patients from Ferrara, Italy, there is evidence that beta mRNA may be present in the cells, because beta chain synthesis can apparently be induced in a cell-free system by adding nonthalassemic (β^A or β^S) reticulocyte supernatant fraction to Ferrara thalassemia ribosomes (95, 96). The data suggest the deficiency, in these patients, of a factor necessary for β^A mRNA translation, or the presence of an inhibitor of β^A synthesis. However, studies of mRNA from other types of beta^0 thalassemia patients have shown no beta chain mRNA in heterologous cell-free systems (69, 88, 90a, 90b, 96a) or by hybridization (96a, 96b).

Environmental factors may influence the translation of preformed globin message in thalassemia. This has been recently suggested by the finding that Hb H (β_4) did not accumulate in the red cells of a patient with Hb H disease (a form of alpha thalassemia) when the patient was iron deficient (96c). In addition, it has been shown that messenger RNA isolated from Hb H disease reticulocytes, when translated in a cell-free system, leads to a much lower α/β synthetic ratio than is observed in intact Hb H disease cells (89). Hybridization studies (91) and primary structure studies of mRNA in Hb H disease (90a, 92) also reveal a lower ratio of α to β mRNA than expected from studies of intact cell globin synthesis. This may be explained in part by feedback inhibition of the rate of release of the normal (β) chain (85).

Pathophysiology of the Anemia

There are many primary and secondary causes of the anemia observed in thalassemia. It is easy to see from the description of the molecular pathology of thalassemia that reduced synthesis of one or another of the globin chains of Hb A will result in the overall synthesis of decreased amounts of Hb A and cause a hypochromic, microcytic anemia with low mean corpuscular hemoglobin of the individual red cells. This is true in both the heterozygous and homozygous states. In the homozygous state, however, another pathophysiologic process worsens the anemia and is responsible for the major clinical manifestations of Cooley's anemia. The continued normal synthesis of the nonaffected globin chain results in the accumulation, within the red cells, of a relative excess of these normal chains. Not finding complementary globin chains with which to bind, these chains form aggregates, precipitate within the cell, and become attached to the cell membrane (60, 97). These precipitates then lead to membrane damage and premature destruction of the red cell (98, 99, 99a). In beta thalassemia, the resulting alpha chain aggregates have no special name and are simply referred to as inclusion bodies or, perhaps improperly, as Heinz bodies. In contrast to true Heinz bodies, which are made up of total precipitated hemoglobin ($\alpha_2\beta_2$), these inclusions have been shown, convincingly, to consist of only alpha globin chains (100), which do

have some attached heme, perhaps in the form of hemichromes (100a). In alpha thalassemia, the resulting beta 4 tetramers constitute Hb H, which is less insoluble than alpha chain aggregates; in the neonatal and fetal periods, gamma 4 tetramers occur and constitute Hb Bart's. This process of inclusion body precipitation occurs in the erythroid precursors as well as in the mature red cells. It is responsible for the marked ineffective erythropoiesis and the hemolytic component seen in both the alpha and beta thalassemia syndromes.

In beta thalassemia, the role of thalassemic inclusions in the pathophysiology of the hemolytic anemia is manifested in the heterogeneous red cell population which is present in this disorder. Fetal hemoglobin is very heterogeneously distributed in the beta thalassemic red cells (see p. 21, Fig. 2–7). Those cells which have the most fetal Hb are those which have the least relative excess of free alpha chain because the gamma chains combine with alpha chains to form Hb F. It has been demonstrated in beta thalassemia that Hb A has a much more rapid turnover than Hb F (101); this suggests that there exist two populations of red cells: one short-lived, which contains less hemoglobin F and hence more inclusions, and the other, which contains much more Hb F and fewer inclusions, and hence has a longer survival (101). Indeed, differential centrifugation of red cells in beta thalassemia reveals that the older, more rapidly sedimenting red cells contain much Hb F and have relatively few alpha chain inclusions, whereas the younger, more slowly sedimenting cells are relatively deficient in Hb F and contain many alpha chain inclusions (98, 99, 102). There is also a good positive correlation between the severity of the disease and the size of the free alpha chain pool in beta thalassemia, and the degree of alpha to nonalpha globin chain imbalance (60, 97).

These findings point out the relationship of the alpha chain inclusions to the hemolytic process, and the beneficial role of gamma chain synthesis in lessening the imbalance of globin chain synthesis, decreasing the formation of alpha chain inclusions, and thus increasing red cell survival. In beta thalassemia, the alpha chain inclusions are found in large quantities in the bone marrow erythroid precursors (103, 104) and are probably the cause of the marked ineffective erythropoiesis or intramedullary destruction of erythroid cells which is observed in homozygous beta thalassemia (105). Prior to splenectomy, these inclusions are practically never seen in peripheral red blood cells, but following splenectomy they appear in large numbers (103) (see p. 21, Fig. 2–9). This observation correlates well with the demonstrated role of the spleen (and reticuloendothelial system) in removing inclusions of the Heinz body type from red cells, thereby damaging or destroying these cells (106–108). This phenomenon can be dramatically observed, under phase microscopy, in wet preparations obtained from fresh beta thalassemic spleens removed at surgery (Fig. 15–6), and is probably the main basis of the hemolytic anemia observed in beta thalassemia. In beta thalassemia the alpha inclusions result from decreased beta chain synthesis. Another inclusion body syndrome has recently been reported in which the inclusions apparently result from an absolute increase in alpha chain production (108a).

In the alpha thalassemia syndrome of Hb H disease, the resulting beta 4 tetramers (Hb H) precipitate more slowly. One does not observe, therefore, marked ineffective erythropoiesis and intramedullary destruction of erythroid cells as seen in beta thalassemia, although some Hb H inclu-

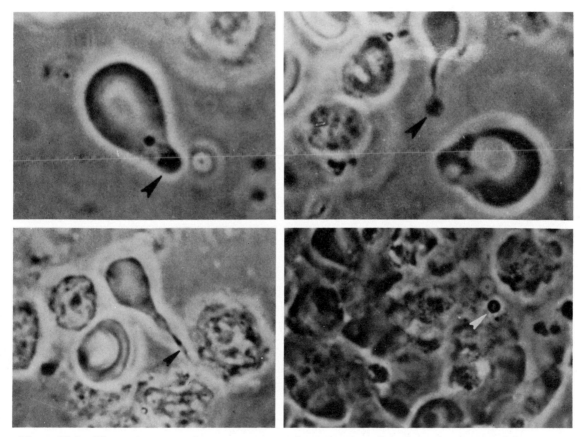

Figure 15–6. Phase microscopy of a wet preparation of scrapings from the spleen of a patient with homozygous beta thalassemia. Note alpha chain inclusion bodies (arrows) within teardrop-shaped red cells, inclusions being pulled out or "pitted" from the red cell by reticuloendothelial cell action (lower left), and inclusions free in the splenic pulp (white arrow).

sions are seen in marrow normoblasts (109). The inclusions form more gradually and occur mainly in mature red cells rather than erythroid precursor cells. The spleen removes these inclusions, thus damaging the red blood cells (98, 99, 107, 110), just as in beta thalassemia. Prior to splenectomy, no preformed Hb H inclusions are seen in the peripheral red blood cell, although soluble Hb H is present and can be made to precipitate in the form of small, stippled inclusions by in vitro incubation of the blood with brilliant cresyl blue (BCB) (Fig. 15–7, A). After splenectomy, large, round, preformed inclusions are also seen in the BCB preparation (2, 98) (as well as with methyl violet and other supravital stains (Fig. 15–7, B), and by phase microscopy. The large inclusions of precipitated β chain are sometimes observed even in the Wright stained blood film of splenectomized hemoglobin H disease patients (see p. 21, Fig. 2–6).

A number of secondary abnormalities occur in thalassemia which can worsen the anemia. Increased iron absorption occurs (111–113a), and because all this iron cannot be utilized owing to the decreased globin synthesis, it accumulates in excess within the erythroid cells and is deposited in the mitochondria of these cells. This may lead to decreased function of mitochondrial enzymes, including those which are necessary for heme synthesis. Decreased heme synthesis may contribute to an even further decrease in Hb A synthesis, but, more likely, the abnormal heme synthesis ob-

served in thalassemia (114–116) is a secondary result of the defect in globin synthesis. Perhaps negative feedback inhibition of heme synthesis occurs as a result of accumulation of heme intermediates. The accumulation of these intermediates could be caused by decreased globin synthesis (116) and also by the impaired mitochondrial enzyme function. The mitochondrial lesion may also be responsible, in part, for decreased red cell ATP synthesis in the face of increased cellular ATP requirements caused by the damaged red cell membrane. More rapid hemolysis of the ATP-deficient red cells might occur.

The anemia of thalassemia may also be aggravated by folic acid deficiency, which can easily develop in the thalassemic homozygote because of the high folic acid requirement resulting from the massive marrow erythroid hyperplasia and cellular turnover (117–119). The splenomegaly invariably associated with homozygous thalassemia also contributes to the anemia either by simply acting as a third space, increasing intravascular volume and causing hemodilution (120), or by causing true hypersplenic destruction of red blood cells. After splenectomy the liver may act in a similar fashion but less effectively. Finally, since fetal hemoglobin has a high oxygen affinity (Chapter 13) and may be quite elevated in some thalassemic patients, tissue hypoxia could theoretically develop, out of proportion to the "anemia" as reflected only in the circulating hemoglobin level.

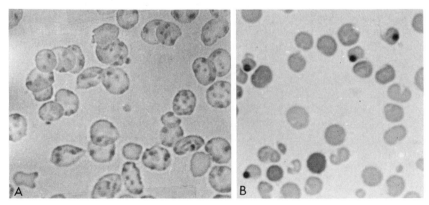

Figure 15–7. Red cell inclusions in Hb H disease. A, Inclusions induced by incubating peripheral blood in 1 per cent brilliant cresyl blue (BCB) and 0.4 per cent citrate for 30 minutes at 37°C (patient not splenectomized). B, Preformed inclusions, in peripheral blood of a splenectomized patient, stained by new methylene blue reticulocyte stain.

CLASSIFICATION OF THE THALASSEMIA SYNDROMES

The thalassemia syndromes are usually classified according to the type of the globin chain which is absent or present in decreased amount. The different types of thalassemia syndromes are listed in Table 15-1. Each type can occur either in the heterozygous or homozygous forms. We will first consider the alpha thalassemia syndromes. Heterozygous alpha thalassemia can occur in two forms: a phenotypically detectable form, referred to as alpha thalassemia 1 trait, and a very mild defect, the alpha thalassemia 2 trait, the existence of which is undetectable except by family studies and by its interaction with the alpha thalassemia 1 gene; it is frequently referred to as the "silent carrier" state of alpha thalassemia. Phenotypically, the heterozygous state for Hb Constant Spring is similar to the alpha thalassemia 2 trait or silent carrier state, except that small amounts (1 to 2 per cent) of the abnormal hemoglobin are detectable. The homozygous state for the alpha thalassemia 1 gene is the hydrops fetalis or Hb Bart's syndrome. The double heterozygous state for the alpha thalassemia 1 and alpha thalassemia 2 genes is the less severe syndrome of Hb H disease.

In the beta thalassemia syndromes, the heterozygous state for beta thalassemia (thalassemia minor or minima) is quite heterogeneous, as indicated by the variations in the amounts of the minor components of hemoglobin present in the affected individual. The various heterozygous states include (1) high Hb A_2 beta thalassemia; (2) delta-beta thalassemia, or F thalassemia characterized by normal Hb A_2 but elevated Hb F; (3) beta thalassemia trait with normal amounts of Hb F and Hb A_2 (? γ-δ-β thalassemia); and (4) Hb Lepore trait, which is phenotypically similar to heterozygous beta thalassemia, but characterized by the presence of small amounts of the abnormal Lepore hemoglobin and some elevation of Hb F but normal Hb A_2. "Homozygous" beta thalassemia (thalassemia major or Cooley's anemia) may result from the combination of any two of these genes. Occasionally, a child will inherit a beta thalassemia gene of standard

TABLE 15-1. CLASSIFICATION OF THE THALASSEMIA SYNDROMES

A. Alpha Thalassemia Syndromes
  1. Heterozygous alpha thalassemia 1
  2a. Heterozygous alpha thalassemia 2, or "silent carrier"
  2b. Hb Constant Spring trait
  3. Hb H disease: the combination of 1 with 2a or 2b
  4. Hydrops fetalis with Hb Bart's: homozygous alpha thalassemia 1
B. Beta Thalassemia Syndromes
  1. Heterozygous beta thalassemia
    a. With elevated Hb A_2 ± elevated Hb F (total absence of or reduced β chain synthesis)
    b. With normal Hb A_2 and elevated Hb F: $\delta\beta$-thalassemia or F-thalassemia (total absence of β chain synthesis)
    c. With normal Hb A_2 and Hb F (? "silent carrier")
    d. Hb Lepore trait
  2. "Homozygous" beta thalassemia or Cooley's anemia
    a. True homozygosity for one or another beta thalassemia gene
    b. Double heterozygosity for any two different beta thalassemia genes
    c. Thalassemia intermedia: certain doubly heterozygous combinations
C. Alpha + Beta Thalassemia
  1. Thalassemia of intermediate severity
D. Rare Forms of Thalassemia
  1. Gamma thalassemia
  2. Delta thalassemia
E. Interacting Thalassemia
  1. Alpha thalassemia + alpha chain variant
    a. Hb Q/alpha thalassemia
  2. Beta thalassemia + beta chain variant
    a. Sickle/beta thalassemia
    b. Hb C/beta thalassemia
    c. Hb E/beta thalassemia
F. Hereditary Persistence of Fetal Hemoglobin (not really a thalassemic disorder)
  1. Heterozygous
  2. Homozygous
  3. In association with beta chain structural variants

severity from one parent and a mild gene (in some cases a "silent carrier" gene) from the other parent. The resulting syndrome is usually termed "thalassemia intermedia." Finally, beta or alpha thalassemia may interact with each other and with a variety of other hemoglobinopathies. These will be discussed in the following sections.

THE ALPHA THALASSEMIA SYNDROMES

Four clinical syndromes are associated with alpha thalassemia:

1. Ordinary heterozygous alpha thalassemia or alpha thalassemia 1.

2a. Mild heterozygous alpha thalassemia or alpha thalassemia 2, ("silent carrier").

2b. Hb Constant Spring trait.

3. Hb H disease: the result of the combination of 1 and 2a or 2b.

4. Hydrops fetalis associated with Hb Bart's: homozygosity for the alpha thalassemia 1 gene.

Two alternate hypotheses have been proposed to explain the two types of alpha thalassemia genes (2, 11, 12, 121–124). In the first theory, it is believed that only one locus on each chromosome controls alpha chain synthesis and that the two types of alpha thalassemia genes are allelic but of different severity, one being associated with absent alpha chain synthesis, the other with mildly decreased synthesis. In the alternate theory, duplication of the alpha chain structural gene is postulated: in alpha thalassemia 2, only one of the four genes would be affected, whereas in alpha thalassemia 1 two genes, usually on the same chromosome (in cis), would be involved. Hemoglobin H disease, therefore, would be the result of alpha thalassemia affecting three of the four alpha chain genes, and hydrops fetalis with Hb Bart's would be the result of alpha thalassemia affecting all four alpha chain genes. The genetic make-up of the various alpha thalas-

semia syndromes, according to both theories, is diagrammatically illustrated in Figure 15–8.

Heterozygous Alpha Thalassemia

Heterozygosity for both types of alpha thalassemia genes is benign. Affected patients are usually of Oriental, African, or Mediterranean descent. These carriers are detected usually on routine hematologic examination or during family studies of patients with the symptomatic thalassemic disorders. In alpha thalassemia 1 trait, there are microcytosis and hypochromia of the red blood cells, usually with some aniso- and poikilocytosis. Usually there is no anemia, the red blood cell count being over 5 million, but occasionally mild anemia is present (Hb of 10 to 12 g. per 100 ml.). Alpha thalassemia 1 trait can be distinguished from beta thalassemia trait by the presence of normal levels of Hb A_2 and Hb F. In the adult, the diagnosis is often difficult; iron deficiency and other causes of hypochromia and microcytosis must be ruled out before the diagnosis can be accepted. In some patients, incubation of the peripheral blood with 1 per cent brilliant cresyl blue (BCB) for twenty

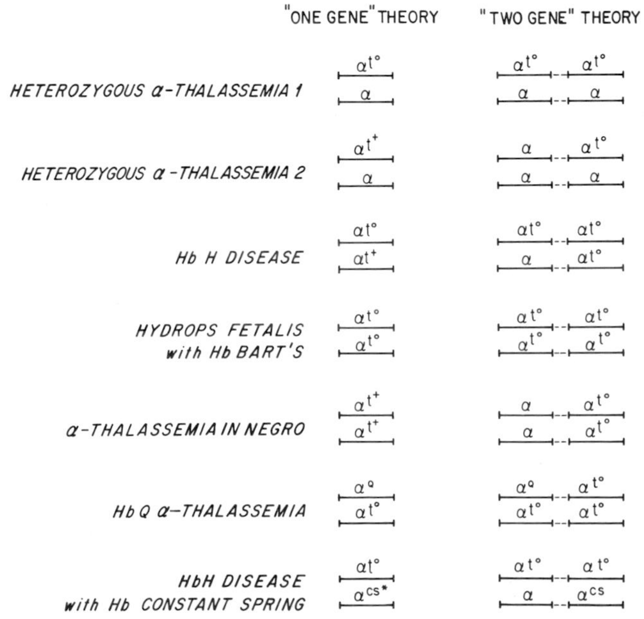

Figure 15–8. The genetics of various alpha thalassemia syndromes according to the "one gene" and "two linked genes" hypotheses. $\alpha =$ Normal alpha chain gene; $\alpha^{t0} =$ alpha thalassemia gene with total absence of alpha chain synthesis; $\alpha^{t+} =$ alpha thalassemia gene with reduced alpha chain synthesis; $\alpha^{Q} =$ gene for alpha chain variant, Hb Q; the "two genes" hypothesis is tenable in this case only if there is an α^{t0} gene always associated in cis with the α^{Q} gene. $\alpha^{CS} =$ Gene for alpha Constant Spring chain; α^{CS*}: the asterisk indicates that the "one gene" hypothesis is tenable in this case only if the suppressor tRNA hypothesis for the origin of α^{CS} is correct and not the chain termination mutation hypothesis (53), or if the alpha thalassemia gene in trans is of the alpha thalassemia 2 type.

minutes reveals occasional red cells (one in several thousand) bearing typical Hb H inclusions of the type seen in Figure 15–7, A. The hematologic findings in patients bearing the alpha thalassemia 2 gene are entirely normal. Diagnosis can only be inferred from family study.

During the neonatal period, the two types of heterozygous alpha thalassemia can be distinguished by the level of Hb Bart's (γ_4) present in cord blood. This has been most thoroughly studied in Thailand (125–128). In patients with alpha thalassemia 1 trait, there is approximately 5 to 6 per cent Hb Bart's, whereas, in those with alpha thalassemia 2 trait, there is only 1 to 2 per cent Hb Bart's. These components disappear by about the sixth month of life. Alpha thalassemia 1 can also be detected with certainty in later life by the study of globin chain synthesis in the peripheral blood reticulocytes of these individuals by the methods previously discussed in the section on globin synthesis in intact thalassemic erythroid cells. In alpha thalassemia 1, there is approximately a 25 per cent reduction in alpha chain synthesis relative to beta chain synthesis (64). A less significant decrease in alpha chain synthesis can be detected by this technique in a group of patients with alpha thalassemia 2; hence, the difference is not great enough for precise identification of individual patients (64).

It should be emphasized that the hemoglobin findings in the newborn period and the synthetic studies apply only to the alpha thalassemia found in the Mediterranean and Oriental populations. The findings in patients of African origin are much less well defined. Although alpha thalassemia trait occurs in the Black, Hb H disease is very rare, and when it occurs it is atypical and mild. Hydrops fetalis with Hb Bart's has never been described in Blacks. Hence, the existence of a different type of alpha thalassemia gene in these individuals has been postulated (2, 11, 66). It has been proposed that in the Black the alpha thalassemia gene is characterized by only slight reduction in alpha chain synthesis and never total absence of alpha chain synthesis. In the two gene theory, "heterozygous" alpha thalassemia would result from two affected genes on opposite chromosomes (in trans) (Fig. 15–8); thus typical

Hb H disease and hydrops fetalis would never occur.

Hemoglobin H Disease

This condition is characterized by a chronic hemolytic anemia of variable severity (110). Most patients have a hemoglobin level of approximately 8 to 10 g. per 100 ml., with moderate reticulocytosis (5 to 10 per cent). However, the variation is wide, and one can see patients either with severe anemia or with very mild anemia. Mongoloid facies similar to that which is associated with homozygous beta thalassemia has occasionally been described. Splenomegaly is usually present, and hepatomegaly is not uncommon. Anemia may become more severe during pregnancy or infection, or after ingestion of oxidant drugs which accelerate the oxidation and precipitation of the Hb H. The peripheral blood typically shows hypochromia, microcytosis, poikilocytosis, polychromasia, and targeting of the red cells (see p. 21, Fig. 2–6). Incubation of blood with one per cent brilliant cresyl blue (BCB) shows finely stippled Hb H inclusions in most of the red cells (Fig. 15–7, A). After splenectomy, large preformed Hb H inclusion bodies can also be seen by supravital staining; they are usually single and round (98, 110) (see Fig. 15–7, B and p. 21). The bone marrow typically shows erythroid hyperplasia. Finely stippled Hb H inclusions can be demonstrated by BCB incubation of the marrow, but large, single, round, preformed inclusion bodies, though present in some late normoblasts (109), are much less abundant in the marrow than the alpha chain inclusions found in homozygous beta thalassemia marrow cells.

The hemoglobin electrophoresis is diagnostic (Fig. 15–9, A). In the newborn, approximately 20 to 40 per cent Hb Bart's (γ_4) is found. This is gradually replaced in older children and adults by Hb H (β_4), the level of which varies between 4 and 30 per cent. Both Hb Bart's and Hb H migrate more rapidly than Hb A when electrophoresis is performed at the usual pH (8.6). Hemoglobin A_2 is reduced to about 1 to 1.5 per cent. Biosynthetic studies have shown that, in peripheral blood reticulocytes, there is approximately a 50 to 75 per cent

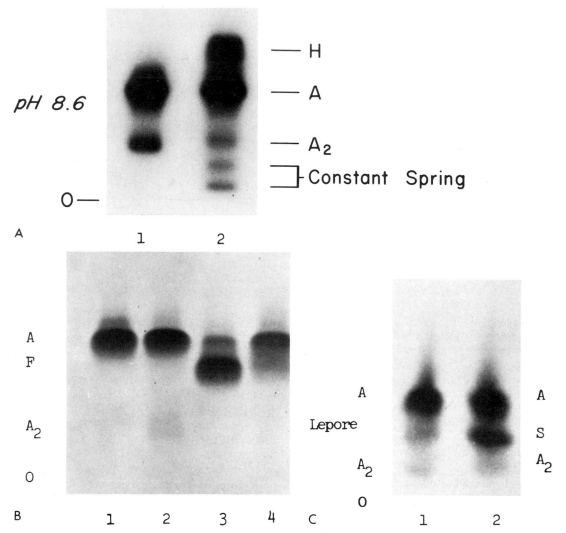

Figure 15–9. Hemoglobin electrophoresis. *A,* Starch gel electrophoresis at pH 8.6; 1: normal; 2: Hb H disease with Hb Constant Spring. *B,* Agarose electrophoresis at pH 8.6; 1: normal; 2: beta thalassemia trait with increased Hb A₂; 3 and 4: homozygous beta thalassemia with different relative amounts of Hb A and Hb F. *C,* Starch gel electrophoresis at pH 8. 6; 1: Hb Lepore trait; 2: sickle cell trait.

   0 indicates the origin. The anode is at the top of the page.

reduction in alpha chain synthesis compared to beta chain synthesis (63, 64).

   Study of the families of such patients with Hb H disease usually reveals that one parent has alpha thalassemia 1, while the other is hematologically normal and is presumably a carrier of the alpha thalassemia 2 gene. Direct transmission of Hb H disease to the offspring of an affected individual has rarely been found, but in such cases presence of an alpha thalassemia 2 gene in the putative normal spouse cannot be ruled out. Usually such offspring of

patients with Hb H disease inherit either alpha thalassemia 1 trait or alpha thalassemia 2 trait (confirmed by analysis of Hb Bart's in cord blood) (128).

   Hemoglobin H has also been described as an acquired defect, usually during the course of erythroleukemia or other myeloproliferative disorders (129–133). In certain cases, the abnormality appears to be clonal or limited to a certain population of red cells (134). The clinical picture of these conditions easily distinguishes them from the hereditary variety of Hb H disease.

Pathophysiology of Hb H Disease

Deficiency of alpha chain synthesis results in overall decreased synthesis of Hb A, hence, in hypochromia and microcytosis. The excess beta chains present form the beta 4 tetramers of Hb H; the latter has a very high oxygen affinity and lacks the Bohr effect as well as heme-heme interaction. Hence, it is a useless pigment for oxygen transport under physiologic conditions. In addition, Hb H is an unstable tetramer; it is easily oxidized and tends to precipitate as the red cells age. These precipitates, as discussed previously, are removed by the spleen and can be demonstrated most abundantly in peripheral blood after splenectomy. They cause disturbances in red cell metabolism and interfere with membrane function and deformability (98, 99). All these factors lead to shortened red cell survival and the hemolytic component of the disease. Because Hb H is relatively stable (soluble) in the younger cells, destruction of bone marrow erythroid precursors (ineffective erythropoiesis) is not a prominent feature of the disease. Shortened ^{51}Cr red cell survival and the apparent splenic trapping of ^{51}Cr-labeled red cells is observed in Hb H disease but should be interpreted with caution: ^{51}Cr binds selectively to the beta chain, and there is evidence that exchange of beta chains can occur between Hb A and Hb H (135). Thus the ^{51}Cr can pass from the labeled Hb A to Hb H, which then precipitates and is removed from the red cells by the spleen without the cell being destroyed; thus the cell loses its label without necessarily being destroyed, and this gives a false impression of the true red cell life span and splenic sequestration (135). More recent studies indicate, however, that ^{51}Cr may be a valid label for the determination of red cell life span in Hb H disease (136).

Hemoglobin Constant Spring Syndromes

In a proportion of patients with Hb H disease, hemoglobin electrophoresis shows, in addition to the usual findings, one or two more slowly migrating components, which amount to 3 to 5 per cent of the total hemoglobin (52, 53) (Fig. 15–9,A). This new hemoglobin is called hemoglobin Constant Spring (Hb CS), and it has been found in patients of Greek (137), Thai (126), and Chinese (52, 53) origin. Hb CS is made up of two normal beta chains and two elongated alpha chains, which have either 28 or 31 additional amino acid residues at their carboxyterminal ends. The shorter Hb CS chain presumably results from proteolytic digestion of the longer CS chain. Typically, one parent of such a patient with Hb H-CS disease carries the alpha thalassemia 1 gene, while the other appears to be hematologically normal, except that hemoglobin electrophoresis shows the presence of approximately 1 per cent Hb Constant Spring. Hence, carriers of the Hb Constant Spring gene resemble patients with the alpha thalassemia 2 gene.

The mechanism of production of Hb Constant Spring is not understood. The currently accepted theory is that of a nucleotide base substitution occurring in the chain termination codon of the alpha chain messenger RNA, from UAA (or UAG) to CAA (or CAG), which would then be translated to give the amino acid glutamine in position 142 of the alpha chain. This phenomenon then would allow the ribosome to continue translating the mRNA until a new termination codon is reached. The final effect is the finding of only a very small amount of the abnormally long alpha chain in the cell. The reduced amount of CS is most likely due to decreased synthesis (53, 137a). This molecular basis of CS has recently been clearly supported by two additional findings:

1. "Fingerprints" of normal globin mRNA contain nucleotide sequences consistent with the theory of a mutant termination codon (92, 92a).

2. Hemoglobin Wayne is a "frame shift" α chain mutant with an abnormally long α chain (see Chapter 13). The sequence of its abnormally long chain of amino acids is consistent with the mRNA sequence proposed for CS when the frame shift is considered (137b, 137c).

The fact that carriers of Hb Constant Spring are phenotypically similar to patients with alpha thalassemia 2 and not alpha thalassemia 1 has been used to support the theory of alpha chain gene duplication (8). Since the contribution of the α-CS gene to the total cell globin is negligible, the absence of hypochromia and other stigmata of thalassemia suggests that there must be more than only one other normal alpha chain gene compensating for the deficiency of normal alpha chains from the α-CS gene. Furthermore, it is difficult to postulate only a single pair of alpha chain genes when Hb CS interacts with alpha thalassemia 1 to give Hb H disease; if there is total absence of alpha chain synthesis from the alpha thalassemia 1 locus, then there must be another normal alpha chain locus in cis with the α-CS locus to account for the presence of some Hb A in these patients (Fig. 15–8). The "one gene" hypothesis in Hb H-CS is tenable only if one postulates (1) that the alpha thalassemia gene in trans to the CS gene is an alpha thalassemia 2 gene (which does not usually fit the clinical or genetic data); or (2) that the chain termination mutation hypothesis for the origin of Hb CS is incorrect. An alternate hypothesis is that the abnormal chain arises because of the presence of an abnormal suppressor tRNA, which reads the chain termination codon as the codon for the amino acid glutamine and allows translation to continue (53). The latter explanation is really quite untenable, since it would lead to termination abnormalities in other globin chains.

Hydrops Fetalis Associated With Hemoglobin Bart's

This is the homozygous state for alpha thalassemia 1. The affected fetus is usually delivered prematurely; it either is stillborn or dies within an hour after birth, grossly hydropic with marked hepatosplenomegaly (138–141). For reasons yet unknown, this syndrome almost exclusively affects people from Southeast Asia. Except for one case in a Greek Cypriot (142), no other cases have been reported from the Mediterranean area. None have been described in people of African origin, perhaps for the reasons presented on page 465.

The hematologic findings are characterized by a severe hypochromic anemia with large numbers of nucleated red blood cells in the peripheral blood. On hemoglobin electrophoresis, the predominant hemo-globin is Hb Bart's (γ_4) (138); a smaller amount of Hb H is present, and, in addition, a minor component, Hb Portland, composed of two gamma and two zeta chains, has been found (65, 143). This hemoglobin is also found in trace amounts in normal cord blood (7). Studies of globin synthesis in one case revealed total absence of alpha chain synthesis in Hb Bart's syndrome (65).

Hemoglobin Bart's has properties similar to Hb H. Thus, not only are the infants anemic, but also their major hemoglobin is poorly functional for oxygen transport. The cause of death is obviously asphyxia. Delivery by cesarean section and exchange transfusion were attempted in one case, but were not successful in prolonging life for more than a few hours (65).

Family studies in such cases usually show the presence of obvious alpha thalassemia trait (alpha thalassemia 1) in both parents. Because of the total absence of alpha chain in these infants, the condition could theoretically be diagnosed by globin synthesis studies of fetal blood early in pregnancy.

THE BETA THALASSEMIAS

Heterozygous Beta Thalassemia

With the increasing use of electronic cell counting equipment, this diagnosis is often suspected first by the discovery of a low MCV and MCH on routine blood counts (144). Beta thalassemia heterozygotes are usually not symptomatic and may not be anemic. Mild anemia, with hemoglobin levels of 10 to 11 g. per 100 ml., usually is present in most patients, and more pronounced anemia may be found in infancy and during pregnancy. The MCH and MCV are usually decreased well below normal, with values of 16 to 20 pg. and 55 to 70 μ^3 typically found. Despite the microcytosis, the MCHC is usually not as low as in iron deficiency. The peripheral blood smear typically shows microcytosis, hypochromia, aniso- and poikilocytosis, with targeting and basophilic stippling of the red cells. (Fig. 15–10, A). The bone marrow shows mild erythroid hyperplasia, with

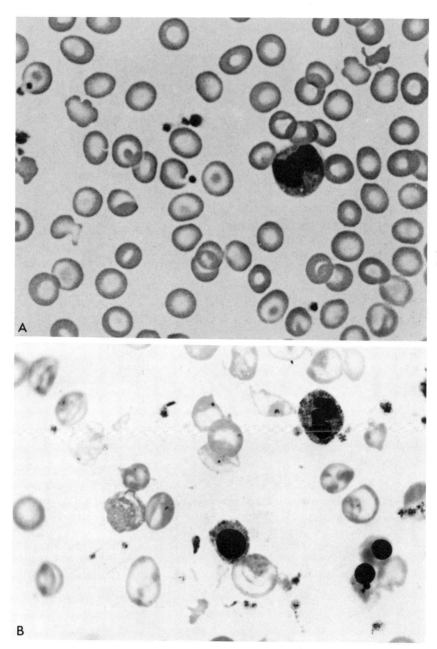

Figure 15-10. Peripheral blood smears in heterozygous beta thalassemia *(A)*, and homozygous beta thalassemia *(B)* following splenectomy. See also p. 21, Figs. 2-4, 2-7, 2-9.

many of the normoblasts showing poor hemoglobinization. Mild to moderate splenomegaly occurs in approximately half the cases.

The differential diagnosis of iron deficiency and alpha or beta thalassemia trait can be difficult in practice. Although, in thalassemia heterozygotes, the MCV tends to be lower when related to the hemoglobin concentration or the red cell count than in iron deficiency (144a,b,c), there is sufficient overlap between the two conditions to require other studies for confirmation. In iron deficiency, the plasma is usually colorless and watery, perhaps owing to reduction of bilirubin and carotene concentrations. In thalassemia heterozygotes, normal plasma pigments are present and are sometimes even slightly increased. Measurement of the serum iron concentration is usually very helpful, and absence of stainable iron in bone marrow aspirates serves to identify individuals with combined thalassemia trait and iron deficiency. This combination is quite common in early childhood and during pregnancy. Iron salts should not be withheld when iron deficiency complicates thalassemia trait.

Moderately severe anemia has occasionally been described in apparent heterozygous beta thalassemia (75a, 75b, 145, 146). However, when this occurs, one should look for associated secondary causes, such as concomitant iron or folic acid deficiency. Such cases should also be distinguished by family studies from the milder forms of homozygous beta thalassemia or double heterozygosity for beta thalassemia genes of different types and severities. The term "thalassemia intermedia" has been used to refer to either severe heterozygous beta thalassemia or mild homozygous beta thalassemia.

There are at least four different types of heterozygous beta thalassemia which can be distinguished on the basis of hemoglobin electrophoresis:

1. Ordinary *beta thalassemia*, or high A_2-thalassemia, by far the commonest variety, characterized by an increased Hb A_2 level of 4 to 6 per cent and usually a normal level of Hb F (Fig. 15–9, *B*), although in approximately half the cases a slightly elevated level of Hb F (1 to 5 per cent) may be present (146a).

2. *Delta-beta thalassemia*, or F-thalassemia, in which the Hb A_2 level is normal or slightly decreased, and the Hb F is increased and varies between 5 and 20 per cent.

3. *Delta-beta thalassemia with normal levels of Hb A_2 and Hb F.* This type of heterozygous beta thalassemia is difficult to distinguish clinically from heterozygous alpha thalassemia. It is usually diagnosed by the finding of beta thalassemia in an offspring. Globin synthesis studies in peripheral blood reticulocytes may be the only laboratory means to make this diagnosis.

4. *Hb Lepore trait,* characterized by normal Hb A_2, slight elevation of Hb F, and the finding of 6 to 15 per cent Hb Lepore (Fig. 15–9, *C*).

The clinical picture in all four types of heterozygous beta thalassemia is rather similar, except perhaps in types 2 and 3, in which anemia and morphologic red blood cell changes may be minimal. The findings in type 3 may be virtually normal, and the term "silent carrier state" has been applied to such cases.

The presence or absence of elevated Hb F in heterozygous A_2-thalassemia is usually of no prognostic significance with regard to the severity of disease in a homozygous offspring. One exception to this rule is a rare variety of A_2-thalassemia in which the heterozygote, in addition to an elevated Hb A_2 level, has an unexpectedly high Hb F level: Hb F of 5 to 15 per cent (147, 148) instead of the 2 to 5 per cent, as observed in approximately half the usual heterozygotes for A_2-thalassemia. The homozygous state for this rare disorder is much milder than homozygosity for the usual A_2-thalassemia (148).

The results of globin biosynthetic studies in heterozygous beta thalassemia have been discussed in the section on the molecular pathology of thalassemia. The beta/alpha synthetic ratio is 0.5 in the peripheral blood reticulocytes. In contrast, the ratio in the bone marrow is close to one. As discussed previously, this finding of apparently balanced globin chain synthesis in the bone marrow is not yet fully explained, but it may be the reason for the absence of hemolysis in beta thalassemia trait. Excess alpha chain precipitates are very inconspicuous in the marrow of patients with heterozygous beta thalassemia (104).

The double inheritance of beta thalassemia and a beta chain structural variant makes it possible to evaluate the amount of β^A chain synthesis directed by the beta thalassemia gene. In high A_2-beta thalassemia, there is some β^A chain synthesis directed by the defective gene in approximately two-thirds of the cases, whereas the other one-third of the cases show totally absent β^A chain synthesis. Total absence of β^A synthesis is especially characteristic of the A_2-beta thalassemia found in Ferrara, Italy (58, 61) and in Thailand (60). In $\delta\beta$-thalassemia, there is almost always total absence of β^A chain synthesis directed by the $\delta\beta$-thalassemia gene.

Homozygous Beta Thalassemia (A_2-Thalassemia)

Clinical Manifestations

The clinical course in most cases is severe. At birth, anemia is not evident, and examination of the peripheral blood smear shows only occasional hypochromic red cells. Diagnosis, however, can be established by study of globin chain synthesis in the cord blood (149). Within a few months, hypochromic, microcytic, hemolytic anemia develops, and a regular transfusion program must be undertaken to maintain an adequate Hb level. The spleen and liver become progressively enlarged. A typical facies develops in many patients, with prominent frontal bossing, prominent cheek bones, and protruding upper jaw, because of expansion of the marrow in the skull and facial bones. Skull x-ray demonstrates the typical "hair-on-end" appearance. The long bones may also become rarefied from the marrow expansion and become subject to repeated pathologic fractures (Fig. 15–11). Occasionally, the expanding marrow extrudes from ribs or vertebrae and forms large intrathoracic masses. Gallstones and leg ulcers are also frequent complications.

Intercurrent infection is extremely common, and, along with neglected anemia, it is the most common cause of death in early childhood. With modern antibiotic therapy and proper transfusion therapy, these causes of death have become less frequent, and many patients survive to their twenties. A benign form of pericarditis with pericardial effusion frequently occurs and is usually self-limited. Secondary hypersplenism may develop in some patients and cause thrombocytopenia, leukopenia, and rapid destruction of transfused cells. This complication may pose a severe management problem, and splenectomy may be required to control it. The incidence of overwhelming infection following splenectomy is significant (150, 151), and careful observation of splenectomized patients is mandatory.

Physical growth and development of these children are usually below normal; menarche and secondary sexual characteristics are usually absent, and the final stature of these patients tends to be short. This problem has been well reviewed by Logothetis et al. (152). Growth retardation begins at approximately 4 years of age and reaches its most significant and noticeable levels at 9 to 10 years of age. There is no associated retardation in intellectual development. No good correlation exists between the degree of anemia (pretransfusion Hb level) and the degree of growth retardation. However, this finding does not rule out the possibility that the degree of anemia in the first few years of life may be related to the degree of growth retardation in later years. Preliminary results of high transfusion programs instituted from an early age suggest that such programs may be beneficial in preventing growth retardation (see Management of the Thalassemia Syndromes). Although growth retardation is more pronounced in splenectomized patients, it is believed that this phenomenon simply reflects the correlation of severity of growth retardation to severity of the clinical course of the disease as manifested by hepatomegaly, cutaneous siderosis, and cephalofacial deformities (152).

Iron absorption is usually increased in thalassemia major (111–113a), and additional iron overload is supplied by the frequent transfusions. Iron overload is probably responsible for damage to the heart, liver, pancreas, and endocrine and other organs. In addition, chronic anemia is believed to play an important role in contributing to the myocardial damage from hemosiderosis (153). Cardiac failure and arrhythmias are the most common causes of death as these patients approach their twenties. Diabetes mellitus (153a) and hepatic insuf-

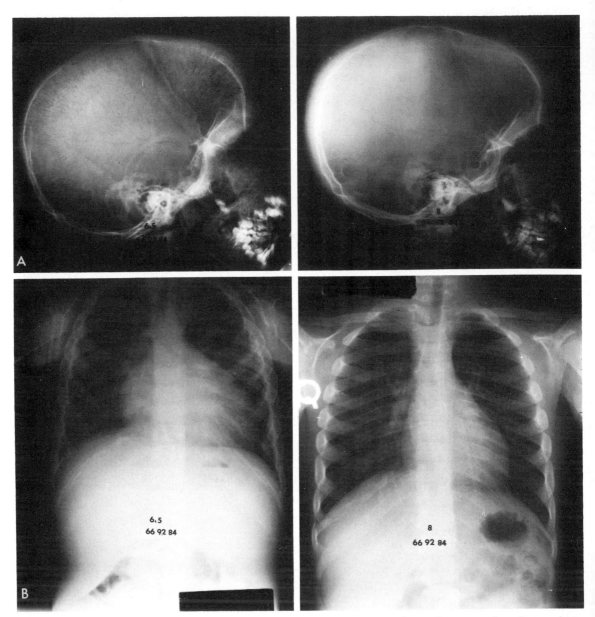

Figure 15–11. Effect of splenectomy and high transfusion regimen on bone changes and cardiomegaly in homozygous beta thalassemia. The x-rays on the left of each set show the patient at age 6½ years before splenectomy and institution of a transfusion program; on the right, x-rays show the patient 1½ years later after splenectomy and institution of high transfusion regimen. Note decrease of "hair-on-end" appearance of skull x-ray (*A*) and decrease of cardiomegaly and recalcification of ribs and shoulder girdle on chest x-ray (*B*).

ficiency may also pose difficult management problems.

Some of the complications and associated manifestations of Cooley's anemia can be prevented or at least lessened by maintaining a near normal hemoglobin level in the children by a high transfusion regimen, as will be discussed in the section on management.

Although the preceding description applies to most patients with homozygous beta thalassemia, a small number of patients have a much milder clinical course and may require few or no blood transfusions. This is especially true of homozygous beta thalassemia in the Black, which appears to be a much milder disease. This is the syndrome of thalassemia intermedia which is discussed later.

Laboratory Findings

Anemia is severe, with marked hypochromia. The findings on peripheral blood smear are striking (Fig. 15-10, *B*): the red cells show severe hypochromia and microcytosis, marked anisocytosis and poikilocytosis, and some polychromasia and basophilic stippling; poorly hemoglobinized normoblasts are found in the peripheral blood, and their number increases markedly following splenectomy. A comparison of the blood smears before and after splenectomy may be found on page 21, Figures 2-4 and 2-8. Even when anemia is severe, the reticulocyte count is usually not very high because of massive destruction of erythroid cells in the marrow, termed "ineffective erythropoiesis."

The red cell osmotic fragility is decreased, a phenomenon explained by the marked hypochromia. The bone marrow is very hypercellular, with marked erythroid hyperplasia characterized by normoblasts which are poorly hemoglobinized (micronormoblastic). Storage cells resembling Gaucher cells are frequently found in the marrow (and spleen) (153b). Examination of the marrow under phase microscopy or stained with methyl violet reveals the presence of many inclusion bodies (alpha globin chain aggregates) in the normoblasts; this finding can be used as a diagnostic test for homozygous beta thalassemia (103–104). These inclusions are also seen in peripheral blood cells after splenectomy (see p. 21, Fig. 2-9).

Increased indirect bilirubin levels and other biochemical evidence of hemolysis can usually be found; dipyrroles resulting from increased heme catabolism give the urine a dark brown color. The hemoglobin electrophoresis findings vary from patient to patient and with the type of thalassemia (Fig. 15-9, *B*). In the homozygous form of the usual variety of beta thalassemia (high A_2-beta thalassemia), there is usually a variable amount of Hb A present. The Hb F is usually elevated and may represent from 10 to 90 per cent of the patient's total hemoglobin. This Hb F is heterogeneously distributed in the red cells (p. 21, Fig. 2-7). The Hb A_2 level may be low, normal, or increased, but the ratio of Hb A_2 to Hb A is usually higher than the normal ratio of 1 to 40, suggesting more efficient synthesis of Hb A_2 relative to Hb A in homozygous beta thalassemia, even if the absolute Hb A_2 level is below normal. Free alpha chains can also be seen in trace amounts as a slow moving component on the hemoglobin electrophoresis (154). Hemoglobin A may be totally absent from some patients with homozygous beta thalassemia, and this type of beta thalassemia has been called the β^0 type. As previously mentioned, it is common in the Ferrara region of Italy and in Thailand. Double heterozygotes for high A_2-beta thalassemia and $\delta\beta$-thalassemia in general have a higher level of Hb F and lower level of Hb A_2 than the simple homozygotes for high A_2-beta thalassemia. The former also tend to have a milder clinical course.

The major pathophysiologic changes, as previously described, can be related to the degree of unbalanced globin chain synthesis. The hypochromia is due to the absent or deficient beta chain synthesis, resulting in overall deficiency of Hb A. The hemolysis is related to the large excess of alpha chains which is present in most of the cells. Since uncombined chains, especially alpha chains, are extremely unstable, they precipitate rapidly and form the inclusion bodies (also called Heinz bodies) previously described. The precipitation of these inclusion bodies is responsible for membrane damage and disturbed cellular metabolism, which lead to the premature destruction of the red cells and red cell precursors, primarily in the marrow (98, 99). There is some correlation between the severity of the disease and the degree of inclusion body formation.

Delta-Beta Thalassemia or F-Thalassemia

Heterozygous F-thalassemia or $\delta\beta$-thalassemia is a condition characterized by mild hypochromia and microcytosis. The changes may be barely noticeable. Hemoglobin electrophoresis reveals low or normal Hb A_2 and elevation of Hb F (5 to 20 per cent). The condition is found mainly in Greeks (155), although it has also been found in Blacks and other racial groups. In association with the usual variety of high A_2-beta thalassemia, a thalassemia intermedia syndrome usually results, characterized by high levels of Hb F and only mild or moderate anemia and hemolysis (155a). The homozygous form of $\delta\beta$-thalassemia is also a relatively mild disorder and may be barely symptomatic (2). The affected individuals have 100 per cent Hb F, with no Hb A or Hb A_2. The relatively benign nature of $\delta\beta$-thalassemia seems to be related to the fact that, although it is associated with totally absent beta and delta chain synthesis, it is also associated with more efficient preservation of gamma chain synthesis than the usual form of beta thalassemia. The overall degree of globin chain imbalance (alpha vs. non-alpha) is presumably not as pronounced; there would, therefore, be less alpha chain inclusion body formation and less hemolysis. Although $\delta\beta$-thalassemia almost always causes absent delta and beta chain synthesis in cis, there is one Black family in which the $\delta\beta$-thalassemia gene was combined with a β^s gene in trans, yet there was some β^A synthesis (156). In a Chinese family with $\delta\beta$-thalassemia, the only type of gamma chain found was $^G\gamma$, suggesting that in that family the thalassemia also affected the $^A\gamma$ gene (157).

Delta-Beta Thalassemia With Normal Levels of Hb A_2 and Hb F

In the study of parents of children with apparent homozygous beta thalassemia, one occasionally encounters a parent in whom both Hb A_2 and Hb F levels are normal. Some of these cases may be heterozygotes for the usual variety of $\delta\beta$- or F-thalassemia in which, for unknown reasons, the Hb F level is only at the upper limits of normal instead of constituting over 5 per cent of the total hemoglobin. Such cases have been well documented (158), and the low level of Hb F is not usually constant within the family. Other members of these families with thalassemia trait usually have the expected elevated Hb F levels (155, 158).

There is a report of a family with children having beta thalassemia of intermediate severity, in which one parent had typical A_2-thalassemia trait, whereas the other parent was hematologically normal, having normal red cell morphology, normal levels of Hb A_2 and Hb F, but an abnormal β/α synthetic ratio of 0.6 characteristic of mild heterozygous beta thalassemia (159). This latter form of heterozygous beta thalassemia was found in a number of relatives of the affected parent and has been termed the "silent carrier" gene for beta thalassemia.

Heterozygous beta thalassemia with normal Hb A_2 and Hb F, however, may also be otherwise phenotypically similar to heterozygous A_2-thalassemia, and the offspring of such an individual and another individual with typical beta thalassemia trait may have homozygous beta thalassemia (thalassemia major) of usual severity instead of a milder thalassemia intermedia syndrome.

Finally, in a family in which heterozygous gamma thalassemia was observed in a neonate in association with beta thalassemia trait, a number of individuals were found to have typical thalassemic red cell morphology, normal levels of Hb A_2 and Hb F, and a β/α synthetic ratio of 0.5 characteristic of heterozygous beta thalassemia (41). The findings suggest that the thalassemia defect in this family may affect the gamma, delta, and beta chain genes on the same chromosome; such an occurrence would explain the normal levels of Hb A_2 and Hb F.

Hemoglobin Lepore Syndrome

Hemoglobin Lepore is composed of two alpha chains and two abnormal non-alpha chains which have the structure of the delta chain at their N-terminus and that of the beta chain at their C-terminus (30). The Lepore chain is believed to have resulted from unequal crossing-over at meiosis of the delta and beta loci, as previously discussed (Fig. 15–3). At least three different Lepore hemoglobins have been described which vary by the point at which the crossing-over occurred between the delta and beta chain structural genes.

Hemoglobin Lepore is produced at a markedly reduced rate, and, in the heterozygote, it accounts for only approximately 6 to 15 per cent of the total hemoglobin. It is detected by electrophoresis and has approximately the same mobility as Hb S (Fig. 15–9, *C*). Clinically, the peripheral blood findings are similar to heterozygous high A_2-beta thalassemia. Hemoglobin electrophoresis, in addition to the abnormal hemoglobin, reveals low or normal Hb A_2 and slight elevation of Hb F. Homozygous Hb Lepore and the combination of heterozygous high A_2-β thalassemia with Hb Lepore are clinically indistinguishable from ordinary homozygous beta thalassemia (2). In homozygous Hb Lepore, there is no normal Hb A or Hb A_2, only Hb F (75 per cent) and Hb Lepore (10 to 20 per cent). These findings indicate that the chromosome bearing the Lepore gene has no normal delta or beta gene associated with it. This confirms the crossing-over hypothesis, and the location of the delta gene at the N-terminus side of the beta gene in the normal chromosome.

The reason for the presence of only small amounts of Hb Lepore in the red cell is not known. There may be decreased synthesis becuase of relative instability of the mRNA for the Lepore chain: globin synthetic studies reveal that synthesis of the Lepore chain, like the δ chain of Hb A_2 (159a, 159b), occurs primarily in marrow cells and is virtually absent in the peripheral blood reticulocyte (74, 159b, 159c). Similar findings have been observed with respect to the α chain of Hb Constant Spring (137a) and the $\beta\delta$ chain of Hb Miyada (anti-Lepore) (159d).

Mild Homozygous Thalassemia (Thalassemia Intermedia)

There is some evidence that certain beta thalassemia genes are milder and produce a less severe clinical syndrome in the homozygous state (2). This is especially true of homozygous beta thalassemia in the Black, which is usually a mild disease (147). The mild beta thalassemia gene, called "silent carrier" gene (159), produces a mild disease in association with the ordinary variety of beta thalassemia. Homozygous $\delta\beta$-thalassemia (F-thalassemia) also tends to be relatively mild because of the higher level of Hb F synthesis in each cell, resulting in less imbalance between alpha and non-alpha chains. Combination of $\delta\beta$- and high A_2-beta thalassemia produces a disease of intermediate severity (155, 155a). In addition, when a patient with homozygous beta thalassemia also inherits an alpha thalassemia gene, the disease will be milder because the associated alpha thalassemia gene results in decreased synthesis of alpha chains and less accumulation of free alpha chains to form inclusion bodies. The end result is less chain imbalance and less hemolysis (160). The reverse is also true; a patient who has the genetic makeup of Hb H disease and who also inherits a beta thalassemia gene has much less hemolysis (160, 161).

It has been proposed that the severity of the disease in homozygous beta thalassemia can be predicted by studying the globin chain synthetic ratio in the peripheral blood reticulocytes of the parents. In those homozygotes who are more mildly affected, one of the parents usually has a β/α synthetic ratio significantly higher than 0.5 (162). In $\delta\beta$-thalassemia, which is usually associated with a milder clinical course than simple beta thalassemia, the $\beta+\gamma/\alpha$ synthetic ratio is significantly higher than in simple beta thalassemia (157).

INTERACTION OF THALASSEMIA WITH ABNORMAL HEMOGLOBINS

When a patient acquires a thalassemia gene for a given globin chain on one chromosome and a gene for a structural variant of the same globin chain on the other chromosome, the percentage of the structurally abnormal hemoglobin observed is increased over the level found in a simple heterozygote for the structural variant. The clinical severity of the condition approaches that of homozygosity for the abnormal hemoglobin (so-called interacting thalassemia). On the other hand, when a patient acquires the combination of thalassemia for one chain and a structural variant for the opposite globin chain, no increase in the abnormal hemoglobin is observed, and the clinical severity of the condition is similar to that of the heterozygous state for the structural variant (noninteracting thalassemia). In fact, when alpha thalassemia is combined with a beta chain structural abnormality, the amount of the abnormal hemoglobin observed is less than in the simple heterozygous state. The common features in all these syndromes are hypochromia and microcytosis of the red cells, as in thalassemia trait, in addition to the finding of the abnormal hemoglobin. Only the clinically important combinations will be briefly described here.

Beta Thalassemia in Association With Beta Chain Structural Variants

Sickle Cell—Beta Thalassemia

This disease primarily affects people of African, Italian, and Greek ancestry. The clinical picture resembles that of sickle cell anemia, but the disease in general tends to run a milder course. Splenomegaly is a common feature and is helpful in differentiating S-thalassemia from sickle cell anemia in the older children and adults. Occasionally, the disease can be extremely mild, and the diagnosis may be discovered as an incidental finding.

Laboratory findings include a variable degree of anemia and targeting, hypochromia, and microcytosis of the red cells. Sickle forms may be observed in the blood smear in the more severely affected cases. The hemoglobin electrophoresis reveals 60 to 90 per cent Hb S, 0 to 30 per cent Hb A, and 1 to 20 per cent Hb F. The clinical severity of the disease cannot be correlated well with the level of Hb A. The condition is discussed at length in Chapter 14.

Hemoglobin C—Beta Thalassemia

This condition occurs mainly in the Black. A mild to moderate hemolytic anemia with splenomegaly is present.

Hemoglobin E—Beta Thalassemia

This is a common disease in Thailand. For reasons not well understood, it is almost as severe as homozygous beta thalassemia. Hemoglobin electrophoresis shows Hb E, a high percentage of Hb F (approximately 50 per cent), and usually no Hb A. It appears that when a β thalassemia gene is present in trans, the β^E gene is unable to compensate, in contrast to the compensatory capacity of the β^A gene and other β structural variants, such as β^S and β^C.

Hemoglobin Q— Alpha Thalassemia

This condition is also found mainly in Thailand and is the double heterozygous state for the alpha thalassemia 1 gene and the alpha chain structural variant, Hb Q. It is of interest mainly because of the associated hemoglobin electrophoresis findings. The affected individuals have total absence of Hb A. This finding is extremely difficult to explain if one assumes the presence of duplicated alpha chain genes. One would expect some alpha chain synthesis from the second alpha chain gene in cis to the Hb Q, even if the two alpha chain genes of the other chromosome are totally inactive. One must postulate, therefore, that the second alpha gene in cis with Hb Q is always affected by alpha thalassemia in the Hb Q heterozygote (Fig. 15–8).

GAMMA THALASSEMIA

An infant with hemolytic anemia at birth was found to have hypochromic, microcytic red cells (41). Heterozygous beta thalassemia, with normal levels of Hb A_2 and Hb F, was found in the father and many of his relatives. Globin chain synthesis studies revealed a decrease in gamma and beta chain synthesis in the reticulocytes of this infant. The disease became self-limited as the baby grew older. The hemolytic anemia disappeared, and the child developed the phenotype of simple heterozygous beta thalassemia. It is believed that this child represents an example of heterozygous γβ(?δ)-thalassemia. The disease should be suspected in cases of hypochromic hemolytic disease in the newborn. Homozygous gamma thalassemia would probably not be compatible with life (163).

HEREDITARY PERSISTENCE OF FETAL HEMOGLOBIN HPFH) AND HEMOGLOBIN KENYA

This condition is found primarily in the Blacks and Greeks (164, 165). The precise nature of the defect is not known, but it results in the absence of beta and delta chain synthesis on the affected chromosome in the Black type, and markedly reduced, if not absent, beta and delta chain synthesis in the Greek type. It differs from thalassemia in that gamma chain production persists at a level equal to alpha chain synthesis (165a), so that no globin chain imbalance or hypochromia of the red blood cells develops. Furthermore, the most important difference is that the fetal hemoglobin is evenly distributed in all the red blood cells, in contrast to the heterogeneous distribution of Hb F observed in thalassemic red cells. In most Blacks with HPFH, the fetal hemoglobin which is present has the typical adult $^G\gamma$:$^A\gamma$ ratio of 2:3 (165b). However, in some Blacks with HPFH, all the Hb F present is of the $^G\gamma$ type, whereas in most Greeks with HPFH, all of the Hb F is of the $^A\gamma$ type; rare Blacks with HPFH may also have predominantly Hb F of $^A\gamma$ type (165b, 165c). These findings indicate that the molecular defect leading to HPFH is quite heterogeneous.

In the heterozygous state, HPFH is asymptomatic. The Hb F level is about 15 to 35 per cent of the total hemoglobin in the Black type, and 5 to 20 per cent in the Greek type. Hemoglobin A_2 is decreased. The homozygous form of HPFH has been found only in Blacks (166). These individuals have 100 per cent fetal hemoglobin and have mild red cell morphologic changes but no anemia. In fact, mild erythrocytosis is present because of the high oxygen affinity of fetal hemoglobin and resulting relative tissue hypoxia.

In association with beta chain structural variants, such as Hb S, HPFH gives hemoglobin electrophoresis findings similar to those found in Hb S–beta^0 thalassemia or homozygous sickle cell anemia, but with an unusually high level of Hb F: absent Hb A, 65 to 85 per cent Hb S, and 15 to 35 per cent Hb F. Clinically, however, this disorder is benign, with no anemia, hemolysis, hypochromia, or painful crises. The benign nature of this disorder is probably related to the fact that the Hb F is evenly distributed among the red cells, and it is known that Hb F inhibits the sickling of Hb S (see Chapter 14).

Hemoglobin Kenya is a newly discovered abnormal hemoglobin (31, 31a) which has permitted more detailed understanding of the linear relationship between the $^G\gamma$, $^A\gamma$, δ, and β chain genes. The non-α chain of Hb Kenya consists of a fusion product containing the N-terminus of the γ chain and the C-terminus of the β chain. The crossover from γ to β sequence occurred before position 136 of the γ chain, so that it is not possible to tell whether it is an $^A\gamma$ or $^G\gamma$ gene which is involved in the fusion product. However, the propositus (who was doubly heterozygous for Hb S and Hb Kenya) had increased levels of Hb F in his red cells, and it was all of the $^G\gamma$ type. If this Hb F came from the γ chain gene(s) in cis to the Kenya gene, and if the $^G\gamma$ $^g\gamma$ $^A\gamma$ $^a\gamma$ model of the γ chain genes is correct (see p. 452), then the crossover must involve either the $^g\gamma$ or $^A\gamma$ gene. In addition, one must conclude from this finding that the $^A\gamma$ gene is situated to the N-terminal side of the δ and β chain genes, and is closer to these genes than is the $^G\gamma$ chain gene. The arrangement of the non-α chain genes would therefore be (going from N- to C-terminus): $^G\gamma$ $^g\gamma$ $^A\gamma$ $^a\gamma$ δ β.

Of additional importance is the fact that Hb Kenya, unlike Hb Lepore, is not associated with a thalassemic state. On the contrary, the gene for Hb Kenya resembles, in many respects, the gene for HPFH. Hb Kenya has been found in the simple heterozygous state as well as in association with Hb S (166a, 166b). In the simple heterozygote, it comprises approximately 10 per cent of the total hemoglobin, but in association with Hb S it accounts for 17 to 19 per cent of the total. All the patients are asymptomatic. There is no hypochromia or microcytosis, and no morphologic changes in the red cells. In all cases, the fetal hemoglobin is elevated (5 to 10 per cent of total hemoglobin), and it is uniformly distributed within the red cells; the Hb F is always of the $^G\gamma$ type (166a, 166b).

DELTA THALASSEMIA

Isolated delta thalassemia has been described as an incidental finding in both the heterozygous (167) and homozygous (168) forms; in the former, there is decreased Hb A_2; in the latter, total absence of Hb A_2. In neither situation are hypochromia, anemia, or red cell morphologic changes observed. The double heterozygous states for delta thalassemia plus $\delta\beta$-thalassemia (169) and delta thalassemia plus HPFH (170) have also been described and are clinically similar to simple heterozygosity for $\delta\beta$-thalassemia or HPFH, except that there is total absence of Hb A_2.

MANAGEMENT OF THE THALASSEMIA SYNDROMES

Prevention

An important step in the prevention of the occurrence of severely affected children with homozygous alpha or beta thalassemia is the detection of the heterozygous state in adults. Physicians should be aware of the possibility of thalassemia trait occurring in individuals with hypochromic anemias, which are refractory to iron therapy, and should perform the necessary diagnostic studies to confirm the diagnosis. In areas where there is a high incidence of thalassemia trait, general population screening surveys probably should be established. Once identified, the affected individuals should be educated about the disease process and its genetics. Two affected heterozygotes contemplating marriage and planning to have a family should be aware of the one-in-four chance of having a severely affected homozygous child.

Prenatal diagnosis of thalassemia is not yet possible, but it may be in the near future. Two major objectives must be met before an accurate prenatal diagnosis of beta thalassemia can be accomplished: (1) development of a safe technique to obtain fetal blood with which to do biosynthetic studies (amniotic fluid alone is not satisfactory because it lacks hemoglobin-synthesizing cells); and (2) the ability to differentiate normal from reduced amounts of fetal beta chain synthesis in a small sample. This is technically complex because of the very small amount of beta chain synthesis which usually occurs in the first trimester (Fig. 15–2) (35–39). Enough beta chain is synthesized, however, so that, with a large number of control studies, it should be possible to determine the normal range of beta chain synthesis and diagnose states of reduced beta chain synthesis in early fetuses. In cases of homozygous beta^0 thalassemia and homozygous alpha thalassemia (Hb Bart's syndrome), the prenatal diagnosis should be fairly simple because of the complete absence of beta or alpha chain synthesis. However, it may be difficult to differentiate the heterozygous from the homozygous state in a beta thalassemic fetus which is producing some beta chain. Nomograms of fetal beta chain synthesis in relation to gestational age are already being established from the study of globin synthesis in abortuses (35a, 39), and techniques for safely obtaining fetal blood samples are under study (38, 170a–e). In fact, the diagnosis of beta thalassemia trait and homozygous beta thalassemia has been suggested in two aborted fetuses (170f). Even when prenatal diagnosis does become routinely available, it is not certain that it will greatly reduce the incidence of homozygous individuals. Such cases will still arise in instances in which the parents are unaware, before the birth of their first affected child, that they have thalassemia trait. Furthermore, some parents may object to abortion, yet wish to attempt having other (hopefully unaffected) children. In individual cases, however, the availability of precise prenatal diagnosis will be greatly appreciated.

Supportive Therapy

There is no specific therapy for the severely affected homozygous thalassemic patient. The treatment is mainly supportive and consists of a regular transfusion program to control the anemia. There are two general types of transfusion programs which can be undertaken. The more standard program consists of transfusing the patient in order to maintain a "safe" hemoglobin level. This usually means transfusing the patient when his hemoglobin drops to a level of 7 or 8 g. per 100 ml., hopefully before the patient becomes symptomatic.

The second type of transfusion program is the so-called high or hypertransfusion (HT) regimen. This consists of transfusing the patient as frequently as necessary to maintain a "normal" hemoglobin level, which is not allowed to drop below a minimum of 10 g. per 100 ml. This usually entails a transfusion of 2 to 3 units of packed red cells at intervals of every two to four weeks. The HT regimen has the obvious disadvantage that the patient receives a much larger total body burden of iron, which cannot be naturally excreted by the body. Calculations of this excess infusion of iron, in comparison with a more standard transfusion regimen, give minimum values in the range of 1 to 2 g. of elemental iron per year (113, 171) for the net increment of iron accumulated. If one does not subtract iron theoretically removed by chelation therapy and the questionable decreased iron absorption from food, the increment may be as high as 3 to 4 g. of elemental iron per year in the HT regimen (172). Since the major cause of death in the second or third decade is probably related to the effects of iron overload, there is a certain reluctance by many to adopt such a program. However, there is good evidence that children who are maintained on an HT regimen do very well, if not better than children maintained on a more standard regimen. The children in the HT group, in general, have fewer intercurrent illnesses and infections, are more active, and lead more normal and happy lives (173, 174). There is

less cardiomegaly and hepatosplenomegaly and fewer bone changes and orthodontic problems (171, 172). There is some dispute as to whether the HT regimen actually improves the growth and development of these children. Some studies claim that hypertransfusion does improve growth (171–173, 175), whereas other studies did not find improved growth (152, 174, 176, 177), and one even found some decrease in growth in the HT group (178). The discrepancy is probably related to the age at which HT is started; HT started after the first few years of life probably does not improve growth and development, but HT started in infancy may prevent growth retardation (171, 172). The most recent follow-up studies on such patients have still not resolved the issue (178a, b).

There is some experimental evidence, in mice, which can be used to support the rationale of HT. In this study (153), mice which were given excess iron parenterally but were not made anemic did not develop cardiac hemosiderosis. However, if the mice were concomitantly made anemic, the iron was deposited in the myocardium. The proponents of hypertransfusion claim, therefore, that hypertransfusion may prevent deposition of iron in parenchymal tissues by preventing the anemia which leads to tissue hypoxia and focal tissue necrosis, which, in turn, may lead to a focus for iron deposition in various organs. If the anemia is prevented, the excess iron accumulated during the hypertransfusion program may be deposited in less harmful sites, such as the reticuloendothelial system, and not in the parenchymal cells of the liver, heart, and other organs (175). It will be some time before one will be able to assess with certainty whether the HT program affects the longevity of the patients who receive it. Thus far, it appears that longevity may not be prolonged (174) but is probably not shortened. The HT regimen seems to contribute to happier lives for the thalassemic children. Certainly one should not limit transfusions in thalassemic children for fear of iron overload. Because the HT regimen does not appear to shorten longevity, it seems reasonable to transfuse a child as frequently as necessary to maintain a minimum hemoglobin of 9 or 10 g. per 100 ml., if the facilities to do so are available. It seems important to institute such a program from an early age if one wishes to lessen the development of severe facial deformities, bony changes, cardiomegaly, and splenomegaly in these patients. The dramatic effects of a good transfusion program (and splenectomy) on the bone changes in a previously untransfused patient are shown in Figure 15–11.

Any transfusion regimen, and especially HT regimen, is associated with a certain incidence of transfusion-related complications. Hepatitis and other viral diseases, such as cytomegalovirus infections, are always a risk and are treated symptomatically. Isoimmunization to minor blood groups (Kell, Duffy, C, K, E), although relatively rare (179), may cause difficulties in crossmatching and in survival time of the transfused red cells. This may be avoided by careful full minor blood group typing of the patient before the institution of transfusions, and careful selection of blood donors. Urticarial reactions usually respond to epinephrine or antihistamines, and may be avoided in some cases by treatment with antihistamines prior to the transfusion. A more difficult problem is the febrile reaction due to prior sensitization of the patient to white blood cell or plasma protein antigens (179). These may be avoided (or prevented) by use of white cell–free blood, which includes frozen red cells or blood passed through Leuko-Pak filters (Fenwal Laboratories). Occasionally, steroids are necessary acutely to treat severe febrile reactions.

Splenectomy

Splenectomy has an important place in the management of thalassemic patients. If a child is maintained on a good hypertransfusion regimen from an early age, marked splenomegaly may not develop (171, 172) because of suppression of extramedullary erythropoiesis. Even established splenomegaly may be reversible following institution of HT (180). However, many patients in spite of adequate transfusions do develop significant splenomegaly, which may cause problems. Progressive splenomegaly usually aggravates the anemia and increases the transfusion requirement by causing a dilutional type of anemia owing to the sequestration of transfused red cells in the large third space provided by the spleen's size. In addition, the spleen may become autonomous, and the patients may develop true hypersplenism, with evidence of destruction in the spleen of red cells and of other formed blood elements, such as white cells and platelets. Rapid onset of splenomegaly and splenic destruction of transfused red cells may be triggered by isoimmunization to minor blood group antigens. Such an occurrence is usually associated with difficulty in crossmatching the blood and development of a positive Coombs' test. In some instances, however, the only sign may be a sudden increase in the child's transfusion requirement and a sudden increase in spleen size. Splenomegaly, on the other hand, may be symptomatic simply by the sheer size of the spleen, causing pressure discomfort in the abdomen or pain from splenic infarcts. In cases in which splenomegaly is symptomatic or causes difficulty in maintaining adequate hemoglobin levels despite appropriate maintenance transfusions, splenectomy should be recommended. Splenectomy will usually result in a lessening of the transfusion requirement and, in combination with a good transfusion program, will usually make it possible to maintain the patient's hemoglobin at a near normal level much more easily than before splenectomy, and achieve the benefits of HT. Splenectomy is rarely necessary before the child reaches the age of 5 or 6 years, but in certain instances splenectomy at an earlier age may be necessary. The decision to perform splenectomy may be aided by doing a ^{51}Cr-tagged red cell survival study, with scanning of the spleen to demonstrate sequestration of labeled red cells. Splenectomy is done reluctantly before the age of 3 or 4 years, because of the demonstration of increased instances of rapidly fatal septicemia in children who have been splenectomized before that age (181). Thalassemic children, in particular, even those over the age of 3 or 4 years, are particularly susceptible to this type of fatal Gram-positive septicemia (150, 151). The reasons for this high incidence are not known. The spleen and the reticuloendothelial (RE) system probably function as bacterial filters of the circulation. In the asplenic thalassemic patient, the loss of splenic filter function is probably aggravated, in addition, by some degree of RE system blockade because of the iron overload. The spleen probably also has a function in antibody synthesis, the absence of which may put the thalassemic patient at a disadvantage in handling infections. Indeed, immunoglobin levels are low in splenectomized thalassemics (182). Because of this increased risk of infection, it is probably advisable, after splenectomy, to maintain thalassemic children on prophylactic doses of penicillin for at least two years, if not indefinitely. Another postsplenectomy complication is the occasional development of marked thrombocytosis with thromboembolic phenomena, which may require anticoagulation.

Use of Iron-Chelating Agents

Because of the marked iron overload which occurs in beta thalassemia, it would be theoretically advantageous to remove the excess iron stores, especially in patients maintained on HT regimens, by the long-term administration of iron-chelating agents. There are two such agents which are available and which have been used extensively in Britain and Europe. The first is desferrioxamine, which is administered by intramuscular injection; the second is diethylenetriamine pentacetate (DTPA), which must be given by intravenous infusion, usually at the time of transfusion (183–185). It is theoretically possible to maintain a near balance of iron stores if one uses the following doses of the two agents concomitantly: 6 mg. of I.V. DTPA with each transfusion and 0.5 to 1.0 g. of desferrioxamine I.M. daily (2). However, studies of urinary iron excretion in response to these drugs have demonstrated that not all patients respond equally well; concomitant use of vitamin C may improve urinary iron excretion in some patients (186), but their iron balance has not yet been studied. Even in patients who are good responders, the amount of iron excretion usually decreases in time, and the drug becomes relatively ineffective (172, 183, 184). The reason for this loss of effectiveness is probably that desferrioxamine can only chelate iron which is in certain labile pools (187); the bulk of the storage iron is probably not chelatable (187). Therefore, in practice, it is

not usually possible to achieve a state of iron balance in most thalassemic patients (2, 172). Rare exceptions may, however, exist; in a child with congenital hypoplastic anemia treated for five years with desferrioxamine, 30 per cent of the amount of transfused iron was recovered in the urine (188). There are additional disadvantages to the use of desferrioxamine: patients may develop allergic reactions to the drug (172); the daily intramuscular injections are associated with some discomfort and can cause more emotional strain than is justified in view of the effectiveness of the drug; finally, cataracts have been described in experimental animals and in three individuals after long-term use (*Physicians' Desk Reference*, 1973, p. 663). For these reasons, the U.S. Food and Drug Administration has discontinued approval of desferrioxamine, except for investigational use, in treatment of transfusion-induced hemosiderosis, although, of course, there are no objections to its use in the treatment of acute iron poisoning. DTPA is generally considered quite toxic, and its usefulness is very limited.

Recently, more optimistic reports have appeared on the use of desferrioxamine in thalassemia (189, 189a, 189b, 210). In summary, these studies have shown that, with higher doses of desferrioxamine, including intravenous desferrioxamine at the time of transfusion, and with concomitant use of vitamin C, sustained high levels of urinary iron excretion and near iron balance can be achieved. These studies clearly show, however, that significant excretion occurs only with increasing age and only after significant iron overload has already occurred, as determined by measurements of liver iron. Desferrioxamine will not prevent the occurrence of this initial iron accumulation. Iron stores reach a level at least ten times above normal before significant chelation is achieved. Although tissue siderosis cannot be prevented or reversed by chelation, it is possible that long-term chelation may be of some benefit by eliminating an additional increment of more reactive and potentially toxic iron, especially in patients on high transfusion regimens.

The role and mode of action of vitamin C in chelation therapy are not clear. Thalassemic patients are usually deficient in vitamin C (and E), both nonspecific, antioxidant substances, presumably because of the oxidant stress of iron overload. It seems, therefore, theoretically advantageous to replenish these vitamins in the thalassemic patient, both to counteract the tissue toxic oxidant stress of iron and to facilitate mobilization of iron. However, it is not clear what role vitamin C may also have on increased gastrointestinal tract absorption of iron in thalassemia.

In conclusion, more carefully controlled, long-term studies are necessary before one can accurately assess the role of desferrioxamine in the treatment of thalassemia.

A new chelator, dihydroxybenzoic acid, is now being evaluated and appears to be very promising (189c).

Other General Measures

The medical management of a child with homozygous beta thalassemia otherwise involves good general pediatric and medical care, which includes a close relationship between physician, patient, and parents, and education of parents and child with regard to seeking early medical attention for any illness, especially at the first sign of fever. Because of the propensity of these children to develop severe and frequently fatal infections, it is probably wise to treat any febrile illness, after the taking of appropriate cultures, with antibiotics until a specific diagnosis becomes apparent. In addition to the fatal septicemias, other infections which these patients develop include a benign pericarditis believed to be of viral etiology (190). However, it may also be the result of streptococcal infection (191), or of iron-induced irritation, analogous to the arthritis of hemochromatosis. It usually subsides spontaneously, although pericardiocentesis may rarely be necessary to relieve tamponade. Other infections include transfusion-related infections, such as hepatitis and cytomegalovirus infection, which must be treated symptomatically. The latter may be avoided by use of blood which is over 48 hours old.

Because of the marked marrow hyperplasia due to the hemolytic component of the disease, thalassemic children should be maintained on daily folic acid replacement (one milligram daily) to prevent the development of relative folic acid deficiency and a megaloblastic crisis, which may aggravate the anemia. Such a crisis may frequently present as thrombocytopenia and a bleeding diathesis.

The consequences of iron overload must be treated as they develop: diabetes, with appropriate diet and insulin therapy; hepatic dysfunction, by dietary and other supportive means. Frequently, thalassemic children may have a prolonged prothrombin time, which, despite its hepatocellular basis, may respond to vitamin K therapy. The most serious and life-threatening complication is that of cardiac hemosiderosis, resulting in arrhythmias and chronic congestive heart failure (190). When these complications develop, the patients must be treated vigorously with low-salt diet, digitalis, diuretics, and antiarrhythmic medications. Fatal Stokes-Adams attacks may occur from arrhythmias which are presumably due to iron deposition in the conducting system of the heart. In a child who develops recurrent arrhythmias, a cardiac pacemaker may be required to prevent a fatal arrhythmia.

As previously discussed in the section on chelation therapy, vitamin C and E supplementation may be beneficial to counteract the oxidant effects of iron overload.

Certain children develop severe cephalofacial deformities and malocclusion because of marrow expansion in the maxilla. This complication can usually be avoided by proper transfusion from an early age and early splenectomy (192). Once the deformity is established, surgical management is possible (193), though difficult.

Finally, androgen therapy (oxymetholone) has been reported to improve the anemia in a case of thalassemia intermedia (194), although secondary causes may have contributed to the anemia in that particular case. Hormonal replacement therapy has been used in certain patients in an attempt to treat various endocrine deficiencies, presumably due to hemosiderosis, and improve development of secondary sexual characteristics. The therapy is usually not effective because sexual retardation seems to be due to target organ unresponsiveness rather than hormone depletion in these patients.

Future Treatment

The future may offer more definitive forms of prevention and therapy of thalassemia. Prenatal diagnosis of thalassemia has been discussed at the beginning of this section in relation to prevention of the disease. Two possible means of therapy may one day become available for the child with established thalassemia major: (1) bone marrow transplantation, and (2) correction of the biochemical defect by genetic engineering and manipulation.

The art of bone marrow transplantation is being developed in a number of centers. It has been successfully carried out in the treatment of aplastic anemia, severe immune deficiency, and in certain cases of acute leukemia, using as a source of bone marrow that of an unaffected sibling who is histocompatible with the patient. The major problem, however, is immunologic; rejection of the graft by the recipient or graft-versus-host reaction have been difficult problems which have led to many failures and fatalities (see Chapter 5). In thalassemia, one would have to destroy the patient's own marrow before such a transplantation, in order to prevent proliferation of the abnormal erythroid cells. This would be impossible to do without destroying the patient's own granulocyte precursors and megakaryocytes as well. Rejection of the marrow graft by the thalassemic patient is very likely, even with proper immunosuppression and good histocompatibility, because of prior sensitization of the patient to various tissue antigens from the many previous blood transfusions. Rejection of the graft would leave the patient totally aplastic. If marrow transplantation is to be successful in thalassemic patients, it should probably be done in infancy before transfusions are initiated. Finally, even if the transplanted marrow becomes engrafted, a graft-versus-host reaction could lead to a rapidly fatal outcome. Until the current problems of bone marrow transplantation are resolved and one can offer the patient a good possibility of a successful outcome, bone marrow transplantation cannot be advised at this time in thalassemia. With good medical management, the patient can be given some 20 or more years of useful life.

If one could suppress the excessive production of the normally produced globin chain in thalassemia, one would eliminate the precipitation of globin chain aggregates which leads to much of the pathophysiology and disability in thalassemia. Research is proceeding to find drugs or other agents which might specifically inhibit the synthesis of one or another globin chain. In beta thalassemia, if one could induce gamma chain synthesis or prevent the neonatal gamma to beta chain switchover, one would increase the relative amount of gamma chain in the thalassemic red cell. This would decrease the disability of the patients by decreasing or eliminating the formation of alpha chain aggregates, which are so important in the development of the hemolytic component of the disease; the gamma chains could combine with the excess alpha chains, and balance would be achieved. Research is also under way in this area.

It is not unrealistic to think that, some day, specific gene therapy for thalassemia may be possible. It is now possible to synthesize a portion of the gene for globin chain synthesis by copying the messenger RNA for globin into a DNA copy, using the RNA-dependent DNA polymerase or reverse transcriptase enzyme of avian myeloblastosis virus (195–197). However, in vitro transcription of this DNA copy does not yield a functional mRNA, presumably because the DNA is not a complete copy of the mRNA, and lacks the information coding for the 5' terminus of the mRNA (198), which contains the initiation sequence for mRNA translation. Another approach to gene therapy would be the isolation of the globin gene from total DNA of non-thalassemic cells and insertion of the gene into thalassemic marrow cells. A general method for specific gene isolation has been described (199), as well as methods for insertion of genetic material into eukaryotic cells (200–206). The ability to isolate pure human globin mRNA could lead to the isolation of the human globin genes from total cellular DNA by preparative DNA-RNA hybridization techniques. The technical and ethical issues involved in gene therapy have been recently reviewed (206–209).

These types of solutions are still far away, but remain possibilities. Once the genetic defect is known more precisely at the messenger RNA and DNA levels, one may have more insight into ways to approach the treatment of thalassemia at the molecular level. In the meantime, the cornerstone of the treatment of thalassemia must remain good general medical care and proper supportive management of the patient in a center which is equipped to provide these.

References

1. Bannerman, R. M.: *Thalassemia. A Survey of Some Aspects.* New York, Grune & Stratton, 1961.
2. Weatherall, D. J., and Clegg, J. B.: *The Thalassemia Syndromes.* 2nd ed. Oxford, Blackwell Scientific Publications, 1972.
3. Wasi, P., Na-Nakorn, S., et al.: Alpha and beta thalassemia in Thailand. Ann. N. Y. Acad. Sci. *165*:60, 1969.
4. Livingstone, F. B.: *Abnormal Hemoglobins in Human Populations.* Chicago, Aldine Publishing Company, 1967.
5. McFadzean, A. J. S., and Todd, D.: The distribution of Cooley's anemia in China. Trans. R. Soc. Trop. Med. Hyg. *58*:490, 1964.
6. Huehns, E. R., Dance, N., et al.: Human embryonic hemoglobins. Cold Spring Harbor Symp. Quant. Biol. *19*:327, 1964.
6a. Lorkin, P. A.: Fetal and embryonic haemoglobins. J. Med. Genet. *10*:50, 1973.
7. Capp, G. L., Rigas, D. A., et al.: Evidence for a new hemoglobin chain (ζ-chain). Nature (Lond.) *228*:278, 1970.
8. Wasi, P.: Is the human globin α-chain locus duplicated? Br. J. Haematol. *24*:267, 1973.
8a. Hollan, S. R., Szelenyi, J. G., et al.: Multiple alpha chain loci for human hemoglobins: Hb J-Buda and Hb G-Pest. Nature (Lond.) *235*:47, 1972.
9. Bernini, L. F., De Jong, W. W. W., et al.: Varianti emoglobiniche nella popolazione tribale dell' Andhra Pradesh. Atti Assoc. Genet. Ital. *15*:191, 1970.
9a. Ostertag, W., von Ehrenstein, G., et al.: Duplicated α chain genes in Hopkins-2-hemoglobin of man and evidence for unequal crossing-over between them. Nature [New Biol.] *237*:90, 1972.
10. Lehmann, H., and Carrell, R. W.: Differences between α and β chain mutants of human hemoglobin and between α and β thalassemia. Possible duplication of the α chain gene. Br. Med. J. *4*:748, 1968.
11. Lehmann, H.: Different types of alpha thalassemia and significance of hemoglobin Bart's in neonates. Lancet *2*:78, 1970.
12. Kattamis, C., and Lehmann, H.: Duplication of alpha thalassemia gene in three Greek families with hemoglobin H disease. Lancet *2*:635, 1970.
13. Lehmann, H., and Carrell, R. W.: Variations in the structure of human hemoglobin with particular reference to the unstable hemoglobins. Br. Med. Bull. *25*:14, 1969.
14. White, J. M.: The synthesis of abnormal hemoglobins. Biochimie *54*:657, 1972.
15. Abramson, R. K., Rucknagel, D. L., et al.: Homozygous Hb J Tongariki: Evidence for only one alpha chain structural locus in Melanesians. Science *169*:194, 1970.
16. Beaven, G. H., Hornabrook, R. W., et al.: Occurence of heterozygotes and homozygotes for the α chain hemoglobin variant Hb J (Tongariki) in New Guinea. Nature (Lond.) *235*:46, 1972.
17. Schroeder, W. A., Huisman, T. J. H., et al.: Evidence for multiple structural genes for the γ chain of human fetal hemoglobin. Proc. Nat. Acad. Sci. USA *60*:537, 1968.
18. Schroeder, W. A., Shelton, J. R., et al.: Worldwide occurence of nonallelic genes for the γ chain of human foetal hemoglobin in newborns. Nature [New Biol.] *240*:273, 1972.
18a. Huisman, T. H. J., Schroeder, W. A., et al.: Evidence for four nonallelic structural genes for the γ chain of human fetal hemoglobin. Biochem. Genet. *7*:131, 1972.
18b. Schroeder, W. A., Bannister, W. H., et al.: Non-synchronized suppression of postnatal activity in non-allelic genes which synthesize the $^G\gamma$ chain in human foetal hemoglobin. Nature [New Biol.] *244*:89, 1973.
19. Price, P. M., Conover, J. H., et al.: Chromosomal localization of human hemoglobin structural genes. Nature (Lond.) *237*:340, 1972.
20. Bishop, J. O., and Jones, K. W.: Chromosomal localization of human hemoglobin structural genes. Nature (Lond.) *240*:149, 1972.
21. Prensky, W., and Holmquist, G.: Chromosomal localization of human hemoglobin structural genes: Techniques queried. Nature (Lond.) *241*:44, 1973.
22. Nance, W. E., Conneally, M., et al.: Genetic linkage analysis of human hemoglobin variants. Am. J. Hum. Genet. *22*:453, 1970.
23. Donahue, R. P., Bias, W. B., et al.: Probable assignment of the Duffy blood group locus to chromosome 1 in man. Proc. Natl. Acad. Sci. USA *61*:949, 1968.
24. Wilson, M. G., Schroeder, W. A., et al.: Hemoglobin variations in D-Trisomy syndrome. New Engl. J. Med. *277*:953, 1967.
25. Bard, H.: Postnatal fetal and adult hemoglobin synthesis in D_1 trisomy syndrome. Blood *40*:523, 1972.
26. Smith, E. W., and Torbert, J. V.: Two abnormal hemoglobins with evidence for a new genetic locus for hemoglobin formation. Bull. Johns Hopkins Hosp. *102*:34, 1958.
27. Wong, S. C., and Huisman, T. H. J.: Further evidence for non-linkage of the Hb α and Hb β structural loci in man. Clin. Chim. Acta *38*:473, 1972.
28. Boyer, S. H., Rucknagel, D. L., et al.: Further evidence for linkage between the β and δ loci governing human hemoglobin and the population dynamics of linked genes. Am. J. Hum. Genet. *15*:438, 1963.
29. Gerald, P. S., and Diamond, L. K.: The diagnosis of thalassemia trait by starch block electrophoresis of the hemoglobin. Blood *13*:61, 1958.
30. Baglioni, C.: The fusion of two peptide chains in hemoglobin Lepore and its interpretation

as a genetic deletion. Proc. Natl. Acad. Sci. USA 48:1880, 1962.

31. Huisman, T. H. J., Schroeder, W. A., et al.: Hemoglobin Kenya, the product of non-homologous crossing-over of γ and β genes. Blood 40:947, 1972.

31a. Huisman, T. H. J., Wrightstone, R. N., et al.: Hemoglobin Kenya, the product of fusion of γ and β polypeptide chains. Arch. Biochem. Biophys. 153:850, 1972.

32. Thompson, R. B., Odom, J., et al.: Hb S, beta thalassemia, and Hb A_2 (B_2) in a family with evidence of a crossover between beta and delta loci. Acta Genet. (Basel) 15:371, 1965.

33. Pearson, H. A., and Moore, M. M.: Human hemoglobin gene linkage: Report of a family with hemoglobin B_2, hemoglobin δ and β-thalassemia, including a probable crossover between thalassemia and delta loci. Am. J. Hum. Genet. 17:125, 1965.

34. Atwater, J., Schwartz, I. R., et al.: Sickling of erythrocytes in a patient with thalassemia-hemoglobin I disease. New Engl. J. Med. 263:1215, 1960.

35. Hollenberg, M. D., Kaback, M. M., et al.: Adult hemoglobin synthesis by reticulocytes from the human fetus at midtrimester. Science 174:698, 1971.

35a. Kazazian, H. H., Jr., and Woodhead, A. P.: Hemoglobin A synthesis in the developing fetus. New Engl. J. Med. 289:58, 1973.

36. Basch, R. A.: Hemoglobin synthesis in short term cultures of human fetal hematopoietic tissues. Blood 39:530, 1972.

37. Pataryas, H. A., and Stamatoyannopoulos, G.: Hemoglobins in human fetuses: Evidence for adult hemoglobin production after the 11th gestational week. Blood 39:688, 1972.

38. Kan, Y. W., Dozy, A. M., et al.: Detection of the sickle gene in the human fetus. Potential for intrauterine diagnosis of sickle cell anemia. New Engl. J. Med. 287:1, 1972.

39. Cividalli, G., Nathan, D. G., et al.: Relation of beta to gamma synthesis during the first trimester: An approach to prenatal diagnosis of thalassemia. Pediatr. Res. 8:553, 1974.

40. Bard, H., Makowski, E. L., et al.: The relative rates of synthesis of hemoglobin A and F in immature red cells of newborn infants. Pediatrics 45:766, 1970.

41. Kan, Y. W., Forget, B. G., et al.: Gamma-beta thalassemia: A cause of hemolytic disease of newborns. New Engl. J. Med. 286:129, 1972.

42. Cooper, H. A., and Hoagland, H. C.: Fetal hemoglobin. Mayo Clin. Proc. 47:402, 1972.

43. Pembrey, M. E., and Weatherall, D. J.: Maternal synthesis of haemoglobin F in pregnancy. Br. J. Haematol. 21:355, 1971.

44. Bard, H.: Etudes préliminaires de la synthèse des hémoglobines foetales et adultes chez le prématuré. Un. Med. Can. 100:1097, 1971.

45. Fraser, I. D.: Adult and foetal haemoglobin in Rh haemolytic disease. Br. J. Haematol. 23:269, 1972.

46. Bhoyroo, S. K., and Storrs, C. N.: Adult and fetal hemoglobin in hemolytic disease of the newborn. Arch. Dis. Child. 46:570, 1971.

47. Guidotti, G.: Thalassemia, In Conference on Hemoglobin. Arden House. New York, Columbia University, 1962.

48. Baglioni, C.: Correlations between genetics and chemistry of human hemoglobins, In Molecular Genetics. Part I. Taylor, J. H. (ed.), New York, Academic Press, 1963, p. 405.

49. Jones, R. T., and Schroeder, W. A.: Chemical characterization and subunit hybridization of human hemoglobin H and associated compounds. Biochemistry 2:1357, 1963.

50. Lehmann, H., and Charlesworth, D.: Observations on hemoglobin P (Congo type). Biochem. J. 119:43, 1970.

50a. Badr, F. M., Lorkin, P. A., et al.: Haemoglobin P-Nilotic containing a β-δ chain. Nature [New Biol.] 242:107, 1973.

51. Ohta, Y., Yamaoka, K., et al.: Hemoglobin Miyada, a β-δ fusion peptide (anti-Lepore) type discovered in a Japanese family. Nature [New Biol.] 234:218, 1971.

52. Milner, P. F., Clegg, J. B., et al.: Haemoglobin H disease due to a unique haemoglobin variant with an elongated α-chain. Lancet 1:729, 1971.

53. Clegg, J. B., Weatherall, D. J., et al.: Hemoglobin Constant Spring—a chain termination mutant? Nature (Lond.) 234:337, 1971.

54. Heywood, J. D., Karon, M., et al.: Amino acids: Incorporation into alpha- and beta-chains of hemoglobin by normal and thalassemic reticulocytes. Science 146:530, 1964.

55. Heywood, J. D., Karon, M., et al.: Asymmetrical incorporation of amino acids into the alpha and beta chains of hemoglobin synthesized in thalassemic reticulocytes. J. Lab. Clin. Med. 66:476, 1965.

56. Weatherall, D. J., Clegg, J. B., et al.: Globin synthesis in thalassemia: An in vitro study. Nature (Lond.) 208:1061, 1965.

57. Bank, A., and Marks, P. A.: Excess alpha chain synthesis relative to beta chain synthesis in thalassemia major and minor. Nature (Lond.) 212:1198, 1966.

58. Bargellesi, A., Pontremoli, S., et al.: Absence of beta-globin synthesis and excess of alpha-globin synthesis in homozygous beta-thalassemia. Eur. J. Biochem. 1:73, 1967.

59. Modell, C. B., Lotter, A., et al.: Haemoglobin synthesis in β-thalassemia. Br. J. Haematol. 17:485, 1969.

60. Weatherall, D. J., Clegg, J. B., et al.: The pattern of disordered haemoglobin synthesis in homozygous and heterozygous β-thalassemia. Br. J. Haematol. 16:251, 1969.

61. Conci, F., Bargellesi, A., et al.: Globin chain synthesis in Sicilian thalassemic subjects. Br. J. Haematol. 19:469, 1970.

61a. Braverman, A., and McCurdy, P. R.: Mild homozygous β-thalassemia in Negroes. Clin. Res. 19:37, 1971.

61b. Friedman, S., Hamilton, R. W., et al.: β-Thalassemia in the American Negro. J. Clin. Invest. 52:1453, 1973.

62. Bank, A., Braverman, S., et al.: Absolute rates of globin chain synthesis in thalassemia. Blood 31:226, 1968.

63. Clegg, J. B., and Weatherall, D. J.: Hemoglobin synthesis in α-thalassemia (hemoglobin H disease). Nature (Lond.) 215:1241, 1967.

64. Kan, Y. W., Schwartz, E., et al.: Globin chain synthesis in alpha thalassemia syndromes. J. Clin. Invest. 47:2515, 1968.

65. Weatherall, D. J., Clegg, J. B., et al.: The hemoglobin constitution of infants with the hemoglobin Bart's hydrops fetalis syndrome. Br. J. Haematol. 18:357, 1970.

66. Schwartz, E., and Atwater, J.: α-Thalassemia in the American Negro. J. Clin. Invest. 51:412, 1972.

67. Braverman, A. S., and Bank, A.: Changing rates of globin chain synthesis during erythroid cell maturation in thalassemia. J. Mol. Biol. 42:57, 1969.

68. Friedman, S., Oski, F. A., et al.: Bone marrow and peripheral blood globin synthesis in an American black family with beta thalassemia. Blood 39:785, 1972.

69. Nienhuis, A. W., Canfield, P. H., et al.: Hemoglobin messenger RNA from human bone marrow: Isolation and translation in homozygous and heterozygous β-thalassemia. J. Clin. Invest. 52:1735, 1973.

70. Shchory, M., and Ramot, B.: Globin chain synthesis in the marrow and reticulocytes of beta thalassemia, hemoglobin H disease, and beta delta thalassemia. Blood 40:105, 1972.

71. Schwartz, E.: Heterozygous beta thalassemia: Balanced globin synthesis in bone marrow cells. Science 167:1513, 1970.

72. Kan, Y. W., Nathan, D. G., et al.: Equal synthesis of α- and β-globin chains in erythroid precursors in heterozygous β-thalassemia. J. Clin. Invest. 51:1906, 1972.

73. Clegg, J. B., and Weatherall, D. J.: Hemoglobin synthesis during erythroid maturation in β-thalassemia. Nature [New Biol.] 240:190, 1972.

74. Gill, F., Atwater, J., et al.: Hemoglobin Lepore trait: Globin synthesis in bone marrow and peripheral blood. Science 178:623, 1972.

75. White, J. M., Long, A., et al.: Compensation of β chain synthesis by the single β chain gene in Hb Lepore trait. Nature [New Biol.] 240:271, 1972.

75a. Friedman, S., Ozsoylu, S., et al.: A new form of β-thalassemia trait of unusual severity. Blood 42:990, 1973.

75b. Stamatoyannopoulos, G., Woodson, R., et al.: Inclusion-body β-thalassemia trait. A form of β-thalassemia producing clinical manifestations in simple heterozygotes. New Engl. J. Med. 290:939, 1974.

76. Watson, J. D.: Molecular Biology of the Gene. 2nd ed. New York, W. A. Benjamin, Inc., 1970.

77. Clegg, J. B., Weatherall, D. J., et al.: Hemoglobin synthesis in beta thalassemia. Nature (Lond.) 220:664, 1968.

77a. Ingram, V. M.: A molecular model for thalassemia. Ann. N.Y. Acad. Sci. 119:485, 1964.

77b. Itano, H. A.: The synthesis and structure of normal and abnormal hemoglobins, In Abnormal Haemoglobins in Africa. Jonxis, J. H. P. (ed.), Oxford, Blackwell Scientific Publications, 1965, p. 3.

78. Rieder, R. F.: Translation of β-globin mRNA in β-thalassemia and the S and C hemoglobinopathies. J. Clin. Invest. 51:364, 1972.

79. Burka, E. R., and Marks, P. A.: Ribosomes active in protein synthesis in human reticulocytes: A defect in thalassemia major. Nature (Lond.) 199:706, 1963.

80. Fuhr, J., Natta, C., et al.: Protein synthesis in cell-free systems from reticulocytes of thalassemic patients. Nature (Lond.) 224:1305, 1969.

81. Bank, A., and Marks, P. A.: Protein synthesis in a cell-free human reticulocyte system: Ribosome function in thalassemia. J. Clin. Invest. 45:330, 1966.

82. Nienhuis, A. W., Laycock, D. G., et al.: Translation of rabbit hemoglobin messenger RNA by thalassemic and non-thalassemic ribosomes. Nature [New Biol.] 231:205, 1971.

83. Gilbert, J. M., Thornton, A. G., et al.: Cell-free hemoglobin synthesis in beta thalassemia. Proc. Natl. Acad. Sci. USA 67:1854, 1970.

84. Nathan, D. G., Lodish, H., et al.: Beta thalassemia and translation of globin messenger RNA. Proc. Natl. Acad. Sci. USA 68:2514, 1971.

85. Cividalli, G., Nathan, D. G., et al.: Translational control of hemoglobin synthesis in thalassemic bone marrow. J. Clin. Invest. 53:955, 1974.

85a. Crystal, R. G., Elson, N. A., et al.: Initiation of globin synthesis in β-thalassemia. New Engl. J. Med. 288:1091, 1973.

86. Nienhuis, A. W., and Anderson, W. F.: Isolation and translation of hemoglobin messenger RNA from thalassemia, sickle cell anemia and normal human reticulocytes. J. Clin. Invest. 50:2458, 1971.

87. Benz, E. J., Jr., and Forget, B. G.: Defect in messenger RNA for human hemoglobin synthesis in beta thalassemia. J. Clin. Invest. 50:2755, 1971.

88. Dow, L. W., Terada, M., et al.: Globin synthesis of intact cells and activity of isolated mRNA in β-thalassemia. Nature [New Biol.] 243:114, 1973.

89. Benz, E. J., Jr., Swerdlow, P. S., et al.: Globin messenger RNA in Hb H disease. Blood 42:825, 1973.

90. Grossbard, E., Terada, M., et al.: Decreased α globin messenger RNA activity associated with polyribosomes in α thalassemia. Nature [New Biol.] 241:209, 1973.

90a. Forget, B. G., Baltimore, D., et al.: Globin messenger RNA in the thalassemia syndromes. Ann. N.Y. Acad. Sci. 232:76, 1974.

90b. Natta, C., Banks, J., et al.: Decreased β-globin mRNA activity in bone marrow cells in homozygous and heterozygous β-thalassemia. Nature [New Biol.] 244:280, 1973.

91. Housman, D., Forget, B. G., et al.: Quantitative deficiency of chain specific globin mRNA in the thalassemia syndromes. Proc. Natl. Acad. Sci. USA 70:1809, 1973.

91a. Kacian, D. L., Gambino, R., et al.: Decreased globin messenger RNA in thalassemia detected by molecular hybridization. Proc. Natl. Acad. Sci. USA 70:1886, 1973.

92. Forget, B. G., Marotta, C. A., et al.: Nucleotide sequences of human globin messenger RNA. Ann. N.Y. Acad. Sci., 1974 (in press).

93. Baglioni, C., Colombo, B., et al.: Chain termination: A test for a possible explanation of

thalassemia. Ann. N.Y. Acad. Sci. *165*:212, 1969.

94. Dreyfus, J. C., Labie, D., et al.: An attempt at demonstrating the existence of a nonsense mutation in β-thalassemia. Eur. J. Biochem. *27*:291, 1972.

95. Conconi, F., Rowley, P. T., et al.: Induction of β-globin synthesis in the β-thalassemia of Ferrara. Nature [New Biol.] *238*:83, 1972.

96. Rowley, P. T., and Kosciolek, B.: Distinction between two types of beta-thalassemia by inducibility of the cell-free synthesis of beta-chains by non-thalassemic soluble fraction. Nature [New Biol.] *239*:234, 1972.

96a. Kan, Y. W., Dozy, A. M., et al.: Absence of functional β-globin mRNA in homozygous β⁰-thalassemia. Blood *42*:991, 1973.

96b. Forget, B. G., Benz, E. J., Jr., et al.: Absence of messenger RNA for beta globin chain in β⁰-thalassemia. Nature (Lond.) *247*:379, 1974.

96c. O'Brien, R. T.: The effect of iron deficiency on the expression of hemoglobin H. Blood *41*:853, 1973.

97. Bargellesi, A., Pontremoli, S., et al.: Excess of alpha globin synthesis in homozygous beta-thalassemia and its removal from the red blood cell cytoplasm. Eur. J. Biochem. *3*:364, 1968.

98. Nathan, D. G., and Gunn, R. B.: Thalassemia: The consequences of unbalanced hemoglobin synthesis. Am. J. Med. *41*:815, 1966.

99. Nathan, D. G., Stossel, T. B., et al.: Influence of hemoglobin precipitation on erythrocyte metabolism in alpha and beta thalassemia. J. Clin. Invest. *48*:33, 1969.

99a. Gunn, R. B., Silvers, D. N., et al.: Potassium permeability in β-thalassemia minor red blood cells. J. Clin. Invest. *51*:1043, 1972.

100. Fessas, P., Loukopoulos, D., et al.: Peptide analysis of the inclusions of erythroid cells in β-thalassemia. Biochim. Biophys. Acta *124*:430, 1966.

100a. Rachmilewitz, E. A., and Thorell, B.: Hemichromes in single inclusion bodies in red cells of beta thalassemia. Blood *39*:794, 1972.

101. Gabuzda, T. G., Nathan, D. G., et al.: The turnover of hemoglobins A, F and A₂ in the peripheral blood of three patients with thalassemia. J. Clin. Invest. *42*:1678, 1963.

102. Loukopoulos, D., and Fessas, P.: The distribution of hemoglobin types in thalassemic erythrocytes. J. Clin. Invest. *44*:231, 1965.

103. Fessas, P.: Inclusions of hemoglobin in erythrocytes of thalassemia. Blood *21*:21, 1963.

104. Yataganas, X., and Fessas, P.: The pattern of hemoglobin precipitation in thalassemia and its significance. Ann. N.Y. Acad. Sci. *165*:270, 1969.

105. Finch, C. A., Deubelbeiss, K., et al.: Ferrokinetics in man. Medicine (Baltimore) *49*:17, 1970.

106. Rifkind, R. A., and Damon, D.: Heinz body anemia—an ultrastructural study. I. Heinz body formation. Blood *25*:885, 1965.

107. Wennberg, E., and Weiss, L.: Splenic erythroclasia: An electronic microscopic study of hemoglobin H disease. Blood *31*:778, 1968.

108. Slater, L. M., Muir, W. A., et al.: Influence of splenectomy on insoluble hemoglobin inclusion bodies in β-thalassemic erythrocytes. Blood *31*:766, 1968.

108a. Weatherall, D. J., Clegg, J. B., et al.: A genetically determined disorder with features both of thalassaemia and congenital dyserythropoietic anaemia. Br. J. Haematol. *24*:681, 1973.

109. Fessas, P., and Yataganas, X.: Intraerythroblastic instability of hemoglobin β₄ (Hb H). Blood *31*:323, 1968.

110. Rigas, D. A., and Koler, R. D.: Decreased erythrocyte survival in hemoglobin H disease as a result of the abnormal properties of hemoglobin H: The benefit of splenectomy. Blood *18*:1, 1961.

111. Erlandson, M. E., Walden, B., et al.: Studies on congenital hemolytic syndromes. IV. Gastrointestinal absorption of iron. Blood *19*:359, 1962.

112. Bannerman, R. M., Callender, S. T., et al.: Iron absorption in thalassemia. Br. J. Haematol. *10*:490, 1964.

113. Necheles, T. F., Allen, D. M., et al.: *Clinical Disorders of Hemoglobin Structure and Synthesis.* New York, Appleton-Century-Crofts, 1969.

113a. Heinrich, H. C., Gabbe, E. E., et al.: Absorption of inorganic and food iron in children with heterozygous and homozygous β-thalassemia. Z. Kinderheilk. *115*:1, 1973.

114. Bannerman, R. M., Grinstein, M., et al.: Haemoglobin synthesis in thalassemia; *in vitro* studies. Br. J. Haematol. *5*:102, 1959.

115. Steiner, M., Baldini, M., et al.: Enzymatic defects of heme synthesis in thalassemia. Ann. N.Y. Acad. Sci. *119*:548, 1964.

116. Bannerman, R. M.: Abnormalities of heme and pyrrole metabolism in thalassemia. Ann. N.Y. Acad. Sci. *119*:503, 1964.

117. Jandl, J. H., and Greenberg, M. S.: Bone marrow failure due to relative nutritional deficiency in Cooley's hemolytic anemia. New Engl. J. Med. *266*:461, 1959.

118. Luhby, A. L., and Cooperman, J. M.: Folic acid deficiency in thalassemia major. Lancet 2:490, 1961.

119. Luhby, A. L., Cooperman, J. M., et al.: Folic acid deficiency as a limiting factor in the anemias of thalassemia major. Blood *18*:786, 1961.

120. Prankerd, T. A. J.: The spleen and anemia. Br. Med. J. 2:517, 1963.

121. Koler, R. D., Jones, R. T., et al.: Genetics of hemoglobin H and α-thalassemia. Ann. Hum. Genet. *34*:371, 1971.

122. Koler, R. D., and Rigas, D. A.: Genetics of hemoglobin H. Ann. Hum. Genet. 25:95, 1961.

123. Wasi, P., Na-Nakorn, S., et al.: Hemoglobin H disease in Thailand: A genetical study. Nature (Lond.) *204*:907, 1964.

124. Wasi, P.: The alpha thalassemia genes. J. Med. Assoc. Thailand, 53:677, 1970.

125. Pootrakul, S., Wasi, P., et al.: Studies on haemoglobin Bart's (Hb-γ₄) in Thailand: The incidence and the mechanism of occurrence in cord blood. Ann. Hum. Genet. *31*:149, 1967.

126. Pootrakul, S., Wasi, P., et al.: Incidence of alpha thalassemia in Bangkok. J. Med. Assoc. Thailand, 53:250, 1970.

127. Na-Nakorn, S., and Wasi, P.: Alpha-thalassemia in Northern Thailand. Am. J. Hum. Genet. 22:645, 1970.

128. Na-Nakorn, S., Wasi, P., et al.: Further evidence for a genetic basis of haemoglobin H disease from newborn offspring of patients. Nature (Lond.) 223:59, 1969.

129. White, J. C., Ellis, M., et al.: An unstable haemoglobin associated with cases of leukemia. Br. J. Haematol. 6:171, 1960.

130. Beaven, G. H., Stevens, B. L., et al.: Occurrence of haemoglobin H in leukemia. Nature (Lond.) 199:1297, 1963.

131. Rosenzweig, A. I., Heywood, J. D., et al.: Hemoglobin H as an acquired defect of chain synthesis: Report of two cases. Acta Haematol. (Basel) 39:91, 1968.

132. Hamilton, R. W., Schwartz, E., et al.: Acquired hemoglobin H disease. New Engl. J. Med. 285:1217, 1971.

133. Andre, R., Najman, A., et al.: Erythro-leucémie avec hémoglobine H acquiré et anomalies des antigènes erythrocytaires. Nouv. Rev. Fr. Hématol. 12:29, 1972.

134. Pagnier, J., Labie, D., et al.: Etude biochimique d'un cas d'erythroleucémie. Nouv. Rev. Fr. Hématol. 12:317, 1972.

135. Gabuzda, T. G., Nathan, D. G., et al.: The metabolism of the individual C^{14}-labelled hemoglobins in patients with H-thalassemia, with observations on radiochromate binding to the hemoglobins during red cell survival. J. Clin. Invest. 44:315, 1965.

136. Tso, S. C.: Red cell survival studies in haemoglobin H disease using [^{51}Cr] chromate and [^{32}P] di-isopropyl phosphofluoridate. Br. J. Haematol. 23:621, 1972.

137. Sofroniadou, K., Kaltsoya, A., et al.: Hemoglobin "Athens": an alpha-chain variant with unusual properties. Abstracts, p. 56, XII International Congress of Haematology, New York. New York, Grune & Stratton, 1968.

137a. Kan, Y. W., Todd, D., et al.: Hemoglobin Constant Spring: Possibly unstable mRNA and evidence for 2 locus theory for α chain production. Clin. Res. 20:471, 1972.

137b. Seid-Akhavan, M., Winter, W. P., et al.: Hemoglobin Wayne: A frameshift variant occurring in two distinct forms. Blood 40:927, 1972.

137c. Laux, B., Dennis, D., et al.: Human α-chain globin messenger: Prediction of a nucleotide sequence. Biochem. Biophys. Res. Commun. 54:894, 1973.

138. Lie-Injo, L. E., and Jo, B. H.: A fast-moving haemoglobin in hydrops foetalis. Nature (Lond.) 185:698, 1960.

139. Lie-Injo, L. E.: Alpha-chain thalassemia and hydrops fetalis in Malaya: Report of five cases. Blood 20:581, 1962.

140. Todd, D., Lai, M. C. S., et al.: Thalassaemia and hydrops foetalis—family studies. Br. Med. J. 3:347, 1967.

141. Kan, Y. W., Allen, A., et al.: Hydrops fetalis with alpha thalassemia. New Engl. J. Med. 276:18, 1967.

142. Diamond, M. P., Cotgrove, I., et al.: Case of intrauterine death due to α-thalassemia. Br. Med. J. 2:278, 1965.

143. Todd, D., Lai, M. C. S., et al.: The abnormal haemoglobins in homozygous α-thalassemia. Br. J. Haematol. 19:27, 1970.

144. Pearson, H. A., O'Brien, R. T., et al.: Screening for thalassemia trait by electronic measurement of mean corpuscular volume (MCV). New Engl. J. Med. 288:351, 1973.

144a. Torlontano, G., Tata, A., et al.: A rapid screening test for thalassemic trait. Acta Haematol. (Basel) 48:234, 1972.

144b. England, J. M., and Fraser,·P. M.: Differentiation of iron deficiency from thalassaemia trait by routine blood count. Lancet 1:449, 1973.

144c. Mentzer, W. C.: Differentiation of iron deficiency from thalassaemia trait. Lancet 1:882, 1973.

145. Aksoy, M.: Thalassemia intermedia: A genetic study in 11 patients. J. Med. Genet. 7:47, 1970.

146. McCarthy, G. M., Temperley, I. J., et al.: Thalassemia in an Irish family. Irish J. Med. Sci. 7:303, 1968.

146a. Pootrakul, P., Wasi, P., et al.: Haematological data in 312 cases of β-thalassaemia trait in Thailand. Br. J. Haematol. 24:703, 1973.

147. Weatherall, D. J.: Biochemical phenotypes of thalassemia in the American Negro population. Ann. N.Y. Acad. Sci. 119:450, 1964.

148. Schokker, R. C., Went, L. N., et al.: A new genetic variant of beta-thalassemia. Nature (Lond.) 209:44, 1966.

149. Gaburro, D., Volpato, S., et al.: Diagnosis of beta thalassemia in the newborn by means of hemoglobin synthesis. Acta Paediatr. Scand. 59:523, 1970.

150. Smith, C. H., Erlandson, M. E., et al.: Postsplenectomy infection in Cooley's anemia. New Engl. J. Med. 266:737, 1962.

151. Smith, C. H., Erlandson, M. E., et al.: Postsplenectomy infection in Cooley's anemia. Ann. N.Y. Acad. Sci. 119:748, 1964.

152. Logothetis, J., Loewenson, R. B., et al.: Body growth in Cooley's anemia (homozygous beta-thalassemia) with a correlative study as to other aspects of the illness in 138 cases. Pediatrics 50:92, 1972.

153. Necheles, T. F., Beard, M. E. J., et al.: Myocardial hemosiderosis in hypoxic mice. Ann. N.Y. Acad. Sci. 165:167, 1969.

153a. Lassman, M. N., Genel, M., et al.: Carbohydrate homeostasis and pancreatic islet cell function in thalassemia. Ann. Intern. Med. 80:65, 1974.

153b. Beltrami, C. A., Bearzi, I., et al.: Storage cells of spleen and bone marrow in thalassemia: An ultrastructural study. Blood 41:901, 1973.

154. Fessas, P., and Loukopoulos, D.: Alpha-chain of human hemoglobin: Occurrence *in vivo*. Science 143:590, 1964.

155. Stamatoyannopoulos, G., Fessas, P., et al.: F-thalassemia: A study of thirty-one families with simple heterozygotes and combinations of F-thalassemia with A$_2$-thalassemia. Am. J. Med. 47:194, 1969.

155a. Kattamis, C., Metaxotou-Mavromati, A. et al.: The clinical and haematological findings in children inheriting two types of thalassemia: high-A$_2$ type β-thalassaemia, and high-F type or δβ-thalassaemia. Br. J. Haematol. 25:375, 1973.

156. Russo, G., and Mollica, F.: Sickle-cell haemoglobin and two types of thalassemia in the same family. Acta Haematol. (Basel) 28:329, 1962.

157. Mann, J. R., MacNeish, A. S., et al.: δβ-thalassemia in a Chinese family. Br. J. Haematol. 23:393, 1972.

158. Fessas, P.: Forms of thalassemia, In *Abnormal Haemoglobins in Africa.* Jonxis, J. H. P. (ed.), Oxford, Blackwell Scientific Publications, 1965, p. 71.

159. Schwartz, E.: The silent carrier of beta-thalassemia. New Engl. J. Med. 281:1327, 1969.

159a. Rieder, R. F., and Weatherall, D. J.: Studies on hemoglobin biosynthesis: Asynchronous synthesis of hemoglobin A and hemoglobin A$_2$ by erythrocyte precursors. J. Clin. Invest. 44:42, 1965.

159b. Roberts, A. V., Weatherall, D. J., et al.: The synthesis of human hemoglobin A$_2$ during erythroid maturation. Biochem. Biophys. Res. Commun. 47:81, 1972.

159c. White, J. M., Lang, A., et al.: Studies of haemoglobin Lepore. Nature [New Biol.] 235:208, 1972.

159d. Roberts, A. V., Clegg, J. B., et al.: Synthesis *in vitro* of anti-Lepore haemoglobin. Nature [New Biol.] 245:23, 1973.

160. Kan, Y. W., and Nathan, D. G.: Mild thalassemia: The result of interaction of alpha and beta thalassemia genes. J. Clin. Invest. 49:635, 1970.

161. Knox-Macauley, H. H. M., Weatherall, D. J., et al.: The clinical and biosynthetic characterization of αβ-thalassemia. Br. J. Haematol. 22:497, 1972.

162. Kan, Y. W., and Nathan, D. G.: Prediction of severity of disease in homozygous β thalassemia. Pediatr. Res. 5:409, 1971.

163. Stamatoyannopoulos, G.: Gamma-thalassemia. Lancet 2:192, 1971.

164. Conley, C. L., Weatherall, D. J., et al.: Hereditary persistence of fetal hemoglobin: A study of 79 affected persons in 15 Negro families in Baltimore. Blood 21:261, 1963.

165. Fessas, P., and Stamatoyannopoulos, G.: Hereditary persistence of fetal hemoglobin in Greece. A study and a comparison. Blood 24:223, 1964.

165a. Natta, C. L., Niazi, G., et al.: Balanced globin chain synthesis in hereditary persistence of fetal hemoglobin (HPFH). Blood 42:991, 1973.

165b. Huisman, T. H. J., Schroeder, W. A., et al.: Hereditary persistence of fetal hemoglobin: Heterogeneity of fetal hemoglobin in homozygotes and in conjunction with β-thalassemia. New Engl. J. Med. 285:711, 1971.

165c. Huisman, T. H. J., Schroeder, W. A., et al.: Nature of fetal hemoglobin in the Greek type of hereditary persistence of fetal hemoglobin, with and without concurrent β-thalassemia. J. Clin. Invest. 49:1035, 1970.

166. Wheeler, J. T., and Krevans, J. R.: The homozygous state of persistent fetal hemoglobin and the interaction of persistent fetal hemoglobin with thalassemia. Bull. Johns Hopkins Hosp. 109:217, 1961.

166a. Kendall, A. G., Ojwang, P. J., et al.: Hemoglobin Kenya, the product of a γ-β fusion gene: Studies of the family. Am. J. Hum. Genet. 25:548, 1973.

166b. Smith, D. H., Clegg, J. B., et al.: Hereditary persistence of foetal haemoglobin associated with a γβ fusion variant, haemoglobin Kenya. Nature [New Biol.] 246:184, 1973.

167. Frazer, G. R., Kitsos, C., et al.: Thalassemias, abnormal hemoglobins, and glucose-6-phosphate dehydrogenase deficiency in the Arta area of Greece: Diagnostic and genetic aspects of complete village studies. Ann. N.Y. Acad. Sci. 119:415, 1964.

168. Ohta, Y., Yamaoka, K., et al.: Two unique structural and synthetical variants, Hb Miyada and homozygous δ-thalassemia, discovered in Japanese. XIII International Congress of Hematology, Munich, Abstracts, p. 233. Munich, J. F. Lehmanns, Verlag, 1970.

169. Fessas, P., and Stamatoyannopoulos, G.: Absence of hemoglobin A$_2$ in an adult. Nature (Lond.) 195:1215, 1962.

170. Thompson, R. B., Warrington, R., et al.: Interaction between genes for delta thalassemia and hereditary persistence of foetal haemoglobin. Acta Genet. (Basel) 15:190, 1965.

170a. Valenti, C.: Antenatal detection of hemoglobinopathies. Am. J. Obstet. Gynecol. 115:851, 1973.

170b. Kan, Y. W., Valenti, C., et al.: Fetal blood—sampling *in utero.* Lancet 1:79, 1974.

170c. Hobbins, J. C., and Mahoney, M. J.: In utero diagnosis of hemoglobinopathies. Technic for obtaining fetal blood. New Engl. J. Med., 290:1065, 1974.

170d. Chang, H., Hobbins, J. C., et al.: In utero diagnosis of hemoglobinopathies. Hemoglobin synthesis in fetal red cells. New Engl. Med., 290:1067, 1974.

170e. Kan, Y. W., Cividalli, G., et al.: Concentration of fetal red blood cells from a mixture of maternal and fetal blood by anti-i serum: An aid to prenatal diagnosis of hemoglobinopathies. Blood 43:411, 1974.

170f. Chang, H., Modell, C. B., et al.: Antenatal diagnosis of the β-thalassemia gene. Pediatr. Res., 8:124, 1974.

171. Piomelli, S., Danoff, S. J., et al.: Prevention of bone malformations and cardiomegaly in Cooley's anemia by early hypertransfusion regimen. Ann. N.Y. Acad. Sci. 165:427, 1969.

172. Beard, M. E. J., Necheles, T. F., et al.: Clinical experience with intensive transfusion therapy in Cooley's anemia. Ann. N. Y. Acad. Sci. 165:415, 1969.

173. Wolman, I. J.: Transfusion therapy in Cooley's anemia: Growth and health as related to long-range hemoglobin levels, a progress report. Ann. N.Y. Acad. Sci. 119:736, 1964.

174. Wolman, I. J., and Ortolani, M.: Some clinical features of Cooley's anemia patients as related to transfusion schedules. Ann. N.Y. Acad. Sci. 165:407, 1969.

175. Kattamis, C., Touliatos, N., et al.: Growth of children with thalassemia: Effect of different transfusion regimens. Arch. Dis. Child. 45:502, 1970.

176. Johnston, F. E., Hertzog, K. P., et al.: Longitudinal growth in thalassemia major. Am. J. Dis. Child. *112*:396, 1966.

177. Wolff, J. A., and Luke, K. H.: Management of thalassemia: A comparative program. Ann. N.Y. Acad. Sci. *165*:423, 1969.

178. Brook, C. G. D., Thompson, E. N., et al.: Growth in children with thalassemia major and effect of two different transfusion regimens. Arch. Dis. Child. *44*:612, 1969.

178a. Necheles, T. F., Sabbah, R., et al.: Intensive transfusion program in thalassemia. Ann. N.Y. Acad. Sci., *232*:179, 1974.

178b. Piomelli, S., Becker, M., et al.: Early hypertransfusion regimen in Cooley's anemia. Ann. N.Y. Acad. Sci., *232*:178, 1974.

179. Economidou, J., Constantoulakis, M., et al.: Frequency of antibodies to various antigenic determinants in polytransfused patients with homozygous thalassemia in Greece. Vox. Sang. *20*:252, 1971.

180. O'Brien, R. T., Pearson, H. A., et al.: Transfusion-induced decrease in spleen size in thalassemia major: Documentation by radioisotopic scan. J. Pediatr. *81*:105, 1972.

181. Eraklis, A. J., Kevy, S. V., et al.: Hazard of overwhelming infection after splenectomy in childhood. New Engl. J. Med. *276*:1225, 1967.

182. Wasi, C., Wasi, P., et al.: Serum-immunoglobin levels in thalassemia and the effect of splenectomy. Lancet *2*:237, 1971.

183. Smith, R. S.: Iron excretion in thalassemia major after administration of chelating agents. Br. Med. J. *2*:1577, 1962.

184. Smith, R. S.: Chelating agents in the diagnosis and treatment of iron overload in thalassemia. Ann. N.Y. Acad. Sci. *119*:776, 1964.

185. Keberle, H.: The biochemistry of desferrioxamine and its relation to iron metabolism. Ann. N.Y. Acad. Sci. *119*:758, 1964.

186. Wapnick, A. A., Lynch, S. R., et al.: The effect of ascorbic acid deficiency on desferrioxamine induced urinary iron excretion. Br. J. Haematol. *17*:563, 1969.

187. Lipschitz, D. A., Dugard, J., et al.: The site of action of desferrioxamine. Br. J. Haematol. *20*:395, 1971.

188. Lukens, J. N., and Neuman, L. A.: Excretion and distribution of iron during chronic desferrioxamine therapy. Blood *38*:614, 1971.

189. Modell, C. B., and Beck, J.: Long-term desferrioxamine therapy in thalassemia. Ann. N.Y. Acad. Sci., *232*:201, 1974.

189a. O'Brien, R. T.: Ascorbic acid enhancement of desferrioxamine-induced urinary iron excretion in thalassemia major. Ann. N.Y. Acad. Sci., *232*:221, 1974.

189b. Constantoulakis, M., Economidou, J., et al.: Combined long-term treatment of hemosiderosis with desferrioxamine and DTPA in homozygous β-thalassemia. Ann. N.Y. Acad. Sci., *232*:193, 1974.

189c. Graziano, J. H., Grady, R. W., et al.: The development of new iron chelating drugs. Blood *42*:1000, 1973.

190. Engle, M. A.: Cardiac involvement in Cooley's anemia. Ann. N.Y. Acad. Sci. *119*:694, 1964.

191. Wasi, P.: Streptococcal infection leading to cardiac and renal involvement in thalassemia. Lancet *1*:949, 1971.

192. Logothetis, J., Economidou, J., et al.: Cephalofacial deformities in thalassemia major (Cooley's anemia). Am. J. Dis. Child. *121*:300, 1971.

193. Jurkiewicz, M. J., Pearson, H. A., et al.: Reconstruction of the maxilla in thalassemia. Ann. N.Y. Acad. Sci. *165*:437, 1969.

194. Craddock, P. R., Hunt, F. A., et al.: The effective use of oxymetholone in the therapy of thalassemia with anemia. Med. J. Aust. *2*:199, 1972.

195. Verma, I. M., Temple, G. F., et al.: *In vitro* synthesis of DNA complementary to rabbit reticulocyte 10S RNA. Nature [New Biol.] *235*:163, 1972.

196. Kacian, D. L., Spiegelman, S., et al.: In vitro synthesis of DNA components of human genes for globins. Nature [New Biol.] *235*:167, 1972.

197. Ross, J., Aviv, H., et al.: *In vitro* synthesis of DNA complementary to purified rabbit globin mRNA. Proc. Natl. Acad. Sci USA *69*:264, 1972.

198. Marotta, C. A., Forget, B. G., et al.: Nucleotide sequences of human globin messenger RNA. Proc. Natl. Acad. Sci. USA, *71*:2300, 1974.

199. Shih, T. Y., and Martin, M. A.: A general method of gene isolation. Proc. Natl. Acad. Sci. USA *70*:1697, 1973.

200. Davidson, R. L., Adelstein, S. J., et al.: Herpes simplex virus as a source of thymidine kinase for thymidine kinase–deficient cells: Suppression and reactivation of the viral enzyme. Proc. Natl. Acad. Sci. USA *70*:1912, 1973.

201. Merril, C. R., Geier, M. R., et al.: Bacterial virus gene expression in human cells. Nature (Lond.) *233*:398, 1971.

202. Qasba, P. K., and Aposhian, H. V.: DNA and gene therapy: Transfer of mouse DNA to human and mouse embryonic cells by polyoma pseudovirions. Proc. Natl. Acad. Sci. USA *68*:2345, 1971.

203. Bakay, B., Croce, C. M., et al.: Restoration of hypoxanthine phosphoribosyl transferase activity in mouse 1R cells after fusion with chick embryo fibroblasts. Proc. Natl. Acad. Sci. USA *70*:1998, 1973.

204. McBride, O. W., and Ozer, H. L.: Transfer of genetic information by purified metaphase chromosomes. Proc. Natl. Acad. Sci. USA *70*:1258, 1973.

205. Rabovsky, D.: Molecular biology: Gene insertion into mammalian cells. Science *174*:933, 1971.

206. Aposhian, H. V.: The use of DNA for gene therapy—The need, experimental approach and implications. Perspectives in Biology and Medicine *14*:98, 1970.

207. Friedman, T., and Roblin, R.: Gene therapy for human genetic disease? Proposals for genetic manipulation in humans raise difficult scientific and ethical problem. Science *175*:949, 1972.

208. Fox, M. S., and Littlefield, J. W.: Reservations concerning gene therapy. Science *173*:195, 1971.

209. Freese, E.: Prospects of gene therapy. Science *175*:1024, 1972.

210. Barry, M., Flynn, D. M., et al.: Long-term chelation therapy in thalassemia major: Effect on liver iron concentration, liver histology, and clinical progress. Br. Med. J. *2*:16, 1974.

II

THE
WHITE
CELL

Chapter 16

Disorders of Leukocyte Function and Development

by Robert L. Baehner

INTRODUCTION

Leukocytes of the peripheral blood play a major role in host defense against infection. Those leukocytes that possess the unique property of phagocytosis protect the host against pyogenic bacterial and fungal infection. Phagocytic cells of the blood include the neutrophil, eosinophil, basophil, and monocyte. In addition, the fixed tissue histiocytes of the reticuloendothelial system are also phagocytic. The phagocytic process was first described by Metchnikoff in 1833, but the specific details of this complex event have come to be better understood over the past 15 years (1). Since infection may occur either within the vascular system or, as more frequently is the case, outside it, the circulating phagocyte must be capable of rapid movement from the bone marrow through the peripheral blood and into extravascular areas to eliminate invading microorganisms. The accumulation of pus in an infected area requires not only leukocytes but also all those factors that contribute to the inflammatory process.

In contrast, circulating lymphocytes are part of the lymphoid system, which includes the thymus and the peripheral and alimentary tract lymph nodes required for the defense against viral as well as bacterial infection. The latter protection is afforded by the B lymphocyte, which contributes to the plasma cell system within lymph nodes responsible for elaboration of antibody in response to bacterial, fungal, and viral anti-

gens. The T lymphocyte, morphologically identical to the B lymphocyte, interacts with the thymus during fetal and neonatal life to confer a lifelong capacity for lymphocytes to become sensitized by a variety of antigens, including microorganisms. T lymphocytes respond to antigenic stimulation in a unique manner called transformation, whereby they proliferate and elaborate substances which act in concert with the macrophage system to protect the host against viral infections.

This chapter will be limited to a consideration of disorders of the development and function of the circulating phagocytes of the peripheral blood. Emphasis will be placed on the polymorphonuclear neutrophil, the major phagocyte of the blood. Diminution in the number of these cells in the peripheral blood and bone marrow or alteration in their phagocytic function produces clinical disorders characterized by chronic and recurrent systemic bacterial or fungal infection.

DEVELOPMENT OF THE BONE MARROW PHAGOCYTES

Myelopoiesis

Present evidence suggests that the phagocytes of the peripheral blood are derived from a common stem cell or colony-forming unit in the bone marrow (2–5). This cell is thought to resemble a small lymphocyte but defies clear-cut identification in bone marrow smears. Two lines of evidence indicate that the stem cell is, in fact, the common precursor cell for myeloid, erythroid, and megakaryocytic lines. First, chronic myelogenous leukemia of the adult type is associated with a chromatid alteration of the G-group chromosome called the Ph[1] or Philadelphia chromosome. The chromosomal defect can be demonstrated in proliferating myeloid and erythroid cells, and megakaryocytes from the bone marrow of affected patients (6). Second, spleen colonies derived from marrow infused into previously lethally irradiated mice, which begin as single stem cell implants, proliferate into colonies containing granulocytic, erythroid, and megakaryocytic forms (7). Preservation of the stem cell pool demands that some of the dividing mother cells provide daughter cells with maturation characteristics identical to the mother (asynchronous cell division) (8).

The bone marrow myeloid mitotic compartment consists of myeloblasts, promyelocytes, and myelocytes — cells that have been shown to be capable of mitotic division both by direct observation in cell cultures (9) and by virtue of their uptake of ^{3}H-thymidine (10). It is generally agreed but not proven that cells in this compartment move from myeloblast to promyelocyte to myelocyte. The number of cell divisions that occur at each morphologic stage is also unknown. The exponential decrease in radioactivity noted in the analysis of the third phase of in vivo di-isopropyl fluorophosphate (DF^{32}P) suggests that there must be at least three cell divisions at the myelocyte stage (11). Furthermore, such a scheme appears to best fit the ^{3}H-thymidine autoradiographic data. A single division has been postulated for the myeloblast and promyelocyte stages. These data indicate that a minimum of five cell divisions occurs during myelopoiesis in man. Since the generation time for each cell division requires about 24 hours, it would appear that a minimum of five to six days is required for the myeloblast to proliferate to the myelocyte stage. The major locus of neutrophil production in man is at the myelocyte stage, since the myelocyte pool is at least four times the size of the preceeding promyelocyte pool.

The bone marrow granulocyte reserve consists of a pool of cells, including the metamyelocytes, band forms, and mature polymorphonuclear leukocytes. In contrast to the mitotic compartment, these cells do not divide but simply mature. This pool of maturing nonproliferating myeloid cells represents approximately 60 per cent of the total myeloid bone marrow cells (12). It has been calculated that the granulocyte reserve in the bone marrow is 7.8×10^9 cells per kg., compared to 3.35×10^9 cells per kg. for the mitotic pool and 0.7×10^9 cells per kg. for the circulating blood pool (13).

Morphology and Function

The myeloblast is the most primitive identifiable cell of the granulocytic series. Less than 5 per cent of myeloid cells are myeloblasts. This cell proliferates into the promyelocyte, the largest myeloid precursor cell. The nucleus is round, the chromatin pattern is fine, and nucleoli are prominent. The promyelocyte develops large azurophilic or reddish-purple granules (indicated as black on Fig. 16–1), which contain myeloperoxidase, several hydrolytic enzymes, bactericidal cationic protein, and sulfated mucopolysaccharides (14–16). The lipid envelope of the granules "buds off" from the plasmalemmal surface of the cell as enzyme protein is synthesized on the concave side of the rough endoplasmic reticulum within the cell. Packaging of the enzyme with the lipid membrane envelope occurs in the region of the Golgi apparatus. These granules are "microbags" of enzymes with physicochemical properties similar to lysosomes of liver and other tissue cells (17, 18). The promyelocyte, in turn, proliferates and gives rise to the myelocyte. The nucleus is smaller but round, the chromatin is slightly clumped, and the nucleoli are no longer present. The myelocyte acquires specific staining granules by which neutrophils, eosinophils, and basophils are so identified (indicated as white on Fig. 16–1). The neutrophilic myelocyte develops specific granules which contain alkaline phosphatase (14, 16). This enzyme is synthesized on the convex surface of the Golgi apparatus (18, 19). Lysozyme and lactoferrin have also been found associated with specific granules of neutrophils (20). Eosinophil granules have a zinc-containing basic protein rich in arginine, peroxidase, and hydrolytic

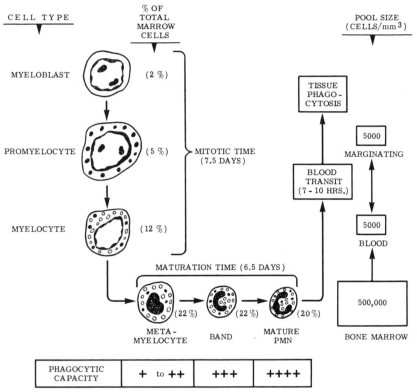

Figure 16–1. Schematic representation of the cellular development and function of the polymorphonuclear leukocyte (PMN). Black granules indicate azurophilic granules, and white granules indicate specific granules. See text for further details.

enzymes, but lack lysozyme and probably alkaline phosphatase (21). The characteristic affinity of eosinophil granules for acid dyes is due to their content of strongly basic protein. Electron microscopic studies reveal both the homogenous granules, as seen in neutrophils, and the characteristic crystalloid granules. Since homogenous granules predominate in young eosinophilic myelocytes, it has been proposed that they transform to crystalloid granules as the cell matures (21, 22). Basophil granules contain abundant sulfated acid mucosubstance but lack acid and alkaline phosphatase (23).

The metamyelocyte, smaller than the myelocyte, has an indented nucleus, clumped chromatin, and many specifically staining cytoplasmic granules. It does not divide but matures to the band form and then to the polymorphonuclear leukocyte (PMN) during a six- to seven-day period (24). Phagocytic capacity is attained at the myelocyte to metamyelocyte stage, but maximal phagocytic efficiency is not attained until the band and PMN stage of

cellular maturation (25). Compared to other blood phagocytes, PMN's appear to phagocytize the most particles and at the fastest rate (26), although precise quantitative methods for measurement of such rates under various conditions have not yet been applied. Coincident with phagocytic capacity, the maturing myeloid cells become more deformable. For example, rigid myeloblasts resist aspiration into 3.5-μ diameter micropipets, whereas progressively less suction is required to move each more mature myeloid form into the pipet. These changes may contribute to the rate of marrow and circulatory egress of granulocytic cells (27). A schematic outline of the cellular development of the myeloid series is illustrated in Figure 16–1.

Myelokinetics

It is estimated that, for every 100 myeloid cells in the bone marrow, one neutrophil circulates in the peripheral blood (circulating granulocyte pool, CGP) in dynamic equilibrium with another neutrophil lodged along the endothelial lining of the vascular tree (marginating granulocyte pool, MGP) (28–30). Radioisotope studies with neutrophils labeled with $DF^{32}P$ have been useful to (a) document the presence of the MGP; (b) establish that the half-life of circulating neutrophils is six to seven hours (31), and that the rate of exit from the circulation is independent of cell age but dependent upon the specific need for such cells in the extravascular tissues; and (c) determine the total blood granulocyte pool (TBGP) and calculate the granulocyte turnover rate (GTR) based upon the equation for first order decay and the two measured parameters, i.e., TBGP and $t_{1/2}$: $GTR = \dfrac{0.693 \times TBGP}{t_{1/2}}$ (32). Neutrophil levels in the blood remain relatively constant but can be perturbed by stress and infection, which increase levels temporarily, or by irradiation and cytotoxic drugs, which depress levels of neutrophils in the blood. From our understanding of neutrophil kinetics, certain loci in the system appear to be likely control points to regulate blood neutrophil levels, i.e., egress of cells from the blood to the tissues, the distribution of blood neutrophils in MGP and CGP, release of neutrophils from the marrow reserve to the blood, the rate of cell production in the mitotic pool, and the inflow of stem cells into the mitotic pool. Very little is known about leukocyte control at any of these possible sites. Epinephrine or exercise-induced granulocytosis studied with the above techniques revealed no change in the TBGP but simply a transient shift of cells from the MGP to the CGP.

There is good evidence to support a neutrophil releasing factor which causes evacuation of the bone marrow granulocyte reserve pool (BMGR). This factor has been found in the plasma of dogs during the leukopenic and recovery phase after vinblastine, nitrogen mustard, or endotoxin injection (33). The leukocytosis in response to acute infection is likely due to mobilization of the bone marrow granulocyte reserve pool to increase the TBGP. In occasional instances, if the infection is massive and demand for neutrophils apparently exceeds the supply (TBGP + BMGR), then neutropenia ensues (34).

In chronic, steady-state neutrophilia (chronic infection, inflammation, or adrenal corticosteroid administration), kinetic studies indicate an increased TBGP and normal GTR but prolonged $t_{1/2}$ of circulating granulocytes. In the latter case, there is also decreased migration of neutrophils into sites of inflammation.

Recent studies indicate that myelopoiesis may be controlled by humoral factors present within granulocytes and monocytes themselves. Human bone marrow blast cells differentiate into mature myeloid and monocyte-macrophage colonies during culture in vitro in soft agar (35). The rate of proliferation and the number of colonies that develop are increased by feeder layers of human peripheral blood cells (36, 37), medium from cultures of peripheral leukocytes (38), and human urine (39). This evidence would indicate that leukocytes, especially monocytes, release a factor which stimulates the further production of committed stem cells to myelopoiesis. The precise mechanisms for the control of this positive feedback mechanism have not yet been clearly defined.

Neutropenia may be defined as a decrease in absolute granulocyte count of the peripheral blood below 1500 per mm.[3] (40, 41). Occasionally, neutropenia may exist despite a total white blood count within the normal range of 5000 to 10,000 per mm[3]. For this reason, Wright's stained blood smears, in addition to total white blood counts, are useful to calculate the absolute granulocyte count during the clinical investigation of infection. The level of granulocytes within the peripheral blood may fluctuate. Some normal individuals have regular fluctuations of total neutrophils every 14 to 23 days that oscillate between 2000 and 4000 per mm.[3] (42). The range for total white blood cell counts as well as the usual distribution of lymphocytes and neutrophilic granulocytes varies during the first eight years of life. Leukocytosis to 40,000 per mm.[3] is present at birth, which decreases to 20,000 per mm.[3] during the first week of life and then gradually returns to the normal range of 5000 to 10,000 per mm.[3] by four years of age. PMN's predominate at birth, but by one week of age, there are equal numbers of mononuclear and polymorphonuclear leukocytes. Lymphocytes predominate until about four years of age, but there is a predominance of polymorphonuclear leuko-cytes in the blood by eight years of age (43).

Development of the Monocyte

The circulating monocyte is derived from a promonocyte present in sparse numbers in the bone marrow (44, 45). In contrast to the granulocyte, there is no appreciable storage reservoir of monocytes in the marrow; how-ever, the number of monocytes increases in the blood during periods of chronic inflam-mation or infection. Similar to PMN's, they leave the circulation at random, but have a maximum intravascular sojourn of about five days (46). The studies by Rebuck have shown that the PMN is the predominant cell contributing to the early phases of inflam-mation; however, within 12 hours following the inflammatory stimulus, the mononuclear cell becomes the predominant cell type within the inflammatory reaction and per-sists within the site of the inflammation for the next 12 hours (47). This mononuclear cell has been clearly shown to be derived from the circulating blood monocyte (48). Early in vivo studies using vital dyes to label blood monocytes and later studies with radiolabeled monocytes have documented that these cells move into the extravascular space, where progressive transformation in-to tissue macrophages takes place. Whether the blood monocyte can give rise to fixed tissue macrophages of the reticuloendothe-lial system, i.e., alveolar macrophage, Kupffer liver cell, spleen and bone marrow histiocyte, remains to be proved. Mono-cytes from animals and from humans cul-tured in vitro can be provoked by various stimuli, including endotoxin, to transform into macrophages (49, 50). During this proc-ess there is a dramatic increase in cell size and an increase in lysosomes and mito-chondria characteristic of macrophages.

Function of Monocytes and Macrophages

The monocyte is one of the phagocytes of the peripheral blood that phagocytizes bac-teria and particulate debris but probably less efficiently than the PMN (51). In addi-tion, human monocytes and macrophages have a surface receptor that is specific for the Fc portion of IgG globulin that can re-sult in the binding of particles coated with these antibodies (53). This process is ex-emplified by incomplete antibodies of the Rh type that lack complement fixing or opsonin activity, but when present on hu-man red cells can induce binding to mono-cytes and macrophages, resulting in red cell sequestration and damage.

The monocyte may also have a role in the processing of antigens in the immune re-sponse, since such cells are necessary for blastic transformation of lymphocytes in mixed leukocyte cultures. Macrophages may defend against viral infection, since peritoneal and pulmonary aveolar macro-phages produce interferon in response to viral infection. Furthermore, they likely play a role in fever production, since en-dogenous pyrogen has been demonstrated within monocytes (52).

DISORDERS DUE TO ALTERED GRANULOCYTE PRODUCTION AND DESTRUCTION

CYCLIC NEUTROPENIA

Patients with cyclic neutropenia have a characteristic clinical course (54). They have periods of well-being for approxi-mately three weeks, punctuated by one-week intervals of fever, malaise, headache, mouth ulcers, and furunculosis. As a rule, severe infections are unusual. Clinical symptoms may be evident during the period of neutropenia. During these intervals the bone marrow demonstrates a lack of granu-locytes beyond the myelocyte stage. Exper-imental models of cyclic neutropenia have been developed by using myelosuppressive drugs, such as cyclophosphamide, which dampen the feedback pool of bone marrow myeloid cells and thus accentuate the nor-mal fluctuation of granulocyte proliferation within the marrow (55). Certain animals, such as the grey collie dog, demonstrate cyclic neutropenia (56) associated with cyclic myelopoiesis and erythropoiesis in the bone marrow (57).

CHRONIC NEUTROPENIAS

Chronic Infantile Agranulocytosis

This is a hereditary disease first described by Kostmann in Sweden in a large family with a history of consanguinity (58). The pattern of inheritance was clearly autosomal recessive. However, since that time, only two of the 24 families in which this disease occurred have had more than one affected child. These patients have a severe disease characterized by chronic and recurrent pyogenic infection of the skin and respiratory tract with onset during the first year of life (59, 60). Eighteen of 28 cases reported in the literature have died of infection. The peripheral blood findings usually reveal marked absolute neutropenia with less than 300 neutrophils per mm³. An associated monocytosis and eosinophilia cause the total white blood count to approach the normal range. Despite the fact that their monocytes and eosinophils phagocytize and kill bacteria normally compared to monocytes from patients with chronic infection, these patients have serious recurrent infections, and death is usual during childhood (60). One patient who lived to young adulthood developed monoblastic leukemia (61). The bone marrow is depleted of the normal reserve of mature granulocytes; a predominance of promyelocytes with large azurophilic granules is evident. In addition, bone marrow monocytes, eosinophilic granulocytes, histiocytes, and reactive plasma cells are increased. A recent study by Barak et al. (62) suggests that the precursors of granulocytes in the bone marrow of these patients are potentially capable of normal proliferation and maturation, since they proliferate and mature normally in vitro in bone marrow soft agar culture. The serum of these patients is not inhibitory to normal bone marrow cultures under the same techniques. Other studies have shown that the proliferative activity of myeloid cells of bone marrow, as measured by ³H-thymidine, is decreased (63).

Chronic Benign Granulocytopenia of Childhood

This disorder may be a mild equivalent of chronic infantile agranulocytosis. The children may have the onset of symptoms of neutropenia by the end of the first year of life. Their clinical course, in contrast to children with congenital infantile agranulocytosis, is characterized by milder infections, mouth ulcers, and stomatitis. The disease tends to be self-limited, usually lasting a few months to a few years (64). The onset may be later than the first few years of life, and frequently no definite incriminating medication or other provocative agent can be implicated. The bone marrow usually contains an adequate supply of maturing granulocytes, since the "arrest" of myeloid development tends to be at the band form of granulocyte development (65, 66).

Pancreatic Insufficiency and Bone Marrow Dysfunction

This is a syndrome of exocrine pancreatic insufficiency, neutropenia, dwarfism, and occasionally metaphyseal dysostosis (67). Thirty-six such cases have been reported. Nine of the 36 cases reported have died in infancy or childhood of infection (68). Although this syndrome appears to be the most common form of exocrine pancreatic insufficiency in infants and children other than cystic fibrosis, Schwachman et al. (69) estimate that the syndrome is found in less than 1 per cent of all their patients with cystic fibrosis. In contrast to patients with cystic fibrosis, the sweat chloride test is normal in these patients. At present, the treatment is completely unsatisfactory. Although in some instances the use of pancreatic preparations may improve the gastrointestinal symptoms, it does not affect the neutropenia. Orthopedic management should be sought in cases of metaphyseal hip dysostosis.

Ineffective Myelopoiesis

A single patient has been reported by Krill et al. (70) and by Zuelzer (71). This patient could develop appropriate leukocytosis during acute infection, but continued to express chronic neutropenia at other times. Myeloid precursors were abundant, and many mature neutrophils were present on bone marrow aspiration. However, the bone marrow PMN's had indistinct granules, increased vacuolization in the cytoplasm, and a dense pyknotic nuclear chromatin, suggesting that these were cells on their way to intermedullary death. The term "myelokathexis" was coined to describe this condition. Splenectomy, corticosteroids, and infusion of fresh plasma did not influence the course of the illness.

Drug-Induced Neutropenias

Certain drugs will occasionally but unpredictably cause profound suppression of myeloid cell formation in the bone marrow (72). The Council on Drugs of the American Medical Association has maintained an up-to-date list of drugs suspected of causing neutropenia. However, certain drugs are more commonly responsible for neutropenia (73). These include antibiotics [novobiocin (74), ristocetin (75), fumagillin (75), methicillin (76)]; sulfonamides [acetazolamide (77), sulfaguanidine (78), sulfamethoxypryridazine (79)]; anticoagulants [phenindione (80)]; antidiabetics [tolbutamide (81), chlorpropamide (82)]; antihistamines [thenaldine (83)]; antihypertensives [chlorothiazide (84), hydrochlorothiazide (85), alpha methyl dopa (86)]; antithyroids [propylthiouracil (87), methimazole (88)]; diuretics [ethacrynic acid (89)]; anti-inflammatory drugs [demecolcine (90), hydroxychloroquine]; penicillamine (91); amodiaquin (92); carbimazole (93); and procainamide (94). Agranulocytosis due to the phenothiazine derivatives is frequently reported, and almost all derivatives except promethazine and methdilazine have been implicated (95). Such drugs act by suppressing DNA synthesis in the bone marrow. In contrast, certain drugs such as amidopyrine may provoke an immunologic reaction in the patient (96). In those cases, the drug acts as a haptene complexed with antigen on the white cell membrane to stimulate the formation of leukocyte antibody by the host. In turn, this causes increased destruction of circulating granulocytes. Agranulocytosis with leukoagglutination demonstrable in vitro has been noted in drugs related to amidopyrine, such as dipyrone (97) and phenylbutazone (98). Sulfapyridine (99), mercurial diuretics (100), and chlorpropamide (101) have all provoked agranulocytosis associated with drug-dependent leukoagglutinins. In the latter cases, the bone marrow will show increased myeloid activity, and no alteration in the development and maturation of myeloid cells will be evident. Of course, drugs regularly used in the treatment of hemopoietic and oncologic disorders (cyclophosphamide, cytosine arabinoside, nitrogen mustard, 6-mercaptopurine, methotrexate), as well as radiation therapy, will produce bone marrow suppression if given in intolerable doses.

Neutropenia With Other Immune System Disorders

Patients with X-linked agammaglobulinemia as well as children with other forms of dysgammaglobulinemia may experience neutropenia (106, 107). Such neutropenia can be either chronic or cyclic in nature; occasionally, it is the initial presenting sign of an underlying antibody deficiency state. Disorders of delayed-type immunity, such as the patient reported by Lux et al. (108), may also be associated with chronic neutropenia. Gitlin and co-workers (109) and de Vaal and Seynhaeve (110) have each reported fatal disease in neonates who had overwhelming bacterial infection, complete lack of granulocytes in the bone marrow, and dysplasia of the thymus.

Aplastic Anemia and Acute Leukemia

The erythropoietic, thrombopoietic, and granulopoietic mechanisms are altered in the bone marrow of patients with aplastic anemia. The major threats to these patients are overwhelming infection and intractable bleeding into vital structures. Children with acute leukemia are also susceptible to bleeding and infection, since the bone marrow becomes infiltrated with lymphoblasts or myeloblasts, or chemotherapy destroys the normal marrow. Infection accounts for 80 per cent of the deaths of children with leukemia.

Nutritional Disorders

Neutropenia is commonly observed as a consequence of vitamin B_{12} or folic acid deficiency. In fact, patients with megaloblastic hemopoiesis may present with severe sepsis due to neutropenia, or bleeding due to thrombocytopenia rather than anemia. Peripheral blood granulocytes usually reveal the deficiency state because of their characteristic polylobulation and deformation of their nuclear chromatin.

Immunoneutropenia

Antibodies against leukocytes as the primary cause for neutropenia are more difficult to define than are antibodies against red blood cells. Some antigens of the leukocyte are common to platelets and solid tissues, whereas other antigens are specific for neutrophils. There are no naturally appearing antibodies to white blood cells. It is estimated that active immunization against these leukocyte-specific antigens requires greater than seven intravenous transfusions of leukocytes. Twenty-five per cent of females with four or more blood transfusions have antibodies in their serum detectable against leukocytes (102). Passively transfused antibodies that develop secondary to blood transfusion disappear rapidly, but postpartum antibodies persist much longer. Such antibodies may be responsible for fever, chills, and transfusion reactions if passively transferred to the recipient and may occasionally cause severe shock and collapse. In this regard, male blood donors are preferred to multiparous female blood donors.

Neonatal isoimmune neutropenia has been described in 12 cases of neonatal neutropenia lasting up to 60 to 70 days because of the passive transfer of maternal leukocyte antibodies (103). However, in most cases, maternal cytotoxic and leukoagglutinating antibodies do not cause neonatal leukopenia (104). Certain drugs stimulate leukocyte antibody production in mothers. Chlorothiazide has produced transient agranulocytosis in the neonate associated with passive transfer of maternal antibody.

Leukoagglutinin-associated neutropenia has been described in association with primary diseases such as lupus erythematosus, rheumatoid arthritis, lymphoma, and infectious mononucleosis (105). The spleen may play an active role in the removal of PMN's in such individuals. Therapy of these patients is directed toward the basic disease, since the neutropenia is usually an asymptomatic incidental finding. However, severe sepsis may occur. Treatment with corticosteroids or splenectomy or both may be required if severe neutropenia ensues.

Congestive Splenomegaly and Neutropenia

Patients with portal hypertension or primary disease of the spleen may develop congestive splenomegaly with the accumulation of "trapped" granulocytes and platelets within the spleen (111). These patients usually develop mild to moderate thrombocytopenia and granulocytopenia. This condition was first described by Wiseman and Doan in 1942, when they reported five cases that achieved a permanent cure by splenectomy (112). The bone marrow of their patients was cellular, and normal myeloid, megakaryocyte, and erythroid proliferation and maturation were evident. This indicated that rapid peripheral blood sequestration was the cause of the pancytopenia. When this condition is encountered, a search should be made for primary active liver disease, cirrhosis, obstruction of the hepatic or portal circulation, and primary splenic disease. Frequently, the neutropenia and thrombocytopenia are improved by bed rest alone. A vascular shunt procedure to divert the portal circulation to the caval circulation or splenectomy should be considered, but only if the neutropenia is associated with severe sepsis. Thrombocytopenia is usually a more significant clinical sequela of congestive splenomegaly than is neutropenia.

LABORATORY INVESTIGATION OF PATIENTS WITH NEUTROPENIA

As mentioned above, the diagnosis of neutropenia is established when the absolute granulocyte count in the peripheral blood is below 1500 per mm^3. The differential diagnosis then lies between decreased production and increased destruction. This differentiation is frequently difficult. In patients suspected of cyclic variations in neutrophil counts, absolute granulocyte counts performed three times a week for two months are necessary. If familial neutropenia is suspected, all of the family members, including grandparents, should have absolute granulocyte counts calculated. A bone marrow aspiration is necessary to establish maturation characteristics of the myeloid series. The term "myeloid arrest," used to describe a maturation hiatus, may be a mismomer, since the granulocytes in these instances are more likely experiencing premature cell death at a fixed point in their maturation, or, in the case of rapid removal in the periphery, a paucity of mature forms may remain in the marrow. Estimation of myeloid cell enzymes, e.g., muramidase excretion in the urine or plasma, may be helpful in establishing this fact (113). The absolute turnover rate of PMN's in peripheral blood may be measured with radioactive labels attached to PMN's, but such procedures are not routine, must be interpreted by experts, and involve radiation exposure (31). The marrow aspirate also permits important observations of the morphology of the myeloid precursors. An estimation of the total proliferative capacity of the myeloid population can be obtained from the mitotic index, i.e., observing the number of mitotic figures in granulocyte precursors relative to the total myeloid cells capable of dividing (114). Radioautography studies measuring ^{3}H-thymidine incorporation into DNA may also be done to assess this (115). An estimation of the available polymorphonuclear neutrophils and band forms (the bone marrow reserve pool) can be obtained from this aspirate.

In order to establish more firmly an accurate estimation of the bone marrow granulocyte reserve pool, a typhoid stimulation test should be done (116). Typhoid vaccine, 0.5 ml., is injected subcutaneously, and absolute granulocyte counts are calculated at 3, 6, 12, and 24 hours. The normal response includes an initial depression in absolute granulocytes over the first three hours, followed by a three- to fourfold stimulation of absolute granulocytes over the next 6 to 12 hours. An epinephrine stimulation test may be done to assess the marginating granulocyte pool, excluding the possibility of splenic pooling of granulocytes (33). In this test, 0.1 ml. of 1:1000 aqueous adrenalin is injected subcutaneously, and the absolute granulocyte counts are monitored at 5, 10, 15, and 30 minutes. Normally the absolute granulocyte count doubles. An estimation of

the inflammatory cycle can be performed by using the cover slip skin window technique, as described by Rebuck (47). Neutrophils appear on the cover slip removed at 3 hours; a mixed population of PMN's and monocytes appears at 6 hours; and by 12 hours the inflammatory cells are predominantly monocytes. A quantitative assessment of the inflammatory cycle can also be done by using specialized plastic chambers for the collection of inflammatory cells (117, 118). However, the cellular response using the skin chamber rather than cover slips collects more granulocytes than mononuclear cells throughout the 24-hour cycle.

Immunoneutropenia should be ruled out, if possible, by appropriate tests which would establish the presence of serum antibody directed against the patient's own granulocytes (119). Leukoagglutinins and cytotoxic antibodies may be present in the serum of these patients. Antinuclear antibody determination using fluorescent antibody techniques and lupus erythematosus cell preparations should also be performed. A thorough inquiry should be made regarding the possibility of drug ingestion as the basis for neutropenia.

MANAGEMENT OF THE NEUTROPENIC PATIENT

Ideally the patient should be kept away from others who have infection and from large crowds within closed environments. This is a goal which is difficult to achieve. If the patient develops an infection, cultures of the infected area should be performed. Antibiotics can then be administered, based upon the culture and antibiotic sensitivity of the microorganism. The response to therapy in cases of neutropenia will be slower and more prolonged because of the lack of adequate granulocytes in the circulation. In the hospital the patient should be treated with reverse isolation techniques in an attempt to combat superinfection with antibiotic-resistant microorganisms transferred from medical personnel. Elaborate and aggressive techniques to control the air environment around the patient and to eradicate microorganisms from the patient's skin and gastrointestinal tract with antibiotics have not yet proved beneficial in these situations, but careful daily cleaning of the isolation room with effective antiseptics and the use of ultraviolet doorway shields are advised. Particular attention to adequate hair and shoe covering, together with masks, gloves, and gowns, should be used to protect severely neutropenic patients from medical personnel and outside visitors. Mouth ulcerations and gingivitis, a frequent problem in patients with cyclic neutropenia, should be treated with appropriate systemic antibiotics if secondary bacterial infection is found. The use of 3 per cent hydrogen peroxide–1 per cent alum mouth wash usually produces symptomatic relief in such cases.

Although platelet concentrates are now available in most blood banks, concentrates of leukocytes with phagocytic capacity are not yet readily available to most patients with neutropenia during periods of overwhelming infection. A commercial centrifugation apparatus or a filtration system is now in use in some medical centers, whereby donors can be leukapheresed in an attempt to harvest adequate numbers of granulocytes (120). The short normal granulocyte survival of six to eight hours necessitates the administration of frequent leukocyte transfusions to patients. In addition, most patients develop leukoagglutinins after repeated transfusions of heterologous leukocytes. Leukocyte-rich plasma obtained from patients with chronic myelogenous leukemia or myeloid metaplasia has been infused into neutropenic patients with sepsis with good results, albeit transient in most cases (121).

The use of steroid compounds is not usually beneficial to patients with neutropenia. Splenectomy has been helpful only in cases of congestive splenomegaly or Felty's syndrome; otherwise, splenectomy has been of little value in the management of patients with neutropenia.

DISORDERS OF GRANULOCYTE MORPHOLOGY

Granule Abnormalities

Application of the lysosome concept (122) to the cellular biology of the polymorphonuclear leukocyte and mononuclear cells has clarified some aspects of their physiologic and pathophysiologic processes. Granules of these cells are lysosomes, since they are membrane-bound organelles that demonstrate stimulation of enzyme activity by destruction of the membrane, i.e., latent activity. Lysosomes of white blood cells are involved in inflammatory reactions leading to tissue necrosis, release of endogenous pyrogens, participation in endotoxic shock, and contribution to the digestion and killing of bacteria. In addition, they may act as storage reservoirs for abnormal metabolites in a variety of inborn errors of metabolism.

Toxic Neutrophils

Morphologic alteration of the neutrophil occurs with severe bacterial infection. "Toxic" neutrophils are characterized by the presence of Döhle bodies, heavy granulation, and cytoplasmic vacuoles (128). Döhle bodies appear as light blue amorphous inclusions by light microscopy; electron microscopy reveals lamellar aggregates of rough endoplasmic reticulum. They have been noted also in the polymorphonuclear leukocytes of pregnant females (123), in familial thrombocytopenia with giant platelets (124), and in patients given cyclophosphamide chemotherapy (125). Toxic granules are identified as heavy azurophilic granules by Romanowsky stains; electron microscopy reveals large, electron-dense, peroxidase-positive granules. PMN's which contain toxic granulations have increased alkaline phosphatase activity, normal beta glucuronidase activity, and normal acid phosphatase activity. Toxic granules have been seen in a variety of disorders characterized by acute and chronic inflammation (126). They can also be induced by prolonged exposure to Wright's stain or following fixation with 2.5 per cent glutaraldehyde which affects lysosomal permeability (127).

Leukocytes in Metabolic Disorders

Vacuolated leukocytes and leukocytes with abnormal granules have been described in a variety of metabolic diseases. Several investigators have described the association of gargoylism with abnormal azurophilic granules in PMN's, lymphocytes, and monocytes. This was first pointed out by Alder in 1939. A few years later, Reilly described four of eight gargoyles with abnormal polymorphonuclear granules. As a consequence of Reilly's association of the Alder anomaly with gargoylism, the term "Reilly bodies" has sometimes been used to describe the abnormal granules of the PMN in this disease. Mittwoch (129) found that all six gargoyles she studied had abnormal inclusions in their lymphocytes. These appeared either as clusters of granules surrounded by vacuoles, as large granular inclusions, or as vacuoles alone. Such granules stained metachromatically with toluidine blue, which differentiates them sharply from the azurophilic granules of normal lymphocytes that do not stain with toluidine blue. In a recent summary of the mucopolysaccharide syndromes (MPS) (130), McKusick and his co-workers pointed out that the bone marrow and peripheral blood PMN's frequently do not contain Reilly bodies. But in 15 cases of either Type I MPS (Hunter's syndrome), Type II MPS (Hurler's syndrome), or Type III MPS (Sanfilippo's syndrome), they noted obvious metachromatic granules in 10 to 60 per cent of lymphocytes. Four cases of Type IV MPS (Morquio's disease) had scattered aggregates of metachromatic granules distinct from Reilly granules in the cytoplasm of polymorphonuclear leukocytes. In contrast, in four cases of Type V MPS (Scheie's syndrome), no lymphocyte or polymorphonuclear leukocyte granules were noted. Vacuolated lymphocytes have also been noted in Wolman's disease, leukemia, bacteremia, lymphogranulomatosis, and infectious mononucleosis. They are a frequent hallmark of Niemann-Pick disease (131), wherein the vacuoles contain lipid cytosomes but require electron microscopy to differentiate them from other vacuoles (132).

Anomalies of granulocyte nuclei are not known to cause functional impairment of these cells. The Pelger-Huet anomaly is inherited as an autosomal dominant disorder in which granulocytic nuclei have no more than two lobes (133). Congenital hypersegmentation of PMN (134) is another benign morphologic abnormality in which 1 to 2 per cent of neutrophils have nuclei with six or more lobes and the cells are twice normal size. This disorder must be differentiated from the hypersegmentation associated with megaloblastic anemias (135).

NORMAL PHYSIOLOGY OF PHAGOCYTE FUNCTION

Phagocytosis in vivo is controlled by both serum and cellular factors and takes place primarily at tissue sites beyond the confines of the vascular tree. The events of phagocytosis by PMN's and monocytes are outlined in six steps in Figure 16–2.

Chemotaxis

The migration of phagocytes from the circulation to tissue sites leads to the accumulation of exudate responsible for the clinical signs of inflammation and infection (136). Inflammatory reactions at tissue sites are provoked initially by local release of histamine and kinins (137) which dilate blood vessels and alter their permeability. PMN's appear to be attracted to sites of inflammation by "chemotactic" factors in the exudates. Certain humoral substances have also been shown to mediate the chemotactic response by PMN's and monocytes (138, 139,

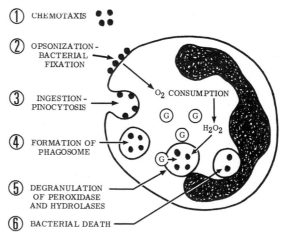

Figure 16–2. Schematic representation of the morphologic and metabolic events of phagocytosis that lead to bacterial killing within the polymorphonuclear leukocyte (PMN). Bacteria are represented as black dots. Granule peroxidase and hydrolases are indicated as G.

140). Filtrates derived from cultures of many species of bacteria are also chemotactic for PMN's and monocytes (141), as is a complex of the fifth, sixth, and seventh components of complement (140), a plasmin-split fragment of the third component of complement (C3), called C3a, which can also be cleaved from C3 during its activation by $\overline{C42}$, and a fragment of the fifth component of complement (C5), called C5a, which is released during activation of C5 (142). On the other hand, PMN's that previously had ingested microorganisms in the blood stream fail to emerge at an inflammatory locus (143). Lymphocytes sensitized by antigen seem to influence migration of monocytes and thus play a role in delayed hypersensitivity. Lymphocytes elaborate macrophage inhibitory factors (MIF) during blastogenic transformation in vitro (144) and seem to direct macrophages to tissue sites impregnated with antigen (145).

Opsonization

The function of opsonins is to react with bacteria and make them more susceptible to ingestion by phagocytes (146). Opsonization of bacteria may occur by three different mechanisms. First, specific antibody alone may act as an opsonin. Presumably, the IgG or IgM antibody combines with the surface antigen of the bacteria through the antibody combining sites located in the F(ab) portion of the molecule. The Fc portion of the molecule is then free to attach to specific receptor sites on the surface of the phagocyte (146a). Specific antibody may also act as an opsonin in concert with complement, by activating C3 via the classic pathway of C1, C4, and C2. Bimolecular $\overline{C42}$ leads to the attachment of hundreds of molecules of C3. Receptor sites for activated C3, called C3b, have been demonstrated on the surface of phagocytes (146b). The C3b on the bacterial surface acts as a ligand between the bacteria and phagocyte. Finally, there is a nonspecific mechanism of opsonization present in nonimmune animals called the heat-labile opsonin system. In the heat-labile opsonin system, immunoglobulin activates C3 via an alternate pathway distinct from C1, C4, and C2. At present the system is thought to consist of factors A and B, properdin, magnesium, and other less well-defined proteins (146c). These different mechanisms may operate concurrently in vivo, but one mechanism may be favored over another, depending on the type of organism, the stage of the infection, and the presence or absence of specific antibody (147, 148, 149).

Ingestion

That portion of the phagocytic cell membrane attached to bacteria invaginates, and bacteria are swept into the phagocyte (150). Ingestion of bacteria by phagocytes requires energy in the form of ATP (151). The demand for energy in the PMN and monocyte is met through anaerobic glycolysis and not by oxidative phosphorylation (152), whereas alveolar macrophages demonstrate brisk oxidative phosphorylation (153). PMN's with impaired anaerobic glycolysis, such as in phosphoglycerate kinase deficiency, shift to oxidative phosphorylation in order to maintain adequate ATP levels for normal phagocytosis (154). Thus efficient ingestion by blood phagocytes occurs in areas of the body with low oxygen saturation as well as in body tissues with normal oxygen saturation.

Formation of Phagosome

The cell wall with an attached organism invaginates and pinches off, and the stoma of the invagination seals, creating the phagosome. A series of complex alterations of lipid metabolism accompanies this process. Membrane phosphatides exhibit accelerated turnover of their phosphorus moieties (155). In the presence of lipophosphatides, fatty acid turnover is increased in phosphatides and unchanged in triglyceride. This shift of fatty acid may be accelerated by the action of a granule lipase, which catalyzes transfer of triglyceride fatty acid to the beta position of phosphatide (156, 157). Recently, methods to isolate phagosomes have been developed (158, 159). Using such techniques, preliminary studies indicate that the ratio of unsaturated fatty acids to saturated fatty acids is lowered in the phagosome membrane because of peroxidation of unsaturated fatty acids during phagocytosis (160).

Degranulation

The phagocytic vacuole containing entrapped bacteria becomes the focal point for the degranulation of lysosomal and peroxidative enzymes (Fig. 16–2, Step 5), which culminates in the death of bacteria (161, 162). The physical transfer of the contents of the lysosomal granules into the phagosome may occur in three ways: (1) fusion of the granule membrane and phagosome membrane, (2) eruption of the intact granule through the phagosome membrane into the vacuole itself, or (3) (less likely) granule rupture prior to fusion with the phagosome, with diffusion across the phagosome membrane into the vacuole (163).

Bacterial Killing

The precise biochemical events that produce bacterial death (Fig. 16–2, Step 6) are still not clearly understood. However, several potential bactericidal systems are present in the phagocyte. One important system involves the generation of hydrogen peroxide. As noted in Figure 16–2, Step 2, particle contact stimulates phagocyte oxidative metabolism, leading to the production of bactericidal hydrogen peroxide within the phagocyte (163). This event is accompanied by increased oxygen consumption and increased pentose shunt activity (164). Two oxidative enzymes, NADH oxidase and NADPH oxidase, have been suggested as the prime oxidative enzymes catalyzing this unique increase in hydrogen peroxide in PMN's (166, 167). Cagan and Karnovsky (166) demonstrated NADH oxidase activity in leukocytes from guinea pigs. They showed that the enzyme catalyzed the reaction between NADH and oxygen to yield H_2O_2. It had a pH optimum of 5.0, a Km for NADH of 1×10^{-3} M, contained FAD, and was insensitive to 1 mM KCN. Comparative studies of human PMN's have also identified NADH oxidase in the soluble subcellular fraction of alkaline KC1 homogenates with sufficient activity to qualify as the prime oxidative enzyme (168). Zatti and Rossi have found a granule-associated NADPH oxidase in guinea pig leukocytes which was cyanide-insensitive and produced hydrogen peroxide (167). A third hydrogen peroxide generating system has been identified which uses

D-amino acids or L-amino acids (provided by ingested bacteria cell walls or by the leukocyte L-amino acids) as substrates (169, 170). In addition to peroxide, it has been suggested that amino acid oxidation leads to the production of a bactericidal aldehyde one carbon less in length than the substrate amino acid (171).

As noted in Figure 16–3, most of the hydrogen peroxide generated within the phagocyte is probably converted to water by catalase present in the soluble portion of the cytoplasm of PMN's and monocytes. However, some hydrogen peroxide is available for the stimulation of the pentose shunt. This stimulation is mediated via the glutathione system. Whether glutathione peroxidase is needed as a catalyst is unclear, since reduced glutathione (GSH) is rapidly oxidized nonenzymatically by H_2O_2 in the presence of trace quantities of metals. The oxidation of GSH to GSSG immediately provides substrate for glutathione reductase (GR), and the required cofactor for GR (NADPH) is provided by the pentose shunt and glucose-6-phosphate dehydrogenase. A 5- to 15-fold increase in pentose shunt activities occurs in phagocytizing PMN's as a result of activation of these pathways (172). About 15 per cent of the hydrogen peroxide diffuses out of the cell (173, 174) or diffuses into the phagocytic vacuole to act there in concert with granule myeloperoxidase (indicated as G on Fig. 16–3) and halide ions, such as chloride or iodide ion (indicated as I

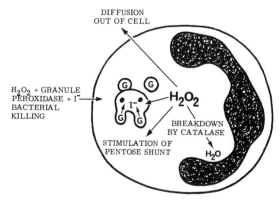

Figure 16–3. Schematic representation of the metabolic activities of hydrogen peroxide (H_2O_2) within a polymorphonuclear leukocyte. The H_2O_2 contributes to a potent bactericidal system in combination with granule peroxidase (G) and iodide ion (I^-). See text for further details. (From Johnston, R. B., Jr., and Baehner, R. L.: Pediatrics 48:732, 1971.)

on Fig. 16–3), to iodinate and kill bacteria (175, 176). The exact mechanism by which oxidation kills bacteria is not established. Lack of either hydrogen peroxide or myeloperoxidase within the phagocytic vacuole leads to diseases characterized by chronic and recurrent infection.

Recently attention has focused on the role of other oxygen derivatives in bacterial killing; these include superoxide anion (O_2^-), hydroxyl radical (OH), and singlet oxygen. Superoxide anion (O_2^-) is a highly reactive radical which is formed by the univalent reduction of oxygen (176a). It can act as a reductant (e.g., in the reduction of ferricytochrome C) or as an oxidant (e.g., in the oxidation of epinephrine), and when the two radicals interact, one is oxidized and the other is reduced as follows: $O_2^- + O_2^- + 2\,H^+ \rightarrow O_2 + H_2O_2$. This dismutation occurs spontaneously with a dissociation rate of 10^2 moles^{-1} sec.$^{-1}$, but is also catalyzed by superoxide dismutase (SOD) which inhibits O_2^--dependent reduction of ferricytochrome C. In a cell-free system that generates O_2^- as well as hydrogen peroxide, xanthine, xanthine oxidase, chloride, and myeloperoxidase are all required for effective killing of E. coli (176b). This system requires hydrogen peroxide because removal of peroxide by catalase inhibits killing, and substitution of xanthine and xanthine oxidase by hydrogen peroxide restores killing to this system. During phagocytosis human PMN's generate O_2^-, as evidenced by the reduction of ferricytochrome C. The latter reduction can be inhibited by SOD (176c). Participation of O_2^- in leukocyte microbicidal activity is suggested by the observation that the killing of bacteria by leukocytes ingesting latex particles coated with SOD is inhibited to a greater extent than it is in leukocytes coated with inactivated protein enzyme (176d).

Singlet molecular oxygen is an electronically excited state of oxygen which emits light (176e). Such chemiluminescence is observed when normal leukocytes are incubated with particles. It is suspected that singlet oxygen may be generated by the oxidation of hypochlorite by myeloperoxidase and hydrogen peroxide (176f). Singlet oxygen can also react with double-bond carbon groups to form electronically excited carbonyl groups which also revert to ground state to produce chemiluminescence. It has been proposed that these reactions may be toxic to microorganisms and, in part, may be responsible for the microbicidal effect of the peroxidase system. It is possible that both singlet oxygen and hydroxyl radicals may also be microbicidal in the absence of myeloperoxidase, but further studies are needed to evaluate properly their role in this regard.

Other potential bactericidal components within the phagocyte include granule lysozyme and a set of granule cationic proteins with specific capacities to kill certain species of bacteria (177). Lactic acid produced as a result of increased cellular glycolysis during phagocytosis may also contribute if it accumulates in the phagosome (178).

Since antibiotics do not diffuse readily into phagocytic cells, bacteria become a potential source of intracellular infection if not killed by the phagocyte (179, 180). Recent studies indicate that lipid-soluble antibiotics, such as rifampin, diffuse into phagocytes and kill intracellular Staphylococcus aureus (181).

Nitroblue Tetrazolium Reduction by Leukocytes

Nitroblue tetrazolium (NBT) has been utilized recently for investigation of leukocyte metabolism and to define clinical diseases due to phagocyte dysfunction. The reduction of tetrazolium salts by PMN's was first noted by Shaffer, Kucera, and Spink (181a). Interpretation of the results of leukocyte studies with NBT must be made in light of the biochemical and physiologic properties of this dye and its interaction with living cells. NBT is a yellow oxidized substance sparingly soluble in neutralized buffer solutions. Because of its positive charge, it does not readily penetrate intact cell membranes (182). Studies of NBT reduction during zymosan ingestion have shown that the NBT reduction occurs in the phagosome (183, 212); however, the means by which all the ingredients necessary to complete the NBT reaction enter the phagosome is not entirely clear. The ingested particle and NBT enter the vacuole together. In fact, the NBT appears to be bound to certain ingested particles. NBT may enter granulocytes spread on glass slides, since the cell membrane is altered by this maneuver. If membrane permeability is altered or disrupted and a source of hydrogen atoms and electrons becomes available, cellular diaphorases reduce NBT to purple formazan precipitate. The reduction of NBT in the phagocytic vacuole apparently occurs because it substitutes for oxygen as a hydrogen acceptor. This property can be shown in vitro by polarographic methods, which indicate that the oxygen consumption induced by leukocyte homogenates in the presence of NADH is inhibited when nitroblue tetrazolium is added. NADH and NADPH generated by leukocytes during glycolysis and glucose oxidation, respectively, are thought to serve as donors of electrons to NBT. Perhaps their reduced pyridine nucleotides become closely associated with the wall of the phagosome, where they interact with the enzyme that can transfer hydrogen to NBT or to oxygen.

Assessment of the reduction of NBT by individual "resting" granulocytes in the whole blood of a variety of patients has been utilized by several workers to assist in the differential diagnosis of bacterial versus viral infection (the so-called NBT test). A recent clinical trial has not confirmed the utility of this procedure (183a, 183b).

PHAGOCYTIC DYSFUNCTION SYNDROMES

Studies of patients with normal or elevated levels of immunoglobulins and recurrent bacterial and fungal infections have identified a group of clinical syndromes related to impaired phagocyte function. The total number of circulating phagocytes is usually normal or elevated. This group of newly defined disorders includes defects of chemotaxis, opsonization, and intracellular bactericidal killing. A comprehensive review of phagocytosis and its abnormalities has recently been published (183c).

Defects of Chemotaxis

Recently, a boy who experienced recurrent cutaneous and respiratory infections due to *Klebsiella* and *E. coli* has been described (184). His leukocytes demonstrated a defect of chemotactic responsiveness in vitro as well as in vivo. The etiology of this defect was thought to be related to an inhibitor of neutrophil chemotaxis that was identified in the serum of this child. The parents' leukocytes had no such abnormality. Subsequently, this child was also found to have a leukocyte defect similar to that of patients with chronic granulomatous disease (185). Yet, other children with chronic granulomatous disease were found to have normal leukotactic responsiveness in vitro. Another male whose PMN's killed bacteria and reduced NBT had a serum inhibitor to chemotaxis. Since normal plasma antagonized the inhibitor in vitro and in vivo but the patient's plasma did not, it is possible that the inhibitor and its antagonist are normal components of human blood and that the basic defect is the absence of the antagonist (185a). A serum inhibitor to chemotaxis in vitro has been identified in cirrhotic patients (185b). Leukocyte mobilization in vivo is reduced in adults with terminal shock and in those given 50 to 75 ml. of 95 per cent alcohol intravenously or orally (186a). In addition, defects of PMN chemotaxis have been reported in diabetic patients (186) and transiently in patients with acute bacterial infection (186a).

Two unrelated children, a 5-year-old girl and a 3-year-old boy, with severe neutropenia and recurrent gingivostomatitis and otitis media were found to have a cellular defect of chemotaxis and random motility. The term "lazy leukocyte syndrome" was coined to describe the inability of their PMN's to traverse millipore filters in response to chemotactic stimuli as well as their poor migration in microhematocrit tubes compared to normals (186b).

Defects of Opsonization

Phagocytosis of bacteria is stimulated by type-specific antibody. This is especially so if the antibody promotes complement fixation to the polymorphonuclear leukocyte membrane (187), or, in the case of monocytes, if it enhances the attachment of particles to the membrane of the phagocyte (188).

Newborn infants are susceptible to gram-negative infection mainly because they lack IgM-specific antibodies which stimulate complement fixation and enhance ingestion of gram-negative bacteria by phagocytes (189).

A patient has been described with increased susceptibility to infection and a subtle disorder of serum complement metabolism (190). This patient had repeated pyogenic infections. His leukocytes were quantitatively and functionally normal, but his serum failed to support ingestion of pneumococci, even though type-specific antibody was present. All complement factors were normal except for the third component of complement, which was reduced to less than 10 per cent of normal. Most of the remainder of the third component of complement was altered to an inactive product. A pseudoglobulin present in normal serum but absent in this patient's serum was thought to be responsible for the lack of stability of the third component of complement. Normal serum corrected this defect in vivo (191).

Two unrelated families with a deficiency of phagocytosis enhancement related to a dysfunction of the fifth component of serum complement have been reported (192, 193). Affected members have been infants with generalized seborrheic dermatitis, intractable diarrhea, local and systemic gram-negative infection, and marked wasting and dystrophy. This defect can be identified by observing faulty ingestion of yeast particles by phagocytes, but normal ingestion of erythrocytes, pneumococci, and latex particles. Apparently, yeast is unique in its requirement for C5 for phagocytosis. Life-saving therapy has been administered to two infants through the use of fresh plasma. Opsonically active C5 is in fresh plasma but not in blood stored longer than five days.

A 15-year-old girl with striking susceptibility to infection by pyogenic organisms was found to have 1/1000th or less of the normal serum concentration of C3. Investigation of members of her family revealed many individuals, including her mother and father, with C3 levels approximately half-normal, and it seems that she is homozygous for C3 deficiency (193a).

Certain patients with sickle cell anemia appear to have deficient heat-labile opsonic function against pneumococci. Since their immunoglobulin levels, total hemolytic complement activity, C3, and C5 are normal, the defect is likely related to a deficiency of one or more enzymes of the alternate pathway of C3 activation (194). Normal activity of their heat-labile opsonin system has been restored with the addition of a 5 to 6S pseu-

doglobulin isolated from normal serum (194a). The sera of patients with agammaglobulinemia and dysgammaglobulinemia also support phagocytosis poorly (195) and this defect may contribute to the increased susceptibility to infections observed in these patients.

Intracellular Defects of Bacterial Killing

Consideration will be given here to those conditions in which a defect in the intraleukocytic microbicidal mechanism results in the prolonged intracellular survival of ingested organisms (196).

CHRONIC GRANULOMATOUS DISEASE OF CHILDHOOD (CGD)

This disease is by far the most common of the functional disorders of leukocyte metabolism (197). A recent review of the world literature describes 92 such patients (198). As indicated in Table 16–1, clinical features include the onset of chronic and recurrent

TABLE 16–1. FREQUENCY OF SIGNS AND SYMPTOMS IN 92 PATIENTS WITH CHRONIC GRANULOMATOUS DISEASE

FINDING	NUMBER OF PATIENTS INVOLVED
Marked lymphadenopathy	87
Pneumonitis	80
Male sex	80
Suppuration of nodes	79
Hepatomegaly	77
Dermatitis	77
Onset by 1 year	72
Splenomegaly	68
Hepatic-perihepatic abscess	41
Death before 7 years of age	34
Osteomyelitis	30
Onset with dermatitis	28
Onset with lymphadenitis	28
Persistent rhinitis	23
Facial-periorofacial dermatitis	22
Conjunctivitis	21
Death from pneumonitis	21
Persistent diarrhea	20
Perianal abscess	17
Ulcerative stomatitis	15

From Johnston, R. B., Jr., and Baehner, R. L.: Pediatrics 48:733, 1971.

infection during the first year of life. Infection is manifested by marked cervical lymphadenitis, pneumonia, hepatosplenomegaly, and dermatitis. Approximately one third of the patients develop osteomyelitis, and about 25 per cent have persistent periorofacial dermatitis, rhinitis, or conjunctivitis. Ulcers of the buccal mucosa, stomatitis, and perianal abscesses are less frequently encountered. The affected organs become the site of abscesses and chronic granulomatous reactions, with the appearance of pigmented histiocytes within them. Approximately one third of these children died before the age of seven. No specific routine laboratory abnormalities have been observed. An appropriate leukocytosis develops during infection. Pulmonary infiltrations, as well as other radiologic evidences of inflammation, are observed. Chronic hypergammaglobulinemia and the anemia of chronic infection are present in the majority of these patients. A bacteriologic review of the microorganisms cultured from purulent foci is given in Table 16–2. It indicates that catalase-positive bacteria, such as *S. aureus*, *Klebsiella-Aerobacter*, *E. coli*, *S. albus*, *Serratia marcescens*, *Pseudomonas*, *Proteus*, and *Salmonella*, have been frequent pathogens. *Candida albicans* and *Aspergillus* have been cultured from some of these pa-

TABLE 16–2. MICROORGANISMS CULTURED FROM PURULENT FOCI

Organism	Number of Patients Involved[*]
Staphylococcus aureus	58
Klebsiella-Aerobacter organisms	22
Escherichia coli	19
Staphylococcus albus	10
Serratia marcescens	9
Candida albicans	7
Pseudomonas organisms	7
Aspergillus organisms	6
Proteus organisms	5
Salmonella organisms	4
Paracolobactrum organisms	4
Streptococci	3
Other enteric bacteria	6
Other organisms[†]	3

[*]Refers to number of different patients from whom that organism was cultured.

[†]*Nocardia* organisms, two: *Actinomyces israelii*, one.

From Johnston, R. B., Jr., and Baehner, R. L.: Pediatrics 48:734, 1971.

tients. It is noteworthy that pneumococci, beta-hemolytic streptococci, and *Hemophilus influenzae* did not cause infection in these patients. These bacteria are catalase-negative and thus effectively produce their own hydrogen peroxide. This is in contrast to those bacteria that did cause infection, which have a potent catalase to convert their own peroxide to water.

Bactericidal studies have shown that the circulating polymorphonuclear leukocytes and monocytes from CGD patients ingest bacteria and fungi adequately but fail to kill those microorganisms that infect them (165, 198, 199). This abnormality has been associated with a failure of bactericidal hydrogen peroxide production within the phagocytic vesicles of these patients' leukocytes (200, 201). Although CGD leukocytes shift their granule contents into the phagocytic vesicles (202, 203), the lack of hydrogen peroxide for peroxidation of bacteria within phagocytic vesicles is thought to be the basis for the bactericidal defect in the CGD phagocyte (204, 205). Superoxide anion is not generated in the leukocytes of patients with CGD (205a), and chemiluminescence is not observed when CGD leukocytes are incubated with particles (205b). Thus the unstable precursors of hydrogen peroxide, i.e., superoxide and singlet oxygen, are not generated by CGD leukocytes. Various hydrogen peroxide–producing enzymes have been studied in an effort to define the enzymatic basis of the disorder. Supernatant from salt solutions of leukocyte homogenates of some patients has been found to be deficient in NADH oxidase, a flavoprotein enzyme that catalyzes the production of hydrogen peroxide from NADH and oxygen (206). The cytolysates of two female patients' PMN's were low in glutathione peroxidase, although other females have had normal activity of this enzyme (207). This enzyme is responsible for peroxide utilization rather than production. Both D- and L-amino acid oxidase activities have been normal in the cytolysates of PMN's from CGD patients (170).

There is a male to female predominance of seven to one. In the majority of male cases, a female carrier state can be determined (208, 209). In contrast, in some male patients and in all of the female patients to date, the carrier state cannot be detected. English workers have found abnormal leukocyte function in both parents of patients and have hypothesized an autosomal recessive mode of inheritance with sex limitations by way of fatality in the female fetus (210). It is probable that the CGD defect can be transmitted as either an autosomal recessive or an X-linked gene, the latter being more common.

Diagnostic Studies for Chronic Granulomatous Disease

Studies of the phagocytic function of a patient's leukocytes will confirm the diagnosis. These tests are listed in Table 16–3. Bactericidal assays utilizing catalase-positive bacteria, such as *S. aureus,* reveal that the patient's granulocytes will phagocytize but not kill such organisms during a two-hour period of incubation compared to control phagocytes (199). Metabolic studies utilizing the response of the phagocyte to latex particles will also prove the diagnosis. Normal leukocytes demonstrate a seven-to tenfold increase in glucose-1-^{14}C oxidation and a three- to fivefold increase in ^{14}C-formate oxidation and in oxygen consumption during phagocytosis, and will bind ^{125}I or ^{131}I. These responses are absent in CGD leukocytes. The quantitative nitroblue tetrazolium test also confirms the diagnosis (208). A simpler screening test has been developed, adapted from the quantitative nitroblue tetrazolium test (211). Furthermore, histochemical slide studies have shown that normal leukocytes reduce nitroblue tetrazolium to purple formazan within the phagocytic vesicles (212). In contrast,

TABLE 16–3.   LEUKOCYTE FUNCTION TESTS THAT ARE ABNORMAL IN CHRONIC GRANULOMATOUS DISEASE

1. Bactericidal Tests
   a. No significant killing of catalase-positive bacteria, e.g., *Staphylococcus aureus.*
   b. Normal killing of catalase-negative bacteria, e.g., beta-hemolytic streptococci.

2. Metabolic Tests
   a. No reduction of nitroblue tetrazolium.
   b. No increase in glucose-1-^{14}C oxidation with phagocytosis.
   c. No increase in oxygen consumption during phagocytosis.
   d. No increase in hydrogen peroxide–dependent ^{14}C-formate oxidation with phagocytosis.
   e. Lack of ^{125}iodide fixation during phagocytosis.

CGD leukocytes fail to reduce NBT to purple formazan; thus this test also provides a convenient and simple method to demonstrate susceptible patients and the carrier of the abnormal X-linked gene (209).

Several mixed defects of phagocytic function similar to those of chronic granulomatous disease have been described. Light-skinned, red-haired female patients with Job's syndrome (213) have had recurrent cold staphylococcal abscesses. Some of these patients' leukocytes have been demonstrated to have metabolic abnormalities similar to those of CGD leukocytes (214). Patients with milder infections and without granulomatous responses in their tissues, such as those described with familial lipochrome histiocytosis (215), also have had metabolic abnormalities of their leukocytes similar to those of CGD leukocytes. One CGD patient had absent serum IgA (216). Four other patients have failed to transform their lymphocytes in response to phytohemagglutinin stimulation (217). Three of these patients were found to have an inhibitor of lymphocyte transformation present in their serum (218). Thus the defect was not due to a specific lymphocyte cellular abnormality in these patients.

Management of the Patient With CGD

No specific therapy has been found. Treatment with methylene blue to increase pentose shunt activity, vitamin A to promote release of lysosomal enzymes, corticosteroids, gamma globulin, and leukocyte transfusions have been unsuccessful. Four hours after administration of normal leukocytes to a patient, there was no increase in the bactericidal activity of his peripheral blood phagocytes (219). Busulfan was given to three patients to induce neutropenia and thus decrease the population of phagocytes available to protect bacteria from serum factors and antibiotics (220). There was possible benefit in one child. Patients' leukocytes were tested for in vitro bactericidal activity in the presence of oxygen in a hyperbaric chamber in an attempt to overcome the oxidative enzyme defect with high intracellular oxygen and thereby to induce peroxide formation and bacterial killing. No such effect was achieved (198). The introduction of a peroxide-generating system into CGD leukocytes has improved their metabolic and bactericidal defects in vitro (200, 204, 221), but it has not yet been possible to adapt such a system for treatment of the patient.

Treatment with bactericidal antibiotics specific for the patient's infecting organism for long periods of time has seemed to prolong the symptom-free intervals between infections in the few patients in which this has been tried (222, 223). Serious infections have still occurred, however. Prompt surgical drainage of abscesses and careful bacteriology must be conscientiously pursued.

MYELOPEROXIDASE DEFICIENCY

Five patients with genetic absence of myeloperoxidase have been described (224). Their leukocytes had decreased fungicidal and bactericidal activity. Genetic study indicates an autosomal recessive mode of inheritance. However, the peroxidase content of eosinophils in these patients was normal. It would appear from these studies that granule myeloperoxidase in neutrophils is essential for the normal and effective killing of bacteria and *Candida* species. This diagnosis can be made by histochemical myeloperoxidase staining of the fresh blood smear. In contrast to CGD phagocytes, the metabolism of ^{14}C-formate and glucose 1-^{14}C oxidation by these phagocytes was found to be greater than normal. It is thought that the inhibition or absence of myeloperoxidase results in the increased utilization of peroxide in nonmyeloperoxidase-mediated, peroxide-dependent reactions, such as formate oxidation and pentose shunt activation (225).

CHEDIAK-HIGASHI DISEASE

This autosomal recessive disorder is characterized by partial oculocutaneous albinism and the presence of giant abnormal lysosomes in most granule-containing cells (226, 227). A similar disorder has been described in mink, cattle, and mice (228). A major clinical manifestation of the disease in affected patients is recurrent bacterial infections, principally with gram-positive organisms. Many patients develop a lymphoma-like accelerated phase, characterized by hepatosplenomegaly, pancytopenia, and lymphadenopathy with generalized lymphocytic and histiocytic proliferation (229). Some patients have manifested a progressive neurologic syndrome resembling spinocerebellar degeneration.

Recent in vitro studies suggest that the giant granules present within phagocytic cells from these patients fail to discharge their lysosomal enzymes and peroxidative enzymes into phagocytic vesicles. There is a delay in the rate of degranulation as well as a total decrease in the overall deposition of granule contents into the phagocyte vesicle (230). Furthermore, in vitro killing of *S. aureus*, beta-hemolytic streptococci, pneumococci, and *Serratia marcescens* was consistently delayed in the leukocytes of these patients. The greatest defect occurred within the first 20 minutes of contact between Chediak-Higashi cells and bacteria (231, 185). In certain patients with granulocytopenia in the progressive form of the disease, frequent infections may be related to the associated decrease in numbers of circulating phagocytes (232).

G6PD-DEFICIENT PMN's

Caucasian G6PD deficiency of the red cells is associated with decreased levels of the enzyme in the PMN (233). In most cases, this does not produce a bactericidal defect in the PMN, since the level of G6PD is between 20 and 50 per cent of normal. In rare cases the enzyme level was less than 1 per cent of normal. These PMN's failed to produce H_2O_2, and a severe disease due to persistent bacterial infection ensued (234, 234a). Although G6PD levels are normal in CGD PMN's, leukocyte homogenates from these patients have revealed a more rapid rate of decay of this enzyme compared to controls (235). NADP and 2-mercaptoethanol corrected the rapid decay. However, both NADP and NAD levels are normal in CGD leukocytes (236), so that the accelerated decay of G6PD cannot be explained on this basis.

Acquired Defects of Phagocytic Function

Certain drugs are known to affect phagocyte function. Steroids in high concentration appear to depress the cellular oxidative enzyme capacity of phagocytes to produce a decrease in intracellular killing (237). NBT reduction by phagocytes was depressed in individuals receiving this therapy for blood dyscrasias or for infection, but the depression was not in the range observed for patients with CGD. Colchicine inhibits microtubule formation in normal phagocytes and alters the rate of degranulation of these cells (238). Vinblastine (Velban) may affect phagocytes in a similar fashion (239).

Patients with acute bacterial infections prior to drug therapy have increased numbers of leukocytes in their peripheral blood which spontaneously reduce NBT (113, 240). It appears that this is a transient response related to humoral or bacterial byproducts, since serum from patients receiving typhoid vaccine or filtrates of bacterial cultures stimulates NBT reduction (116). The test appears to be of some use in differentiating bacterial from nonbacterial infection and also as a screening test for chronic granulomatous disease.

Phagocyte Response of the Neonate

Newborn infants, especially infants of low birth weight, are unduly susceptible to infection. It is not clear whether intracellular defects are present in neonatal phagocytes. As previously noted, newborn serum has less opsonic activity for *E. coli* and yeast (241, 242) because of a deficiency of 19S antibodies. Those studies that report diminished gram-negative microbicidal activity of newborn PMN's in vitro could be explained by diminished uptake of viable bacteria rather than by an intrinsic cellular defect (243, 244). Indeed, other investigators have observed normal killing of *E. coli* and *S. aureus* in vitro by phagocytes of newborns (242). Leukocytes of newborn infants manifest an activated metabolic state with increased resting oxygen consumption, pentose shunt activity, and spontaneous reduction of NBT compared to normal adult controls (245, 246). It is of interest that the increased spontaneous NBT reduction by neonatal leukocytes is diminished in the blood of premature infants with bacterial infection (247).

References

1. Metchnikoff, E.: Untersuchungen über die mesodermalen Phagocyten einiger Wirbeltiere. Biol. Z. *3*:560, 1883.
2. Loutit, J. F.: Biocycles in the reticuloendothelial system. Ann. N.Y. Acad. Sci. *88*:122, 1960.
3. Becker, A. J., McCulloch, E. A., et al.: Cytological demonstration of the clonal nature of spleen colonies derived from transplanted mouse marrow cells. Nature (Lond.) *197*:452, 1963.
4. Nowell, P. C., and Cole, L. J.: Clonal repopulation in reticular tissues of x-irradiated mice: Effect of dose and limb-shielding. J. Cell. Physiol. *70*:37, 1967.
5. Hellman, S., and Grate, H. E.: Enhanced erythropoiesis with concomitant diminished granulopoiesis in pre-irradiated recipient mice. Evidence for a common stem cell. J. Exp. Med. *127*:605, 1968.
6. Whang, J., Frei, E., III, et al.: The distribution of the Philadelphia chromosome in patients with chronic myelogenous leukemia. Blood *22*:664, 1963.
7. Till, J. E., and McCulloch, E. A.: A direct measurement of radiation sensitivity of normal mouse bone marrow cells. Radiation Res. *14*:213, 1961.
8. Osgood, E. E.: Regulation of cell proliferation, In *The Kinetics of Cellular Proliferation.* Stohlman, F., Jr. (ed.), New York, Grune & Stratton, 1959, p. 282.
9. Boll, I., and Kühn, A.: Granulocytopoiesis in human bone marrow cultures studied by means of kinematography. Blood *26*:449, 1965.
10. Bond, V. P.: Cell turnover in blood and blood forming tissues studied with tritiated thymidine, In *The Kinetics of Cellular Proliferation.* Stohlman, F., Jr. (ed.), New York, Grune & Stratton, 1959, p. 188.
11. Warner, H. R., and Athens, J. W.: An analysis of granulocyte kinetics in blood and bone marrow. Ann. N. Y. Acad. Sci. *113*:523, 1964.
12. Donohue, D. M., Gabrio, B. W., et al.: Quantitative measurements of hematopoietic cells of the marrow. J. Clin. Invest. *37*:1567, 1958.
13. Athens, J. W.: Neutrophilic granulocyte kinetics and granulocytopoiesis, In *Regulation of Hematopoiesis.* Vol. II. Gorden, A. S. (ed.), New York, Appleton-Century-Crofts, 1970, p. 1143.
14. Ackerman, G. A.: Ultrastructure and cytochemistry of the developing neutrophil. Lab. Invest. *19*:290, 1968.
15. Bainton, D. F., and Farquhar, M. G.: Differences in enzyme content of azurophil and specific granules of polymorphonuclear leukocytes. I. Histochemical staining of bone marrow smears. J. Cell. Biol. *39*:286, 1968.
16. Bainton, D. F., Ullyot, J. L., et al.: The development of neutrophilic polymorphonuclear leukocytes in human bone marrow. Origin and content of azurophil and specific granules. J. Exp. Med. *134*:907, 1971.
17. Baggiolini, M., Hirsch, J. G., et al.: Resolution of granules from rabbit heterophil leukocytes

into distinct populations by zonal sedimentation. J. Cell. Biol. *40*:529, 1969.

18. Cohn, Z. A., and Hirsch, J. G.: The isolation and properties of the specific cytoplasmic granules of rabbit polymorphonuclear leukocytes. J. Exp. Med. *112*:983, 1960.

19. Bainton, D. F., and Farquhar, M. G.: Origin of granules in polymorphonuclear leukocytes. Two types derived from opposite faces of Golgi complex in developing granulocytes. J. Cell. Biol. *28*:277, 1966.

20. Baggiolini, M., deDuve, C., et al.: Association of lactoferrin with specific granules in rabbit heterophil leukocytes. J. Exp. Med. *131*:559, 1970.

21. Archer, G. T., and Hirsch, J. G.: Isolation of granules from eosinophil leukocytes and study of their enzyme content. J. Exp. Med. *118*:227, 1963.

22. Dunn, W. B., Hardin, J. H., et al.: Ultrastructural localization of myeloperoxidase in human neutrophil and rabbit heterophil and eosinophil leukocytes. Blood *32*:935, 1968.

23. Zucker-Franklin, D.: Electron microscopic study of human basophils. Blood *29*:878, 1967.

24. Cronkite, E. P., and Fliedner, T. M.: Granulocytopoiesis. New Engl. J. Med. *270*:1347, 1964.

25. Brandt, L.: Studies on the phagocytic activity of neutrophilic leukocytes with special reference to chronic myeloproliferative conditions and megaloblastic anemia. Scand. J. Haematol. (Suppl.) *2*:1, 1967.

26. Baehner, R. L., and Johnston, R. B., Jr.: Monocyte function in children with neutropenia and chronic infections. Blood *40*:31, 1972.

27. Lichtman, M. A.: Cellular deformability during maturation of the myeloblast. Possible role in marrow egress. New Engl. J. Med. *283*:943, 1970.

28. Cartwright, G. E., Athens, J. W., et al.: The kinetics of granulopoiesis in normal man. Blood *24*:780, 1964.

29. Athens, J. W., Raab, S. O., et al.: Leukokinetic studies. III. The distribution of granulocytes in blood of normal subjects. J. Clin. Invest. *40*:159, 1961.

30. Craddock, G. G., Jr., Perry, S., et al.: Evaluation of marrow granulocyte reserves in normal and disease states. Blood *15*:840, 1960.

31. Mauer, A. M., Athens, J. W., et al.: Leukokinetic studies. II. A method for labeling granulocytes *in vitro* with radioactive diisopropyl fluorophosphate (DFP^{32}). J. Clin. Invest. *39*:1481, 1960.

32. Athens, J. W.: Granulocyte kinetics in health and disease in human tumor cell kinetics. National Cancer Institute Monograph, No. 30, 1963, pp. 135–155.

33. Boggs, D. R., Marsh, J. C., et al.: Neutrophil releasing activity in plasma of human subjects injected with endotoxin. Proc. Soc. Exp. Biol. Med. *127*:689, 1968.

34. Marsh, J. C., Boggs, D. R., et al.: Neutrophil kinetics in acute infection. J. Clin. Invest. *461*:943, 1967.

35. Bradley, T. R., and Metcalf, D.: The growth of mouse bone marrow cells *in vitro*. Aust. J. Exp. Biol. Med. Sci. *44*:287, 1966.

36. Boggs, D. R.: The kinetics of neutrophilic leuko-

37. Pike, B. L., and Robinson, W. A.: Human bone marrow colony growth in agar gel. J. Cell. Physiol. *76*:77, 1970.

38. Iscove, N. N., Senn, J. S., et al.: Colony formation by normal and leukemic human marrow cells in culture: Effect of conditioned medium from human leukocytes. Blood *37*:1, 1971.

39. Robinson, W. A., and Pike, B. L.: Leukopoietic activity in human urine. New Engl. J. Med. *282*:1291, 1970.

40. Davidson, W. M.: Inherited variations in leukocytes. Semin. Hematol. *5*:255, 1968.

41. Kauder, E., and Mauer, A. M.: Neutropenias of childhood. J. Pediatr. *69*:147, 1966.

42. Morley, A. A.: A neutrophil cycle in healthy individuals. Lancet *2*:1220, 1966.

43. Kato, K.: Leukocytes in infancy and childhood. A statistical analysis of 1,081 total and differential counts from birth to fifteen years. J. Pediatr. *7*:7, 1935.

44. Van Furth, R., and Cohn, Z. A.: The origin and kinetics of mononuclear phagocytes. J. Exp. Med. *128*:241, 1966.

45. Volkman, A.: The origin and turnover of mononuclear cells in peritoneal exudate in rats. J. Exp. Med. *124*:241, 1966.

46. Whitelaw, D. M.: The intravascular life span of monocytes. Blood *28*:455, 1966.

47. Rebuck, J. W., and Crowley, J. H.: A method of studying leukocyte function *in vivo*. Ann. N.Y. Acad. Sci. *59*:757, 1951.

48. Trepel, F., and Begemann, H.: On the origin of the skin window macrophages. Acta. Haematol. (Basel) *36*:386, 1966.

49. Cohn, Z. A., and Benson, B.: The differentiation of mononuclear phagocytes. Morphology, cytochemistry, and biochemistry. J. Exp. Med. *121*:153, 1965.

50. Cohn, Z. A., and Benson, B.: The *in vitro* differentiation of mononuclear phagocytes. II. The influence of serum on granule formation, hydrolase production, and pinocytosis. J. Exp. Med. *121*:835, 1965.

51. Cline, M. J., and Lehrer, R. I.: Phagocytosis by human monocytes. Blood *32*:423, 1968.

52. Van Furth, R.: Origin and kinetics of monocytes and macrophages. Semin. Hematol. *7*:125, 1970.

53. LoBuglio, A., Cotran, R., et al.: Red cells coated with immunoglobulin G: Binding and sphering by mononuclear cells in man. Science *158*:1582, 1967.

54. Page, A. R., and Good, R. A.: Studies in cyclic neutropenia. A clinical and experimental investigation. Am. J. Dis. Child. *94*:623, 1957.

55. Morley, A. A., and Stohlman, F., Jr.: Cyclophosphamide-induced cyclical neutropenia. An animal model of a human periodic disease. New Engl. J. Med. *282*:643, 1970.

56. Lund, J. E., Padgett, G. A., et al.: Cyclic neutropenia in grey collie dogs. Blood *29*:452, 1967.

57. Dale, D. C., Kimball, H. R., et al.: Studies of cyclic neutropenia in grey collie dogs. Clin. Res. *18*:402, 1970.

58. Kostman, R.: Infantile genetic agranulocytosis

(agranulocytosis infantilis heriditaria). A new recessive lethal disease in man. Acta. Paediatr. (Suppl.) *105*:45, 1956.

59. Krill, C. E., Jr., Smith, H. D., et al.: Chronic idiopathic granulocytopenia. New Engl. J. Med. *270*:973, 1964.

60. Miller, D. R., Freed, B. A., et al.: Congenital neutropenia. Report of a fatal case in a Negro infant with leukocyte function studies. Am. J. Dis. Child. *115*:337, 1968.

61. Gilman, P. A., Jackson, D. P., et al.: Congenital agranulocytosis: Prolonged survival and terminal acute leukemia. Blood *36*:576, 1970.

62. Barak, Y., Paran, M., et al.: *In vitro* induction of myeloid proliferation and maturation in infantile genetic agranulocytosis. Blood *38*: 74, 1971.

63. Wriedt, K., Kauder, E., et al.: Defective myelopoiesis in congenital neutropenia. New Engl. J. Med. *283*:1072, 1970.

64. Salomonsen, L.: Granulocytopenia in children. Acta. Paediatr. *35*:189, 1948.

65. Stahlie, T. D.: Chronic benign neutropenia in infancy and early childhood. Report of a case with a review of the literature. J. Pediatr. *48*: 710, 1956.

66. Zuelzer, W. W., and Bajoghli, M.: Chronic granulocytopenia in childhood. Blood *23*:359, 1964.

67. Schwachman, H., Diamond, L. K., et al.: The syndrome of pancreatic insufficiency and bone marrow dysfunction. J. Pediatr. *65*:645, 1964.

68. Shmerling, D. H., Prader, A., et al.: The syndrome of exocrine pancreatic insufficiency, neutropenia, metaphyseal dysostosis and dwarfism. Helv. Paediatr. Acta *24*:547, 1969.

69. Schwachman, H., Holsclaw, D., et al.: Comments to editors, In *1971 Year Book on Pediatrics*. Gellis, S. S. (ed.), Chicago Year Book Medical Publishers, 1971, p. 291.

70. Krill, C. E., Jr., Smith, H. D., et al.: Chronic idiopathic granulocytopenia. New Engl. J. Med. *270*:973, 1964.

71. Zuelzer, W. W.: "Myelokathexis"—A new form of chronic granulocytopenia. Report of a case. New Engl. J. Med. *270*:699, 1964.

72. Hugeley, C. M., Jr.: Drug-induced dyscrasias. II. Agranulocytosis. J.A.M.A. *118*:817, 1964.

73. Pisciotta, A. V.: Agranulocytosis induced by certain phenothiazine derivatives. J.A.M.A. *208*: 1862, 1969.

74. Simon, A. J., and Rogers, D. E.: Agranulocytosis associated with novobiocin administration: Report of a case. Ann. Intern. Med. *46*:778, 1957.

75. Newton, R. M., and Ward, V. G.: Leukopenia associated with ristocetin (Spontin) administration. J.A.M.A. *166*:1956, 1958.

76. Levitt, B. H., Gottlieb, A. H., et al.: Bone marrow depression due to methicillin, a semisynthetic penicillin. Clin. Pharmacol. Ther. *5*: 301, 1965.

77. Underwood, L. C.: Fatal bone marrow depression after treatment with acetazolamide (Diamox). J.A.M.A. *161*:1477, 1956.

78. Stevens, A. R.: Agranulocytosis induced by sulfaguanidine. The danger of an antibacterial drug in a symptomatic remedy. Arch. Intern. Med. *123*:428, 1969.

79. Schwartz, M. J., and Norton, W. S., II.: Thrombocytopenia and leukopenia associated with use of sulfamethoxypyridazine. J.A.M.A. *167*: 457, 1958.

80. Tashjian, A. H., Jr., and Leddy, J. P.: Agranulocytosis associated with phenindione. A case report with review of the literature. Arch. Intern. Med. *105*:121, 1960.

81. Brod, R. C.: Blood dyscrasias associated with tolbutamide therapy. J.A.M.A. *171*:296, 1959.

82. Karilin, H.: Fatal agranulocytosis following chlorpropamide treatment of diabetes. New Engl. J. Med. *262*:1076, 1960.

83. Adams, D. A., and Perry, S.: Agranulocytosis associated with thenalidine (Sandostene) tartrate therapy. J.A.M.A. *167*:1207, 1958.

84. Zuckerman, A. J., and Chazam, A. A.: Agranulocytosis with thrombocytopenia following chlorothiazide therapy. Br. Med. J. *11*:1338, 1958.

85. Schotland, M. G., and Crumback, M. M.: Neutropenia in an infant secondary to hydrochlorothiazide: With a new review of hematologic reactions to "thiazide" drugs. Pediatrics *31*: 754, 1963.

86. Hallwright, G. P.: Agranulocytosis caused by alpha methyl dopa (Aldomet). New Zealand Med. J. *60*:567, 1961.

87. McGavack, T. H., and Chevalby, J.: Untoward hematologic responses to the antithyroid compounds. Am. J. Med. *17*:36, 1954.

88. Croke, A. R., and Berry, J. W.: Agranulocytosis occurring during methimazole (Tapazole) therapy. J.A.M.A. *148*:45, 1952.

89. Walker, J. G.: Fatal agranulocytosis complicating treatment with ethacrynic acid. Ann. Intern. Med. *64*:1303, 1966.

90. Dittman, W. A., and Ward, J. R.: Demecolcine toxicity. A case report of severe hematopoietic toxicity and a review of the literature. Am. J. Med. *27*:519, 1959.

91. Corcos, J. M., Soler-Bechara, J., et al.: Neutrophilic agranulocytosis during administration of penicillamine. J.A.M.A. *189*:265, 1964.

92. Booth, K., Larkin, K., et al.: Agranulocytosis coincident with amodiaquine therapy. Br. Med. J. *3*:32, 1967.

93. Tait, G. B.: Fatal agranulocytosis during carbimazole therapy. Lancet *1*:303, 1957.

94. Wang, R. I. H., and Schuller, G.: Agranulocytosis following procainamide administration. Am. Heart. J. *78*:282, 1969.

95. Pisciotta, A. V.: Agranulocytosis induced by certain phenothiazine derivatives. J.A.M.A. *208*: 1862, 1969.

96. Moeschlin, S.: Leukocyte auto-antibodies. Acta. Haematol. (Basel) *20*:167, 1958.

97. Huguley, C. M.: Agranulocytosis induced by dipyrone. A hazardous antipyretic and analgesic. J.A.M.A. *189*:938, 1964.

98. Weisman, G., and Xefteris, E. D.: Phenylbutazone leukopenia. Arch. Intern. Med. *103*: 957, 1959.

99. Moeschlin, S.: Immunoleukopenies et immunoagranulocytosis. Rev. Hematol. *8*:249, 1953.

100. Koszewski, B. J., and Hubbard, T. F.: Immunologic agranulocytosis due to mercurial diuretics. Am. J. Med. *20*:958, 1956.

101. Stein, J. H., Hamilton, H. E., et al.: Agranulocy-

tosis caused by chorpropamide. Arch. Intern. Med. *113*:186, 1964.

102. Lalezari, P.: Lecture on leukocyte antibodies. Boston, 1968.

103. Lalezari, P., and Bernard, G. E.: An isologous antigen-antibody reaction with human neutrophils related to neonatal neutropenia. J. Clin. Invest. *45*:1741, 1966.

104. Overweg, J., and Engelfriet, C. P.: Cytotoxic leukocyte iso-antibodies formed during the first pregnancy. Vox Sang. *16*:97, 1969.

105. Tullis, J. L.: Prevalence, nature, and identification of leukocyte antibodies. New Engl. J. Med. *258*:569, 1958.

106. Good, R. A., and Zak, S. J.: Disturbances in gamma globulin synthesis as "experiments of nature." Pediatrics *18*:109, 1964.

107. Lonsdale, D., Deodhar, S. D., et al.: Familial granulocytopenia and associated immunoglobulin abnormality. J. Pediatr. *71*:790, 1967.

108. Lux, S. E., Johnston, R. B., Jr., et al.: Chronic neutropenia and abnormal cellular immunity in cartilage-hair hypoplasia. New Engl. J. Med. *282*:231, 1970.

109. Gitlin, D., Vawter, G., et al.: Thymic alymphoplasia and congenital aleukocytosis. Pediatrics *33*:184, 1964.

110. de Vaal, O. M., and Seynhaeve, V.: Reticular dysgenesia. Lancet *2*:1123, 1959.

111. Crosby, W. H.: Hypersplenism. Ann. Rev. Med. *13*:127, 1962.

112. Wiseman, B. K., and Doan, C. A.: Primary splenic neutropenia. A newly recognized syndrome closely related to congenital hemolytic icterus and essential thrombocytopenic purpura. Ann. Intern. Med. *16*:1097, 1942.

113. Zucker, S., Hanes, D. J., et al.: Plasma muramidase: A study of methods and clinical applications. J. Lab. Clin. Med. *75*:83, 1970.

114. Japa, J.: A study of the mitotic activity of normal human bone marrow. Br. J. Exp. Pathol. *23*: 272, 1942.

115. Rubini, J. R.: *In vitro* DNA labeling of bone marrow and leukemic blood leukocytes with tritiated thymidine. II. H³-thymidine biochemistry *in vitro*. J. Lab. Clin. Med. *68*: 566, 1966.

116. Marsh, J. C., and Perry, S.: The granulocyte response to endotoxin in patients with hematologic disorders. Blood *23*:581, 1964.

117. Senn, H., Holland, J. F., et al.: Kinetic and comparative studies on localized leukocyte mobilization in normal man. J. Lab. Clin. Med. *74*:742, 1969.

118. Southam, C. M., and Levin, A. G.: A quantitative Rebuck technique. Blood *27*:734, 1966.

119. Payne, R.: Agglutination technique for demonstration of leukocyte iso-antigens in man. Meth. Med. Res. *10*:27, 1964.

120. Buckner, D., Graw, R. G., Jr., et al.: Leukapheresis by continuous flow centrifugation (CFC) in patients with chronic myelocytic leukemia (CML). Blood *33*:353, 1969.

121. Shohet, S. B.: Morphologic evidence for the *in vivo* activity of transfused chronic myelogenous leukemia cells in a case of massive staphylococcal septicemia. Blood *32*:111, 1968.

122. deDuve, D., Pressman, B. C., et al.: Tissue fractionation studies. VI. Intracellular distribution patterns of enzymes in rat-liver tissue. Biochem. J. *60*:604, 1955.

123. Abernathy, M. R.: Döhle bodies associated with uncomplicated pregnancy. Blood *27*:380, 1966.

124. Hegglin, R.: Simultaneous constitutional changes in neutrophils and platelets. Helv. Med. Acta *12*:439, 1945.

125. Itaga, T., and Laszlo, J.: Döhle bodies in other granulocytic alterations during chemotherapy with cylcophosphamide. Blood *20*:668, 1962.

126. Gordin, R.: Toxic granulation of leukocytes. Acta Med. Scand. (Suppl.) *143*:270, 1962.

127. Allison, A. C., and Malluci, L.: Histochemical studies of lysosomes and lysosomal enzymes in the virus infected cultures. J. Exp. Med. *121*:463, 1965.

128. McCall, C. E., Katayama, I., et al.: Lysosomal and ultrastructural changes in human "toxic" neutrophils during bacterial infection. J. Exp. Med. *129*:267, 1969.

129. Mittwoch, V.: Abnormal lymphocytes in gargoylism. Br. J. Haematol. *5*:365, 1959.

130. McKusick, V. A., Kaplan, D., et al.: The genetic mucopolysaccharidoses. Medicine (Baltimore) *44*:445, 1965.

131. Abta, F., and Bloom, W. E.: Essential lipoid histiocytosis (Type· Niemann and Pick). J.A.M.A. *90*:2076, 1928.

132. Snyder, R. A., and Brady, R. O.: The use of white cells as a source of diagnostic material from lipid storage disease. Clin. Chim. Acta *25*: 331, 1969.

133. Klein, A., Hussor, A. E., et al.: Pelger-Huet anomaly of the leukocytes. New. Engl. J. Med. *253*:1057, 1955.

134. Davidson, W. M., Milner, R. D. G., et al.: Giant neutrophil leukocytes: An inherited anomaly. Br. J. Haematol. *6*:339, 1960.

135. Mauer, A. M.: White blood cell disorders. Pediatr. Clin. North Am. *9*:739, 1962.

136. Hersh, E. M., and Bodey, G. P.: Leukocytic mechanism in inflammation. Ann. Rev. Med. *21*:105, 1970.

137. Lewis, G. P.: The role of peptides in the first stages of inflammation, In *Injury, Inflammation, and Immunity.* Baltimore, Williams and Wilkins, 1964.

138. Boyden, S.: The chemotactic effect of mixtures of antibody and antigen on polymorphonuclear leukocytes. J. Exp. Med. *115*:453, 1962.

139. Ward, P. A., Lepow, I., et al.: Bacterial factor chemotactic for polymorphonuclear leukocytes. Am. J. Pathol. *52*:725, 1968.

140. Ward, P. A.: Chemotaxis of polymorphonuclear leukocytes. Biochem. Pharmacol. (Suppl.) *110*:99, 1968.

141. Horwitz, D. A., and Garrett, M. A.: Use of leukocyte chemotaxis *in vitro* to assay mediators generated by immune reactions. J. Immunol. *106*:649, 1970.

142. Ward, P. A., and Hill, J. H.: C5 chemotactic fragments produced by an enzyme in lysosomal granules of neutrophils. J. Immunol. *104*: 535, 1970.

143. Williams, K. E., and Walters, M. N. I.: Inhibition

of leukocytic emigration after phagocytosis. J. Pathol. Bacterial. 98:167, 1968.

144. David, J.: Macrophage migration. Fed. Proc. 27:6, 1962.

145. MacKaness, G. B.: The influence of immunologically committed lymphoid cells on macrophage activity *in vivo.* J. Exp. Med. 129:973, 1969.

146. Wood, W. B., Jr.: Studies on the cellular immunology of acute bacterial infections. Harvey Lectures 47:72, 1951.

146a. Messner, R. P., and Jelinek, J.: Receptors for human gamma G globulin on human neutrophils. J. Clin. Invest. 49:2165, 1970.

146b. Lay, W. H., and Nussenzweig, V.: Receptors for complement on leukocytes. J. Exp. Med. 128:991, 1968.

146c. Alper, C. A., Goodkofsky, I., et al.: Studies of glycine-rich B-glycoprotein (GBG), properdin Factor B, and C3 proactivator (C3PA). Fed. Proc. 31:787, 1972.

147. Hirsch, J. G., and Strauss, B.: Studies in heat-labile opsonin in rabbit serum. J. Immunol. 92:145, 1964.

148. Johnston, R. B., Jr., Klemperer, M. R., et al.: The enhancement of bacterial phagocytosis by serum. The role of complement components and two cofactors. J. Exp. Med. 129:1275, 1969.

149. Rabinovitch, M.: Phagocytosis: The engulfment stage. Semin. Hematol. 5:134, 1968.

150. Zucker-Franklin, D., and Hirsch, J. G.: Electron microscope studies on the degranulating rabbit peritoneal leukocytes during phagocytosis. J. Exp. Med. 120:569, 1964.

151. Sbarra, A. J., and Karnovsky, M. L.: The biochemical basis of phagocytosis. I. Metabolic changes during the ingestion of particles by polymorphonuclear leukocytes. J. Biol. Chem. 234:1355, 1959.

152. Karnovsky, M. L.: Metabolic basis of phagocytic activity. Physiol. Rev. 42:143, 1962.

153. Oren, R., Farnham, A. E., et al.: Metabolic patterns in three types of phagocytizing cells. J. Cell. Biol. 17:487, 1963.

154. Baehner, R. L., Feig, S. A., et al.: Metabolic, phagocytic and bactericidal properties of phosphoglycerate kinase–deficient (PGK) polymorphonuclear leukocytes (PMN) (abstract). Blood 38:833, 1971.

155. Karnovsky, M. L., and Wallach, D. F. H.: The metabolic basis of phagocytosis. III. Incorporation of organic phosphate into various classes of phosphatides during phagocytosis. J. Biol. Chem. 236:1895, 1961.

156. Shohet, S. B.: Changes in fatty acid metabolism in human leukemic granulocytes during phagocytosis. Lab. Clin. Med. 75:659, 1970.

157. Elsbach, P.: Increased synthesis of phospholipid during phagocytosis. J. Clin. Invest. 47:2217, 1968.

158. Wetzel, M. G., and Korn, E. D.: Phagocytosis of latex beads by *Acahamoeba castellanii* (Neff). III. Isolation of the phagocytic vesicles and their membranes. J. Cell. Biol. 43:90, 1969.

159. Stossel, T. P., Pollard, T. D., et al.: Isolation and properties of phagocytic vesicles from polymorphonuclear leukocytes. J. Clin. Invest. 51:604, 1972.

160. Smolen, J. E., Shohet, S. B., et al.: Lipid composition changes in human polymorphonuclear cell fractions after phagocytosis (abstract). Submitted to 1971 American Soc. Clin. Invest., May 3, Atlantic City, N.J.

161. Cohn, Z. A., and Hirsch, J. G.: The influence of phagocytosis on the intracellular distribution of granule-associated components of polymorphonuclear leukocytes. J. Exp. Med. 112:983, 1960.

162. Hirsch, J. G.: Cinemicrophotographic observation of granule lysis in polymorphonuclear leukocytes during phagocytosis. J. Exp. Med. 116:827, 1962.

163. Nathan, D. G., and Baehner, R. L.: Disorders of phagocytic cell function, In *Progress in Hematology.* Vol. VII. Brown, E. B., and Moore, C. V. (eds.), New York, Grune & Stratton, 1971, p. 250.

164. Baehner, R. L., and Nathan, D. G.: Leukocyte oxidase: Defective activity in chronic granulomatous disease. Science 155:835, 1967.

165. David, W. C., Douglas, S. D., et al.: A selective neutrophil dysfunction syndrome: Impaired killing of staphylococci. Ann. Intern. Med. 69:1237, 1968.

166. Cagan, R. H., and Karnovsky, M. L.: Enzymatic basis of the respiratory stimulation during phagocytosis. Nature (Lond.) 204:255, 1964.

167. Zatti, M., and Rossi, F.: Mechanism of respiratory stimulation in phagocytosing leukocytes. The KCN-insensitive oxidation of $NADPH_2$. Experiencia 22:758, 1966.

168. Baehner, R. L., Gilman, N., et al.: Respiration and glucose oxidation in human and guinea pig leukocytes—Comparative studies. J. Clin. Invest. 49:692, 1970.

169. Cline, M. J., and Lehrer, R. I.: D-amino acid oxidase in leukocytes: A possible D-amino acid–linked antimicrobial system. Proc. Natl. Acad. Sci. USA 62:756, 1969.

170. Eckstein, M. R., Baehner, R. L., et al.: Amino acid oxidase activity in leukocytes from guinea pigs, humans with acute infections and children with chronic granulomatous disease. J. Clin. Invest. 50:1985, 1971.

171. Paul, B. B., Jacobs, R. R., et al.: The role of the phagocyte in host-parasite interaction. XXIV. Aldehyde·generation by the myeloperoxidase-chloride antimicrobial system. A possible *in vivo* mechanism of action. Infection and Immunity 2:414, 1970.

172. Reed, P. W., and Tepperman, J.: Phagocytosis-associated metabolism and enzymes in the rat polymorphonuclear leukocyte. Am. J. Physiol. 216:223, 1969.

173. Baehner, R. L., Nathan, D. G., et al.: Oxidant injury of caucasian glucose-6-phosphate dehydrogenase–deficient red blood cells by phagocytosing leukocytes during infection. J. Clin. Invest. 50:2466, 1971.

174. Paul, B., and Sbarra, A. J.: The role of phagocyte in host-parasite interactions. XIII. The direct quantitative estimation of H_2O_2 in phagocytizing cells. Biochem. Biophys. Acta 156:168, 1968.

175. Klebanoff, S. J.: Myeloperoxidase: Contribution to the microbicidal activity of intact leukocytes. Science 169:1095, 1970.

176. Klebanoff, S. J.: Myeloperoxidase–halide–hydrogen peroxide antibacterial system. J. Bacteriol. 95:2131, 1968.

176a. Fridovich, I.: Superoxide radical and superoxide dismutase. Acc. Chem. Res. 5:321, 1972.

176b. Klebanoff, S. J.: Role of the superoxide anion in the myeloperoxidase mediated antimicrobial system. J. Biol. Chem., 1974 (in press).

176c. Babior, B. M., Kipnes, R. S., et al.: Biological defense mechanisms. The production by leukocytes of superoxide, a potential bactericidal agent. J. Clin. Invest. 52:741, 1973.

176d. Johnston, R. B., Jr., Keele, B., et al.: Inhibition of phagocytic bactericidal activity by superoxide dismutase: A possible role for superoxide anion in the killing of phagocytized bacteria. J. Clin. Invest. 52:44a, 1973.

176e. Allen, R. C., Stjernholm, R. L., et al.: Evidence for the generation of an electronic excitation state(s) in human polymorphonuclear leukocytes and its participation in bactericidal activity. Biochem. Biophys. Res. Commun. 47:679, 1972.

176f. Allen, R. C., and Steele, R. H.: The functional generation of electronic excitation states by myeloperoxidase. Red. Proc. 32:478, 1973.

177. Zeya, H. I., and Spitznagel, J. K.: Antimicrobicidal specificity of leukocyte lysosomal cationic proteins. Science 154:1049, 1966.

178. Mandell, G. L.: Intraphagosomal pH of human polymorphonuclear neutrophils. Proc. Soc. Exp. Biol. Med. 134:447, 1970.

179. Alexander, J. W., and Good, R. A.: Effect of antibiotics on the bactericidal activity of human leukocytes. J. Lab. Clin. Med. 71:971, 1968.

180. Holmes, B., Quie, P. G., et al.: Protection of phagocytized bacteria from killing action of antibiotics. Nature (Lond.) 210:1131, 1966.

181. Mandell, G. L., and Vest, T. K.: Killing of intraleukocytic staphylococcus aureus by rifampin in vitro and in vivo studies. J. Infect. Dis. 125:486, 1972.

181a. Shaffer, J. M., Kucera, C. J., et al.: The protection of intracellular Brucella against therapeutic agents and the bactericidal action of serum. J. Exp. Med. 97:77, 1953.

182. Pearse, A. G. E.: Histochemistry, Theoretical and Applied. 2nd ed. Boston, Little, Brown and Company, 1960, p. 536.

183. Presig, E., and Hitzig, W. H.: Nitroblue tetrazolium test for the detection of chronic granulomatous disease—Technical modification. Eur. J. Clin. Invest. 1:409, 1971.

183a. Steigbigel, R. T., Johnson, P. K., et al.: Hematologic tests versus NBT test in diagnosis of bacterial infection. New Engl. J. Med. 290:235, 1974.

183b. Nathan, D. G.: NBT reduction by human phagocytes. New Engl. J. Med. 290:280, 1974.

183c. Stossel, T. P.: Phagocytosis. New Engl. J. Med. 290:717, 1974.

184. Ward, P. A., and Schlegel, R. J.: Impaired leukotactic responsiveness in a child with recurrent infections. Lancet 2:344, 1969.

185. Root, R. K., Rosenthal, A. S., et al.: Abnormal bactericidal, metabolic, and lysosomal functions of Chediak-Higashi syndrome leukocytes. J. Clin. Invest. 51:649, 1972.

185a. Smith, C. W., Hollers, J. C., et al.: A serum inhibitor of leucotaxis in a child with recurrent infections. J. Lab. Clin. Med. 79:878, 1972.

185b. DeMeo, A. N., and Anderson, B. R.: Defective chemotaxis associated with a serum inhibitor in cirrhotic patients. New Engl. J. Med. 286:735, 1972.

186. Mowat, A. G., and Baum, J.: Chemotaxis of polymorphonuclear leukocytes from patients with diabetes mellitus. New Engl. J. Med. 284:621, 1971.

186a. Brayton, R. G., Stokes, P. E., et al.: Effect of alcohol and various diseases on leukocyte mobilization, phagocytosis, and intracellular bacterial killing. New Engl. J. Med. 282:123, 1970.

186b. Miller, M. E., Oski, F. A., et al.: Lazy leukocyte syndrome. A new disorder of neutrophil function. Lancet 1:665, 1971.

187. Ward, H. K., and Enders, J. F.: An analysis of the opsonic and tropic action of normal and immune sera based on experiments with the pneumococcus. J. Exp. Med. 51:517, 1933.

188. Abramson, N., Gelfand, E. W., et al.: The interaction between human monocytes and red cells: Specificity for IgG subclasses and IgG fragments. J. Exp. Med. 132:1207, 1970.

189. Michael, J. G., and Rosen, F. S.: Association of "natural" antibodies to gram-negative bacteria with the 1-macroglobulins. J. Exp. Med. 118:619, 1963.

190. Alper, C. A., Abramson, N., et al.: Increased susceptibility to infection associated with abnormalities of complement-mediated functions and of the third component of complement (C3). New Engl. J. Med. 282:349, 1970.

191. Alper, C. A., Abramson, N., et al.: Studies in vivo and in vitro on an abnormality in the metabolism of C3 in a patient with increased susceptibility to infection. J. Clin. Invest. 49:1975, 1970.

192. Jacobs, J. D., and Miller, M. E.: Fatal familial "Leiner's Disease": A deficiency of the opsonic activity of serum complement. Pediatrics 49:225, 1972.

193. Miller, M. E., and Nilsson, V. R.: A familial deficiency of the phagocytosis enhancing activity of serum related to a dysfunction of the fifth component of complement (C5). New Engl. J. Med. 282:354, 1970.

193a. Alper, C. A., Colten, H. R., et al.: Homozygous deficiency of C3 in a patient with repeated infections. Lancet 2:1179, 1972.

194. Winkelstein, J. A., and Drachman, R. H.: Deficiency of pneumococcal serum opsonizing activity in sickle cell disease. New Engl. J. Med. 279:459, 1968.

194a. Johnston, R. B., Jr., Struth, A., et al.: Deficient serum opsonins in sickle cell disease. Pediatr. Res. 6:381, 1972.

195. Stossel, T. P.: Evaluation of opsonic and leukocyte function with a spectrophotometric test in patients with infection and with phagocytic disorders. Blood 42:121–130, 1973.

196. Klebanoff, S. J.: Intraleukocytic microbicidal defects. Ann. Rev. Med. 22:39, 1971.

197. Berendes, H., Bridges, R. A., et al.: A fatal granulomatosis of childhood. Minn. Med. 40:309, 1957.

198. Johnston, R. B., Jr., and Baehner, R. L.: Chronic granulomatous disease: Correlation between pathogenesis and clinical findings. Pediatrics 48:730, 1971.

199. Quie, P. G., White, J. G., et al.: *In vitro* bactericidal capacity of human polymorphonuclear leukocytes: Diminished activity in chronic granulomatous disease of childhood. J. Clin. Invest. 46:668, 1967.

200. Baehner, R. L., Nathan, D. G., et al.: Correction of metabolic deficiencies in the leukocytes of patients with chronic granulomatous disease. J. Clin. Invest. 49:865, 1970.

201. Holmes, B., Page, A. R., et al.: Studies of the metabolic activity of leukocytes from patients with a genetic abnormality of phagocytic function. J. Clin. Invest. 46:1422, 1967.

202. Baehner, R. L., Karnovsky, M. T., et al.: Degranulation of leukocytes in chronic granulomatous disease. J. Clin. Invest. 47:187, 1969.

203. Kauder, E., Kahle, L. L., et al.: Leukocyte degranulation and vacuole formation in patients with chronic granulomatous disease of childhood. J. Clin. Invest. 47:1753, 1968.

204. Johnston, R. B., Jr., and Baehner, R. L.: Improvement of leukocyte bactericidal activity in chronic granulomatous disease. Blood 35:350, 1970.

205. Klebanoff, S. J., and White, L. R.: Iodinating defect in the leukocytes of a patient with chronic granulomatous disease of childhood. New Engl. J. Med. 280:460, 1969.

205a. Curnutte, J. T., Whitten, D. M., et al.: Defective leukocyte superoxide production in chronic granulomatous disease. New Engl. J. Med. 290:593, 1974.

205b. Stjernholm, R. L., Allen, R. C., et al.: Impaired chemoluminescence during phagocytosis of opsonized bacteria. Infect. Immun. 7:313, 1973.

206. Baehner, R. L., and Karnovsky, M. L.: Deficiency of reduced nicotinamide adenine dinucleotide oxidase in chronic granulomatous disease. Science 162:1277, 1968.

207. Holmes, B., Park, B. H., et al.: Chronic granulomatous disease in females: Deficiency of leukocyte glutathione peroxidase. New Engl. J. Med. 282:217, 1970.

208. Baehner, R. L., and Nathan, D. G.: Quantitative nitroblue tetrazolium test in chronic granulomatous disease. New Engl. J. Med. 278:971, 1968.

209. Windhorst, D. B., Holmes, B., et al.: A newly defined X-linked trait in man with demonstration of the Lyon effect in carrier females. Lancet 1:737, 1967.

210. Chandra, R. W., Cope, W. A., et al.: Chronic granulomatous disease. Evidence for an autosomal mode of inheritance. Lancet 2:71, 1969.

211. Johnston, R. B., Jr.: Screening test for the diagnosis of chronic granulomatous disease. Pediatrics 43:122, 1969.

212. Nathan, D. G., Baehner, R. L., et al.: Failure of nitroblue tetrazolium reduction in the phagocytic vacuoles of leukocytes in chronic granulomatous disease. J. Clin. Invest. 48:1895, 1969.

213. Davis, S. D., Schaller, J., et al.: Job's syndrome: Recurrent "cold" staphylococcal abscesses. Lancet 1:1013, 1966.

214. Bannatyne, R. M., Skowron, P. N., et al.: Job's syndrome—A variant of chronic granulomatous disease. J. Pediatr. 75:236, 1969.

215. Rodey, G. E., Park, B. H., et al.: Defective bactericidal activity of peripheral blood leukocytes in lipochrome histiocytosis. Am. J. Med. 49:322, 1970.

216. Douglas, S. D., Davis, W. C., et al.: Granulocytopathies: Pleomorphism of neutrophil dysfunction. Am. J. Med. 46:901, 1969.

217. Barnes, R. D., Bishun, N. P., et al.: Impaired lymphocyte transformation and chromosomal abnormalities in fatal granulomatous disease of childhood. Acta. Paediatr. (Stockholm) 59:403, 1970.

218. Berkel, I., and Gelfand, E. W.: Personal communication.

219. Quie, P. G.: Chronic granulomatous disease of childhood. Adv. Pediatr. 16:287, 1969.

220. Thompson, E. N., and Soothill, J. F.: Chronic granulomatous disease: Quantitative clinicopathological relationships. Arch. Dis. Child. 45:24, 1970.

221. Buckley, R., Hochstein, P., et al.: A study of the defect in septic granulomatosis. J. Reticuloendothel. Soc. 4:430, 1967.

222. Lischner, H. W., and Lammot, T. R., III: Antibiotic therapy in chronic granulomatous disease of childhood (CGDC) (abstract). Soc. Pediatr. Res., 1968, p. 48.

223. Philippart, A. I., Colodny, A. H., et al.: Chronic granulomatous disease of childhood. J. Pediatr. Surg. 4:85, 1969.

224. Lehrer, R. I., and Cline, M. J.: Leukocyte myeloperoxidase deficiency and disseminated candidiasis: The role of myeloperoxidase in resistance to Candida infection. J. Clin. Invest. 48:1478, 1969.

225. Klebanoff, S. J., and Pincus, S. H.: Hydrogen peroxide utilization in myeloperoxidase deficient leukocytes: A possible microbicidal control mechanism. J. Clin. Invest. 50:2226, 1971.

226. Chediak, M.: Nouvelle anomalie leucocytaire de caractère constitutionel et familial. Rev. Hématol. 7:362, 1952.

227. Higashi, O.: Congenital abnormality of peroxidase granules. A case of "congenital gigantism of peroxidase granules," a preliminary report. Tohuku J. Exp. Med. 58:246, 1953.

228. Padgett, G. A., Reiquan, C. W., et al.: Comparative studies of susceptibility to infection in the Chediak-Higashi syndrome. J. Pathol. Bacteriol. 95:509, 1968.

229. Dent, P. B., Fish, L. A., et al.: Chediak-Higashi syndrome: Observations on the nature of the associated malignancy. Lab. Invest. 15:1634, 1966.

230. Stossel, T. P., Root, R. K., et al.: Phagocytosis in

chronic granulomatous disease and the Chediak-Higashi syndrome. New Engl. J. Med. *286*:120, 1972.

231. Clawson, C. C., Repine, J. E., et al.: Chediak-Higashi syndrome: Quantitative defect in bacterial capacity. Abstract presented to Fourteenth Annual Meeting American Society of Hematology. Dec. 5–7, 1971, San Francisco, Calif.

232. Blume, R. S., Bennett, J. M., et al.: Defective granulocyte regulation in the Chediak-Higashi syndrome. New Engl. J. Med. *279*:1009, 1968.

233. Baehner, R. L., Nathan, D. G., et al.: Oxidant injury of Caucasian glucose-6-phosphate dehydrogenase–deficient red blood cells by phagocytizing leukocytes during infection. J. Clin. Invest. *50*:12, 1971.

234. Cooper, M. R., DeChatelet, L. R., et al.: Complete deficiency of leukocyte G6PD with defective bactericidal activity. J. Clin. Invest. *51*:769, 1972.

234a. Gray, G. R., Klebanoff, S. J., et al.: Neutrophil dysfunction, chronic granulomatous disease, and non-spherocytic haemolytic anaemia caused by complete deficiency of glucose-6-phosphate dehydrogenase. Lancet *1*:530, 1973.

235. Bellanti, J. A., Cantz, B. E., et al.: Accelerated decay of glucose-6-phosphate dehydrogenase activity in chronic granulomatous disease. Pediatr. Res. *4*:405, 1970.

236. Baehner, R. L., Johnston, R. B., Jr., et al.: Comparative study of the metabolic and bactericidal characteristics of severe glucose-6-phosphate dehydrogenase–deficient polymorphonuclear leukocytes and leukocytes from children with chronic granulomatous disease. J. Reticuloendothel. Soc., 1974 *12*:150, 1972.

237. Mandell, G. L., Rubin, W., et al.: The effect of an NADH oxidase inhibitor (hydrocortisone) on polymorphonuclear leukocyte bactericidal activity. J. Clin. Invest. *49*:1381, 1970.

238. Malawista, S. E., and Bodel, P. T.: The dissociation by colchicine of phagocytosis from increased oxygen consumption in human leukocytes. J. Clin. Invest. *46*:786, 1967.

239. Malawista, E. E.: Vinblastine: Colchicine-like effects on human blood leukocytes during phagocytosis. Blood *37*:519, 1971.

240. Feigen, R. D., Shackelford, P. G., et al.: Nitroblue tetrazolium dye test as an aid in the differential diagnosis of febrile disorders. J. Pediatr. *78*:230, 1971.

241. Miller, M. E.: Phagocytosis in the newborn infant: Humoral and cellular factors. J. Pediatr. *74*:255, 1969.

242. Dossett, J. H., Williams, R. C., et al.: Studies on interaction of bacteria, serum factors, and polymorphonuclear leukocytes in mothers and newborns. Pediatrics *44*:49, 1969.

243. Cocchi, P., and Marianelli, L.: Phagocytosis and intracellular killing of *Pseudomonas aeruginosa* in premature infants. Helv. Paediatr. Acta *22*:100, 1967.

244. Coen, R., Grush, O., et al.: Studies of bactericidal activity and metabolism of the leukocyte in full-term neonates. J. Pediatr. *75*:400, 1969.

245. Park, B. H., Holmes, B., et al.: Metabolic activities in leukocytes of newborn infants. J. Pediatr. *76*:237, 1970.

246. Humbert, J. R., Kurtz, M. L., et al.: Increased reduction of nitroblue tetrazolium by neutrophils of newborn infants. Pediatrics *45*:125, 1970.

247. Cocchi, P. Mari, S., et al.: NBT tests in premature infants. Lancet *2*:1426, 1969.

Chapter 17

Infectious Mononucleosis and Other Disorders With Atypical Lymphocytes

by Robert L. Baehner

INTRODUCTION

Knowledge concerning the biology of the circulating lymphocyte and its role in infection has undergone rapid evolution since the early investigations of Maximow, Dominici, Pappenhein, and Downey. Until recently, circulating lymphocytes were viewed as "short-lived" cells with limited biological activity. Currently, the lymphocyte pool is known to be composed of cells with varying life spans, fates, fine structural features, and capabilities to mediate various immunologic functions. More than a decade ago, Nowell (1) reported that phytohemagglutinin prepared as crude extracts of red kidney bean *Phaseolus vulgaris*, caused small normal lymphocytes from the peripheral blood to undergo a series of morphologic changes to produce "blastlike" cells in tissue culture. This finding clearly indicated that circulating small lymphocytes were not "end-stage" but rather were resting cells capable of undergoing further differentiation, a process now referred to as lymphocyte transformation.

Striking morphologic similarities between atypical lymphocytes seen in the peripheral blood of patients with infectious mononucleosis and other viral infections and the spectrum of cell types present after transformation of the small lymphocyte by phytohemagglutinin in vitro have suggested that infectious mononucleosis is a disease involving transformed lymphocytes (2).

MORPHOLOGIC FEATURES OF ATYPICAL LYMPHOCYTES

The atypical lymphocyte of infectious mononucleosis was described in the classic paper by Downey and McKinlay (3). They recognized three types of atypical lymphocytes stained with Romanowsky dyes and visualized by light microscopy. Type I contained dark basophilic cytoplasm with vacuoles, an indented mature nucleus with dense nuclear chromatin, and a perinuclear clear zone. Type II contained lighter blue cytoplasm with less vacuoles, giving a "washed out" or "ground glass" appearance. The cell was larger; the nucleus was usually round, and the nuclear chromatin was coarse. The Type III cell was large with basophilic vacuolated cytoplasm; azurophilic rods were present in some of the large vacuoles, and the indented nucleus was immature with fine chromatin and prominent nucleoli. The latter type of cell was seen frequently in patients with leukemia, whereas the other two types of cells were not.

Further refinement of morphologic characteristics using the electron microscope (4) showed that the atypical lymphocyte had a greater cell and cytoplasmic area, greater cell length, more nucleoli than the normal lymphocyte, and was characterized by prominent polyribosomes and vacuoles in the cytoplasm. One of the most striking differences between normal lymphocytes and infectious mononucleosis lymphocytes was the number and appearance of free ribosomes in the latter cell type. When ribosomes did occur in normal lymphocytes, they were usually isolated, but in mononucleosis lymphocytes they occurred in clusters and rosettes considered to be polyribosomes. Lymphocytes stimulated by antigenic provocation called "immunoblasts" (5) also demonstrate increased free ribosomes with the appearance of polyribosomes.

Cells with the morphologic appearance of atypical lymphocytes have been observed in long-term cultures of lymphocytes obtained from the peripheral blood of patients with infectious mononucleosis as well as of patients with lymphoblastic leukemia (6), myelogenous leukemia (7), Hodgkin's lymphoma, lymphosarcoma, and multiple myeloma (8); rarely, atypical lymphocytes have been observed in the blood of healthy individuals. Infectious mononucleosis cell lines had one consistent fine structural feature not reported previously in cell lines derived from peripheral blood (9). Unusual cytoplasmic structures, consisting of a reticular array of 22-millimicron particles in association with rough endoplasmic reticulum, were present in a high percentage of cells. These small intracellular particles were viruslike and formed by an outer unit membrane structure containing central material of medium density. The significance of these cytoplasmic aggregates must still be established, since the electron microscopic identification of viruslike particles in cell cultures is only suggestive evidence of virus infection. They may represent cellular alterations resulting from infection with herpes-like virus. The ability to harvest these long-term cultures of lymphocytes from the peripheral blood of patients with infectious mononucleosis has been found to disappear when the clinical and laboratory parameters of the patient return toward normal (10–12).

Atypical lymphocytes of patients with infectious mononucleosis include a population of cells that are synthesizing DNA (13), as indicated by incorporation of ^{3}H-thymidine into nuclei. It has been estimated that 1 of 100 such cells in DNA synthesis divides per hour, whereas only one peripheral acute leukemia cell per 1000 cells divides per hour in vitro (14). Quantitation of DNA synthesis of lymphocytes from patients with infectious mononucleosis was found to be significantly greater than it was in other cells of lymphoid origin as well as in lymphocytes of normals and of patients with other illnesses. However, RNA and protein synthesis were not different from that of control cells (15).

Investigation of the biosynthetic capacities of continuous cell lines of infectious mononucleosis lymphocyte cultures revealed that they synthesize immunoglobulins with IgG, IgA, and IgM heavy polypeptide chain specificity. Infectious mononucleosis atypical lymphocytes that exhibit immunofluorescence with IgM antibodies are thought to be T cells (15a). The remainder are B cells (15b). Five to 20 per cent of the cells that reacted with fluorescent antiserum directed against antigenic determinants of human IgG also cross-reacted with the determinants common to IgA and IgM. Heterophil and heteroagglutinin activity for sheep, horse, and beef red cells could not be detected in the concentrated supernatants from these cell lines, even when individual cells were plaqued and examined for localized hemolysis in gel; neither 10S nor 7S hemolytic activity for sheep, pig, horse, or beef red cells could be detected (16).

These cells have a predominant diploid mode in chromosome analysis. About 50 per cent of the cells contained secondary constrictions of one or both long arms of Group C chromosomes. A smaller percentage of similar anomalies have been detected in long-term cultures of cells from patients with leukemia and Burkitt's lymphoma. It has not been determined whether these abnormalities are artifacts of long-term tissue culture or whether they represent the oncologic potential of the cells involved. The salient properties of the circulating atypical lymphocyte are listed in Figure 17–1.

LYMPHOID RESPONSE IN INFECTIOUS MONONUCLEOSIS

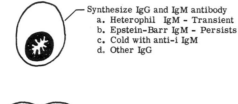

CIRCULATING
ATYPICAL
LYMPHOCYTE

— Increased polyribosomes
— Active DNA synthesis
— Replicating
— Easily grown in tissue culture
    a. Synthesize IgG, IgA, IgM
    b. Chromosomal changes
    c. Contain ? virus particles

TISSUE
PLASMA
CELL

— Synthesize IgG and IgM antibody
    a. Heterophil IgM - Transient
    b. Epstein-Barr IgM - Persists
    c. Cold with anti-i IgM
    d. Other IgG

Figure 17-1. Schematic representation of the lymphoid response in infectious mononucleosis. See text for further details.

LYMPH
NODE

Variable
Pattern

— Lymphoid hyperplasia
— Reticulum cell hyperplasia
— Rare Reed-Sternberg-like cell

DISORDERS CHARACTERIZED BY ATYPICAL LYMPHOCYTES

Infectious Mononucleosis

Clinical Manifestations

The course of illness may be divided into three distinct periods. During the first week or prodromic period, irregular fever, mild sore throat, headache, and nonspecific malaise predominate. By the second week, fever is more regular, cervical nodes become enlarged, and pharyngitis may be marked. Less than 10 per cent of the patients have anorexia, jaundice, and abdominal discomfort related to liver involvement. This phase of the illness usually lasts one to two weeks and is followed by a period of convalescence. Ninety per cent of the patients note that their symptoms have receded by the end of six weeks. In general, children have a shorter convalescent phase than adults.

A summary of the physical findings of children with infectious mononucleosis is listed in Table 17-1. Fever and lymphadenopathy are the hallmarks of this disease. The cervical lymph nodes, especially the posterior chains, are most always involved, and generalized adenopathy is noted frequently. The nodes are moderately tender, and moderate degrees of enlargement persist for several weeks after the symptoms subside. Exudate associated with pharyngitis is seen in approximately one-half the cases. Pharyngeal inflammation may produce disturbing subjective symptoms; mild edema of the uvula frequently occurs, and the gums may become swollen and tender with occasional bleeding. Multiple small petechiae may occur near the junction of the hard and soft palates. Often liver function abnormalities will reveal hepatic involvement when the liver is not palpable. There may be edema of the eyelids. Skin rash, jaundice, and neurologic

TABLE 17-1. PHYSICAL FINDINGS IN CHILDREN WITH INFECTIOUS MONONUCLEOSIS

Lymphadenopathy	83%
Cervical	46%
Generalized	34%
Fever	86%
Pharyngitis	57%
Exudate	29%
Splenomegaly	47%
Hepatomegaly	28%
Edema of eyelids	10%
Rash	8%
Jaundice	5%
Neurologic symptoms	1%

From Baehner, R. L., and Shuler, S. E.: Clin. Pediatr. 6:393, 1967.

symptoms are found in less than 10 per cent of the cases. Splenomegaly may be present more frequently than suspected if repeated examinations are performed (17). However, liver enlargement is not as frequent as spleen enlargement in most individual series. In general, the frequency of physical abnormalities is similar for adults and children. Skin rash, jaundice, and neurologic symptoms are also infrequent in the adult age group. Rashes may be attributed to drugs, since drugs are frequently administered to these patients during their infection (18). The neurologic abnormality may range from acute meningoencephalitis to facial diplegia, mononeuritis, and the Guillian-Barré syndrome. Electrocardiographic abnormalities have been reported in 4 of 39 children without cardiac symptoms. These returned to normal following recovery. Occasionally, children may have otitis media following their illness. Spontaneous rupture of the spleen occurs infrequently, but may occur at any phase of the illness (19, 20).

Laboratory Manifestations

Leukopenia due to reduction in total numbers of circulating granulocytes may be present at the onset and throughout the illness (21), but the total white blood count usually rises during the febrile stage of the illness. A range from 5000 to 25,000 per mm.³ is usual; total leukocyte counts above 40,000 per mm.³ are unusual. During the early phase of the illness, leukocyte alkaline phosphatase is normal in infectious mononucleosis but is elevated in bacterial pharyngitis (22). Following the first 48 hours of illness in which polymorphonuclear leukocytes predominate, there is a gradual increase in the number of mononuclear cells, so that by the end of the first week there is a mononuclear leukocytosis, with the development of many atypical lymphocytes. These cells are suggestive of, but not diagnostic of, infectious mononucleosis. They have been seen with other viral diseases, such as viral hepatitis, viral pneumonia, herpes zoster, herpes simplex, roseola, rubeola, rubella, and influenza Type B. They also have been encountered in patients with lymphoma, leukemia, rickettsial pox, undulent fever, and certain allergic diseases, and even occasionally in normal persons (23). In all these conditions, however, there are usually fewer atypical lymphocytes than in infectious mononucleosis. Patients with infectious mononucleosis have more than 25 per cent atypical lymphocytes on at least one blood smear examination, whereas patients with the other viral illnesses tend to have less than 15 per cent atypical lymphocytes. Atypical lymphocytes in the bone marrow of individuals with infectious mononucleosis are rarely noted (24).

Anemia directly related to infectious mononucleosis is rare, but a few patients have developed autoimmune hemolytic anemia with jaundice, a positive Coombs' reaction, and increased concentrations of cold agglutinins and anti-i antibody (25). Although severe hemolysis is rare, 25 per cent of patients with proven infectious mononucleosis may have an increased rate of red cell destruction, and 80 per cent exhibit some degree of spherocytosis on peripheral blood smear (26). Thus evidence for occult hemolysis may be obtained in a large percentage of such patients. Symptomatic thrombocytopenia is rare in this disease. Slight platelet depression has been noted in approximately 25 per cent of the patients during the third week of illness (27). Most instances of mild thrombocytopenia are probably related to redistribution of platelets secondary to enlargement of the spleen. However, in some patients thrombocytopenia results from immune destruction.

The immunopathology of mononucleosis has been recently reviewed (27a). Pathologic examination of the lymph nodes from patients with infectious mononucleosis shows a variable pattern. In general, the node is enlarged, and the architecture is preserved. At times, considerable distortion may result from either hyperplasia of cortical follicles or, more strikingly, engorgement by pleomorphic reticulum cells in the paracortical (thymus-dependent) areas (27b). Occasionally, the node contains giant cells not distinguishable from Reed-Sternberg cells (28, 29). Hence the diagnosis of Hodgkin's disease may be seriously entertained. With the use of immunofluorescent techniques, IgM macroglobulin and IgG globulin synthesis has been localized to plasmacytoid cells present in lymph nodes and bone marrow (30). These responses of the lymphoid system in infectious mononucleosis are summarized in Figure 17–1.

Determination of Heterophil Antibodies

The original serologic test for infectious mononucleosis was based upon the observation that sera from patients with infectious mononucleosis contained high concentrations of an antibody capable of agglutinating suspensions of sheep erythrocytes (31). Davidson demonstrated that antibody specific for infectious mononucleosis differed from other heterophil antibodies by being absorbed completely by beef erythrocytes (32). A presumptive agglutination test using unabsorbed serum and sheep erythrocytes may be positive in sera of patients with viral hepatitis, viral pneumonia, lymphoma, leukemia, tuberculosis, serum sickness, and after immunizations with A and B blood group antigens. However, these antibodies will be absorbed completely by Forssman antigens. Heterophil titer readings generally accepted as positive are 1:56 or higher for the presumptive or Paul-Bunnell titer, and 1:28 or higher after guinea pig absorption (33).

In addition to heterophil antibodies, sera from patients with infectious mononucleosis may contain an unusual diversity of antibodies, such as cold agglutinins with anti-i specificity (34), cardiolipin flocculating antibodies causing biological false-positive tests for syphilis (35), anti-IgG macroglobulins resembling rheumatoid factor (36), and antinuclear antibodies (37). More than 35 years ago, Belk (38) predicted that a heterogeneous array of antibodies would be found in this disease. Only 5 per cent of the elevated IgM immunoglobulin can be accounted for by the heterophil antibody; the remainder are likely general cold antibodies to red cells (39). Kostinas and Cantow have found that virtually all their patients studied had red cell antibodies other than heterophil antibody detectable in their sera. The majority of these antibodies were cold antibodies reacting at less than body temperature (40). IgM and IgA antibody levels peak in the serum earlier than IgG antibodies, with a delay of

approximately two to three weeks noted for the latter. Cryoglobulinemia has been consistently identified with the elevation in IgM antibody (41). Thus, in infectious mononucleosis, there appears to be a generalized immunoproliferation characterized by an increased variety of serum antibodies, especially of the IgM type.

Recent Development in Clinical Testing for the Detection of Antibody in Infectious Mononucleosis

Lee and co-workers have recently described a simple but sensitive slide test for the diagnosis of infectious mononucleosis. They had shown previously that horse erythrocytes contributed to higher sensitivity and specificity than did sheep erythrocytes for the serologic diagnosis of infectious mononucleosis if the appropriate absorption tests were done (42). It is now possible to confirm the diagnosis of infectious mononucleosis serologically in just two minutes. The spot test requires mixing two separate drops of the patient's serum with different antigens before adding the serum to horse erythrocytes. One drop of serum is mixed with a suspension of guinea pig kidney, which removes human antibodies to horse erythrocytes; antibodies specific for mononucleosis are not absorbed. Any agglutination with horse red cells would then indicate a positive test. The other drop of serum is added to beef erythrocytes, which absorb infectious mononucleosis antibodies, so that no agglutination occurs when it is added to horse erythrocytes. This differential procedure makes the test highly specific, simple to perform, and suitable for large scale studies and for testing individual patients in small hospital laboratories.

Evidence for Viral Etiology

Infectious mononucleosis remains one of the few common infectious diseases in which the causative agent has yet to be conclusively identified. Although infections caused by agents such as cytomegalovirus, adenovirus, and *Toxoplasma gondii* may occasionally produce an infectious mononucleosis-like syndrome, infections by these organisms do not result in the development of heterophil antibodies.

Recent studies indicate that a member of the herpes group of viruses, the Epstein-Barr (EB) virus, is closely associated with infectious mononucleosis, although it is not yet possible to determine conclusively whether it is the cause. The EB virus was first detected by Epstein in continuous lymphoblastic cell cultures originally derived from a child with Burkitt's East African lymphoma, a malignant tumor involving lymphoid tissue, most often affecting children and occurring in East Africa and tropical areas in the West Indies, New Guinea, and parts of South America (43). Although this virus possesses morphologic characteristics of the herpes group, it lacks antigens common to the other herpes groups which infect both man and other animals. Although Burkitt's tumor is rare in the United States, antibody to EB virus was encountered frequently (44). The sera of 80 per cent of adults and 50 per cent of children, ages 2 to 4 years, were positive. In 1967, a technician in Dr. Henle's laboratory, who had previously been shown to have serum devoid of antibodies to EB virus and in whom attempts to culture leukocytes had been unsuccessful, developed infectious mononucleosis. Following her illness, not only did she develop EB virus antibodies, but it became possible to culture her leukocytes. One to 3 per cent of these cultured leukocytes contained EB virus antigen (45). This chance observation led to examination of sequentially collected sera obtained from freshmen at Yale University and stored in the expectation that some of these students would develop infectious mononucleosis. Following their illness, all developed significant rises in antibody titer to the EB virus, ranging from a titer of 1:40 to 1:640. Furthermore, EB virus antibody and heterophil antibody developed and reached peak levels at approximately the same time, but heterophil antibodies usually declined to undetectable levels within two to three months, whereas the EB virus antibodies persisted. Absorption studies showed that heterophil and EB antibodies were quite distinct from one another. Further investigations at Yale showed that some patients with clinical and hematologic features consistent with infectious mononucleosis, but whose sera were persistently heterophil antibody–negative, had rising or high antibody titers to EB virus, suggesting that they were true cases of infectious mononucleosis (46).

Antibody to EB virus is generally detected by employing an indirect immunofluorescence test using continuous EB virus–containing lymphoblastic cell cultures as an antigen. Dilutions of patients' sera and a potent antihuman IgG conjugate are added. The cells fluoresce if EB virus antibody is present in patients' sera (47). Antibody to EB virus may also be detected by a complement fixation test, and these antibodies parallel those detected by immunofluorescence (48). Whether EB virus itself directly causes infectious mononucleosis may be resolved by recovering virus from patients in the acute stage of infection and transmitting it to healthy volunteers who in turn develop illness or at least excrete the virus and develop serologic evidence of infection. Toward that end, lymphocytes from a donor negative for Epstein-Barr virus have been transformed with throat swab material taken from a case of infectious mononucleosis. These cells contain herpes virus particles only after they have been transformed. It is likely that EB virus present in oral secretions provoked these changes (49).

Infectious Mononucleosis and Acute Leukemia

Despite speculation that infectious mononucleosis could be an abortive form of acute lymphocytic leukemia, nine cases that developed both diseases concurrently have now been reported in the literature. In some cases, infectious mononucleosis preceded the onset of acute leukemia, and in others it occurred at various times during hematologic remission. This suggests that infectious mononucleosis is an intercurrent illness which is etiologically unrelated to acute leukemia (50).

Other Infections with Atypical Lymphocytes

Postperfusion Syndrome

The advent of the cardiopulmonary bypass technique employed in open heart surgery has resulted in the recognition of an infectious mononucleosis–like syndrome characterized by fever, splenomegaly, and atypical lymphocytes three to six weeks after operation. Atypical lymphocytes in the blood of patients after extracorporeal circulation was first described in 1958 (51, 52). The postperfusion syndrome has been diagnosed in 3 to 11 per cent of patients submitted to open heart surgery. Biological studies have recovered cytomegalovirus from these patients. Complement fixing antibodies to cytomegalovirus can also be detected in these patients (53). Furthermore, antibodies to Epstein-Barr virus have been found in 8 per cent of patients undergoing open heart surgery with or without extracorporeal circulation. No overt illness developed in 6 of 18 of these patients with anti-EB virus antibody who previously lacked the antibody prior to their perfusion operation (54).

Acquired Cytomegalic Inclusion Disease (C.I.D.)

Until recently, little has been known about the clinical manifestations of postnatally acquired C.I.D. infection. Although most C.I.D. infections may be inapparent, there is now good evidence that acquired C.I.D. infection not uncommonly produces various clinical symptoms, especially in young children. Clinical manifestations in children include hepatitis, hepatosplenomegaly, and chronic liver disease (55–57), as well as a pertussis-like illness, bronchitis, and pneumonia (58). Pneumonia has been found to be a common manifestation of C.I.D. infection in patients of all ages after renal homotransplantation. Acquired C.I.D. infection is sometimes manifested clinically as an acute febrile illness with the hematologic features of infectious mononucleosis with tonsillitis or enlargement of the lymph nodes but without a positive heterophil agglutination test. Involvement of the liver, sometimes with jaundice as a presenting sign, seems to be a regular feature of this disease which occurs in previously healthy individuals, particularly adults, but also after massive blood transfusions in which fresh blood has been used (59). On the other hand, Starr et al. have reported 26 infants born during 12 months at a general hospital who had congenital cytomegalovirus infection. Clinically apparent signs of cytomegalic inclusion disease were present in only one infected infant. The birth weight of nine infected infants was less than 2500 g., but the occurrence of neonatal problems, such as jaundice and hepatosplenomegaly, was similar to that found among unaffected control infants. During a mean follow-up of eight months, unfavorable clinical outcome was observed in three infected infants with low birth weights, and no unfavorable outcome was observed in the controls. However, it is unlikely that inapparent congenital cytomegalovirus infection will explain a high percentage of neonatal problems, such as jaundice, organomegaly, and congenital anomalies (60).

Other Infectious and Noninfectious Causes of Atypical Lymphocytes

A parasitic infection, toxoplasmosis (61, 62), may resemble infectious mononucleosis in all respects. Infectious and serum hepatitis may be associated with atypical lymphocytes. Noninfectious systemic diseases, such as the hypersensitivity reaction, serum sickness (63), and diphenylhydantoin toxicity (64), may produce peripheral blood findings similar to those in infectious mononucleosis. Atypical lymphocytes as well as plasma cells appear in the blood.

Clinical Management of the Patient With Infectious Mononucleosis

Specific treatment is not required for most patients with mononucleosis or the other mononucleosis-like illnesses. Bed rest appropriate to the degree of morbidity and antipyretics will suffice in most instances. It is important to recognize the development of secondary bacterial infection or unusually severe manifestations or complications of the illness for which specific treatment would be mandatory. Superimposed beta-hemolytic streptococcal pharyngitis has been associated with infectious mononucleosis. Severe respiratory distress due to lymphoidal hypertrophy of the nasal airway occurs in some cases and seems to respond rather dramatically to steroid therapy. Although steroid therapy may shorten the duration of fever, it is not indicated except for treatment of specific complications, such as hemolytic anemia and thrombocytopenia (65, 66), and the above described airway obstruction.

References

1. Nowell, P. C.: Phytohemagglutinin: An initiator of mitosis in cultures of normal human leukocytes. Cancer Res. 20:462, 1960.

2. Chessin, L. N.: The circulating lymphocyte—Its role in infectious mononucleosis. Ann. Intern. Med. 69:333, 1968.

3. Downey, H., and McKinlay, C. A.: Acute lymphadenosis compared with acute leukemia. Arch. Intern. Med. 32:82, 1923.

4. Schumacher, H. R., McFeeley, A. E., et al.: The mononucleosis cell. III. Electron microscopy. Blood 33:6, 1969.

5. Dameshek, W.: "Immunoblasts" and "immunocytes" in an attempt at a functional nomenclature. Blood 21:243, 1963.

6. Moore, G. E., Ito, E., et al.: Culture of human leukemic cells. Cancer 19:713, 1966.

7. Iwakata, S., and Grace, J.: Cultivation in vitro of myeloblasts from human leukemia. N.Y. State J. Med. 64:2279, 1964.

8. Moore, G. E., Grace, J. T., et al.: Leukocyte cultures of patients with leukemia and lymphomas. N.Y. State J. Med. 66:2757, 1966.

9. Moses, H. L., Glade, P. R., et al.: Infectious mononucleosis: Detection of herpes-like virus and reticular aggregates of small cytoplasmic particles in continuous lymphoid cell lines derived from peripheral blood. Proc. Natl. Acad. Sci. USA 60:489, 1968.

10. Glade, P. R., Hirshaut, Y., et al.: Infectious mononucleosis: In vitro evidence from limited lymphoproliferation. Blood 33:292, 1968.

11. Epstein, L. B., and Brecher, G.: DNA and RNA synthesis of circulating atypical lymphocytes in infectious mononucleosis. Blood 25:197, 1965.

12. Hale, A. J., and Cooper, E. H.: DNA synthesis in infectious mononucleosis and acute leukemia. Acta Haematol. (Basel) 29:257, 1963.

13. MacKinney, A. A.: Division of leukocytes already in DNA synthesis from patients with acute leukemia and infectious mononucleosis. Acta Haematol. (Basel) 38:163, 1967.

14. Besser, G. M., Davis, J., et al.: Glandular fever and specific viral infections: Uptake of tritiated thymidine by circulating leukocytes. Br. J. Haematol. 13:189, 1967.

15. Burns, C. P., and Stjernholm, R. L.: Metabolism of the lymphocyte in infectious mononucleosis. J. Reticuloendothel. Soc. 9:323, 1971.

15a. Thomas, D. B.: Antibodies to membrane antigen(s) common to thymocytes and a subpopulation of lymphocytes in infectious-mononucleosis sera. Lancet 1:399, 1972.

15b. Thomas, D. B., and Phillips, B.: Evidence for membrane antigen(s) specific for human B lymphoblasts. Clin. Exp. Immunol. 14:91, 1973.

16. Chessen, L. N., et al.: The circulating lymphocyte: Its role in infectious mononucleosis. Ann. Intern. Med. 69:333, 1968.

17. MacIntyre, O. R., and Ebahl, F. G., Jr.: Palpable spleens in college freshmen. Ann. Intern. Med. 66:301, 1967.

18. Baehner, R. L., and Shuler, S. E.: Infectious mononucleosis in childhood. Clinical expressions, serologic findings, complications, and prognosis. Clin. Pediatr. 6:393, 1967.

19. Hoagland, R.J., and Henson, H. M.: Splenic rupture in infectious mononucleosis. Ann. Intern. Med. 46:1184, 1957.

20. Dalrymple, W.: Systemic effects of mononucleosis. Postgrad. Med. 43:158, 1968.

21. Cantow, E. F., and Kostinas, J. E.: Studies on infectious mononucleosis. IV. Changes in the granulocytic series. J. Clin. Pathol. 46:43, 1966.

22. Sramkova, L., Kouba, K., et al.: Alkaline phosphatase in neutrophil leukocytes of patients with infectious mononucleosis and the effect of corticosteroid therapy. Blood 26:479, 1965.

23. Litwins, J., and Leibowitz, S.: Abnormal lymphocytes ("virocytes") in virus diseases other than infectious mononucleosis. Acta Haematol. (Basel) 5:225, 1951.

24. Lenzarne, L. R., Paul, J. T., et al.: Blood and bone marrow in infectious mononucleosis. J. Lab. Clin. Med. 31:1079, 1946.

25. Deagon, J. G., Skaggs, H., Jr., et al.: Acute hemolytic anemia complicating infectious mononucleosis: The mechanism of hemolysis. Tex. Rep. Biol. Med. 25:309, 1967.

26. Kostinas, J. E., and Cantow, E. F.: Studies on infectious mononucleosis. II. Autohemolysis. Am. J. Med. Sci. 252:296, 1966.

27. Cantow, E. F., and Kostinas, J. E.: Studies on infectious mononucleosis. III. Platelets. Am. J. Med. Sci. 251:64, 1966.

27a. Immunopathology of infectious mononucleosis. Lancet, 2:712, 1973.

27b. Carter, R. L., In Oncogenesis and Herpes Viruses. Biggs, P. M., deThe, G., and Payne, L. N. (eds.), Lyon, I.A.R.C. Scientific Publications No. 2, 1972, p. 230.

28. Lukes, J., Tindle, B. H., et al.: Reed-Sternberg-like cells in infectious mononucleosis. Lancet 2:1003, 1969.

29. McMahon, N. J., Gordon, H. W., et al.: Reed-Sternberg cells in infectious mononucleosis. Am. J. Dis. Child. 120:148, 1970.

30. Carter, R. L.: Infectious mononucleosis: Some observations on the cellular localization of immune globulin synthesis. Am. J. Clin. Pathol. 45:574, 1966.

31. Paul, J. R., and Bunnel, W. W.: The presence of heterophil antibodies in infectious mononucleosis. Am. J. Med. Sci. 183:90, 1932.

32. Davidson, I.: Serologic diagnosis of infectious mononucleosis. J.A.M.A. 108:289, 1937.

33. Hoagland, R. J.: The clinical manifestations of infectious mononucleosis: A report of 200 cases. Am. J. Med. Sci. 240:21, 1960.

34. Jenkins, H. J., Koster, H. G., et al.: Infectious mononucleosis: An unsuspected source of anti-i. Br. J. Haematol. *11*:480, 1965.

35. Bernstein, A.: False-positive Wasserman reactions in infectious mononucleosis. Am. J. Med. Sci. *196*:79, 1938.

36. Carter, R. L.: Antibody formation in infectious mononucleosis. II. Other 19S antibodies and false-positive serology. Br. J. Haematol. *12*: 268, 1966.

37. Kaplan, M. E., and Tan, E. M.: Antinuclear antibodies in infectious mononucleosis. Lancet *1*:651, 1968.

38. Belk, W. P.: Minor hemagglutinins: Study of a single human blood containing autoagglutinin, heteroagglutinins, hemolysins and a rouleaux-forming substance. J. Lab. Clin. Med. *20*:1035, 1935.

39. Wollhein, F. A., and Williams, R. C., Jr.: Studies on the macroglobulins of human serum. I. Polyclonal immunoglobulin class M (IgM) increase in infectious mononucleosis. New Engl. J. Med. *274*:61, 1966.

40. Kostinas, J. E., and Cantow, E. F.: Studies on infectious mononucleosis. I. Antibodies. Am. J. Med. Sci. *252*:125, 1966.

41. Kaplan, M. E.: Cryoglobulinemia in infectious mononucleosis: Quantitation and characterization of the cryoproteins. J. Lab. Clin. Med. *71*:754, 1968.

42. Lee, C. L., Davidson, I., et al.: Horse agglutinins in infectious mononucleosis. II. The spot test. Am. J. Clin. Pathol. *49*:12, 1968.

43. Epstein, M. W., Barr, Y. M., et al.: Studies with Burkitt's lymphoma. Wistar Inst. Symp. Monogr. *4*:69, 1965.

44. Henle, G., and Henle, W.: Immunofluorescence: Interference and complement fixation techniques in the detection of herpes-type virus in Burkitt tumor cell lines. Cancer Res. *27*: 2442, 1967.

45. Henle, G., Henle, W., et al.: Relation of Burkitt's tumor–associated herpes-type virus to infectious mononucleosis. Proc. Natl. Acad. Sci. USA *59*:94, 1968.

46. Evans, A. S., Niederman, J. C., et al.: Seroepidemiological studies of infectious mononucleosis with EB virus. New Engl. J. Med. *279*: 1121, 1968.

47. Banatvala, J. E.: Infectious mononucleosis: Recent developments. Br. J. Haematol. *19*:129, 1970.

48. Gerber, P., Hamredmoy, R. A., et al.: Infectious mononucleosis: Complement fixing antibodies to herpes-like virus associated with Burkitt lymphoma. Science *169*:173, 1968.

49. Perqua, M. S., Blake, J. M., et al.: Evidence for viral excretion of EB virus in infectious mononucleosis. Lancet *1*:710, 1972.

50. Freedman, M. H., Gilchrist, G. S., et al.: Concurrent infectious mononucleosis and acute leukemia. J.A.M.A. *214*:1677, 1970.

51. Kreel, I., Zaroff, L. I., et al.: A syndrome following total body perfusion. Surg. Gynecol. Obstet. *111*:317, 1960.

52. Battle, J. E., Jr., and Hewlett, J. S.: Hematologic changes observed after extracorporeal circulation during open-heart surgery. Cleve. Clin. Q. 25:112, 1958.

53. Lang, D. J., and Henshaw, J. B.: Cytomegalic virus infection in the post-perfusion syndrome. Recognition of primary infections in four patients. New Engl. J. Med. *280*:1145, 1969.

54. Henle, W., Henle, G., et al.: Antibody responses to the Epstein virus and cytomegaloviruses after open-heart and other surgery. New Engl. J. Med. *282*:1068, 1970.

55. Row, R., Rhode, W. P., et al.: Detection of human salivary gland virus in the mouth and urine of children. Am. J. Hyg. 67:57, 1958.

56. Henshaw, J. B., Betts, R. F., et al.: Acquired cytomegalovirus infection: Association with hepatosplenomegaly and abnormal liver function tests. New Engl. J. Med. *272*:602, 1965.

57. Stern, H.: Isolation of cytomegalovirus and clinical manifestations of infection at different ages. Br. J. Haematol. *1*:665, 1968.

58. Henshaw, J. B.: Congenital acquired cytomegalovirus infection. Pediatr. Clin. North Am. *13*: 279, 1966.

59. Klemola, E., Von Essen, R., et al.: Cytomegalovirus mononucleosis in previously healthy individuals. Five new cases and follow-up of 13 previously published cases. Ann. Intern. Med. *71*:11, 1969.

60. Starr, J. G., Bart, R. D., Jr., et al.: Inapparent congenital cytomegalovirus infection. Clinical and epidemiologic characteristics in early infancy. New Engl. J. Med. *282*:1075, 1970.

61. Remington, J. S., Barnett, C. G., et al.: Toxoplasmosis and infectious mononucleosis. Arch. Intern. Med. *110*:744, 1962.

62. Eshchar, J., Warren, M., et al.: Syndromes of acute fever. J.A.M.A. *195*:390, 1966.

63. Schmidt, J. J., Robinson, H. J., et al.: Peripheral plasmacytosis serum sickness. Ann. Intern. Med. 59:542, 1963.

64. Holland, P., and Maurer, A. M.: Diphenylhydantoin-induced hypersensitivity reaction. J. Pediatr. 66:322, 1965.

65. Schumacher, H. R., Jacobson, W. A., et al.: Treatment of infectious mononucleosis. Ann. Intern. Med. 58:217, 1963.

66. Bender, C. E.: The value of cortical steroids in the treatment of infectious mononucleosis. J.A.M.A. *199*:529, 1967.

Chapter 18

The Primary Immunodeficiencies and the Serum Complement Defects

by Fred S. Rosen, Chester A. Alper, and Charles A. Janeway

Immunity results from many interacting mechanisms which may be specific or non-specific. The failure of one or another *specific* immunity mechanism results in immunodeficiency disease. It has been known for two decades that there is a clear-cut dichotomy between cellular and humoral immunity. This division of labor in the immune response has a cellular and architectural basis (Fig. 18–1), and very recently methods have been developed to identify the various lymphoidal cells which are responsible for humoral or cellular immunity. Those lymphocytes which mediate cellular immunity are called T lymphocytes, because they are *t*hymus-dependent for their competence. Cells which differentiate to synthesize and secrete immunoglobulins are designated B cells, as they are derived from the *b*one marrow or the *b*ursa of Fabricius in avian species. The cells tend to differ with respect to their morphology (Fig. 18–2). Immunodeficiencies may be classified according to their B or T cell deficits or both (1).

B lymphocytes have membrane-bound immunoglobulins and receptors for aggregated IgG and the third component of complement (C3). Between 15 and 25 per cent of circulating lymphocytes have these surface markers. If blood lymphocytes are incubated in the cold with fluorescein-labeled antiserum to one of the immunoglobulins, speckled fluorescence appears on the surface of the B cells bearing that immunoglobulin. Approximately 8 to 14 per cent are positive with anti-IgG, 3 to 7 per cent with anti-IgM, and 0.5 to 2 per cent with anti-IgA. The surface immunoglobulins of B cells can be removed with trypsin, but the B cells replenish the surface immunoglobulin in approximately six hours in in vitro cultures (2). B cells form rosettes with sheep red cells (E) coated with antibody (A) and the first four reacting components of complement, EAC1423 (3). The number of rosette-forming cells is equivalent to the total number of lymphocytes with surface immunoglobulins as detected with immunofluorescence. Heat-aggregated IgG, labeled with fluorescein or rhodamine, also adheres to B cells.

B cells can be separated from T cells on density gradients because the former are more dense (4). B cells isolated from the blood can be forced in vitro to synthesize and secrete immunoglobulins following mitotic provocation by pokeweed mitogen or the mitogen produced by normal T cells upon their contact with antigen (5).

It has already been pointed out that T cells are less dense than B cells, more numerous, and lacking in surface immunoglobulins and surface receptors for C3 and aggregated IgG. On the other hand, T cells form rosettes with unsensitized sheep erythrocytes (E). In the cold, 55 to 75 per cent of blood lymphocytes form E rosettes (6). In mice, specific antisera have been pro-

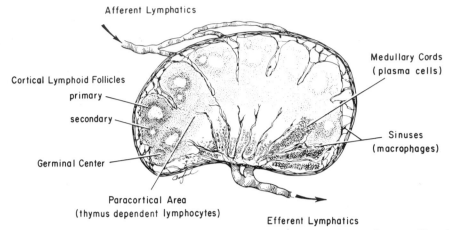

Figure 18–1.   Schematic diagram of a lymph node. Note the different sites for B (plasma cell) and T cell production.

duced to T cells or the so-called theta (θ) antigen of T cells (7). Nothing analogous to θ antigen has been found in human T lymphocytes, but several groups of markers have been used to make antisera specific for human T cells. T cells enlarge and convert to blast-like cells, and divide under a variety of conditions. Nonspecific mitogens, such as phytohemagglutinin and concanavalin A, are specific for T cells, whereas pokeweed mitogen stimulates both B and T cells. Antigens such as PPD, *Candida*, trichophytin, or streptokinase will also provoke mitosis in T cells from sensitized individuals. Allogeneic cells also stimulate T cell mitosis—the so-called mixed lymphocyte reaction (8). Responses to all these mitotic stimuli can be quantitated by assay of ^{3}H-thymidine incorporation into newly synthesized DNA.

Stimulated T cells release a variety of mediators which are generally low molecular weight proteins. Among them are the aforementioned mitogen for B cells, a factor which arrests macrophage migration (MIF), chemotaxins for PMN's and monocytes, interferon, and yet other poorly defined substances. Any one of these factors can be assayed in vitro as a measure of cellular immunity (9). However, nothing has replaced the skin test as a simple and reliable measure of cellular immunity.

Sensitized lymphocytes can turn into killer cells upon exposure to allogeneic cells. It is not yet clear whether these killer cells are T cells, B cells, or from another subpopulation of lymphoidal elements.

THE IMMUNOGLOBULINS

The secretory products of terminally differentiated B lymphocytes are the immunoglobulins. They comprise the most heterogeneous group of proteins in the blood, but nonetheless a great deal is known about their structure. The Nobel prize in medicine was awarded in 1972 to Rodney Porter and Gerald Edelman for their pioneering contributions to the elucidation of immunoglobulin structure (10, 11). All immunoglobulins share a common structural plan. They are composed of two light or L chains and two heavy or H chains. The molecules are symmetrical about their long axis. Immunoglobulins can be divided into five classes, designated IgG, IgA, IgM, IgD, and IgE. Some of their physical and biological characteristics are shown in Tables 18–1 and 18–2. Each class has a unique heavy chain, designated γ for IgG, α for IgA, μ for IgM, δ for IgD, and ϵ for IgE. Light chains are of only two types, kappa (κ) and lambda (λ). An immunoglobulin is composed of two identical H and two identical L chains. Thus molecular formulas can be written for all possible immunoglobulins, as for hemoglobin, *sic* $\gamma_2\kappa_2$ or $\delta_2\lambda_2$, or $\alpha_2\kappa_2$, and so forth. Subclasses of IgG and IgA are now recognized. There are four for IgG and two for IgA. Thus there are $\gamma1$, $\gamma2$, $\gamma3$, and $\gamma4$ chains, and $\alpha1$ and $\alpha2$ chains. To be more precise, an IgG molecule might be written: $\gamma4_2\kappa_2$ or $\gamma2_2\lambda_2$. Similarly, an IgA molecule might be $\alpha2_2\kappa_2$, and so forth.

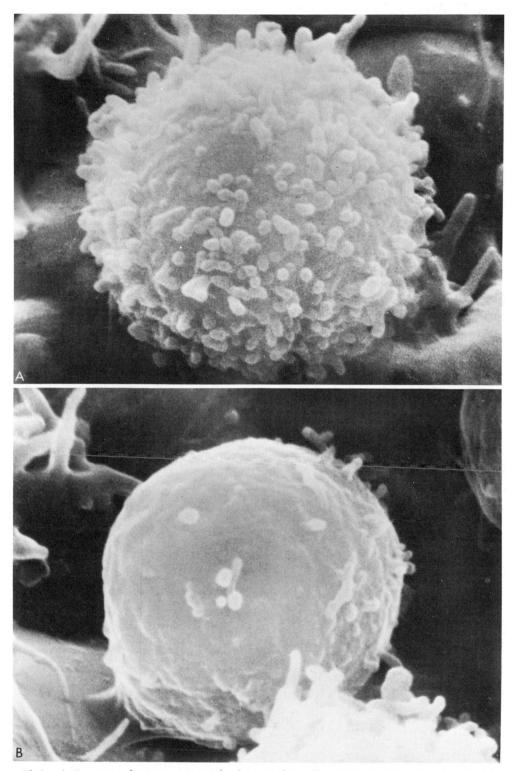

Figure 18–2. *A*, Scanning electron micrograph of a typical B cell, with its fimbriated surface. *B*, A typical T cell, with its relatively smooth surface. (From Bentalich, Z., Siegel, F. P., et al.: J. Exp. Med. *138*:607, 1973.)

TABLE 18–1. QUANTITATION AND METABOLISM OF IMMUNOGLOBULINS IN MAN

IMMUNOGLOBULIN	SERUM CONCENTRATION, MG./100 ML.	% TOTAL BODY POOL IN PLASMA	$t_{1/2}$ DAYS	% PLASMA POOL CATABOLIZED PER DAY	SYNTHETIC RATE, MG./KG./DAY
IgG	600–1500	45	23	6.7	33
IgA	200–300	42	5.8	25	24
IgM	75–150	76	5.1	18	6.7
IgD	0–3	75	2.8	37	0.4
IgE	~0.05	51	2.5	89	0.016

From Rosen, F. S., and Merler, E.: Genetic defects in gamma-globulin synthesis, In *The Metabolic Basis of Inherited Disease*. 3rd ed. Stanbury, J. B., Wyngaarden, J. B., et al. (eds.), New York, McGraw-Hill, 1972, p. 1645.

Light chains are composed of 220 amino acid residues and are attached to the N-terminal half of heavy chains (440 residues) by a single interchain disulfide bond (Fig. 18–3). Heavy chains are joined to each other at their center by two to five interchain disulfide bonds, depending on their class or subclass. The center of the heavy chain is called the hinge region and is susceptible to proteolysis. IgG molecules can be cleaved by pepsin into three fragments, two of which are designated Fab fragments, and one an Fc fragment (10). Fab fragments are composed of one light chain and one N-terminal half of a heavy chain. Fc fragments are composed of the C-terminal halves of the two heavy chains. The antibody combining sites reside in the two Fab fragments and not in the Fc fragment.

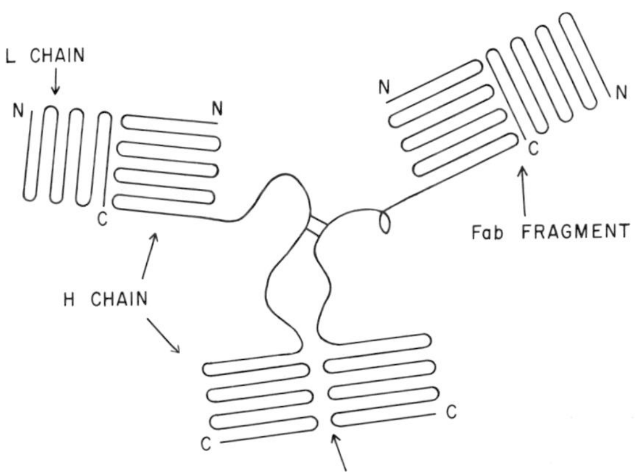

To be more precise, the combining site lies in the N-terminal half of the L and H chains of the Fab fragment. These are called the variable regions and constitute the first 110 amino acid residues of the N-termini of H and L chains. Two hypervariable regions can be located on each H and L chain in the variable region, and these four hypervariable regions must constitute the combining site which renders the immunoglobulin specific (12). The C-terminal half of L chains and the C-terminal three quarters of H chains are remarkably similar in antibodies within any class or subclass. They are thus called the constant regions. At least two genes, then, are required for immunoglobulin synthesis, a V gene and a C gene for the variable and constant segments.

The sites responsible for the genetic functions of immunoglobulins, such as complement fixation, transplacental transport, or macrophage interaction, reside in the Fc fragment. None of these functional sites has been precisely localized. Genetic markers for IgG1, IgG2, IgG3, and IgA2 are also known on their respective Fc fragments. They are discussed in Chapter 27.

IgG constitutes 80 per cent of the serum antibody. It is the only immunoglobulin which crosses from the maternal to the fetal circulation. Most antibody to viruses, gram-positive bacteria, bacterial exotoxins, and the capsular polysaccharides of *Neisseria* and *Hemophilus* belong to the IgG class. So also do "warm" hemolysins.

IgM molecules, which are pentamers of $\mu_2\kappa_2$ or $\mu_2\lambda_2$, have a molecular weight of 1,000,000. IgM antibodies comprise ap-

Figure 18–3. Schematic diagram of an IgG molecule.

TABLE 18–2. BIOLOGICAL AND PHYSICOCHEMICAL CHARACTERISTICS OF THE CLASSES OF IMMUNOGLOBULINS (NORMAL ADULT HUMAN)

	IgM	IgA SERUM	IgA SECRETORY (IgAsec)	IgG	IgD	IgE
Molecular weight	880,000	155,000	350,000	144,000	165,000	188,000
Plasma concentration (mg%)	50–150	75–400	Detectable but very low	900–1900	0.5–50	5–150×10^{-3}
Colostral concentrations (mg%)	40–50	None detected	200–500	90	None detected	None detected
Respiratory secretions (mg%)	0.1	Detectable but very low	4.0	Detectable but very low	None detected	1–20×10^{-3}
Lacrimal secretions (mg%)	Detectable	Detectable but very low	0.6	Detectable but very low	None detected	Not done
Gastrointestinal secretions (mg%)	Detectable but very low	None detected	1.2	Detected	Not done	Not done
Degradation rate ($t_{1/2}$ in days)	5.1	5.8	Not done	23.0	2.8	2.3
Antigen combining sites	10	2	Presumed to be ≥ 9	2	?	2
Complement fixation	4+ for one subclass	None	None	Detectable for 3 subclasses	None	None
Bactericidal reaction	4+ for one subclass	None	None	Detectable for 3 subclasses	None	Not done
Skin fixation	None	None	None	None	None	4+
Non-cytotoxic histamine release	None	None	None	None	None	4+
Antiviral activity	None detected	None	None	Present	None detected	Not done
Anti gram-negative bacilli activity	4+	Present but? positive value	Present but? positive value	Present	None detected	Not done
Anti-bacterial toxin activity	Little or none	Present	Not done	4+	None detected	Not done
Placental transmission	Little or none	Little or none	None	4+	Little or none	Little or none
Body compartment	Predominantly intravascular	Predominantly intravascular	External exocrine secretions	Intravascular and E.C.F.°	Predominantly intravascular	Intravascular and in external secretions
Site of biosynthesis	Much in spleen, other lymphoid tissue	Spleen, lymphoid tissue	Submucosa	All lymphoid tissue	Spleen, lymph nodes	Predominantly in submucosa
Carbohydrate concentration	7%	4%	4%	0–1%	4%	

°Extracellular fluid.
Key: 4+ accounts for most or all of whole serum activity
    1+ accounts for little of whole serum activity
From Robbins, J. B.: Immunologic mechanism. In *Pediatrics*. 15th ed. Barnett, H., and Einhorn, A. H. (eds.), New York, Appleton-Century-Crofts, 1972, p. 433.

proximately 10 per cent of serum antibodies directed against the macromolecular lipopolysaccharide antigens, such as the endotoxins of gram-negative bacteria, the Wassermann and Forssman antigens, and the I antigen of erythrocytes. "Natural" antibodies and isohemagglutinins are of the IgM class. So too are the "cold" agglutinins and hemolysins.

No group of antibody specificities is peculiar to IgA or IgD classes. However, IgA is found to predominate in all the body secretions, such as colostrum, saliva, succus entericus, and respiratory tract secretions. So called secretory IgA is usually present as dimers of $\alpha_2\kappa_2$ or $\alpha_2\lambda_2$. It is formed locally by plasma cells subjacent to the secretory surfaces.

The anaphylactic or reaginic antibodies are of the IgE class. Although present in only trace amounts in the blood, they are of paramount importance in allergic disease (13, 14).

The normal levels of all immunoglobulins vary with age. Normal values are given by Stiehm and others (15, 16).

PRIMARY B CELL DEFICIENCIES

The outstanding clinical manifestation of patients with quantitative or qualitative defects of B cell function is recurrent, invasive infection with pyogenic bacteria. These infections are not different from those observed in normal individuals of the same age—pyoderma, pharyngitis, sinusitis, otitis media, pneumonia, sepsis, and meningitis. They respond normally to antimicrobial therapy, but are notable for their frequency and often for their severity. There is a diminished or absent antibody response to injected antigens or to infection, which has given rise to the term introduced by the Swiss workers—the *antibody deficiency syndrome.* Since this basic pathogenetic defect results in failure of phagocytosis, an essential step in the control of invasion by pyogenic bacteria, it is not surprising that an indistinguishable clinical picture has been observed in patients with deficiency of the third component of complement (C3) described later in this chapter. Cellular immune responses of the T cells being preserved, these patients respond to most viral, fungal, or mycobacterial infections normally. A number of different primary disorders can give rise to the antibody deficiency syndrome (Table 18–3).

TABLE 18–3. PRIMARY IMMUNODEFICIENCIES

	SUGGESTED CELLULAR DEFECT			INHERITANCE		
	B Cells					
	Circulating Ig-bearing B lymphocytes					
TYPE	(a)°	(b)°°	T cells	X-Linked	Autosomal Recessive	Other‡
X-linked agammaglobulinemia	X	(X)†		X		
Thymic hypoplasia			X			X
Severe combined immunodeficiency	X	(X)	X	X	X	X
with dysostosis	X	?	X		X	
with adenosine deaminase deficiency	X		X		X	
with generalized hemopoietic hypoplasia	X		X		X	
Selective Ig deficiency						
IgA	?	X	(X)			X
Others		?				X
X-linked immunodeficiencies with increased IgM		X		X		
Immunodeficiency with ataxia telangiectasia		X	X		X?	
Immunodeficiency with thrombocytopenia and eczema (Wiskott-Aldrich syndrome)			X	X		
Immunodeficiency with thymoma	X°		X			X
Immunodeficiency with normo- or hypergammaglobulinemia	X	X	(X)			X
Transient hypogammaglobulinemia of infancy		X				X
Varied immunodeficiencies (largely unclassified and common)	X	X	(X)		(X)	X

°Absent or very low.
°°Easily detectable or increased.
†Some cases with circulating B lymphocytes without detectable surface Ig have been found.
‡Implies multifactorial or unknown genetic basis or no genetic basis.
X Common.
(X) Low frequency.
? Uncertain.
Reprinted by permission from Cooper, M. D., Faulk, W. P., et al.: New Engl. J. Med. 288:966, 1973.

Transient Hypogammaglobulinemia of Infancy

Normally, the synthesis of immunoglobulins in response to infection and other antigenic stimuli begins after birth. However, if the fetus is infected in utero after the 20th week of gestation by rubella virus, cytomegalovirus, *Toxoplasma*, or syphilis, he (or she) can mount an impressive antibody response to the invasive pathogen. This antibody response, consisting largely of IgM and to a lesser extent of IgA and IgG antibodies, can be helpful in the diagnosis of prenatal infection. A cord or neonatal serum level of IgM in excess of 20 mg. per 100 ml. is considered presumptive evidence of intrauterine infection (17). The level of IgG globulin, which is passively acquired by transplacental passage, falls rapidly during the first month of life, levels off during the second month, and soon begins to rise. Rarely, there is delay in the maturation of B cells and their immunologic function; the level of IgG globulins received by passive transfer from the mother continues to fall and is not adequately raised by immunoglobulins synthesized by the infant, so that within a few months the total gamma globulin level is much lower than usual for that age. The infants have overt infections, unexplained episodes of fever, and often bronchitis with wheezing. Regular injections of gamma globulin (see below) will protect them from severe, invasive infections. The injections may be discontinued when the IgG globulins begin to rise toward normal levels, usually before the age of 3 years. The cause of this transient hypogammaglobulinemia is not known. Normal numbers of B cells are present in the circulation of affected infants.

X-linked Agammaglobulinemia (Congenital Agammaglobulinemia; Bruton's Disease)

X-linked agammaglobulinemia usually manifests itself in the second year of life, although the onset of the characteristically severe, recurrent infections may begin at any age from 8 months to 3 years. The infections are those caused by the common pyogenic organisms—*Staphylococcus aureus*, pneumococci, meningococci, *Hemophilus influenzae*, and less often beta-hemolytic streptococci or *Pseudomonas*. They differ from infections in normal children only in their frequency, severity, and the tendency for infection with the same organism to occur more than once. Pyoderma, purulent conjunctivitis, pharyngitis, otitis media, sinusitis, bronchitis, pneumonia, empyema, purulent arthritis, meningitis, and sepsis occur with surprising frequency and may be associated with unusually high fever and unexpected elevation or depression of the leukocyte count. A rather indolent rheumatoid-like arthritis with sterile effusion into one of the large joints develops in about one-third of patients and may be the presenting complaint. The children usually, but not always, handle most viral infections normally (18).

There should be a high index of suspicion about this diagnosis on the basis of the history of repeated severe bacterial infections. A careful family history may uncover instances of death from overwhelming infection or multiple severe infections in other male siblings, maternal uncles, or male offspring of maternal aunts. Examination reveals little except the signs of infection, evidence of joint involvement if present, and unusually small, smooth tonsils. Lateral films of the pharynx fail to reveal an adenoid shadow. Lymph nodes are small but palpable; regional nodes may be swollen and tender during episodes of infection. Immunochemical assay reveals a marked diminution of IgM, IgA, and IgG globulins in the serum. It is important to remember that, because of individual variations and the low levels of immunoglobulins normally found in the early months of life, the diagnosis cannot be firmly established by immunoelectrophoresis until 6 to 8 months of age (see Fig. 18–4). However, failure of IgM or IgA to appear in significant concentration and a steady fall in IgG during the first 3 to 4 months of life should suggest the diagnosis, especially in the presence of a positive family history. Isohemagglutinins are usually absent or in very low titer. Injection of vaccines is not followed by an adequate antibody rise, and

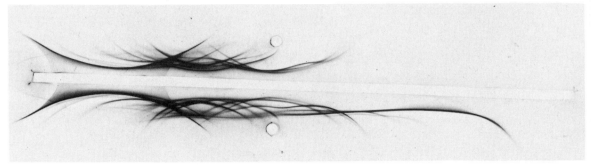

Figure 18–4. Immunoelectrophoresis of normal (bottom) and agammaglobulinemic (top) sera. The anode is to the left. The pattern was developed with horse antihuman serum.

removal of a stimulated regional lymph node discloses absence of the expected germinal centers, secondary follicles, and plasma cells.

The thymus is normal, but lymph nodes and spleen lack the usual follicular architecture. Germinal centers are absent, and there are few if any plasma cells in the medullary cores or red pulp. Although the number of lymphocytes in the tissues appears diminished, they are present in the thymus-dependent areas of lymphoid tissue, and normal numbers are found in the blood. Plasma cells are absent from the bone marrow. However, plasma cells may be normally absent from the bone marrow in children under 5 years of age, so that this is an unhelpful finding (19). Study of the circulating lymphocytes has revealed normal numbers of T cells but complete absence of B cells. We have found normal numbers of B cells in only one case of proved X-linked agammaglobulinemia. These B cells are abnormal in that they are unresponsive to the T cell mitogen and pokeweed mitogen and do not synthesize immunoglobulins in vitro (4).

Provided the diagnosis is made before repeated infections have produced serious anatomic damage (e.g., bronchiectasis, pulmonary insufficiency, middle ear deafness), the immediate prognosis for these children is excellent, and they gain and grow normally. However, in later childhood, adolescence, or early adult life, complications may develop in some of these patients. Slowly progressive neurologic disease, suggesting a "slow virus" infection, accompanies a dermatomyositis-like syndrome with brawny edema, perivascular mononuclear infiltrates, and, terminally, severe systemic symptoms and death. Thus far, no consistent cause for these complications has been found. An enterovirus was repeatedly isolated from blood, stool, and spinal fluid in the last patient to succumb with the dermatomyositis-like picture.

Vigorous antimicrobial therapy is indicated for individual infections which respond to treatment as in normal individuals. Regular injections of gamma globulin, which is almost pure IgG, in doses adequate to maintain a plasma concentration of IgG globulin above 200 mg. per 100 ml. are essential. Maintenance therapy is initiated with a loading dose of 0.3 g. (1.8 ml.) per kg. of IgG globulin. This may be given in divided doses over a period of a week in order to minimize discomfort. Thereafter, an average dose of 0.1 g. (0.6 ml.) per kg. per month (the volume of the injection may be scaled down if injections are given every two or three weeks) is required to maintain a protective level of antibody. Intramuscular administration is necessary to avoid reactions with the standard preparation. A preparation satisfactory for intravenous administration has been shown to be effective in preventing infections in these patients and is being developed for clinical trials (20). Prophylaxis with gamma globulin is usually effective in preventing invasive bacterial infection and communicable disease, and its institution generally cures hydrarthrosis. It does not control localized superficial infection of skin or respiratory tract; in a few instances, antimicrobial drugs may have to be given in addition to control chronic sinusitis, most frequently due to *H. influenzae*. Infections may be prevented for considerable periods by the administration of broad-spectrum antibiotics without gamma globulin.

Once a case of X-linked agammaglobu-

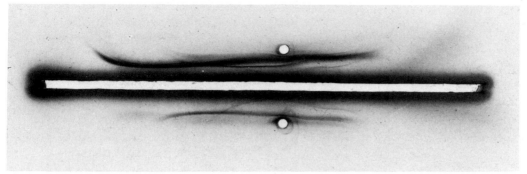

Figure 18–5. Immunoelectrophoresis of normal (top) and dysgammaglobulinemic (bottom) sera. The anode is to the left. The pattern was developed with goat antihuman immunoglobulins.

linemia has been identified in a family, each subsequent male sibling or male offspring of a maternal aunt should be followed up carefully, with clinical examination and serial immunoelectrophoretic analyses of the serum at intervals of every two months from birth through the first year. Infants so detected and given prophylactic gamma globulin before severe infections have occurred seem to thrive particularly well.

X-linked Immunodeficiency with Increased IgM

In a few instances, patients are observed with manifestations similar to those in X-linked agammaglobulinemia, but with higher levels of immunoglobulins, which, when analyzed, turn out to reflect a marked deficiency of serum IgA and IgG but an elevation in the concentration of IgM. The congenital form of this disease seems to occur almost entirely in males and has a suggestive X-linked pattern of inheritance. Except for a greater frequency of "autoimmune" hematologic disorders (neutropenia, hemolytic anemia, thrombocytopenia), the clinical course in these patients resembles that of X-linked agammaglobulinemia (21). Histologically, there is disorganization of the follicular architecture of the lymphoid tissues, but PAS-positive plasmacytoid cells containing IgM are present, and even tonsillar hypertrophy due to these cells has been observed. Only B cells with IgM surface fluorescence are found. No B cells with surface IgA or IgG

are present. Similar disturbances of the immunoglobulin picture associated with the antibody deficiency syndrome have been seen in adults with frequent respiratory tract infections and bronchiectasis, and in some infants with congenital rubella.

Selective Immunoglobulin Deficiencies (Dysgammaglobulinemia)

This term is used to describe cases in which there are consistent deficiencies of one or more of the recognizable plasma immunoglobulins. Although often associated with the clinical manifestations of the antibody deficiency syndrome, some instances of selective immunoglobulin deficiency may be chance laboratory findings in otherwise apparently normal individuals (Fig. 18–5).

Selective deficiency of IgG subclasses may occur, in which the patient is unable to synthesize one or more of the IgG subclasses and thus fails to produce antibodies in one or more of the four presently identified IgG subclasses. This results in failure to respond to particular types of antigens, in increased susceptibility to a limited spectrum of bacterial infections, and in a reduction in total serum IgG concentration proportional to the percentage of the total IgG pool accounted for by the deficient IgG subclass. Of course, a deficiency in IgG1 is most severe, since this subclass contitutes over 70 per cent of the IgG (22, 23).

Selective IgA deficiency is observed with considerable frequency (3 to 7 per 1000 population). In a few patients, this may portend the development of ataxia telangiectasia, but an appreciable number of such individuals remain healthy throughout life. However, a high incidence of rheumatoid arthritis, systemic lupus erythematosus, and malabsorption syndrome has been observed among this group of patients (24, 25). A significant number of IgA-deficient individuals have circulating antibodies to IgA and have anaphylactic reactions upon receiving whole blood or plasma (26).

Deficiency of secretory IgA may well play a role in undue susceptibility to certain infections, particularly viral, of the respiratory and gastrointestinal tracts. Secretory IgA is the form of antibody synthesized in plasma cells closely related to the mucous membranes and secreted into colostrum, saliva, and respiratory and intestinal secretions as two subunits of IgA in combination with a "secretory piece" synthesized by the epithelial cells and another polypeptide chain which stabilizes the polymer (J chain). Thus deficiency of this type of local immunity may contribute to the clinical picture of agammaglobulinemia and ataxia telangiectasia, as well as to the tendency to recurrent otitis media or to chronic diarrhea in some patients with selective IgA deficiency. Likewise, the efficacy of certain respiratory viral vaccines when administered intranasally or of oral poliomyelitis vaccine may depend more upon the establishment of local immunity than upon the stimulation of systemic antibody formation (24a). It is difficult to assess "secretory" immunity.

Rare cases of *immunodeficiency with normal or increased immunoglobulins* have been observed, in which the classic picture of the antibody deficiency syndrome was accompanied by a normal or even increased level of immunoglobulins and the presence of plasma cells in the tissues, but a failure to form specific antibodies to a variety of antigens. These have not been adequately studied with modern methods to provide an adequate explanation (25a).

Immunodeficiency in Gastrointestinal Disease

Malabsorption, inflammatory bowel disease, and protein-losing enteropathy may be associated with a variety of immunologic disturbances. As mentioned above, certain cases of nontropical sprue are accompanied by deficiency of IgA, the predominant immunoglobulin in intestinal secretion that is normally produced in the lymphoid cells of the lamina propria (25b). Agamma-A-globulinemia has also been observed in a few cases of tropical sprue. Crabbe and Hermans have pointed out that there is a second type of patient with malabsorption characterized by diffuse hypogammaglobulinemia (and nearly absent IgA). These patients are particularly susceptible to respiratory infections and often harbor intestinal *Giardia* (see below). In these patients nodular lymphoid hyperplasia may be noted in small bowel biopsies (25c).

Severe hypoalbuminemia due to gastrointestinal exudate has been observed in patients with Milroy's disease and in patients with intestinal lymphangiectasia (25d). Correction of lymphangiectasia by selected small bowel resection can be accomplished in some cases.

In some patients with intestinal lymphangiectasia, the serum protein loss is so massive as to involve immunoglobulins and even lymphocytes. In such patients hypoalbuminemia, hypogammaglobulinemia, lymphocytopenia, and T cell insufficiency with susceptibility to viral and fungal infection as well as delayed homograft rejection may occur (25e, 25f).

Variable Unclassified Immunodeficiency (Acquired Hypogammaglobulinemia)

This is the most common form of immunodeficiency with serious clinical consequences and probably includes a number of entities; it occurs in either sex at any age without any known causative factor, either genetic or acquired, although a predisposition may be inherited since its development has been reported in siblings or among relatives.

The picture is that of the antibody deficiency syndrome associated with immunoglobulin deficiency, which may be somewhat less severe than in the X-linked form of agammaglobulinemia. Pathologically, there is necrobiotic change in the follicular architecture of the lymph nodes and spleen, or lymphadenopathy and splenomegaly due to reticulum cell hyperplasia. The predominant infections are sinusitis and pneumonia, often leading to bronchiectasis unless intensively treated. Although the rheumatoid arthritis-like complications are occasionally seen, a spruelike malabsorption syndrome and pernicious anemia are more common. Recent work has demonstrated that this malabsorption syndrome is often due to *Giardia lamblia* demonstrated either in aspirates of duodenal fluid or in biopsy specimens of duodenal mucosa (26a).

Management is the same as for X-linked agammaglobulinemia: substitution therapy with regular injections of large doses of immune serum globulin for prophylaxis and intensive antimicrobial therapy for acute infections. The chronic diarrhea and malabsorption due to giardiasis, which may give a picture of protein-losing enteropathy, usually respond promptly to metronidazole (Flagyl) in doses of 0.25 g. t.i.d. for five days.

Patients with "acquired" agammaglobulinemia may have no B cells, but, more commonly, normal numbers of B cells or even increased numbers of B cells are found (27). In some patients the B cells do not synthesize immunoglobulin; in others, immunoglobulin synthesis is normal, but there is no secretion of the immunoglobulin formed. We have studied one patient whose B cells functioned normally in vitro when cultured in normal AB+ serum, but did not in the patient's serum. Obviously a whole spectrum of B cell maturation failure is presented by these patients. In some patients, T cell function deteriorates progressively. This is particularly true of patients who have an associated thymoma.

PRIMARY T CELL DEFICIENCIES

Patients with T cell deficiency have much more serious susceptibility to infection than patients with complete or partial B cell defects. In its most severe forms, T cell deficiency results in an inability to terminate opportunistic infections with organisms that are ordinarily innocuous. Consequently, varicella, vaccinia, and herpes and measles viruses can be fatal infections. The enterobacilli are invasive, and infection with *Monilia* is common. Malignancy of both the lymphoreticular organs and other viscera is also a common complication of the T cell disorders.

Severe Combined Immunodeficiency

Severe combined immunodeficiency (Swiss type agammaglobulinemia, alymphocytosis, thymic alymphoplasia) is the most profound of the cellular defects. Affected patients usually have no T or B cells; the disease is invariably fatal. It is genetically determined, and there is clear evidence of autosomal recessive and X-linked recessive transmission of the disease. The clinical and laboratory findings may be quite variable from case to case, even among affected members of a single family (Fig. 18–6).

The onset of persistent infection of the lungs; monilial infection of the oropharynx, esophagus, and skin; chronic diarrhea; and wasting and runting begins in the early months of life and progresses with monotonous regularity to a fatal termination despite all attempts at routine therapy. Affected infants usually do not survive the first year or two of life. Examination usually reveals absence of tonsils, very small or absent lymph nodes despite chronic infection, chronic pneumonitis evidenced by a pertussis-like cough, inspiratory retractions of the chest, rales, a somewhat distended abdomen with wasting, and oral thrush (28).

Roentgenographic signs include pulmonary infiltration and absence of a thymic shadow. There is usually an absolute decrease in the number of circulating lymphocytes, and occasionally neutropenia. In typical cases, the immunoglobulins are markedly decreased, but variants have been described in which circulating immunoglobulins are normal or there is selective immunoglobulin deficiency. M components may be present in the circulation (29). Plasma cells have been found in the tissues of such patients, but antibody formation is almost always impaired or absent. Tests of delayed hypersensitivity give negative results: sensitization cannot be induced with dinitrochlorobenzene, cultured lymphocytes do not respond to phytohemagglutinin, and skin allografts are not rejected. T cells are almost always absent from the circulation, and the few lymphocytes pres-

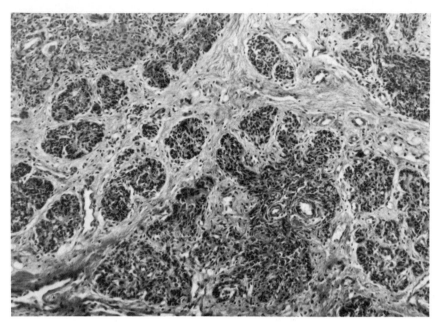

Figure 18–6. Photomicrograph of thymus from a patient with severe combined immunodeficiency (× 400). No Hassall's bodies are present, the blood vessels are small, and islets of fetal spindle cells are seen without lymphoidal elements.

ent in the blood usually have the characteristics of B cells.

Recently, several but not all infants with the autosomal recessive form of the disease have been found to lack the enzyme adenosine deaminase (ADA) from their red cells and other tissues. These ADA-deficient infants frequently have a dyschondroplasia, most noticeable on x-rays of ribs. Heterozygosity was detectable in the parents by their half-normal levels of ADA (30). The accumulation of adenosine in these infants may be lymphocytotoxic or interfere with pyrimidine biosynthesis (30a). Other interesting ideas stemming from this observation remain to be explored, but the causative association between the ADA deficiency and the immunodeficiency is at present obscure.

Treatment of the infections in these patients must be specific. Pulmonary infection is frequently due to *Pneumocystis carinii*, requiring pentamidine or pyrimethamine and sulfadiazine. Routine antimicrobial therapy, fungistatic drugs, or human gamma globulin are only temporarily effective and do not prevent the inexorable fatal course of the disease if the immunologic deficiency is not overcome. The use of attenuated viral or BCG vaccines must be avoided, since the attenuated viruses or mycobacteria can produce fatal generalized disease, and natural infection with herpes, varicella, or measles virus is uniformly and progressively fatal.

The establishment of immunologic competence with transplants of bone marrow in these infants is still experimental and should only be carried out in those centers with adequate manpower, clinical and laboratory experience, and physical facilities for what is an exacting ordeal for patient, family, nurses, and physicians. Success depends upon attention to a number of factors (31–34):

For an index case in a family, the diagnosis is seldom made until infection is already established. Every subsequent sibling should be carefully watched for early signs of the disease—absence of clinically demonstrable thymic tissue at birth, low peripheral lymphocyte count, absence of serum IgM and IgA, and failure of cultured lymphocytes from cord blood or subsequent blood samples to respond to phytohemagglutinin. Affected infants can be maintained in a sterile environment or laminar flow apparatus. They require exquisite care in administration of systemic and topical antibiotics.

A donor of bone marrow whose cells are HL-A identical and can be shown to be

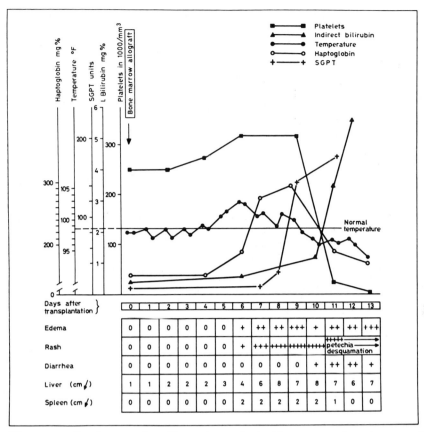

Figure 18–7. The course of graft-versus-host disease in a patient with severe combined immunodeficiency who received histoincompatible bone marrow (5 × 10⁶ cells). The patient died on day 13.

histocompatible in vitro by mixed lymphocyte culture (MLC) should be identified. In practice, this almost always means a sibling. However, a successful transplant from an MLC-identical maternal uncle has been accomplished despite HL-A nonidentity between donor and recipient (Figs. 18–7 and 18–8). Administration of a suitable dose of bone marrow cells from the donor when the infant is as free of infection as possible is accomplished with 50 × 10⁶ nucleated cells per kg. intravenously. More cells are optimal for intraperitoneal injection, perhaps 50 × 10⁷. Evidence that the graft has become established and that immunologic reconstitution (T cell function as shown by phytohemagglutinin responses, B cell function by immunoglobulin synthesis) has occurred usually requires three to eight weeks (Fig. 18–9).

In skilled hands, patients with this hitherto fatal disease have been cured and appear normal. Nevertheless, success is not universal, there is much to learn, and the treatment is heroic. Intrauterine diagnosis of this disorder has not been accomplished, but might ultimately lead to its prevention in affected families. The possibility of finding ADA deficiency in amnion cells remains to be explored.

Variant forms of severe combined immunodeficiency have been described. These include cases with dysostosis (short-limbed dwarfism) and rare cases with generalized hemopoietic hypoplasia. The latter has been called reticular dysgenesis; infants with this type of immunodeficiency also lack granulocytic precursors in the bone marrow and granulocytes in peripheral blood and survive for only a short time after birth (35). Nezelof syndrome, which is severe combined immunodeficiency with normal immunoglobulins, is a specious diagnosis, and the term should be dropped. This variant is included in the term severe combined immunodeficiency.

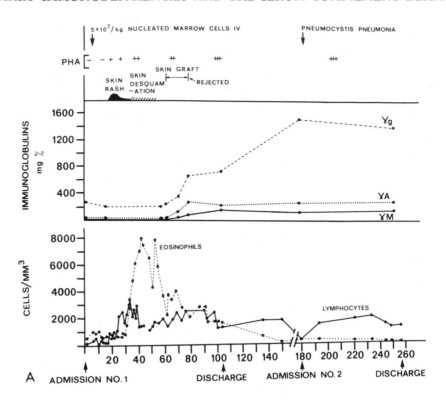

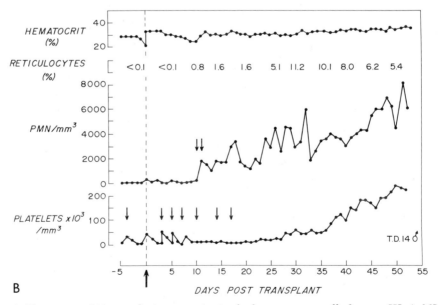

Figure 18-8. *A,* The course of immunologic reconstitution by bone marrow cells from an HL-A, MLC identical donor in a patient with severe combined immunodeficiency. *B,* The course of hemopoietic reconstitution by bone marrow cells from an HL-A, MLC identical donor in a patient with aplastic anemia. (From Camitta, B., et al.: Posthepatitic severe aplastic anemia—an indication for early bone marrow transplantation. Blood *43:*473, 1974.)

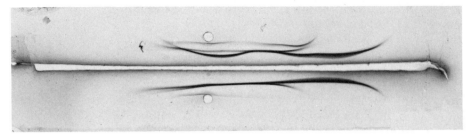

Figure 18–9. Immunoelectrophoresis of serum from a normal individual (bottom) and from a patient with severe combined immunodeficiency (top) following bone marrow transplantation. A number of M components are visible.

Immunodeficiency with Ataxia Telangiectasia

This is an autosomal recessive disease in which abnormalities of the thymus have been found at postmortem examination. Gradually progressive cerebellar ataxia begins in early childhood. This is associated with increasing telangiectasia, which first becomes apparent as a rather inconspicuous dilatation of small blood vessels in the bulbar conjunctivae and ultimately is visible in the skin at about 5 years of age. Gonadal dysgenesis and failure of sexual maturation may be present in those who survive into the second decade. In late childhood, recurrent sinobronchial infections begin in many patients, often leading to bronchiectasis. There is also a tendency to the development of malignant tumors, particularly of the lymphoid system. These reflect an immunologic disturbance affecting T cell function, as shown by blunting of delayed hypersensitivity reactions, failure to reject allografts normally, and reduced response of the lymphocytes to phytohemagglutinin. At postmortem examination late in the disease, the thymus is abnormally small and has a decreased number of lymphocytes; there is a poor differentiation between cortex and medulla and decided diminution in Hassall's corpuscles. The number of circulating lymphocytes and the architecture of the lymph nodes vary considerably and do not always correlate well with the patient's history. The most consistent B cell defect is a low level or absence of IgA globulin in the serum, which occurs in about 70 per cent of affected persons and may precede clinical evidence of immunologic deficiency by a number of years (36).

Immunodeficiency with Thrombocytopenia and Eczema (Wiskott-Aldrich Syndrome)

The Wiskott-Aldrich syndrome is an X-linked recessive disorder which is usually manifested by eczema, thrombocytopenia, and a wide variety of infections beginning late in the first year, although it may present rarely as thrombocytopenia alone. Death may occur from hemorrhage, infection, or the development of a malignant process similar to the Letterer-Siwe type of reticuloendotheliosis.

The infections may be caused by a wide variety of micro-organisms, including viruses, bacteria, fungi, and *Pneumocystis carinii*. Transient episodes of arthritis have been observed.

Results of studies of the pathogenesis of the Wiskott-Aldrich syndrome are confusing. The lymphoid tissues appear normal early in the course of the disease, but as it progresses there may be a loss of lymphocytes from the thymus and paracortical areas of the lymph nodes. The peripheral lymphocyte count may decrease, and there is a variable loss of cellular immunity, resulting in increased susceptibility to viral or fungal disease. Studies of immunoglobulin production in these patients suggest normal responses to a variety of antigens. IgM values are often low, and isohemagglutinins and Forssman antibodies, normally present as "natural" antibodies, are usually lacking. The failure of these patients to respond to pneumococcal polysaccharides has led to the postulation that they have a general inability to respond to polysaccharide antigens, as opposed to normal responses to protein antigens (37, 38). Whether this failure resides in the recognition system of the lymphocytes, in a deficit of the macrophages in processing such antigens, or in a qualitative deficiency of plasma cell function is not clear. Since polysaccharides are widely distributed and important constituents of bacteria and fungi, it is reasonable that such a selective immunologic deficiency might have a serious impact upon resistance. Transfer factor has been tried and found to induce cellular immunity and clinical improvement in some patients with this disease (39).

Congenital Thymic Aplasia (DiGeorge Syndrome)

Congenital thymic aplasia (DiGeorge syndrome, third and fourth pharyngeal pouch syndrome) results from a failure of the normal embryogenesis of the thymus and parathyroid glands, which are derived from the third and fourth pharyngeal clefts. The syndrome is not genetically determined but appears rather to result from some intrauterine accident before the eighth week of gestation. Affected infants invariably have neonatal tetany. Anomalies of the great blood vessels are very frequently encountered, usually right-sided aortic arch, as is tetralogy of Fallot (40, 41). These cardiac complications are the cause of late death in these children (42). Mental subnormality also accompanies this syndrome.

The T cell defect in children with congenital thymic aplasia varies from the most profound to the barely discernible. In any case, T cell function improves in these children with age, so that by 5 years of age no T cell deficit can be ascertained. It is not clear how this grossly retarded T cell maturation occurs in the absence of a thymus gland. Some children may have a small thymic remnant, but T cell maturation may occur at sites other than the thymus.

Transplants of fetal thymus into these infants results in a rapid acquisition of T cell function (43–45). A hormonelike substance is thought to be secreted by the thymic epithelium. It has been called "thymosin," and it is presumed to effect T cell maturation (46). It has thus far eluded isolation.

Infection Following Splenectomy

The risk of death from overwhelming sepsis following splenectomy is well established (47). The young are more at risk than those who have been splenectomized at a later age (i.e., after 5 years of age). Children with congenital asplenia and Ivemark's syndrome (asplenia and partial situs inversus) have the greatest mortality from septic infection (48). Fatal bloodstream infection results presumably from bacteria to which the splenectomized child has no pre-existent antibody (see p. 248).

The pathophysiology of this immunologic deficit may be multifactorial, but is quite straightforward. The spleen has two important roles. It is the lymph node of the blood stream and thus the site of antibody response to antigens presented via that route. Secondly, it has an important phagocytic function in the absence of antibody. That is, the granulopectic activity of the liver is adequate for clearing immune complexes, but in the absence of antibody the accessary phagocytic function of the spleen is required to clear the bloodstream of foreign or bacterial particles (49). When mice were injected intravenously with small doses of killed pneumococci and then splenectomized eight or more hours later, they were resistant to a challenge of live pneumococci of the same type which was fatal to a control group of mice which were simply splenectomized. In other words, the opportunity to synthesize some antibody to the challenging bacteria was absolutely protective (50).

COMPLEMENT

It was almost a century ago that the ability of fresh serum to destroy certain bacteria was noted. This bactericidal capacity was soon resolved into a heat-stable substance, bactericidin, bacteriolysin, i.e., specific antibody, and a heat-labile substance called complement. At the turn of this century, Ehrlich and Morgenroth found similar requirements for the immune lysis of sheep red cells. Since the release of hemoglobin could be quantitated, the sheep cell (E), amboceptor or antibody (A), and complement (C) model system provided a powerful tool for the further study of complement and its actions.

The complement system is now known to consist of nine sequentially interacting proteins (Fig. 18–10). In the presently accepted nomenclature, they are numbered, in order of their sequential reaction, C1, 4, 2, 3, 5, 6, 7, 8, 9, (51). It is now clear that certain substances and particles can "by-pass" the first three components, C1, C4, and C2, and can activate C3 and subsequent components by an alternate pathway. Such a pathway was first described by Pillemer and his co-workers, who called it the properdin system, and it is currently being intensively reinvestigated (52). In addition to the components of complement themselves, the complement system also contains at least three inhibitors or inactivators at the C1, the C3, the C6, and the properdin Factor B steps. A list of the complement proteins, including synonyms, is given in Table 18–4.

All of the complement components and related macromolecules thus far studied are glycoproteins and contain between 3 and 43 per cent carbohydrate. C1 exists in native serum as a macromolecular complex of three separate molecules, C1q, C1r, and C1s, perhaps bonded through Ca^{2+} as a ligand (53). The complex is dissociable by chelation of the Ca^{2+} with EDTA. Dissociation is also favored by relatively high ionic strength. The C1 complex has a sedimentation coefficient of 18S, whereas the subcomponents are 11S, 7S, and 4S, respectively. There is evidence that the complex occurs naturally as 1C1q:2C1r:4C1s.

C1q has a molecular weight of about 400,000, and it consists of five or six similar subunits of 57,000 daltons in noncovalent attachment. Since five or six IgG molecules can be bound maximally to one C1q molecule, it may be that there is a combining site for immunoglobulins on each of the subunits. C1q is sufficiently large to visualize by electron microscopy. Such ultrastructural studies suggest that the molecule is a 200-Å diameter disk with five or six subunits arranged around a central core. Another form of the molecule, a 400-Å rod structure containing the same subunits, has also been observed and suggests that C1q may undergo extensive conformational change, perhaps relevant to C1r and C1s activation (54). C1q, with its hydroxylysine, hydroxyproline, and high glycine content, is collagen-like, and it is, therefore, of great interest in that its biological activity is destroyed by collagenase (55).

C1r and C1s have been isolated in both zymogen and activated ($\overline{C1r}$ and $\overline{C1s}$) forms. The zymogen form of C1r can be activated by proteolytic enzymes such as trypsin. $\overline{C1r}$ and $\overline{C1s}$ are esterases, the activities of which can be blocked by diisopropylfluorophosphate. C1s may consist of a single subunit, whereas $\overline{C1s}$ consists of two subunits of 36,000 and 77,000 daltons. It may be that $\overline{C1r}$ cleaves $\overline{C1s}$ and that the active enzymatic center on $\overline{C1s}$ is on the 36,000 molecular weight fragment. C1s cleaves esters containing a positively charged amino acid (N-acetylglycyl-L-lysine methyl ester and tosyl-L-arginine methyl ester, for example), as well as compounds containing an aromatic amino acid, such as acetyl-L-tyrosine ethyl ester or N-carbobenzoxy-L-tyrosine p-nitrophenyl ester. There is evidence that the active center of

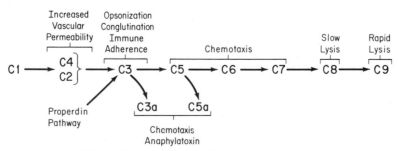

Figure 18–10. Scheme of complement system.

TABLE 18–4.   PHYSICOCHEMICAL PROPERTIES OF HUMAN COMPLEMENT
AND PROPERDIN PROTEINS

	C1q	C1r	C1s	C2	C3	C4	C5	C6
APPROXIMATE MEAN NORMAL SERUM CONCENTRATION (MG./100 ML.)	18	10	3	1	150	40	7	6
RELATIVE ELECTROPHORETIC MOBILITY	γ_2	β	α_2	β_1	β_1-β_2°	β_1	β_1	β_2
APPROXIMATE MOLECULAR WEIGHT	400,000	170,000	110,000	117,000	185,000	240,000	200,000	95,000
SEDIMENTATION COEFFICIENT ($S_{20.w}$)	11	7	4	6	9.5	10	9	6
CARBOHYDRATE (%)	15	–	–	–	2.7	14	19	–
SYNONYMS	11S component; C'O	–	C1 esterase	–	β_{1C}-globulin; properdin Factor A	β_{1E}-globulin	β_{1F}-globulin	–

°Dependent on divalent cation concentration.

C$\overline{1s}$ contains an anionic as well as hydrophobic binding site in accord with these specificities (56).

C4 is a molecule of about 240,000 daltons which, when cleaved by C$\overline{1s}$, yields two fragments, C4a of about 10,000 daltons and C4b of about 230,000 daltons. C4b binds to the red cell surface and participates in further complement activation (57).

C2 has a molecular weight of 117,000. It is acted upon by C$\overline{1s}$ to produce two fragments, C2a (83,000 daltons) and C2b (34,000 daltons). C2a attaches to the antibody-C$\overline{14}$ site (58). Preliminary electrophoretic evidence suggests that C2 is a tetramer-type molecule.

Studies of C3 structure by SDS polyacrylamide gel electrophoresis in the presence of reducing agent suggest that it consists of two kinds of subunits: an alpha chain with a molecular weight of 110,000, and a 70,000 molecular weight beta chain. Enzymatic cleavage of C3 by C$\overline{42}$ or trypsin appears to cleave a fragment, C3a, with a molecular weight of 6800, from the alpha chain, leaving C3b (around 180,000 daltons) (59). On interaction of C3 with EAC$\overline{142}$, C3b attaches to the red cell membrane at multiple sites which may be remote from the antibody-C$\overline{142}$ site. Further degradation of C3b occurs in whole serum, partly

as the result of the proteolytic action of the C3 inactivator, to C3c (7S) and C3d (around 27,000 daltons). Cell-bound C3b may be attached via its C3d portion, so that C3c is released by the action of the C3 inactivator on cell-bound C3b (60).

Preliminary studies of C5 indicate that it, like C3, contains two polypeptide chains. The alpha chain has a molecular weight of 120,000, and the beta chain 80,000. Cleavage of C5 to C5a (10,000 to 15,000 daltons) and C5b by trypsin or EAC$\overline{1423}$ appears also to occur on the alpha chain. Structural studies of the remaining complement proteins are incomplete.

Aggregated forms of IgG or IgM, particularly in antigen-antibody complexes, bind to C1q in macromolecular C1. It is presumed that this binding, which occurs in a minimal molar ratio of one IgM or two IgG molecules to one molecule of C1q, produces a conformational change in the C1q such that activation of C1r and C1s as proteolytic enzymes ensues. Of the IgG subclasses, IgG1 and IgG3 are most potent in activating C1; IgG2 is less active, and IgG4 does not do so at all. The activated form of C1s, designated C$\overline{1s}$, then cleaves C4 and C2 to yield C$\overline{4}$ and C$\overline{2}$ which, in turn, form a bimolecular complex, C$\overline{42}$ (61). This complex (C3 convertase) is capable of

TABLE 18–4. PHYSICOCHEMICAL PROPERTIES OF HUMAN COMPLEMENT AND PROPERDIN PROTEINS *(Continued)*

C7	C8	C9	C$\overline{1}$ Inhibitor	C3 Inactivator	C6 Inactivator	Properdin	GBG	GBGase
6.5	5	0.2	18	1	—	2.5	35	—
β_2	β_1	α_2	α_2	β	β	γ†	β_2	α_2
120,000	150,000	79,000	90,000	100,000	—	185,000†	100,000	—
5	8	4.5	4	5	6	5†	6	3
—	—	—	42	—	—	9.8†	10.6	—
—	—	—	C1 esterase inhibitor; α_2 neuramino-glycoprotein	C3b inactivator; conglutinogen activating factor (KAF)	—	—	C3 proactivator (C3PA); properdin Factor B; heat-labile factor (HLF); unknown factor (UF)	C3PAase; Factor D

†These values are for properdin isolated in activated forms. Native properdin is a β-globulin which has not yet been isolated. From Alper, C. A.: Complement, In *Structure and Function of Plasma Proteins.* Vol. 1. Allison, A. C. (ed.), New York, Plenum Publishing Corporation, 1974 (in press).

cleaving C3 enzymatically into C3a, a fragment of about 6800 daltons, and C3b, only slightly smaller than native C3. C3b produced in this fashion on cell surfaces is designated C$\overline{3}$ and is capable, in conjunction with C$\overline{42}$, of activating C5. The subsequent sequential activation of C6 and C7 allows the formation of a stable trimolecular complex, C$\overline{567}$ in the fluid phase and presumably on the cell surface as well. The addition of C8 to red cells sensitized by antibody and the first seven complement components (EAC$\overline{1-7}$) may result in slow lysis of such cells. Rapid lysis accompanies the addition of C9 to EAC$\overline{1-8}$. The mechanism by which the fully activated complement system produces membrane damage and cell lysis is not understood; it may be that the terminal multimolecular complex acts as a detergent or, in some other nonenzymic way, alters membrane structure so that damage results.

The properdin system (Fig. 18–11), as originally defined, consisted of properdin itself and two other proteins, designated Factors A and B (62, 62a). Factor A was known to be destroyed by incubation with hydrazine, and Factor B by heating serum at 50°C. Properdin itself has been isolated and char-

acterized but only in activated form (63). It is now clear that Factor A is C3 and that activated Factor A is probably the major cleavage fragment of C3, C3b. Factor B has also been isolated and characterized as glycine-rich beta-glycoprotein (GBG), C3 proactivator (C3PA), heat-labile factor (HLF), and unknown factor (UF) (64, 65). An enzyme, variously designated GBGase, C3PAase, or Factor D, has recently been found to be part of the system and has the

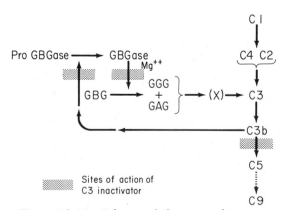

Figure 18–11. Scheme of the properdin system. GBG is synonymous with Factor B or C3PA, and GBGase is synonymous with Factor D or C3PAase.

capacity to cleave GBG and destroy Factor B activity (66, 67). An activated fragment of GBG has the ability, probably through its action on an unidentified intermediary protein(s), to cleave C3 into C3a and C3b. Remarkably, C3b is necessary for the activation of proGBGase and possibly for the activity of GBGase as well. A positive feedback loop is thereby formed, in which generation of a product (C3b) activates a system capable of producing further cleavage of C3 and generation of more C3b. The C3 inactivator acts as a brake on this process by cleaving C3b in such a fashion that it is no longer able to activate proGBGase and by inactivating GBGase already formed (68).

There is now considerable evidence that the C3-converting enzymes of the classic and alternate pathways, and probably of certain other pathways as well, whether assembled on surfaces or in the fluid phase, are able to produce a kind of innocent bystander reaction. For example, $EAC\overline{(1)42}$ or $C\overline{(1)42}$ can act on C3 so that there is transient activation of a combining site on $C\overline{3}$ for red cells unsensitized by antibody or early complement components. Zymosan, on interaction with serum, causes the activation of C3 and the assembly of $C\overline{567}$ in the fluid phase, which can then attach components C8 and C9. The latter phenomenon has been termed reactive hemolysis (69).

Complement contributes essentially to the inflammatory response and to host defense against invasion by pathogenic organisms. In certain pathologic states, complement appears to play a role in mediating tissue injury. Although earlier studies of complement emphasized immune cell lysis with its requirement for all components, it is now abundantly established that many of the important biological activities of the complement system become manifest early in the activation sequence. Neutralization of certain viruses may be accomplished by the properdin pathway or by IgM antibody, C1 and C4, or by IgM antibody, C1, C4, C2, and C3. The properdin pathway, the classic pathway, and all the proteins of the common pathway are probably required for the bactericidal properties of serum for smooth gram-negative bacteria.

Both C3a and C5a are anaphylatoxins; that is to say, they both cause contraction of smooth muscle and an increase in vascular permeability (70, 71). They both cause degranulation of mast cells with attendant histamine release. Both C3a and C5a are chemotactic for leukocytes. The anaphylatoxin properties of these fragments are rapidly destroyed in whole serum by the action of an enzyme called anaphylatoxin inactivator, probably identical with carboxypeptidase B (72). There is evidence that another enzyme, chemotactic factor inactivator, destroys the chemotactic activity of C3a, C5a, and $C\overline{567}$. As was pointed out earlier, C3a and C5a may be generated by noncomplement proteolytic enzymes, such as plasmin, trypsin, and tissue and bacterial proteases, as well as by classic or alternate pathway activation. Evidence has been presented that such noncomplement enzymes may play a role in the local inflammatory response to nonimmune injury.

Activation of the classic sequence through C3 is required for the enhancement by serum of the phagocytosis of antibody-sensitized erythrocytes or encapsulated pyogenic bacteria, such as pneumococci (73, 74). For the latter, maximal enhancement also requires proteins of the alternate pathway. Endotoxin particles in a paraffin oil emulsion are phagocytosed only with the aid of the alternate pathway, providing a model for nonantibody properdin-dependent opsonization of gram-negative bacteria (75). The enhancement of phagocytosis would seem to be one of the most important biological functions of complement and of particular importance for defense against infection by pyogenic bacteria.

Immune adherence is the property of $EAC\overline{(1)4(2)3}$ to attach to primate red cells, mammalian B lymphocytes, macrophages, monocytes, polymorphonuclear cells, and rabbit platelets. Particles other than erythrocytes acted upon by antibody and the first four complement components also exhibit immune adherence. This function of complement may be of importance in the clearance from the blood of bacteria and other pathogenic organisms (76).

The measurement of whole serum hemolytic complement is a useful screening test for the integrity of the complete system. However, decreases in the concentration of individual components to 50 per cent or less of the normal level may have little or no effect in this test. The test is based on the ability of sheep red cells properly sensitized by rabbit antibody to sheep erythrocytes to be lysed by the complete classic complement sequence. Hemoglobin released by such lysis can be measured spectrophotometrically with great precision and related to the percentage of cells lysed.

The measurement of complement proteins in highly complex mixtures such as human serum requires antibodies of very high specificity. Antibodies have now been produced against the majority of the complement proteins, and most precipitate with their respective antigens in whole serum. Quantitative immunochemical techniques are therefore available for the quantitation of complement proteins in serum and other biological fluids.

The measurement of the serum concentration of complement proteins in patients provides some information about the participation of complement in disease. However, this information, by its very static quality, is limited and ambiguous. The serum concentrations of all proteins, including those of the complement system, are determined by a dynamic equilibrium between synthesis and catabolism. A normal serum level may reflect a balance between abnormally accelerated synthesis and catabolism (77).

Deposition of complement proteins (usually along with immunoglobulins) in tissues such as kidney and skin has been taken as evidence for complement activation in disease. Such deposition is detected by the fluorescent antibody technique, using antibodies to individual proteins, such as C3, C4, and properdin (78). From studies in animals, it is clear that such deposition may result either from filtration and trapping of immune complexes within small blood vessels, as in the renal glomeruli, or from antibody reacting directly with kidney or other tissue antigens.

Metabolic studies with radioisotopically labeled purified complement proteins have yielded important information about complement protein metabolism. Although intuitively one might expect that rapid clearance of labeled complement proteins would attend complement activation in vivo, this is not necessarily true. It is only the case if fluid phase conversion products are cleared at a more rapid rate than the native molecule. Such is true of C3b and C4b, which

are removed from the circulation at rates five or more times those of the native proteins (77). No information is yet available for fragments of other complement proteins.

Hereditary Angioneurotic Edema

Hereditary angioneurotic edema results from a genetically determined deficiency of the C1 inhibitor. The defect is transmitted as an autosomal dominant. The serum of affected patients contains anywhere from 5 to 30 per cent of the normal concentration of C1 inhibitor (18 mg. per 100 ml. (79).

Patients with this disease are prone to recurrent episodes of swelling (Fig. 18–12). The edema fluid accumulates rapidly in the affected part, which becomes tense but not discolored; no itching, no pain, and no redness are associated with the edema. Laryn-

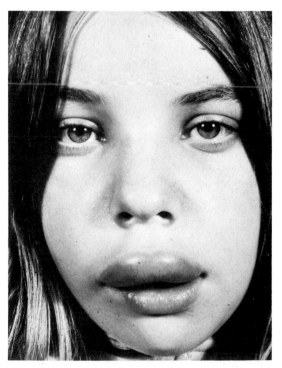

Figure 18–12. Face of a girl with hereditary angioneurotic edema during an attack. [From Rosen, F. S., and Alper, C. A.: Disorders of the complement system, In *Immunologic Disorders in Infants and Children.* Stiehm, E. R., and Fulginiti, V. A. (eds.), Philadelphia, W. B. Saunders Company, 1973, p. 291.]

geal edema may be fatal because of airway obstruction and consequent pulmonary edema. If the intestinal tract is involved, most often the jejunum, severe abdominal cramps and bilious vomiting ensue. Diarrhea, which is clear and watery in character, occurs when the colon is affected. The attacks last 48 to 72 hours. Although they are often unheralded, they may occur subsequent to trauma, menses, excessive fatigue, and mental stress. Attacks of angioedema are infrequent in early childhood; the disease exacerbates at adolescence and tends to subside in the sixth decade of life. In children especially a mottling of the skin reminiscent of erythema marginatum may be frequently noticed unassociated with the angioedema (80).

Attacks of angioedema are associated with the generation of activated C1 ($\overline{\text{C1}}$) in the plasma, an event which cannot be measured in normal plasma (81). The natural substrates of C1, C4, and C2 are consumed so that their serum concentration falls precipitously as the attack progresses. The terminal components of the complement system remain unaffected. Highly purified $\overline{\text{C1}}$ or $\overline{\text{C1s}}$, when injected into normal skin or into patients intradermally, induces angioedema. This reaction does not occur in people genetically deficient in C2, or in guinea pigs genetically deficient in C4, thus suggesting that the interaction of $\overline{\text{C1}}$ with C4 and C2 generates one or more factors which enhance vascular permeability — the effect is on the postcapillary venule (82). A polypeptide kininlike substance which has vasopermeability-inducing properties has also been generated in the plasma of the patients. Its origin from C2 appears likely but is not proved (83).

The activation of C1 in hereditary angioneurotic edema may occur via fibrinolysin, the intrinsic clotting mechanism, or the kallikrein system (84). In any case, the fibrinolytic inhibitors, epsilon-aminocaproic acid and its cyclic analog, tranexamic acid, provide effective prophylaxis against recurrent episodes of angioedema (85). Methyltestosterone is also effective in many patients when taken prophylactically as a daily 5-mg. linguet.

The autosomal dominant inheritance of hereditary angioneurotic edema remains an interesting puzzle. Obviously affected individuals are heterozygous for the abnormality. Despite this, their serum contains very little C1 inhibitor (average 17 per cent of normal), and liver biopsies can be shown to contain a markedly reduced number of hepatic parenchymal cells engaged in C1 inhibitor synthesis. In 15 per cent of affected kindred, sera of patients contain normal or elevated amounts of a cross-reacting, immunologically nonfunctional protein. There is no difference in the clinical picture in the CRM+ and CRM− patients (86).

Hereditary C2 Deficiency

In several species there appears to be a commonly occurring genetic defect of one of the complement components. Many strains of mice are deficient in C5; C6 deficiency is common in outbred rabbits (87, 88). Recently C4 deficiency has been encountered in guinea pigs at the N.I.H. (89). None of these animal strains appears to be at obvious risk for increased susceptibility to infection or other pathologic phenomena.

A sizable number of kindred have been discovered to be deficient in C2, apparently the common complement component deficiency in man (90, 91). The defect is transmitted as an autosomal recessive trait, but heterozygotes are easily detected by their having half the normal C2 concentration by functional or immunochemical measurements (92). Homozygous C2-deficient individuals do not have increased susceptibility to infection; this may be owing to the intact functioning of their alternate pathway or properdin system. However, several C2-deficient individuals have been found to have "collagen" disease, such as polymyositis and lupuslike illness (93). Whether or not there is increased connective tissue disease in C2-deficient individuals may reflect the mode of ascertainment of this deficiency.

Hereditary C3 Deficiency

C3 deficiency has been found in three kindreds recently. Homozygotes contain no C3 in their serum by immunochemical measurement and less than 0.1 per cent of normal by sensitive functional assay (94).

These children are subject to recurrent pyogenic infections, and their clinical history has a striking resemblance to agammaglobulinemia. C3-deficient serum is unable to sustain opsonization of bacterial particles.

C3 or the β_{1C} globulin has two common allelic forms, designated S for the electrophoretically slow variant, and F for the electrophoretically fast variant. The former is more common than the latter and has a gene frequency of 0.7, while the F variant has a gene frequency of 0.3 Several rare alleles have been discovered (95). In any case, individuals who are heterozygous for C3 deficiency appear homozygous because one allelic form is not expressed (96). Informative segregation of the nonexpressed allele can be seen in such heterozygotes in an affected kindred.

One family has been described to have a hypomorphic form of C3F designated C3f (97).

Miscellaneous Defects

Very recently a family in Rochester has been found to have C6 deficiency. The heterozygous state is readily detected, and the defect is transmitted as an autosomal recessive (98). A family with C7 deficiency has been found in Arizona. No data have as yet been published on this kindred. A family with C1r deficiency has been reported. Two affected homozygotes have a lupuslike syndrome, and two siblings were reported to have died of infection in infancy (99).

A significant number of patients with immunodeficiency have marked depressions in serum C1q levels (100). The significance of this association is not known, and the finding is not consistent in immunodeficiency. The C1q deficiency may result from increased consumption of this protein (101). Sporadic cases of C1s and C1r deficiency have been reported without genetic information.

C3 Hypercatabolism

As previously described, the alternate pathway of C3 activation or the properdin system operates by a positive feedback in that the generation of small amounts of C3b accelerates the pathway and results in considerable conversion of C3 to C3b. The C3 inactivator is a β-globulin of the serum which inhibits this alternate pathway at two points. It enzymatically cleaves C3b to C3c, thereby inactivating C3b, and it inhibits GBGase (C3PAase), an α-euglobulin enzyme involved in C3 activation by the alternate pathway. A patient homozygous for C3 inactivator deficiency has been found to have recurrent pyogenic infection due to the influenza bacillus, meningococci, and pneumococci, including mastoiditis, otitis, pneumonia, and septicemia (102). The consequence of his genetic deficiency is a spontaneous activation of the alternate pathway at all times, so that his serum contains C3b and GBGase but no GBG (or Factor B) and very little C3. The catabolic rate of C3 is four times normal, as ascertained by injection of ^{125}I-radiolabeled C3. As a consequence of the accelerated C3 destruction, he releases increased amounts of the C3 anaphylatoxin or C3a, so that he has massive histaminuria and occasional showers of hives (103). The urticaria is particularly pronounced when he is exposed to hot or cold water. Infusions of plasma halt the in vivo C3 hypercatabolism and cause the disappearance of C3b from his circulation. Ordinarily C3b produced in his circulation by the alternate pathway activation adheres to his erythrocytes so that they are C3 Coombs' positive (104). This phenomenon disappears transiently following the normal plasma infusion. Despite C3b on his red cells, their survival is normal, and he has no hemolytic anemia.

Several patients with endogenous C3 hypercatabolism have been described recently with partial lipodystrophy (105, 106). The mechanism of C3 cleavage in vivo in these patients is not understood, but it appears not to involve the alternate pathway but rather another mechanism of fluid phase C3 cleavage.

C5 Dysfunction

A familial disorder which may involve a dysfunctional C5 molecule has been reported in several families. Affected persons have eczema and increased susceptibility to infection by staphylococci and gram-negative bacteria during the first year of life. Their clinical picture resembles Leiner's disease. Their serum exhibits decreased enhancement of phagocytosis of yeast by normal peripheral blood leukocytes. The concentration of C5 is normal by immunochemical estimation and by hemolytic assay. Inheritance patterns are unclear (107).

Acquired Defects in the Complement System

It is generally considered that a decrease in serum complement results from in vivo "complement fixation." This is, on further reflection, a naive notion, for the serum level of any one or all the complement components reflects the rate of synthesis as well as the rate of catabolism of these proteins. In recent years it has been most convenient to assay for the serum concentration of C3 or the β_{1C}-globulin. By aforementioned immunochemical techniques, this measurement is readily available in most clinical laboratories. C3 levels in serum may decrease to very low concentrations in the presence of hepatocellular damage, for the hepatic parenchymal cell is the site of C3 synthesis. On the other hand, decreased serum C3 levels in lupus erythematosus reflect in vivo consumption of this protein by antigen-antibody interaction. This can be confirmed by studying the catabolic rate of ^{125}I-labeled C3 in patients with S.L.E. or mixed cryoglobulinemia.

C3 levels are very low in sera of children with acute poststreptococcal glomerulonephritis or membranoproliferative glomerulonephritis. In both instances, the lowered C3 level is due to a combination of decreased synthesis and increased catabolism. In acute poststreptococcal glomerulonephritis, there is initially a marked fall in all classic complement components, but within two or three days of the onset of symptoms most of the components return to normal (108). The concentrations of C3 and C5, however, remain low for three or four weeks. Evidence from metabolic studies with purified ^{125}I-labeled C3 suggests that, in the initial phase, the C3 concentration is lowered as part of the activation of the complement system, presumably by antigen-antibody complexes. Circulating conversion

products of C3 can sometimes be demonstrated during this initial phase. Studies performed two or three days after the onset of symptoms suggest that depressed C3 synthesis is responsible for the prolonged lowering of the level of C3 (and perhaps of C5 as well) after the initial activation phase.

The situation in membranoproliferative glomerulonephritis is far less clear (109). In this disorder, particularly as it occurs in children and adolescents, lowered hemolytic complement is a usual finding. This is almost always the result of markedly reduced levels of C3 and C5, with normal levels of most other complement components. Serum concentrations of GBG or properdin Factor B are usually normal in these patients, or at most slightly reduced. By immunofluorescent techniques using antibodies to immunoglobulins and C3, the latter proteins are demonstrable on the glomeruli in most patients. The sera of some patients with membranoproliferative glomerulonephritis contain circulating C3d and also may contain a protein termed nephritic factor which, when a normal serum protein, presumably deficient in the nephritic serum, is added, is capable of cleaving C3 in vitro (110). The nature of the nephritic factor is uncertain, with some investigators claiming that it is antibody of the IgG3 class, and others that it is a nonimmunoglobulin serum protein. The relevance of the lytic-nephritic interaction with C3 to the lowered C3 levels observed in vivo is cast into doubt by metabolic studies with labeled C3 in patients with membranoproliferative glomerulonephritis. The latter studies have shown normal or near-normal plasma disappearance curves of the injected C3, so that the low levels of C3 in some of these patients, at least, including those with nephritic factor, are primarily the result of depressed synthesis. Depressed synthesis of C3 in vitro by liver obtained from such patients has also been demonstrated.

There is some evidence that complement activation may occur in severe disseminated intravascular coagulation with fibrinolysis. In this clinical situation, it may be that the generated plasmin and possibly also thrombin attack C3 directly. Serum levels of the latter protein may be lowered. The lowered C3 serum concentrations observed in patients with advanced hepatic cirrhosis or other hepatocellular disease may result from associated disseminated intravascular coagulation and fibrinolysis, or from interference with C3 synthesis in this organ, which is its site of synthesis. We have observed marked elevations of C3 serum concentration in patients with severe biliary obstruction. The mechanisms for this elevation are unknown.

In certain cases of acquired hemolytic anemia, C3 is detected on erythrocytes by a Coombs antiglobulin reagent specific for this protein. General Coombs reagents vary in their content of anti-C3 and for the most part are anti-IgG. The presence of C3 on patients' red cells may indicate an antierythrocyte antibody which has "fixed complement," activation of C3 by other means with C3 deposition as part of the innocent bystander reaction, or an unusual abnormality of the red cell membrane, making it more "susceptible" to C3 uptake, as in paroxysmal nocturnal hemoglobinuria.

Total serum hemolytic complement and the levels of individual complement proteins are normal or elevated in patients with rheumatoid arthritis, and there is no evidence in serum of complement activation. However, the joint space is relatively sequestered from the circulating plasma, and there is now considerable evidence that complement participates locally in rheumatoid joint inflammation. Hemolytic complement is reduced in joint fluid from patients with rheumatoid arthritis, particularly those with rheumatoid factor and with nodules, when compared with joint effusions from patients with other disease. There is a reduction in the relative concentrations in the rheumatoid joint effusions of several complement proteins, including C4, C2, C3, and properdin Factor B, and conversion products of the latter two proteins are often found. Chemotactic factors, thought to consist of C5a and $C\overline{567}$, are found in the majority of rheumatoid joint effusions. By immunofluorescence, C3 and C4 have been identified in the lining cells, blood vessels, and intercellular connective tissue of rheumatoid synovial membranes. Incubation of normal leukocytes with joint fluid from patients with seropositive rheumatoid arthritis, but not seronegative disease, caused the development of intracellular inclusions containing IgG, IgM, and C3. It is not clear whether complement activation in joints affected by rheumatoid arthritis results from the presence of complexes of IgG antibody with an unknown, possibly viral, antigen, of complexes of IgM rheumatoid factor with aggregated gammaglobulin, of proteolytic enzymes from leukocytes, or of some combination of these factors (111).

Tests for paroxysmal nocturnal hemoglobinuria (PNH) depend upon the unusual susceptibility of red cells in this disease to complement lysis. In the Ham test, the test red cells are incubated in acidified (pH 6.7) fresh serum from an ABO-compatible person or from the patient. The minimal complement activation that occurs at somewhat acid pH will produce lysis of PNH cells but not normal erythrocytes. An important control consists of incubating the patient's red cells with serum heated at 56°C prior to acidification. With destruction of total hemolytic complement, such serum will not lyse PHN cells. The sugar water test for PNH depends upon minimal complement activation, probably attendant upon euglobulin precipitation. In this test patient's whole blood is mixed with 9 volumes of a 10 per cent solution and incubated. All tests for PNH lysis depend on the integrity of the properdin system in the lytic reagent. PNH cells, for unknown reasons, take up much more $\overline{C3}$ than normal erythrocytes.

References

1. WHO Committee: Primary immunodeficiencies. Report of WHO Organization Committee. Pediatrics 47:927, 1971.
2. Raff, M. C.: Surface antigenic markers for distinguishing T and B lymphocytes in mice. Transplant. Rev. 6:52, 1971.
3. Bianco, C. R., and Nussenzweig, U.: A population of lymphocytes bearing a membrane receptor of antigen-antibody-complement complexes. I. Separation and characterization. J. Exp. Med. 132:702, 1970.
4. Geha, R. S., Rosen, F. S., et al.: Identification and characterization of subpopulations of lymphocytes in human peripheral blood after fractionation on discontinuous gradients of albumin: The cellular defect in X-linked agammaglobulinemia. J. Clin. Invest. 52:1725, 1973.
5. Geha, R. F., Schneeberger, E., et al.: Interaction of human thymus-derived and non-thymus-derived lymphocytes in vitro. Induction of proliferation and antibody synthesis in B lymphocytes by a soluble factor released from antigen-stimulated T lymphocytes. J. Exp. Med. 138:1230, 1973.
6. Bach, J. F., Muller, J. Y., et al.: In vivo specific antigen recognition by rosette forming cells. Nature (Lond.) 227:1251, 1970.

7. Reif, A. E., and Allen, J. M. V.: Mouse thymic iso-antigens. Nature (Lond.) 209:521, 1966.

8. Amos, D. B., and Bach, F. H.: Phenotypic expressions of the major histocompatibility locus in man (HL-A): Leukocyte antigens and mixed leukocyte culture reactivity. J. Exp. Med. 128:623, 1968.

9. David, J. R.: Lymphocyte mediators and cellular hypersensitivity. New Engl. J. Med. 288:143, 1973.

10. Porter, R. R.: Structural studies of immunoglobulins. Science 180:713, 1973.

11. Edelman, G. M.: Antibody structure and molecular immunology. Science 180:830, 1973.

12. Fleischman, J. B.: Amino acid sequences in the Fd of a rabbit antibody heavy chain. Immunochemistry 10:401, 1973.

13. Bennich, H., and Johansson, S. G. O.: Structure and function of human immunoglobulin E, In *Advances in Immunology*. Vol. 13. Dixon, F. J., Jr., and Kunkel, H. G. (eds.), New York, Academic Press, 1971, pp. 1–51.

14. Ishizaka, K., Ishizaka, T., et al.: Physicochemical properties of reaginic antibody. VI. Effect of heat on γE–γG, and γA-antibodies in the sera of ragweed sensitive patients. J. Immunol. 99:610, 1967.

15. Stiehm, E. R., and Fudenberg, H. H.: Serum levels of immune globulins in health and disease. A survey. Pediatrics 37:715, 1966.

16. Buckley, R. H., Dees, S. C., et al.: Serum immunoglobulins. I. Levels in normal children and in uncomplicated childhood allergy. Pediatrics 41:600, 1968.

17. Alford, C. A., Schaefer, J., et al.: Correlative immunolysis, microbiologic and clinical approach to diagnosis of acute and chronic infections in newborn infants. New Engl. J. Med. 277:437, 1967.

18. Rosen, F. S., and Janeway, C. A.: The gamma globulins. III. The antibody deficiency syndromes. New Engl. J. Med. 275:709, 1966.

19. Steiner, M. L., and Pearson, H. A.: Bone marrow plasmacyte values in childhood: Morphologic correlation in developmental immunology. J. Pediatr. 68:652, 1966.

20. Janeway, C. A., Merler, E., et al.: Intravenous gamma globulin: Metabolism of gamma globulin fragments in normal and agammaglobulinemic persons. New Engl. J. Med. 278:919, 1968.

21. Rosen, F. S., Kevy, S. V., et al.: Recurrent bacterial infections and dysgammaglobulinemia: Deficiency of 7S gamma globulins in the presence of elevated 19S gamma globulins. Report of two cases. Pediatrics 28:182, 1961.

22. Schur, P., Borel, H., et al.: Selective gamma G globulin in patients with recurrent pyogenic infections. New Engl. J. Med. 283:631, 1970.

23. Yount, W. S., Hong, R., et al.: Imbalances of gamma globulin subgroups and gene defects in patients with primary hypogammaglobulinemia. J. Clin. Invest. 49:1957, 1970.

24. Crabbe, P. A., and Heremans, J. F.: Selective IgA deficiency with steatorrhea. Am. J. Med. 42:319, 1967.

24a. Ogra, P. L., Karzan, D. T., et al.: Immunoglobulins in serum and secretions after poliovaccine infection. New Engl. J. Med. 279:893, 1968.

25. Amman, A. J., and Hong, R.: Selective IgA deficiency and autoimmunity. Clin. Exp. Immunol. 7:833, 1970.

25a. Giedion, A., and Scheidegger, J. J.: Kongenitale immunparese bei Fehlen spezifischer β₂-Globuline und quantitativ normalen γ-Globulinen. Helv. Paediatr. Acta 12:241, 1957.

25b. Gelzayd, E. A., McCleery, J. L., et al.: Intestinal malabsorption and immunoglobulin deficiency. Arch. Intern. Med. 127:141, 1971.

25c. Hermans, J. F., and Crabbe, P. A.: IgA deficiency: General considerations and relation to human disease, In *Immunologic Deficiency Diseases in Man*. Bergsma, D., and Good, R. A. (eds.), New York, National Foundation — March of Dimes, 1968, pp. 298–307.

25d. Rosen, F. S., Smith, D. H., et al.: The etiology of hypoproteinemia in a patient with congenital chylous ascites. Pediatrics 30:696, 1962.

25e. Strober, W., Wochner, R. D., et al.: Intestinal lymphangiectasia: A protein-losing enteropathy with hypogammaglobulinemia, lymphocytopenia and impaired homograft rejection. J. Clin. Invest. 46:1643, 1967.

25f. Weiden, P. L., Blaese, R. M., et al.: Impaired lymphocyte transformation in intestinal lymphangiectasia: Evidence for at least two functionally distinct lymphocyte populations in man. J. Clin. Invest. 51:1319, 1972.

26. Vyas, G. N., Perkins, H. A., et al.: Anaphylactoid transfusion reactions associated with anti-IgA. Lancet 2:312, 1968.

26a. Ochs, H. D., Ament, M. E., et al.: Giardiasis with malabsorption in X-linked agammaglobulinemia. New Engl. J. Med. 287:341, 1972.

27. Geha, R., Schneeberger, E., et al.: On the heterogeneity of the common variable form of agammaglobulinemia. New Engl. J. Med., 1974, (in press).

28. Rosen, F. S., and Janeway, C. A.: The gamma globulins. III. The antibody deficiency syndromes. New Engl. J. Med. 275:769, 1966.

29. Geha, R. S., Schneeberger, E., et al.: Synthesis of an M component by circulating B lymphocytes in severe combined immunodeficiency (SCID). New Engl. J. Med. 290:726, 1974.

30. Giblett, E. R., Anderson, J. E., et al.: Adenosine-deaminase deficiency in two patients with severely impaired cellular immunity. Lancet 2:1067, 1972.

30a. Green, H., and Chan, T.-S.: Pyrimidine starvation induced by adenosine in fibroblasts and lymphoid cells: Role of adenosine deaminase. Science 182:836, 1973.

31. Gatti, R. A., Meuwissen, H. J., et al.: Immunological reconstitution of sex-linked lymphopenic immunologic deficiency. Lancet 2:1366, 1968.

32. DeKoning, J., van Bekkum, D. W., et al.: Transplantation of bone marrow cells and foetal thymus in an infant with lymphopenic immunological deficiency. Lancet 1:1223, 1969.

33. Levey, R. H., Gelfand, E. W., et al.: Bone marrow transplantation in severe combined immunodeficiency syndrome. Lancet 2:571, 1971.

34. Stiehm, M. E., Lawlor, G. J., Jr., et al.: Immunologic reconstitution in severe combined immunodeficiency without bone-marrow

chromosomal chimerism. New Engl. J. Med. 286:797, 1972.

35. Gitlin, D., Vawter, G., et al.: Thymic alymphoplasia and congenital aleukocytosis. Pediatrics 33:184, 1964.

36. Peterson, R. D. A., Kelly, W. D., et al.: Ataxia-telangiectasia, its association with defective thymus, immunologic deficiency disease, and malignancy. Lancet 1:1189, 1964.

37. Blaese, R. M., Brown, R. S., et al.: The Wiskott-Aldrich syndrome. Lancet 1:1056, 1968.

38. Cooper, M. D., Chase, H. P., et al.: Wiskott-Aldrich syndrome. Am. J. Med. 44:499, 1968.

39. Spitler, L. E., Levin, A. S., et al.: The Wiscott-Aldrich syndrome: Results of transfer factor therapy. J. Clin. Invest. 51:3216, 1972.

40. Kretschmer, R., Say, B., et al.: Congenital aplasia of the thymus gland. New Engl. J. Med. 279:1275, 1968.

41. DiGeorge, A. M.: Congenital absence of thymus and its immunologic consequences: Concurrence with congential hypoparathyroidism, In Immunologic Diseases in Man. Bergsma, D. (ed.), New York, National Foundation (Birth Defects: Orig. Art. Ser. 4:116, 1968).

42. Freedom, R. M., Rosen, F. S., et al.: Congenital cardiovascular disease and anomalies of the third and fourth pharyngeal pouch. Circulation 16:165, 1972.

43. August, C. S., Rosen, F. S., et al.: Implantation of a fetal thymus, restoring immunological competence in a patient with thymic aplasia (DiGeorge's syndrome). Lancet 2:1210, 1968.

44. Cleveland, W. W., Fogel, B. J., et al.: Foetal thymic transplant in a case of DiGeorge's syndrome. Lancet 2:1211, 1968.

45. August, C. S., Levey, R. H., et al.: Establishment of immunologic competence in a child with congenital thymic aplasia by a graft of fetal thymus. Lancet 1:1080, 1970.

46. Goldstein, A. L., Guha, A., et al.: Purification and biological activity of thymosin, a hormone of the thymus gland. Proc. Natl. Acad. Sci. USA 69:1800, 1972.

47. Eraklis, A. J., Kevy, S. V., et al.: Hazard of overwhelming infection after splenectomy in childhood. New Engl. J. Med. 276:1225, 1967.

48. Kevy, S. V., Tefft, M., et al.: Hereditary splenic hypoplasia. Pediatrics 42:752, 1968.

49. Benacerraf, B., Sebestyen, M., et al.: A quantitative study of the kinetics of blood clearance of P^{32}-labelled Escherichia coli and staphylococci by the reticuloendothelial system. J. Exp. Med. 110:27, 1959.

50. Schulkind, M. L., Ellis, E. F., et al.: Effect of antibody upon clearance of I^{125}-labelled pneumococci by the spleen and liver. Pediatr. Res. 1:178, 1967.

51. WHO Committee on complement: Nomenclature of complement. Bull. WHO 39:935, 1968.

52. Pillemer, L., Blum, L., et al.: The properdin system and immunity. I. Demonstration and isolation of a new serum protein, and properdin, and its role in immune phenomena. Science 120:279, 1954.

53. Lepow, I. H., Naff, G. B., et al.: Chromatographic resolution of the first component of human complement into three activities. J. Exp. Med. 117:983, 1963.

54. Polley, M. J.: Ultrastructural studies of Clq and of complement-membrane interaction. Progr. Immunol. 1:597, 1971.

55. Calcott, M. A., Müller-Eberhard, H. J., et al.: Clq protein of human complement. Biochemistry. 11:3443, 1972.

56. Bing, D.: Nature of the active site of a subunit of the first component of human complement. Biochemistry 8:4503, 1969.

57. Patrick, R. A., Taubman, S. B., et al.: Cleavage of the fourth component of human complement (C4) by activated Cls. Immunochemistry 7:217, 1970.

58. Müller-Eberhard, H. J.: Complement. Ann. Rev. Biochem. 38:389, 1969.

59. Dias da Silva, W., Eisels, J. W., et al.: Complement as a mediator of inflammation. III. Purification of the activity with anaphylatoxin properties generated by interaction of the first four components of complement and its identification as a cleavage product of C'3. Pediatrics 37:1017, 1966.

60. Abramson, N., Alper, C. A., et al.: Deficiency of C3 inactivator in man. J. Immunol. 107:19, 1971.

61. Müller-Eberhard, H. J., Polley, M. J., et al.: Formation and functional significance of a molecular complex derived from the second and the fourth components of human complement. J. Exp. Med. 125:359, 1967.

62. Blum, L., Pillemer, L., et al.: The properdin system and immunity. XIII. Assay and properties of a heat-labile serum factor (Factor B) in the properdin system. Z. Immunitätsforsch. Allerg. Klin. Immunol. 118:349, 1959.

62a. Pensky, J., Wurz, L, et al.: The properdin system and immunity. XII. Assay, properties and partial purification. Z. Immunitätsforsch. Allerg. Klin. Immunol. 118:329, 1959.

63. Pensky, J., Hinz, C. F., Jr, et al.: Properties of highly purified human properdin. J. Immunol. 100:142, 1968.

64. Boenisch, T., and Alper, C. A.: Isolation and properties of a glycine-rich β glycoprotein of human serum. Biochim. Biophys. Acta 221:529, 1970.

65. Götze, O., and Müller-Eberhard, H. J.: The C3-activator system: An alternate pathway of complement activation. J. Exp. Med. 134:90s, 1971.

66. Müller-Eberhard, H. J., and Götze, O.: C3 proactivator convertase and its mode of action. J. Exp. Med. 135:1003, 1972.

67. Alper, C. A., and Rosen, F. S.: Genetic aspects of the complement system, In Advances in Immunology. Vol. 14. Dixon, F. J., and Kunkel, H. G. (eds.), New York, Academic Press, 1971, pp. 252–290.

68. Alper, C. A., Rosen, F. S., et al.: Inactivator of the third component of complement as an inhibitor in the properdin pathway. Proc. Natl. Acad. Sci. USA 69:2910, 1972.

69. Lachmann, P. J., and Thompson, R. A.: Reactive lysis: The complement-mediated lysis of unsensitized cells. II. The characterization of activator reactor as C56 and the participation of C8 and C9. J. Exp. Med. 131:643, 1970.

70. Lepow, I. H.: Biologically active fragments of complement. Progr. Immunol. 1:579, 1971.

71. Cochrane, C. G., and Müller-Eberhard, H. J.: The

derivation of two distinct anaphylatoxin activities from the third and fifth components of human complement. J. Exp. Med. *127*:371, 1968.

72. Bokisch, V. A., and Müller-Eberhard, H. J.: Anaphylatoxin inactivator of human plasma: Its isolation and characterization as a carboxypeptidase. J. Clin. Invest. *49*:2427, 1970.

73. Johnston, R. B., Jr., Klemperer, M. R., et al.: The enhancement of bacterial phagocytosis by serum. The role of complement and two cofactors. J. Exp. Med. *129*:1275, 1969.

74. Smith, M. R., and Wood, B. W., Jr.: Heat-labile opsonins to Pneumococcus. I. Participation of complement. J. Exp. Med. *130*:1209, 1969.

75. Stossel, T. P., Alper, C. A., et al.: Serum-dependent phagocytosis of paraffin oil emulsified with bacterial lipopolysaccharide. J. Exp. Med. *137*:690, 1973.

76. Nelson, R. A.: The immune-adherence phenomenon. Proc. R. Soc. Med. *49*:55, 1956.

77. Alper, C. A., and Rosen, F. S.: Studies of the *in vivo* behavior of human C'3 in normal subjects and patients. J. Clin. Invest. *46*:2021, 1967.

78. Cochrane, C. G., and Koffler, D.: Immune complex disease in experimental animals and man. In *Advances in Immunology*. Vol. 16. Dixon, F. J., and Kunkel, H. G. (eds.), New York, Academic Press, 1973, pp. 185–264.

79. Donaldson, V. H., and Evans, R. R.: A biochemical abnormality in hereditary angioneurotic edema: Absence of serum inhibitor of C'1 esterase. Am. J. Med. *35*:37, 1963.

80. Donaldson, V. H., and Rosen, F. S.: Hereditary angioneurotic edema: A clinical survey. Pediatrics *37*:1017, 1966.

81. Donaldson, V. H., and Rosen, F. S.: Action of complement in hereditary angioneurotic edema. The role of C'1-esterase. J. Clin. Invest. *43*:2204, 1964.

82. Klemperer, M. R., Donaldson, V. H., et al.: Effect of C'1 esterase on vascular permeability in man: Studies in normal and complement-deficient individuals and in patients with hereditary angioneurotic edema. J. Clin. Invest. *47*:604, 1968.

83. Donaldson, V. H., Ratnoff, O. D., et al.: Permeability-increasing activity in hereditary angioneurotic edema plasma. J. Clin. Invest. *48*: 642, 1969.

84. Donaldson, V. H.: Blood coagulation and related plasma enzymes in inflammation. Ser. Haematol. *3*:39, 1970.

85. Sheffer, A. L., Austen, K. F., et al.: Tranexamic acid therapy in hereditary angioneurotic edema. New Engl. J. Med. *287*:452, 1972.

86. Rosen, F. S., Alper, C. A., et al.: Genetically determined heterogeneity of the C1 esterase inhibitor in patients with hereditary angioneurotic edema. J. Clin. Invest. *50*:2143, 1971.

87. Cinader, B., and Dubiski, S.: Suppression of murine allotypic specificities in animals with a complement system. J. Immunol. *101*: 1236, 1968.

88. Rother, K., Rother, U., et al.: Deficiency of the sixth component of complement in rabbits with an inherited complement defect. J. Exp. Med. *124*:773, 1966.

89. Frank, M. M., May, J., et al.: In vitro studies of complement function in sera of C4-deficient guinea pigs. J. Exp. Med. *134*:176, 1971.

90. Klemperer, M. R., Woodworth, H. C., et al.: Hereditary deficiency of the second component of complement (C'2) in man. J. Clin. Invest. *45*:880, 1966.

91. Klemperer, M. R., Austen, K. F., et al.: Hereditary deficiency of the second component of complement (C'2) in man: Further observations on a second kindred. J. Immunol. *98*:72, 1967.

92. Klemperer, M. R.: Hereditary deficiency of the second component of complement in man: An immunochemical study. J. Immunol. *102*: 168, 1969.

93. Agnello, V., DeBracco, M. M. E., et al.: Hereditary C2 deficiency with some manifestations of systemic lupus erythematosus. J. Immunol. *108*:837, 1972.

94. Alper, C. A., Colten, H. R., et al.: Homozygous deficiency of the third component of complement (C3) in a patient with repeated infections. Lancet *2*:1179, 1972.

95. Alper, C. A., and Rosen, F. S.: Studies of the *in vivo* behavior of human C'3 in normal subjects and patients. J. Clin. Invest. *47*:2181, 1967.

96. Alper, C. A., Propp, R. P., et al.: Inherited deficiency of the third component of human complement. J. Clin. Invest. *48*:553, 1969.

97. Alper, C. A., and Rosen, F. S.: Studies of a hypomorphic variant of human C3. J. Clin. Invest. *50*:324, 1971a.

98. Leddy, J. P., Frank, M. M., et al.: Hereditary deficiency of sixth component of complement (C6) in man (Abstract No. 182). J. Clin. Invest. *52*:50a, 1973.

99. Day, N. K., Geiger, H., et al.: C1r deficiency: An inborn error associated with cutaneous and renal disease. J. Clin. Invest. *51*:1102, 1972.

100. Gewurz, H., Pickering, R. J., et al.: Decreased C'1q protein concentration and agglutinating activity in agammaglobulinemia syndromes: An inborn error reflected in the complement system. Clin. Exp. Immunol. *3*:437, 1968.

101. Kohler, P. F., and Müller-Eberhard, H. J.: Complement-immunoglobulin relation: Deficiency of C'1q associated with impaired immunoglobulin G synthesis. Science *163*: 474, 1968.

102. Alper, C. A., Abramson, N., et al.: Complement defect associated with increased susceptibility to infection. New Engl. J. Med. *282*: 349, 1970a.

103. Alper, C. A., Abramson, N., et al.: Studies *in vivo* and *in vitro* on an abnormality in the metabolism of C3 in a patient with increased susceptibility to infection. J. Clin. Invest. *49*: 1975, 1970.

104. Abramson, N., Alper, C. A., et al.: Deficiency of C3 inactivator in man. J. Immunol. *107*:19, 1971.

105. Alper, C. A., Bloch, K. J., et al.: Increased susceptibility to infection in a patient with type II essential hypercatabolism of C3. New Engl. J. Med. *288*:601, 1973.

106. Peters, D. K., Williams, D. G., et al.: Mesangiocapillary nephritis, partial lipodystrophy, and hypocomplementaemia. Lancet *2*:535, 1973.

107. Miller, M. E., and Nilsson, U. R.: A familial deficiency of the phagocytosis-enhancing activity of serum related to a dysfunction of the fifth component of complement (C5). New Engl. J. Med. 282:354, 1970.

108. Klemperer, M. R., Gotoff, S. P., et al.: Estimation of the serum beta-1-C globulin concentration. Pediatrics 35:765, 1965.

109. Gotoff, S. P., Fellers, F. X., et al.: The beta-1-C globulin in childhood nephrotic syndrome. Laboratory diagnosis of progressive glomerulonephritis. New Engl. J. Med. 273:524, 1965.

110. West, C. D., Winter, S., et al.: Evidence for in vivo breakdown of beta-1-C globulin in hypocomplementemic glomerulonephritis. J. Clin. Invest. 46:539, 1967.

111. Schur, P. H., and Austen, K. F.: Complement in human disease. Ann. Rev. Med. 19:1, 1968.

III

COAGULATION

Chapter 19

Blood Coagulation in Hemostasis

by Virginia H. Donaldson
and C. Thomas Kisker

In man, hemostasis depends upon the state of the vasculature, the quality, quantity, and functional capacity of the platelets, and the rather complex coagulation mechanisms of the blood plasma. Each of two pathways for generating clot-promoting activity in plasma is important, for sufficient deficiency of a single component of either pathway is usually associated with a bleeding tendency. Present knowledge of human blood coagulation, which has come largely from studies of plasma from persons with hereditary defects of plasma clotting factors or with acquired inhibitors of coagulation, permits us to summarize mechanisms of coagulation in a fashion which meaningfully correlates laboratory science with clinical observation.

PHYSIOLOGY OF COAGULATION

One mechanism of generating coagulant activity in plasma is initiated when blood contacts substances in tissues, as when an injury occurs, and is called the *extrinsic clotting mechanism* (Fig. 19–1). The other pathway can become active in plasma free of blood cells by exposure to a foreign surface, such as a glass test tube (1–5). This mechanism, known as the *intrinsic pathway*, seems to act independently of the extrinsic pathway. When either is activated, a series of events follows in which pro-

coagulant plasma proteins are converted into active forms, some of which are enzymes (6,7). Ultimately thrombin, a proteolytic enzyme responsible for the conversion of fibrinogen to fibrin, is generated. Even though a small amount of enzymatic activity may theoretically be amplified enormously by subsequent enzymatic steps in coagulation, the presence of inhibitors in the blood, the formation of complexes, and the inactivation of components of these coagulant complexes seem to limit clot-promoting activity.

Intrinsic Clotting Mechanism

The reasons for the prompt clotting of cell-free plasma upon transfer to a glass vessel (3, 4) were clarified when a specific property of plasma was found lacking from the plasma of Mr. John Hageman (5). Although he had no hemorrhagic symptoms, Mr. Hageman's blood clotted only after an extraordinarily long time in a glass test tube. The property lacking from his plasma has been called Hageman factor (Factor XII) (see Table 19–1), and it resides in a protein which has since been found in most mammalian plasmas. When normal plasma comes in contact with a glass-like surface, Hageman factor is activated and appears to acquire enzymatic activity, enabling it to then interact with another clotting factor,

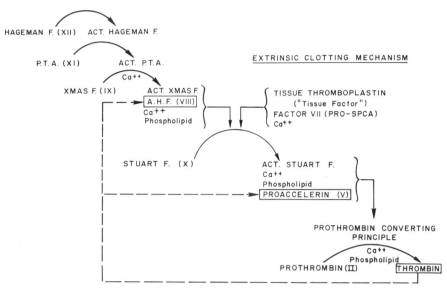

Figure 19–1. The production of thrombin during blood clotting.

plasma thromboplastin antecedent (PTA or Factor XI) (8). Hageman factor has been called "surface factor" or "contact factor," and it may be activated by numerous insoluble substances not normally present in the body (9), as well as by a soluble chemical called ellagic acid (10). An important common characteristic of activating substances seems to be their net negative charge (9). In the body,

several tissue constituents can activate Hageman factor. Because of their ability to activate Hageman factor, collagen (11, 12) and sebaceous secretions (13, 14) may perform important hemostatic functions when blood vessels or the skin are injured.

In addition to its coagulant action, activated Hageman factor can induce pathophysiologic changes characteristic of in-

TABLE 19–1.   GLOSSARY OF TERMS COMMONLY USED

Term	International Nomenclature	Other
Fibrinogen	Factor I	—
Prothrombin	Factor II	—
Thromboplastin	Factor III	Thrombokinase
Proaccelerin	Factor V	Ac-globulin
Stuart factor	Factor X	
Activated Stuart factor	Factor Xa	Autoprothrombin C, thrombokinase
Pro SPCA	Factor VII	Co-thromboplastin
Antihemophilic factor	Factor VIII	AHF, antihemophilic Factor A.
Christmas factor	Factor IX	Plasma thromboplastin component (PTC), Christmas Factor, antihemophilic Factor B
Plasma thromboplastin antecedent	Factor XI	PTA, antihemophilic Factor C
Hageman factor	Factor XII	"Contact factor"*
Plasmin	—	Fibrinolysin
Plasminogen	—	Profibrinolysin

*Activated PTA is sometimes also referred to as "contact factor."

flammation by initiating a series of enzymatic changes in plasma which culminate in the release of inflammatory polypeptides, known as kinins (15–17). These polypeptides in turn can cause vasodilatation, increased vascular permeability, and pain, thus producing signs of inflammation. Activated Hageman factor may contribute to the inflammation of gout or pseudogout, for microcrystalline monosodium urate crystals (18) and calcium pyrophosphate (18) can induce its activation. L-homocystine, also an activator of Hageman factor (19), perhaps contributes to the thromboembolic tendency often fatal to individuals with homocystinuria (20), but platelet alterations are probably more important in the etiology of this tendency (21). Cartilage and heparin, known for their anticoagulant action at later stages of coagulation, can cause release of kinin polypeptides in plasma in vitro, probably by first activating Hageman factor (22).

The precise mechanism of activation of Hageman factor by negatively charged substances is unclear. Hageman factor may be activated by insoluble substances during adsorption to their surfaces, but the nature of its reaction with soluble activators is not known. When purified Hageman factor is activated in solutions of ellagic acid, it behaves as if it were rendered relatively insoluble, as judged by its sedimentation and gel filtration behavior (23). These alterations may indicate exposure of hydrophobic portions of the molecule which are obscured in the precursor, or the formation of large polymers (23, 24). Speer and Ridgway (25) thought that activation with barium stearate was reversible, but the apparent reversibility may instead have resulted from residual unactivated Hageman factor in experimental mixtures. Following different means of activation in vitro, Hageman factor–like activity more effective in promoting kinin formation than clotting was found in low molecular weight components (16, 17).

The reaction between activated Hageman factor and PTA (see Fig. 19–1) is apparently enzymatic in nature, but is not inhibited by diisopropylfluorophosphate (DFP) or soybean trypsin inhibitor (8, 26). In spite of its enzymatic behavior with respect to PTA, activated Hageman factor has not been found to hydrolyze artificial substrates (9). Once activated, PTA may promote clotting while complexed with activated Hageman factor on a surface (27, 28), but it acts separately from activated Hageman factor in solution (23, 29). Both the coagulant and esterolytic properties of activated PTA are blocked by DFP (30), attesting to its enzymatic nature. Activated PTA interacts with Christmas factor (Factor IX, plasma thromboplastin component, or PTC) in the presence of calcium, or certain other divalent metal ions (30). During activation, the electrophoretic mobility of Christmas factor activity changes, suggesting that hydrolysis of the molecule may have occurred (31). Once active, Christmas factor is readily inhibited by heparin (32, 33).

In the next event in intrinsic coagulation, a complex with coagulant activity forms which is composed of activated Christmas factor, phospholipid, AHF (antihemophilic factor or Factor VIII), and calcium (34, 35). Calcium is critical to the maintenance of this complex, for Hougie et al. (34) found that preparations of AHF or Christmas factor and lipid were excluded from large pore gels when mixed with calcium, as if a large complex formed, but in the absence of calcium, components of the complex were eluted separately from the gel column. Even in the absence of calcium, AHF may combine with phospholipid (34). In other experiments, antiserum to either AHF or Christmas factor neutralized the coagulant activity of a preformed complex consisting of purified preparations of these two factors with lipid and calcium (35).

The activated complex of AHF, Christmas factor, phospholipid, and calcium then activates Stuart factor (Factor X) (Fig. 19–1). Apparently coincidentally, AHF becomes inactive (36), possibly because of its involvement in a complicated feedback mechanism involving thrombin. Once a small amount of thrombin is generated during clotting, it can interact with AHF, rendering it more active in formation of a complex which activates Stuart factor (37, 38). With the formation of larger amounts of thrombin, however, the activity of AHF is destroyed (36). Thus, AHF behaves as a cofactor and a substrate, and theoretically may effectively regulate the activation of Stuart factor.

Activated Stuart factor (Xa) has been called "thrombokinase" by Milstone (39), and "autoprothrombin C" by Seegers and his associates (45). Its capacity to act upon prothrombin requires the formation of another complex, consisting of activated Stuart factor, phospholipid, proaccelerin (Factor V), and calcium (40–42). Again, calcium behaves as an essential ligand in the formation of the active complex. Factor V may become attached to the lipid in the absence of calcium (40), but lacks the capacity for prothrombin conversion in its own right (41). Today there is considerable unanimity in the view that the activated Stuart factor complexed with proaccelerin on a phospholipid micelle with calcium is the active prothrombin-converting principle (43) (see Fig. 19–1).

The enzymatic nature of activated Stuart factor is further indicated by its ability to hydrolyze certain synthetic amino acid esters (44), and by its inhibition by PMSF (phenylmethanesulfonyl fluoride) (45), DFP, and soybean trypsin inhibitor (46, 47). Stuart factor may also be activated in vitro by the venom of Russell's viper (48), allowing its identification in plasma through the coagulant effect of the venom.

The formation of thrombin by a catalytic mechanism was postulated by Morawitz (49) long before the chemical identification of prothrombin. When the prothrombin molecule is attacked by the prothrombin-converting principle containing activated Stuart factor, it is hydrolyzed, releasing two or more fragments (50), one of which has the coagulant properties of thrombin. Thrombin itself may also catalyze the conversion of prothrombin to thrombin by a proteolytic action distinct from that of activated Stuart factor (51).

Extrinsic Clotting Mechanism

When tissues are injured, "thromboplastic" substances released from cells can initiate clotting. A thromboplastic substance in tissues such as brain and lung induces clotting by forming a complex with Factor VII (pro-SPCA) in the plasma in an instantaneous, and perhaps stoichiometric, reaction (52). The enzymatic activity of the complex of Factor VII, calcium, and tissue thromboplastin is inhibited by DFP and soybean trypsin inhibitor (52), but neither component of the complex alone can acti-

vate Stuart factor nor be altered by either protease inhibitor (52). The site responsible for the catalytic activation of Stuart factor may reside on the Factor VII molecule, for Østerud et al. (53) separated activated Factor VII from such a complex following its exposure to phospholipase C. The activated Factor VII so separated was probably still combined with phospholipid, but free of the protein portion of thromboplastin (53).

The thromboplastic material, called "tissue factor" by Nemerson and his colleagues, has been found in fractions of lung, placenta, and brain cells which contain microsomes (54–57). Nemerson and Pitlick (58, 59) have isolated and characterized tissue factor from bovine lung and find it to be a complex of a protein apoenzyme and lipid. This apoenzyme interacts with Factor VII to generate Stuart factor converting activity if it is first combined with an appropriate phospholipid, for apoprotein can bind to certain lipids but then fail to develop coagulant activity (59). The solubilized apoprotein portion of tissue factor has peptidase activity (60), but it is not yet certain if this property is also related to its coagulant activity.

The electrophoretic mobility of bovine Stuart factor gradually changes following its activation with Russell's viper venom (47), as if the molecule were hydrolyzed, but the fact that coagulant activity attributable to activated Stuart factor develops before the change in its charge suggests that activation involves a minor molecular alteration. After Stuart factor has been activated through the extrinsic pathway just described, it in turn derives its prothrombin converting activity through the formation of a complex with phospholipid, calcium, and proaccelerin, functionally identical to that arising during intrinsic clotting (Fig. 19–1).

The prothrombin converting complex resembles the complex of activated Christmas factor, AHF, phospholipid, and calcium which activates Stuart factor. The activity of both AHF and proaccelerin is enhanced by thrombin. Both AHF and proaccelerin are relatively thermolabile, are inactivated during clotting, presumably through further action of thrombin (61, 62), and are consequently not identifiable as coagulant substances in serum. Thus here, too, the rate of formation of thrombin generating activity is probably regulated by the amount of thrombin, which has already formed as if to facilitate clotting initially and promote hemostasis, but to prevent generation of excessive amounts of thrombin favoring thrombosis. One proaccelerin preparation, however, was only inactivated by thrombin (63), as if a substance required for activation might have been removed during purification.

Although the intrinsic and extrinsic pathways of coagulation are considered to function separately until a prothrombin-converting principle is formed, there are hints that reactions involving Factor VII and factors concerned with contact activation of the intrinsic pathway may occur. On the one hand, contact activation of Factor VII–deficient plasma may be defective (64), and on the other hand plasma from some individuals with Christmas factor deficiency demonstrates impaired formation of activated Stuart factor following contact with tissue thromboplastin (65). Reasons for the suggested relationship between contact activation and Factor VII are not entirely clear, but there are chemical similarities between Factor VII and Christmas factor (see p. 568).

Fibrin Formation

Fibrinogen is a complex molecule consisting of three pairs of polypeptide chains, designated alpha (A), beta (B), and gamma (66), which are linked together in disulfide bonds near their N-terminal portions (67). Thrombin, once generated, has remarkably specific proteolytic activity, for it readily catalyzes the transformation of fibrinogen to insoluble fibrin (68, 69), releasing two pairs of acidic polypeptide fragments, fibrinopeptides A and B, from the alpha (A) and beta (B) chains of fibrinogen, respectively (70), by hydrolyzing certain arginylglycine bonds in these two chains (21). Fibrinopeptide A is released more rapidly than is fibrinopeptide B. Following release of fibrinopeptides A, end-to-end polymerization of residual soluble intermediates occurs (Fig. 19–2) (72). The slower release of fibrinopeptide B may facilitate some later stages of polymerization, perhaps involving side-to-side polymerization reactions between fibrin monomers.

Fibrinopeptides A are chemically heterogeneous. One form, fibrinopeptide AP, is a phosphorylated fibrinopeptide A, and another, fibrinopeptide AY, lacks the N-terminal alanine usually present in fibrinopeptide A (72). While the reasons for this heterogeneity are unclear, it probably does not reflect genetically determined differences, because all three species of fibrinopeptide A were found in blood drawn from a large number of individuals (72). Conceivably, they result from in vivo degradation of fibrinogen or fibrinopeptides.

Fibrin Stabilization

Fibrin formed by polymerization of fibrin monomers released by thrombin has limited tensile strength. Another reaction, initiated by thrombin, induces stabilization of this fibrin. Thrombin activates a plasma enzyme called fibrin stabilizing factor (Factor XIII or fibrinase) in the presence of calcium (Fig. 19–2) (73). Activated fibrin stabilizing factor is a transamidase which

THE FINAL STAGE OF CLOTTING

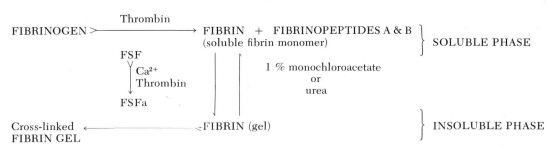

Figure 19–2. The soluble and insoluble phases of fibrinogen production.

establishes cross-linkages between adjacent fibrin monomers. The chemical reaction introduces a chemical bond between the gamma amide of a glutamine residue of one monomer and the epsilon amino group of a lysine residue of an adjacent monomer (74–76) coincident with the release of ammonia (74). The chemical stability of fibrin is thereby increased (77), for unstabilized fibrin is soluble in solutions of urea or 1 per cent monochloracetic acid, but stabilized fibrin is not. Although cross-linking between gamma chains induced by fibrin stabilizing factor occurs quickly and renders the fibrin insoluble in urea or monochloroacetic acid, extensive cross-linking between alpha chains occurs more slowly and may make fibrin resistant to fibrinolytic activity (77). The change in solubility of fibrin was reported before fibrin stabilizing factor was identified in plasma when Robbins (78) noted that the fibrin formed in the test tube was soluble in monochloroacetic acid if calcium was not included in the clotting mixture.

Fibrin stabilizing activity is probably a primitive coagulation mechanism, for fibrinogens of certain crustaceans coagulate by this means rather than by polymerization of fibrin monomers released by thrombin (79). It is not known if such a mechanism is involved in species lacking plasma coagulation mechanisms, but in which coagulation is accomplished by cells called amebocytes (80).

Inhibitors of Clotting

Several plasma inhibitors can regulate clot-promoting activity by blocking activated clotting factors. When plasma comes in contact with glass, activity attributable to activated Hageman factor gradually decays (4), as if enzymatic destruction had occurred (81). Both activated Hageman factor and activated PTA may be inhibited by an α-globulin in plasma (82, 83). An α-neuraminoglycoprotein (84), known principally for its inhibition of an esterase derived from the first component of complement (inhibitor of C1 esterase, or C$\bar{1}$ inactivator) (85), can impair the action of activated Hageman factor and activated PTA in experimental mixtures utilizing purified preparations of enzymes and inhibitor (85). However, its role in regulating the early

stages of clotting in vivo is obscure. Purified preparations of inhibitor of C1 esterase did not delay clotting of normal plasma, and plasma genetically deficient in inhibitor of C1 esterase still inhibits activated PTA (86).

Inhibitors of thrombin have been described through various experimental manipulations. *Antithrombin I* is a term applied to the inactivation of thrombin coincident with its adsorption to fibrin (87). *Antithrombin II*, a plasma protein which reacts with heparin (heparin cofactor) to inhibit clotting of plasma by thrombin, now seems identical with *antithrombin III*, gradually effective in blocking thrombin even in the absence of heparin (*vide infra*). Progressive antithrombin activity which is said to develop when prothrombin is converted to thrombin is called *antithrombin IV* (80).

Preparations of heparin cofactor inhibit plasmin as well as thrombin (88a, 88b). Heparin accelerates a stoichiometric reaction of this antithrombin with thrombin by inducing a conformational change that exposes a critical arginine residue, which enhances binding to thrombin (88c).

Recent definitive studies of Yin, Wessler, and Stoll (89, 90) provide convincing experimental support for the identity of *antithrombin III* with *antithrombin II* (heparin cofactor) (91, 92), for during extensive purification these inhibitory properties were inseparable (89). More important, this purified antithrombin seemed much more effective as an inhibitor of activated Stuart factor than of thrombin (91). Heparin markedly enhanced the inhibition of both thrombin and activated Stuart factor by purified preparations of this inhibitor (90), but, again, blockade of activated Stuart factor far exceeded that of thrombin. While both the coagulant and esterolytic properties of activated Stuart factor were blocked, only the coagulant activity of thrombin preparations was inhibited (90). Protamine sulfate did not reverse heparin-induced total blockade of activated Stuart factor by this inhibitor (90), although it did neutralize heparin blockade of thrombin-induced clotting. Thus, the mechanisms of reaction of this inhibitor with activated Stuart factor and thrombin differ. Its importance in clotting may rest mainly in its inhibition of activated Stuart factor, for this action provides a mechanism for regulating the function of both intrinsic and extrinsic mechanisms of coagulation before thrombin forms. Activated Hageman factor and activated PTA were not blocked by preparations of "antiactivated Factor X" (89), nor did it affect inactive Stuart factor (90).

In animal experiments, clot-promoting complexes containing activated Stuart factor are inactivated by the liver (93). Serum itself can inactivate tissue thromboplastin (94, 95), provided calcium ions are present, perhaps by interfering with Factor VII activity. As mentioned above, the adsorption of thrombin by fibrin is associated with loss of its activity (87).

The gradually emerging body of in vitro experimental evidence indicates that there are multiple inhibitors of clotting in plasma, and, in addition, one coagulant substance may be subject to inhibition by more than one inhibitory substance. Conversely, a single inhibitory substance may interfere with the function of more than one coagulant, as demonstrated by the effects of inhibitor of C1 esterase (α_2-neuraminoglycoprotein) and of "antiactivated Factor X." Additional clues as to the physiologic importance of naturally occurring plasma inhibitors will doubtless soon be reported.

FIBRINOLYSIS

Plasma has the capacity to dissolve fibrin clots. In freshly drawn plasma, the fibrinolytic property is normally inactive. Under a number of circumstances, plasminogen, the precursor of a fibrinolytic enzyme, may be converted to its active form, plasmin. In the test tube, plasmin can digest fibrin clots, and, while best known for this property, it can also digest fibrinogen; proaccelerin; AHF; Christmas factor; the first, third, and fifth components of the complement system (an immune mechanism of the body discussed elsewhere in this volume); and some other proteins of the body. Plasmin is a proteolytic enzyme of broad specificity; its action can also be measured upon several proteins not normally present in the body, and upon synthetic esters of arginine, lysine, and histidine. Since plasminogen exists in high concentrations in plasma, the potential exists for plasmin to form in concentrations harmful to the body if left

uncontrolled. The natural in vivo function of plasmin is usually considered to be fibrinolytic, but since it can also affect a number of other plasma enzyme systems, such as complement, it is possible that it participates in defense mechanisms involved in immunologic injury. Several plasma inhibitors of plasmin regulate its action.

Plasminogen may be activated in vitro during incubation with chloroform (96) by exposure to streptokinase (97), a product of certain beta-hemolytic streptococci, or by limited digestion with urokinase, an activator of plasminogen found in normal urine (98). In addition, certain substances in tissues, particularly vascular tissue, can activate plasminogen (99). Blood drawn from persons who have been strenuously exercised (100) or alarmed (100), who have received adrenaline injections (101) or electroshock therapy (102), or who have sustained shock because of hemorrhage (103) is likely to have fibrinolytic activity. Although the exact means through which fibrinolytic activity evolves is not understood, one or more substances capable of activating plasminogen may be released from the vascular endothelium. Through a complex mechanism, activated Hageman factor can interact with certain other plasma components called "Hageman factor cofactors" to generate a property which can activate plasminogen (104). In addition, the fibrinolytic mechanism is apparently more readily activated upon a fibrin surface. Thus, plasmin is likely to evolve as a result of clotting, as if its teleologic designation were to defend against thrombosis.

Hemorrhage due primarily to spontaneous fibrinolysis is extremely rare. When fibrinolytic activity, or its consequences, is identified in blood from a person with a hemorrhagic syndrome, it nearly always results from an episode of intravascular coagulation (see pp. 600–610). However, a rare patient has been thought to have fibrinolytic purpura, in which hemorrhage seems to have been the result of primary fibrinolysis (112). The capacity of plasmin to hydrolyze fibrinogen and fibrin has been utilized to identify its effects in blood, for incoagulable fragments of fibrinogen and fibrin may be identified in serum by immunochemical tests utilizing monospecific antibody to fibrinogen.

Inhibition of Fibrinolysis

Several plasma components can inhibit fibrinolytic activity, either by blocking the action of plasmin or by inhibiting the activation of plasminogen. Aoki and Von Kaulla (105) have chromatographically separated plasma inhibition directed against plasmin from that directed against preparations of plasminogen activator derived from vascular tissue. Antiactivator activity was also separated from α_1-antitrypsin (105). Alpha$_2$-macroglobulin can inhibit plasmin (106), and although the proteolytic action of plasmin is blocked when it is complexed with α_2-macroglobulin, esterolytic activity persists (107). Alpha$_2$-antiplasmin reacts immediately with plasmin, forming a dissociable complex (108), but α_1-inhibitor reacts slowly and irreversibly with plasmin (108). Other in vitro maneuvers have defined the multiplicity of inhibitors of plasmin in plasma, for a component of antiplasmin activity is labile at 56°C, and another component stable at this temperature (109). Additionally, part of the heat-stable antiplasmin is inactivated by primary amines (hydrazine, for example), while part remains stable (109). Serum inhibitor of C1 esterase, also effective in blocking plasmin (110), may be a significant component of heat-labile antiplasmin activity in plasma. Rimon and his associates (111) described other evidence of the broad specificity of plasma antiplasmin, for purified preparations of α_1-antiplasmin also blocked trypsin, chymotrypsin, and thrombin.

Fibrinolysis in the Neonate

The usual in vivo function of plasmin in the infant is as obscure as it is in older age groups. The concentration of plasminogen in the plasma of the newborn is significantly lower than that in adults (113) and is unrelated to the level in maternal plasma; premature infants are even more deficient (114). This deficiency may persist for six weeks or longer (115). The concentration of inhibitory activity in plasma directed against streptokinase-activated fibrinolytic activity is also low in premature and full-term infants (114). The fact that fibrinolytic activity may be evident in blood obtained from the newborn infant, or even the premature infant, suggests that an equilibrium exists at lowered concentrations of components of this system, which allows activation of plasminogen to occur upon such provocation as anoxia sustained during delivery. It has been proposed that inadequate fibrinolytic mechanisms may lead to pathophysiologic changes in the respiratory distress syndrome (116), but other factors may be more important.

VITAMIN K AND THE SYNTHESIS OF CERTAIN CLOTTING FACTORS

Some clotting factors important to both the intrinsic and extrinsic coagulation pathways are synthesized by the liver, provided adequate vitamin K is available. Christmas factor, Stuart factor, prothrombin, and Factor VII are dependent on vitamin K for their biosynthesis, but fibrinogen and proaccelerin, also synthesized by the liver, do not require vitamin K. Vitamin K–dependent clotting factors are chemically similar, for all are largely removed from plasma which has been adsorbed with barium sulfate or aluminum hydroxide, and, except for prothrombin, they are not inactivated or "consumed" during clotting, for their coagulant activity may be identified in fresh serum. Concentrations of vitamin K–dependent clotting factors in plasma from pregnant women are elevated, while in cases of hepatic injury, they are decreased (117). Moreover, coumarin drugs, used as indirectly acting anticoagulants, exert their effects by interfering with the synthesis of these vitamin K–dependent clotting factors by the liver. Dr. Seegers and his associates believe that vitamin K–dependent clotting substances are actually derivatives of a parent prothrombin molecule (118). The inherited deficiencies of isolated factors in this group of coagulants suggest that they are at least partially synthesized in vivo as separate proteins.

Direct evidence of the influence of vitamin K upon synthesis of vitamin K–dependent clotting factors in the liver came from in vitro experiments in which livers isolated from rats given a coumarin drug were then perfused with solutions containing sufficient vitamin K to induce synthesis of these proteins (119). Vitamin K appears to act at a synthetic step after the formation of specific messenger RNA, but before release of functional coagulant proteins (120). Rats and humans, genetically resistant to the effects of coumarin drugs, have provided important clues as to the interrelated actions of coumarin anticoagulants and vitamin K in vivo. Humans resistant to anticoagulant effects of coumarins on the basis of an inherited autosomal dominant trait are coincidentally extremely sensitive to the effects of vitamin K (121), but rats genetically resistant to warfarin are also resistant to vitamin K (122, 123). Conceivably, an inherited alteration in cellular receptor sites in humans may favor the binding of vitamin K but discourage the binding of coumarin compounds, while in rats such a receptor may be altered in a manner limiting binding of both substances. Resistance to coumarin compounds could not be attributed to altered catabolism or increased excretion rates.

In support of the predictions made by Hemker, which were based on kinetic studies of the coagulant properties of plasma from persons treated with coumarin-like anticoagulants (124), inactive prothrombin-like protein, or "preprothrombin," has been detected in such plasma by immunochemical means (125). This protein interferes with the conversion of prothrombin to thrombin, and seems to represent one or more precursor molecules which may bind to other plasma coagulants but then fail to function. The term "protein induced by vitamin K antagonists," or "PIVKA" (124), has been applied to this protein, and it is absent from plasma of patients deficient in vitamin K–dependent clotting factors because of hepatocellular disease. Therefore, its presence offers another means of distinguishing hepatic failure from other causes of impaired synthesis of these clotting factors. The electrophoretic mobility of prothrombin in normal plasma (125) differs from that of prothrombin-like protein in plasma from patients given vitamin K antagonist (126), when examined by immunoelectrophoretic means with antisera to human prothrombin.

It is likely that the action of vitamin K in the synthesis of clotting factors is directed at a step in which carbohydrate is attached to a polypeptide backbone of the molecule already synthesized (127–129). Inhibitors of protein synthesis did not block synthesis of vitamin K–dependent clotting factors in in vivo and in vitro studies of rats (127, 128). Intracellular localization of ^{3}H–vitamin K mainly to the microsomal fractions rather than to mitochondria, ribosomes, or purified nuclei of rats' liver cells was not significantly altered in animals given warfarin (130), as if the site of action of vitamin K were at the microsome.

The lipid solubility of vitamin K governs its absorption from the gastrointestinal tract. Faulty biliary function, malabsorption, or steatorrhea may induce a deficiency of vitamin K–dependent clotting factors because the vitamin is not available to the liver. Once absorbed, the vitamin may be inadequately utilized by the liver if hepatocellular injury or disease is present or this organ is immature, as in the prematurely born. Salicylates and *Cinchona* alkaloids can antagonize vitamin K (131, 132). Intrauterine anoxia may block the use of vitamin K by the newborn liver. The normal bacterial flora of the large intestine, responsible for synthesis of much of the vitamin K used, is not present in the newborn, so that the infant may be deficient in this source of vitamin K. Vitamin K may be absorbed by the large intestine of the infant (133), but experimental evidence that this may occur in adults is inadequate. Prolonged parenteral alimentation and the effect of antibiotics given during the newborn period upon colonic flora may further interfere with this source of vitamin K and place the infant at risk of hemorrhage (163).

COAGULATION IN THE NEWBORN PERIOD

Although a number of plasma proteins in maternal plasma may cross the placenta and reach the fetal circulation, insignificant amounts of most clotting proteins cross this barrier. Concentrations of vitamin K–dependent clotting factors, fibrinogen, and AHF in maternal plasma are elevated late in pregnancy, but much lower concentrations are found in plasma of the newborn, and there is apparently no relationship between titers of clotting factors in maternal and fetal blood following a normal delivery (134). When Gitlin and his associates injected radioactively labeled preparations of purified plasma proteins intravenously into pregnant women about to deliver, only traces of labeled fibrinogen appeared in fetal plasma (135). However, its rate of disappearance from maternal plasma was slightly more rapid than in other normal persons. In other experiments in which fetal tissues were evaluated for their capacity to incorporate radioactive amino acids into proteins then identified with monospecific antisera (136), fetuses of 5.5 weeks' gestation or more could synthesize fibrinogen. Plasminogen could not be synthesized unless the fetus was of 10 weeks' gestation or more (136).

Several factors contribute to the physiologic deficiency of vitamin K–dependent clotting factors in the newborn. Inadequate reserves of vitamin K exist in tissues of the infant, and other sources of this important vitamin are inadequate, for the appropriate intestinal flora, apparently responsible for synthesis of much of the vitamin K needed, is not established in the first few days of life. Moreover, human breast milk contains inadequate amounts of vitamin K. Even when vitamin K is made available, immaturity of liver function may impair its utilization, particularly in the premature infant (137). Thus, a physiologic state of vitamin K deficiency and inadequate levels of vitamin K–dependent clotting factors in plasma of infants in the first few days of life leave them susceptible to hemorrhage. The clotting defect in plasma increases after birth, and is greatest at two or three days of life. Concentrations of these clotting factors usually return to levels found in cord blood by the end of the first week of life, but adult levels are not reached until many weeks later (138). Transplacental transfer of coumarin compounds taken by the mother can interfere with the use of vitamin K by the fetus or neonate, and has caused fetal and neonatal demise (139, 140). Heparin, however, does not appear to cross the placenta and is apparently without risk to the fetus (141). Maternal ingestion of antiepileptic medications, including barbiturates (142), may similarly affect hemostatic mechanisms of the fetus; vitamin K administration will correct the defect. Salicylates taken in large doses by the mother may lead to prolongation of the plasma prothrombin time of her newborn infant (143).

Plasma concentrations of clotting factors which do not require vitamin K for their synthesis are variable during the first few days of life. Antihemophilic factor concentrations in plasma from newborn infants are similar to those in plasma from normal adults, even though the maternal plasma contains elevated concentrations (144). Proaccelerin levels, somewhat low during the first two days of life, resemble those in normal adult plasma by six days of life (145), and fibrinogen concentrations, only occasionally low at birth, then reach normal levels by three days of life (146). Fibrinogen in plasma from umbilical cord blood may clot slowly with thrombin (147), and fibrin then formed is unusually resistant to physical compression (148). Fibrinogen synthesized by the fetus may differ from that synthesized by the adult. The kinetics of the polymerization reaction of fibrin monomers derived from cord plasma fibrinogen differ from those of adult fibrin monomers (148a). This "fetal fibrinogen" is isoelectric at a different pH than adult fibrinogen (148b) and has a higher phosphorous content (148c); peptide maps of tryptic digests of "fetal fibrinogen" differ slightly from those of adult fibrinogen (148d). The unusual behavior of fetal fibrinogen, however, may result from fragments split from fibrinogen by fibrinolytic enzymes after the blood is drawn, for when blood was drawn from umbilical cord vessels directly into an inhibitor of fibrinolysis, the coagulation abnormalities were usually not observed (149).

Plasma concentrations of Hageman factor, also slightly low at birth, spontaneously reach levels found in normal adult plasma by 14 days (150), but PTA concentrations reach normal adult levels only after about 60 days of life (151). Their deficiencies in the newborn require no therapy.

In infants born in an anoxic state, the capacity of the liver to utilize vitamin K is further compromised. In addition, the bleeding time of such infants is likely to be prolonged (152), thus placing added burdens upon the already limited hemostatic competence of early life.

Hemorrhagic Disease of the Newborn

A hemorrhagic syndrome, known to occur most frequently between the second and seventh days of life, is apparently due to a deficiency of vitamin K–dependent clotting factors (153–156). Dam recognized that breast-feeding may lead to a rapid fall in plasma prothrombin (156), and there is clearly an increased risk of hemorrhagic disease of the newborn in the breast-fed newborn, probably because human milk contains less vitamin K than cows' milk (157). Further, the intestinal flora established during breast-feeding differs from that induced during cows' milk feeding, perhaps contributing to the risk of hemorrhage in breast-fed infants (157).

This hemorrhagic syndrome most commonly begins precipitously with spontaneous bleeding from the gastrointestinal tract, and less often from the umbilical stump, into the skin or even intracranially. The incidence of hemorrhagic disease varies widely in different populations between 0.1 and 1 per cent of live births; infant feeding customs are probably important in determining its incidence. The reasons for its increased incidence in winter and spring are not clear. If not treated, as many as one-third of affected infants may succumb (158).

Establishment of a correct diagnosis is, as always, important. In addition to a typical clinical syndrome, the infant with hemorrhagic disease of the newborn has a hemostatic defect characterized by a long prothrombin time and long whole blood or plasma clotting time. The fact that the concentration of platelets is normal, and fibrinogen levels are usually normal by the time this syndrome is manifest, aids in its distinction from some other bleeding disorders associated with intravascular coagulation. Specific assays to measure concentrations of clotting factors will demonstrate low levels of those factors requiring vitamin K for their synthesis.

Treatment is curative. In the full-term infant, a parenteral dose of 100 micrograms of water-soluble vitamin K should result in significant shortening of the 1-stage prothrombin time within four to eight hours. Even feeding cows' milk may be effective treatment (159). If hemorrhage is severe or if the infant was prematurely born, blood transfusion, in accordance with the infant's weight, will be necessary to replace loss and to provide coagulant proteins, for vitamin K may not be utilized by the premature liver. The blood need not be freshly drawn, as the vitamin K–dependent clotting factors are stable during storage at low temperatures.

Preferably, vitamin K prophylaxis should be given to the newly born in small amounts of between 100 micrograms and 1.0 milligram. High doses of water-soluble synthetic vitamin K are to be avoided, as they may interfere with conjugation of bilirubin by the liver and, more importantly, cause rapid hemolysis owing to the oxidant effects of the drug (160, 160a). The resulting hyperbilirubinemia may have serious consequences. Doses of over 5 mg. daily of water-soluble vitamin K were recognized as playing a role in hyperbilirubinemia in prematures (161), but doses of 1 mg. were therapeutically effective and without this risk (162). Aballi and de Lamerens (138) found 25 micrograms to be a satisfactory prophylactic dose. Since some infant diet preparations used as substitutes for milk are deficient in vitamin K, supplementation of these formulas with vitamin K, 100 micrograms per liter, has been recommended recently (162). This should provide the young infant with sufficient reserves of vitamin K that, should an illness, such as one diarrheal in nature, interfere with intestinal absorption, a symptomatic hemostatic defect could be avoided. Young infants receiving antibiotic therapy are also likely to develop vitamin K deficiency (163).

Other Causes of Hemorrhage in the Newborn

The trauma associated with difficult birth may induce ugly hematomata, particularly of the cranium, even without undue hemostatic incompetence. Toxic damage to the liver of various causes may induce deficiencies of vitamin K–dependent clotting factors and a hemorrhagic syndrome not amenable to treatment with vitamin K. Thrombocytopenia, because of infectious processes or of maternal antibody which has crossed the placenta and then reacted with platelets of the fetus, is discussed elsewhere in this volume (Chap. 21).

When intravascular coagulation occurs, it often leads to a hemorrhagic syndrome. Intravascular clotting and subsequent loss of plasma clotting factor activities usually "consumed" during clotting in vitro have been implicated as causes of hemorrhage in the survivor of monochorionic twins, the other of which succumbed in utero (164). Thromboplastic substances from the macerated twin probably reached the circulation of the surviving twin through vascular anastomoses in the placenta (164). In addition, a syndrome of intravascular clotting has been identified in infants surviving abruptio placentae (165) and born of a woman with toxemia of pregnancy (166). Experiments done with pregnant sheep using living exteriorized fetuses support the concept that a coagulant episode on one side of the placenta can be reflected on the other side (167). Infections with cytomegalic inclusion virus (168), herpes simplex virus (169), and doubtless other viral and bacterial agents may lead to intravascular coagulation in this age group, as well as in older individuals. A detailed discussion of the mechanism of intravascular coagulation and its consequences is presented later in this chapter (see pp. 600–610).

PRINCIPLES OF DIAGNOSTIC LABORATORY PROCEDURES

As in establishing any diagnosis, the laboratory is used to obtain confirmatory evidence of pathologic changes suspected from information obtained from a patient's history and physical findings. Persons with hereditary bleeding syndromes are likely to have indisputable histories of hemorrhagic episodes, if they are sufficiently deficient in a coagulation factor. A notable exception is in those with Hageman trait, in whom Hageman factor is virtually absent from plasma, for such individuals are nearly always free of hemorrhagic tendency. Those deficient in PTA may have sufficiently mild symptoms that they do not attract notice (see p. 580).

Care must be taken to heed evidence of a hemorrhagic tendency described by a patient who, at first laboratory investigation, may have a normal whole blood clotting time, for this is an insensitive test of hemostatic function. The hemophiliac who is only partially deficient in antihemophilic factor activity may live comfortably with the trauma presented by ordinary daily life. Once the competence of his hemostatic mechanisms is truly challenged, however, as by surgery or dental extraction, many transfusions may be needed to stop the consequent hemorrhage. Therefore, knowledge that certain relatives have clear evidence of a bleeding tendency, or have required transfusion in situations where this would ordinarily not be necessary, should justify a search for partial deficiency of a clotting factor with appropriate laboratory tests or consultation. Possible alterations in vascular function and in platelet numbers and functions should also be sought.

Precise diagnosis, a prerequisite for appropriate therapy of hemostatic disorders, can be accomplished only with proper laboratory studies. Numerous descriptions of suitable methods for identifying and quantifying deficiencies of coagulation factors have already been published (170–175), and only brief descriptions of the principles involved follows. A tabular summary of alterations in laboratory tests characterizing disordered hemostasis is shown in Table 19–2. Most of the tests used will not be abnormal unless the concentration of one or more clotting factors is reduced to less than 10 per cent of normal, and in some instances to less than 5 per cent of the normal level. Therefore, when the patient's history warrants it, specific assays for deficient clotting factors should be performed to rule out partial defects despite a normal clotting time.

Clotting Time

The clotting of venous blood is delayed if any clotting factor, with the exceptions of Factor VII and fibrin stabilizing factor, is sufficiently deficient, or if an inhibitory substance acts as an anticoagulant. Factor VII is not required for normal coagulation unless it is initiated by tissue substances (tissue thromboplastins), and stabilization of fibrin is not a requirement for its insolu-

TABLE 19–2. LABORATORY ABNORMALITIES OF SOME HEREDITARY COAGULATION DISORDERS

Defect	Clotting Time	Prothrombin Time	Thrombin Time	Partial Thrombo-plastin Time	Serum Prothrombin Activity	Bleeding Time	Other
Classical hemophilia	Normal or long	Normal	Normal	Long	Normal or high	Normal	Adsorbed plasma° corrects
Christmas disease	Normal or long	Normal	Normal	Long	Normal or high	Normal	Serum corrects
PTA deficiency	Normal or long	Normal	Normal	Long	Normal or high	Normal or long	Adsorbed plasma° or serum corrects
Hageman trait	Long	Normal	Normal	Long	High	Normal	Adsorbed plasma° or serum corrects
Stuart factor deficiency	Normal or long	Long	Normal	Long	High	Normal	Serum corrects
Proaccelerin deficiency	Normal or long	Long	Normal	Long	High	Normal	Adsorbed plasma° corrects
Factor VII deficiency	Normal	Long	Normal	Normal	Normal	Normal	Russell's viper venom corrects
Hypoprothrombinemia or dysprothrombinemia	Normal or long	Normal or long	Normal	Normal or long	Normal	Normal	Aged plasma corrects
Afibrinogenemia	Infinite	Infinite	Infinite	Infinite	Normal	Normal or long	No clotting with thrombin
Dysfibrinogenemia	Long or normal	Normal or long	Usually long	Normal or long	Normal	Normal or long	Thrombin clotting usually delayed
Fibrin stabilizing factor deficiency	Normal	Normal	Normal	Normal	Normal	Normal	Clot dissolves in 1% monochloroacetic acid
Von Willebrand's disease	Varies	Normal	Normal	Varies	Normal or high	Long	AHF titer may be low
Fletcher trait	Long	Normal	Normal	Long	Normal	Normal	Prolonged exposure to activating surface corrects

°Fresh citrated plasma adsorbed with aluminum hydroxide, or fresh oxalated plasma adsorbed with barium sulfate.

bility, which represents the end point in measuring the clotting time. When the blood has developed fibrinolytic activity, it may be incoagulable because fibrin is digested as it forms.

Partial Thromboplastin Time

When plasma is allowed to clot in the presence of added phospholipid and calcium, a more sensitive assessment of the intrinsic coagulation mechanism is provided (see Table 19–2). This assay is usually standardized by adding kaolin, celite, or a similar substance to the clotting mixture to provide optimal activation of Hageman factor (activated partial thromboplastin time) and to avoid variability in clotting times due to variable suboptimal activation of this factor. Even though relatively sensitive to mild deficiencies, the partial thromboplastin time can be normal in the presence of a minor defect.

One-Stage Prothrombin Time

This tests the effect of tissue thromboplastin upon the recalcified clotting time of plasma, and is a measure of the overall efficiency of the extrinsic pathway of coagulation. Therefore, if either Factor VII, proaccelerin, Stuart factor, prothrombin, or fibrinogen is sufficiently deficient, or an anticoagulant substance interferes with their function, the one-stage prothrombin time may be prolonged.

Another measure of the later steps in coagulation can be made with Russell's viper venom (RVV), which activates Stuart factor without first interacting with Factor VII. The Russell's viper venom time is normal in plasma deficient in Factor VII, as participation of this clotting factor is circumvented. The RVV time is prolonged if Stuart factor is truly deficient, or when concentrations of prothrombin, proaccelerin, or fibrinogen are sufficiently low.

Thrombin Time

When a solution of thrombin is added to normal plasma, it acts upon fibrinogen so that visible fibrin forms. Thus, one can directly measure fibrinogen by chemical or gravimetric methods by converting it to fibrin with thrombin. When fibrinogen is qualitatively or quantitatively abnormal, or an anticoagulant substance interferes with its interaction with thrombin or with polymerization of fibrin monomers released by thrombin, the thrombin time—that is, the time required for formation of a visible clot when a standardized amount of thrombin is added to plasma—is prolonged. Fibrin stabilizing factor does not affect the thrombin time. A frequent cause of a prolonged thrombin time is the presence of therapeutically administered anticoagulant, heparin, which delays this step in coagulation. The presence of digestion products of fibrinogen or fibrin also prolongs the thrombin time, largely by delaying polymerization of fibrin monomers.

Fibrin Stabilizing Factor

One can identify this enzyme indirectly by using a modification of the technique which led to its discovery. When plasma has clotted following recalcification, it is then incubated in 1 per cent monochloroacetic acid or 5 M urea. If the clot dissolves, fibrin stabilizing factor has not functioned and is presumably deficient. Neither urea nor monochloroacetic acid will disrupt the chemical bonds established between fibrin monomers by fibrin stabilizing factor.

Serum Prothrombin Activity (Prothrombin Consumption Test)

When blood has clotted for a given period of time, a certain amount of prothrombin in plasma will have been converted to thrombin by any prothrombin-converting principle which has formed. Therefore, the reactions leading to the formation of prothrombin converting activity can be roughly evaluated by measuring the prothrombin remaining in serum after a given time interval. Prothrombin can be specifically measured by using a modification of a one-stage prothrombin time in which Factor VII, Stuart factor, and proaccelerin and fibrinogen are present in optimal concentrations, so that the assay is therefore sensitive only to variations in prothrombin concentration (174). When any of the clotting factors active in the intrinsic pathway other than prothrombin are sufficiently deficient, the concentration of prothrombin in serum will be high, because this protein is used suboptimally since the generation of prothrombin converting activity is deficient. Prothrombin consumption is also poor when inadequate numbers of platelets are present, or if these cells are qualitatively abnormal, as well as when an anticoagulant substance retards generation of prothrombin converting activity. A normal serum prothrombin activity does not rule out partial defects in the intrinsic pathway, for it is not a sufficiently sensitive measure to exclude minor defects.

Thromboplastin Generation Test

Upon incubating a mixture of serum (normally deficient in antihemophilic factor activity, proaccelerin, prothrombin, and fibrinogen) and plasma which has been adsorbed with barium sulfate or aluminum hydroxide (deficient in Christmas factor, Stuart factor, Factor VII, and prothrombin), phospholipid, and calcium, prothrombin converting activity is generated. The intensity of this activity can then be measured by adding samples from this mixture to recalcified plasma (170). The prothrombin in the second plasma will be converted to thrombin if prothrombin converting activity has formed in the preliminary incubation mixture. Thus, a deficiency in a clotting factor normally found in adsorbed plasma or in serum may be tentatively identified using this method. In addition, coagulant function of platelets can be tested by substituting them for the phospholipid preparation in the incubation mixture. Exact identification of a defect using this method can be made only if plasma or serum from an individual known to be deficient in the factor in question is included in the incubation mixture to measure the ability of serum or adsorbed plasma from the patient to correct the defect.

Specific Clotting Factor Assays

These measurements are best done in a laboratory where defects in appropriate substrate plasma samples have been clearly identified. The coagulant activity deficient in a patient's plasma can be quantified by testing its capacity to correct the defect measured by the activated partial thromboplastin or the prothrombin times of plasma known to be deficient in the specific clotting factors being examined. When the test plasma is deficient in the same activity, its ability to shorten the clotting time of the deficient plasma is limited.

Inhibitors (Circulating Anticoagulants)

When plasma contains an inhibitor of normal clotting (circulating anticoagulant), it will delay the clotting of normal plasma. If the plasma clotting time is prolonged because of a deficiency, addition of a small amount of normal plasma will hasten clotting. Therefore, when equal volumes of the abnormal plasma are mixed with normal plasma and the partial thromboplastin time measured, the clotting time will be longer than normal if an inhibitor is present. If the inhibitor is particularly potent, one part of the patient's plasma in nine parts of normal plasma will delay clotting of the mixture. It should be remembered that some inhibitors function optimally at 37°C and act slowly. Therefore, to avoid missing a circulating anticoagulant in a plasma sample, the mixtures should be incubated at 37°C, preferably for one or several hours before performing the clotting assay. If an inhibitor is present, one can designate its effect upon specific clotting factors by measuring the residual concentrations of each clotting factor in an assay specific for that factor.

Bleeding Time

To evaluate the efficiency of combined hemostatic mechanisms, the time required for an incised wound to stop bleeding can be measured. In an attempt to eliminate some of the numerous variables in measurement of the bleeding time, Harker and Slichter have devised a calibrated template to hold disposable blades which will provide a standard puncture in performing the Ivy test (170a). The method for measuring the bleeding time described by Ivy determines the time required for cessation of bleeding from standard wounds to the forearm under the stress of increased venous pressure. The method of Duke merely measures the time for bleeding to stop after a standard wound to the ball of the finger. The earlobe should not be used to measure bleeding times, especially in a subject with a history of a bleeding tendency, because it is difficult to achieve hemostasis in this area with local pressure, and, should bleeding persist, there may be permanent damage to the external ear. The bleeding time may be prolonged in most persons with von Willebrand's disease, thrombocytopenia, qualitative defects of platelets, and thrombocytosis, and in some with congenital afibrinogenemia, uremia, and possibly deficiency in PTA. Abnormal serum proteins may interfere with vascular or platelet function or both to prolong the bleeding time. Reasons for a prolonged bleeding time may seem obscure, and a search into the nature of drugs used by the patient may provide helpful information, since aspirin and certain other drugs commonly exacerbate this abnormality.

Platelet functions are discussed elsewhere in this volume (Chs. 20 and 21).

DEFECTIVE COAGULATION DUE TO DEFICIENCIES

Hereditary Disorders of Coagulation

The inherited defects of coagulation are rare and represent deficient or defective synthesis of one or more coagulant substances necessary for normal hemostasis; most are inherited as autosomal recessive traits. Others, such as classical hemophilia, are inherited as recessive traits linked to the X chromosomes (X-linked recessive), or exhibit variable inheritance patterns.

Classical Hemophilia

This disorder and Factor IX deficiency are by far the commonest of the inherited factor deficiencies. The hemophiliac usually suffers repeated hemorrhages into joints and soft tissues. Since this disease is inherited as an X-linked recessive trait, its victims with rare exceptions are male. The disorder may not be recognized in the first year of life unless circumcision is performed (175a). The young infant with hemophilia may gradually develop hemorrhagic episodes as he begins to crawl. The incidence of unusual bleeding is surprisingly low in the hemophiliac under 1 year of age (175a). Once he begins to walk, he may bleed repeatedly into the joint spaces, often leading to permanent disability. Although eruption of primary teeth is rarely accompanied by significant bleeding, eruption of secondary teeth may be. Dental extraction is risky and requires preventive prophylaxis (see p. 597). In the newborn, hemorrhage may occur from the umbilical stump or following circumcision, should an unsuspected propositus be subjected to this procedure. A Talmudic awareness of such a disorder allowed exemption of a male from the rite of circumcision if brothers so challenged had bled excessively (176).

Otto (177), though he had not actually cared for a hemophiliac, related its peculiar inheritance pattern in telling of a woman, who, though not subject to hemorrhage herself, transmitted a bleeding tendency to some but not all of her sons. Despite long-standing awareness of the hereditary nature of hemophilia and like disorders, reasons for tendencies to bleed have emerged from the experiments and observations of the past 50 or more years. Wright (178) was perhaps the first to report that blood from a hemophiliac clotted very slowly, but not until later did Addis (179) provide the important clue that the clotting time of plasma from an individual with a hemophilia-like disease could be shortened by mixing it with some normal plasma. Thus, a deficiency in the blood clotting mechanism, correctable with normal plasma, was associated with the bleeding tendency. Plasma from those with classic hemophilia is deficient in antihemophilic factor activity (180), and, consequently, the hemophiliac has a defect in the intrinsic pathway of coagulation (see Fig. 19–1). Some descriptions of hemophilia prior to 1952 may actually have referred to Christmas disease, a similar syndrome inherited as an X-linked recessive, not until then shown to represent a deficiency of a substance distinct from AHF.

Antihemophilic factor is a glycoprotein of high molecular weight (181, 182), with the electrophoretic mobility of a slow beta or fast gamma globulin. The logical view that this protein is absent from plasma of hemophiliacs has been successfully challenged through immunochemical studies of hemophilic plasma. Antisera to crude preparations of antihemophilic factor (183) are neutralized by hemophilic plasma. Moreover, a precipitating rabbit antibody to AHF demonstrated entirely normal concentrations of AHF protein in plasma of hemophiliacs, using electroimmunodiffusion techniques (184). Hints that there is an AHF-like protein which lacks normal function in some hemophilic plasmas are also found in earlier studies of Hoyer and Breckenridge (185). They observed that plasma from some, but not all, hemophiliacs neutralized a naturally occurring anticoagulant substance known to destroy AHF activity in normal plasma. Such an anticoagulant, which occasionally develops in hemophilic patients and rarely in non-hemophiliacs, probably represents antibody directed against AHF. Heterogeneity may exist among AHF-like proteins in plasma from different hemophiliacs, for only plasma from certain hemophiliacs neutralized the anticoagulant. It may be an antibody which detects an alteration of a very restricted portion of the AHF molecule, the remainder of which is homologous with other human AHF proteins (186). Antibody raised in an alien species may be insensitive to such a minor alteration, being induced instead by another portion of the molecule having extensive homology among humans, but differing from AHF in the species challenged. Gralnick (187) found that plasma from some hemophiliacs lacked antigen detectable with goat antiserum to human AHF, also suggesting that different AHF-like proteins may occur in different hemophiliacs. Goat antiserum may recognize a portion of the molecule which varies among humans and is not detected by the rabbit antiserum used by Zimmerman and his colleagues (184). None of these observations really elucidate the nature of the AHF-like molecule in hemophilia; it may be a distorted or precursor form of functional AHF. While the pattern of inheritance of classic hemophilia may suggest that a single gene regulates synthesis of appropriately active AHF, this may be misleading. In addition to the immunochemical studies cited here, the autosomal inheritance of AHF deficiency in von Willebrand's disease suggests involvement of a non–X-linked gene in synthesis of this protein.

The severity of the bleeding tendency in hemophilia is related to the degree of deficiency of AHF activity. Those with 10 per cent or more of the normal level of AHF activity in their plasma may, with care, live relatively free of bleeding episodes, unlike most of those with 1 per cent or less of the normal level. Generally, affected members of a kindred with hemophilia suffer similar degrees of disability and bleeding tendency. Why episodes of bleeding occur even when the patient is unaware that he has sustained trauma is not entirely clear, but emotional factors may be important. When adolescence heralds escape from parental overprotectiveness, the bleeding tendency is likely to lessen in severity, despite the characteristic risk-taking behavior of many bleeders (188). The physiologic mechanisms of this emotionally related change are still obscure. Exercise (189) or injections of adrenaline (190) may increase the titer of antihemophilic factor activity in the plasma of a mild hemophiliac, as in plasma of normal persons, but not in severe hemophiliacs. Decreased severity of hemophilic bleeding in adult life cannot be attributed to increased levels of AHF activity in plasma (177).

The management of hemophilia requires numerous supportive measures involving orthopedic, dental, and educational personnel, in addition to intravenously administered replacement therapy with fractions of plasma rich in AHF early in bleeding episodes, to be discussed further on pages 594–600 (see Table 19–3).

The Carrier State in Hemophilia

The daughters of a hemophiliac must inherit from their father the X chromosome which bears a gene for hemophilia. Thus, all daughters of a hemophiliac will be hemophilia carriers. Usually, however, they are not themselves subject to hemorrhage

TABLE 19–3. THERAPY OF HEMOSTATIC DEFECTS

Factor	Available Preparations	Half-Life, Hours	Increase in Plasma After 1 U./kg.	Hemostatic Level: Minor Trauma	Hemostatic Level: Major Trauma or Surgery	Level for Maintenance Hemostasis	Reference
VIII	Fresh frozen plasma, cryoprecipitate, concentrate (commercial)	8–12	2%	20–30%	50%	10%	216, 460, 461, 462
IX	Plasma concentrate, or stored plasma	24	1–1½%	15%	25%	5–10%	216, 463, 464
von Willebrand's disease	Cryoprecipitate, fresh frozen plasma	24–48	3%	20–30%	50%	10%	465, 466
XI	Plasma	40–80	2%	10–15%	20%	10%	467
VII	Plasma, commercial concentrate	5	1%	5–10%	10%	5%	468, 469, 470
V	Fresh frozen plasma, less than 1 month old	36	1½%	10%	25%	5%	471, 472, 473
X	Plasma, commercial concentrate	24–60	1%	10%	15%	5%	474
II	Plasma, commercial concentrate	72	1%	15%	25%	10%	475
I	Plasma, commercial concentrate, cryoprecipitate	72	1–1½ mg. per 100 ml.	150 mg. per 100 ml.	200 mg. per 100 ml.	100 mg. per 100 ml.	476
XIII	Plasma	72	1%	2–3%	2–3%	2–3%	477

because the normal X chromosome derived from their mothers directs synthesis of sufficient functional AHF to maintain hemostasis. A female with hemophilia may result from mating of a female carrier with a hemophiliac, for she may derive abnormal X chromosomes from each parent; only half of the daughters of such a mating would be affected, the other half being carriers. Half of the daughters born of a normal male and carrier female will be carriers; half of their sons will have the disease.

Despite their usual asymptomatic state, females who carry the gene for hemophilia have on the average only about half the normal concentration of AHF activity in their plasma (191). This is usually adequate for normal hemostasis. According to the hypothesis described by Beutler et al. (192), and by Lyon (193), one X chromosome in each cell of a female is inactivated at random early in embryonic life. From this, one would predict that the individual would have about half the normal levels of AHF activity, for half of her cells would be derived from cells with a normally functioning X chromosome, while half would be derived from cells in which the abnormal X chromosome is functional. Since these events occur in random fashion, an individual carrier may have more or less than half normal plasma concentrations of AHF activity, and it is therefore difficult to designate a carrier by quantifying AHF activity in her plasma with an assay to measure its coagulant properties. In addition, the normal range is wide and may include levels of 40 per cent of the normal mean (191, 194), making this measure of the carrier state a difficult basis for decision.

Zimmerman, Ratnoff, and Littell (195, 195a) described a characteristic ratio of nonfunctional AHF protein to functional protein in the carrier state. As one would anticipate, the carrier state is characterized by production of entirely normal amounts of AHF protein detectable immunochemically, since both the abnormal and the normal X chromosomes direct synthesis of AHF-like antigens. Only half, or less, of this material has coagulant activity in a suitable assay to measure AHF. Therefore, the concentration of AHF antigen is about twice what one would predict from the concentration of functional AHF in plasma of a carrier. This approach to diagnosis of the

carrier state may eventually simplify the problem of the physician asked for genetic counseling in regard to risk in pregnancy of a possible carrier.

Christmas Disease

To describe the bleeding syndrome associated with the inherited deficiency of Christmas factor (PTC, Factor IX), which was first described in the Christmas family, would be to repeat a description of symptoms of those deficient in AHF. Both are inherited as X-linked recessive traits, and the nature of the hemorrhagic syndrome is identical. Christmas disease was not distinguished from classic hemophilia until 1952, when several groups reported that, in certain cases of a hemophilia-like disease, there was a deficiency of a plasma clotting factor distinct from AHF. Christmas factor is in the α_2-globulin fraction of plasma (196). At first, a functional deficiency of Christmas factor was thought to reflect absence of the procoagulant protein from plasma, but several recent observations indicate that at least some cases of Christmas disease are an expression of genetically determined alterations of Christmas factor molecules which interfere with their coagulant function (194). As in the case of hemophilia, plasma from some patients with Christmas disease will neutralize a naturally occurring acquired circulating anticoagulant directed against Christmas factor, as if such a plasma contained a dysproteinemic form of Christmas factor (197), while plasma from other patients lacks this property, as if they failed to synthesize Christmas factor.

Nonfunctional Christmas factor proteins are heterogeneous. The prothrombin time of plasma from certain persons with Christmas disease was prolonged under certain conditions (65, 201) and inhibited extrinsic clotting. Such plasma apparently contained a protein similar to Christmas factor which lacked coagulant activity, while it in some way inhibited the extrinsic pathway. This variant of Christmas disease was dubbed hemophilia B_M because Christmas disease is also known as hemophilia B. Densen found that a circulating anticoagulant which inhibited Christmas factor activity was neutralized by plasma from those with hemophilia B_M (198). In addition, rabbit antiserum to bovine Christmas factor gave a precipitin reaction with hemophilia B_M plasma, and the antibody was neutralized by the plasma (198). Thus, a plasma protein with some properties of Christmas factor seems to exist in hemophilia B_M. In other kindred, the plasma of affected individuals may contain nonfunctional Christmas factor differing from that in hemophilia B_M in that it fails to interfere with coagulation initiated through the extrinsic pathway (199). Some patients with Christmas disease experience notable remission of their bleeding tendency, as well as a parallel increase in plasma concentration of functional and antigenic Christmas factor with increasing age (200).

Information regarding the carrier state is scanty, but carriers are probably also variably affected. Carriers of hemophilia B_M originally described had low plasma levels of functional Christmas factor activity, but more significantly, their plasma prothrombin times were prolonged (201).

Christmas disease may be identified with certainty when the plasma of a suspected propositus fails to shorten the clotting time of plasma from one known to have this defect, provided both are free of inhibitors of clotting. A presumptive laboratory diagnosis can be made when the coagulation defect is repaired by serum, but not by plasma depleted of vitamin K–dependent clotting factors by adsorption with aluminum hydroxide or barium sulfate. The platelet count and bleeding time are normal, and if the defect is mild, the whole blood clotting time will also be normal, and only more sensitive measures, such as an activated partial thromboplastin time, may reveal a defect. Specific assays to quantify plasma coagulants must be used to define the defect where the patient's history demands it.

The management of Christmas disease is analogous to that of hemophilia. The stability of Christmas factor in plasma during storage allows use of older plasma for replacement therapy, but plasma fractions rich in Christmas factor may be necessary to restore plasma activity to satisfactory levels at times of injury or for surgery. The incidence of serum hepatitis has been significant following the use of such fractions.

Details of replacement therapy are discussed on pp. 594–596.

Christmas deficiency may be acquired in association with certain endocrinopathies, such as hypopituitarism (202). It is not known if there is a Christmas factor-like protein lacking function in plasma from such a patient.

Plasma Thromboplastin Antecedent (PTA, Factor XI) Deficiency

PTA deficiency is inherited as an autosomal recessive trait (203), but heterozygous individuals may be detected with appropriate tests. Most affected kindred are Jewish. The bleeding tendency is relatively mild, but significant bleeding may occur after injury or surgical procedures, tonsillectomy, and dental extraction, and some affected patients are troubled with epistaxis. Menorrhagia and postpartum hemorrhage may sometimes be severe; hysterectomy has occasionally seemed necessary because of menorrhagia (204).

It is likely that PTA deficiency does not represent a dysproteinemia, for the degree of deficiency in coagulant activity parallels that of antigen in plasma reacted with antiserum to this protein. Forbes and Ratnoff (194) were able to neutralize heterologous PTA antibody activity to only a limited degree with plasma from some individuals partially deficient in PTA. This infrequent trait may have yet undescribed variants.

The coagulation defect in PTA deficiency is one of impaired intrinsic generation of prothrombin converting activity. The prolonged clotting time of sufficiently deficient plasma can be shortened by the addition of normal serum or of adsorbed plasma, but a firm diagnosis requires demonstration that such plasma fails to correct the clotting defect in plasma from one known to be deficient in PTA.

Persons with PTA deficiency seldom require specific replacement therapy, for the defect is incomplete and the tendency to bleed impressively mild. In preparation for surgery, fresh plasma might be given, but its effectiveness is difficult to assess because many affected patients withstand surgery without undue bleeding.

Hageman Trait

This rare familial hemostatic defect is nearly always asymptomatic. Propositi are detected by chance through incidental discovery of extraordinarily long plasma or whole blood clotting times. Deficient function of Hageman factor is transmitted as an autosomal recessive trait, in which there is apparently a failure to synthesize Hageman factor protein. Heterologous antiserum which neutralized the coagulant activity of Hageman factor in normal plasma could not be neutralized by plasma from persons severely deficient in Hageman factor activity, nor did it give a precipitin band when reacted with Hageman trait plasma in double agar diffusion, even though a precipitin reaction developed with normal plasma (205).

Since only the intrinsic pathway is grossly defective when Hageman factor is deficient, the prothrombin time of such plasma is normal, but the consumption of prothrombin during clotting of whole blood is poor, leading to higher than normal concentrations of residual prothrombin in serum. Persons with Hageman trait generally require no special therapy for their hemostatic defect and, with rare exceptions, can withstand surgery, injury, and dental extractions without bleeding excessively. Occasionally an individual with Hageman trait has required transfusion for excessive bleeding following childbirth or dental extraction, and affected persons with frequent epistaxes and easy bruising have been reported (206). Therefore, it is wise for the physician to have blood available for use following surgery on those with Hageman trait, should it become necessary.

Hageman factor is a remarkably thermostable plasma protein with a molecular weight of about 75,000 (23), which has the electrophoretic behavior of a gamma globulin once partially purified (207).

Even though Hageman factor acquires potent coagulant properties when activated in vitro, its physiologic in vivo role is unclear, largely because of the strikingly asymptomatic nature of Hageman trait. Perhaps its role in generating polypeptide kinins and vascular changes characterizing inflammation is more important in human pathophysiology than its coagulant function.

Proaccelerin (Factor V) Deficiency or Parahemophilia

In 1947, Owren (208) found that the plasma of a female with a lifelong hemorrhagic tendency was deficient in clotting activity not previously shown necessary for normal hemostasis. This procoagulant, called proaccelerin, or Factor V, is unstable, as noted by Quick (209), and acts in vitro with activated Stuart factor, calcium ions, and phospholipid to form a prothrombin-converting principle. The clotting and prothrombin times are prolonged if plasma is sufficiently deficient in proaccelerin. Presumptive evidence of proaccelerin deficiency may be obtained if the prothrombin time of the plasma in question is shortened by the addition of plasma which has been depleted of the vitamin K clotting factors by adsorption with aluminum hydroxide gel or barium sulfate. This presumption assumes that the mixture contains adequate fibrinogen. The diagnosis may be confirmed if the prothrombin time of plasma from an individual with parahemophilia, or one artificially depleted of proaccelerin, is not corrected by the plasma in question.

Sporadic spontaneous bleeding may affect the gastrointestinal tract, skin, or nervous system, but hemarthrosis is atypical of parahemophilia. In those less deficient in proaccelerin, bleeding may be limited to times of challenge, as after surgery, dental extractions, or injury, but epistaxis or menorrhagia may be a problem. Proaccelerin deficiency is inherited as an autosomal recessive trait, in which heterozygous individuals may be detected by quantifying plasma proaccelerin. Studies to date indicate that proaccelerin deficiency results from failure of synthesis of this plasma protein (210, 211), because antisera against human proaccelerin were not neutralized by proaccelerin-deficient plasma, including that from Owren's original patient.

Treatment of bleeding episodes or prophylaxis for essential surgery requires intravenous infusion of freshly drawn plasma or plasma frozen for less than one month. A plasma concentration of 25 per cent of that in normal plasma is probably adequate for uncomplicated surgery (see Table 19–3).

Deficiencies of Other Vitamin K–Dependent Clotting Factors

Stuart Factor (Factor X) Deficiency

The bleeding tendency associated with congenital deficiency of Stuart factor activity may begin in infancy with umbilical bleeding. Affected females may develop menorrhagia, which may be severe at the time of the menarche but then lessen in severity after the first few cycles (212); postpartum bleeding may be severe.

Stuart factor deficiency, inherited as an autosomal recessive trait, may reflect a variety of errors in protein biosynthesis. Several abnormal Stuart factor–like proteins have been described which may be identified with antiserum to normal Stuart factor. For example, Girolami (213), Densen (214), and their associates found that, despite a deficiency in Stuart factor coagulant activity in affected members of an Italian kindred, the plasma neutralized heterologous antibody to this factor. Thus, plasma contained antigens related to Stuart factor, and, in addition, these antigens could not be distinguished immunologically from normal Stuart factor, and were in normal concentrations in plasma. Although this plasma substance failed to act normally during clotting, the Russell's viper venom clotting time of this defective plasma was normal, as if the abnormal "Stuart factor" were activated by the venom. Plasma from affected members of two other kindred and from the original patient, Mr. Stuart, failed to neutralize antibody against normal Stuart factor, as if deficient in Stuart factor protein (215). Plasma from affected members of three additional kindreds contained Stuart factor–like protein which was immunologically deficient with respect to that in normal plasma. Thus, Stuart factor deficiency may result from apparent failure of synthesis, synthesis of an abnormal protein with a normal complement of antigenic determinants or one deficient in antigenic determinants, or synthesis of a partially functional protein unreactive during blood clotting but normally reactive with Russell's viper venom, and is identifiable immunologically.

Since Stuart factor is stable during storage, treatment of hemorrhagic episodes need not require fresh plasma. Levels of 15 per cent of normal are probably adequate for dental extraction or surgery (216) (see Table 19–3).

Factor VII (Pro-SPCA) Deficiency

The hemorrhagic tendency associated with Factor VII deficiency is clinically indistinguishable from that of Stuart factor deficiency; in the newborn, bleeding from the umbilicus may occur, and both sexes are affected. Epistaxis is often troublesome, and menorrhagia may necessitate artificial suppression of menstruation. The coagulation defect is characterized only by a long prothrombin time, for Factor VII is unique in its participation with tissue factor in coagulation via the extrinsic mechanism. Since Russell's viper venom directly activates Stuart factor without interacting with Factor VII, plasma deficient only in Factor VII clots normally upon adding this venom, whereas plasma deficient in Stuart factor activity often, but not always, clots poorly.

Factor VII deficiency is inherited as an autosomal recessive trait (217) through at least two types of error in biosynthesis. Some affected persons have a nonfunctional protein in their plasma detectable immunologically, while others have neither functionally nor immunologically detectable Factor VII in their plasma (194, 210).

Treatment of bleeding episodes requires plasma transfusion, but since Factor VII is stable during storage, plasma need not be freshly drawn. Effective hemostasis may be accomplished with lower levels of Factor VII in plasma than are required for other clotting factors, for concentrations as low as 5 per cent of normal may be adequate for surgical procedures (216). The rate of disappearance of Factor VII from plasma following intravenous administration is remarkably rapid (Table 19–3).

Deficient Prothrombin (Factor II) Activity

Defective hemostasis because of deficient prothrombin function occurs rarely; the tendency to hemorrhage is related to the severity of the deficiency. Affected persons are likely to sustain hemorrhage after injury, surgery, and dental extraction, and they may have menorrhagia, but spontaneous bleeding is not characteristic of this disorder. The one-stage prothrombin time may be only slightly prolonged, despite a significant deficiency of plasma prothrombin activity. The Russell's viper venom clotting time may be only a few seconds longer than that of normal plasma, since prothrombin is only partially deficient. Specific assays for plasma prothrombin function are necessary to identify this defect; the one-stage prothrombin time is influenced to a greater degree by partial deficiencies of Factor VII, Stuart factor, and proaccelerin than of prothrombin.

Either defective prothrombin molecules or a true deficiency of prothrombin is inherited as an autosomal trait (194). Shapiro et al. described dysprothrombinemia in a kindred (218) in which abnormal prothrombin molecules could not be fully converted to thrombin. The plasma of heterozygous individuals contained both normal and abnormal prothrombins. Josso and his associates (219, 220) described another kindred with dysprothrombinemia distinct from Shapiro's kindred in that prothrombin-like molecules were abnormally electropositive, and also failed to be fully converted to thrombin, even though able to react with prothrombin converting principle. However, this counterfeit prothrombin could interact with staphylocoagulase to generate thrombin, just as normal prothrombin does. Josso et al. (221) also found congenital hypoprothrombinemia due to deficient synthesis of a prothrombin-like protein, since reported in several other kindred. The plasma from the patient originally described by Quick (222) lacked prothrombin-like protein from a fraction of plasma normally rich in this material (223).

Dysprothrombinemic or hypoprothrombinemic bleeding may be treated with normal plasma or fractions thereof rich in prothrombin, and since prothrombin is stable, outdated plasma is satisfactory. The amount of plasma required may be estimated as suggested for treatment of hemophilia with plasma (see Table 19–3). Plasma depleted of cryoprecipitable materials is satisfactory for replacement therapy in patients with inherited deficiencies of vitamin K–dependent clotting factors, for these factors are excluded from the cryoprecipitate. The administration of vitamin K is useless, for those congenitally deficient in these factors cannot use the vitamin in the defective biosynthetic pathway.

Congenital Afibrinogenemia and Dysfibrinogenemia

Congenital Afibrinogenemia

Infrequently, a patient is found to have no detectable plasma fibrinogen throughout life, and may have severe or even fatal hemorrhage when injured or subjected to surgery. Somewhat surprisingly, persons with congenital afibrinogenemia are unlikely to bleed spontaneously, and females need not have menorrhagia, attesting to the importance of vascular and platelet factors in hemostasis. Even though hemorrhage into joint spaces may occur, this is unlikely to result in residual damage, perhaps because of failure to deposit fibrin. In infancy, the syndrome may announce itself with bleeding from the umbilicus or from ammoniacal dermatitis of the diaper area. Later, there is typical re-bleeding from wounds, for initial bleeding may cease in a short time to be followed by recurrence when the wound is disrupted by stress, as if the hemostatic "seal" were inadequate. Although plasma fibrinogen may be undetectable in congenital afibrinogenemia, traces in association with platelets may be important to hemostasis through their enhancing effect upon adhesive properties of platelets (224). In some cases there are traces of fibrinogen in plasma (225).

Congenital afibrinogenemia reflects failure of the liver to synthesize fibrinogen, and when fibrinogen is given intravenously, its duration of survival in vascular compartments is normal (225). The defect is inherited as an autosomal recessive trait, a consanguineous mating frequently providing a proband. Heterozygous individuals are often undetectable (226), but parents or siblings may have subnormal fibrinogen levels (227, 228). Some patients given fibrinogen for this defect have developed antibodies to fibrinogen (229), suggesting its recognition as a foreign protein by the recipient.

The clotting time of whole blood and plasma is infinite when fibrinogen is absent, but the steps leading to thrombin formation function normally, and when purified fibrinogen is mixed with such plasma, coagulation will occur at a normal rate. The viscosity of plasma is reduced, and erythrocytes sediment very slowly, as both phenomena are largely dependent upon plasma fibrinogen.

Replacement therapy with intravenously administered plasma fractions rich in fibrinogen is necessary to perform surgery or after injury. Cohn fraction I or cryoprecipitates from normal plasma may be used, but the risk of hepatitis from cryoprecipitated fibrinogen of individual plasma is much less than with fractions prepared from pooled plasma (230). The concentration of fibrinogen in unfractionated plasma is inadequate for replacement therapy (see Table 19–3).

Congenital Dysfibrinogenemia

Since plasma fibrinogen from normal persons behaves as if heterogeneous during column chromatography (231), it is not surprising that a number of functionally abnormal fibrinogens have been found. Some persons with dysfibrinogenemia have a bleeding tendency (231a), some are subject to thrombosis (232), while most affected persons are relatively free of symptoms despite an easily detectable coagulation defect. Several patients, however, have sustained wound dehiscence postoperatively. Dysfibrinogenemia is inherited as an autosomal dominant trait.

In dysfibrinogenemia, the thrombin clotting time of plasma is characteristically delayed, and the prothrombin time is often prolonged. The whole blood clotting time may be normal, but the clot which forms may be easily disrupted and appear abnormal (232, 233). When clotting was measured with thromboelastrographic techniques in which the resistance provided by fibrin as it forms is measured, some dysfibrinogenemic bloods behaved normally, while in others, clotting was delayed, qualitatively abnormal, or absent (234). The actual concentration of fibrinogen in plasma measured immunologically, by salt or heat precipitin or electrophoretically, is usually normal (Table 19–4). The amount of fibrinogen ultimately included in a clot is usually normal or slightly depressed, but in some dysfibrinogenemics, no coagulable protein was detectable (235).

The abnormal fibrinogens have been named according to the city in which the studies were done; fibrinogens Baltimore and Vancouver may be identical (194). Some abnormal fibrinogens fail to interact with thrombin normally, so that the release of fibrinopeptides is delayed, as in the cases of fibrinogens Baltimore (236) and Bethesda (237). Others are apparently hydrolyzed normally by thrombin, but fibrin monomers formed polymerize into visible fibrin more slowly than normal monomers. The electrophoretic mobility of some abnormal fibrinogens is distinctive, for fibrinogens Bethesda, Baltimore, Vancouver, and Louvain are abnormally electronegative, and fibrinogens Cleveland and Amsterdam are abnormally electropositive (see Table 19–4). In heterozygous individuals, including most cases reported, both normal and abnormal fibrinogens are found in plasma. Hampton (238) described a dysfibrinogenemia in which the fibrin formed could not be cross-linked by fibrin stabilizing factor. This appeared to be inherited through the X chromosome (239), and was named fibrinogen Oklahoma.

One recently described abnormal fibrinogen (fibrinogen Philadelphia) is catabolized more rapidly than normal (239a), and the propositus with fibrinogen Bethesda II demonstrated increased fractional catabolic rates of intravenously administered, radioactively labeled, autologous and homologous fibrinogen (239b). The release of fibrinopeptide A from fibrinogen Giessen (239c) apparently failed to occur during incubation with thrombin; polymerization of monomers was delayed, and this fibrinogen was partially resistant to digestion by plasmin. Fibrinogen Montreal (243d) has an abnormality of the alpha (A) chain, but fibrinopeptide release by thrombin appeared unimpaired. Fibrinogen Iowa City (239e) clots abnormally slowly because of impaired polymerization of fibrin monomers, despite the fact that the affected person is completely asymptomatic and apparently homozygous for the defect. Fibrinogen Los Angeles (239f), isolated from the plasma of a young physician, also demonstrated abnormal polymerization of

TABLE 19–4. SOME DISTINGUISHING FEATURES OF ABNORMAL FIBRINOGENS IN DYSFIBRINOGENEMIA

MAJOR FUNCTIONAL ABNORMALITY	DEAE CHROMATOGRAPHIC BEHAVIOR	ELECTROPHORETIC MOBILITY OF ANTIGENIC DETERMINANTS (COMPARED TO NORMAL)	EFFECT ON NORMAL PLASMA FIBRINOGEN CLOTTING	THROMBO-ELASTOGRAPHIC BEHAVIOR
Abnormal Fibrinogen-Thrombin Interaction:				
Fibrinogen Baltimore°	Abnormal	Anodal	0	Abnormal
Fibrinogen Bethesda I	Normal	Anodal	Inhibits	–
Abnormal Aggregations of Fibrin Monomers:				
Fibrinogen Zurich I°	–	Normal	Inhibits	Normal
Fibrinogen Zurich II	–	Normal	Inhibits	–
Fibrinogen Paris II°	Normal	Normal	Inhibits	Abnormal
Fibrinogen Weisbaden	–	Normal	Inhibits	–
Fibrinogen Cleveland I°	–	Cathodal	Inhibits	Abnormal
Fibrinogen Amsterdam	–	Cathodal	Inhibits	–
Fibrinogen Nancy	Abnormal	Abnormal	Inhibits	–
Fibrinogen St. Louis	Normal	–	–	–
Fibrinogen Iowa City°	–	Normal	0	–
Fibrinogen Montreal	–	Normal	Inhibits	–
Fibrinogen Los Angeles°	–	Abnormal	Inhibits	–
Fibrinogen Philadelphia°	Abnormal	Anodal	Inhibits	–
Abnormal Fibrinogen-Thrombin Interaction and Aggregation of Fibrin Monomers:				
Fibrinogen Detroit	(Abnormal)†	Normal & anodal	Inhibits	Abnormal
Fibrinogen Giessen°	Normal	Normal	Inhibits	–
Fibrinogen Bethesda II°	Normal	Slightly anodal	Inhibits	–
Fibrinogen Cleveland II°	Normal	Normal	Inhibits	–
Other:				
Fibrinogen Paris I°	–	Abnormal	Inhibits	Abnormal
Fibrinogen Vancouver	–	Anodal	0	–
Fibrinogen Louvain	–	Anodal	Inhibits	–
Fibrinogen Metz	–	Abnormal	0	–
Fibrinogen Troyes°	–	–	–	–
Fibrinogen Parma	–	–	0	Abnormal
Fibrinogen Oklahoma	(Defective fibrin stabilization)			
Fibrinogen Oslo (clots rapidly)	–	–	–	–

°Defects partially corrected by calcium.
†Amberlite CG50 chromatography.

fibrin monomers. Fibrinogen Cleveland II (239g) exists in the plasma of a homozygous propositus with a mild bleeding tendency, and in several asymptomatic relatives. The defect in this molecule resides in the alpha (A) chain, resulting in delayed release of fibrinopeptide A by thrombin and defective polymerization of thrombin-released monomers. All these defects are apparently the result of autosomally inherited traits (239h).

Egeberg (240) described apparently enhanced coagulability and thromboembolism in persons with a species of fibrinogen molecules which clotted more rapidly than normal. Both sexes were affected. This has been called fibrinogen Oslo.

The sensitivity of fibrinogen function to minor structural alteration has been exemplified by fibrinogen Detroit, in which an amino acid substitution in the alpha (A) chain of this molecule, presumed responsible for its defective coagulability, is associated with a lowered carbohydrate content of the molecule and secondary conformational changes (241, 242). Fibrinogen Detroit clots abnormally slowly when reacted with the venom of *Bothrops jararaca*, known to release only the A peptides from alpha chains of fibrinogen (243).

Treatment of dysfibrinogenemia associated with impaired hemostasis involves intravenous administration of normal fibrinogen, but less is required than for replacement therapy in the afibrinogenemic patient, and most patients do not ordinarily require such therapy (216). The appropriate management of the dysfibrinogenemic individual consequently disposed to thrombosis is not yet clear.

Fibrin Stabilizing Factor (Factor XIII) Deficiency

When blood is deficient in fibrin stabilizing factor, it will clot readily, but the fibrin clot formed is friable. The fibrin formed in recalcified plasma is soluble in 5 M urea or 1 per cent monochloroacetic acid, enabling diagnosis of this defect. Infants with a congenital deficiency of fibrin stabilizing factor may have umbilical bleeding in the first week of life, and later sustain repeated bouts of severe bleeding after injury. Typically, the bleeding occurs 24 or more hours after the injury and apparent initial hemostasis. Too frequently, hemorrhage involves the central nervous system, and delayed wound healing leads to disfiguring scar formation. The activity of the fibrin stabilizing enzyme may be measured directly by testing its transamidating activity (aminoacyl transferase activity) by quantifying the incorporation of ^{14}C-glycine methyl ester into casein (244). Alternatively, it can be measured in an assay in which monodansyl cadaverine is incorporated into casein by plasma containing fibrin stabilizing factor activity (245).

The phenotypes of fibrin stabilizing factor "deficiency" states vary, for while affected members of several kindred reported have nonfunctional material which is antigenically related to normal fibrin stabilizing factor in their plasma (246), another patient (247) lacked antigenic as well as functional properties of the enzyme from his blood. The pattern of inheritance of fibrin stabilizing factor deficiency gives the appearance of variance from one kindred to another. In some kindreds it appears to be transmitted as an autosomal trait, while in others only males appear to be affected, as if the trait might be X-linked (248). If appropriately tested, heterozygous individuals can be identified in some instances.

Because fibrin stabilizing factor activity is stable during storage and present in both plasma and serum, therapy with intravenously administered plasma stored in a blood bank or fibrinogen-rich fractions is permissible. Levels of only 2 to 3 per cent of normal may be adequate for hemostasis (216) (see Table 19–3).

von Willebrand's Disease

Persons with this autosomal dominant inherited disorder have a mild lifelong bleeding tendency, but may have prolonged epistaxis, gingival and gastrointestinal bleeding, and easy bruising. Hemarthroses are rare, but females may be seriously troubled by menorrhagia. Easy bruising may be a presenting symptom in early childhood, and bleeding from sites of injury or dental extractions may be protracted. The severity of the disease can vary impressively from one affected patient to another, even within the same kindred.

Von Willebrand first described this disorder in persons living in the Åland Islands who had a prolonged bleeding time (249, 250). Later a delay in blood clotting in such individuals was reported (251, 252), which was attributed to a deficiency of antihemophilic factor (AHF) activity in both males and females (252–254). Although platelet adhesion to glass is diminished in many cases, there is no firm evidence of an intrinsic abnormality of platelets in von Willebrand's disease (255).

In contrast to the normal concentrations of AHF antigen despite low AHF coagulant activity in plasma of persons with classic hemophilia, the concentration of AHF antigen and coagulant activity parallel one another in plasma from persons with von Willebrand's disease, as if this autosomally inherited deficiency reflected failure of synthesis of antihemophilic globulin (195). The effects of transfusion, however, revealed additional biosynthetic complexities in this disease. When normal plasma or plasma fractions rich in AHF antigen and coagulant activity are given intravenously to patients with von Willebrand's disease, the plasma concentration of AHF coagulant activity increases progressively to levels exceeding those predicted from the dose given, and then persists beyond the time at which it would have disappeared from the plasma of a hemophiliac (254–256). Moreover, when *hemophilic* plasma or normal *serum* (each deficient in AHF coagulant activity, but containing AHF antigen) is infused into a person with von Willebrand's disease, the AHF coagulant activity in the recipient's plasma also increases for about eight hours to levels resembling those obtained when normal plasma was given (257). This apparent induction of synthesis of functional AHF in vivo does not occur in vitro, and is not associated with comparable increases in concentration of AHF antigen. The AHF antigen in the recipient's plasma only reaches levels which one could predict from the amount given, and then decreases rapidly (257a). Although the effects of transfusion suggest that de novo synthesis of AHF may be initiated by some component of normal or hemophilic plasma, the possibility that hypercatabolism of AHF occurs in von Willebrand's disease and is arrested by a substance in the administered plasma has not been rigorously excluded.

The prolonged bleeding time and impaired retention of platelets in columns of glass beads, common in cases of von Willebrand's disease, can also be transiently corrected by blood or plasma transfusion. Bouma and his associates (258) have found that partially purified preparations of AHF, rich in AHF antigen, corrected the defect in platelet adhesiveness. Similarly prepared "AHF" from hemophilic plasma, containing AHF antigen but deficient in coagulant activity, can also repair platelet adhesiveness when mixed with blood of persons with von Willebrand's disease (258a). Therefore, some property associated with AHF antigen, but independent of its coagulant activity, seems to correct the defective platelet adhesiveness. Aggregation of platelets, which is normally induced by the antibiotic ristocetin, was also defective in some cases of von Willebrand's disease (258a) and could be improved upon increasing the concentration of AHF antigen in the test mixture by adding hemophilic or normal platelet-deficient plasma to platelet-rich von Willebrand's plasma (258b).

The relationship of the prolonged bleeding time to plasma concentrations of AHF coagulant and antigenic properties is less clear. The bleeding time is normal in severe hemophilia. In addition, when some patients with von Willebrand's disease were stressed by infection, hemorrhage, or pregnancy, the plasma concentrations of both the coagulant and antigenic properties of AHF reached normal levels without transfusion, but the bleeding times remained prolonged (258c). Defective platelet adhesiveness was improved in one case tested, as if the substance in plasma which is responsible for repairing defective platelet adhesiveness might differ from that which shortens the bleeding time. Conceivably a "von Willebrand's factor," necessary for a normal bleeding time and distinct from the coagulant and antigenic properties of the AHF molecule, is also at fault in this syndrome.

Despite the complexity of the von Willebrand defects, a reasonable diagnosis can be made upon identification of low concentrations of plasma AHF activity, a prolongation of the bleeding time, and often impaired platelet adhesiveness, particularly when an autosomal mode of inheritance of a bleeding tendency associated with these alterations affecting the sexes equally can be identified in the kindred. When the family history is negative and the AHF titer is near the normal range, establishing the diagnosis is more difficult, and an intrinsic platelet defect which may be responsible for the prolonged bleeding time must be excluded (255). When therapeutically justifiable, the effect of a plasma transfusion upon the concentration of AHF coagulant activity in the patient's plasma can give diagnostic assistance, for a progressive increase in this activity should follow over several hours. When available, the immunochemical quantitation of AHF antigen and its correlation with AHF coagulant activity can, if carefully done, demonstrate a parallel between these two measurements, but a disparate elevation of functional activity as compared to antigen concentration several hours following transfusion. Even though hemophilic plasma induces formation of AHF-like material in plasma of a von Willebrand patient, the reverse does not occur (257).

Treatment of this disorder is relatively simple, for the component of plasma which induces production of AHF in vivo is relatively stable and present in stored plasma; fresh plasma contains higher concentrations (216). The prolonged bleeding time is less likely to pose postoperative problems than the AHF deficiency (216). A plasma level of AHF activity 30 per cent of normal, adequate for some procedures, may be achieved with as little as 10 ml. per kg. per day (216); this may be initiated one day before planned surgery. A satisfactory hemostatic state may be produced simply by increasing the AHF levels to those desired (see Table 19–3). There is no indication for platelet transfusion in von Willebrand's disease, since there is no evidence of an intrinsic platelet defect; substances in normal plasma seem responsible for improving platelet adhesiveness.

An "acquired von Willebrand's syndrome" has been reported in association with systemic lupus erythematosus (258d), acquired dysgammaglobulinemias (258e, 258f), and intoxication with a pesticide (258g). Plasma concentrations of AHF coagulant activity were diminished in proportion to antigen (258h), but a typical delayed and exaggerated rise in plasma AHF activity following transfusion is unlikely to occur (258f–258h). Nonetheless, depressed platelet adhesiveness could be corrected with cryoprecipitate in vitro (258f), and strenuous exercise of one patient induced a rise in his plasma AHF activity from 20 per cent to 100 per cent of the normal (258f). The bleeding time, prolonged despite normal numbers of platelets, was normal following transfusion (258g). During treatment of the underlying lupus syndrome with corticosteroids, the clinical and laboratory alterations of this acquired von Willebrand's syndrome remitted (258d). It is not certain that adequate diagnostic studies of others in the kindred of some of these patients have been done to exclude the possibility that the patient was a mildly affected member of a kindred with inherited von Willebrand's disease.

Studies of the von Willebrand problem will doubtless provide further insights into the vascular mechanisms of hemostasis and the biosynthesis of AHF. This defect, along with that of classic hemophilia and of an autosomally inherited combined deficiency of proaccelerin and AHF in which nonfunctional AHF antigen is synthesized (194), implies that at least two autosomal genes and one X-linked gene are involved in the synthesis of the normal AHF molecule.

Fletcher Factor Deficiency

In 1955, Hathaway and his associates reported that four offspring of a consanguineous marriage had prolonged plasma clotting times despite normal concentrations of known clotting factors (259). This completely asymptomatic defect was thought to be due to an abnormality in the initial phases of the intrinsic pathway of coagulation, perhaps because of a deficiency of a substance participating in the activation of Hageman factor by glasslike surfaces (260), given the name Fletcher factor. However, the partial thromboplastin time of "Fletcher-deficient" plasma progressively shortens during its incubation with kaolin, and Hathaway's suggestion that the defect might conceivably reflect the action of a substance which interferes with the activation of Hageman factor by kaolin or like substances was not excluded (259). Recent studies by Saito et al. favor the view that plasma from persons with "Fletcher defect" contains an agent which blocks the activation of Hageman factor by glass (261), but this inhibition may have been revealed secondarily to a deficiency of a plasma component which functions in surface-induced reactions (261a). Such a deficiency does exist in Fletcher trait plasma and involves the kinin releasing mechanism (261b). Kallikreins are proteolytic enzymes which release vasoactive polypeptides, such as bradykinin. In functional and immunologic assays, a plasma prekallikrein was markedly deficient in Fletcher trait plasma (261b–261d). Fletcher factor, then, appears to be a prekallikrein. The prekallikrein was initially considered to be essential to the surface activation of Hageman factor (261b), but recent studies indicate that the activated form of prekallikrein (kallikrein) probably enhances the function of already activated Hageman factor (261c). Other plasma mechanisms which depend upon activated Hageman factor for their action are also defective in Fletcher trait plasma. There is a striking delay in the generation of fibrinolytic activity, permeability-enhancing activity, arginine esterase activity, and chemotactic activity (261c–261e). Despite the fact that kinin could not be released when Fletcher trait plasma was treated with substances known to activate Hageman factor and kallikrein (261b, 261c), certain fractions were isolated from

Fletcher trait plasma which had kallikrein-like activity, as if there may be more than one prekallikrein in normal plasma. Alternatively, the kallikrein-like activity isolated from Fletcher trait plasma may reside in a markedly distorted variant of the normal plasma kallikrein molecule.

Although Fletcher trait, like Hageman trait, is not associated with a bleeding tendency, explorations of its biochemical mechanisms have provided many clues to the interrelated functions of blood coagulation and other plasma enzymes.

DEFECTIVE COAGULATION DUE TO IMPAIRED UTILIZATION: CIRCULATING ANTICOAGULANTS OR INHIBITORS

In a number of pathologic states substances develop in the plasma which interfere with normal coagulation. These circulating anticoagulants by definition inhibit the clotting of normal plasma and are identifiable when the plasma in question delays the clotting of normal plasma. Their existence often leads to a bleeding tendency. Circulating anticoagulants have been described as having inhibitory activity directed against each of the stages of coagulation, and this characterization may provide a clue to the underlying disease process when a diagnosis has not been clarified. Margolius et al. reviewed this subject extensively in 1961 (262), and Feinstein and Rapaport have recently summarized current knowledge of circulating anticoagulants (263).

Circulating Anticoagulants Directed Against AHF

Acquired hemophilia due to interference with the function of AHF may occur in women within a few months of delivery of a child, and in middle-aged or elderly persons of either sex who may or may not have obvious disease. Hemophiliacs can also develop an anticoagulant against AHF and become refractory to transfusion, making the problems of management desperate. Although the nature of anticoagulants against AHF has been disputed, largely because of experimental evidence of their enzymelike behavior (264), a large literature now attests

to the antibody nature of these substances, for they are composed of polypeptide chains identifiable as immunoglobulin components. The reason that hemophiliacs may develop these inhibitors could lie in their recognition of the foreign nature of the normal AHF protein transfused. An incidence of 21 per cent among hemophiliacs tested (262, 265) indicates the need for concern as to their presence. They may occur in children of one year, but the mean age of onset in one series was eight years (265). Although more frequent in severe hemophiliacs, they may occur in milder cases as well (265). While most circulating anticoagulants against AHF are apparently 7S gamma globulins, an unusual variety was an IgA myeloma protein which formed a complex with AHF, which dissociated in the presence of penicillin (266). Another was a macroglobulin (267).

The anticoagulant responsible for the rare occurrence of acquired hemophilia in women post partum could conceivably reflect a maternal immune response to an AHF protein in the developing fetus which differs from maternal AHF and gains access to maternal circulation at delivery. Since antigenically different nonfunctional AHF molecules exist, it is likely that some functionally normal AHF proteins also differ from others. While maternal 7S antibody to AHF may cross the placenta and affect the fetus and newborn infant (268), it is unlikely that maternal AHF molecules would do so, for AHF in plasma is of very large molecular weight.

Other varieties of acquired hemophilia due to circulating anticoagulants occur in such disease states as pemphigus, erythema multiforme, rheumatoid arthritis, penicillin reactions, and reticulum cell sarcoma (262, 269). It is difficult to identify incitants except in those patients who have been transfused.

Treatment of these anticoagulants may be urgent and difficult. Recognizing that an anamnestic antibody response may increase the titer of anticoagulants in hemophiliacs given AHF-rich plasma, Green (270) reasoned that clones of cells producing the antibody might be made extremely susceptible to cytotoxic agents following infusion of AHF immunogen. Accordingly, some success followed infusion of sufficient quantity of cryoprecipitated AHF to neutralize circulating anticoagulant followed by a single

large dose of cyclophosphamide. Any residual anticoagulant will gradually disappear
over a month or more if its production has
ceased. Apparently, only limited success
has come from this therapeutic approach
(270a). Other therapeutic measures must
include whole blood if indicated; corticosteroids and prolonged use of low doses of
cytotoxic drugs have been disappointing in
the management of patients with this type
of circulating anticoagulant (271). Exchange
transfusion has been used as a means of
removing anticoagulant while replacing
AHF (272). Infusion of AHF-rich concentrates in sufficient quantity to neutralize
anticoagulant may then allow additional
AHF to be effective until the titer of anticoagulant rises again.

Circulating Anticoagulant Against Christmas Factor

In about 12 per cent of a series of cases of
Christmas factor deficiency, circulating
anticoagulants were detected (262). The
titer of anticoagulant activity in plasma may
fall over a period of months to rise again
after transfusion, as in the case of anticoagulants directed against AHF in some hemophiliacs (271). Christmas factor is inactivated by the anticoagulant (271), and this
effect is more readily demonstrated if the
patient's plasma is incubated with normal
plasma before assay. Therapy is difficult
because of inactivation of infused Christmas factor by the anticoagulant, but concentrated plasma fractions rich in Christmas
factor may be infused in sufficient quantity
to neutralize the anticoagulant and thus
repair the hemostatic defect. George and
his colleagues have reported a familial
tendency in affected members of a kindred
with Christmas disease to develop circulating anticoagulants of this type (273). The
anticoagulant property resided in plasma
components with properties of 7S immunoglobulins which reacted only with activated Christmas factor (273, 274).

Circulating Anticoagulants in Other Inherited Coagulation Defects

Rare instances of circulating anticoagulants directed against PTA (275), proaccelerin (276, 277), and Factor VII (278) have

been noted. Circulating anticoagulants
against proaccelerin developed in a patient
with acute pancreatitis and in another with
carcinoma of the colon (211), even though
neither was deficient in proaccelerin initially. The anticoagulants behaved like 7S immunoglobulins, and progressively inhibited
prothrombin converting activity during incubation with normal plasma. A possible
role of streptomycin used in antituberculous
therapy in the induction of some circulating
anticoagulants directed against proaccelerin
has been reported (263).

Inhibitors of Fibrin Formation

Paraproteins may interfere with the last
stage of clotting by obstructing the polymerization of fibrin monomers released by the
action of thrombin upon fibrinogen. Thus, a
number of adult patients with myeloma proteins have been shown to have long thrombin times due to defective polymerization of
fibrin monomers. These defects are not
necessarily associated with a hemorrhagic
syndrome. The structure of the fibrin clot
which forms may be grossly abnormal (279).
In some instances, the inhibitory effect of
IgG myeloma proteins may reflect an antigen-antibody reaction, for Fab and F(ab′)$_2$
fragments but not Fc fragments of the isolated protein exerted this effect (280).

When fibrinogen or fibrin has been digested by the fibrinolytic enzyme plasmin,
fragments can be released into the circulation which have anticoagulant actions. They
affect the last stage of clotting mainly by
interference with polymerization of fibrin
monomers (281). Incoagulable fragments of
fibrinogen may also interact with thrombin,
so competing with normal fibrinogen and
delaying clotting (281a). Plasmin can further
increase a hemostatic defect by inactivating
proaccelerin, AHF, and Christmas factor
(282), and in very rare instances it may be
responsible for a bleeding tendency, because a state of primary fibrinolysis exists,
and fibrin is digested by fibrinolytic enzymes as it forms.

Anticoagulants in Systemic Lupus Erythematosus (S.L.E.)

Circulating anticoagulants occur in 10 to
25 per cent of adult patients with S.L.E.
(283, 284). Ecchymoses, mucosal bleeding,

epistaxis, and menorrhagia may be troublesome, but usually symptoms are mild, and hemarthroses are conspicuously absent (263).

Typically, the coagulation defect is an expression of impaired conversion of prothrombin, with a long prothrombin time and long clotting time. If the anticoagulant is mild, the use of a 1/100 dilution of tissue thromboplastin in a one-stage prothrombin time may reveal its presence. Most significantly, the patient's plasma delays the clotting of normal plasma.

The anticoagulant resides in the gamma globulin fraction of plasma (284), and may cross the placenta to be detectable in the blood of the infant for several weeks or months after birth (285). The mechanism of action of this circulating anticoagulant, long disputed because of technical difficulties in its definition, seems to reside in blockade of action of a prothrombin-converting principle (286) by inhibition of activated Stuart factor (287) or the lipid component of the active complex (263), rather than by interfering with the interaction of tissue thromboplastin with plasma as suggested by earlier studies (288). In some patients with S.L.E. this anticoagulant may also be associated with a deficiency of prothrombin (263). When bleeding occurs, it is more likely to be due to concomitant thrombocytopenia or possibly to prothrombin deficiency than to the circulating anticoagulant, which may be present in the absence of hemorrhagic symptoms (263).

Adequate treatment of the underlying disease with corticosteroids may reduce the titer of anticoagulant. The anticoagulant may be an early symptom of S.L.E. and therefore helpful in diagnosis. Certain drugs can induce a syndrome closely resembling S.L.E. (289, 290), which may be complicated by a circulating anticoagulant (290a). Although more common in adults than in children, the syndrome is otherwise remarkably similar in older and younger age groups (291).

NONTHROMBOCYTOPENIC PURPURA

Hereditary

Hereditary Hemorrhagic Telangiectasia

Near the turn of the century, Osler (292), Weber (293), and Rendu (294) each described patients with a hemorrhagic syndrome due to vascular lesions. This disorder is inherited as an autosomal dominant trait and characterized by multiple telangiectatic lesions of skin and mucous membranes. The nasal and gastrointestinal mucosal lesions are particularly prone to hemorrhage, but lesions may occur in the lung, spleen, liver, and kidney as well. Skin lesions may be nodular or macular, or resemble the vascular spider of cirrhosis of the liver. They are actually composed of defective vessels with deficient muscular coats; aneurysmal dilatation and arteriovenous fistulas may exist within the lesions, particularly in the lung. Tests of coagulation function are normal; the bleeding time is prolonged only if a lesion is punctured, but not when normal vessels are punctured.

Telangiectases gradually develop on the skin of the palms, soles, and scalp, as well as on other more exposed areas, during the second to fifth decades of life (295), but are inapparent in infancy. The initial symptom in childhood is likely to be epistaxis from mucosal telangiectases, which may abate during adolescence and worsen again in adult life. Severe, even fatal, nasal or gastrointestinal bleeding may occur. Chronic anemia and disabling bouts of epistaxis may plague those who live a normal life span, for the disease worsens with age. Treatment of local areas of involvement with electrocoagulation and irradiation is not helpful (295), but grafting of the nasal mucosa with skin has arrested disabling epistaxis in certain cases (295a). Estrogens may lessen the bleeding tendency (296), and acute blood loss and anemia due to chronic blood loss require conventional replacement therapy. Nearly continuous treatment with oral iron salts or parenteral iron preparations or both may be necessary.

With Hereditary Disorders of Connective Tissue

The Ehlers-Danlos syndrome (cutis hyperelastica) is characterized by hyperelasticity of connective tissue of the skin, hyperextensible joints, dissecting aneurysm of the aorta, and retinal detachment. A hemorrhagic tendency apparently results from the poor connective tissue support provided to vascular tissues. The disease is transmitted as an autosomal dominant trait, but may be inapparent until adolescence or early adult life. The tourniquet test is often positive, and platelets may be decreased (297). Coincident deficiency of Christmas factor in related patients with Ehlers-Danlos syndrome (298) and possible mild defects in platelet function in affected individuals in another kindred (299) may add to their bleeding tendency. In some cases of Ehler-Danlos syndrome, the conversion of procollagen to collagen by fibroblasts was deficient, leading to accumulations of excessive amounts of procollagen in connective tissues. This defect seems to be due to decreased procollagen peptidase activity (299a).

Individuals with osteogenesis imperfecta may have ecchymosis, epistaxis, melena, and subconjunctival and preretinal hemorrhages as major features of the disease. Although defective supporting connective tissues allow easy injury of the vasculature, leading to bleeding, defective platelet function may add to this disability (297, 300). Bleeding apparently due to degenerative changes of the vessels of submucosal tissues and skin (301) may be a serious complication of this familial disorder. Therapy of these syndromes and associated bleeding is unsatisfactory.

Pseudoxanthoma elasticum is a rare syndrome inherited most often as an autosomal recessive trait (302) with partial limitation to the female; rarely, it appears as an autosomal dominant trait (302). Changes in skin, connective tissue, and arteries are the result of alterations in collagen, making it elastin-like, perhaps through a degenerative process. Thus, the dermis and arteries contain less collagen than normal, but large amounts of elastin-like material. Deposits of calcium in the dermis and arteries may be the result of interaction between soluble calcium and the large amounts of acid mucopolysaccharides in these areas (303). Although the majority of cases become clinically apparent between the ages of 30 and 50 years because of the peculiar laxity of the skin and yellowish plaques which occur in the skin and mucous membranes, some cases are apparent in childhood (304). The arterial disease provoked by this elastin-like material results in syndromes of diminished tissue perfusion, including angina pectoris, myocardial infarction, and cerebrovascular accidents, as well as hypertension and pronounced psychic disturbances. Arterial hemorrhage into the gastrointestinal tract can be severe. Angioid streaks and central chorioretinitis also reflect the vascular component of this disease. Transfusion may be necessary when gastrointestinal bleeding complicates pseudoxanthoma elasticum, but there is no presently known therapy for the basic disease.

Acquired

Anaphylactoid Purpura (Schönlein-Henoch) Purpura

This purpuric syndrome actually reflects the effect of systemic vasculitis, the cause of which is unclear. It is likely to follow shortly after an acute infectious illness, possibly an etiologic factor, which may have been treated with antibiotics and other medications, conceivably able to incite vascular lesions. The possibility that immunologic or hypersensitivity reactions cause the vasculitis is unproven, but, as Osler suggested (305), it may resemble serum sickness. Even so, hemolytic complement titers are usually normal in the acute phase of this disease (306), as if immune reactions utilizing complement may not have occurred. In about 40 per cent of cases, the acute syndrome recurs, and involvement of the kidney results in persistent renal lesions in 25 to 35 per cent of cases (307, 308).

This relatively common disorder occurs most often in children under seven years of age, who develop skin lesions at some time during the illness which are so characteristic as to be pathognomonic in both type and distribution. Initially, lesions are likely to be urticarial and soon develop central red areas which expand and may become hemorrhagic. Scattered petechiae also occur. The legs, buttocks, and perineal areas are involved, but the thorax is peculiarly exempt from the petechial, wheal-like rash. Even so, there may be diffuse edema, which frequently involves the face and scalp, giving a grotesque appearance. The skin lesions in adults may be less typical, often lacking the wheal-like component, making the diagnosis difficult. Painful joint involvement probably reflects periarticular swelling, which is prominent but unassociated with erythema (307). Abdominal colic may be severe, and gross gastrointestinal bleeding can complicate this already serious and frequent component of the disease. Intussusception may occur in the course of the abdominal syndrome of anaphylactoid purpura. Thus, the consequences of this vasculitis with endothelial damage and increased vascular permeability are widespread.

Treatment of this syndrome is generally supportive in nature, with a watchful eye to the complications of abdominal and renal involvement. While corticosteroid therapy in sufficiently high doses may relieve pain in the joints or abdomen, leading to dramatic improvement, it does not alter the course or duration of the disease (309). Its use in combination with cytotoxic agents in the later nephritic phase of the disease may lead to improvement (310), but pre-existing hypertension may be potentiated by corticosteroids (311).

Scurvy

The hemorrhagic syndrome due to vitamin C deficiency is now uncommon. Humans, other primates, and guinea pigs are uniquely susceptible to scurvy, for they are unable to synthesize ascorbic acid de novo from its precursor, L-gulonolactone (312), and therefore rely upon exogenous sources for this substance. Ascorbic acid is essential for the formation and stabilization of intercellular material, hyaluronic acid, and collagen (313), and inadequate ascorbic acid intake results in symptoms owing to disruption of, or failure of formation of, such materials. Since vascular structures are weakened by incompetent "intercellular cement" or collagen, bleeding may occur.

Although adults are likely to have cutaneous bleeding, scorbutic infants characteristically present with subperiosteal hemorrhages, usually of the femur and humerus. The onset is most often between the second and twelfth months of life. particularly in infants never breast-fed (314), and bleeding from the gums, bowel, and nose, into the central nervous system, and retrobulbar hemorrhage may occur. There is no coagulation abnormality, and the bleeding time is normal in scurvy. Slight thrombocytopenia is rarely present (314). Defective release of platelet contents in scurvy may contribute to the bleeding tendency (315). Treatment with ascorbic acid, 100 to 200 mg. daily, leads to cessation of bleeding and dramatic improvement within 24 hours (314).

Autoerythrocyte Sensitization

Painful ecchymoses characteristic of autoerythrocyte sensitization occur in crops, the onset of which is heralded by a stinging sensation. Gardner and Diamond (316), noting that this illness often followed shortly after significant physical trauma, believed symptoms reflected an acquired sensitization to the patient's own erythrocytes. Moreover, intracutaneous injections of the patient's erythrocytes could reproduce a typical lesion, so lending support to the hypothesis of autosensitization. The lesion itself is distinctive because of the prominent inflammatory component, for these ecchymoses have angry, hot red halos about them but do not become necrotic. There is no abnormality of coagulation or platelet function.

Ratnoff and Agle (317) have studied this syndrome extensively and clearly indicated the emotional component of the disorder. Affected persons are all females with severe emotional problems. They are beset with hysterical and masochistic character traits, cannot adequately deal with their hostilities, and suffer from anxiety and depressive states. Moreover, they are extremely suggestible, and lesions have been induced through hypnotic suggestion, even to designation of the site of the lesion so induced (317). Self-inflicted trauma is impossible to exclude as an initiating factor in spontaneously occurring lesions, and the pathophysiology of this psychosomatic syndrome and its unique lesion is unclear. Although typically an affliction of women in their third and fourth decades, it has been known in late teenagers, and in about 25 per cent of cases symptoms began between 14 and 20 years of age. In treatment, judicious abstention from extensive diagnostic procedures may avoid reinforcing the physical aspects of the problem. These are inseparable from the emotional aspects of the disease, and cautious supportive psychotherapy may have an important therapeutic role. Early, more intensive psychotherapy of the young patient as soon as possible after diagnosis may meet with significant success (317).

MANAGEMENT OF HEMOPHILIA AND CHRISTMAS DISEASE

In 1937, Carol Burch outlined a grim prognosis for hemophiliacs in that 82 of a group of 98 hemophilic boys died by the age of 15 (318). With modern methods of replacement of deficient clotting factors, life expectancy may be relatively normal, and progressive permanent crippling defects may be avoided. Thus, the major emphasis in management must be prevention of both orthopedic and psychologic crippling. This is only possible when medical and paramedical personnel work together to provide the medical needs and the support and guidance to assure a normal home, school, and work experience.

Transfusion Therapy

In 1840 (319) Samuel Lane first described the successful transfusion of blood into a child with probable hemophilia. The boy had had a surgical procedure to correct strabismus and bled following the procedure. The bleeding ceased following transfusion of fresh blood.

When a deficient factor is replaced, the hemostatic defect due to the deficiency is repaired, and hemostasis can be maintained for prolonged periods of time with repeated transfusions, allowing even major surgical procedures. The quantity of deficient factor to be transfused and the interval between transfusions depends upon the severity and type of deficiency, the half-life of the deficient factor, and the nature of the bleeding episode.

The average increases in concentrations of factors following transfusion, their half-lives, and the minimal concentrations of factors necessary to achieve hemostasis following minor trauma and major surgery are shown in Table 19–3. For example, one unit (the amount in 1 ml. of normal plasma) of Factor VIII per kg. body weight given intravenously can increase the plasma concentration 2 per cent. The administration of one unit of Factor IX (Christmas factor or PTC) per kg. body weight, however, only increases the deficient factor level from 1 to $1\frac{1}{2}$ per cent, because of the large extra-

vascular reservoir of this protein. Thus, approximately 15 units per kg. are necessary to obtain a 15 per cent level of Factor IX. In order to maintain a particular level, one half the initial amount of factor can be given at each half-life interval. For example, ten units per kg. of body weight of Factor IX given every 20 to 24 hours will maintain a minimal hemostatic level of 5 per cent of normal Factor IX concentration. In the case of Factor VIII, to maintain a minimal hemostatic level of at least 10 per cent, 10 units per kg. should be given every 8 to 12 hours. In von Willebrand's disease, plasma transfusion apparently stimulates in vivo production of Factor VIII activity which lasts 20 to 30 hours (320), and replacement need be given only once daily or less often, depending on individual response.

The response of any individual to replacement is variable. Table 19–3 provides useful guidelines and specific references relating to therapy, but adequate laboratory control of the replacement is necessary in managing a hemophiliac, particularly with major trauma or when undergoing surgery. The products available for the replacement of deficient factors are also listed in Table 19–3. Unfractionated plasma can be used for treatment of all the deficiencies. Plasma should be freshly frozen or drawn just prior to transfusion for treating Factor VIII deficiency or von Willebrand's disease, and must be frozen for less than one month for treating Factor V deficiency. The major limitation in the use of plasma is in the excessive expansion of intravascular volume which may occur if large amounts of a factor are required. "Cryoprecipitate," a fraction of plasma extracted by freezing and slowly thawing plasma (321), contains high concentrations of both Factor VIII and fibrinogen, so that adequate levels of these factors can be achieved without harmful increase in intravascular volume. Severe anaphylactic reactions have been reported in patients receiving cryoprecipitate, but these are exceedingly rare (322). Cryoprecipitate also contains the factor which shortens the bleeding time in patients with von Willebrand's disease and is therefore useful for treatment of this condition.

Commercial concentrates are available for treatment of deficiency of factors VIII, IX, VII, and X, and of prothrombin and fibrinogen deficiencies. These preparations have the advantage of high concentrations of factors in small volumes, allowing repeated replacement for prolonged periods of time without excessive volume expansion. The commercial preparations are, however, obtained from large pools of plasma, and therefore must be assumed to be contaminated with hepatitis virus. In addition, the recovery and half-life of Factor VIII may be variable, depending on the preparation (323).

Soft Tissue Bleeding and Lacerations

The management of a soft tissue hematoma or laceration in a child with hemophilia depends upon its location, the degree of discomfort, and its size. Small hematomas and lacerations can often be managed at home with local pressure, ice, and observation for increasing size or continued bleeding. A soft tissue hematoma which is increasing in size or a laceration which continues to bleed for a period of hours despite local measures can usually be managed on an outpatient basis by giving a single intravenous injection of a preparation of the deficient factor to provide a hemostatic level, followed by continued observation. Soft tissue bleeding in a vital region, such as the pharyngeal or subglottic area, however, always requires replacement of deficient factor to a hemostatic level for 48 to 72 hours and in-hospital observation for continued bleeding.

Lacerations of the tongue and frenulum, though not usually life-threatening, are in an area where maintenance of the hemostatic clot is difficult. These lacerations, although small, usually require four to five days of replacement infusions to maintain hemostasis, or bleeding will recur.

Acute Hemarthrosis

Although minor soft tissue bleeding can sometimes be adequately treated by local measures, hemarthrosis is the most frequent cause of permanent crippling and demands special attention if crippling is to be prevented.

The onset of bleeding into a joint of a hemophiliac is heralded by pain or stiffness or both in the affected joint. On physical examination, there is discomfort associated with movement, often significant limitation of motion, and increased warmth over the joint. Periarticular swelling with detectable effusion into the joint is frequently absent unless bleeding has been present for a prolonged time or effusion into the joint was present before the acute bleeding episode. Increased distention of the capsule of the joint and increased pressure within the joint will occur if bleeding continues. Although bleeding may occur into any joint, certain ones are more frequently involved than others, the most common in order of frequency being the knee, elbow, ankle, shoulder, and wrist. Bleeding in the vertebral column is most unusual. Since the development of degenerative arthritis in hemophilia is related to the number and severity of hemarthroses, establishment of immediate hemostasis is the most important therapeutic consideration.

The importance of prompt transfusion of sufficient Factor VIII or IX to establish hemostasis in an acute hemarthrosis cannot be overemphasized. Ali et al. (324) found that 72 per cent of 39 hemophilic boys given a transfusion of a preparation of the factor deficient at the onset of acute hemarthrosis returned to full activity after less than one week, whereas 52 per cent of 44 boys who did not receive transfusion of the factor were unable to return to full activity for two weeks or longer. A significant joint deformity occurred in every seven hemarthroses in boys of similar age and severity of hemophilia who did not receive adequate replacement therapy.

For the treatment of an acute hemarthrosis, the transfusion of the factor which is deficient, in the form of either plasma or a plasma fraction in amounts sufficient to increase the patient's level to 20 to 25 per cent of normal, will achieve hemostasis. To maintain hemostasis, the level of deficient factor should be maintained at approximately 10 per cent of normal for a period of 48 to 72 hours. Recently, Honig et al. (325) successfully treated 47 of 51 episodes of acute hemarthrosis in boys with Factor VIII deficiency by administering a single dose of Factor VIII concentrate sufficient to achieve a level of approximately 50 per cent of normal. In addition to this infusion, the involved joints were immobilized to minimize further trauma, and the immobilization was followed by a period of progressive ambulation. Similar results were obtained *without* immobilization in hemarthrosis, the symptoms of which were present for 24 hours or less, by adding a five-day course of prednisone to the single infusion of a Factor VIII preparation (326). Prednisone was given orally, 1 mg. per lb. for three days to a maximum dose of 80 mg., followed by 0.5 mg. per lb. for two days to a maximum of 40 mg. (326). Examinations of the joints five to seven days after treatment showed that only 7 of 62 joints (11 per cent) treated with the combination of a single injection of 25 units per kg. of Factor VIII and a five-day course of prednisone had failed to return completely to normal function, whereas 34 per cent of patients treated only with factor replacement remained abnormal. A single transfusion with 16 units per kg. of Factor IX and a five-day course of prednisone is also effective for treating acute hemarthrosis in Factor IX–deficient patients. If symptoms of bleeding have been present longer than 24 hours, or significant clinical improvement is not apparent 24 hours after transfusion, repeated transfusion of Factor VIII or IX should be given to maintain the 10 per cent hemostatic level for 48 to 72 hours.

Routine aspiration of the joints is recommended by some (327, 328); others recommend aspiration of only larger hemarthrosis (328, 329). The small amount of blood in the joint early during an acute bleeding episode cannot be totally removed, so that the risk of increased bleeding, further trauma to the joint, and the possibility of introducing an infection rule against routine aspiration of early hemarthroses. If there is distention of the capsule under pressure with a large hemarthrosis, aspiration can be done after replacement of the deficient clotting factor, giving significant relief of pain.

Immobilization of the affected joint with a splint or other appliance is also frequently recommended in the treatment of acute hemarthrosis (325, 327, 330), but splinting and immobilization, even for a short period of time, cause notable muscular weakness and wasting in the extremity. Passive and active physical therapy are then necessary before a complete range of motion returns and weight-bearing can begin, and time lost from school or employment is often excessive. This is eliminated by restricting weight-bearing without splinting for the first 24 to 36 hours only, followed by gradual return to full ambulation.

Chronic Synovitis

With repeated hemorrhages into joints, inflammation occurs with hypertrophy of synovial tissues, and a form of chronic synovitis develops. The synovitis is often accompanied by recurrent effusion into the joint, frequently without pain, limitation of motion, or clinical evidence of acute bleeding. The chronic synovitis leads eventually to erosion of the cartilage of the joint and is usually associated with an increased frequency of acute hemarthrosis. It may be possible to delay the onset of chronic synovitis by transfusion of deficient factor at the earliest onset of an acute hemarthrosis, but the hemarthroses studied by Van Creveld et al. (330a), which were treated with adequate replacement of deficient factor, nevertheless showed significant synovial changes. The long-term benefits of a brief course of corticosteroids with the transfusion of deficient factor can be judged only after further follow-up. The intra-articular injection of corticosteroids for the treatment of chronic synovitis has been disappointing. Poulain and Josso (331) reported an initial reduction in synovitis following the intra-articular injection of corticosteroids, but it was not lasting. Our experience has been similar to theirs, and because of the possible detrimental effects on joint cartilage from intra-articular corticosteroid injections, this form of therapy has been discontinued.

Jordan (332) has given 800 R. of deep X-ray therapy to joints with chronic synovitis and reports good but somewhat delayed improvement. The possible hazards of X-ray therapy to developing ossification centers must be carefully considered when contemplating the use of this form of therapy.

The irreversible damage to tissues of the joint due to prolonged synovitis has prompted Storti et al. (333) to recommend synovectomy. His results, though very encouraging, must be confirmed before a general recommendation for synovectomy can be given.

Contractures

The outcome of chronic synovitis is loss of cartilage and the development of fibrosis, fibrous adhesions with reduction of joint mobility, and contractures. The correction of contractures, most commonly flexion contractures of the knee, may be accomplished in a number of ways. The use of a plaster spica cast, hinged at the knee with subluxation hinges, has been very satisfactory. With this method, as described by Jordan (332), the tightening of a cord by means of a short stick (the Quingel) gradually stretches the knee into extension.

Another approach to the treatment of contractures involves active and resistive physical therapy exercises administered by a well-trained physical therapist, while plasma concentrations of the deficient factor are maintained at adequate levels (334). The resistive exercises are performed daily with the physical therapist after the patient has been transfused with deficient factor to achieve a plasma level of 15 per cent normal.

The advantage of active and resistive physical therapy over casting is that the exercises increase the strength of the supporting structures of the joint simultaneously with the increasing range of motion. The limitations of the method are the necessity for a well-trained physical therapist, a cooperative patient, and the transfusion of deficient factor during the treatment.

Dental Complications

Most dental procedures can be managed with a minimum of hospitalization (336). Historically, local anesthesia has been omitted or used sparingly for restorative dentistry in the hemophilic child. Local infiltration anesthesia can be given without replacement of deficient factor. However, this approach is not applicable to mandibular and posterosuperior alevolar nerve block anesthesia, for it has initiated dissecting cervical hematomas and respiratory embarrassment in one case, leading to death (337).

Careful mandibular or posterosuperior alveolar nerve block anesthesia may be used following replacement of the deficient factor to a level of 25 per cent of normal. Then, after local infiltration anesthesia or mandibular and posterosuperior alveolar nerve block, comprehensive, painless restorative dentistry is possible for a hemophilic child even on an outpatient basis. Replacement therapy with preparations of the deficient factor should be continued at repeated intervals if needed, but in our hands, ordinary restorative dental procedures have been uncomplicated and have usually not required a second infusion. If signs of bleeding or of inflammation persist near the time when the plasma level of deficient factor is becoming inadequate, additional replacement should be given.

Dental extractions are best accomplished on an in-patient basis. The preoperative replacement of deficient factor is given as for surgery, and plasma samples are tested before and after the administration to assure adequate plasma concentrations. Anesthesia is given by an anesthesiologist through an oral tracheal tube. The surgical procedure includes complete curettage of the alveolus to remove granulation tissue, the placement of sutures if needed, and packing of the socket with adsorbable gelatin sponge (Gelfoam), of which the layer in contact with tissue is soaked in topical thrombin. Replacement of the deficient clotting factor is continued for five to seven days after the operation, depending upon the extent of the surgery involved. The level of deficient factor concentration should be maintained above 10 per cent of normal throughout this period. Some centers have found it possible to decrease the amount of replacement therapy following surgery by local systemic administration of antifibrinolytic agents, such as epsilon aminocaproic acid (337a). Renal obstruction due to clot formation in the renal pelvis can occur if epsilon aminocaproic acid is given to a child with hemophilia and concurrent hematuria. Thus, frequent examination of the urine for blood is indicated before and during this therapy.

Exfoliating deciduous teeth can present a problem for both patient and doctor. Most patients do not require hospitalization but are treated with local pressure, powdered topical thrombin applied to the bleeding area, and a soft or liquid diet. Sporadic bleeding often occurs, and repeated prolonged applications of pressure to the area may be necessary. If hemorrhage is severe enough to cause a significant drop in hemoglobin despite local measures, extraction of the tooth and maintenance of hemostatic levels of deficient factor for two to three days is indicated. Because of the shallowness of the exfoliation site, allowing comparatively rapid wound healing, the duration of replacement therapy need only be for two or three days.

Many dental emergencies can be prevented if a meaningful preventive program is initiated in the dental office. Our patients are seen in a dental office every four months, when a routine dental examination is performed and a topical fluoride is applied. Diagnostic bite-wing dental X-ray films are taken twice yearly for the detection of new caries. Oral hygiene instruction is given with the aid of disclosing tablets, which stain dental plaque a bright red and therefore provide a useful visual aid in the instruction of proper tooth brushing. One milligram of supplemental sodium fluoride per day is prescribed for children eight years of age and younger. After eight years of age, the crowns of all the permanent teeth except third molars have calcified, and supplemental fluoride is no longer needed. Dietary limitation of refined carbohydrates is also discussed.

The benefits of such a preventive dentistry program are evident in a review of the clinical results of Steinle and Kisker (336). From July, 1968, to July, 1970, 14 teeth were extracted from new patients who had not been followed with the preventive program, whereas no teeth were extracted because of decay from the original 34 patients on the preventive program.

Hematuria

Prentice and co-workers reported a 77 per cent incidence of renal abnormalities in 34 hemophilic patients studied (338). Most of these abnormalities were believed to result from clot formation in the renal tract. Hematuria, a frequent complication of hemophilia, particularly in the older child and adult, is complicated by the danger of a clot formation in the renal tract if a normal hemostatic mechanism is established. Hematuria, per se, does not seem to be harmful to renal tissues, whereas clot forma-

tion with subsequent obstruction is clearly detrimental. In hemophilic patients with inadequate hemostasis, the presence of urokinase, an activator of the fibrinolytic system, probably contributes to the inability of hemophilic patients to establish a stable hemostatic plug. For this reason, a number of investigators (339, 340) attempted the use of epsilon aminocaproic acid (EACA), a potent inhibitor of fibrinolysis, in the management of persistent hematuria, and with some success. The use of EACA cannot be recommended, however, because of several reports of renal obstruction following its administration (341, 342). Abildgaard and co-workers recommend a trial of corticosteroids in patients with hematuria and report control of the hematuria without complications in 80 per cent so treated (343). To date, no confirmatory studies are available, but this form of therapy seems worthy of trial before intravenous administration of the deficient clotting factor. Because of the possibility of clot formation in the renal pelvis with subsequent obstruction, any replacement therapy should be administered in sufficient quantity to establish immediate hemostatic levels. Correction of the plasma deficiency to levels required for surgery and maintenance above that effective in minor trauma until gross and microscopic hematuria have ceased is therefore indicated.

Major Surgery

Major surgical procedures can be performed on severe hemophiliacs, but should be carried out in a center in which levels of clotting factors can be accurately measured, so that hemostasis can be maintained during and following the operative procedures. A search for a possible circulating inhibitor described earlier (p. 589) should always be made prior to considering any surgical procedure. In the absence of inhibitors, levels of factors required for safe surgery, as presented in Table 19–3, can be obtained with relative ease, particularly with high-potency plasma concentrates. Plasma concentrations of deficient factors should be maintained above those recommended for minor trauma for a period of seven days postoperatively during the early stages of wound healing, after which they can be reduced to usual maintenance levels for another seven days or until complete healing occurs. Examples of successful surgical maintenance for the various factor deficiencies are given in the references of Table 19–3.

Pseudotumor

Continued subperiosteal hemorrhage, with an expanding hematoma gradually eroding the adjacent bone, is an uncommon but difficult complication to manage. Pseudotumors are estimated to occur in 1 to 2 per cent of severe hemophiliacs (344). Tumor formation follows recurrent bleeding into the subperiosteal area or rarely intraosseously over a period of months. Surgical management is possible if sufficient surrounding uninvolved tissue is resectable and adequate replacement of clotting factor is provided (345). Van Creveld and Kingma (346) and Krill and Mauer (347) described successful management of pseudotumor with replacement therapy alone. X-ray therapy has also been reported to be effective (348).

Central Nervous System Bleeding

Bleeding into the central nervous system, the most serious complication of hemophilia, is said to be the leading cause of death (349). Silverstein reported a mortality of 71 per cent due to this complication in his review of the world literature in 1960 (350). With present therapeutic materials for obtaining hemostatic levels of deficient clotting factors, there is no longer justification for an excessively conservative approach to diagnosis and therapy once recommended by Fessey and Meynell (351). A lumbar puncture should be performed after replacement of the deficient clotting factor, and other neurosurgical diagnostic and therapeutic procedures, including angiography and evacuation of a subdural hematoma, can also be safely carried out (352, 353).

The onset of severe headache and vomiting with or without a history of head trauma should alert the physician to the possibility of central nervous system bleeding, particu-larly if followed by progressive neurologic signs.

Gastrointestinal Hemorrhage

Gastrointestinal bleeding is uncommon in the child with hemophilia, but the incidence of duodenal ulcer in patients with hemophilia is significantly increased as they enter the third decade (354, 354a). Other forms of gastrointestinal bleeding, particularly intramural bleeding, can occur in childhood, and symptoms vary from mild abdominal pain to intestinal obstruction. The hematoma usually ruptures into the intestinal tract; thus blood is often present in the stool. Rupture into the peritoneal cavity has also been reported (355). A recent report by Dodds and co-workers (356) of the roentgenographic changes with intramural bleeding demonstrates the usefulness of X-ray contrast studies in delineating an intramural hematoma. These bleeding episodes can generally be managed with replacement therapy and without surgical intervention.

Psychiatric Aspects

Hemophilia, like any chronic illness, exerts a profound influence on the life of the individual concerned and his family. Agle has described a variety of psychiatric syndromes in patients with hemophilia (188). Some of these, such as excessive risk-taking behavior, passive dependent behavior, and possible psychophysiologic responses which increase bleeding, may be directly detrimental to the survival of the patient. Other family members may also develop inappropriate responses which disrupt the family unit, isolate the patient, and for numerous reasons lead indirectly to more frequent hemorrhages. The mother's guilt concerning genetic transmission may be expressed either by over-protectiveness or by actual desertion (188, 357). A father's attitude of denial toward his son can lead to further risk-taking behavior by the child who grasps for paternal attention. The disappointment of having a son with hemophilia can result in a form of rejection whereby the father assumes the role of an uninterested bystander.

School experience is likely to be counter-productive for the hemophilic child. The practice of segregating hemophiliacs in special schools, common in Europe, should be avoided so that the hemophiliac may learn to adjust to normal children. Even in public school, the teacher's fear of the disease often segregates the hemophiliac from his classmates psychologically or physically. Frequent absences due to bleeding episodes further restrict his ability to gain social acceptance. With continued surveillance and frequent conferences between teachers and concerned medical and paramedical personnel, an excellent learning experience is possible (358).

Prophylaxis

Prompt transfusion of Factor VIII at the onset of a bleeding episode is paramount if chronic disability is to be retarded or prevented. The prevention of continued bleeding and its consequences is the ultimate goal of management, and therefore prophylactic administration of deficient factor to prevent hemorrhage has been explored. This form of therapy has been of some value in those patients with rapidly recurring hemarthrosis of a single joint (359). However, the expense of this form of treatment, the amount of deficient factor required, and the difficulties encountered with daily or three times weekly transfusions make it unrealistic for many children over a prolonged period. Kasper et al. (360) administered preparations of Factor VIII three times a week in a quantity sufficient to achieve a level of 65 to 70 per cent and showed a significant decrease in the frequency of hemarthrosis, though it was not totally prevented. In our experience, weekly administration of preparations of the deficient factor sufficient to achieve levels in excess of 50 per cent failed even to reduce the incidence of acute hemarthrosis (361). Other forms of therapy have been used to lessen the frequency and severity of hemarthrosis. Although studies by Mainwaring and Keidan (362), Katsumi (363), and Reid (364) suggested some benefit from the use of EACA, a double-blind study by Strauss et al. (365) did not show any beneficial effects, and the use of this agent in hemophiliacs has caused serious complications (341, 342).

A short course of therapy with corticosteroids was effective in reducing the amount of replacement needed (326). Long-term administration of corticosteroids, however, is not recommended because of the concomitant complications (366).

A continuing program of physical therapy and physical education to maintain joint mobility and to provide protection to the joints through increased muscular strength has seemed of value in decreasing the number of acute hemarthroses and in providing some of the psychologic needs of a growing boy.

Home Therapy

The administration of transfusions of deficient factor at home by either the hemophiliac or a member of his family allows immediate treatment of a bleeding episode and should thereby decrease the amount of bleeding and subsequent deformity. Furthermore, home transfusion will reduce the cost of treatment and should decrease the time lost from school or employment. When the patient and his family can be adequately trained and surveillance of a home transfusion program carried out, this approach to management of acute hemarthrosis and minor injuries has been shown to have many advantages (366a, 366c).

ACCELERATED UTILIZATION

Introduction

Although unproved, a theoretical balance between continuous formation of fibrin and its removal by fibrinolysis has been an attractive hypothesis to explain the homeostatic mechanism for blood coagulation in normal individuals. Whether an imbalance due to triggering of a normally inactive coagulation mechanism or acceleration of continually active coagulation explains localized and disseminated intravascular coagulation is unclear. Nevertheless, both localized venous and arterial thrombosis and disseminated intravascular coagulation do occur, and their diagnosis and management are of concern.

Localized Intravascular Coagulation

Venous Thrombosis and Pulmonary Embolism

A thrombus is formed in flowing blood, and therefore its appearance is different from that of the usual blood clot formed in a test tube. The intravascular thrombus is composed of a "head," containing platelets and white cells stabilized by fibrin strands at its point of attachment to a vessel, followed by a "tail," consisting of fibrin and red cells with only a few platelets.

Thrombi may occur when circulating thrombogenic substances are localized and activated. Venous thrombosis may occur in valve pockets and at vein junctures, the points of maximum stasis along the venous channels (367). Stasis predisposes to thrombosis, for in areas of stasis activated clotting factors can accumulate, protected from removal by the liver and inhibition by circulating anticoagulants and inhibitors. Because local generation of coagulant activity may occur in areas of stasis, thrombosis often occurs in shock, congenital heart disease, obesity, and dehydration where there is relative circulatory stasis.

When there is an increase in concentrations of circulating thrombogenic substances or a decrease in circulating inhibitors, there may be thrombosis. For example, it has been suggested that an increased incidence of thrombosis may occur in patients with abnormally high concentrations of Factor V (368) and Factor VIII (369), and with an abnormal fibrinogen with increased reactivity to thrombin (240), decreased concentration of antithrombin (370), accelerated thromboplastin generation (371), increased platelet adhesiveness (372), or increased inhibition of fibrinolysis (373). A causal relationship between elevated concentrations of clotting factors in plasma and thrombosis has not been established, however. Increased coagulant activity in plasma may in fact be the result rather than the cause of thrombosis.

In children, thromboembolic disease is usually a complication of another disease. A tendency to thrombosis, for example, is evident in patients with the nephrotic syndrome (374, 375), severe trauma (376), burn injury (377, 378), homocystinuria, and paroxysmal nocturnal hemoglobinuria (379, 379a). Although continuous activation of the clotting mechanism has been suggested as the cause of thrombosis in patients with cyanotic congenital heart disease (380), chronic intravascular coagulation in such patients is unproved (381). It is theoretically possible that the combined effects of increased blood viscosity, an abnormal endothelial surface, tissue hypoxia, activation of the clotting mechanism, and decreased erythrocyte deformability may all contribute to thrombosis in these patients. Decreased red cell deformability occurs in patients with hemoglobinopathies S and C, and conceivably may favor thrombosis because of impaired blood flow. With trauma or infection, such as osteomyelitis (382), primary injury to the vascular endothelium is a probable cause of thrombosis.

The characteristic clinical findings of venous thrombosis in children include pain, swelling, discoloration of the involved extremity, fever, and tachycardia. As mentioned, a history of trauma or other disease conditions predisposing to thrombosis is the rule. Tenderness and localized increased temperature along the course of the involved vein is usual, and in the lower extremity, dorsiflexion of the foot is impaired on the affected side as compared to the unaffected (Homans' sign) (383). Homans' sign is, of course, nonspecific; it may be produced by other local inflammatory or neoplastic conditions (384). Marks and Sussman have recommended venography in establishing a diagnosis of venous thrombosis in children (385). However, the utility of this procedure (386) and of other diagnostic approaches to venous thrombosis, including the injection of ^{131}I-labeled fibrinogen (387), measurement of plasmin digestion products of fibrinogen and fibrin (388), and the Doppler effect (389), have not been adequately explored in children.

Two sites of venous thrombosis are of particular interest to pediatricians because of their frequent occurrence in infants. Portal vein thrombosis may occur in the newborn period as a result of the spread of phlebitis from the umbilical vein (390), or as the result of an umbilical catheterization (406). The occluded vein may remain completely blocked, causing portal hypertension. It may recanalize or it may be re-placed by multiple tortuous vessels (cav-ernous transformation). In infancy, the renal vein may also be a site of thrombosis, par-ticularly in infants of diabetic mothers (390a) and in association with severe infec-tion or dehydration. If the thrombosis is acute, hemorrhagic infarction and rupture of the kidney may lead to death. If it occurs gradually, the kidney may remain viable, but a clinical and pathologic syndrome re-sembling membranous glomerulonephritis may result. While surgical treatment of thrombosis of the portal or renal vein has usually been recommended, conservative medical management of renal vein throm-bosis during the acute stage has been in-creasingly accepted (391).

Pulmonary thromboembolism in children, as in adults, is usually associated with some underlying condition, such as a hemoglo-binopathy, a congenital heart lesion, or thrombosis of a deep vein. The symptoms of pulmonary thromboembolism are also similar, including dyspnea, tachypnea, chest pain, cough, hemoptysis, unilateral localized wheezing, a friction rub, rales, splinting of the chest, dullness, tachy-cardia, increased jugular venous pressure, and accentuation of the pulmonic compo-nent of the second heart sound. The inci-dence of electrocardiographic changes in children with pulmonary embolism is un-known, but right-sided T wave inversion, right bundle-branch block, and the pattern of acute cor pulmonale are found in only 10 to 20 per cent of adult patients (392). Increased activity of serum lactic dehydro-genase and of bilirubin concentration with normal glutamic-oxaloacetic transaminase activity may be helpful on occasion (393). Roentgenographic demonstration of local-ized reduction or absence of vascular mark-ings with relative radiolucency in patients with acute pulmonary embolism, or of a radio-opaque area of consolidation resem-bling a truncated cone in patients with hemorrhagic infarction, is helpful if pres-ent. If the chest X-ray is normal, lung scan-ning with a radioisotope may be useful in demonstrating a perfusion defect (394). Angiography has been used in adults (395) to localize embolism by outlining it with contrast material, but because of difficulties in its interpretation and possible induction

of thromboembolism, angiography is sel-dom used in children.

Medical treatment of thromboembolism involves the use of anticoagulants. Heparin, a highly negatively charged sulfated muco-polysaccharide, has several anticoagulant properties, including interference with the function of activated Factor IX (30), inhibi-tion of activated Factor X or thrombin (89), and interference with the polymerization of fibrin monomers. Coumarin compounds act as anticoagulants indirectly by com-peting with vitamin K in the synthesis of Factors II, VII, IX, and X, as previously discussed (p. 568). Though commonly recom-mended, there are few satisfactorily con-trolled trials establishing the usefulness of heparin for treatment of deep thrombosis of the lower extremity; anticoagulants may be contraindicated in patients with central nervous system thrombosis, because hemor-rhage may result from their use. Prophy-lactic anticoagulation of patients with the nephrotic syndrome has been suggested (375), but controlled trials have not been done. Barritt and Jordan (396) reported benefit from the use of heparin and cou-marin in adults with pulmonary embolism, and we recommend this approach in the treatment of children.

For initial anticoagulation, heparin should be used because its action is immediate and direct, and it is easily reversible with protamine sulfate. Therapeutic levels of heparin can usually be obtained by inject-ing 100 units per kg. body weight intra-venously, and anticoagulant levels can then be maintained by continuous infusion, preferably with a constant infusion pump, giving 100 units per kg. of heparin over each succeeding four-hour period. The whole blood clotting time may thereby be kept between 20 and 30 minutes with little adjustment. The activated PTT can also be used to follow heparin therapy. In uncom-plicated cases, sufficient heparin is given to double the baseline PTT. This level of he-parinization should be continued for eight to ten days, the time required for firm ad-herence of a thrombus to the vessel wall un-der experimental conditions (397). Couma-rin should be started five days before heparin is discontinued, since two to three days are required for adequate prolongation of the prothrombin time, and it may be as long as five to seven days before there is an optimal anticoagulant effect from coumarin.* An initial dose of three to four times the maintenance dose will usually provide a therapeutic reduction of clotting activity to approximately 20 per cent of normal. In patients with normal hepatic function, the maintenance dose of coumarin is usually 0.05 to 0.1 mg. per kg., but there is extreme variability between individuals, and repeated prothrombin times are necessary to adjust the dose for each patient. Since the individual response to coumarin is quite variable, coumarin therapy must be monitored daily during the initial period of anticoagulation. Three to six months of therapy is recommended for adults with thromboembolic disease, as it is during this period of time that the risk of recurrent thromboembolism is greatest. In children, the duration of therapy should be determined by the nature and duration of the underlying condition which predisposed to the development of the thromboembolic complication.

Serious bleeding can occur during the administration of anticoagulants. Reversal of the bleeding tendency from heparin is relatively simply carried out by rapid neutralization with protamine sulfate. The dose of protamine to be given can be calculated by estimating the amount of heparin remaining and giving 1 to 1.5 mg. of protamine for each 100 units of heparin. Protamine in excess is itself an anticoagulant. Vitamin K should be given parenterally to reverse the anticoagulant effects of coumarin. One-half milligram per kilogram of body weight of vitamin K_1 is sufficient to reverse the effects. In an emergency, transfusion of plasma or concentrate will be of immediate benefit.

Drugs which affect platelet aggregation and adhesion should be most effective in preventing thrombosis, since platelet aggregation seems to be a primary event in thrombosis. Dipyridamole, which decreases the rate of platelet aggregation and

possibly platelet adhesiveness, has not been tested in children, and its clinical effectiveness in adults has been variable (398, 399). Aspirin can abolish the release of endogenous ADP from the platelets and prevent the second wave of aggregation (400), but its usefulness in the treatment of thromboembolic states is unclear. Dextran 70 may have an antithrombotic effect because it inhibits both ADP-induced platelet aggregation and adhesiveness, and is said to be effective in treating patients with thromboembolic disease (401). Fibrinolytic activators, such as streptokinase and urokinase, have been used in adults with thromboembolism (402), but have not been tested in children except in the hemolytic-uremic syndrome (403), where benefit was suggested in an uncontrolled study.

Valve Prosthesis Biomaterials

Thromboembolism is the leading cause of postoperative morbidity after implantation of artificial heart valves (398). Thrombosis is also a complication of ventricular shunt procedures for hydrocephalus (404), shunt procedures for renal dialysis (405), and indwelling catheters (406). Thromboembolic complications following the introduction of biomaterials into the blood stream result predominantly from the interaction of platelets with the foreign surface. Harker and co-workers demonstrated increased platelet turnover in the face of normal duration of survival of fibrinogen in patients with prosthetic heart valves (407). These findings indicate increased platelet utilization without significant fibrin formation. The nature of the interaction between platelets and the foreign surface is unclear. Adhesion of platelets to many surfaces appears related to the protein interface or bridge between the surface and the platelets, and there are many proteins which can serve as this interface (408). Though investigation of biomaterials and surface coatings is under way, no suitably nonthrombogenic material is presently available. Until such material is available, drugs which inhibit platelet aggregation and adhesion (398) may help control the thromboembolic complications of biomaterials in the blood stream.

*The initial effect of coumarin is to decrease Factor VII activity without influence on Factors V, IX, or X, because their half-lives are longer than that of Factor VII. Hence, during the first day or two of treatment, the prothrombin time may be increased without effect on the intrinsic coagulation system.

Renal Disease

Intravascular coagulation may contribute to the genesis and progression of chronic renal disease. Wardle and Taylor found cryofibrinogen, low platelet counts, and increased serum levels of fragments presumed to be split from fibrinogen or fibrin by plasmin (fibrinogen-related antigen) in patients with acute renal failure of varying causes (409), suggesting chronic intravascular coagulation. Fibrinogen-related antigens were found in the serum of patients with persistent glomerulonephritis and were thought to correlate with histologic evidence of disease activity in patients with persistent glomerulonephritis (410). Stiehm and co-workers (411) found increased concentrations of fibrinogen-related antigens in the urine of 60 per cent of 89 patients with various renal diseases, but this need not have reflected fibrin deposition in the kidney. Some patients, particularly those with the nephrotic syndrome, excrete molecules as large as IgM, and there is markedly increased glomerular permeability which could also allow fibrinogenuria. In the absence of proteinuria, however, fibrinogen-related antigens in the urine may represent increased fibrin deposition and lysis within the kidney.

Further support for the involvement of coagulation mechanisms in renal disease comes from studies of experimental nephritis. Humair and co-workers (412) produced lesions similar to those of glomerulonephritis in mice by injection of "Liquoid" (sodium polyanetholesulfonate) (412), a substance which promotes blood coagulation. Lesions were prevented by pretreatment of the animals with heparin or urokinase (413). Anticoagulants, however, did not alter the progression of nephrotoxic serum nephritis induced in mice by injecting immune complexes (414). The authors concluded that fibrinogen or fibrin deposition played a role in the nephritis, but was not the primary cause. Thirteen children with progressive renal disease were treated with anticoagulants by Herdman and co-workers (415), who reported significant improvement in two patients with rapidly progressive nephritis. Cade (416) found improvement in eight of ten patients with chronic proliferative glomerulonephritis given prolonged therapy with depo-heparin

in a controlled study. Priscilla Kincaid-Smith and her co-workers, however, did not find any improvement with heparin therapy in six patients with acute renal failure due to glomerulonephritis (417), nor did Freedman and his associates in seven patients with various forms of chronic renal disease (418). Freedman reported complications related to heparin therapy, including gastrointestinal bleeding, alopecia, and muscular weakness. Thus, the use of heparin cannot be recommended.

Intravascular coagulation has been implicated in renal transplant rejection. Lowenhaupt and Nathan (419) and Rosenberg et al. (420) found that the platelets in the effluent renal vein blood decreased precipitously coincident with the development of platelet aggregates in the small renal arteries and glomeruli during accelerated acute homotransplant rejection in dogs. In addition, there was apparent consumption of fibrinogen, prothrombin, and Factors V and VIII, and the liberation of fibrin split products. Braun (421) found fibrinogen fragments D and E in the urine at various times following renal homotransplantation in humans. Antoine and co-workers (422) reported fibrinuria in 54 per cent of 22 patients following renal transplantation, but the suspected causes other than intrarenal coagulation included surgical ischemia, intravascular fibrinolysis without coagulation, and increased glomerular permeability. Thus, though all these findings suggest that localized intravascular coagulation may occur during transplantation rejection, treatment with heparin may not influence the rejection phenomenon.

Localized intravascular coagulation is thought to be of etiologic significance in patients with the hemolytic-uremic syndrome, an illness characterized by renal failure, anemia, and thrombocytopenia, first described by Gasser and co-workers (423). The syndrome occurs primarily in children under the age of two years, but older children and adults have been affected (424, 425). It is usually preceded by three to ten days of gastroenteritis or, occasionally, an upper respiratory infection. This prodrome is followed by acute hemolytic anemia, thrombocytopenia, and renal failure, with hypertension, heart failure, and, in some cases, an encephalitic syndrome. In addition to thrombocytopenia, the red cells are fragmented, with helmet and burr-shaped cells present in the blood smear. Other coagulation tests are not consistently abnormal. Avalos and co-workers (426) and Katz et al. (427) studied 26 and 16 infants, respectively, and found frequent prolongation of the prothrombin time, normal or decreased concentrations of Factor X, and normal or increased concentrations of Factors V, VII, IX, XI, and XIII. Fibrinogen concentration was frequently increased, and fibrinogen and fibrin split products were found in the sera of some patients.

Numerous agents have been implicated in the etiology of the syndrome, but none has been proved. Although the primary cause of the renal lesion is not known, it is thought to be the result of localized glomerular intravascular coagulation. Wehinger and Kunzer (428) suggested that the initial insult may be hemolysis, with release of thromboplastin-like substances from the red cell stroma, thus initiating intravascular clotting. Others believe that local endothelial damage caused by some unknown agent leads to activation of the coagulation system with platelet and fibrin deposition in the glomerular vessels (429). Regardless of the mechanism, patchy renal cortical necrosis occurs. Continued hemolysis and thrombocytopenia may be the result of trauma to platelets and red cells during their passage through a meshwork of fibrin and damaged endothelium in the renal microvasculature.

Because the initiating events are unclear, therapy is controversial. Corticosteroids have not been beneficial (430, 431). Gilchrist and co-workers (432) found improvement with heparin therapy in seven of eight consecutive patients treated, whereas Katz et al. (427) reported an increased mortality in patients treated with heparin; the dosage was difficult to regulate in anuric patients. In a review of the problem, Kaplan (433) found no difference in mortality in patients treated with heparin compared to those receiving only supportive measures, and Vitacco and co-workers did not find any benefit from heparin therapy in a controlled study of a series of 30 patients (433a). Brain and his associates demonstrated increased fibrinogen turnover in a patient

with the hemolytic-uremic syndrome (434), suggestive of active intravascular coagulation. Harker, however, was unable to show increased fibrinogen turnover in four patients with hemolytic-uremic syndrome (435). We were also unable to detect active intravascular clotting as measured by the presence of "soluble circulating fibrin" in patients with the hemolytic-uremic syndrome. Mandal and McNulty (436) reported benefit from phenformin and ethyloestrenol, two drugs which reduce platelet adhesiveness and aggregation, and Bergstein et al. (403) believed that streptokinase administered intravenously to patients with the hemolytic-uremic syndrome was therapeutically advantageous. The value of inhibition of platelet function and of fibrinolytic therapy in this disease is yet to be confirmed. Thus, confusion reigns in the debate over the efficacy of anticoagulant and fibrinolytic therapy for this disease, but all agree that supportive measures, including control of hypertension and peritoneal dialysis (401a), are critical in the management of patients with the hemolytic-uremic syndrome.

Hemangioma

Kasabach and Merritt (437) first described an infant with a capillary hemangioma who developed a bleeding disorder. Though numerous reports have appeared since their original description, excessive bleeding associated with hemangioma is uncommon. The majority of capillary hemangiomas increase in size for four to six months after birth and then gradually decrease in size over the next two years without the development of a bleeding tendency. Straub and associates (438) found a shortened plasma half-life of ^{131}I-labeled fibrinogen and preferential accumulation of radioactivity at the site of a hemangioma. This supports the view that a hemorrhagic tendency might result from local clotting in the hemangioma.

Hoak and his co-workers (439) found localized thrombi and increased consumption of fibrinogen and platelets in mice with hemangiomata, an animal model of the Kasabach-Merritt syndrome. The apparent consumption was not altered by heparin.

Successful treatment of severe intravascular coagulation associated with a secondary bleeding disorder requires treatment of the hemangioma itself. Surgery may be possible if the hemangioma is well localized. In massive hemangiomas which were not easily resectable, Goldberg and Fonkalsrud (440) and Brown and co-workers (441) induced significant regression in size by the use of corticosteroids. This effect of steroids was first noted by Zarem and Edgerton (441a). When corticosteroids are not effective, radiation therapy has been useful (442, 443).

Disseminated Intravascular Coagulation

Diagnosis

Disseminated intravascular coagulation may occur if widespread in vivo activation of the clotting mechanism leads to intravascular fibrin formation. Three factors may theoretically influence in vivo activation. First, damage to the endothelium of vessels with exposure of collagen could lead to activation of Hageman factor and to platelet aggregation with subsequent release of platelet factor 3, a phospholipid which then may help to promote generation of thrombin. Second, introduction of thromboplastic substances into the circulation may generate thrombin through the extrinsic pathway. Third, decreased concentrations of circulating inhibitors and anticoagulants and impairment of the reticuloendothelial system may potentiate the effects of circulating active clotting factors and indirectly contribute to disseminated intravascular coagulation. Although fibrin may form complexes with fibrinogen and other plasma proteins and remain soluble in plasma, with increasing concentrations of fibrin, polymerization ultimately occurs and can lead to fibrin deposits in the microcirculation. When fibrin is deposited, tissue ischemia and necrosis may lead to the release of thromboplastic substances into the blood stream and increased thrombin generation. Thrombin can also activate Factors V and VIII, which may provide further clotting activity. With the activation of the clotting mechanism, activation of the fibrinolytic system also occurs.

In a patient with intravascular coagulation and secondary fibrinolysis, profound alterations of the hemostatic mechanism may develop. Platelets, Factors V, VIII, prothrombin, and fibrinogen are normally consumed in the process of coagulation. If the consumption of these factors exceeds their production, deficiencies result which are reflected by prolongation of the prothrombin time, the partial thromboplastin time, and the thrombin time. Factor XIII (fibrin stabilizing factor) and Factor X concentrations may also be reduced (444). Fibrinolysis may cause a reduction in plasma plasminogen levels, and its proteolytic action on fibrinogen and fibrin results in circulating fibrinogen and fibrin degradation products. These products prolong the thrombin time by interfering with fibrin polymerization and can be measured directly as fibrinogen-related antigen in the serum by immunochemical means (410). Because plasmin digests not only fibrinogen and fibrin but also Factors V, VIII, and IX, further reduction in these factors may occur. Thus, the patient with disseminated intravascular coagulation will classically have a reduction in platelet numbers, decreased concentrations of Factors V, VIII, prothrombin, and fibrinogen, and the presence of fibrinogen-related antigen in his serum.

A number of conditions known to be associated with disseminated intravascular coagulation are listed in Table 19–5, with

TABLE 19–5. CONDITIONS ASSOCIATED WITH DISSEMINATED INTRAVASCULAR COAGULATION

Malignancy (478, 478a)
Intravascular hemolysis (479, 480)
Snake bite (481)
Hemorrhagic pancreatitis (482)
Severe birth asphyxia (483)
Hepatitis (484)
Abruptio placentae (165)
Intrauterine fetal death (485)
Respiratory distress syndrome (486)
Pulmonary embolism (487)
Heat stroke (448)
Purpura fulminans (488, 489)
Infections
　Viral (490, 491)
　Bacterial (452, 492, 493)
　Rickettsial (494, 494a)
　Fungal (495)
　Sepsis with asplenia (496, 497)

appropriate references. The diagnosis of disseminated intravascular coagulation should be suspected in a patient with one of these underlying conditions in whom an acute deficiency of clotting factors develops. Among the pitfalls in establishing this diagnosis, however, is the fact that increased consumption of clotting factors may not cause a decreased concentration if production is correspondingly accelerated. Despite normal clotting factor levels, evidence of active fibrinolysis detected by increased fibrinogen-related antigen in the serum is usually present when measured by sensitive immunochemical methods (445). Once thrombin generation has ceased, restoration of plasma clotting factors and the removal of fibrin degradation products proceed at variable rates. Thus, decreased levels of certain factors and the presence of fibrinogen-related antigen in the serum do not necessarily indicate *active* disseminated intravascular coagulation. Fibrinogen-related antigen in the serum, for example, may persist for as long as 72 hours (446). The platelet count may also increase slowly over a period of days after an episode of disseminated intravascular coagulation (447). Labeling fibrinogen with ^{131}I and measuring its rate of disappearance from the plasma has been useful in defining consumption of fibrinogen in the absence of severe abnormalities of other clotting factor activities (455). An accelerated disappearance of fibrinogen is not a specific measure of thrombin activity, because plasmin as well as thrombin may digest fibrinogen, thus increasing the rate of fibrinogen clearance from the vascular compartment. Protamine sulfate may selectively precipitate complexes of fibrinogen and thrombin and plasmin-altered fibrinogen and fibrin. Thus, the serial dilution protamine sulfate test may be useful in establishing a diagnosis (448a); however, false-positive tests can be found in a number of conditions (448b). We have devised a more specific assay which allows detection of thrombin-altered fibrinogen, but it is time-consuming and thus not useful at the bedside (449). Another direct measure of thrombin activity is an immunologic assay developed by Nossel and co-workers (450) for measuring the A peptide released from fibrinogen by thrombin. Fletcher and associates have developed a method based on

the formation of high molecular weight complexes of fibrin and fibrinogen when thrombin activity is present (451). Each of these methods may be useful in defining conditions in which active intravascular coagulation is occurring, thus permitting initiation of proper therapy and evaluation of its effectiveness.

Even though hemorrhage is not always a manifestation of disseminated intravascular coagulation, an acute, severe episode of disseminated intravascular coagulation, as may occur in meningococcal sepsis, can result in a significant hemorrhagic tendency and anemia (452). The anemia is believed to be the result of destruction of red blood cells which were traumatized as they passed through vessels partially occluded with fibrin strands (453). The appearance of fragmented and burred red cells on the blood smear suggests the effect of this trauma. When an episode of disseminated intravascular coagulation is mild and transient, such as may occur with abortions induced by intrauterine injections of hypertonic saline, there may be no apparent bleeding and no anemia (454).

Treatment

The basic treatment of intravascular coagulation is aimed at amelioration of the underlying condition which precipitated the episode. In addition, the use of heparin to inhibit thrombin formation should be considered. If, as has been suggested, fibrin deposition may lead to irreversible shock because of decreased blood flow through the microvasculature, then the early institution of heparin therapy prior to the development of deficiencies in clotting factors might prevent this complication. There is, however, no controlled experimental proof of the efficacy of heparin in human diseases associated with intravascular coagulation prior to the development of abnormal clotting tests. If a bleeding disorder occurs as a result of clotting factor deficiencies with an episode of disseminated intravascular coagulation, heparin anticoagulation may be helpful (455). The clinical benefit of heparin therapy in brief endotoxemic conditions in addition to treatment with specific antibiotics and supportive measures is, however, questionable (447, 456).

The effectiveness of heparin in controlling an episode of disseminated intravascular coagulation may also be variable, for where there may be continued release of tissue thromboplastin, as in patients with acute promyelocytic leukemia (457), prolonged heparinization may be necessary. Heparin also may not be particularly effective in reversing platelet consumption in patients presenting with the hemolytic-uremic syndrome and thrombotic thrombocytopenic purpura.

Despite the lack of controlled experimental proof, it is generally accepted that a brief course of heparin should be given as treatment of intravascular coagulation in those patients with low plasma concentrations of Factors V, VIII, and fibrinogen. Adequate anticoagulation can be achieved and maintained by giving an initial dose of 100 units per kg. of heparin intravenously, followed by 100 units per kg. each four hours thereafter given by constant infusion. This will usually delay the whole blood clotting time to approximately 20 to 30 minutes. In those patients in whom the clotting time is initially prolonged because of lowered concentrations of clotting factors, the effect of heparin may be judged by testing the effect of the patient's plasma upon the partial thromboplastin time of normal plasma. In this test, the patient's plasma is diluted 1:2 with normal plasma and the partial thromboplastin time measured. Prolongation of this mixed partial thromboplastin time to 70 to 90 seconds (normal 34 ± 4 seconds) demonstrates adequate heparin effect and allows reasonable control of treatment. The duration of anticoagulation is primarily dependent upon control of the initiating disease. Some laboratory guidelines to evaluate the progress of therapy are helpful. If heparin is effective and fibrinogen synthesis is unimpaired, increased concentrations of fibrinogen should be apparent within 24 hours and may be measured in the presence of heparin by a heat precipitation method (458). Colman and co-workers have found the prothrombin time useful in assessing the effectiveness of heparin, for when intravascular clotting subsided, the prothrombin time returned to normal or was shortened by at least five seconds (459), probably because of rapid regeneration of Factor V. In patients with meningococcal sepsis treated with antibiotics and heparin, soluble circulating fibrin disappeared when sepsis was controlled with antibiotics, usually within 15 hours (456). Should the coagulation defects fail to improve, it is important to determine whether heparinization was adequate. Replacement of fibrinogen and other clotting factors with fresh plasma or concentrates can be given once a patient is adequately heparinized, but may not then be necessary. In the occasional patient with severe liver disease, replacement therapy may be necessary to restore the concentration of the plasma clotting factors after an episode of disseminated intravascular coagulation has ceased. It is important, however, to maintain adequate anticoagulation if replacement is given; otherwise, replacement may increase the severity of disseminated intravascular coagulation by adding needed factors. Antifibrinolytic agents, such as EACA, should not be given to patients with disseminated intravascular coagulation, because fibrinolysis is an important mechanism for removal of fibrin deposits present in the microcirculation.

Disseminated Intravascular Coagulation in the Newborn

Intravascular coagulation in the newborn is often more difficult to identify than that in the older child. As in the older child, it is often associated with, or actually caused by, another illness, commonly sepsis or shock. However, because of the normally low concentrations of vitamin K–dependent clotting factors in plasma of the newborn, the laboratory confirmation of suspected intravascular coagulation in the neonate is not readily clear. The partial thromboplastin time and prothrombin time of plasma from premature and normal neonates may be prolonged. Normally, a full-term infant will respond readily to as little as 0.1 mg. of vitamin K administered intramuscularly, and the prothrombin time will be shortened to the normal range within hours or a day of its administration. If, however, the infant is premature, has been in shock, or is anoxic, he may be unable to respond to the vitamin K because these conditions have compromised the capacity of the liver to utilize this vitamin in the synthesis of vitamin K–dependent clotting factors. Therefore, the failure to respond to parenterally administered vitamin K in the predicted fashion is not certain evidence of disseminated intravascular coagulation, but more likely represents an immature liver or significant liver disease. Plasma Factor V and fibrinogen concentrations are independent of vitamin K synthetic mechanisms. Though the liver is the source of both Factor V and fibrinogen, their concentrations, even in the premature infant, approach adult levels (134). Thus, a decreased concentration of Factor V or fibrinogen suggests intravascular coagulation or a serious liver disorder as opposed to vitamin K deficiency.

Normally, platelets are in excess of 100,000 per mm.³ in the newborn, and a significant decrease, may be caused by increased consumption as a result of intravascular coagulation, immunothrombopenia, defective production associated with a viral illness, hereditary deficiency, or drug depression (498). The presence of fibrinogen-related antigen in the serum of an infant may not be a reliable measure of intravascular clotting, for the process of birth itself may provoke sufficient fibrinolytic activity to cause the appearance of fibrinogen-related antigen in the infant's serum. If an assay for the identification of thrombin-hydrolyzed fibrinogen ("circulating fibrin") in plasma is employed (440), disseminated intravascular clotting may be identified with fair certainty. Regrettably, this kind of assessment is not available at the bedside. Thus, the diagnosis of disseminated intravascular coagulation must be based on the clinical appreciation that some underlying condition (birth asphyxia, abruptio placentae, sepsis, respiratory distress syndrome, dead twin fetus) known to be associated with intravascular clotting is present and is associated with a significant reduction of platelets, fibrinogen, and Factors V and VIII.

As a useful guide, the results of various laboratory tests, as shown in Table 19–6, should aid the clinician in differentiating disseminated intravascular coagulation from liver disease and vitamin K deficiency. Should the diagnosis of intravascular clotting in the neonate be established and proper management of its underlying cause initiated, further therapy of the hemostatic defect may not be necessary, for the normal synthetic mechanism can replace plasma clotting factors, provided that vitamin K has been made available. The use of a directly acting anticoagulant, such as heparin, may aid in the alleviation of a bout of intravascular clotting, though there is little published evidence justifying its use. If it is effective, heparin should exert its therapeutic action reasonably quickly, and only brief administration of this drug should be necessary. Therefore, it has been our custom to infuse heparin intravenously at a rate of 100 units per kg. every four hours by constant infusion for a 24-hour period. Fresh plasma (10 mg. per kg. of body weight) or cryoprecipitated fractions of plasma are given if the clotting factor deficiencies are severe. Occasionally, the infusion of platelet concentrates is given, should their concentration be significantly

TABLE 19–6. USUAL LABORATORY FINDINGS IN LIVER DISEASE, VITAMIN K DEFICIENCY, AND INTRAVASCULAR COAGULATION

	LIVER DISEASE	VITAMIN K DEFICIENCY	INTRAVASCULAR COAGULATION
Red cells	Targeting	Normal	Fragmented
Platelets	Normal or decreased	Normal	Decreased
Fibrinogen	Decreased	Normal	Decreased
Factor V	Decreased	Normal	Decreased
Factor VIII	Normal	Normal	Decreased
Prothrombin	Decreased	Decreased	Decreased
Fibrin degradation products	Normal or increased	Normal	Increased

less than 50,000 per mm.³ Exchange transfusion using fresh blood has also been reported effective in treating apparent intravascular clotting in newborn infants with intravascular hemolysis, sepsis, shock, and the respiratory distress syndrome (498, 499).

The clinician faced with the emergent problem of a hemorrhagic newborn, having made the diagnosis of disseminated intravascular coagulation, must bear in mind that significant intravascular clotting is secondary to, or symptomatic of, an ongoing pathologic process needing identification and treatment. Thus, the treatment of the underlying disorder, such as shock or sepsis, should receive primary attention, and the use of heparin and replacement therapy be undertaken only if the need is apparent.

LIVER DISEASE

Inasmuch as the liver is the site of synthesis of fibrinogen and proaccelerin (V) as well as vitamin K–dependent clotting factors, if the synthetic capacity of hepatic cells is sufficiently impaired by disease, the concentrations of these clotting factors in plasma may become deficient. When the biliary tract is obstructed, the absorption of lipids, and therefore vitamin K, will be impaired. The hemostatic defect in the case of biliary obstruction can be corrected with parenterally administered vitamin K, whereas that resulting from hepatic failure is resistant to vitamin K administration.

Liver disease may also be complicated by consumption of clotting factors and platelets because of associated intravascular coagulation. This may be seen in young patients with fulminant hepatitis and acute hepatic necrosis, and complicates the therapy of the other hemostatic problems associated with hepatitis (500, 501). The diagnosis and therapy of a patient with parenchymal liver disease is, therefore, similar to that of the newborn with a hemorrhagic syndrome. Defective blood coagulation with severe parenchymal liver disease associated with a bleeding tendency requires replacement with blood plasma or fractions thereof. In certain adults with cirrhosis of the liver, heparin therapy may induce spontaneous replenishment of circulating platelets and fibrinogen (501), as if intravascular coagulation had occurred. In such cases,

it would be important to avoid providing coagulant proteins without giving a directly acting anticoagulant, such as heparin.

Fibrinolytic activity of blood has been repeatedly reported as increased in various types of liver disease. A circulating "activator" of plasminogen may participate in this enhancement of fibrinolysis (502), but it is not certain if this reflects coincident or prior generation of clot-promoting activity in the blood of the patient. Enhanced fibrinolysis alone need not be associated with hemorrhage and is unlikely to require therapy, and antifibrinolytic agents may be dangerous if the fibrinolytic activity is a consequence of intravascular coagulation.

The use of certain plasma concentrates to replace vitamin K–dependent clotting factors in a patient whose liver is unable to synthesize these proteins is a rational approach to restoring adequate hemostasis. Unfortunately, such preparations may generate sufficient clot-promoting activity in vivo to induce a syndrome of intravascular coagulation (503).

Thus, the safest replacement therapy for patients with severe liver disease is exchange transfusion with fresh whole blood. Heparin anticoagulation should also be given if intravascular coagulation is suspected.

References

1. Lister, J.: On the coagulation of the blood. Proc. R. Soc. Med. 12:580, 1862–63.
2. Bordet, J., and Gengou, O.: Recherches sur la coagulation du sang et les sérums anticoagulants. Ann. Inst. Pasteur (Paris) 15:129, 1901.
3. Shafir, E., and deVries, A.: Studies on the clot promoting activity of glass. J. Clin. Invest. 35:1183, 1956.
4. Margolis, J.: Glass surface and blood coagulation. Nature (Lond.) 178:805, 1956.
5. Ratnoff, O. D., and Colopy, J.: A familial hemorrhagic trait associated with a deficiency of a clot-promoting fraction of plasma. J. Clin. Invest. 34:602, 1955.
6. MacFarlane, R. G.: The enzyme cascade in the blood clotting mechanism and its function as a biochemical amplifier. Nature (Lond.) 202:498, 1964.
7. Davie, E. W., and Ratnoff, O. D.: Waterfall sequence for intrinsic blood coagulation. Science 145:1310, 1964.
8. Ratnoff, O. D., Davie, E. W., et al.: Studies on the action of Hageman factor. Evidence that activated Hageman factor in turn activates plasma thromboplastin antecedent. J. Clin. Invest. 49:803, 1961.

9. Ratnoff, O. D.: The biology and pathology of the initial stages of blood coagulation. Prog. Hematol. 4:204, 1966.

10. Ratnoff, O. D., and Crum, J. D.: Activation of Hageman factor by solutions of ellagic acid. J. Lab. Clin. Med. 63:359, 1964.

11. Niewiarowski, S., Bankowski, E., et al.: Adsorption of Hageman factor (XII) on collagen. Experientia 20:367, 1964.

12. Wilner, G. D., Nossel, H. L., et al.: Activation of Hageman factor by collagen. J. Clin. Invest. 47:2608, 1968.

13. Nossel, H. L.: Activation of Factor XII (Hageman) and XI (PTA) by skin contact. Proc. Soc. Exp. Biol. Med. 122:16, 1969.

14. Ogston, D., Ogston, C. M., et al.: Studies on the clot-promoting effect of skin. J. Lab. Clin. Med. 73:70, 1969.

15. Margolis, J.: Activation of plasma by contact with glass: Evidence for a common reaction which releases plasma kinin and initiates coagulation. J. Physiol. 144:1, 1958.

16. Kaplan, A. P., and Austen, K. F.: A pre-albumin activator of pre-kallikrein. J. Immunol. 105:802, 1970.

17. Wuepper, K. D., Tucker, E. S., et al.: Plasma kinin system: Proenzyme components. J. Immunol. 105:1307, 1970.

18. Kellermeyer, R. W., and Breckenridge, R. T.: Inflammatory process in acute gouty arthritis. I. Activation of Hageman factor by sodium urate crystals. J. Lab. Clin. Med. 65:307, 1965.

19. Ratnoff, O. D.: Activation of Hageman factor by L-homocystine. Science 162:1007, 1968.

20. Schimke, R. N., McKusick, V. A., et al.: Homocystinuria. J.A.M.A. 193:87, 1965.

21. Harker, L., Slichter, S. J., et al.: Platelet thromboembolism and its prevention in homocystinuria (abstract) Proc. Am. Soc. Hematol., Miami, Fla., Dec. 3–6, 1972, p. 46.

22. Moskowitz, R. W., Schwartz, H. J., et al.: Generation of kinin-like agents by chondroitin sulfate, heparin, chitin sulfate, and human articular cartilage: Possible pathophysiologic implications. J. Lab. Clin. Med. 76:790, 1970.

23. Donaldson, V. H., and Ratnoff, O. D.: Hageman factor: Alterations in physical properties during activation. Science 150:754, 1965.

24. Vroman, L.: Effects of hydrophobic surfaces upon blood coagulation. Thromb. Diath. Haemorrh. 18:259, 1967.

25. Speer, R. J., and Ridgway, H.: The formation and "decay" of XIIa. Thromb. Diath. Haemorrh. 18:259, 1967.

26. Nossel, H. L.: The early stages of blood coagulation, In Recent Advances in Blood Coagulation. Poller, L. (ed.), Boston, Little, Brown and Co., 1969.

27. Haanen, C., Morselt, G., et al.: Contact activation of factor XII. Thromb. Diath. Haemorrh. 17:307, 1967.

28. Haanen, C.: The nature of the factor IX activating principle, In Human Blood Coagulation. Hemker, H. C., Loeliger, E. A., et al. (eds.), Heidelberg, Springer-Verlag, 1969, pp. 58–76.

29. Ratnoff, O. D.: Studies on the product of the reaction between activated Hageman factor and plasma thromboplastin antecedent. J. Lab. Clin. Med. 80:704, 1972.

30. Ratnoff, O. D., and Davie, E. W.: The activation of Christmas factor (factor IX) by activated plasma thromboplastin antecedent (factor XI). Biochemistry (Wash.) 1:677, 1962.

31. Schiffman, S., Rapaport, S. I., et al.: Starch block electrophoresis of clotting factors. Clin. Res. 12:110, 1964.

32. Kingdon, H. S., Davie, E. W., et al.: The reaction between activated plasma thromboplastin antecedent and diisopropylphosphofluoridate. Biochemistry (Wash.) 3:166, 1964.

33. Pitlick, F.: Thesis. University of Washington, 1968; cited by Davie, E. W., In Recent Advances in Blood Coagulation. Poller, L. (ed.), Boston, Little, Brown and Co., 1969, pp. 13–28.

34. Hougie, C., Denson, K. W. E., et al.: A study of the reaction product of factor VIII and factor IX by gel filtration. Thromb. Diath. Haemorrh. 18:211, 1967.

35. Densen, K.: The interaction of Factors VIII, IX and X, In Human Blood Coagulation. Hemker, H. C., Loeliger, E. A., et al. (eds.), Heidelberg, Springer-Verlag, 1969, pp. 48–53.

36. Alexander, B., Goldstein, R., et al.: Congenital afibrinogenemia. A study of some basic aspects of coagulation. Blood 9:843, 1954.

37. Rapaport, S. I., Schiffman, S., et al.: The importance of activation of antihemophilic globulin and proaccelerin by traces of thrombin in the generation of intrinsic prothrombinase activity. Blood 21:221, 1963.

38. Lundblad, R. L., Pitlick, R., et al.: Activation of antihemophilic factor and the role of proteolytic enzymes. Fed. Proc. 25:317, 1966.

39. Milstone, J. H.: Thrombokinase of the blood as trypsin-like enzyme. J. Gen. Physiol. 45:103, 1962.

40. Papahadjopoulos, D., and Hanahan, D. J.: Observations on the interaction of phospholipids and certain clotting factors in prothrombin activator formation. Biochem. Biophys. Acta 90:436, 1964.

41. Jobin, F., and Esnouf, M. P.: Studies on the formation of the prothrombin converting complex. Biochem. J. 102:666, 1967.

42. Hemker, H. C., Esnouf, M. P., et al.: Formation of prothrombin converting activity. Nature (Lond.) 215:248, 1967.

43. Davie, E. W., Hougie, C., et al.: Mechanisms of blood coagulation, In Recent Advances in Blood Coagulation. Poller, L. (ed.), Boston, Little, Brown and Co., 1969, pp. 13–28.

44. Esnouf, M. P., and Williams, W. J.: The isolation and purification of a bovine plasma protein which is a substrate for the coagulant action of Russell's viper venom. Biochem. J. 84:62, 1962.

45. Seegers, W. H., Marciniak, E., et al.: Note on the inactivation of autoprothrombin C with diisopropylfluorophosphate or phenylmethanesulfonyl fluoride. Thromb. Diath. Haemorrh. 22:32, 1969.

46. Breckenridge, R. T., and Ratnoff, O. D.: The role

of proaccelerin in human blood coagulation. Evidence that proaccelerin is converted to a prothrombin converting principle by activated Stuart factor: With notes on the anticoagulant action of soybean trypsin inhibitor, protamine sulfate and hexadimethrine bromide. J. Clin. Invest. 44:302, 1965.

47. Jackson, C. M., and Hanahan, D. J.: Studies on bovine Factor X. II. Characterization of purified Factor X. Observations on some alterations in zone electrophoretic and chromatographic behavior occurring during purification. Biochemistry (Wash.) 7:4506, 1968.

48. MacFarlane, R. G.: The coagulant action of Russell's viper venom: The use of antivenom in defining its reactions with a serum factor. Br. J. Haematol. 7:496, 1961.

49. Morawitz, P.: Die Chemie de Blutgerinnung. Ergebn. Physiol. 4:307, 1905. Translated by Hartmann, R. C., and Guenther, P. F., In Chemistry of Blood Coagulation. Springfield, Ill., Charles C Thomas, Publisher, 1967.

50. Shapiro, S. S.: Human prothrombin activation: Immunochemical study. Science 162:127, 1968.

51. Stenn, K. S., and Blout, E. R.: Mechanism of bovine prothrombin activation by an insoluble preparation of bovine factor Xa (thrombokinase). Biochemistry (Wash.) 11:4502, 1972.

52. Nemerson, Y.: The reaction between bovine brain tissue factor and factors VII and X. Biochemistry (Wash.) 5:601, 1966.

53. Østerud, B., Berre, S., et al.: Activation of the coagulation factor VII by tissue thromboplastin and calcium. Biochemistry (Wash.) 11:2853, 1972.

54. Chargaff, E., Benditt, A., et al.: The thromboplastic protein: Structure, properties, disintegration. J. Biol. Chem. 156:161, 1944.

55. Straub, W., and Duckert, F.: The formation of extrinsic prothrombin activator. Thromb. Diath. Haemorrh. 5:402, 1961.

56. Williams, W. J.: The activity of lung microsomes in blood coagulation. J. Biol. Chem. 239:933, 1964.

57. Nemerson, Y., and Spaet, T. H.: The activation of Factor X by extracts of rabbit brain. Blood 22:657, 1964.

58. Nemerson, Y., and Pitlick, F. A.: Purification and characterization of the protein component of tissue factor. Biochemistry (Wash.) 9:5105, 1970.

59. Pitlick, F. A., and Nemerson, Y.: Binding of the protein component of tissue factor to phospholipids. Biochemistry (Wash.) 10:5100, 1970.

60. Pitlick, F. A., Nemerson, Y., et al.: Peptidase activity associated with tissue factor of blood coagulation. Biochemistry (Wash.) 10:2650, 1971.

61. Ware, A. G., Murphy, R. C., et al.: A function of Ac-globulin in blood clotting. Science 106:618, 1947.

62. Prentice, C. R. M., Ratnoff, O. D., et al.: Experiments on the nature of the prothrombin-converting principle: Alteration of proaccelerin by thrombin. Br. J. Haematol. 13:898, 1967.

63. Surgenor, D. M., Wilson, N. A., et al.: Factor V

64. Hemker, H. C.: Factor VII in the intrinsic system. In Human Blood Coagulation. Hemker, H. C., Loeliger, E. A., et al. (eds.), Heidelberg, Springer-Verlag, 1969, p. 82.

65. Hougie, C., and Twomey, J. J.: Haemophilia B$_m$: A new type of factor IX deficiency. Lancet 1:698, 1967.

66. Blomback, B.: Nomenclature of fibrinogen and fibrin chains and other derivatives of fibrinogen and fibrin. Thromb. Diath. Haemorrh. (Suppl.) 35:161, 1969.

67. Blomback, B., Blomback, M., et al.: N-terminal disulfide bond of human fibrinogen. Nature (Lond.) 218:130, 1968.

68. Bailey, K., Bettelheim, F. R., et al.: Action of thrombin in clotting of fibrinogen. Nature (Lond.) 167:233, 1951.

69. Lorand, L.: Fibrinopeptide. New aspects of fibrinogen-fibrin transformation. Nature (Lond.) 167:992, 1951.

70. Blomback, B.: Fibrinogen to fibrin transformation, In Blood Clotting Enzymology, Seegers, W. H. (ed.), New York, Academic Press, 1967, pp. 143–215.

71. Lorand, L., and Yudkin, E. R.: The effect of arginyl peptides on the clotting of fibrinogen with thrombin. Biochem. Biophys. Acta 25:437, 1957.

72. Blombäck, B., and Vestermark, A.: Isolation of fibrinopeptides by chromatography. Arkiv. Kemi. 12:173, 1958.

73. Lorand, L., and Konishi, K.: Activation of the fibrin stabilizing factor of plasma by thrombin. Arch. Biochem. 105:58, 1964.

74. Loewy, A. G.: Enzymatic control of insoluble fibrin formation, In Fibrinogen. Laki, K. (ed.), New York, Marcel Dekker, Inc., 1968, pp. 185–223.

75. Fuller, G. M., and Doolittle, R. F.: The formation of cross-linked fibrins: Evidence for the involvement of lysine ε-amino groups. Biochem. Biophys. Res. Commun. 25:694, 1966.

76. Pisano, J. J., Finlayson, J. S., et al.: Cross link in fibrin polymerization by factor XIII: Epsilon (gamma glutamyl) lysine. Science 160:892, 1968.

77. Schwartz, M-L., Pizzo, S. V., et al.: The effect of fibrin stabilizing factor on the subunit structure of human fibrin. J. Clin. Invest. 50:1506, 1971.

78. Robbins, K. C.: A study on the conversion of fibrinogen to fibrin. Am. J. Physiol. 142:581, 1944.

79. Lorand, L., Doolittle, R. F., et al.: A new class of blood coagulation inhibitors. Arch. Biochem. Biophys. 102:171, 1963.

80. Levin, J., and Bang, F.: Description of cellular coagulation in the limulus. Bull. Johns Hopkins Hosp. 115:337, 1964.

81. Ratnoff, O. D.: An enzyme in plasma inactivating Hageman factor. J. Clin. Invest. 37:923, 1958.

82. Nossel, H. L., and Niemetz, J.: A normal inhibitor of blood coagulation contact reaction product. Blood 25:712, 1965.

83. Forbes, C. D., Pensky, J., et al.: Inhibition of activated Hageman factor and activated plasma thromboplastin antecedent by purified serum

CĪ inactivator. J. Lab. Clin. Med. 76:809, 1970.

84. Pensky, J., and Schwick, H. G.: Human serum inhibitor of C1 esterase: Identity with alpha-2 neuraminoglycoprotein. Science 163:698, 1959.

85. Pensky, J., Levy, L. R., et al.: Partial purification of a serum inhibitor of C1 esterase. J. Biol. Chem. 236:1674, 1964.

86. Ratnoff, O. D., Pensky, J., et al.: The inhibitory properties of plasma against activated plasma thromboplastin antecedent (Factor XIa) in hereditary angioneurotic edema. J. Lab. Clin. Med. 80:803, 1972.

87. Quick, A. J., and Favre-Gilly, J. E.: Fibrin factor influencing consumption of prothrombin in coagulation. Am. J. Physiol. 158:387, 1947.

88. Seegers, W. H., Johnson, J. F., et al.: An antithrombin reaction related to prothrombin activation. Am. J. Physiol. 176:97, 1954.

88a. Abildgaard, U.: Highly purified antithrombin III with heparin cofactor activity prepared by disc electrophoresis. Scand. J. Clin. Lab. Invest. 21:89, 1968.

88b. Highsmith, R. F., and Rosenberg, R. D.: Inhibition of plasmin by human antithrombin-heparin cofactor. Fed. Proc. 33:209, 1974.

88c. Rosenberg, R. D., and Damus, P. S.: The purification and mechanism of action of human antithrombin-heparin cofactor. J. Biol. Chem. 248:6490, 1973.

89. Yin, E. T., Wessler, S., et al.: Identity of plasma-activated factor X inhibitor with antithrombin III and heparin co-factor. J. Biol. Chem. 246:3712, 1971.

90. Yin, E. T., Wessler, S., et al.: Biological properties of the naturally occurring plasma inhibitor to activated factor X. J. Biol. Chem. 246:3703, 1971.

91. Biggs, R., Denson, K. W. E., et al.: Antithrombin III and antifactor Xa. Br. J. Haematol. 19:283, 1970.

92. Seegers, W. H., and Marciniak, E.: Inhibition of autoprothrombin C activity with plasma. Nature (Lond.) 193:1188, 1962.

93. Spaet, T.: Studies on the in vivo behavior of blood coagulation product I in rats. Thromb. Diath. Haemorrh. 8:276, 1962.

94. Thomas, L.: Studies on intravascular thromboplastic effect of tissue suspensions in mice; factor in normal rabbit serum which inhibits the effects of sedimentable tissue component. Bull. Johns Hopkins Hosp. 81:26, 1947.

95. Hjort, P.: Natural inhibitor of tissue thromboplastin. Thromb. Diath. Haemorrh. (Suppl. 7) 1:41, 1962.

96. Denis, J., and de Marbaix, J.: Sur les peptonizations provoquées par le chloroforme et quelques autres substances. Cellule 5:197, 1889.

97. Tillett, W. S., and Garner, R. L.: The fibrinolytic activity of hemolytic streptococci. J. Exp. Med. 58:545, 1933.

98. Williams, J. R. B.: The fibrinolytic activity of urine. Br. J. Exp. Pathol. 32:530, 1951.

99. Astrup, T., and Permin, P.: Fibrinolysis in the animal organism. Nature (Lond.) 159:681, 1947.

100. Biggs, R., Macfarlane, R. G., et al.: Observations on fibrinolysis. Experimental activity produced by exercise or adrenaline. Lancet 1:402, 1947.

101. Macfarlane, R. G., and Biggs, R.: Observations on fibrinolysis. Spontaneous activity associated with surgery, trauma, etc. Lancet 2:862, 1946.

102. Fantl, P., and Simon, S. E.: Fibrinolysis following electrically induced convulsions. Aust. J. Exp. Biol. Med. Sci. 26:521, 1948.

103. Tagnon, H., Levenson, S. M., et al.: The occurrence of fibrinolysis in shock, with observations on the prothrombin times and the plasma fibrinogen during shock. Am. J. Med. Sci. 211:88, 1946.

104. Ogston, D., Ogston, C. M., et al.: Studies on a complex mechanism for the activation of plasminogen by kaolin or chloroform. The participation of Hageman factor and additional cofactors. J. Clin. Invest. 48:1786, 1969.

105. Aoki, N., and Von Kaulla, K. N.: Human serum plasminogen antiactivator: Its distinction from antiplasmin. Am. J. Physiol. 220:1137, 1971.

106. Ganrot, P. O.: Inhibitor of plasmin activity by α-2 macroglobulin. Clin. Chim. Acta 16:328, 1967.

107. Harpel, P., and Mossesson, M.: Degradation of human fibrinogen by α-2 macroglobulin: One mechanism for the metabolism of circulating fibrinogen (abstract). Proc. Am. Soc. Hematol., Miami, Fla., Dec. 3–6, 1972, p. 83.

108. Norman, P. S., and Hill, B. M.: Studies of the plasmin system. III. Physical properties of the two plasmin inhibitors in plasma. J. Exp. Med. 108:639, 1958.

109. Ratnoff, O. D., Lepow, I. H., et al.: The multiplicity of plasmin inhibitors in human serum demonstrated by the effect of primary amino compounds. Bull. Johns Hopkins Hosp. 94:169, 1954.

110. Ratnoff, O. D., Pensky, J., et al.: The inhibition of plasmin, plasma kallikrein, plasma permeability factor and the C1r subcomponent of the first component of complement by serum C1 esterase inhibitor. J. Exp. Med. 129:315, 1969.

111. Rimon, A., Shamash, Y., et al.: The plasmin inhibitor of human plasma. J. Biol. Chem. 241:5102, 1966.

112. Ratnoff, O. D.: Bleeding Syndromes. Springfield, Ill., Charles C Thomas, Publisher, 1960, pp. 88–90.

113. Boisvert, P. L.: The streptococcal antifibrinolysin test in clinical use. J. Clin. Invest. 19:65, 1940.

114. Phillips, L. L., and Skrodelis, J.: A comparison of the fibrinolytic enzyme system in maternal and umbilical cord blood. Pediatrics 22:715, 1958.

115. Quie, P. G., and Wannamaker, W. L.: The plasminogen-plasmin system of newborn infants. Am. J. Dis. Child. 100:836, 1960.

116. Lieberman, J.: Clinical syndromes associated with deficient lung fibrinolytic activity. I. A new concept of hyaline membrane disease. New Engl. J. of Med. 260:619, 1959.

117. Smith, H. P., Warner, E. D., et al.: Prothrombin deficiency and the bleeding tendency in liver injury (chloroform intoxication). J. Exp. Med. 66:891, 1937.

118. Seegers, W. H.: *Prothrombin*. Cambridge, Harvard University Press, 1962.
119. Olson, J. P., Miller, L. L., et al.: Synthesis of clotting factors by the isolated perfused rat liver. J. Clin. Invest. 45:690, 1960.
120. Suttie, J. W.: Control of prothrombin and factor VII biosynthesis by vitamin K. Arch. Biochem. Biophys. 118:166, 1967.
121. O'Reilly, R. A., Pool, J. G., et al.: Hereditary resistance to coumarin anticoagulant drugs in man and rat. Ann. N.Y. Acad. Sci. 151:913, 1968.
122. Greaves, H. H., and Ayres, P.: Heritable resistance to warfarin in rats. Nature (Lond.) 215:877, 1967.
123. Hermodson, M. A., Suttie, J. W., et al.: Warfarin metabolism and vitamin K requirement in the warfarin resistant rat. Am. J. Physiol. 217:1316, 1969.
124. Hemker, H. C., Veltkamp, J. J., et al.: Kinetic aspects of the interaction of blood clotting enzymes. III. Demonstration of an inhibitor of prothrombin conversion in vitamin K deficiency. Thromb. Diath. Haemorrh. 19:346, 1968.
125. Nilehn, J. E., and Ganrot, P. O.: Plasma prothrombin during treatment with dicumarol II. Scand. J. Clin. Lab. Invest. 22:23, 1968.
126. Josso, F., LaVergne, J. M., et al.: Différents états moléculaires du facteur II (Prothrombine). Leur étude à l'aide de la staphycoagulase et d'anticorps anti-facteur II. I. Thromb. Diath. Haemorrh. 20:88, 1968.
127. Babior, B. M.: The role of vitamin K in clotting factor synthesis. I. Evidence for the participation of vitamin K in the conversion of a polypeptide precursor of factor VII. Biochim. Biophys. Acta 123:606, 1966.
127a. Hill, R. B., Gaetani, S., et al.: Vitamin K and biosynthesis of protein and prothrombin. J. Biol. Chem. 243:3930, 1968.
128. Pereira, M., and Couri, D.: Studies on the site of action of dicumarol on prothrombin synthesis. Biochem. Biophys. Acta 237:348, 1971.
129. Woolf, I. L., and Babior, B. M.: Vitamin K and warfarin. Metabolism, function and interaction. Am. J. Med. 53:261, 1972.
130. Bell, R. G., and Matschiner, J. T.: Intracellular distribution of vitamin K in the rat. Biochim. Biophys. Acta 184:597, 1969.
131. Pirk, L. A., and Engelberg, R.: Hypoprothrombic action of quinine sulfate. J.A.M.A. 128:1093, 1945.
132. Shapiro, A.: Studies on prothrombin. VI. The effect of synthetic vitamin K from the colon in the newborn infant. J. Pediatr. 68:305, 1966.
133. Aballi, A. J., Howard, C. E., et al.: Absorption of vitamin K from the colon in the newborn infant. J. Pediatr. 68:305, 1966.
134. Cade, J. F., Hirsh, J., et al.: Placental barrier to coagulation factors: Its relevance to the coagulation defect at birth and to haemorrhage in the newborn. Br. Med. J. 2:281, 1969.
135. Gitlin, D., Kumate, J., et al.: The selectivity of the human placenta in the transfer of plasma protein from mother to fetus. J. Clin. Invest. 43:1938, 1964.
136. Gitlin, D., and Biasucci, A.: Development of γG, γA, γM, β1C/β1A, C'1 esterase inhibitor, ceruloplasmin, transferrin, hemopexin, haptoglobin, fibrinogen, plasminogen, α_1-antitryp-

sin, orosomucoid, β-lipoprotein, α_2-macroglobulin, and prealbumin in the human conceptus. J. Clin. Invest. 48:1433, 1969.
137. Aballi, A. J., Lopez-Banus, V., et al.: Coagulation studies in the newborn period. Alterations of thromboplastin generation and effects of vitamin K in full term and premature infants. A.M.A. J. Dis. Child. 94:489, 1957.
138. Aballi, A. J., and de Lamerens, S.: Coagulation changes in the neonatal period and in early infancy. Pediatr. Clin. North Am. 9:785, 1962.
139. Fillmore, S. J., and McDevitt, E.: Effects of coumarin compounds on the fetus. Ann. Intern. Med. 73:731, 1970.
140. Bloomfield, D. K.: Fetal deaths and malformations associated with the use of coumarin derivatives in pregnancy. Am. J. Obstet. Gynecol. 107:883, 1970.
141. Flessa, H., Kapstrom, A. B., et al.: Placental transport of heparin. Am. J. Obstet. Gynecol. 93:570, 1965.
142. Kohler, H. G.: Hemorrhage in the newborn of epileptic mothers (Letter to the editor). Lancet 1:267, 1966.
143. Earle, R., Jr.: Congenital salicylate intoxication. Report of a case. New Engl. J. Med. 265:1003, 1965.
144. Ratnoff, O. D., and Holland, T. R.: Coagulation components in normal and abnormal pregnancies. Ann. N.Y. Acad. Sci. 75:626, 1959.
145. Israels, L. G., Zipursky, A., et al.: Factor V levels in the neonatal period. Pediatrics 15:180, 1966.
146. Taylor, P. M.: Concentration of fibrinogen in the plasma of normal newborn infants. Pediatrics 19:233, 1957.
147. Biggs, R.: *Prothrombin Deficiency*. Oxford, Blackwell Scientific Publications, 1951.
148. Burstein, M., Lewi, S., et al.: Sur l'existence du fibrinogène foetal. Sang. 25:102, 1956.
148a. Guillin, M.- C., and Ménaché, D.: Study on the polymerization of human and bovine and foetal fibrinogen. Proc. Third Congress, Int. Soc. on Thrombosis and Haemostasis. Washington, D.C., 1972, p. 98.
148b. Aguercif, M., Giacometti, N., et al.: Existe-t-il un fibrinogene foetal? Pediatrie 38:381, 1973.
148c. Witt, I., and Müller, H.: Phosphorous and hexose content of human foetal fibrinogen. Biochim. Biophys. Acta. 221:402, 1970.
148d. Witt, I., Müller, H., et al.: Evidence for the existence of foetal fibrinogen. Thromb. Diath. Haemorrh. 22:101, 1969.
149. Larrieu, M. J., Soulier, J. P., et al.: Le sang du cordon ombilical: Etude complète de sa coagulabilité, comparison avec le sang maternel. Etudes Néo-natales 1:1, 1952.
150. Kurkcougla, M., and McElfrish, A.: The Hageman factor: Determination of its concentration during the neonatal period and presentation of a case of Hageman factor deficiency. J. Pediatr. 47:61, 1960.
151. Hilgartner, M. W., and Smith, C. H.: Plasma thromboplastin antecedent (factor XI) in the neonate. J. Pediatr. 66:747, 1965.
152. Aballi, A. J., Lopez-Banus, V., et al.: Coagulation studies in the newborn period. III. Hemorrhagic disease of the newborn. A.M.A. J. Dis. Child. 97:524, 1959.
153. Brinkhous, K. M., Smith, H. P., et al.: Plasma

prothrombin level in normal infancy and in hemorrhagic disease of the newborn. Am. J. Med. Sci. *193*:475, 1937.

154. Dam, H., Tage-Hansen, E., et al.: Vitamin K lack in normal and sick infants. Lancet *2*:1157, 1939.

155. Hartmann, J. R., Howell, D. A., et al.: Disorders of blood coagulation during the first week of life. A.M.A. J. Dis. Child. *90*:594, 1966.

156. Dam, H., Dyggve, H., et al.: The relation of vitamin K deficiency to hemorrhagic disease of the newborn. Adv. Pediatr. *5*:129, 1952.

157. Keenan, W. J., Jewett, T., et al.: Role of feeding and vitamin K in hypothrombinemia of the newborn. Am. J. Dis. Child. *121*:171, 1971.

158. Ratnoff, O. D.: *Bleeding Syndrome.* Springfield, Ill., Charles C Thomas, Publisher, 1960, Chapter 7.

159. Sutherland, J. M., Glueck, H. I., et al.: Hemorrhagic disease of the newborn. Breast feeding as a necessary factor in the pathogenesis. Am. J. Dis. Child. *113*:524, 1967.

160. Allison, A. C.: Danger of vitamin K to newborn. Lancet *1*:669, 1955.

160a. Zinkham, W. H., and Childs, B.: Effect of vitamin K and naphthalene metabolites on glutathione metabolism of erythrocytes from normal newborns and patients with naphthalene hemolytic anemia. Am. J. Dis. Child. *94*:420, 1957.

161. Bound, J. P., and Telfer, J. P.: Effect of vitamin K dosage on plasma bilirubin levels in premature infants. Lancet *1*:720, 1956.

162. Committee on Nutrition, American Academy of Pediatrics: Vitamin K supplementation for infants receiving milk substitute infant formulas and for those with fat malabsorption. Pediatrics *48*:483, 1972.

163. Goldman, H. I., and Depositio, F.: Hypoprothrombinemic bleeding in young infants. Am. J. Dis. Child. *11*:430, 1966.

164. Benirshke, K.: Twin placenta in perinatal mortality. N.Y. State J. Med. *61*:149, 1961.

165. Edson, J. R., Blaese, R. M., et al.: Defibrination syndrome in an infant born after abruptio placentae. J. Pediatr. *72*:342, 1968.

166. Leissring, J. C., and Vorlicky, L. N.: Disseminated intravascular coagulation in a neonate. Am. J. Dis. Child. *115*:100, 1968.

167. Bishop, A. J., Israels, L. G., et al.: Placental transfer of intravascular coagulation between mother and fetus. Pediatr. Res. *5*:113, 1971.

168. Midulla, M., Marzetti, G., et al.: Generalized cytomegalic inclusion disease, hypergammaglobulinemia, and antithrombin activity in a newborn infant. Helv. Paediatr. Acta *23*:205, 1968.

169. Mauer, A. M.: *Pediatric Hematology.* New York, McGraw-Hill, 1968, Chapter 27.

170. Biggs, R., and Macfarlane, R. G.: *Human Blood Coagulation and its Disorders.* 3rd ed., Oxford, Blackwell Scientific Publications, 1969.

170a. Harker, L. A., and Slichter, S. J.: The bleeding time as a screening test for evaluation of platelet function. New Engl. J. Med. *287*:155, 1972.

171. Hardisty, R. M., and Ingram, G. I. C.: *Bleeding Disorders. Investigation and Management.* Philadelphia, F. A. Davis Co., 1965.

172. Quick, A. J.: *Hemorrhagic Diseases and Thrombosis.* 2nd ed. Philadelphia, Lea and Febiger, 1966.

173. Stefanini, M., and Damashek, W.: *The Hemorrhagic Disorders.* 2nd ed. New York, Grune & Stratton, 1962.

174. Tocantins, L. M., and Kazal, L. A. (eds.), *Blood Coagulation, Hemorrhage and Thrombosis. Methods of Study.* New York, Grune & Stratton, 1964.

175. Biggs, R. (ed.), *Human Blood Coagulation, Haemostasis and Thrombosis.* Oxford, Blackwell Scientific Publications, 1972.

175a. Baehner, R. L., and Strauss, H. S.: Hemophilia in the first year of life. New Engl. J. Med. *275*:524, 1966.

176. *The Babylonia Talmud.* Epstein, I. (ed.), Yebamoth, Sect. 64 B. Vol. 1, p. 431. London, Soncino Press, 1936.

177. Ratnoff, O. D.: Hereditary disorders of hemostasis, In *The Metabolic Basis of Inherited Disease.* 3rd ed. Stanbury, J. B., Wyngaarden, J. B., et al. (eds.), New York, McGraw-Hill, 1966, pp. 1137–1175.

178. Wright, A. E.: On a method for determining the condition of blood coagulability for clinical and experimental purposes, and on the effect of the administration of calcium salts in hemophilia and actual or threatened hemorrhage. Br. Med. J. *2*:223, 1893.

179. Addis, T.: The pathogenesis of hereditary hemophilia. J. Pathol. Bacteriol. *15*:427, 1911.

180. Patek, A. J., Jr., and Taylor, F. H. L.: Hemophilia: Some properties of substance obtained from normal plasma effective in coagulation of hemophilic blood. J. Clin. Invest. *16*:113, 1937.

181. Lundblad, R. L., and Davie, E. W.: The activation of antihemophilic factor (Factor VIII) by activated Christmas factor (activated Factor IX). Biochemistry (Wash.) *3*:1720, 1964.

182. Ratnoff, O. D., Kass, L., et al.: Studies on purification of antihemophilic factor (factor VIII). II. Separation of partially purified antihemophilic factor by gel filtration of plasma. J. Clin. Invest. *48*:957, 1969.

183. Shanberge, J. N., and Gore, I.: Studies on the immunologic and physiologic activities of antihemophilia factor (AHF). J. Lab. Clin. Med. *50*:954, 1957.

184. Zimmerman, T. S., Ratnoff, O. D., et al.: The immunologic differentiation of classic hemophilia (factor VIII deficiency) and von Willebrand's disease with observations on combined deficiencies of antihemophilic factor and proaccelerin (factor V) and on an acquired anticoagulant against antihemophilic factor. J. Clin. Invest. *40*:224, 1971.

185. Hoyer, L., and Breckenridge, R. T.: Immunologic studies of antihemophilic factor (AHF) (factor VIII): Cross-reacting material in a genetic variant of hemophilia. Blood *32*:962, 1968.

186. Cinader, B., Dubuski, S., et al.: Distribution, inheritance and properties of an antigen, MUBI, and its relation to hemolytic complement. J. Exp. Med. *120*:897, 1964.

187. Gralnick, H. R., Abrell, E., et al.: Immunological studies of factor VIII (antihemophilic globulin) in hemophilia A. Nature [New Biol.] *230*:16, 1971.

188. Agle, D. P.: Psychiatric studies of patients with

hemophilia and related states. Arch. Intern. Med. *114*:76, 1964.

189. Rizza, C. R.: The effect of exercise on the level of antihemophilic globulin in human blood. J. Physiol. *156*:128, 1961.

190. Ingram, G. I. C.: Increase in antihemophilic globulin activity following infusion of adrenaline. J. Physiol. *156*:217, 1961.

191. Rapaport, S. I., Patch, M. J., et al.: Antihemophilic globulin levels in carriers of hemophilia A. J. Clin. Invest. *39*:1619, 1960.

192. Beutler, E., Yeh, M., et al.: The normal human female as a mosaic of X-chromosome activity: Studies using the gene for G-6-PD deficiency as a marker. Proc. Natl. Acad. Sci. USA *48*:9, 1962.

193. Lyon, M. F.: Chromosomal and subchromosomal inactivation. Ann. Rev. Genet. 2:31, 1968.

194. Ratnoff, O. D.: The molecular basis of hereditary clotting disorders, In *Progress in Hemostasis and Thrombosis*. Vol. 1. Spaet, T. (ed.), New York, Grune & Stratton, 1972, pp. 39–74.

195. Zimmerman, T. S., Ratnoff, O. D., et al.: Detection of carriers of classic hemophilia using an immunologic assay for antihemophilic factor (factor VIII). J. Clin. Invest. *50*:235, 1971.

195a. Ratnoff, O. D., and Bennet, B.: The genetics of hereditary disorders of blood coagulation. Science *179*:1291, 1973.

196. Lewis, J. H., Walters, D., et al.: Application of continuous flow electrophoresis to the study of the blood coagulation proteins and the fibrinolytic system. I. Normal human materials. J. Clin. Invest. 37:1323, 1958.

197. Fantl, P., Sawers, R. J., et al.: Investigation of hemorrhagic disease due to beta-thromboplastin deficiency complicated by a specific inhibition of thromboplastin formation. Australas. Ann. Med. 5:163, 1956.

198. Densen, K. W. E., Biggs, R., et al.: An investigation of three patients with Christmas disease due to an abnormal type of factor IX. J. Clin. Pathol. *21*:160, 1968.

199. Roberts, H. R., Grizzle, J. E., et al.: Genetic variants of hemophilia B: Detection by means of a specific PTC inhibitor. J. Clin. Invest. *47*:360, 1968.

200. Veltkamp, J. J., Meilof, J., et al.: Another genetic variant of hemophilia B: Hemophilia B$_{Leyden}$. Scand. J. Haematol. 7:82, 1970.

201. Twomey, J. J., Corliss, J., et al.: Studies on the inheritance and nature of haemophilia B$_M$. Am. J. Med. *46*:372, 1969.

202. Brown, C. H., Krols, L. K., et al.: Factor IX deficiency and bleeding in a patient with Sheehan's syndrome. Blood *39*:650, 1972.

203. Rosenthal, R. L., Dreskin, O. H., et al.: New hemophilia-like disease caused by deficiency of third plasma thromboplastin factor. Proc. Soc. Exp. Biol. Med. *82*:171, 1953.

204. Ratnoff, O. D.: *Bleeding Syndromes*, Springfield, Ill., Charles C Thomas, Publisher, 1960, Chapter 6.

205. Smink, M. M., Daniel, T. M., et al.: Immunologic demonstration of a deficiency of Hageman factor–like material in Hageman trait. J. Lab. Clin. Med. *69*:819, 1967.

206. Ratnoff, O. D.: *Bleeding Syndromes*. Springfield,

Ill., Charles C Thomas, Publisher, 1960, Chapter 8.

207. Speer, R. J., Ridgway, H., et al.: Activated human Hageman factor (factor XII). Thromb. Diath. Haemorrh. *14*:1, 1965.

208. Owren, P. A.: Coagulation of blood: Investigation of a new clotting factor. Acta Med. Scand. (Suppl.) *194*:1, 1947.

209. Quick, A. J.: On the constitution of prothrombin. Am. J. Physiol. *140*:212, 1943.

210. Denson, K. W. E.: *The Use of Antibodies in the Study of Blood Coagulation*. Philadelphia, F. A. Davis Co., 1967.

211. Feinstein, D. I., Rapaport, S. I., et al.: Factor V anticoagulants: Clinical, biochemical and immunological observations. J. Clin. Invest. *49*:1578, 1970.

212. Ratnoff, O. D.: *Bleeding Syndromes*. Springfield, Ill., Charles C Thomas, Publisher, 1960, Chapter 7.

213. Girolami, A., Molaro, G., et al.: "New" congenital hemorrhagic condition due to presence of an abnormal factor X (factor X$_{Friuli}$): Study of a large kindred. Br. J. Haematol. *19*:179, 1970.

214. Denson, K. W. E., Lurie, A., et al.: The factor X defect: Recognition of abnormal forms of factor X. Br. J. Haematol. *18*:317, 1970.

215. Prydz, H., and Gladhaug, Å.: Factor X. Immunologic studies. Thromb. Diath. Haemorrh. 25:157, 1971.

216. Shulman, N. R.: Surgical care of patients with hereditary disorders of blood coagulation, In *Treatment of Hemorrhagic Disorders*. Ratnoff, O. D. (ed.), Hagerstown, Md., Harper & Row, Publishers, 1968, pp. 61–84.

217. Alexander, B., Goldstein, R., et al.: Congenital SPCA deficiency: A hitherto unrecognized coagulation defect with hemorrhage rectified by serum and serum fractions. J. Clin. Invest. *30*:596, 1951.

218. Shapiro, S. S., Martinez, J., et al.: Congenital dysprothrombinemia: An inherited structural disorder of human prothrombin. J. Clin. Invest. *48*:2251, 1969.

219. Josso, F., LaVergne, J. M., et al.: Les dysprothrombinémies constitutionelles et acquieses. Nouv. Rev. Fr. Hematol. *10*:633, 1970.

220. Josso, F., Monasterio de Sanches, J., et al.: Congenital abnormality of the prothrombin molecule (Factor II) in four siblings: Prothrombin Barcelona. Blood 38:9, 1971.

221. Josso, F., Prou-Wartelle, O., et al.: Etude d'un cas d'hypoprothrombinémie congénitale. Nouv. Rev. Fr. Hematol. 2:647, 1962.

222. Quick, A. J.: *The Physiology and Pathology of Hemostasis*. Philadelphia, Lea and Febiger, 1951, p. 57.

223. Lanchantin, G. F., Hart, D. W., et al.: Amino acid composition of human plasma prothrombin. J. Biol. Chem. 243:5479, 1968.

224. Gugler, E., and Luscher, E. F.: Platelet function in congenital afibrinogenemia. Thrombosis Diath. Haemorrh. *14*:361, 1965.

225. Gitlin, D., and Borges, W.: Studies in the metabolism of fibrinogen in two patients with congenital afibrinogenemia. Blood 8:679, 1953.

226. Vandenbroucke, J., Verstraete, M., et al.: L'afi-

brinogénémie congénitale: Présentation d'un nouveau cas et revue de la litterature. Acta Haematol. *12*:87, 1954.

227. Lawson, H. A.: Congenital afibrinogenemia. Report of a case. New Engl. J. Med. *248*:551, 1953.

228. Yamagata, S., Mori, K., et al.: A case of congenital afibrinogenemia and review of reported cases in Japan. Tohoku J. Exp. Med. *95*:15, 1968.

229. De Vries, A., Rosenberg, T., et al.: Precipitating antifibrinogen antibody appearing after fibrinogen infusion in a patient with congenital afibrinogenemia. Am. J. Med. *30*:486, 1961.

230. Breckenridge, R. T., and Ratnoff, O. D.: In *Treatment of Hemorrhagic Disease*. Ratnoff, O. D. (ed.), Hagerstown, Md., Harper & Row, Publishers, 1968, Chapter 2.

231. Finlayson, J. S., and Mossesson, M. W.: Heterogeneity of human fibrinogen. Biochemistry (Wash.) *2*:42, 1963.

231a. Imperato, C., and Dettori, A. G.: Ipofibrinogenemia congenita con fibrinoasternia. Helv. Acta *13*:380, 1958.

232. Beck, E. A., Charache, P., et al.: A new inherited coagulation disorder caused by an abnormal fibrinogen (fibrinogen Baltimore). Nature (Lond.) *208*:143, 1965.

233. Samama, M. Soria, J., et al.: Dysfibrinogénémie congénitale et familiale sans tendance hémorragique. Nouv. Rev. Fr. Hematol. *9*:817, 1969.

234. Menaché, D.: Les dysfibrinogénémies congénitales. Nouv. Rev. Fr. Hematol. *10*:653, 1970.

235. Mammen, E. F., Prasad, A. S., et al.: Congenital dysfibrinogenemia: Fibrinogen Detroit. J. Clin. Invest. *48*:235, 1969.

236. Beck, E. A., Shainoff, J., et al.: Functional evaluation of an inherited abnormal fibrinogen: "fibrinogen Baltimore." J. Clin. Invest. *50*:1874, 1971.

237. Gralnick, H. R., Givelbar, K. M., et al.: Fibrinogen Bethesda: A congenital dysfibrinogenemia with delayed fibrinopeptide release. J. Clin. Invest. *50*:1819, 1971.

238. Hampton, J. W.: Qualitative fibrinogen defect associated with abnormal fibrin stabilization. J. Lab. Clin. Med. *72*:882, 1968.

239. Hampton, J. W., Cunningham, G. R., et al.: The pattern of inheritance of defective fibrinase (Factor XIII). J. Lab. Clin. Med. *67*:914, 1966.

239a. Martinez, J., Holburn, R. R., et al.: Fibrinogen Philadelphia. A hereditary hypodysfibrinogenemia characterized by fibrinogen hypercatabolism. J. Clin. Invest. *53*:600, 1974.

239b. Gralnick, H. R., Givelber, H. M., et al.: A new congenital abnormality of human fibrinogen. Fibrinogen Bethesda II. Thromb. Diath. Haemorrh. *29*:562, 1973.

239c. Krause, W. H., Heene, D. L., et al.: Congenital dysfibrinogenemia (Fibrinogen Giessen). Thromb. Diath. Haemorrh. *29*:547, 1973.

239d. Lacombe, M., Soria, J., et al.: Fibrinogen Montreal. A new case of congenital dysfibrinogenemia with defective aggregation of monomers. Thromb. Diath. Haemorrh. *29*:536, 1973.

239e. Jacobsen, C. D., and Hoak, J. C.: Fibrinogen Iowa City: An abnormal fibrinogen with no clinical symptoms. Thromb. Res. *2*:261, 1973.

239f. Zietz, B. H., and Scott, J. L.: An inherited defect in fibrinogen polymerization: Fibrinogen Los Angeles (abstract). Clin. Res. *18*:179, 1970.

239g. Crum, E. D., Shainoff, J. R., et al.: Fibrinogen Cleveland II: An abnormal fibrinogen with defective release of fibrinopeptide A. J. Clin. Invest. *53*:1308, 1974.

239h. Gralnick, H. R., and Finlayson, J. S.: Congenital dysfibrinogenemias. Ann. Intern. Med. *77*: 472, 1972.

240. Egeberg, O.: Inherited fibrinogen abnormality causing thrombophilia. Thromb. Diath. Haemorrh. *17*:176, 1967.

241. Blomback, M., Blomback, B., et al.: Fibrinogen Detroit: A molecular defect in the N-terminal disulphide knot of human fibrinogen. Nature (Lond.) *218*:134, 1968.

242. Blomback, M., and Blomback, B.: Fibrinogen Detroit: A molecular defect in the N-terminal disulphide knot, In *Hemophilia and New Hemorrhagic States*. Brinkhous, K. M. (ed.), Chapel Hill, University of North Carolina Press, 1970, p. 242.

243. Laurent, T. C., and Blomback, B.: On the significance of the release of two different peptides from fibrinogen during clotting. Acta Chem. Scand. *12*:187, 1968.

244. Loewy, A. G.: Enzymatic control of insoluble-fibrin formation, In *Fibrinogen*. Laki, K. (ed.), New York, Marcel Dekker, 1968, p. 185.

245. Lorand, L., Uragama, T., et al.: Diagnostic and genetic studies on fibrin-stabilizing factor with a new assay based on amine incorporation. J. Clin. Invest. *48*:1054, 1969.

246. Duckert, F.: Le facteur XIII et la proteine XIII. Nouv. Rev. Fr. Hematol. *10*:685, 1970.

247. Kiesselbach, T. H., and Wagner, R. H.: Fibrin-stabilizing factor: A thrombin labile platelet protein. Am. J. Physiol. *211*:1472, 1966.

248. Ratnoff, O. D., and Steinberg, A. G.: Inheritance of fibrin-stabilizing factor deficiency. Lancet *1*:25, 1968.

249. Von Willebrand, E. A.: Hereditare pseudohamophilie. Finska Läk.-Sälsk. Handl. *68*:87, 1926.

250. Von Willebrand, E. A.: Ueber hereditare pseudohamophilie. Acta Med. Scand. *76*:54, 1931.

251. Alexander, B., and Goldstein, R.: Dual hemostatic defect in pseudohemophilia. J. Clin. Invest. *32*:551, 1953.

252. Larrieu, M. J., and Soulier, J. P.: Déficit en facteur antihémophilique A, chez une fille associé à un trouble du saignement. Rev. Hematol. *8*:361, 1953.

253. Jurgens, R., Lehmann, W., et al.: Mitteilung uber den Mangel an antihamophilen Globulin (Faktor VIII) bei der Aalandischen Thrombopathie (von Willebrand-Jurgens). Thromb. Diath. Haemorrh. *1*:257, 1957.

254. Nilsson, I. M., Blomback, M., et al.: Von Willebrand's disease and its correction with human plasma fraction 1-0. Acta Med. Scand. *159*:179, 1957.

255. Weiss, H. J.: Von Willebrand's disease — Diagnostic criteria. Blood *32*:668, 1968.

256. Nilsson, I. M., Blomback, M., et al.: Von Willebrand's disease in Sweden. Its pathogenesis

and treatment. Acta Med. Scand. *164*:263, 1959.

257. Cornu, P., Larrieu, M. J., et al.: Transfusion studies in von Willebrand's disease: Effect on bleeding time and Factor VIII. Br. J. Haematol. *9*:189, 1963.

257a. Bennett, B., Ratnoff, O. D., et al.: Immunologic studies in von Willebrand's disease. Evidence that the antihemophilic factor (AHF) produced after transfusion lacks an antigen associated with normal AHF and the inactive material produced by patients with classic hemophilia. J. Clin. Invest. *51*:2597, 1972.

258. Bouma, B. N., von Mourik, J. A., et al.: Immunochemical characterizations of von Willebrand factor and antihemophilic factor A. Abstracts, Second Congress Intern. Soc. Thromb. and Haemostasis, 1971, p. 6.

258a. Howard, M. A., Sawers, R. J., et al.: Ristocetin: A means of differentiating von Willebrand's disease into two groups. Blood *41*:687, 1973.

258b. Weiss, H. J., Rogers, J., et al.: Defective ristocetin-induced platelet aggregation in von Willebrand's disease and its correction by factor VIII. J. Clin. Invest. *52*:2697, 1973.

258c. Ratnoff, O. D., and Bennett, B.: Clues to the pathogenesis of bleeding in von Willebrand's disease. New Engl. J. Med. *289*:1182, 1973.

258d. Simone, J. V., Cornet, J. A., et al.: Acquired von Willebrand's syndrome with systemic lupus erythematosus. Blood *3*:806, 1968.

258e. Ingram, G. I. C., Kingston, P. J., et al.: Four cases of acquired von Willebrand's syndrome. Br. J. Haematol. *21*:189, 1971.

258f. Mant, M. J., Hirsh, J., et al.: Von Willebrand's syndrome presenting as an acquired bleeding disorder in association with a monoclonal gammopathy. Blood *42*:429, 1973.

258g. Veltkamp, J. J., Stevens, P., et al.: Production of bleeding factor. Thromb. Diath. Haemorrh. *23*:412, 1970.

258h. Ingram, G. I. C., Prentice, C. R. M., et al.: Low factor VIII–like antigen in acquired von Willebrand's syndrome and response to treatment. Br. J. Haematol. *25*:137, 1973.

259. Hathaway, W. E., Belhasen, L. P., et al.: Evidence for a new plasma thromboplastin factor. I. Case report, coagulation studies and physicochemical properties. Blood *26*:521, 1965.

260. Hathaway, W. E., and Alsever, J.: The relation of "Fletcher factor" to factors XI and XII. Br. J. Haematol. *18*:161, 1970.

261. Saito, H., Ratnoff, O. D., et al.: Letter regarding the nature of Fletcher defect. Blood *39*:745, 1972.

261a. Saito, H., Ratnoff, O. D., et al.: Inhibition of the adsorption of Hageman factor (factor XII) to glass by normal human plasma. J. Lab. Clin. Med., 1974 (in press).

261b. Wuepper, K. D.: Biochemistry and biology of components of the plasma kinin-forming system, In *Inflammation: Mechanisms and Control.* Lepow, I. H., and Ward, P. A. (eds.), New York, Academic Press, 1972, p. 93.

261c. Weiss, A. S., Gallin, J. I., et al.: Fletcher factor deficiency. A diminished rate of Hageman factor activation caused by absence of prekallikrein with abnormalities of coagulation,

fibrinolysis, chemotactic activity, and kinin-generation. J. Clin. Invest. *53*:622, 1974.

261d. Saito, H., Ratnoff, O. D., et al.: Defective activation of clotting, fibrinolytic and permeability-enhancing systems in human Fletcher trait plasma. Circ. Res., 1974 (in press).

261e. Donaldson, V. H., Saito, H., et al.: Defective esterase and kinin-forming activity in Fletcher trait plasma; a fraction rich in kallikrein-like activity. Circ. Res., 1974 (in press).

262. Margolius, A., Jr., Jackson, D. P., et al.: Circulating anticoagulants. A study of forty cases and a review of the literature. Medicine (Baltimore) *40*:145, 1961.

263. Feinstein, D. I., and Rapaport, S. I.: Acquired inhibition of blood coagulation, In *Progress in Hemostasis and Thrombosis.* Spaet, T. (ed.), New York, Grune & Stratton, 1972, pp. 75–95.

264. Breckenridge, R. T., and Ratnoff, O. D.: Studies on the nature of the circulating anticoagulant directed against antihemophilic factor. Blood *20*:137, 1962.

265. Strauss, H. S.: Acquired circulating anticoagulants in hemophilia A. New Engl. J. Med. *281*:866, 1969.

266. Glueck, H. I., Hong, R., et al.: A circulating anticoagulant in multiple myeloma: Its modification by penicillin. J. Clin. Invest. *44*:1866, 1965.

267. Castaldi, P. A., and Penny, R.: A macroglobulin with inhibitory activity against coagulation factor VIII. Blood, *35*:370, 1970.

268. Frick, P. G.: Hemophilia-like disease following pregnancy with transplacental transfer of an acquired circulating anticoagulant. Blood *8*:598, 1953.

269. Ratnoff, O. D.: *Bleeding Syndromes*, Springfield, Ill., Charles C Thomas. Publisher, 1960, Chapter XI.

270. Green, D.: Suppression of an antibody to factor VIII by a combination of factor VIII and cyclophosphamide. Blood *37*:381, 1971.

270a. Hruby, M. A., and Schulman, I.: Failure of combined factor VIII and cyclophosphamide to suppress antibody to factor VIII in hemophilia. Blood *42*:919, 1973.

271. Lewis, J. H., Ferguson, J. H., et al.: Hemorrhagic disease with circulating inhibitors of blood clotting: Anti-AHF and anti-PTC in eight cases. Blood *11*:846, 1956.

272. Hall, M.: Haemophilia complicated by an acquired circulating anticoagulant: A report of three cases. Br. J. Haematol. *7*:340, 1961.

273. George, J. N., Miller, G. M., et al.: Studies in Christmas disease: Investigation and treatment of familial acquired inhibitor of factor IX. Br. J. Haematol. *21*:333, 1971.

274. Hardisty, R. M.: A naturally occurring inhibitor of Christmas factor (factor IX). Thromb. Diath. Haemorrh. *8*:67, 1962.

275. Lisker, R., Josephson, A. M., et al.: The correction of a hemorrhagic diathesis in preparation for surgery. The correction of plasma thromboplastin antecedent deficiency. A.M.A. Arch. Intern. Med. *100*:474, 1957.

276. Horder, M. H.: Isolierter Factor V-Mangel bedingt durch einenspezifischen Hemmkorper. Acta Haematol. *13*:235, 1955.

277. Ferguson, J. H., Johnson, C. L., Jr., et al.: A circulating inhibitor (Anti-Ac-G) specific for the labile factor-V of the blood clotting mechanism. Blood 13:382, 1958.

278. Chevallier, P., Bernard, J., et al.: Deux cas d'hypoconvertinémie familiale. Sang 26:650, 1955.

279. Lackner, H., Hunt, V., et al.: Abnormal fibrin ultrastructures, polymerization, and clot retraction in multiple myeloma. Br. J. Haematol. 18:625, 1970.

280. Coleman, M., Vigliano, E. M., et al.: Inhibition of fibrin monomer polymerization by lambda myeloma globulin. Blood 39:210, 1972.

281. Fletcher, A. P., Alkjaersig, N., et al.: Pathogenesis of the hemorrhagic diathesis developing during "fibrinolytic" states: The significance of defective fibrin polymerization. J. Clin. Invest. 39:1005, 1959.

281a. Wallen, P., and Bergstrom, K.: Action of thrombin on plasmin-digested fibrinogen. Acta Chem. Scand. 12:574, 1958.

282. Donaldson, V. H.: Effect of plasmin in vitro upon clotting factors in plasma. J. Lab. Clin. Med. 561:644, 1960.

283. Harvey, A. M., Shulman, L. E., et al.: Systemic lupus erythematosus. Review of the literature and clinical analysis of 138 cases. Medicine (Baltimore) 33:291, 1954.

284. Lee, S. L., and Sanders, M. A.: A disorder of blood coagulation in systemic lupus erythematosus. J. Clin. Invest. 34:1814, 1965.

285. Frick, P. G.: Acquired circulating anticoagulants in "collagen" disease. Autoimmune thromboplastin deficiency. Blood 10:691, 1955.

286. Yin, E. T., and Gaston, L. W.: Purification and kinetic studies on a circulating coagulant in a suspected case of lupus erythematosus. Thromb. Diath. Haemorrh. 14:87, 1965.

287. Breckenridge, R. T., and Ratnoff, O. D.: Studies on the site of action of circulating anticoagulant in disseminated lupus erythematosus. Am. J. Med. 35:813, 1963.

288. Conley, C. L., Hartmann, R. C., et al.: II. Circulating anticoagulants: A technique for their detection and clinical studies. Bull. Johns Hopkins Hosp. 84:255, 1949.

289. Dustan, H. P., Taylor, R. D., et al.: A syndrome elicited by prolonged administration of large doses of hydralazine. J. Lab. Clin. Med. 42:801, 1953.

290. Parker, C. W.: Drug reactions, In Immunological Diseases. Samter, M. (ed.), Boston, Little, Brown and Co., 1965, p. 676.

290a. Alarcon-Segovia, D., Wakim, K., et al.: Clinical and experimental studies on the hydralazine syndrome and its relationship to systemic lupus erythematosus. Medicine (Baltimore) 46:1, 1967.

291. Meislin, A. G., and Rothfield, N.: Systemic lupus erythematosus in childhood. Analysis of 42 cases with comparative data on 200 adult cases followed concurrently. Pediatrics 42:37, 1968.

292. Osler, W.: On a familial form of recurring epistaxis associated with multiple telangiectases of the skin and mucous membranes. Bull. Johns Hopkins Hosp. 12:333, 1901.

293. Weber, F. P.: A case of multiple hereditary developmental angiomata (telangiectases) of the skin and mucous membranes associated with recurring hemorrhages. Lancet 2:160, 1907.

294. Rendu, M.: Epistaxis répétées chez un sujet porteur de petits angiomes cutanés et muqueux. Bull. Mem. Soc. Med. Hôp. Paris 13:731, 1896.

295. Ratnoff, O. D.: Bleeding Syndromes. Springfield, Ill., Charles C Thomas, Publisher, 1960, Chapter 19.

295a. Saunders, W. H.: Hereditary hemorrhagic telangiectasia. Arch. Otolaryngol. 76:65, 1962.

296. Koch, H. J., Jr., Escher, G. C., et al.: Hormonal management of hereditary hemorrhagic telangiectasia. J.A.M.A. 149:1376, 1952.

297. Ratnoff, O. D.: Bleeding Syndromes. Springfield, Ill., Charles C Thomas, Publisher, 1960, Chapter 18.

298. Lisker, R., Nogueron, A., et al.: Plasma thromboplastin component deficiency in the Ehler-Danlos syndrome. Ann. Intern. Med. 53:388, 1960.

299. Goodman, R. M., Levitsky, J. M., et al.: The Ehler-Danlos syndrome and multiple neurofibromatosis in a kindred of mixed derivation with special emphasis on hemostasis in the Ehler-Danlos syndrome. Am. J. Med. 32:976, 1962.

299a. Lichtenstein, J. R., Martin, G. R., et al.: Defect in conversion of procollagen to collagen in a form of Ehlers-Danlos syndrome. Science 182:298, 1973.

300. Gautier, P., and Guinand-Doniol, J.: Un cas de maladie de Lobstein associée à une thrombasthénie héréditaire et familiale de Glanzmann. Bull. Mem. Soc. Med. Hôp. Paris 68:577, 1952.

301. Kaplan, L., and Hartmann, W. W.: Elastica disease. Case of Gronblad-Strandberg syndrome with gastro-intestinal hemorrhage. A.M.A. Arch. Intern. Med. 94:489, 1954.

302. McKusick, V. A.: Heritable Disorders of Connective Tissue. St. Louis, Mo., C. V. Mosby Co., 1956, Chapter 6.

303. Smith, J. G., Jr., Sams, W. M., Jr., et al.: Pseudoxanthoma elasticum. Arch. Dermatol. 86:729, 1962.

304. Eddy, D. D., and Farber, E. M.: Pseudoxanthoma elasticum. Internal manifestations. Arch. Dermatol. 86:741, 1962.

305. Osler, W.: The visceral lesions of purpura and allied conditions. Br. Med. J. 1:517, 1914.

306. Wedgwood, R. J. P., and Janeway, C. A.: Serum complement in children with "collagen disease." Pediatrics 11:569, 1953.

307. Wedgwood, R. J. P., and Klaus, M. H.: Anaphylactoid purpura (Schoenlein-Henoch syndrome)—A long-term followup study with special reference to renal involvement. Pediatrics 16:196, 1955.

308. Allen, D. M., Diamond, L. K., et al.: Anaphylactoid purpura in children (Schoenlein-Henoch syndrome). A.M.A. J. Dis. Child. 99:147, 1960.

309. Mauer, A. M.: Pediatric Hematology. New York, McGraw-Hill, 1968, p. 431.

310. Michael, A. F., Vernier, R. L., et al.: Immunosuppressive therapy of chronic renal disease. New Engl. J. Med. 276:817, 1967.

311. Wedgwood, R. J.: Diseases of mesenchymal tissues. In Textbook of Pediatrics. Nelson, W. E. (ed.), Philadelphia, W. B. Saunders Co., 1969, pp. 993–995.

312. Burns, J. J.: Biosynthesis of L-ascorbic acid: Basic defect in scurvy. Am. J. Med. 26:740, 1959.

313. Wolbach, S. B., and Bessey, O. A.: Tissue changes in vitamin deficiencies. Physiol. Rev. 22:233, 1942.

314. Ratnoff, O. D.: Bleeding Syndromes. Springfield, Ill., Charles C Thomas, Publisher, 1960, Chapter 20.

315. Wilson, P. A., McNicol, G. P., et al.: Platelet abnormality in human scurvy. Lancet 1:975, 1967.

316. Gardner, F. H., and Diamond, L. K.: Autoerythrocyte sensitization: A form of purpura producing painful bruising following autosensitization to red cells in certain women. Blood 10:674, 1955.

317. Ratnoff, O. D., and Agle, D. P.: Psychogenic purpura: A reevaluation of the syndrome of autoerythrocyte sensitization. Medicine (Baltimore) 47:475, 1968.

318. Birch, C. L.: Hemophilia, Clinical and Genetic Aspects. Illinois Medical Monographs, Vol. No. 4. Urbana University of Illinois, 1937.

319. Lane, S.: Haemorrhagic diathesis: Successful transfusion of blood. Lancet 1:185, 1840.

320. Biggs, R., and Matthews, J. M.: Treatment of haemorrhage in von Willebrand's disease and the blood level of factor VIII. Br. J. Haematol. 9:203, 1963.

321. Pool, J. E., Hershgold, E. J., et al.: High-potency antihaemophilic factor concentrate prepared from cryoglobulin precipitate. Nature (Lond.) 203:312, 1964.

322. Ahrons, S., Glavind-Kristensen, S., et al.: Severe reactions after cryoprecipitated human factor VIII. Vox Sang. 18:182, 1970.

323. Smith, C. M., Miller, G. E., et al.: Factor VIII concentrates in outpatient therapy. J.A.M.A. 220:1352, 1972.

324. Ali, A. M., Gandy, R. H., et al.: Joint haemorrhage in haemophilia: Is full advantage taken of plasma therapy? Br. Med. J. 3:828, 1967.

325. Honig, G. R., Forman, E. N., et al.: Administration of single doses of AHF (Factor VIII) concentrates in the treatment of hemophilic hemarthroses. Pediatrics 43:26, 1969.

326. Kisker, C. T., and Burke, C.: Double-blind studies on the use of steroids in the treatment of acute hemarthrosis in patients with hemophilia. New Engl. J. Med. 282:639, 1970.

327. Biggs, R., and Matthews, J. M.:The treatment of spontaneous bleeding in hemophilia, In The Treatment of Haemophilia and Other Coagulation Disorders. Biggs, R., and MacFarlane, R. G. (eds.), Philadelphia, F. A. Davis, 1966, p. 129.

328. Wanken, J. J., Eyring, E. J., et al.: Should haemophiliac haemarthroses be aspirated? Lancet 2:1253, 1969.

329. Britten, A. F.: Treatment of haemarthrosis in hemophilia. New Engl. J. Med. 283:375, 1970.

330. Dormandy, K. M., and Madgwick, J. C. A.: The management of acute haemarthrosis and muscle haemorrhages. Bibl. Haematol. 34:164, 1970.

330a. Van Creveld, S., Hoedemaeker, P. S., et al.: Degeneration of joints in hemophiliacs under treatment by modern methods. J. Bone Joint Surg. 53B:296, 1971.

331. Poulain, M., and Josso, F.: La fonction des hemarthroses du genou chez l'hémophile. Hemostase 4:363, 1964.

332. Jordan, H. H.: Conservative orthopaedic approach to rehabilitation of the severely crippled hemophiliac. Wiederherstellungschir. Traum. 9:95, 1967.

333. Storti, E., Traldi, A., et al.: Synovectomy, a new approach to haemophilic arthropathy. Acta Haematol. 41:193, 1969.

334. Kisker, C. T., Perlman, A. W., et al.: Arthritis in hemophilia. Semin. Arthritis Rheum. 1:220, 1971.

335. Tavenner, R. W. H.: Use of tranexamic acid in control of hemorrhage after extraction of teeth in haemophilia and Christmas Disease. Br. Med. J. 2:314, 1972.

336. Steinle, C. J., and Kisker, C. T.: Pediatric dentistry for the child with hemophilia. New Engl. J. Med. 283:1325, 1970.

337. Archer, W. H., and Zubrow, H. J.: Fatal hemorrhage following regional anesthesia for operative dentistry in hemophilia. Oral Surg. 7:464, 1954.

337a. Walsh, P. W., Rizza, C. R., et al.: Epsilon aminocaproic acid therapy for dental extractions in hemophilia and Christmas disease: A double blind controlled trial. Br. J. Haematol. 20:463, 1971.

338. Prentice, C. R. M., Lindsay, R. M., et al.: Renal complications in haemophilia and Christmas disease. Quart. J. Med. 40:47, 1971.

339. Barkham, P.: Haematuria in haemophiliac treated with epsilon aminocaproic acid. Lancet 2:1061, 1964.

340. Tsevrenis, H., and Mandalaki, T.: Hematuria in a haemophiliac treated with E-aminocaproic acid. Lancet 1:610, 1965.

341. McNicol, G. P., Fletcher, A. P., et al.: The use of epsilon aminocaproic acid, a potent inhibitor of fibrinolytic activity in the management of postoperative hematuria. J. Urol. 86:829, 1961.

342. Gobbi, F.: Use and misuse of aminocaproic acid. Lancet 2:472, 1967.

343. Abildgaard, C. F., Simone, J. V., et al.: Steroid treatment of hemophilic hematuria. J. Pediatr. 66:117, 1965.

344. Gunning, A. J.: The surgery of hemophiliac cysts, In Treatment of Hemophilia and Other Coagulation Disorders. Biggs, R., and MacFarlane, R. G. (eds.), Philadelphia, F. A. Davis Company, 1966, p. 262.

345. Shulman, N. R., Cowan, D. H., et al.: The physiologic basis for therapy of classic hemophilia (factor VIII deficiency) and related disorders. Ann. Intern. Med. 67:856, 1967.

346. Van Creveld, S., and Kingma, M. J.: Subperiosteal hemorrhage in haemophilia A and B. Acta Paediatr. Scand. 50:291, 1961.

347. Krill, C. E., Jr., and Mauer, A. M.: Pseudotumor of calcaneus in Christmas disease. J. Pediatr. 77:848, 1970.

348. Lazarovits, P., and Griem, M. L.: Radiotherapy of hemophilia in pseudotumors. Radiology, 91:1026, 1968.

349. Kerr, C. B.: Intracranial haemorrhage in hemophilia. J. Neurol. Neurosurg. Psychiat. 27:166, 1964.

350. Silverstein, A.: Intracranial bleeding in hemophilia. Arch. Neurol. 3:141, 1960.

351. Fessey, B. M., and Meynell, M. S.: Hemorrhage involving the central nervous system in haemophilia—Account of the management of five cases. Br. Med. J. 2:211, 1966.

352. Davies, S. H., Turner, J. V., et al.: Management of intracranial haemorrhage in haemophilia. Br. Med. J. 2:1627, 1966.

353. Ferguson, G. G., Barton, W. B., et al.: Subdural hematoma in hemophilia; successful treatment with cryoprecipitate—Case report. J. Neurosurg. 29:524, 1968.

354. Stuart, J., Davies, S. H., et al.: Haemorrhagic episodes in haemophilia—A 5-year prospective survey. Br. Med. J. 2:1624, 1966.

354a. Forbes, C. D., Burr, R. D., et al.: Gastrointestinal bleeding in haemophilia. Quart. J. Med. 42: 503, 1973.

355. Lautkin, A., Karelitz, B. I., et al.: Roentgen findings in colon in a hemophiliac with melena. J. Mt. Sinai Hosp. 23:319, 1956.

356. Dodds, W. J., Spitzer, R. M., et al.: Gastrointestinal roentgenographic manifestations of hemophilia. Am. J. Roentgenol. Radium Ther. Nucl. Med. 110:413, 1970.

357. Agle, D., and Mattsson, A.: Psychiatric and social care of patients with hereditary hemorrhagic disease. In *Treatment of Hemorrhagic Disorders.* Ratnoff, O. D. (ed.), Hagerstown, Md., Harper and Row, 1968, pp. 111–125.

358. Burke, C.: Working with parents of children with hemophilia. Nursing Clin. North Am. 7:787, 1972.

359. Van Creveld, S.: Prophylaxis of joint hemorrhages in hemophilia. Acta Haematol. (Basel) 41:206, 1969.

360. Kasper, C. K., Dietrich, S. L., et al.: Hemophilia prophylaxis with factor VIII concentrate. Arch. Intern. Med. 125:1004, 1970.

361. Kisker, C. T., and Burke, C.: Double-blind study on weekly prophylaxis in hemophilia. In preparation.

362. Mainwaring, D., and Keidan, S. E.: Fibrinolysis in haemophilia. The effect of E-aminocaproic acid. Br. J. Haematol. 11:682, 1965.

363. Katsumi, O.: New aspects on the treatment of hemophilia. Nagoya J. Med. Sci., 28:179, 1966.

364. Reid, W. O., Hodge, S. M., et al.: The use of EACA in preventing or reducing hemorrhages in the hemophiliac. Thromb. Diath. Haemorrh. 18:179, 1967.

365. Strauss, H. S., Kevy, S. V., et al.: Ineffectiveness of prophylactic epsilon aminocaproic acid in severe hemophilia. New Engl. J. Med. 273: 301, 1965.

366. Bennett, A. E., and Ingram, G. I. C.: A controlled trial of longterm steroid treatment in haemophilia. Lancet 1:967, 1967.

366a. Rabiner, F. S., and Telfer, M. C.: Home transfu-sion for patients with hemophilia A. New Engl. J. Med. 283:1011, 1970.

366b. Lazerson, J.: Hemophilia home transfusion program: Effect on school attendance. J. Pediatr. 81:330, 1972.

366c. Levine, P. H., and Britten, A. F. H.: Supervised patient management of hemophilia: A study of 45 patients with hemophilia A and B. Ann. Intern. Med. 78:195, 1973.

367. Sevitt, S., and Gallagher, N.: Venous thrombosis and pulmonary embolism. A clinico-pathologic study in injured and burned patients. Br. J. Surg. 48:475, 1961.

368. Gaston, L. W.: Studies on a family with elevated plasma level of factor V (proaccelerin) and a tendency to thrombosis. J. Pediatr. 68:367, 1966.

369. Penick, G. D., Dejanov, I. L., et al.: Predisposition to intravascular coagulation. Thromb. Diath. Haemorrh. (Suppl.) 21:543, 1966.

370. Koszewski, B. J., and Vahbzadeh, H.: Hypercoagulability syndrome due to heparin cofactor deficiency. A case report and review of the literature. Thromb. Diath. Haemorrh. 11:485, 1964.

371. DeCamp, P. T., Carrera, A. E., et al.: The hypercoagulable state. Surgery 63:173, 1968.

372. Bobek, K., and Cepelak, V.: Laboratory diagnosis of venous thrombosis. Acta. Med. Scand. 60:121, 1958.

373. Brakman, P., Mohler, E. R., et al.: A group of patients with impaired plasma fibrinolytic system and selective inhibition of tissue activator-induced fibrinolysis. Scand. J. Haematol. 3:389, 1966.

374. Scheinman, J. I., and Stiehm, E. R.: Fibrinolytic studies in the nephrotic syndrome. Pediatr. Res. 5:206, 1971.

375. Kendall, A. G., Lohmann, R. C., et al.: Nephrotic syndrome; a hypercoagulable state. Arch. Intern. Med. 127:1021, 1971.

376. Innes, D., and Sevitt, S.: Coagulation and fibrinolysis in injured patients. J. Clin. Pathol. 17:1, 1964.

377. Arturson, G., and Wallenius, G.: Hypercoagulability of blood after burn trauma in rats. Acta Chir. Scand. 128:340, 1964.

378. Nelson, G. D., and Paletta, F. X.: Burns in children. Surg. Gynecol. Obstet. 128:518, 1969.

379. Gilder, S. S.: Homocystinuria. Can. Med. Assoc. J. 99:1013, 1968.

379a. Crosby, W. H.: Paroxysmal nocturnal hemoglobinuria. A classic description by Paul Strubing in 1882, and a bibliography of the disease. Blood 6:270, 1951.

380. Dennis, L. H., Stewart, J. L., et al.: A consumption coagulation defect in congenital cyanotic heart disease and its treatment with heparin. J. Pediatr. 71:407, 1967.

381. Abildgaard, C. F., and Shulman, I.: Absence of coagulation abnormalities in children with cyanotic congenital heart disease. Lancet 2:660, 1968.

382. Horvath, F. L., Brodeu, A. E., et al.: Deep thrombophlebitis associated with acute osteomyelitis. J. Pediatr. 79:815, 1971.

383. Homans, J.: Disease of the veins. New Engl. J. Med. 231:51, 1944.

384. Moses, W. R.: The early diagnosis of phle-

bothrombosis. New Engl. J. Med. *234*:388, 1946.

385. Marks, J. G., and Sussman, S. J.: Thrombophlebitis in an 8-year old girl. J. Pediatr. *80*:336, 1972.

386. Rogoff, S. M., and DeWeese, J. A.: Phlebography of the lower extremity. J.A.M.A. *172*:1599, 1960.

387. Palko, P. D., Nanson, E. M., et al.: Early detection of deep venous thrombosis using I¹³¹ tagged human fibrinogen. Can. J. Surg. 7:215, 1964.

388. Ruekley, C. V., Das, P. C., et al.: Serum fibrin/fibrinogen degradation products associated with post-operative pulmonary embolus and venous thrombosis. Br. Med. J. *4*:395, 1970.

389. Sigel, B., Popky, G. L., et al.: Augmentation flow sounds on the ultrasonic detection of venous abnormalities. Invest. Radiol. 2:256, 1967.

390. Hsia, D. Y., and Gellis, S. S.: Portal hypertension in infants and children. Am. J. Dis. Child. *90*:290, 1955.

390a. Oppenheimer, E. G., and Esterly, J. R.: Thrombosis in the newborn: Comparison between infants of diabetic and nondiabetic mothers. J. Pediatr. *67*:549, 1965.

391. Seller, R. A., Pravin, K., et al.: Nonsurgical management of thrombosis of bilateral renal veins and inferior vena cava in a newborn. Clin. Pediatr. 9:543, 1970.

392. Littman, D.: Observations on the electro-cardiographic changes in pulmonary embolism, In *Pulmonary Embolic Disease*, Sasahara, A. A., and Stein, M. (eds.), New York, Grune & Stratton, 1965.

393. Wacker, W. E. C., Rosenthal, M., et al.: A triad for the diagnosis of pulmonary embolism and infarction. J.A.M.A. *178*:8, 1961.

394. Sutherland, J. D., DeNardo, L., et al.: Lung scans with I¹³¹ labeled macroaggregated human serum albumin (maa). Am. J. Roentgenol. Radium Ther. Nucl. Med. 98:416, 1966.

395. Williams, J. R., Wilcox, W. C., et al.: Angiography in pulmonary embolism. J.A.M.A. *184*:473, 1968.

396. Barritt, D. W., and Jordan, S. C.: Anticoagulant drugs in treatment of pulmonary embolism. A controlled trial. Lancet *1*:1309, 1960.

397. Wessler, S., Freiman, D. G., et al.: Experimental pulmonary embolism with serum induced thrombi. Am. J. Pathol. 38:89, 1961.

398. Sullivan, J. M., Harken, D. E., et al.: Pharmacological control of thromboembolic complications of cardiac valve replacement. A preliminary report. New Eng. J. Med. 279:576, 1968.

399. Browse, N. L., and Hale, J. H.: Effect of dipyridamole on the incidence of clinically detectable deep vein thrombosis. Lancet 2:718, 1969.

400. Weiss, H. J., Aledort, L. M., et al.: The effect of salicylates on the hemostatic properties of platelets in man. J. Clin. Invest. 47:2169, 1968.

401. Bygdeman, S.: Prevention and therapy of thromboembolic complications with dextran. Progr. Surg. 7:114, 1969.

401a. Kaplan, B. S., Katz, J., et al.: An analysis of the results of therapy in 67 cases of the hemolytic-uremic syndrome. J. Pediatr. 78:420, 1971.

402. Kakker, V. V., Flanc, C., et al.: Treatment of deep vein thrombosis. A trial of heparin, streptokinase and arvin. Br. Med. J. *1*:896, 1969.

403. Bergstein, J. M., Edson, J. R., et al.: Fibrinolytic treatment of the haemolytic-uremic syndrome. Lancet *1*:448, 1972.

404. Gabriele, O. F., and Clark, D.: Calcified thrombus of the superior vena cava. Complication of ventriculoatrial shunt. Am. J. Dis. Child. *117*:327, 1969.

405. Lytton, B., Goffinet, J. A., et al.: Experience with arteriovenous fistula in chronic hemodialysis. J. Urol. *104*:512, 1970.

406. Wigger, H. J., Bransilver, B. R., et al.: Thrombosis due to catheterization in infants and children. J. Pediatr. 76:1, 1970.

407. Harker, L. A., and Slichter, S. J.: Studies of platelet and fibrinogen kinetics in patients with prosthetic heart valves. New Eng. J. Med. 283:302, 1970.

408. Lymon, D. S., and Kim, S. W.: Interactions at the blood polymer interface. Conference on mechanical surface gas layer effects on moving blood, San Diego, California, Jan. 13–15, 1971, Fed. Proc. 30:1658, 1971.

409. Wardle, E. N., and Taylor, G.: Fibrin breakdown products and fibrinolysis in renal disease. J. Clin. Pathol. *21*:140, 1962.

410. Chirawong, P., Nanra, R. S., et al.: Fibrin degradation products and the role of coagulation in "persistent" glomerulonephritis. Ann. Intern. Med. 74:853, 1971.

411. Stiehm, E. R., Kuplic, L. S., et al.: Urinary fibrin split products in human renal disease. J. Lab. Clin. Med. 77:843, 1971.

412. Humair, L., Potter, E. V., et al.: The role of fibrinogen in renal disease. I. Production of experimental lesions in mice. J. Lab. Clin. Med. 74:60, 1969.

413. Humair, L., Potter, E. V., et al.: The role of fibrinogen in renal disease. II. Effects of anticoagulants and urokinase on experimental lesions in mice. J. Lab. Clin. Med. *74*:72, 1969.

414. Briggs, J. D., Potter, E. V., et al.: The role of fibrinogen in renal disease. III. Fibrinolytic and anticoagulant treatment of nephrotoxic serum nephritis in mice. J. Lab. Clin. Med. 74:715, 1969.

415. Herdman, R. C., Edson, R., et al.: Anticoagulants in renal disease. Am. J. Dis. Child. *119*:27, 1970.

416. Cade, J. R., De Quesada, A. M., et al.: Effect of long term high dose heparin treatment on the course of chronic proliferative glomerulonephritis. Nephron 8:67, 1971.

417. Kincaid-Smith, P., Saker, E. M., et al.: Anticoagulants in "irreversible" acute renal failure. Lancet 2:1360, 1968.

418. Freedman, P., Meister, H. P., et al.: The clinical, functional and histologic response to heparin in chronic renal disease. Invest. Urol. 7:398, 1970.

419. Lowenhaupt, R., and Nathan, P.: Platelet accumulation observed by electron microscopy in the early phase of renal allotransplant rejection. Nature (Lond.) *220*:822, 1968.

420. Rosenberg, J. C., Broersma, R. J., et al: Relation-

ship of platelets, blood coagulation, and fibrinolysis to hyperacute rejection of renal xenografts. Transplantation 8:152, 1969.

421. Braun, W. E., and Merrill, J. P.: Urine fibrinogen fragments in human renal allografts. A possible mechanism of renal injury. New Engl. J. Med. 278:1366, 1968.

422. Antoine, B., Nevev, T., et al.: Fibrinuria during renal transplantation. Transplantation 8:98, 1969.

423. Gasser, C., Gautier, F., et al.: Hämolytisch-urämische Syndrome: Bilateral Nierenrindenekrosen bei akuten erworbenen hämolytischen Anämien, Schweiz. Med. Wochenschr. 85:905, 1955.

424. Waddell, A. J., and Matz, L. R.: Haemolytic-uremic syndrome: A report of two cases in adults. Med. J. Aust. 2:893, 1966.

425. King, L. R., Wulsin, J. H., et al.: Hemolytic-uremic syndrome in older children and adults. J. Urol. 101:273, 1969.

426. Sanchez Avalos, J., Vitacco, M., et al.: Coagulation studies in the hemolytic-uremic syndrome. J. Pediatr. 76:538, 1970.

427. Katz, J., Lurei, A., et al.: Coagulation findings in the hemolytic-uremic syndrome of infancy. Similarity to hyperacute renal allograft rejection. J. Pediatr. 78:426, 1971.

428. Wehinger, H., and Kunzer, W.: Haemolytic uraemic syndrome. Lancet 2:1085, 1968.

429. Gervais, M., Richardson, J. B., et al.: Immunofluorescent and histologic findings in the hemolytic uremic syndrome. Pediatrics 47:352, 1971.

430. Giantonio, C., Vitacco, M., et al.: The hemolytic-uremic syndrome. J. Pediatr. 64:478, 1964.

431. Javett, S. N., and Senior, B.: Syndrome of hemolysis, thrombopenia and nephropathy in infancy. Pediatrics 29:209, 1962.

432. Gilchrist, G. S., Ekert, H., et al.: Heparin therapy in the haemolytic uraemic syndrome. Lancet 1:1123, 1967.

433. Kaplan, B. S., Katz, J., et al.: An analysis of the results of therapy in 67 cases of the hemolytic-uremic syndrome. J. Pediatr. 78:420, 1971.

433a. Vitacco, M., Sanchez Avalos, J., et al.: Heparin therapy in the hemolytic uremic syndrome. J. Pediatr. 83:271, 1973.

434. Brain, M. C., Baker, L. R., et al.: Heparin therapy in the haemolytic-uremic syndrome. Quart. J. Med. 36:608, 1967.

435. Harker, L. A., and Slichter, S. J.: Platelet and fibrinogen consumption in man. New Engl. J. Med. 287:999, 1972.

436. Mandal, B. K., and McNulty, M.: Treatment of haemolytic-uremic syndrome with phenformin and ethyloestrenol. Lancet 2:1036, 1971.

437. Kasabach, H. H., and Merritt, K. K.: Capillary hemangioma with extensive purpura. Am. J. Dis. Child. 59:1063, 1940.

438. Straub, P. W., Kessler, S., et al.: Chronic intravascular coagulation in Kasabach-Merritt syndrome. Preferential accumulation of fibrinogen I^{131} on a giant hemangioma. Arch. Intern. Med. 129:475, 1972.

439. Hoak, J. C., Warner, E. D., et al.: Hemangioma with thrombocytopenià and microangiopathic anemia (Kasabach-Merritt syndrome):

An animal model. J. Lab. Clin. Med. 77:941, 1971.

440. Goldberg, S. J., and Fonkalsrud, E.: Successful treatment of hepatic hemangioma with corticosteroids. J.A.M.A. 208:2473, 1969.

441. Brown, S. H., Jr., Neerhout, R. C., et al.: Prednisone therapy in the management of the large hemangiomas in infants and children. Surgery 71:168, 1972.

441a. Zarem, H. A., and Edgerton, M. T.: Induced resolution of cavernous hemangiomas following prednisolone therapy. Plast. Reconstr. Surg. 39:76, 1967.

442. Lampe, I., and Latourette, H. B.: Management of hemangiomas in infants. Pediatr. Clin. North Am. 6:511, 1959.

443. Park, W. C., and Phillips, R.: The role of radiation therapy in the management of hemangiomas of the liver. J.A.M.A. 212:1496, 1970.

444. Merskey, C., Johnson, A. J., et al.: The defibrination syndrome: Clinical features and laboratory diagnosis. Br. J. Haematol. 13:528, 1967.

445. Merskey, C., Kleiner, G. J., et al.: Quantitative estimation of split products of fibrinogen in human serum, relation to diagnosis and treatment. Blood 28:1, 1966.

446. Niemetz, J., and Nossel, H. L.: Activated coagulation factors: In vivo and in vitro studies. Br. J. Haematol. 16:337, 1969.

447. Corrigan, J. J., Jr., and Jordan, C. M.: Heparin therapy in septicemia with disseminated intravascular coagulation. Effect on mortality and on correction of hemostatic defects. New Engl. J. Med. 283:778, 1970.

448. Stefanini, M., and Spicer, D. D.: Hemostatic breakdown, fibrinolysis, and acquired hemolytic anemia in a patient with fatal heatstroke. Pathogenetic mechanisms. Am. J. Clin. Pathol. 55:180, 1971.

448a. Gruewich, V., and Hutchinson, E.: Detection of intravascular coagulation by a serial dilution protamine sulfate test. Ann. Intern. Med. 75:895, 1971.

448b. Yip, M. L. B., Lee, S., et al.: Nonspecificity of the protamine test for disseminated intravascular coagulation. Amer. J. Clin. Pathol. 57:487, 1972.

449. Kisker, C. T., and Rush, R.: Detection of intravascular coagulation. J. Clin. Invest. 50:2235, 1971.

450. Nossel, H. L., Younger, L. R., et al.: Radioimmunoassay of human fibrinopeptide A. Proc. Natl. Acad. Sci. USA 68:2350, 1971.

451. Fletcher, A. P., Alkjaersig, N., et al.: Blood hypercoagulability and thrombosis. Trans. Assoc. Am. Phys. 83:159, 1970.

452. Winkelstein, A., Songster, C. L., et al.: Fulminant meningococcemia and disseminated intravascular coagulation. Arch. Intern. Med. 124:55, 1969.

453. Bull, B. S., and Kuhn, I. N.: The production of schistocytes by fibrin strands (a scanning electron microscope study). Blood 35:104, 1970.

454. Stander, R. W., Flessa, H. C., et al.: Changes in maternal coagulation factors after intraamniotic injection of hypertonic saline. Obstet. Gynecol. 37:660, 1971.

455. Lo, S. S., Hitzig, W. H., et al.: Clinical experience

with anticoagulant therapy in the management of disseminated intravascular coagulation therapy in children. Acta Haematol. (Basel) 45:1, 1971.

456. Kisker, C. T., and Rush, R.: Circulating fibrin in meningococcemia. J. Pediatr. 82:787, 1973.

457. Gralnick, H. R., Bagley, J., et al.: Heparin treatment for the hemorrhagic diathesis of acute promyelocytic leukemia. Am. J. Med. 52:167, 1972.

458. Foster, J. B. T., DeNatale, A., et al.: Determination of plasma fibrinogen by means of centrifugation after heating. Am. J. Clin. Pathol. 31:42, 1959.

459. Colman, R. W., Robboy, S. J., et al.: Disseminated intravascular coagulation (DIC): An approach. Am. J. Med. 52:679, 1972.

460. Ahlberg, A.: Orthopedic surgery in bleeders. Bibl. Haematol. 34:170, 1970.

461. McMillan, C. W., Webster, W. P., et al.: Continuous intravenous infusion of factor VIII in classic hemophilia. Br. J. Haematol. 18:659, 1970.

462. Mazza, J. J., Bowie, E. J. W., et al.: Antihemophilic factor VIII in hemophilia. J.A.M.A. 211:1318, 1970.

463. Dike, G. W. R., Bidwell, E., et al.: The preparation and clinical use of a new concentrate containing factor IX, prothrombin and factor X and of a separate concentrate containing factor VII. Br. J. Haematol. 22:469, 1972.

464. Gilchrist, G. S., Ekert, H., et al.: Evaluation of a new concentrate for the treatment of factor IX deficiency. New Engl. J. Med. 280:291, 1969.

465. Bennett, E., and Dormandy, K.: Pool's cryoprecipitate and exhausted plasma in the treatment of von Willebrand's disease and factor XI deficiency. Lancet 2:731, 1966.

466. Ponka, J. L., Monto, R. W., et al.: Operative treatment of gastric hemorrhage in a patient with von Willebrand's disease. Ann. Surg. 165:318, 1967.

467. Rosenthal, R. L., and Sloan, E.: PTA (factor XI) levels and coagulation studies after plasma infusion in PTA-deficient patients. J. Lab. Clin. Med. 66:709, 1965.

468. Hoag, S. M., Aggeler, P. M., et al.: Disappearance rate of concentrated proconvertin extracts in congenital and acquired hypoproconvertinemia. J. Clin. Invest. 39:554, 1960.

469. Owen, C. A., Amundsen, M. A., et al.: Congenital deficiency of factor VII. Ann. J. Med. 37:71, 1964.

470. Marder, V. J., and Shulman, N. R.: Clinical aspects of congenital factor VII deficiency. Am. J. Med. 37:182, 1964.

471. Borchgrevink, C. F., and Owren, P. A.: Surgery in a patient with factor V (proaccelerin) deficiency. Acta Med. Scand. 170:743, 1961.

472. Rush, B., and Ellis, H.: The treatment of patients with factor V deficiency. Thromb. Diath. Haemorrh. 14:74, 1965.

473. Webster, W. P., Roberts, H. R., et al.: Hemostasis in factor V deficiency. Am. J. Med. Sci. 248:194, 1964.

474. Roberts, H. R., Lechler, E., et al.: Survival of transfused factor X in patients with Stuart disease. Thromb. Diath. Haemorrh. 13:305, 1965.

475. Biggs, R., and Denson, K. W. E.: Fate of

476. Biggs, R.: The treatment of patients with congenital deficiency of factors I, II, V, VII, X, XI, and XIII, In Treatment of Haemophilia and Other Coagulation Disorders. Biggs, R., and Macfarlane, R. G. (eds.), Philadelphia, F. A. Davis Company, 1966, p. 240.

477. Ikkala, E., Myllya, G., et al.: Transfusion therapy in factor XIII deficiency. Scand. J. Haematol. 1:308, 1962.

478. Didisheim, P., Bowie, E. J., et al.: Intravascular coagulation fibrinolysis (ICF) syndrome and malignancy: Historical review on report of two cases with metastatic carcinoid and with acute myelomonocytic leukemia, In Transactions of the Seventeenth Annual Symposium on Blood, Wayne State University School of Medicine, Jan. 17, 18, 1969.

478a. Peck, S. D., and Reiquam, C. W.: Disseminated intravascular coagulation in cancer patients. Supportive evidence. Cancer 31:1114, 1973.

479. Rock, R. C., Bove, J. R., et al.: Heparin treatment of intravascular coagulation accompanying hemolytic transfusion reactions. Transfusion 9:57, 1969.

480. Mannucci, P. M., Lobina, G. F., et al.: Effect on blood coagulation of massive intravascular haemolysis. Blood 33:207, 1969.

481. Reid, H. A., Chan, K. E., et al.: Prolonged coagulation defect (defibrination syndrome) in Malayan viper bite. Lancet 1:621, 1963.

482. Kwaan, H. C., Anderson, M. C., et al.: A study of pancreatic enzymes as a factor in the pathogenesis of disseminated intravascular coagulation during acute pancreatitis. Surgery 69:663, 1971.

483. Chessis, J. M., and Wigglesworth, J. S.: Coagulation studies in severe birth asphyxia. Arch. Dis. Child. 46:252, 1971.

484. Rake, M. O., Pannell, G., et al.: Intravascular coagulation in acute hepatic necrosis. Lancet 1:533, 1970.

485. Moore, C. M., McAdams, A. J., et al.: Intrauterine disseminated intravascular coagulation: A syndrome of multiple pregnancy with a dead twin fetus. J. Pediatr. 74:523, 1969.

486. Karpatkin, M., Sacker, I., et al.: Respiratory-distress syndrome and disseminated intravascular coagulation in two siblings. Lancet 1:102, 1972.

487. McKay, D. G., Franciosi, R., et al.: Symposium on thrombohemorrhagic phenomena. Part II. Pulmonary embolism and disseminated intravascular coagulation. Am. J. Cardiol. 20:374, 1967.

488. Mallen, D.: Heparin therapy of purpura fulminans. Pediatrics 38:211, 1966.

489. Hattersley, P. G.: Purpura fulminans. Complete recovery with intravenously administered heparin. Am. J. Dis. Child. 120:467, 1970.

490. McKay, D. G., and Margaretten, W.: Disseminated intravascular coagulation in virus diseases. Arch. Intern. Med. 120:129, 1967.

491. Shershow, L. W., Ekert, H., et al.: Intravascular coagulation in generalized herpes simplex infection of the newborn. Acta Paediatr. Scand. 58:535, 1969.

492. Goldenfarb, P. B., Zucker, S., et al.: The coagula-

tion mechanism in acute bacterial infection. Br. J. Haematol. *18*:643, 1970.

493. McCracken, G. H., and Dickerman, J. D.: Septicemia and disseminated intravascular coagulation. Am. J. Dis. Child. *118*:431, 1969.

494. Trigg, J. W., Jr.: Hypofibrinogenemia in Rocky Mountain spotted fever. New Engl. J. Med. *270*:1042, 1964.

494a. Ognibene, A. S., O'Leary, D. S., et al.: Myocarditis and disseminated intravascular coagulation in scrub typhus. Am. J. Med. Sci. *262*:233, 1971.

495. Prochazka, J. V., Lucas, R. N., et al.: Systemic candidiasis with disseminated intravascular coagulation. A complication of total parenteral alimentation. Am. J. Dis. Child. *122*:255, 1971.

496. Adner, M. M., Kauff, R. E., et al.: Purpura fulminans in a child with pneumococcal septicemia two years after splenectomy. J.A.M.A. *213*:1681, 1970.

497. Bisno, A. L., and Freeman, J. C.: The syndrome of asplenia, pneumococcal sepsis, and disseminated intravascular coagulation. Ann. Intern. Med. *72*:389, 1970.

498. Oski, F. A., and Naiman, J. L.: Thrombocytopenia in the newborn, In *Hematologic Problems in the Newborn.* Philadelphia, W. B. Saunders Co., 1972, p. 273.

499. Gross, S., and Melhorn, D. K.: Exchange transfusion with citrated whole blood for disseminated intravascular clotting. J. Pediatr. *78*:415, 1971.

500. Rake, M. O., Flute, P. T., et al.: Intravascular coagulation in acute hepatic necrosis. Lancet *1*:533, 1970.

501. Tytgat, G. N., Collen, D. J., et al.: La diathèse hémorragique en cas de cirrhose du foie. Nouv. Rev. Fr. Hematol. 8:123, 1968.

502. Fletcher, A. P., Biederman, O., et al.: Abnormal plasminogen-plasmin system activity (fibrinolysis) in patients with cirrhosis: Its cause and consequences. J. Clin. Invest. *43*:681, 1964.

503. Cedarbaum, A. I., and Roberts, H. R.: Complications of the use of prothrombin concentrate in liver disease. Clin. Res. *21*:92, 1973.

Chapter 20

Platelet Physiology

by Scott Murphy
and Frank H. Gardner

ANATOMY

The platelet, as its name implies, circulates as a thin disk. This shape, which is characteristic of the cell in vivo, is frequently lost in vitro because multiple physical and chemical stimuli, most notably glass contact, cause it to assume a spherical configuration with frequent protrusions of cytoplasm in the form of veils or dendrites. Thus the student's concept of the cell's shape is often derived from study of the activated cells seen on routine peripheral blood smears rather than the resting cell, as seen in Figure 20–1. A marginal bundle of microtubules traverses the circumference of the disk close to the inner surface of the plasma membrane (1). These apparently rigid structures act as a cytoskeleton, maintaining the cell in its disk shape. Thus the cell appears to be relatively rigid and inflexible in the resting state. As will be discussed subsequently, much of the cell's function is mediated through its responses to adenosine diphosphate (ADP), which causes platelets to aggregate in hemostatic plugs. The first manifestation of response to ADP is an almost instantaneous conversion from discoid to spherical shape (2); this shape change precedes aggregation. Thus when the cell functions, it does so as a sphere. There is as yet no known functional purpose served by the nonspherical configuration of the resting cell. Furthermore, upon exposure to cold temperatures, the microtubules disappear and the cell assumes a spherical configuration with mul-

tiple dendritic projections. If such exposure is prolonged, as when platelets are stored for transfusion, this change becomes irreversible, and the cell's viability upon transfusion is reduced (3).

When thin sections are viewed with the electron microscope, the cell's complex and highly specialized internal structure becomes apparent. Aside from the microtubules mentioned above, a typical plasma membrane, apparent vacuoles, granules of variable density, mitochondria, and fields of glycogen are prominent. Many or all of the apparent vacuoles are in reality fingerlike projections of extracellular space into the depths of the cell; their connection with extracellular space is not apparent in thin-section preparations (4). Since this so-called "surface-connecting system" or "open canalicular system" is lined with plasma membrane, the quantity of membrane possessed by each cell is very great relative to its volume. Since it has been proposed that the cell membrane contains the platelet's procoagulant activity, which will be discussed in detail below, this abundance of membrane lipid may be of crucial physiologic importance. Although the cell membrane has many highly specialized functions, its appearance by electron microscopy is indistinguishable from that of membranes of other cells.

As far as is known, platelet mitochondria are not unique; they carry on the respiratory function typical of mitochondria in many cell types. Platelet granules display a wide variation in electron density. Cell fractiona-

626

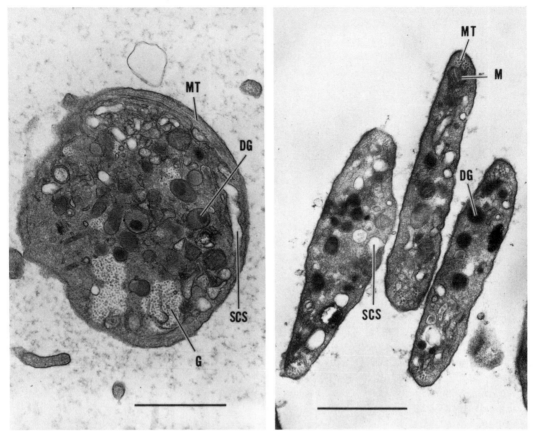

Figure 20–1. Platelet ultrastructure. When the platelet's disk shape is well preserved in thin sections, one sees the cell sectioned through (left) or perpendicular to (right) the plane of the disk. Code: MT, circumferential bundle of microtubules; DG, dense granules; G, glycogen; SCS, surface-connecting system or open canalicular system; M, mitochondria; horizontal line, one micron.

tion studies (5) have shown that they contain lysosomal enzymes, calcium, potassium, adenosine diphosphate (ADP), adenosine triphosphate (ATP), and serotonin, all in high concentration. The extremely dense granules contain a relatively high concentration of potassium, calcium, adenine nucleotides, and serotonin, while the less dense granules are proportionately higher in lysosomal enzymes. When the "release reaction" is stimulated by thrombin or connective tissue, the contents of these granules are secreted into the extracellular space. The physiologic function of this secretory process is discussed below. The abundant fields of glycogen provide a ready source of carbohydrate from which the cell can derive energy for this secretion and the contractile process which it will subsequently undergo.

BIOCHEMISTRY— CARBOHYDRATE, LIPID, AND PROTEIN METABOLISM

Much is known concerning the metabolic pathways available to the platelet for synthesis of high-energy phosphate bonds and macromolecules. The following have been identified: glycogen synthesis, glycogen breakdown, hexose monophosphate shunt, glycolysis, citric acid cycle capable of metabolizing both pyruvate and fatty acids to CO_2, amino acid (alanine, glutamate, aspartate) synthesis, fatty acid synthesis, phospholipid synthesis, and protein synthesis. Far less is known of the extent to which the cell uses these pathways in vivo and to what extent it depends on them for viability and functional integrity. Some, such as protein synthesis, may be vestigial remnants of pathways critical for the cell's development within the megakaryocyte but of little importance after release from the marrow.

In vitro, glucose metabolism proceeds almost entirely to lactate, with considerably less than 5 per cent going to CO_2 through the hexose monophosphate shunt and the citric acid cycle (6). It is likely, therefore, that the resting cell in the circulation derives most of its energy from glycolysis. During aggregation and the release of granular contents, there is rapid breakdown of glycogen to glucose and a burst of glucose metabolism to lactate through glycolysis (7) and to CO_2 through the hexose monophosphate shunt (8). This acute response subsides in several minutes, and, coinciding with retraction of the platelet aggregate, there ensues a substantial increase in glucose metabolism to CO_2 through the citric acid cycle which persists, in vitro at least, for several hours (9). Although these in vitro experiments are highly artificial, it appears that the energy for the initial events of aggregation is derived from ATP stores, glycolysis, and oxidative phosphorylation, while subsequent contractile activity of the aggregate relies to a greater extent on oxidative phosphorylation. The platelet can also use free fatty acids as substrate for the citric acid cycle (10). We do not know to what extent fatty acids are used relative to glucose, but they may be critical for resting and stimulated metabolism.

During coagulation in vivo, platelets provide phospholipid ("platelet factor 3") which accelerates the generation of thrombin and therefore fibrin at the site of bleeding. This knowledge has stimulated active study of platelet lipid metabolism during the past ten years. Furthermore, the platelet membrane functions in a highly specialized fashion in its response to thrombin, collagen, and ADP. Since lipid makes up a considerable portion of plasma membrane substance, interest in membrane lipid has been particularly intense. Platelet membrane lipid content is quite similar to that of other cells; 90 per cent of the neutral lipids is cholesterol, and the major phospholipids are lecithin, phosphatidyl ethanolamine, phosphatidyl serine, phosphatidyl inositol, and sphingomyelin (11). The cholesterol: phospholipid ratio is 0.53, and the phospho-

lipid:protein ratio is 0.39. These values are not unique, and even detailed analysis of fatty acid components have yielded results similar to those found in other cells. Futhermore, after hemolysis, red cell membranes can substitute for platelet phospholipid as procoagulants (12). Therefore, it seems quite likely that an understanding of the unique functions of the platelet membrane will be derived from a study of membrane protein rather than membrane lipid.

The platelet is the only formed element of the blood which possesses both acetyl CoA carboxylase and fatty acid synthetase, the two enzymes necessary for de novo fatty acid synthesis (13). Furthermore, the cell can utilize plasma fatty acids to acylate lysocompounds as well as synthesize most of the major phospholipids from glycerol. Again, nothing is known of the extent to which the cell depends on these synthetic capacities to maintain viability and function; they may be vestigial capacities of little importance to the mature cell. However, Lewis and Majerus (14) have shown that thrombin elicits a marked increase in phosphatidyl serine synthesis from glycerol relative to phosphatidyl choline synthesis, suggesting a functional role for lipid synthesis. How the cell uses the phosphatidyl serine synthesized is unknown. Furthermore, it has recently been shown (15) that human platelets are capable of synthesizing prostaglandins (specifically PGE_2 and $PGF_{2\alpha}$), that aggregating agents such as thrombin, collagen, ADP, and epinephrine stimulate this synthesis (16), and that aspirin blocks the stimulating effect of these agents (17). Since PGE_2 (18) enhances the platelet aggregation which occurs in response to the release of endogenous ADP (see below), its synthesis after exposure to thrombin may play an important role in the formation of the hemostatic plug.

The platelet contains no DNA but does contain ribosomes and a stable messenger RNA which directs the de novo synthesis of protein. Protein synthesis is more active in young platelets, recently released from the marrow, a finding analogous to erythrocyte maturation (19). A contractile protein, which has been called thrombosthenin, makes up approximately 15 per cent of the total platelet protein. By electron microscopy, partially purified thrombosthenin displays a fibrillar structure, which resembles the myofilaments of smooth muscle and the microfibrils which become apparent in platelet cytoplasm after exposure to hypotonic solutions (20). Thrombosthenin also resembles smooth muscle actomyosin in its biochemical reactivity (21). Seen from this perspective, one might naively say that the platelet is a circulating smooth muscle cell awaiting its chance to play its role in hemostasis by contracting and tightening the platelet plug which forms at the site of vessel injury.

The platelet contains several plasma proteins which are inseparable from the cell and not merely absorbed to surface membrane. Prominent among these are fibrinogen, albumin, Factor V, Factor XI, and Factor XIII (22). The physiologic role of these proteins is unknown, but platelet fibrinogen, normally constituting 10 per cent of platelet protein (23), is consistently decreased in the inherited disorder of platelet function, thrombasthenia (24).

Several investigators have studied platelet protein, particularly membrane protein, in an attempt to understand the uniquely specific response of the cell to exogenous thrombin, connective tissue, and ADP. For example, Jamieson et al. (25) have described a platelet membrane enzyme, collagen-glucosyltransferase, which transfers glucose from platelet uridine diphosphate-glucose to collagen. They propose that this enzyme mediates the adhesive interaction of the platelet membrane with connective tissue. These observations are obviously preliminary, but they point the way to a more detailed understanding of the platelet's response to surface stimuli.

THE RELEASE REACTION AND ADENINE NUCLEOTIDE METABOLISM

Figure 20–2 offers a scheme for the formation of a hemostatic platelet plug in response to vessel injury. When a vessel is severed, flowing blood is exposed to subendothelial tissue which contains components to which platelets adhere. Collagen has been the most extensively studied of the components, although there is no doubt that subendothelial tissue constituents other than collagen are capable of activating platelets (26). Adhesion of platelets to collagen results in the selective release of platelet constituents, most importantly ADP, and the exposure of platelet phospholipid which catalyzes the generation of thrombin through both the intrinsic and extrinsic coagulation pathways. Both ADP and thrombin cause platelet aggregation and the further release of ADP from these platelets "recruited" to the scene of injury. In this way, a porous platelet plug is formed which can then undergo contraction through the activation of thrombosthenin. Meanwhile, the thrombin generated converts fibrinogen to fibrin strands which are intermingled with the platelet aggregates, adding strength to the platelet plug.

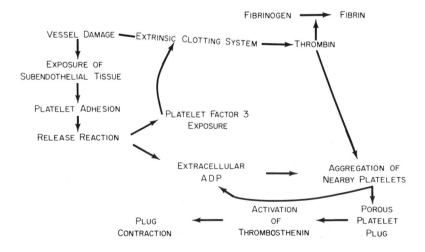

Figure 20–2. Events leading to formation of hemostatic platelet plug. Vessel damage (upper left) initiates the series of reactions.

The release of platelet constituents, the so-called release reaction, plays a central role in these events. Until recently it was assumed that platelet plug formation was accompanied by a nonspecific leakage of all platelet constituents and essentially cellular disintegration. It is now known that the release process is highly selective and that the cell continues to function in an organized way long after release has occurred and the plug has formed. Holmsen and colleagues have shown that platelet nucleotides become labeled when incubated with ^{32}P, ^{14}C-adenosine, or ^{14}C-adenine, but that only unlabeled ADP and ATP are released if the release reaction is induced by any of a variety of stimuli, such as collagen, thrombin, or ADP (27). From their data, they inferred the existence of two major nucleotide pools, a storage (unlabeled) pool, making up 60 per cent of the cell's ADP and ATP content, and a metabolic (labeled) pool (40 per cent). During release, 10 to 20 per cent of the metabolic ATP is converted to hypoxanthine to provide the energy for release, while the rest of the cell's metabolic nucleotides continue to serve the cell's needs. The importance of these concepts is emphasized by the recent description of a series of patients who have bleeding tendencies and decreased quantities of nucleotides in the storage pool (28).

Cell fractionation studies have shown that the storage pool of nucleotides is located within the dense granules of the resting platelet. The less dense α-granules contain a variety of acid hydrolases, such as β-N-acetylglucosaminidase, β-galactosidase, β-glucuronidase, cathepsin, and aryl sulfatase, which are released during the release reaction induced by thrombin but not by ADP or epinephrine (29). The role that these enzymes play in the cell's physiologic function is unknown. In contrast to the acid hydrolases, cytoplasmic enzymes, such as lactic dehydrogenase, and mitochondrial enzymes, such as cytochrome c oxidase, are not released, attesting to the specificity of the release process.

Striking morphologic changes have been observed during the release reaction by electron microscopy (30). In response to most release inducers, the platelet becomes spherical and throws out several pseudopods. Granules are crowded together in the center of the cell and appear to fuse. Final-ly, they disappear as their contents are secreted into the extracellular space. It is assumed that the granule contents pass through the surface-connecting or open-canalicular system as they move from the center of the cell to the extracellular space.

The mechanism by which exogenous or released ADP produces platelet aggregation is under intensive study, but no widely accepted concept has evolved as yet. Much recent interest has been directed to the function of cyclic 3',5'-adenosine monophosphate (cAMP). In many cell types cAMP acts as an intracellular messenger, mediating response to extracellular stimuli. Cyclic AMP is synthesized from ATP by adenyl cyclase, an enzyme in the cell membrane, and is inactivated by a second enzyme, phosphodiesterase, which converts it to 5'AMP. Salzman (31) has proposed the generalization that substances which inhibit aggregation are associated with increased cAMP levels (prostaglandin PGE_1, caffeine, theophylline), while those that enhance aggregation are associated with decreased cAMP (ADP, epinephrine, thrombin, collagen, kaolin, prostaglandin PGE_2). Cyclic AMP and its acylated derivative, dibutyryl cyclic AMP, inhibit aggregation when added to platelet-rich plasma (PRP)—a fact consistent with the above hypothesis. Other investigators (32) have presented data in conflict with this attractive concept. Further developments in this area are awaited with interest.

Phospholipid accelerates the speed with which fibrin is generated by acting as a catalyst at two sites in the intrinsic clotting system: the conversion of Factor X to activated Factor X in the presence of Factor VIII, activated Factor IX, and calcium, and the conversion of prothrombin to thrombin in the presence of activated Factor X, Factor V, and calcium. This phospholipid activity has been called platelet factor 3 (PF 3), although phospholipid from many sources is equally as effective as platelet phospholipid. No single phospholipid has unique activity, and many types are able to function. As the cell circulates, PF 3 activity is "buried" within the cell and not available. Most evidence (33) suggests that it is a component of the plasma membrane which becomes exposed on the surface of the cell during the membrane changes coincident with the release reaction. The platelet plug, therefore, offers a catalytic surface upon which clotting factors can interact to generate fibrin. This would appear to be most physiologic in localizing fibrin formation to the site of vessel injury.

IN VITRO AND IN VIVO STUDY OF PLATELET FUNCTION

In 1963, Born and Cross (34) described a technique by which the investigator could continuously monitor platelet aggregation in vitro. When citrated whole blood is centrifuged at slow speeds, platelet-rich plasma (PRP) is formed as a supernatant relatively free of white cells and red cells. In an "aggregometer," PRP can be stirred at a constant temperature of 37° C and its optical density (O.D.) continuously recorded. When platelet aggregation occurs, O.D. decreases. Both stirring and the small amount of free, unbound calcium present in citrated plasma are necessary for aggregation to occur with most agents. The precise cause for the O.D. fall has not been defined completely. Born and Hume (35) have shown that early after ADP addition the formation of many small aggregates, each containing two to six platelets, results in little or no O.D. change, while later a relatively large O.D. change occurs when aggregates contract without increase in the number of platelets included in the aggregate. Thus the aggregometer clearly measures more than simply aggregate formation.

The most commonly used aggregating agents for in vitro study have been ADP, connective tissue or collagen, and epinephrine. At concentrations of ADP less than 0.2 μM (Fig. 20–3), the initial wave of aggregation is followed by disaggregation. In most normal individuals (36), at some critical concentration between 0.2 μM and 1.4 μM the initial wave of aggregation will be followed by a secondary wave of nearly complete aggregation which shows no tendency to reversal. This secondary wave coincides with the occurrence of the release reaction, during which the storage pool of endogenous ADP is secreted in concentrations high enough to cause irreversible aggregation. Concentrations of ADP much greater than the critical concentration are

high enough to produce one irreversible wave of aggregation. Similarly, beginning at concentrations of 0.1 to 1.0 μM, epinephrine also produces a primary wave of aggregation which is almost invariably followed by an irreversible second wave. In general, epinephrine produces an easily recognized second wave over a much wider concentration range than ADP, so that it is the best agent to use for screening purposes when looking for a defect in the release reaction in patients. When connective tissue suspensions are used as aggregating agents, a lag period of approximately one minute is followed by rapid, complete, and irreversible aggregation. Again, aggregation coincides with the release of the storage pool of adenine nucleotides.

In the hereditary disease, thrombasthenia, the patient's platelets do not aggregate with ADP and other aggregating agents, even at very high concentrations. In the group of patients with so-called "storage-pool disease" (28), the amount of ADP in the storage pool is reduced. In these patients, the primary wave of aggregation with ADP is normal, but there is no response to the usual concentrations of connective tissue and diminutive secondary waves with ADP and epinephrine. Finally, some drugs produce a relative inhibition of the release reaction; aspirin has been the most intensively studied. A few patients (37) have

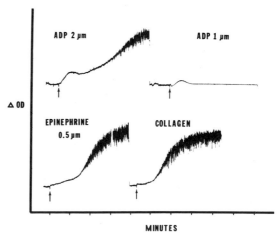

Figure 20–3. Platelet aggregation with ADP, epinephrine, and collagen. Arrows indicate time of the addition of the agent. Concentrations refer to final concentrations. A rise in the tracing reflects a decrease in the optical density (O.D.).

been described whose platelets have an "aspirin-like defect" in the absence of drug ingestion. In these patients and in normal individuals who ingest aspirin, the storage pool of ADP is present but is released only by exceptionally strong stimuli. Usually, the primary response to ADP is intact, but secondary waves with ADP and epinephrine are absent. There is no response to routine concentrations of connective tissue, but release will occur with concentrated solutions which are able to overcome the drug's inhibitory effects.

An enormous volume of literature dealing with platelet aggregation has accumulated during the past decade. In much of it, attempts at quantitation have been made in order to detect small differences between different patient populations. For example, the rate of the initial fall in O.D. or the total percentage change in O.D. have been recorded. Suffice it to say that no general agreement has been reached as to the best method of quantitation, and it is probably best at this time to consider only large differences significant. Currently, the authors merely record whether a primary or secondary wave is present or absent. With this reservation that the method yields a relatively gross measurement, aggregation studies have been and should continue to be of great clinical importance.

Another widely used method is the measurement of platelet adhesiveness, more precisely the percentage of platelets retained by a glass bead column when a sample of blood is passed through it. The original method of Salzman has been modified so that in some dedicated laboratories a quite reproducible measurement can be made. Coller and Zucker (38) have pointed out many technical pitfalls; the degree of retention can be significantly altered by the volume of blood introduced into the column, the type of anticoagulant used, the speed of transit, the number of and size of the beads and how tightly they are packed, the type of plastic tubing used, and whether or not the blood is agitated prior to its introduction. Furthermore, the platelet count of the first milliliter of blood exiting from the column will be much higher than that of the last milliliter. Therefore, minute attention to technical detail is mandatory.

The percentage retention is significantly decreased in many patients whose studies

of platelet aggregation are also abnormal; in these patients, the technique has little additional to offer. However, in von Willebrand's disease, studies of platelet aggregation have been normal in most laboratories, while reduced retention is a consistent finding. The test is often useful when the bleeding time and Factor VIII are not diagnostic of the illness (39).

Although these in vitro measurements have been very helpful in evaluating platelet function, the single most useful test for evaluating patients has been the template bleeding time, a modification of the original Ivy technique (40). Since it assesses all those platelet functions which are involved in the formation of the platelet plug at the site where a small blood vessel has been severed, significant platelet defects of any type should be reflected in an abnormal study. Since the test becomes abnormal when the platelet count falls below 100,000 per mm^3 and in normal individuals after aspirin ingestion, it can be considered quite sensitive and the most valuable tool for screening for platelet function. We currently believe that a repeatedly normal bleeding time excludes a platelet function abnormality of clinical significance. The study can be performed quite adequately in children over the age of one year.

PLATELET PRODUCTION AND LIFE SPAN IN THE CIRCULATION

The circulating platelet represents a fragment of the cytoplasm of the megakaryocyte—a large, granulated, polyploid cell with hypersegmented nucleus found in the bone marrow. A great deal of information about this cell is now available, but the reader should keep in mind that the summary to follow is derived almost entirely from data from experimental animals and that human data are very scarce.

There is little doubt that the megakaryocyte arises from the same pluripotential stem cell that produces the other blood cells (41). The pluripotential stem cell gives rise to a compartment of so-called committed stem cells which proliferate by cell division (Fig. 20–4). Since it has been demonstrated that no cell which is differentiated enough to be recognizable as a megakaryocyte is

Figure 20-4. Model for megakaryocytopoiesis in the rat. Proliferating pluripotential and committed stem cells give rise to morphologically unrecognizable polyploid cells, capable of nuclear replication but not cell division. These polyploid precursors then mature into recognizable megakaryocytes, which retain the capacity for DNA synthesis during the megakaryoblast stage prior to nuclear and cytoplasmic maturation. Code: open nuclei are 2N cells, lightly stippled nuclei are 4N, crosshatched nuclei are 8N, heavily stippled nuclei are 16N, and solid nuclei are 32N. [From Ebbe, S., In *Regulation of Hematopoiesis.* Vol. 2, 1970. Gordon, A. S. (ed.). Courtesy of Appleton-Century-Crofts, Publishing Division of Prentice-Hall, Englewood Cliffs, N.J.; copyright 1970 by Meredith Corporation.]

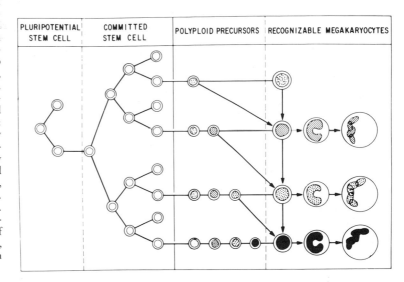

capable of cell division, it is evident that all the proliferating cells in the committed stem cell compartment are too undifferentiated for morphologic identification. The megakaryoblasts, which make up approximately 20 per cent of megakaryocytic cells, have a large nuclear:cytoplasmic ratio, basophilic cytoplasm, and a large, immature nucleus. They already have from four to 32 times the normal, diploid content of DNA and are capable of further DNA synthesis but not of cell division. Because megakaryoblasts are already polyploid, it is necessary to hypothesize the existence of a compartment of morphologically unrecognizable polyploid precursors, in which cells from the committed stem cell compartment synthesize DNA but do not divide. This process of DNA synthesis without cell division, which continues through the megakaryoblast stage, has been called "endomitosis."

More mature megakaryocytes do not synthesize DNA. As maturation occurs, the cell enlarges, the cytoplasm develops characteristic granulation, the nucleus develops multiple lobes, and the nuclear:cytoplasmic ratio decreases. By electron microscopy, the megakaryocyte membrane undergoes multiple invaginations, which then fuse within the cell to form the so-called "demarcation membrane system" (42). This membrane system separates the cytoplasm into thousands of fragments which will be released

as platelets (4,000 per megakaryocyte in the rat). The membrane of the circulating platelet is, therefore, derived from that of the megakaryocyte. This maturation process occurs in about ten days in man. The formation of the "demarcation membrane system" begins after DNA synthesis has been completed, and seems analogous to the invagination of membrane which occurs after DNA synthesis when cells of normal chromosome content divide. It has been proposed that the megakaryocyte's polyploid DNA content triggers and controls the enormous synthesis of new membrane which the cell must achieve, just as DNA synthesis in diploid cells triggers and controls membrane synthesis in dividing cells.

In the rodent, electron microscopy has demonstrated extensions of mature megakaryocyte cytoplasm into marrow sinusoids (43). From these extensions, individual platelets may be released or larger portions of cytoplasm may break off to fragment subsequently into individual platelets in the venous circulation or perhaps in the small vessels of the lung. Apparently some megakaryocytes escape into the circulation as whole cells to release their platelets elsewhere, presumably in the lung. The percentage of megakaryocytes which migrate in this fashion to produce platelets outside the marrow is unknown.

As is true with other blood elements, homeostatic control mechanisms exist to regulate the rate of platelet production. If an animal is made acutely thrombocytopenic either by injection of antiplatelet antibody or by exchange transfusion with platelet-poor blood, there is a lag period before platelet production increases (44). The lag period occurs because the control mechanisms exert their activity by influencing the stem cells and those precursors of the megakaryoblast which cannot be recognized morphologically. After that lag period, increasing numbers of stem cells have differentiated into megakaryocytes, and these megakaryocytes mature to produce platelets at a faster than normal rate. These megakaryocytes have an increased degree of ploidy and larger size. It seems likely that these two changes are related; the volume of mature megakaryocyte cytoplasm is proportional to the degree of ploidy achieved when the cell is immature. These large megakaryocytes apparently produce a large platelet with increased hemostatic capability; this fact will be considered subsequently. The reverse occurs when thrombocytosis is induced artificially with platelet transfusions (45). Decreased numbers of small megakaryocytes with decreased ploidy are produced.

The mechanisms by which this homeostatic control is achieved have not yet been clarified. The plasma of animals made thrombocytopenic has in it material which stimulates platelet production by animals who receive it intravenously. This effect can be detected with certainty only when the recipient animals have been made thrombocytotic by platelet transfusion and when platelet production is monitored by detecting the incorporation of a radioactive precursor, such as ^{35}S-sulfate (46) or ^{75}Se-selenomethionine (47), into circulating platelets. Lesser amounts of this material are present in normal plasma and plasma from thrombocytotic animals. This material has been called "thrombopoietin," but its chemical nature, site of synthesis, and mode of action are unknown. Studies in this field are complicated by nonspecific, nonhomeostatic mechanisms by which platelet production is influenced. For example, thrombocytosis is common in patients with a wide variety of inflammatory states and malignancy, while platelet production is decreased during some viremias.

Most current evidence suggests that the

human platelet, newly released from the marrow, is destined to survive in the circulation for eight to ten days (Fig. 20–5). After this time, it is removed from the circulation because of its senescence; i.e., it dies of "old age." The sites of removal are not known with certainty, but body surface scanning after infusion of ^{51}Cr-labeled platelets suggests that the liver and spleen are primarily responsible (48). The critical factors in the aging process are unknown. There is considerable evidence that the platelet decreases in size and in hemostatic capacity as it circulates (49); it seems certain that other metabolic capacities related to viability are lost as well. Several investigators have taken advantage of the large size of young platelets by using an increase in platelet size to suggest a shortened platelet life span in patients (50). In the future, it is hoped that other metabolic measurements characteristic of platelet youth can be used in a similar fashion. Superimposed upon this aging process, there is almost certainly a component of random loss, independent of age, as platelets are consumed to meet the day-to-day hemostatic needs of the body (51). In normal humans, the proportion of

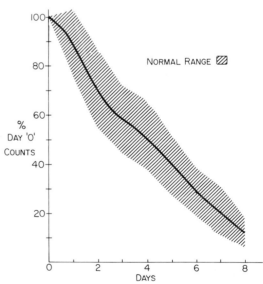

Figure 20–5. Platelet life span in normal man. After in vitro labeling with sodium chromate (^{51}Cr) and reinfusion, platelet-bound radioactivity disappears from the circulation over the next eight to ten days. The pattern of linear decay suggests that most platelets leave the circulation because they age and become nonviable. Undoubtedly, there is a small component of random loss due to utilization in ongoing hemostasis.

the platelet mass which is consumed in this fashion is disputed, since different methods of measuring platelet life span suggest differing values for the amount of random loss. This dispute cannot be resolved with the techniques currently available.

The role of the spleen in platelet kinetics is complex (52). Of the total body platelet mass in normal humans, 65 per cent is in the circulating blood volume, while platelets residing temporarily in the spleen are there in addition to what one would predict on the basis of splenic blood volume. They remain viable and interchange freely and frequently with platelets in the general circulation. In patients with splenomegaly, the percentage of the total body platelet mass which resides in this splenic pool increases in proportion to the size of the spleen. This phenomenon accounts in part for the peripheral thrombocytopenia seen in these patients.

There is suggestive evidence that the splenic pool (53) is relatively rich in younger and larger platelets when compared to the general circulating population. Studies in experimental animals suggest that this is particularly true for the large platelet produced prematurely by the large megakaryocyte under the stress of thrombocytopenia. A teleologic purpose for these splenic functions is not apparent at this time.

Unlike leukocytes, platelets do not marginate near the endothelium in the microcirculation, and there is no pool of platelets in the marrow. Thus, aside from the splenic pool, there is no platelet reserve to compensate for peripheral depletion.

THE THROMBOCYTOPENIC STATE

As discussed previously, the bleeding time is the most reliable and sensitive method for assessing in vivo platelet function. If platelet production is depressed, as in aplastic anemia (Fig. 20–6), the bleeding time becomes prolonged at platelet counts of less than 100,000 per mm³ and markedly prolonged below 20,000 per mm³ (40). Therefore, platelet plug formation is measurably defective with platelet counts in the range of 20,000 to 100,000 per mm³, but cli-

nicians recognize that spontaneous hemorrhage is rare in this range, and major surgical procedures, such as splenectomy, can be carried out without difficulty and without the support of platelet transfusions. Clinicians also agree that the patient with a platelet count of less than 5,000 per mm³ is at a very great risk from life-threatening hemorrhage, while the patient at 20,000 per mm³ is, in general, quite safe in spite of the fact that platelet plug formation as measured by the bleeding time is markedly defective at both levels. This clinical finding has led to the hypothesis that platelets perform a function beyond that of forming plugs, the so-called "endothelial supporting function" (54). The best experimental evidence for this concept comes from work with isolated, perfused organs which develop endothelial damage and edema if the perfusate is plasma containing no platelets (55). When the perfusate is plasma containing platelets, these changes are markedly delayed, and the preservation of organ integrity is prolonged. Plasma with platelet counts as low as 10,000 per mm³ adequately performs this function. The nature of this function has not been further defined.

Another important parameter in the understanding of the thrombocytopenic state is the relative age of the circulating platelet population. If thrombocytopenia is due to a thrombocytolytic process, or if the platelet count is rising after a period of marrow sup-

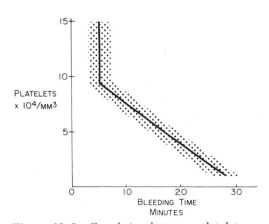

Figure 20–6. Correlation between platelet count and bleeding time in aplastic anemia. The template Ivy bleeding time is the most sensitive index of impaired platelet function. As the platelet count falls, the bleeding time is progressively prolonged. (From Harker, L. A., and Slichter, S. J.: New Engl. J. Med. 287:155, 1972.)

pression, the circulating platelet population will be relatively young, and at any level of platelet count, the bleeding time will be shorter and the hemorrhagic tendency less than if the platelet count is falling or stable at a low level due to marrow suppression (40, 53).

PLATELET IMMUNOLOGY

The platelet surface membrane contains multiple antigens which fix complement in the presence of appropriate specific antibodies. These include the histocompatibility antigens (the HL-A series), shared with many other cell types, and other antigens found only on platelets. Traditionally, HL-A typing has been carried out by lymphocyte cytotoxicity assays, but it is now clear that platelet complement fixation assays can be used as well (56). This finding has had an important clinical application. Thrombocytopenic patients, isoimmunized and refractory to platelet transfusions after multiple transfusions from random donors, will respond to platelet transfusions from HL-A-matched siblings (57). We assume from this fact that the antibodies responsible for isoimmunization in these patients are directed against histocompatibility antigens.

The antigen, P1^{A1}, found only on platelets, has considerable clinical importance. Approximately 2 per cent of the population lacks this antigen. Most of the patients with post-transfusion purpura have had a circulating, complement fixing antibody against P1^{A1} in their sera during the thrombocytopenic phase of their illness, and all have had P1^{A1}-negative platelets after recovery (58). One half of the mothers of infants with isoimmune neonatal thrombocytopenia are P1^{A1}-negative, while the affected infants are P1^{A1}-positive (58). Antibodies against this antigen cross the placenta to produce thrombocytopenia in the infant. These antibodies do not fix complement themselves, but they can be detected because they block complement fixation by the antibodies found in patients with post-transfusion purpura. We assume that P1^{A1} must be a particularly strong antigen, since it accounts for such a large percentage of these cases.

Other antigens unique to platelets have been described, but they have not been of great clinical significance.

Unfortunately, only one in vitro technique for demonstrating the interaction between antibody and platelet antigens has stood the test of time. This technique detects the fixation of complement by the subsequent inhibition of lysis of sensitized sheep red cells (58). Using these methods, antibodies can be detected in most of the patients with post-transfusion purpura and quinidine purpura, 50 per cent of mothers of newborns with isoimmune thrombocytopenia, and approximately 10 per cent of multiply transfused patients (59). Unfortunately, complement fixing antibodies are not found in most patients refractory to platelet transfusions, and they are never found in idiopathic thrombocytopenic purpura or in thrombocytopenic patients with lymphoma or systemic lupus erythematosus. To further our understanding of the latter states, there is a great need for other types of assays based on immunologic principles other than complement fixation which will reproducibly detect the antiplatelet factors which mediate these pathologic processes. One assay based on the capacity of antibody-coated platelets to stimulate lymphocyte division may have broad applicability (60).

PLATELETS IN CHILDREN

Platelet number and function are similar in children and adults, with the exception of observations in the newborn period. It has been reported (61) that platelet counts are often normally very low in premature infants weighing less than 1700 g, but more recent studies suggest that counts under 100,000 per mm^3 are unusual and suggest pathology (62). Although platelet numbers are normal in full-term newborns, there are several reports of abnormal in vitro function. Corby and Schulman (63) reported that newborn platelets aggregated poorly with epinephrine and collagen, suggesting a defective release reaction. They also pointed out that the antenatal administration to pregnant women of drugs such as aspirin and promethazine hydrochloride (Phenergan) markedly impaired newborn platelet aggregation.

References

1. White, J. G., and Krivit, W.: An ultrastructural basis for the shape changes induced in platelets by chilling. Blood 30:625–635, 1967.
2. Born, G. V. R.: Observations on the change in shape of blood platelets brought about by adenosine diphosphate. J. Physiol. (Lond.) 209:487–511, 1970.
3. Murphy, S., and Gardner, F. H.: Platelet preservation; effect of storage temperature on maintenance of platelet viability—deleterious effect of refrigerated storage. New Engl. J. Med. 280:1094–1098, 1969.
4. White, J. G.: Interaction of membrane systems in blood platelets. Am. J. Pathol. 66:295–342, 1972.
5. Day, H. J., Holmsen, H., et al.: Subcellular particles of human platelets. Scand. J. Haematol. (Suppl. 7):1–35, 1969.
6. Murphy, S., and Gardner, F. H.: Platelet storage at 22° C; metabolic, morphologic, and functional studies. J. Clin. Invest. 50:370–377, 1971.
7. Karpatkin, S., and Langer, R. M.: Biochemical energetics of simulated platelet plug formation; effect of thrombin, adenosine diphosphate, and epinephrine on intra- and extracellular adenine nucleotide kinetics. J. Clin. Invest. 47:2158–2168, 1968.
8. Chaudhry, A. A., Meta, E. E., et al.: Effect of aggregating agents on the pentose phosphate pathway (PPP) of human platelets. Am. Soc. Hematol., Thirteenth Annual Meeting, Abstract 87, 1970.
9. Warshaw, A. L., Laster, L., et al.: The stimulation by thrombin of glucose oxidation in human platelets. J. Clin. Invest. 45:1923–1934, 1966.
10. Cohen, P., and Wittels, B.: Energy substrate metabolism in fresh and stored human platelets. J. Clin. Invest. 49:119–127, 1970.
11. Marcus, A. J., Ullman, H. L., et al.: Lipid composition of subcellular particles of human blood platelets. J. Lipid Res. 10:108–114, 1969.
12. Cohen, P.: Relationship between membrane function and permeability. I. Similarity of "platelet factor-3" availability in pure erythrocyte and pure platelet suspensions. Br. J. Haematol. 13:739–745, 1967.
13. Majerus, P. W., Smith, M. B., et al.: Lipid metabolism in human platelets. I. Evidence for a complete fatty acid synthesizing system. J. Clin. Invest. 48:156–164, 1969.
14. Lewis, N., and Majerus, P. W.: Lipid metabolism in human platelets. II. De novo phospholipid synthesis and the effect of thrombin on the pattern of synthesis. J. Clin. Invest. 48:2114–2123, 1969.
15. Clausen, J., and Srivastava, K. C.: The synthesis of prostaglandins in human platelets. Lipids 7:246–250, 1972.
16. Silver, M. J., Smith, J. B., et al.: Human blood prostaglandins: Formation during clotting. Prostaglandins 1:429–436, 1972.
17. Smith, J. B., and Willis, A. L.: Aspirin selectively inhibits prostaglandin production in human platelets. Nature [New Biol.] 231:235–237, 1971.
18. Shio, H., and Ramwell, P.: Effect of prostaglandin E$_2$ and aspirin on the secondary aggregation of human platelets. Nature [New Biol.] 236:45–46, 1972.
19. Booyse, F. M., Hoveke, T. P., et al.: Studies on human platelets. II. Protein synthetic activity of various platelet populations. Biochim. Biophys. Acta 157:660–663, 1968.
20. Zucker-Franklin, D., and Grusky, G.: The actin and myosin filaments of human and bovine blood platelets. J. Clin. Invest. 51:419–430, 1972.
21. Nachman, R. L., Marcus, A. J., et al.: Platelet thrombosthenin: Subcellular localization and function. J. Clin. Invest. 46:1380–1389, 1967.
22. Walsh, P. N.: Albumin density gradient separation and washing of platelets and the study of platelet coagulant activities. Br. J. Haematol. 22:205–217, 1972.
23. Nachman, R. L., Marcus, A. J., et al.: Immunologic studies of proteins associated with subcellular fractions of normal human platelets. J. Lab. Clin. Med. 69:651–658, 1967.
24. Nachman, R. L., and Marcus, A. J.: Immunological studies of proteins associated with the subcellular fractions of thrombasthenic and afibrinogenaemic platelets. Br. J. Haematol. 15:181–189, 1968.
25. Jamieson, G. A., Urban, C. L., et al.: Enzymatic basis for platelet:collagen adhesion as the primary step in haemostasis. Nature [New Biol.] 234:5–7, 1971.
26. Baumgartner, H. R., and Haudenschild, C.: Adhesion of platelets to subendothelium. Ann. N.Y. Acad. Sci. 201:22–36, 1972.
27. Holmsen, H., Day, H. J., et al.: Adenine nucleotide metabolism of blood platelets. VI. Subcellular localization of nucleotide pools with different functions in the platelet release reaction. Biochim. Biophys. Acta 186:254–266, 1969.
28. Holmsen, H., and Weiss, H. J.: Further evidence for a deficient storage pool of adenine nucleotides in platelets from some patients with thrombocytopathia—"storage pool disease." Blood 39:197–209, 1972.
29. Holmsen, H., and Day, H. J.: The selectivity of the thrombin-induced platelet release reaction: Subcellular localization of released and retained constituents. J. Lab. Clin. Med. 75:840–855, 1970.
30. White, J. G.: Fine structural alterations induced in platelets by adenosine diphosphate. Blood 31:604–622, 1968.
31. Salzman, E. W.: Cyclic AMP and platelet function. New Engl. J. Med. 286:358–363, 1972.
32. Droller, M. J., and Wolfe, S. M.: Thrombin-induced increase in intracellular cyclic 3′,5′-adenosine monophosphate in human platelets. J. Clin. Invest. 51:3094–3103, 1972.
33. Marcus, A. J., Zucker-Franklin, D., et al.: Studies of human platelet granules and membranes. J. Clin. Invest. 45:14–28, 1966.
34. Born, G. V. R., and Cross, M. J.: The aggregation of blood platelets. J. Physiol. (Lond.) 168:178–195, 1963.
35. Born, G. V. R., and Hume, M.: Effects of the

numbers and sizes of platelet aggregates on the optical density of plasma. Nature (Lond.) 215:1027–1029, 1967.

36. Hardisty, R. M., Hutton, R. A., et al.: Secondary platelet aggregation: A quantitative study. Br. J. Haematol. 19:307–319, 1970.

37. Weiss, H. J., and Rogers, J.: Thrombocytopathia due to abnormalities in platelet release reaction—Studies on six unrelated patients. Blood 39:187–196, 1972.

38. Coller, B. A., and Zucker, M. B.: Reversible decrease in platelet retention by glass bead columns (adhesiveness) induced by disturbing the blood. Proc. Soc. Exp. Biol. Med. 136:769–771, 1971.

39. Weiss, H. J.: von Willebrand's disease—Diagnostic criteria. Blood 32:668–679, 1968.

40. Harker, L. A., and Slichter, S. J.: The bleeding time as a screening test for evaluation of platelet function. New Engl. J. Med. 287:155–159, 1972.

41. Ebbe, S.: Megakaryocytopoiesis, In Regulation of Hematopoiesis. Vol. 2. Gordon, A. S. (ed.), New York, Appleton-Century-Crofts, 1970, pp. 1587–1610.

42. Behnke, O.: An electron microscope study of the megacaryocyte of the rat bone marrow. I. The development of the demarcation membrane system and the platelet surface coat. J. Ultrastruct. Res. 24:412–433, 1968.

43. Behnke, O.: An electron microscope study of the rat megacaryocyte. II. Some aspects of platelet release and microtubules. J. Ultrastruct. Res. 26:111–129, 1969.

44. Ebbe, S., Stohlman, F., Jr., et al.: Megakaryocyte size in thrombocytopenic and normal rats. Blood 32:383–392, 1968.

45. Harker, L. A.: Kinetics of thrombopoiesis. J. Clin. Invest. 47:458–465, 1968.

46. Harker, L. A.: Regulation of thrombopoiesis. Am J. Physiol. 218:1376–1380, 1970.

47. Shreiner, D. P., and Levin, J.: Detection of thrombopoietic activity in plasma by stimulation of suppressed thrombopoiesis. J. Clin. Invest. 49:1709–1713, 1970.

48. Aster, R. H.: Studies of the fate of platelets in rats and man. Blood 34:117–128, 1969.

49. Karpatkin, S.: Heterogeneity of human platelets. I. Metabolic and kinetic evidence suggestive of young and old platelets. J. Clin. Invest. 48:1073–1082, 1969.

50. Garg, S. K., Amorosi, E. L., et al.: Use of the megathrombocyte as an index of megakaryocyte number. New Engl. J. Med. 284:11–17, 1971.

51. Murphy, E. A., and Francis, M. E.: The estimation of blood platelet survival. II. The multiple hit model. Thromb. Diath. Haemorrh. 25:53–80, 1971.

52. Jandl, J. H., and Aster, R. H.: Increased splenic pooling and the pathogenesis of hypersplenism. Am. J. Med. Sci. 253:383–397, 1967.

53. Shulman, N. R., Watkins, S. P., Jr., et al.: Evidence that the spleen retains the youngest and hemostatically most effective platelets. Trans. Assoc. Am. Physicians 81:302–313, 1968.

54. Wojcik, J. D., Van Horn, D. L., et al.: Mechanism whereby platelets support the endothelium. Transfusion 9:324–335, 1969.

55. Gimbrone, M. S., Aster, R. H., et al.: Preservation of vascular integrity in organs perfused in vitro with a platelet rich medium. Nature (Lond.) 222:33, 1969.

56. Svejgaard, A., and Kissmeyer-Neilsen, F.: Complement-fixing platelet isoantibodies. Vox Sang. 18:12–20, 1970.

57. Yankee, R. A., Grumet, F. C., et al.: Platelet transfusion therapy; the selection of compatible platelet donors for refractory patients by lymphocyte HL-A typing. New Engl. J. Med. 281:1208–1212, 1969.

58. Shulman, N. R., Marder, V. J., et al.: Platelet and leukocyte isoantigens and their antibodies: Serologic, physiologic and clinical studies, In Progress in Hematology. Vol. IV. Moore, C. V., and Brown, E. B. (eds.), New York, Grune & Stratton, 1964, pp. 222–304.

59. Aster, R. H., Levin, R. H., et al.: Complement-fixing platelet iso-antibodies in serum of transfused persons. Correlation of antibodies with platelet survival in thrombocytopenic persons. Transfusion 4:428–440, 1964.

60. Handin, R. I., Piessens, W. F., et al.: Stimulation of non-immunized lymphocytes by platelet-antibody complexes in idiopathic thrombocytopenic purpura. New Engl. J. Med. 289:714–718, 1973.

61. Medoff, H. S.: Platelet counts in premature infants. J. Pediatr. 64:287–289, 1964.

62. Aballi, A. J., Puapondh, Y., et al.: Platelet counts in thriving premature infants. Pediatrics 42:685–689, 1968.

63. Corby, D. G., and Schulman, I.: The effects of antenatal drug administration on aggregation of platelets of newborn infants. J. Pediatr. 79:307–313, 1971.

Chapter 21

Clinical Disorders of the Platelets

by Irving Schulman

THROMBOCYTOPENIAS

Thrombocytopenia Due to Excessive Platelet Destruction

Idiopathic Thrombocytopenic Purpura

The term "idiopathic thrombocytopenic purpura" (ITP) has traditionally been used to define an acquired hemorrhagic state due to a marked reduction of the circulating platelet count in the presence of a normal marrow and the absence of associated systemic disease. Continuing observations have indicated the validity of identifying two major groups: (1) acute ITP, characterized by an abrupt onset and a very high rate of rapid, complete, and permanent recovery, occurring primarily in children (1–7); and (2) chronic ITP, characterized by a relatively insidious onset and a very low rate of spontaneous recovery, occurring primarily in adults (8–12). The finding, by recently developed techniques, that the majority of individuals with chronic ITP has demonstrable antiplatelet antibodies (13, 14) has suggested that this group should no longer be designated as "idiopathic" but rather diagnosed as having "autoimmune thrombocytopenic purpura" (15). At present, immunologic data relating to ITP in childhood are insufficient to warrant such a designation. Moreover, while studies of large groups of children with ITP have provided firm statistics concerning prognosis, it is not possible to predict in the individual child, at the outset of the disease, whether the disorder will follow the acute or chronic course.

AGE, SEX, AND RACE. ITP in children may occur at any age, but is most frequent between the ages of two and six years. The disorder occurs with equal frequency in boys and girls in contrast to the situation in adults, in whom there is a 3:1 predominance in women. In childhood, ITP appears to be less common in black than in white children, even when the fact that purpura is more difficult to observe in the former group is taken into account.

PRECEDING ILLNESS. Antecedent febrile illness has been reported in 50 per cent to 85 per cent of children with ITP, with the incidence depending upon the definition of "significant" illness, the effort expended in history taking, and the interval of time between the previous illness and the onset of ITP that the investigator accepts as indicating a possible relationship. Of those with prior illnesses, approximately one-third have had definite exanthemata (rubella, rubeola, varicella). The remaining two-thirds usually have demonstrated symptoms of upper respiratory infections or vaguely defined febrile illness. Prior immunization, gastroenteritis, and bacterial infections have also been implicated in rare instances. While the reported interval of time between the prior illness and the onset of ITP has ranged from a few days to as long as six weeks, the most common interval is two to three weeks.

Both the frequency of ITP and the seasonal incidence appear to vary considerably from year to year and from one locale to another, presumably representing the occurrence rate of viral illness in the community. In most large series, the disorder has been most frequent in winter and spring.

CLINICAL MANIFESTATIONS. Easy bruising and the sudden spontaneous development of cutaneous petechiae and ecchymoses are the presenting manifestations in the majority of children. Approximately one-third of patients present with epistaxis, usually in association with purpura. Hematuria, melena, and bleeding from oral mucous membranes may also be seen, but are relatively infrequent in children. Central nervous system hemorrhage is exceedingly rare, occurring in less than 1 per cent of patients in several large series (6, 7, 16). When it does occur, it is likely to appear during the first week of illness.

Physical examination is usually normal apart from the skin and mucous membranes, and the child rarely appears ill. Hepatosplenomegaly of significant degree does not occur in ITP, and the finding of enlargement of these organs should immediately suggest an alternative diagnosis. The tip of the spleen has been found to be palpable in 5 to 10 per cent of children with ITP, a frequency similar to that which may be detected in normal children of similar age examined with equal care.

LABORATORY FINDINGS. At the time of onset, when spontaneously developing petechiae and ecchymoses are evident, platelet counts are usually less than 20,000 per mm.³ On peripheral smear, platelet clumps are rarely found, and the single platelets are commonly large and bizarre in shape. The total leukocyte count is usually normal, and a mild to moderate lymphocytosis is frequent. Slight eosinophilia has been noted in some series, but is not a constant finding and appears to bear no relationship to etiology or prognosis. The degree of anemia is related to the amount of blood loss.

Marrow examination is essential to exclude other causes of thrombocytopenia. In ITP, megakaryocytes are numerous and on occasion appear to be enormously increased. They appear round and smooth and seem to be devoid of surrounding collars of platelets. This appearance, which in the past was interpreted as signifying impaired platelet production, is now believed to represent an increase in the pool of young megakaryocytes involved in the rapid platelet turnover in response to peripheral platelet destruction.

Other laboratory tests (bleeding time, clot retraction, tourniquet test) merely reflect the thrombocytopenia and are rarely needed. Recent observations by Harker and Slichter (17) have demonstrated that, for any given platelet count, the bleeding time in ITP tends to be shorter than that found in patients whose thrombocytopenia results from failure of production of platelets. This presumably results from the fact that in ITP young, large, and functionally more active platelets are released in response to the thrombopenia.

CLINICAL COURSE, NATURAL HISTORY, AND PROGNOSIS. The natural history of ITP in childhood must be appreciated if indications for, and results of, various forms of treatment are to be judged. At least 80 per cent of children with ITP will achieve a complete and permanent recovery in the absence of any specific treatment. In a large series reported by Lusher and Zuelzer, 92.6 per cent of children recovered completely (6). Of those who recover, 50 per cent do so within four weeks from the time of onset, and 85 per cent within four months. Most of the remainder (of those who will ultimately recover) achieve remission within a year, although individual instances of recovery occurring as long as several years after onset have been reported. A small percentage of children demonstrate recurrent episodes of thrombocytopenia and purpura after achieving a normal platelet count. The recurrences commonly follow infections and usually remit spontaneously. Some episodes, considered to represent recurrent purpura, may in fact be the result of a fall in platelet count coincident with cessation of steroid therapy (see below). In other words, the initial disease process still existed, but the platelet count had been raised by the steroid therapy.

It is the general experience that the bleeding tendency in ITP is most severe during the first days or week after onset and then abates markedly, even though the platelet count has not changed significantly. This amelioration of the bleeding tendency may result from the production of younger and functionally more active platelets, as described previously.

As indicated earlier, central nervous hemorrhage is very rare, and overall mortality in recent large series has been significantly less than 1 per cent.

The definition of when ITP in childhood should be designated as chronic is, at best, arbitrary. As described above, at least 85 to 90 per cent of children will recover completely within a year, and the disease is traditionally classified as chronic after that time. However, although spontaneous recovery after one year is relatively rare, instances of complete cure as long as 3½ years after onset have been reported (16).

TREATMENT. In view of the extremely favorable outlook for children with ITP, the indications for any mode of therapy must be considered carefully. Most controversy centers about the use of corticosteroids, despite the fact that most workers are in accord about results obtained when they are employed. There is complete agreement that the use of corticosteroids does not improve the prognosis for complete and permanent recovery. There is also agreement that their use does not accelerate the rate at which recovery occurs. On the other hand, there is evidence to indicate that corticosteroid therapy may elevate the platelet count in children with ITP, albeit temporarily. The frequency with which steroid therapy is followed by a significant rise in platelet count is difficult to estimate, since marked variation in dosage and regimen is to be found in most reported studies. Available data suggest that, when prednisone in a dose of 1 to 2 mg. per kg. per day is utilized early in the disease, approximately 60 per cent of children will demonstrate a substantial rise in platelet count within one to three weeks. In one-third of these, elevation of platelet count persists, and complete recovery is evident when steroids are discontinued (doubtless due to spontaneous recovery). In the other two-thirds, the platelet count returns to thrombocytopenic levels when steroids are discontinued. There is no correlation between the response to the prednisone therapy, at the doses indicated, and the ultimate prognosis for complete recovery. There is now evidence to suggest that the major effect of corticosteroids is to block removal of antibody-coated platelets from the circulation by the reticuloendothelial system (18), and that children whose platelet counts are not raised by 1 to 2 mg. per kg. per day of prednisone may, in fact, show a response to a higher dose. Thus, in a recent small series we have observed a rise in platelet count in one week in 80 per cent of children given 4 mg. per kg. per day of prednisone for three days, followed by 2 mg. per kg. per day thereafter (19). That these responses did not represent spontaneous remission was indicated by the return of thrombocytopenia when prednisone was discontinued after three weeks. In addition to their effects on platelet number, there is some evidence to indicate that corticosteroids ameliorate the bleeding tendency in thrombocytopenic states by a direct effect on the vasculature (20–22).

On the other hand, a specific hazard accompanies the use of corticosteroids in ITP, apart from their general side effects (23). Cohen and Gardner (23a) demonstrated, in adults, that sustained high-dose corticosteroid therapy could suppress platelet formation and prevent remission from occurring; we have seen similar instances in children, in whom presumed chronic ITP was "cured" by the cessation of steroid therapy which had been administered for several months. We have not seen this complication when prednisone therapy has been given for one month or less.

It would appear that the decision to utilize corticosteroid therapy in ITP of childhood should stem from the desire to decrease the bleeding tendency in the early days of the disease, either by raising the platelet count or by improving vascular integrity, while avoiding the possibility of inducing suppression of platelet formation. It is our present policy to employ prednisone, 2 mg. per kg. per day for one week, followed by 1 mg. per kg. per day for two additional weeks, with tapering of the dose and discontinuance of treatment in the fourth week. In the absence of gross bleeding, treatment is halted whether or not a rise in platelet count has occurred. As described before, the platelet count which has risen in response to steroid therapy very commonly falls again when therapy is stopped, and petechiae may reappear. This per se should not prompt reinstitution of therapy, since a rise in platelet count may then occur spontaneously. Unless significant bleeding is seen, it is our policy to withhold additional steroid therapy. Should thrombocytopenia and purpura persist beyond three months, a second course of corticosteroid therapy may be tried, again limited to four weeks. The interval between courses and the limitation in dose and duration of therapy are necessary to avoid the suppressive effects of steroids.

Platelet transfusions are rarely indicated, and their use should be reserved for control of severe bleeding. The platelet count alone should not be used as an indication for platelet transfusion. The in vivo survival of transfused platelets is very short, usually limited to several hours.

While careful observation is necessary during the initial days after the onset of ITP, return to fairly normal activity is permissible when the tendency toward spontaneous hemorrhage abates, despite persisting thrombocytopenia. Body-contact sports should be avoided, but early return to school is desirable.

CHRONIC ITP. Persistence of thrombocytopenia after one year usually indicates chronicity, and spontaneous recovery after this time, while possible, is rare. Although antecedent infection is less common, insidious onset more common, and the incidence in girls slightly greater than in boys in those children who develop chronic ITP when compared with those who recover, no prognostic indices are available for the individual child. The treatment of choice for chronic ITP is splenectomy, and over 70 per cent of children so treated recover completely (6, 7, 16). It is rare that the severity of hemorrhagic manifestations prompts splenectomy; rather it is the ongoing fear of serious hemorrhage, on the part of parent and physician, and the desire to return the child to a more normal life, that finally recommends the operation. While there is some evidence to suggest that children who have responded to prior steroid therapy are more likely to achieve lasting benefit from splenectomy than those who have not, exceptions in both groups are sufficiently common to preclude use of the response to steroids as a criterion for operation. Other methods seeking to predict benefit or failure from splenectomy have involved body surface scanning after infusion of isotopically labeled platelets in order to determine whether the spleen or the liver is the major site of platelet destruction. Here, too, the predictability of the test has not been exacting enough to warrant its routine use in selecting patients for surgery (18, 24, 25).

Following splenectomy, a postoperative rise in platelet count is seen in virtually every patient, with the peak rise occurring in 4 to 14 days. Patients whose platelet counts reach 500,000 per mm.[3] in the post-operative period tend to have a better likelihood of permanent benefit than those whose maximum rise fails to reach this level. Some children may develop a postoperative thrombocytosis exceeding one million per mm.[3], but this is transient and anticoagulation is not needed.

The risk of postsplenectomy sepsis and meningitis is very low in ITP (26), and routine prophylaxis with penicillin is not recommended. However, febrile illnesses in the splenectomized child must be observed and treated promptly, and alertness to the possibility of septicemia and meningitis, predominantly pneumococcal, must be maintained.

The children whose platelet counts fail to return to normal levels after splenectomy may, nevertheless, demonstrate significant improvement in the bleeding tendency after the operation. This may result from an actual increase in platelet count over preoperative levels, and also from the fact that removal of the spleen permits a younger and more active population of platelets to circulate.

Immunosuppressive therapy has been used in treatment of children whose thrombocytopenia persists despite splenectomy (27–30). Most trials have utilized azathioprine and corticosteroids in combination, and approximately one-third of children so treated were considered to have shown benefit. In most studies, many months of treatment were necessary before a rise in platelet count was evident, and in the majority a return to prior levels was seen as immunosuppressive therapy was discontinued. Actinomycin C (31), cyclophosphamide (32), and, most recently, vinblastine (33) have been used in the treatment of chronic ITP refractory to splenectomy, with some benefit reported with each. In view of the growing concern about an increased incidence of malignancies in patients subjected to long-term immunosuppression, and of the evidence of gonadal damage attributed to cyclophosphamide therapy (34), use of immunosuppressive drugs in the management of chronic ITP should at present be restricted to those rare children who fail to respond to splenectomy and continue to show a significant bleeding tendency thereafter.

ETIOLOGY AND PATHOGENESIS OF ITP. Studies by Harrington et al. in 1951 demonstrated conclusively the existence, in the plasma of patients with ITP, of a humoral factor capable of inducing thrombocytopenia when transfused into normal individuals (35). The transmission of this factor across the placenta could explain the clinical observations of the occurrence of neonatal thrombopenia in the infants of mothers with a history of ITP. Many investigations have since demonstrated that the factor is an IgG immunoglobulin, which may be detected by in vitro tests in a high proportion of adults with ITP, as well as systemic lupus erythematosus, rheumatoid arthritis, and other disorders generally classified as autoimmune (13–14). There is no longer any doubt that the thrombocytopenia in ITP results from accelerated platelet destruction. The latter results from accelerated removal of antibody-coated platelets from the circulation by the reticuloendothelial system (18). In most cases the spleen is the major site of sequestration of antibody-coated platelets; in situations in which heavy coating of the platelets by antibody occurs, the liver becomes the primary organ of platelet destruction (18, 25, 36, 37). Splenectomy is beneficial in those circumstances in which the spleen is the primary site of platelet removal, and it may fail to provide improvement when hepatic sequestration is predominant. Corticosteroid therapy in ITP acts to impede removal of antibody-coated platelets from the circulation by suppressing reticuloendothelial function (18).

In adults, in whom the occurrence of ITP is rarely preceded by a precipitating infection, spontaneous recovery is rare, antibody may be detected for many years, and antiplatelet antibody appears capable of coating all platelets, the evidence suggests that the fundamental process is one of autoimmunity. In children with acute ITP, the pathogenesis is not entirely clear. The fact that the thrombocytopenia in children also results from accelerated platelet destruction, rather than from interference with production, is unquestioned (18). However, no systematic study of the incidence of antiplatelet antibodies has as yet been conducted with current techniques in children with acute ITP. The high frequency of antecedent infection in childhood ITP and the very high rate of spontaneous, complete, and permanent recovery indicate fundamental differences between the childhood and adult forms of the disease. The fact that acute ITP onset commonly develops several weeks after antecedent infection suggests that platelet destruction due to direct effect of viruses on platelets is unlikely. On the other hand, the time interval is consistent with the hypothesis that the antibody generated in response to infection may play a role in the pathogenesis of the thrombocytopenia. Experimental studies have demonstrated that a variety of soluble antigen-antibody complexes may induce agglutination, aggregation, and release of constituents in platelets of animals and man (38, 39). In addition, sera of children with postrubella thrombocytopenic purpura have been shown by Myllylä et al. (40) to induce platelet agglutination in the presence of "small-size" rubella antigen in high dilution, whereas sera of children with prior rubella but no subsequent thrombocytopenia demonstrated low titers of the platelet-agglutinating antibody in the presence of the antigen. These workers postulate that both small-size virus antigen and the antibody against it are required to induce postrubella thrombocytopenia purpura, and that the disorder is a result of a "hyperimmune state." Since both small-size antigens and antibody are required, the duration of thrombocytopenia would depend upon the continued presence of both. It is of interest that antibodies capable of inducing platelet aggregation in the presence of small virus antigens were not found in several cases of congenital rubella with thrombocytopenia.

Whether all types of acute ITP are the result of the development of antigen-antibody complexes, which subsequently attach to platelets and thereby cause them to be rapidly removed from the circulation, requires further study.*

Immune Neonatal Thrombocytopenic Purpura

Thrombocytopenia, in the absence of any other systemic disease, may occur in new-

---

*Editor's Note: Recently Handin and Stossel and their co-workers have developed tests for the detection of platelet antibodies in children with ITP. The results show that such antibodies are present in a high proportion of patients (40a, b).

borns of mothers who themselves have had ITP or in those of mothers with no prior history of thrombocytopenic purpura. In the former group, thrombocytopenia in the infant results from transplacental passage of the antiplatelet antibody which produced ITP in the mothers; in the latter group, antiplatelet antibody apparently results from isoimmunization of the mother to the infant's platelets, thus leading to thrombocytopenia in the offspring, but no disorder in the mother.

The incidence of neonatal thrombocytopenia in offspring of mothers who have had ITP appears to depend upon the maternal status at the time of delivery. Thus, thrombocytopenia at birth has been reported in 0 per cent to 20 per cent of infants whose mothers had achieved a normal platelet count following splenectomy and were not thrombocytopenic at time of delivery. On the other hand, the incidence of neonatal thrombocytopenia is 50 per cent to 85 per cent if the mother has remained thrombocytopenic despite splenectomy (41–47). It is likely that both the incidence of thrombocytopenia in the newborns and the response to splenectomy in the mothers represent an index of severity of the maternal disease (i.e., antibody titer).

Isoimmune neonatal thrombocytopenic purpura was estimated by Pearson et al. (48) to occur in approximately one in every 5000 births. The mother is immunized by an antigen present in the fetus's (and the father's) platelets and absent from her own. The firstborn infant is affected in 50 per cent of reported cases. Thrombocytopenia may occur in each succeeding infant. However, instances have been reported in which a subsequent infant has been unaffected despite apparently having the same platelet type as a sibling who was born thrombocytopenic.

In both forms of immune neonatal thrombocytopenia, the infant may appear normal at the moment of birth, but then begin to exhibit petechiae and purpura within minutes to hours after birth. In most instances, hemorrhagic manifestations are limited to the skin; however, large cephalhematomas and bleeding from the nose, gastrointestinal tract, urinary tract, umbilical cord, and skin punctures and into the central nervous system may occur. In general, hemorrhagic manifestations tend to be most severe in the first days of life, then abate despite persistence of thrombocytopenia.

Thrombocytopenia may be documented in the cord blood of affected infants, and platelet counts are usually below 30,000 per mm.³ if spontaneous hemorrhage is evident. White cell and red cell counts are usually normal. Hyperbilirubinemia may develop after 24 hours and is believed to result from breakdown of blood in areas of occult and enclosed hemorrhage. The bilirubin is predominantly unconjugated and may reach levels requiring exchange transfusion for prevention of kernicterus.

Bone marrow examination in the newborn period may create diagnostic difficulties. In most cases, normal or increased numbers of megakaryocytes are seen. However, decreased or even absent megakaryocytes may occur and raise the possibility of congenital amegakaryocytic thrombocytopenia (see below) (48). There is no apparent correlation between the number of megakaryocytes seen in the marrow in immune neonatal thrombocytopenia and the severity or ultimate prognosis of the disease.

Since both forms of immune neonatal thrombocytopenia result from passively acquired antibody, complete recovery from the thrombocytopenia is to be expected. It is generally stated that the duration of thrombocytopenia is shorter in infants with the isoimmune form than in those whose mothers have had ITP. However, there is great variation within each group, so that significant increases in platelet counts may be observed in days or delayed for several months. Most infants with isoimmune neonatal thrombocytopenia reach normal platelet counts within three weeks; those with disease resulting from maternal ITP usually have subnormal platelet counts for more than six weeks (41, 48, 49). Persistence of thrombocytopenia for more than four months should raise questions about the original diagnosis.

The reported prognosis in immune neonatal thrombocytopenia varies considerably in different series. Thus, while the mortality of infants whose mothers have had ITP has been calculated to be about 10 per cent in collected series, Anthony and Krivit have reported 14 consecutive cases with no mortality (47). In isoimmune neonatal thrombocytopenia, the mortality has been estimated to be 14 per cent (48), most due to intracra-

nial hemorrhage. While there is no doubt that
the majority of infants will recover completely in the absence of specific therapy,
the understandable fear of central nervous
system hemorrhage and the reports of significant mortality in some series has
prompted attempts to ameliorate the hemorrhagic tendency. As with ITP, there is
no firm evidence that corticosteroids short-
en the disease in the newborn and very little indication that they promote a significant
rise in platelet count in the infant. That they
decrease the tendency to bleed in the absence of a change in platelet count is
suggested, but certainly not proved. It has
been our policy to employ corticosteroid
therapy in all but the mildest cases. When
purpura appears in the immediate neonatal
period, hydrocortisone, 10 mg. every 12
hours intravenously, has been used for the
first few days, followed by prednisone, 1 to
2 mg. per kg. per day, in divided doses
orally thereafter. Corticosteroid therapy is
limited to three weeks, independent of the
response in platelet count. Pearson et al.
have reported that, in a small series of infants with isoimmune disease, corticosteroids appeared to shorten the duration of
thrombocytopenia when compared to an untreated group (48). They also suggested that
antepartum treatment of the mother may be
of value.

In the event of active bleeding, more vigorous therapy is indicated. Transfusion of
platelet concentrates appears valuable,
even though the in vivo longevity of the
donor platelets is very short in the presence
of antiplatelet antibody. Newborn infants
may be given two platelet packs (i.e., platelets from 1000 ml. of blood), with the transfusion repeated every six to eight hours as
needed. It should be emphasized that
bleeding, not the platelet counts, is an indication for such treatment. In instances of
severe and life-threatening hemorrhage,
and in instances in which prior infants have
manifested serious bleeding, exchange
transfusion with fresh blood has been performed in an attempt to remove antibody
and supply platelets (48, 49). Because of the
variability in the course of infants with neonatal thrombocytopenia, the specific benefit
of exchange transfusion is difficult to evaluate; all observers agree, however, that it
should be reserved for the very severe
cases. In isoimmune neonatal thrombocyto-

penia, washed maternal platelets, obtained
by plasmapheresis, may be of value (50).*

Familial Thrombocytopenic Purpuras

A variety of inherited forms of thrombocytopenia has been described in families. In
general, these have been characterized by
the presence of normal numbers of megakaryocytes in the marrow, shortened survival of autologous platelets, but normal
survival of homologous platelets. Thus, the
thrombocytopenia is probably the result of
the production of intrinsically defective
platelets which have decreased survival in
the circulation. Some of the familial thrombocytopenias are associated with striking morphologic abnormalities of the platelets,
while in others platelet morphology appears
normal. Studies of platelet function indicate
that in some of the inherited thrombocytopenias the platelets which circulate are
functionally impaired, so that the bleeding
tendency may be greater than anticipated
from the platelet count. In general, corticosteroids are of no value, and splenectomy
will, at best, result only in partial improvement in the familial thrombocytopenias. In
some (e.g., Wiskott-Aldrich syndrome), the
hazard of postsplenectomy infection clearly
outweighs any benefit from splenectomy.

SEX-LINKED THROMBOCYTOPENIAS. The
Wiskott-Aldrich syndrome is an immunologic disorder characterized by thrombocytopenia, eczema, and recurrent infections (51–53). Decreased levels of isohemagglutinins are characteristic (54).
Melena commonly occurs during the first
few months of life and may appear in the
neonatal period. Circulating platelets are
abnormally small, and both platelets and
megakaryocytes are structurally abnormal
when examined by electron microscopy
(55). Autologous platelets have a strikingly
short survival, while homologous platelets
survive normally (55–57). Corticosteroids
are of no value, and splenectomy imposes a

*Editor's Note: Our practice is to utilize washed
maternal platelets rather than corticosteroids. There
is strong belief in some quarters that subsequent infants of mothers who have had a previous baby with
isoimmune neonatal thrombocytopenia should be
delivered by cesarean section to avoid possible cerebral bleeding. It is not possible to be dogmatic with
regard to such a recommendation. Clinical data are
not sufficient to permit firm guidelines.

severe risk of overwhelming infection without significantly modifying the thrombocytopenia (57). Sex-linked thrombocytopenia associated with decreased isohemagglutinins and increased IgA, but without eczema and recurrent infections, has been described (58), as has sex-linked thrombocytopenia with normal platelet morphology and without any other manifestations of the Wiskott-Aldrich syndrome (59–61). Finally, a family with sex-linked thrombocytopenia, elevated serum IgA levels, and renal disease has also been reported (62). Whether all of the sex-linked thrombocytopenias represent variants of the Wiskott-Aldrich syndrome remains to be clarified.

AUTOSOMAL DOMINANT THROMBOCYTOPENIA. The *May-Hegglin anomaly* is a form of familial thrombocytopenia associated with giant, often bizarre, platelets and large basophilic inclusion bodies (Döhle bodies) within the cytoplasm of granulocytes (63–65). There are indications that there may be an associated quantitative defect in platelet production and some functional impairment of circulating thrombocytes. Only about one-third of patients demonstrating the May-Hegglin anomaly develop thrombocytopenia and a hemorrhagic state. Familial thrombocytopenia transmitted through autosomal dominant inheritance has also been described with giant platelets, but no granulocyte inclusion bodies (66–68), and with normal platelet morphology (69–73).

AUTOSOMAL RECESSIVE THROMBOCYTOPENIA. Families have been described in whom the thrombocytopenia has been associated with normal platelet morphology (74) and with giant platelets (74). A specific form of familial thrombocytopenia transmitted as an autosomal recessive disorder is the Bernard-Soulier syndrome (75–80). In this disorder, platelets are extremely large and characterized by coalescence of platelet granules to produce a "pseudonucleus," thus causing the platelets to appear "lymphocytoid." Platelet counts may be normal or mildly to severely decreased. A defect in platelet Factor 3 activity has been described (79–80).

Thrombocytopenia Associated with Giant Hemangioma

The association between giant hemangioma and thrombocytopenia was de-

scribed by Kasabach and Merritt in 1940 (81) and has been confirmed on numerous occasions since (82–86). Studies demonstrating accumulation of radioactivity in the hemangiomas following transfusion of ^{51}Cr-labeled platelets have supported the concept that thrombocytopenia results from sequestration and destruction of platelets within the vascular tumor (84, 85, 87, 88). More recent findings of associated depletions of fibrinogen, Factor V, and Factor VIII in some cases indicate that extensive clotting may occur in the vessels of the hemangioma, with resulting consumption of those circulating coagulation factors which are similarly depressed in disseminated intravascular clotting (83, 89–91).

Since the hemangiomas are congenital, bleeding, secondary to thrombocytopenia, may appear in the first days or weeks of life or be delayed for months or even years. Hemangiomas leading to thrombocytopenia are most commonly solitary and large. However, instances have been reported in which the hemangiomas have been relatively small and multiple. Giant hemangiomas are most frequently located on the surface of the body, but may occur anywhere. The pathogenesis of thrombocytopenia in association with visceral hemangiomas may elude detection for significant periods of time until the presence of the vascular tumor is appreciated.

In observing the course of an infant with a giant hemangioma, a fairly typical series of events may be noted which indicates the advent of the associated hemorrhagic state. The hemangioma may suddenly grow much larger, become very hard, develop a purplish hue, and demonstrate ecchymoses in the overlying skin and petechiae in adjacent skin. Shortly thereafter, petechiae may appear at sites distant from the tumor, and marked thrombocytopenia with or without associated coagulation factor depletion will be present on laboratory examination. Recovery from the thrombocytopenia associated with giant hemangioma depends upon shrinkage of the tumor through natural regression or in response to radiation therapy, or its removal by surgery. Since both radiation and surgery pose hazards to young infants, conservative management is to be desired. Therefore, thrombocytopenia in the absence of significant hemorrhagic manifestations need not be taken as an indication for vigorous treatment. Severe bleeding, hemorrhagic enlargement, or rapid enlargement of the tumor in an area (e.g., neck, thorax) where compression of the airway may occur demand that steps be taken to shrink or remove the tumor. Recent reports of the beneficial effects of large doses of corticosteroids in promoting shrinkage of the hemangiomas (92, 93) and the elevation of the platelet count and depleted coagulation factors (94) offer the hope that a relatively conservative form of treatment may permit control of tumor size and hemorrhagic complications in some cases. Heparin therapy has been employed in instances in which laboratory evidence of consumption coagulopathy has been detected (89, 90). While significant elevation of the depleted coagulation factors following adequate heparin dosage is usually seen, the effect on the low platelet count is much less striking. Moreover, the abnormalities in the hemostatic mechanism will almost invariably return to pretreatment levels as soon as heparin is discontinued. These considerations, plus the fact that very large doses of heparin are sometimes required to promote improvement in laboratory values, suggest that heparinization should be employed only on rare occasions (severe hemorrhage with clear-cut evidence of consumption coagulapathy) and with great caution.

Thrombocytopenia With Splenic Enlargement

Thrombocytopenia may be associated with splenomegaly of virtually any cause. While the mechanism of the "hypersplenism" has long been debated, it now seems probable that increased splenic pooling of platelets is the cause of the thrombocytopenia. This conclusion has been suggested by studies which have revealed a very low recovery of transfused ^{51}Cr-labeled platelets, but a normal or only slightly decreased survival of the platelets in the circulation (95, 96). It has been calculated that, in thrombocytopenia resulting from splenomegaly, as much as 90 per cent of the total platelet mass may be pooled in the spleen at any one time, as contrasted with the normal state, in which about one-third of the platelets may be found in the spleen. Following transfusion, only 10 to 30 per cent of labeled

normal platelets may be recovered in recipients with significant splenomegaly, in comparison with 60 to 75 per cent recovery in normal recipients. In asplenic individuals, 90 to 100 per cent of transfused platelets can be recovered (96, 97). Studies have indicated that the thrombocytopenia associated with splenomegaly does not result from excessive destruction of platelets in the large splenic pool but rather from their very slow passage through the enlarged organ.

In children, conditions likely to lead to "hypersplenic" thrombocytopenia include portal hypertension due to cirrhosis or portal vein thrombosis; infiltrative diseases, such as Gaucher's disease, Niemann-Pick disease, and Hand-Schüller-Christian disease; lymphomas; congenital hemolytic syndromes (sickle cell disease, thalassemia, spherocytosis); splenic vein thrombosis; and myeloproliferative disease (98, 99).

Thrombocytopenia due to splenic enlargement is likely to be associated with neutropenia and hemolytic anemia of variable degree. The thrombocytopenia tends to be moderate in degree (usually greater than 50,000 per mm.³) and rarely produces significant hemorrhagic symptoms. Anemia and increased transfusion requirement, rather than hemorrhage, usually prompt consideration of splenectomy. Removal of the enlarged spleen will usually correct the thrombocytopenia completely, but the operation should be considered in terms of the underlying cause of the splenomegaly, the jeopardy of subsequent infection, and the overall benefit or lack thereof to the patient.

Drug-related Immune Thrombocytopenias

Acute thrombocytopenia may occur in individuals following reexposure to drugs to which they previously have been sensitized. This phenomenon was first described following oral ingestion of quinine (100), but the list of drugs believed to be associated with accelerated platelet destruction on an immunologic basis has enlarged rapidly and now includes quinidine, digitoxin, chlorothiazide derivatives, sulfonamide derivatives, meprobamate, phenylbutazone, and para-aminosalicylic acid, among many others (101). It was originally postulated that sensitization followed fixation of the offending drug to the platelet and the development of an antibody directed against the platelet-drug antigenic complex (102). More recent studies indicate that the platelet itself is not involved in the genesis of the antibody but rather is the specific cell to which the drug-antibody complex becomes affixed (103–106). Damage to the platelets through subsequent complement fixation, agglutination, or lysis leads to their ultimate accelerated destruction (106–113). Thrombocytopenia develops only in the presence of the drug in an immunized individual, and normal platelet counts will return when the drug is completely eliminated, even though the specific antibody may be shown to persist. The interaction between the offending drug-specific antibody (in the patient's serum) and normal platelets forms the basis of a variety of in vitro tests whereby drug-related immunologic purpura may be diagnosed. Various tests have been described which depend upon the demonstration of some alteration of the normal platelets or their function in the presence of the drug and the specific antibody—e.g., impaired clot retraction, platelet agglutination, lysis or aggregation, complement fixation, or platelet injury (platelet Factor 3 release) (107, 110, 113–118). Skin tests for detection of specific drug sensitivity are unreliable. Administration of the suspected drug, even as a challenge, may be extremely dangerous since severe thrombocytopenia may develop within hours, even after a very small dose.

Once drug-related immune thrombocytopenia develops, the most important aspect of treatment is removal of the offending agent. Corticosteroids may ameliorate the bleeding manifestations during the acute phase but have no influence on the rate of recovery, which depends upon the rapidity with which the involved drug is eliminated. Platelet transfusions are of little benefit, since the donor platelets are affected by the drug-antibody complex, as are the patient's own platelets, and thus they are removed rapidly from the circulation.

Post-transfusion Purpura

Post-transfusion purpura is a rare complication of blood transfusion in which thrombocytopenic purpura develops about one week after transfusion (119–124). Studies have shown that the basic mechanism is sensitization of a patient to a platelet antigen (Pl^{A1}) present in the donor blood but absent in the recipient (121, 122). Evidence suggests that the complex formed by the Pl^{A1} antigen and the specific antibody attaches to the recipient's (Pl^{A1}-negative) platelets and leads to their subsequent destruction by agglutination and lysis associated with complement fixation (121). The syndrome has thus far been reported only in women who had prior pregnancies.

Thrombocytopenia with Disseminated Intravascular Clotting and Related Syndromes

Severe thrombocytopenia is a hallmark of the syndrome of disseminated intravascular clotting, which has been described elsewhere in this volume. The association of thrombocytopenia, hemolytic anemia associated with fragmented and irregularly contracted erythrocytes, and a characteristic pattern of "consumption coagulopathy" in the presence of circulating fibrin split products identifies the syndrome of DIC. Two other syndromes which also present the combination of thrombocytopenia and microangiopathic hemolytic anemia are thrombotic purpura (TTP) and the hemolytic-uremic syndrome (HUS). These syndromes have much in common with each other and may, in fact, be variants of the same basic pathologic process. Despite the fact that both TTP and HUS only very rarely give clear-cut evidence of consumption coagulopathy, they are often regarded as variants of DIC, an assumption which does not appear justified on the basis of evidence now at hand.

Thrombotic thrombocytopenic purpura is predominantly a disease of young adults, but it certainly occurs in children as well. Thrombocytopenic purpura, microangiopathic hemolytic anemia, fever, and severe neurologic symptoms (convulsions, paresthesias, personality changes, stupor, and coma) constitute the typical syndrome (125). The characteristic pathologic finding is a widespread abnormality of arterioles and capillaries, in which there is occlusion of these vessels by a hyaline material which has been shown to be composed mainly of platelets and fibrin (126–131). Hyaline material has also been identified in the subendothelial areas of affected vessels, and endothelial proliferation in proximity to the hyaline thrombi has been noted frequently (130). The pathologic findings have led most workers to conclude that TTP is a widespread disease of the microcirculation causing destructive lesions of the small vessels, followed by the formation of platelet-fibrin thrombi at the sites of injury, leading, in turn, to microangiopathic hemolytic anemia and symptoms resulting from vascular occlusion in many organs (132). Although the etiology of TTP cannot be identified in most cases, it has occurred in association with immune disorders characterized by diffuse vasculitis of the microcirculation (e.g., lupus, polyarteritis, rheumatoid arthritis).

While neurologic symptoms predominate, laboratory signs pointing to severe renal involvement (hematuria, proteinuria, azotemia) may be found in almost all patients. Although fibrin-split products have been found in the sera of some patients, significant depletion of Factors II, V, VIII, and fibrinogen almost never occurs (133, 134). Positive lupus preparations have been reported in 10 to 20 per cent of cases (134).

Although the mortality rate in TTP is very high, recoveries have been reported with increasing frequency following treatment with large doses of corticosteroids together with other therapeutic maneuvers designed to ameliorate the thrombocytopenia and the anemia, to interefere with fibrin formation, and to inhibit platelet aggregation. Thus, corticosteroid therapy has been accompanied by splenectomy (135–138), heparinization (139–141), fibrinolytic therapy (142), and administration of aspirin and dipyridamole (143, 144). Of the various treatment regimens, the combination of corticosteroids and splenectomy appears, at present, to have been most effective. Studies employing drugs which inhibit platelet aggregation are underway in many centers, and the results will be awaited with interest.

The *hemolytic-uremic syndrome* is discussed in Chapters 7 and 19. The disorder has many features in common with TTP, and the pathologic changes in the microcirculation are virtually identical with those found in TTP. The major difference is that in HUS the lesions are usually limited to the kidneys. As in TTP, fibrin deposition is characteristic in the affected vessels, but laboratory evidence of typical consumption coagulopathy is rarely found, thus making the assumption that HUS is a disorder of disseminated intravascular coagulation tenuous at best.

HUS has been considered a disease of very young infants (usually under 24 months of age), associated with a very high mortality rate and a high incidence of residual renal disease and hypertension. More recent experience has demonstrated that the disorder is not uncommon in older infants and children, and that there is a wide range in severity among affected patients (145–151). There is also evidence to suggest that both age distribution and severity may vary in different locales where the disorder is endemic (146–151) and in different epidemics (152, 153). Such observations suggest varying etiologies of the syndrome, with the final common pathway being damage to the microcirculation, either by the infectious agents or by immune complexes formed in response to the agents. The kidney is the major target organ.

HUS in children is usually preceded by prodromal manifestations, of which diarrhea (often bloody), vomiting, and abdominal pain are most frequent, while symptoms of upper respiratory infection are decidedly less common. The duration of the prodromata is variable, and a "silent interval" between the initial signs of illness and the onset of hemolytic anemia, purpura, and uremia has been described. Presenting symptoms usually relate to the complications of acute renal insufficiency and include edema, heart failure, pallor, seizures, stupor, and coma. Hematuria, oliguria, and anuria may also represent presenting manifestations.

Anemia associated with reticulocytosis and microangiopathic changes in red cell morphology is present in all cases. Thrombocytopenia, with platelet counts less than 150,000 per mm.^{3}, is present in more than 85 per cent of cases. As with TTP, the pathologic finding of fibrin thrombi in renal arterioles and glomerular capillaries has prompted studies of the coagulation mechanism. A great variety of changes has been reported in various studies, many suggesting a "hypercoagulable" state, with elevations of fibrinogen and Factor VIII levels and a shortening of the activated partial thromboplastin time. These have, on occasion, been associated with depletion of the various components of the prothrombin complex. Fibrin-split products have been reported in some patients, as has prolongation of the thrombin time (154–157). It is extremely rare that evidence of consumption coagulopathy is found at the time that patients are first seen. In fact, fibrinogen turnover, which is increased in DIC, is normal in HUS (157a). Some investigators have surmised that the "hypercoagulable" state represents a rebound phenomenon from an initial episode of disseminated intravascular clotting. Others believe that the primary event is damage to the microcirculation, which is followed by localized platelet-fibrin deposition, and that the observed changes in coagulation parameters are the result of, not the cause of, the syndrome. Thus, while some patients do indeed demonstrate the classic finding of DIC in the course of the illness, this must be considered rare. Therefore, the hypothesis that the HUS is a manifestation of disseminated intravascular clotting has little to support it at present.

Recommendations for treatment of the HUS must be weighed against recent reports which demonstrate remarkable improvement in mortality as a result of meticulous attention to the treatment of the renal failure and the increasing use of early and repeated peritoneal dialysis. Thus, Gianantonio et al. have reported a 5 per cent mortality in their last 100 patients since the introduction of peritoneal dialysis (147). Heparin therapy has still not been subjected to controlled study and poses the danger of serious complications (150, 157, 159, 160). As in TTP, the value of agents which inhibit platelet aggregation requires further study. While some patients who demonstrate persistent or progressive involvement of the coagulation mechanism may benefit from heparinization, routine use of this mode of therapy does not appear justified at present. Similarly, the value of heparin, other anticoagulants, or antiplatelet aggregating agents in reducing the incidence of chronic renal disease [9.5 per cent reported by Tune et al. (146), 30 per cent by Gianantonio et al. (158)] has yet to be demonstrated.

Miscellaneous Causes of Accelerated Platelet Destruction

Thrombocytopenia may occur in association with systemic infections of viral, bacterial, or rickettsial origin. It is unlikely that a single mechanism can be ascribed to any particular organism, and it is probable that multiple mechanisms may produce thrombocytopenia in the face of severe infection. The degree to which a direct effect of the microorganism on platelets may result in accelerated in vivo destruction is not known, but this may be one mechanism. The effects of the organisms or their toxins in producing diffuse vascular damage, leading to disseminated platelet aggregation, may be another. Since many systemic infections are associated with splenomegaly, platelet sequestration in the spleen may also play a role. Virtually any form of sepsis may lead to intravascular coagulation, as discussed elsewhere in this volume, of which thrombocytopenia is a hallmark. In the newborn period, toxoplasmosis (161), cytomegalic inclusion disease (162, 163), disseminated herpes (164, 165), congenital syphilis (166, 167), and gram-negative septicemia (168–170) are commonly associated with thrombocytopenia. In older children, thrombocytopenia may accompany tuberculosis (171, 172), typhoid (173), measles (174), rubella (175), varicella, scarlet fever, and many types of bacterial sepsis (174–176). In all, the possibility of DIC must be kept in mind if the thrombocytopenia occurs during the acute phase of the infections (177).

Thrombocytopenia is a common manifestation of systemic lupus erythematosus, and may occur with autoimmune acquired hemolytic anemia (Evans' syndrome) and severe erythroblastosis fetalis.

Thrombocytopenia Due to Impaired Platelet Production

Thrombocytopenia on the basis of diminished platelet production stems, in virtually all instances, from reduction in the number of megakaryocytes in the marrow. This may follow replacement of the marrow, as in leukemia, lymphomas, reticuloendotheliosis, metastatic neuroblastoma, other malignancies, and granulomatous diseases; or hypoplasia or aplasia of the marrow, whether congenital, idiopathic, or secondary to drugs, chemical toxins, or ionizing radiation (see Ch. 5).

Congenital amegakaryocytic thrombocytopenia is a rare cause of neonatal thrombocytopenia, in which the marrow content of megakaryocytes is strikingly reduced and which is most commonly associated with bilateral absence of the radii (178–183). Hemorrhagic manifestations tend to be most common in the early weeks of life, then abate to a significant degree, even though thrombocytopenia persists. A frequent associated feature is a striking leukemoid reaction in the neonatal period, which may suggest congenital leukemia (180–183). The leukemoid reaction resolves, however, in the absence of any specific therapy. Should the affected infants escape serious hemorrhage, they tend to do surprisingly well. Long-term observations have revealed a slow but steady increment in platelet count, so that levels may be reached which, while subnormal, are compatible with effective hemostasis.

While drugs which cause thrombocytopenia usually do so on an immunologic basis, as described before, or by leading to aplastic anemia, several agents appear to have a specific effect on platelet production. Among the best studied are thiazide diuretics which, after maternal ingestion, have been implicated as a cause of neonatal thrombocytopenic purpura, associated with diminution of megakaryocytes (184). Estrogens (185, 186), and alcohol (187, 188) have also been implicated. In these situations, megakaryocytes and platelet levels return to normal after elimination of the drugs.

Congenital rubella, which is associated with thrombocytopenia in 30 per cent of affected infants (189–191), and live-virus measles immunization, which is followed by reduced platelet levels in 85 per cent of recipients (192), appear to produce damage to and diminution in the number of megakaryocytes.

Cyanotic congenital heart disease is frequently associated with thrombocytopenia when arterial oxygen saturations are below 65 per cent and hematocrits over 65 per cent in children past one year of life (193). The improvement in platelet counts after corrective surgery or multiple phlebotomies suggests that the thrombocytopenia results from decreased platelet production secondary to impaired oxygenation of the marrow (194), but a short platelet life span has been defined in several patients. The latter fact suggests the possiblity that platelets may be consumed or sequestered in congested organs.

Congenital thrombopoietin deficiency is a very rare cause of severe congenital thrombocytopenia unresponsive to steroids and splenectomy, but strikingly responsive to infusions of fresh or fresh-frozen plasma (195). One patient studied for over 15 years still requires and responds to plasma infusions given every two to three weeks (196, 197). In this disorder, megakaryocytes are plentiful, but appear to require "thrombopoietin" for megakaryocyte maturation and platelet release.

FUNCTIONAL ABNORMALITIES OF PLATELETS

A hemorrhagic state, congenital or acquired, may occur when the platelets, though normal in number, are functionally abnormal. In essence, the abnormality may involve any step in the platelet hemostatic mechanism, i.e., the formation of the platelet plug, the participation in coagulation through availability of platelet Factor 3, and clot retraction. In terms of platelet function, the defect may involve adhesion, release of nucleotides, aggregation, and platelet Factor 3 "exposure." In general, functional abnormalities of the platelets produce symptoms similar to those encountered in the presence of thrombocytopenia, i.e., bleeding primarily from skin and mucous membranes — recurrent epistaxis, excessive bleeding after trauma or surgery (particularly after tonsillectomy and adenoidectomy), menorrhagia, and gastrointestinal hemorrhage. Bleeding elsewhere may also occur, and in severe instances of functional abnormality, central nervous system hemorrhage is a definite threat.

Prolongation of the bleeding time is characteristic of all functional abnormalities of the platelets. The specific defects may be identified in most cases by presently available techniques.

Congenital

VON WILLEBRAND'S DISEASE. This has been described in detail elsewhere in this volume. The basic defect leading to prolongation of the bleeding time and to the predominant hemorrhagic symptoms is believed to be a failure of platelet adhesion, which, in turn, appears to result from a congenital deficiency of a plasma factor needed for this step in hemostasis (198–201). Aggregation of the platelets in response to addition of collagen and ADP is normal, as is platelet Factor 3 availability and clot retraction (202–204). Apart from the bleeding time, the in vitro test most likely to demonstrate the platelet defect is one which tests the adhesiveness of the platelets to glass beads under controlled conditions (205). Available evidence suggests that the plasma factor required for normal platelet adhesiveness is not identical with the factor required for Factor VIII synthesis. Recent studies by Holmberg and Nilsson (206) suggest the possibility of two genetic variants of von Willebrand's disease, one autosomal dominant, the other sex-linked recessive.

THROMBASTHENIA. Thrombasthenia is a congenital, lifelong bleeding disorder transmitted as an autosomal recessive and characterized by failure of platelets to aggregate in response to ADP (207–210) (Fig. 21–1). Upon exposure of the platelets to collagen, ADP is released normally, but in

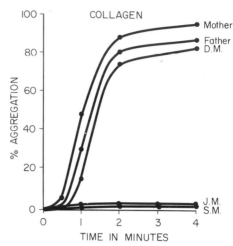

Figure 21–2. Platelet aggregation in response to collagen in same family as in Figure 21–1. (From Corby, D. G., Zirbel, C. L., et al.: Am. J. Dis. Child. *121*:140, 1971.)

view of the basic defect, aggregation does not occur (Fig. 21–2). Secondary to the basic defect, platelet adhesion to glass and platelet Factor 3 availability are usually abnormal. Deficient platelet fibrinogen has also been found (211–213). Bleeding manifestations will usually respond to transfusion of normal platelets. However, repeated transfusions may be followed by immunization, thus suggesting that selection of donors on the basis of similarity in histocompatibility antigens is advisable (214).

PLATELET STORAGE POOL DEFICIENCY. Families have been described with a mild, recessive, hemorrhagic disease, characterized by decreased aggregation of platelets in response to collagen and epinephrine. Analysis of the platelets has revealed a greatly reduced content of platelet ADP as the probable basic abnormality (215, 216).

DEFECTIVE PLATELET NUCLEOTIDE RELEASE. Patients having clinical manifestations similar to those with platelet storage pool deficiency and similarly impaired aggregation in response to collagen and ADP, but with normal content of platelet ADP, have also been described (217–221). In these individuals the basic defect is presumed to be in the release mechanism itself.

DEFECTIVE PLATELET FACTOR 3 CONTENT AND AVAILABILITY. Cases have been described in which the hemorrhagic state has been ascribed to reduced content (222, 223) or abnormal availability of PF 3

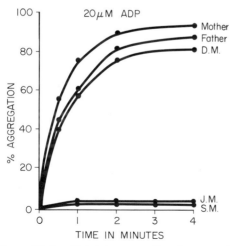

Figure 21–1. Platelet aggregation in response to ADP in two siblings with thrombasthenia and in unaffected family members. (From Corby, D. G., Zirbel, C. L., et al.: Am. J. Dis. Child. *121*:140, 1971.)

(224). Whether these are, in fact, specific defects in the PF 3 mechanism or secondary to an underlying defect in aggregation is not entirely clear.

THE NEWBORN. The platelets of newborn infants have been found to aggregate normally in response to ADP, but subnormally in response to collagen and epinephrine (225, 226). Preliminary studies indicate that the defect is greater in prematurely born infants. Investigations have also suggested that the defect in the neonate relates to impaired release rather than to reduced content of platelet ADP. Of importance is the fact that many sedative and analgesic drugs commonly used in labor may greatly exaggerate the impaired aggregation of newborn platelets (225) (see below). The significance of the observed abnormalities of platelet function of the newborn in the pathogenesis of hemorrhage in the neonatal period is unknown.

Acquired

DRUGS. An increasingly large number of drugs has been shown to impair platelet function in vitro. The vast majority exert their effect by impairing aggregation in response to collagen and low molar ADP, thus indicating that the effect is on the release reaction. A variety of pharmacologic agents has been identified which induce release and promote aggregation (227) (Table 21–1). The effect of most of these drugs on the bleeding time has not been critically evaluated. The in vitro effect may not be clinically significant.

Of commonly available drugs which impair aggregation, aspirin has received most study (228–231). Normal therapeutic doses are capable of inducing marked reduction of platelet aggregation in response to collagen, with the effect becoming apparent within hours after ingestion and remaining demonstrable for several days. Platelets which have been subject to aspirin effect remain so affected throughout their life span. It has been estimated that only 10 to 20 per cent of unaffected platelets are required for normal hemostasis, and thus the clinical effect of a single dose of aspirin is probably lost within only a few days (232). Large single doses of aspirin or continuing therapy may promote a significant prolongation of bleeding time

TABLE 21–1. PHARMACOLOGIC AND PHYSIOCHEMICAL AGENTS AFFECTING PLATELET FUNCTION

A. Inducers of Release and/or Aggregation
   Adenosine diphosphate (ADP)
   Epinephrine
   Serotonin
   Collagen
   Thrombin
   Trypsin
   Gamma globulin (antigen-antibody complexes)
   Viruses
   Endotoxin
   Triethyl tin
   Polylysine
   Polystyrene particles
   Estrogens
   Fatty acids

B. Inhibitors of Release and/or Aggregation
   Adenosine
   Adenosine monophosphate (AMP)
   Adenosine triphosphate (ATP)
   Cylic AMP
   Prostaglandin E_1
   Antihistamines
   Local anesthetics
   Alpha-adrenergic agents (phentolamine)
   Chlorpromazine
   Imipramine
   Diphenhydramine
   Pyrimidopyrimidine (Persantine)
   Ethacrynic acid
   Acetylsalicylic acid (aspirin)
   Phenylbutazone
   Indomethacin
   Guanidosuccinic acid
   Arginyl esters
   Prednisolone
   Glyceryl guaiacolate
   Atropine
   Heparin
   Dextran
   Azathioprine
   Vincristine
   Fibrinogen degradation products
   Colchicine

Adapted from "Platelet Function," by Hathaway, W. E., In *Advances in Pediatrics*. Volume 19, by Schulman, I. (ed.). Copyright © 1972 by Year Book Medical Publishers, Inc., Chicago. Used by permission.

(228), and purpura in a child attributed to aspirin has been reported (233). Aspirin was suspected as a probable cause for post-tonsillectomy hemorrhage in 1945 (234), and it is quite possible that instances of post-tonsillectomy and postdental extraction hemorrhage may be attributed to the use of aspirin for pain. Cases of protracted menstrual bleeding in some girls may also be the result of this mechanism. In the presence of an underlying hemorrhagic state (the hemophilias, the thrombocytopenias, von Willebrand's disease, and so forth), the use of drugs causing impaired platelet function is definitely hazardous and may increase the severity of the bleeding tendency (235, 236).

PLATELET ABNORMALITIES ASSOCIATED WITH DISEASE STATES. Numerous disease entities have been identified in which there is an associated abnormality of platelet function. These have recently been reviewed by Hathaway (227). The exact mechanism in many of these disorders is not clear and may involve a defect in the platelet membrane, a coexisting defect in platelet metabolism, or an acquired metabolic defect due to malnutrition secondary to the underlying disease. Hemorrhagic manifestations are usually mild, if at all present, but occasionally may be significant, as in glycogen storage disease (237, 238) and uremia (238–243).

THROMBOCYTOSIS

Abnormal elevation of the platelet level is said to exist when the count exceeds 400,000 per mm.^{3} by direct counting methods. In children, thrombocytosis is most commonly encountered as a component of chronic inflammatory diseases, such as rheumatoid arthritis, regional enteritis, ulcerative colitis, tuberculosis, sarcoidosis, chronic hepatitis, chronic osteomyelitis, and others (244–246). Significant elevations of the platelet count may also occur with a wide variety of neoplastic diseases (247). In children, thrombocytosis is commonly associated with neuroblastoma. Mild to moderate degrees of thrombocytosis may occur with iron deficiency of moderate severity (hemoglobin concentrations of 6 to 8 g. per 100 ml.) (248).

Surgical procedures are usually followed by a moderate thrombocytosis during the first postoperative week, with a return to normal levels in the second or third week (249–253). The thrombocytosis which follows splenectomy usually reaches a peak in seven to ten days, at which time levels of 500,000 to 1 million per mm.^{3} may be found in about one-half the patients. Counts exceeding 1 million may occur in about 10 per cent of patients. While a return to normal platelet levels is usually achieved by two months after splenectomy, about one-third of patients will demonstrate a persistent significant elevation of platelet count (250).

In children, postsplenectomy thrombocytosis, even of marked degree, is not associated with thrombotic complications and is not an indication for anticoagulation therapy.

Essential thrombocythemia is a myeloproliferative disorder which, although primarily a disease of adults, does occur in children (254, 255). Platelet counts usually exceed 1 million per mm.^{3} and may be severalfold higher. The peripheral blood film contains masses of platelets which are even more dramatically evident in the marrow, where abundant megakaryocytes are found. A combination of both thrombotic and hemorrhagic manifestations occurs, the latter attributed to interference with the coagulation mechanism and to qualitative abnormalities of platelet function (256, 257). Strokes and myocardial infarctions have occurred in children; bleeding manifestations include purpura, epistaxis, gastrointestinal hemorrhage, and hematuria. Therapy is usually directed at reducing the platelet count by agents causing destruction of megakaryocytes in the marrow. Busulfan, melphalan, and uracil mustard have been used (258, 259). Drugs which suppress platelet function may prove to be of value in preventing thrombotic complications.

References

1. Newton, W. A., Jr., and Zuelzer, W. W.: Idiopathic thrombocytopenic purpura in childhood. New Engl. J. Med. 245:879, 1951.
2. Clement, D. H., and Diamond, L. K.: Purpura in infants and children. Its natural history. A.M.A. J. Dis. Child. 85:259, 1953.
3. Komrower, G. M., and Watson, G. H.: Prognosis in idiopathic thrombocytopenic purpura of childhood. Arch. Dis. Child. 29:502, 1954.
4. Walker, J. H., and Walker, W.: Idiopathic thrombocytopenic purpura in childhood. Arch. Dis. Child. 36:649, 1961.
5. Schulman, I.: Diagnosis and treatment: Management of idiopathic thrombocytopenic purpura. Pediatrics 33:979, 1964.
6. Lusher, J. M., and Zuelzer, W. W.: Idiopathic thrombocytopenic purpura in childhood. J. Pediatr. 68:971, 1966.
7. Choi, S. I., and McClure, P. D.: Idiopathic thrombocytopenic purpura in childhood. Can. Med. Assoc. J. 97:562, 1967.
8. Baldini, M.: Idiopathic thrombocytopenic pur-

pura. New Engl. J. Med. *274*:1245, 1302, 1360, 1966.

9. Harrington, W. J., Minnich, V., et al.: The autoimmune thrombocytopenias. Progr. Hematol. *1*:166, 1956.

10. Carpenter, A. F., Wintrobe, M. M., et al.: Treatment of idiopathic thrombocytopenic purpura. J.A.M.A. *171*:1911, 1959.

11. Doan, C. A., Bouroncle, B. A., et al.: Idiopathic and secondary thrombocytopenic purpura: Clinical study and evaluation of 381 cases over a period of 28 years. Ann. Intern. Med. *53*:861, 1960.

12. Lozner, E. L.: The thrombocytopenic purpuras. Bull. N.Y. Acad. Med. *30*:184, 1954.

13. Karpatkin, S., and Siskind, G. W.: In vitro detection of platelet antibody in patients with idiopathic thrombocytopenic purpura and systemic lupus erythematosus. Blood *33*:795, 1969.

14. Karpatkin, S., Strick, N., et al.: Cumulative experience in the detection of anti-platelet antibody in 234 patients with idiopathic thrombocytopenic purpura, systemic lupus erythematosus and other clinical disorders. Am. J. Med. *52*:776, 1972.

15. Karpatkin, S.: Autoimmune thrombocytopenic purpura. Am. J. Med. Sci. *261*:127, 1971.

16. Lammi, A. T., and Lovric, V. A.: Idiopathic thrombocytopenic purpura: An epidemiologic study. J. Pediatr. *83*:31, 1973.

17. Harker, L., and Slichter, S. J.: Bleeding time as screening test to evaluate platelet function. New Engl. J. Med. *287*:155, 1972.

18. Shulman, N. R., Marder, V. J., et al.: Similarities between known antiplatelet antibodies and the factor responsible for thrombocytopenia in idiopathic purpura: Physiologic, serologic and isotopic studies. Ann. N.Y. Acad. Sci. *124*:499, 1965.

19. Schulman, I.: Unpublished observations.

20. Labram, C.: Etude de l'action vaso-constrictrice de la prednisone. Rev. Fr. Etud. Clin. Biol. *8*:765, 1963.

21. Robson, H. N., and Duthie, J. J. R.: Capillary resistance and adrenocortical activity. Br. Med. J. *2*:971, 1950.

22. Faloon, W. W., Greene, R. W., et al.: The hemostatic defect in thrombocytopenia as studied by the use of ACTH and cortisone. Am. J. Med. *13*:12, 1952.

23. Weisberger, A. S., and Suhrland, L. G.: Massive corticosteroid therapy in the management of resistant thrombocytopenic purpura. Am. J. Med. Sci. *236*:425, 1958.

23a. Cohen, P., and Gardner, F. H.: Thrombocytopenic effect of sustained high dosage prednisone. Therapy in thrombocytopenic purpura. New Engl. J. Med. *265*:611, 1961.

24. Najean, Y., Ardaillou, N., et al.: The platelet destruction site in thrombocytopenic purpuras. Br. J. Haematol. *13*:409, 1967.

25. Aster, R. H., and Keene, W. R.: Sites of platelet destruction in idiopathic thrombocytopenic purpura. Br. J. Haematol. *16*:61, 1969.

26. Diamond, L. K.: Splenectomy in childhood and the hazard of overwhelming infection. Pediatrics *43*:886, 1969.

27. Reiquiam, C. W., and Prosper, J. C.: Chronic idiopathic thrombocytopenia: Treatment with prednisone, 6-mercaptopurine, vincristine, and fresh plasma transfusions. J. Pediatr. *68*:885, 1966.

28. Lo, S. S., Hitzig, W. H., et al.: Management of chronic ITP in children with particular reference to immunosuppressive therapy. Acta Haematol. (Basel) *41*:1, 1969.

29. Kuzemko, J. A., and Keidan, S. E.: Treatment of chronic idiopathic thrombocytopenic purpura with azathioprine and prednisolone: A clinical trial with three children. Clin. Pediatr. (Bologna) *7*:216, 1968.

30. Hilgartner, M. W., Lanzkowsky, P., et al.: The use of azathioprine in refractory idiopathic thrombocytopenic purpura in childhood. Acta Paediatr. Scand. *59*:409, 1970.

31. Martin, H., Nowicki, L., et al.: Behandlung des Morbus Werlhof mit Actinomycin C. Dtsch. Med. Wochenschr. *92*:1061, 1967.

32. Laros, R. K., and Penner, J. A.: "Refractory" thrombocytopenic purpura treated successfully with cyclophosphamide. J.A.M.A. *215*:445, 1971.

33. Marmont, A. M., Damasio, E. E., et al.: Vinblastine sulphate in idiopathic thrombocytopenic purpura. Lancet *2*:94, 1971.

34. Miller, J. J., III, Williams, G. F., et al.: Multiple late complications of therapy with cyclophosphamide, including ovarian destruction. Am. J. Med. *50*:530, 1971.

35. Harrington, W. J., Minnich, V., et al.: Demonstration of a thrombocytopenic factor in the blood of patients with thrombocytopenic purpura. J. Lab. Clin. Med. *38*:1, 1951.

36. Najean, Y., and Ardaillou, N.: The sequestration site of platelets in idiopathic thrombocytopenic purpura: Its correlation with the results of splenectomy. Br. J. Haematol. *21*:153, 1971.

37. Aster, R. H., and Jandl, J. H.: Platelet sequestration in man. II. Immunological and clinical studies. J. Clin. Invest. *43*:856, 1964.

38. Movat, H. Z., Mustard, J. R., et al.: Platelet aggregation and release of ADP, serotonin, and histamine associated with phagocytosis of antigen-antibody complexes. Proc. Soc. Exp. Biol. Med. *120*:232, 1965.

39. Muller-Eckhardt, C., and Luscher, E. F.: Immune reactions of human blood platelets. I. A comparative study on effects on platelets of heterologous anti-platelet anti-serum, antigen-antibody complexes, aggregated gamma globulin and thrombin. Thromb. Diath. Haemorrh. *20*:155, 1968.

40. Myllylä, G., Vaheri, A., et al.: Interaction between human blood platelets, viruses, and antibodies. IV. Post-rubella thrombocytopenic purpura and platelet aggregation by rubella antigen-antibody interaction. Clin. Exp. Immunol. *4*:323, 1969.

40a. Handin, R. E., Piessens, W. F., et al.: Stimulation of non-immunized lymphocytes by platelet-antibody complexes in idiopathic thrombocytopenic purpura. New Engl. J. Med. *283*:714, 1973.

40b. Handin, R. E., and Stossel, T. P.: Phagocytosis of antibody-coated platelets by human granulocytes. New Engl. J. Med. *290*:989, 1974.

41. Harrington, W. J., Sprague, C. C., et al.: Immunologic mechanisms in idiopathic and neonatal thrombocytopenic purpura. Ann. Intern. Med. 38:433, 1953.

42. Peterson, O. H., and Larson, P.: Thrombocytopenic purpura in pregnancy. Obstet. Gynecol. 4:454, 1954.

43. Tancer, M. L.: Idiopathic thrombocytopenic purpura and pregnancy: Report of 5 new cases and review of the literature. Am. J. Obstet. Gynecol. 79:148, 1960.

44. Heys, R. F.: Steroid therapy for idiopathic thrombocytopenic purpura during pregnancy. Obstet. Gynecol. 28:532, 1966.

45. Goodhue, P. A., and Evans, T. S.: Idiopathic thrombocytopenic purpura in pregnancy: Report of a case and review of the literature. Obstet. Gynecol. Surv. 18:671, 1963.

46. Heys, R. F.: Child-bearing and idiopathic thrombocytopenic purpura. J. Obstet. Gynaecol. Br. Cwlth. 73:205, 1966.

47. Anthony, B., and Krivit, W.: Neonatal thrombocytopenic purpura. Pediatrics 30:776, 1962.

48. Pearson, H. A., Shulman, N. R., et al.: Isoimmune neonatal thrombocytopenic purpura: Clinical and therapeutic considerations. Blood 23:154, 1964.

49. Shulman, N. R., Marder, V. J., et al.: Platelet and leukocyte isoantigens and their antibodies: Serologic, physiologic and clinical studies. Progr. Hematol. 4:222, 1964.

50. Adner, M. M., Fisch, G. R., et al.: Use of "compatible" platelet transfusions in treatment of congenital isoimmune neonatal thrombocytopenic purpura. New Engl. J. Med. 280:244, 1969.

51. Wiskott, A.: Familiärer, angeborener Morbus Werlhofii? Mschr. Kinderheilk. 68:212, 1937.

52. Aldrich, R. A., Steinberg, A. G., et al.: Pedigree demonstrating a sex-linked recessive condition characterized by draining ears, eczematoid dermatitis and bloody diarrhea. Pediatrics 13:133, 1954.

53. Krivit, W., and Good, R. A.: Aldrich's syndrome (thrombocytopenia, eczema, and infection in infants). Am. J. Dis. Child. 97:137, 1959.

54. Wolff, J. A.: Wiskott-Aldrich syndrome: Clinical, immunologic, and pathologic observations. Arch. Dis. Child. 42:604, 1967.

55. Grottum, K. A., Hovig, T., et al.: Wiscott-Aldrich syndrome: Qualitative platelet defects and short platelet survival. Br. J. Haematol. 17:373, 1969.

56. Kuramoto, H., Steiner, M., et al.: Lack of platelet response to stimulation in the Wiscott-Aldrich syndrome. New Engl. J. Med. 282:475, 1970.

57. Pearson, H. A., Shulman, N. R., et al.: Platelet survival in Wiscott-Aldrich syndrome. J. Pediatr. 68:755, 1966.

58. Canales, L., and Mauer, A. M.: Sex-linked hereditary thrombocytopenia as a variant of Wiskott-Aldrich syndrome. New Engl. J. Med. 277:899, 1967.

59. Schaar, F. E.: Familial idiopathic thrombocytopenic purpura. J. Pediatr. 62:546, 1963.

60. Vestermark, B., and Vestermark, S.: Familial sex-linked thrombocytopenia. Acta Paediatr. 53:365, 1964.

61. Ata, M., Fisher, O. D., et al.: Inherited thrombocytopenia. Lancet 1:119, 1965.

62. Gutenberger, J., Trygstad, C. W., et al.: Familial thrombocytopenia, elevated serum IgA levels and renal disease. Am. J. Med. 49:729, 1970.

63. Wassmuth, D. R., Hamilton, H. E., et al.: May-Hegglin anomaly. Hereditary affection of granulocytes and platelets. J.A.M.A. 183:737, 1963.

64. Oski, F. A., Naiman, J. L., et al.: Leukocytic inclusions—Döhle bodies—associated with platelet abnormality (the May-Hegglin anomaly). Report of a family and review of the literature. Blood 20:657, 1962.

65. Jordan, S. W., and Larsen, W. E.: Ultrastructural studies of the May-Hegglin anomaly. Blood 25:921, 1965.

66. Kurstjens, R., Bolt, C., et al.: Familial thrombopathic thrombocytopenia. Br. J. Haematol. 15:305, 1968.

67. Niewiarowski, S., Poplawski, A., et al.: Abnormalities of platelet function and ultrastructure in macrothrombocytic thrombopathia. Scand. J. Haematol. 6:377, 1969.

68. Baadenhuijsen, H., Hirschhäuser, C., et al.: Metabolic observations on platelets from patients with familial thrombopathic thrombocytopenia. Br. J. Haematol. 20:417, 1971.

69. Woolley, E. J. S.: Familial idiopathic thrombocytopenic purpura. Br. Med. J. 1:440, 1956.

70. Seip, M.: Hereditary hypoplastic thrombocytopenia. Acta Paediatr. 52:370, 1963.

71. Bithell, T. C., Didisheim, P., et al.: Thrombocytopenia inherited as an autosomal dominant trait. Blood 25:231, 1965.

72. Myllylä, G., Pelkonen, R., et al.: Hereditary thrombocytopenia: Report of three families. Scand. J. Haematol. 4:441, 1967.

73. Murphy, S., Oski, F. A., et al.: Hereditary thrombocytopenia with an intrinsic platelet defect. New Engl. J. Med. 281:857, 1969.

74. Cullum, C., Cooney, D. P., et al.: Familial thrombocytopenic thrombocytopathy. Br. J. Haematol. 13:147, 1967.

75. Bernard, J., and Soulier, J. P.: Sur une nouvelle varieté de dystrophie thrombocytaire hemorragipare congénitale. Sem. Hôp. Paris 24:3217, 1948.

76. Bernard, J., Caen, J., et al.: La dystrophie thrombocytaire hemorragipare congénitale. Rev. Hematol. 12:222, 1957.

77. Alagille, D., Josso, F., et al.: La dystrophie thrombocytaire hemorragipare: Discussion nosologique. Nouv. Rev. Fr. Hematol. 4:755, 1964.

78. Kanska, B., Niewiarowski, S., et al.: Macrothrombocytic thrombopathia: Clinical, coagulation and hereditary aspects. Thromb. Diath. Haemorrh. 10:88, 1963.

79. Ulutin, O. N.: Primary thrombocytopathy. Isr. J. Med. Sci. 1:857, 1965.

80. Gröttum, K. A., and Solum, N. O.: Congenital thrombocytopenia with giant platelets: A defect in the platelet membrane. Br. J. Haematol. 16:277, 1969.

81. Kasabach, H. H., and Merritt, K. K.: Hemangioma with extensive purpura. Am. J. Dis. Child. 59:1063, 1940.

82. Good, T. A., Carnazzo, S. F., et al.: Thrombocy-

topenia and giant hemangioma in infants. Am. J. Dis. Child. *90*:260, 1955.

83. Blix, S., and Aas, K.: Giant hemangioma, thrombocytopenia, fibrinogenopenia, and fibrinolytic activity. Acta Med. Scand. *169*:63, 1961.

84. Kontras, S. B., Green, O. C., et al.: Giant hemangioma and thrombocytopenia in a newborn infant treated by irradiation therapy. Am. J. Dis. Child. *105*:188, 1963.

85. Propp, R. P., and Scharfman, W. B.: Hemangioma-thrombocytopenia syndrome associated with microangiopathic hemolytic anemia. Blood *28*:623, 1966.

86. Shin, W. K. T.: Hemangiomas of infancy complicated by thrombocytopenia. Am. J. Surg. *116*:896, 1968.

87. Brizel, H. E., and Raccuglia, G.: Giant hemangioma with thrombocytopenia: Radioisotopic demonstration of platelet sequestration. Blood *26*:751, 1965.

88. Kontras, S. B., Green, O. C., et al.: Giant hemangioma and thrombocytopenia in a newborn infant treated by irradiation therapy. Am. J. Dis. Child. *105*:188, 1963.

89. Verstraete, M., Amery, A., et al.: Heparin treatment of bleeding. Lancet *1*:446, 1963.

90. Hillman, R. S., and Phillips, L. L.: Clotting and fibrinolysis in a cavernous hemangioma. Am. J. Dis. Child. *113*:649, 1967.

91. Williams, O. K., Van Buskirk, F. W., et al.: Giant hemangioendothelioma with thrombocytopenia and hypofibrinogenemia. Am. J. Roentgenol. *106*:204, 1969.

92. Fost, N. C., and Esterly, N. B.: Successful treatment of juvenile hemangiomas with prednisone. J. Pediatr. *72*:351, 1968.

93. Goldberg, S. J., and Fonkalsrud, E.: Successful treatment of hepatic hemangioma with corticosteroids. J.A.M.A. *208*:2473, 1969.

94. Schneider, H. J., and Lascari, A. D.: Consumption coagulopathy in an infant with Kasabach-Merritt syndrome. Helv. Paediatr. Acta *23*:674, 1968.

95. Aster, R. H.: Pooling of platelets in the spleen: Role in the pathogenesis of "hypersplenic" thrombocytopenia. J. Clin. Invest. *45*:645, 1955.

96. Cohen, P., Gardner, F. H., et al.: Reclassification of the thrombocytopenias by the ^{51}Cr-labeling method for measuring platelet lifespan. New Engl. J. Med. *264*:1294, 1961.

97. Penny, R., Rozenberg, M. C., et al.: The splenic platelet pool. Blood *27*:1, 1966.

98. Amorosi, E. L.: Hypersplenism. Semin. Hematol. *2*:249, 1965.

99. Cooney, D. P., and Smith, B. A.: The pathophysiology of hypersplenic thrombocytopenia. Arch. Intern. Med. *121*:332, 1968.

100. Vipan, W. H.: Quinine as a cause of purpura. Lancet *2*:37, 1865.

101. Aster, R. H., In *Hematology.* Williams, W. J., Beutler, E., et al. (eds.), New York, McGraw-Hill, 1972, p. 1141.

102. Ackroyd, J. F.: The immunological basis of purpura due to drug hypersensitivity. Proc. R. Soc. Med. *55*:30, 1962.

103. Miescher, P., and Miescher, R.: Die Sedormid-Anaphlaxie. Schweiz. Med. Wochenschr. *82*:1279, 1952.

104. Miescher, P., and Straessle, R.: Experimentelle Studien über den Mechanismus der Thrombocyten Schadigung durch Antigen-antikorper Reacktionen. Vox Sang. *1*:83, 1956.

105. Croft, J. D., Jr., Swisher, S. N., Jr., et al.: Coombs'-test positivity induced by drugs: Mechanisms of immunologic reactions, and red cell destruction. Ann. Intern. Med. *68*:176, 1968.

106. Shulman, N. R.: Mechanism of blood cell damage by adsorption of antigen-antibody complex, In *Immunopathology.* Third International Symposium. Grabar, P., and Miescher, P. A. (eds.), Basel, Schwabe, 1964, p. 338.

107. Shulman, N. R.: Immunoreactions involving platelets. III. Quantitative aspects of platelet agglutination, inhibition of clot retraction, and other reactions caused by the antibody of quinidine purpura. J. Exp. Med. *107*:697, 1958.

108. Shulman, N. R.: Immunoreactions involving platelets. IV. Studies on the pathogenesis of thrombocytopenia in drug purpura using test doses of quinidine in sensitized individuals: Their implications in idiopathic thrombocytopenic purpura. J. Exp. Med. *107*:711, 1958.

109. Shulman, N. R.: A mechanism of cell destruction in individuals sensitized to foreign antigens and its implications in autoimmunity. Ann. Intern. Med. *60*:506, 1964.

110. Ackroyd, J. F.: The pathogenesis of thrombocytopenic purpura due to hypersensitivity to Sedormid. Clin. Sci. *7*:249, 1949.

111. Ackroyd, J. F.: The role of complement in sedormid purpura. Clin. Sci. *10*:185, 1951.

112. Shulman, N. R.: Immunoreactions involving platelets. I. A steric and kinetic model for formation of a complex from a human antibody, quinidine as a haptene, and platelets, and for fixation of complements by the complex. J. Exp. Med. *107*:665, 1958.

113. Van der Weerdt, C. M.: Thrombocytopenia due to quinidine or quinine: Report on a series of 28 patients. Vox Sang. *12*:265, 1967.

114. Aster, R. H., and Enright, S. E.: A platelet and granulocyte membrane defect in paroxysmal nocturnal hemoglobinuria: Usefulness for the detection of platelet antibodies. J. Clin. Invest. *48*:1199, 1969.

115. Horowitz, H. I., Rappaport, H. I., et al.: Change in platelet Factor 3 as a means of demonstrating immune reactions involving platelets: Its use as a test for quinidine-induced thrombocytopenia. Transfusion *5*:336, 1965.

116. Horowitz, H. I., and Nachman, R. L.: Drug purpura. Semin. Hematol. *2*:287, 1965.

117. Karpatkin, S., Strick, N., et al.: Cumulative experience in the detection of anti-platelet antibody in 234 patients with idiopathic thrombocytopenic purpura, systemic lupus erythematosus and other clinical disorders. Am. J. Med. *52*:776, 1972.

118. Deykin, D., and Hellerstein, L. J.: The assessment of drug-dependent and isoimmune antiplatelet antibodies by the use of platelet aggregometry. J. Clin. Invest. *51*:3142, 1972.

119. Shulman, N. R., Marker, V. J., et al.: Platelet and leukocyte isoantigens and their antibodies: Serologic, physiologic and clinical studies. Progr. Hematol. *4*:222, 1964.

120. Van Loghem, J. J., Dorfmeijer, H., et al.: Serological and genetical studies on a platelet antigen (Zw). Vox Sang. 4:161, 1959.

121. Shulman, N. R., Aster, R. H., et al.: Immunoreactions involving platelets. V. Post-transfusion purpura due to a complement-fixing antibody against a genetically-controlled platelet antigen: A proposed mechanism for thrombocytopenia and its relevance in "autoimmunity." J. Clin. Invest. 40:1597, 1961.

122. Morrison, F. S., and Mollison, P. L.: Post-transfusion purpura. New Engl. J. Med. 275:243, 1966.

123. Svejgaard, A, Pedersen, M. F., et al.: Post-transfusion purpura caused by a specific platelet isoantibody. Danish Med Bull. 14:41, 1967.

124. Morse, E. E.: Post-transfusion thrombocytopenic purpura. Johns Hopkins Med. J. 121:365, 1967.

125. Casale, A.: Thrombotic thrombocytopenic purpura: Report of a case and review of 157 cases. Hawaii Med. J. 25:93, 1965.

126. Moschcowitz, E.: An acute febrile pleiochromic anemia with hyaline thrombosis of terminal arterioles and capillaries: An undescribed disease. Arch. Intern. Med. (Chicago) 36:89, 1925.

127. Baehr, G., Klemperer, P., et al.: An acute febrile anemia and thrombocytopenic purpura with diffuse platelet thromboses of capillaries and arterioles. Trans. Assoc. Am. Physicians 51:43, 1936.

128. Altschule, M. D.: A rare type of acute thrombocytopenic purpura: Widespread formation of platelet thrombi in capillaries. New Engl. J. Med. 227:477, 1942.

129. Gore, I.: Disseminated arteriolar and capillary platelet thrombosis: A morphological study of its histogenesis. Am. J. Pathol. 26:155, 1950.

130. Feldman, J. D., Mardiney, M. R., et al.: The vascular pathology of thrombotic thrombocytopenic purpura: An immunohistochemical and ultrastructural study. Lab. Invest. 15:927, 1966.

131. Craig, J. M., and Gitlin, D.: The nature of the hyaline thrombi in thrombotic thrombocytopenic purpura. Am. J. Pathol. 33:251, 1957.

132. Brain, M. C., Dacie, J. V., et al.: Microangiopathic haemolytic anemia: The possible role of vascular lesions in pathogenesis. Br. J. Haematol. 8:358, 1962.

133. Lerner, R. G., Rapaport, S. I., et al.: Thrombotic thrombocytopenic purpura: Serial clotting studies, relation to the generalized Shwartzman reaction, and remission after adrenal steroid and dextran therapy. Ann. Intern. Med. 66:1181, 1967.

134. Amorosi, E. L., and Ultmann, J. E.: Thrombotic thrombocytopenic purpura: Report of 16 cases and review of the literature. Medicine (Baltimore) 45:139, 1966.

135. Moorhead, J. F.: Thrombotic thrombocytopenic purpura: Recovery after splenectomy. Arch. Intern. Med. (Chicago) 117:284, 1966.

136. Distenfeld, A., and Oppenheim, O.: The treatment of acute thrombotic thrombocytopenic purpura with corticosteroids and splenectomy: Report of 3 cases. Ann. Intern. Med. 65:245, 1966.

137. Hill, J. B., and Cooper, W. M.: Thrombotic throm-

138. Bernard, R. P., Bauman, A. W., et al.: Splenectomy for thrombotic thrombocytopenic purpura. Ann. Surg. 169:616, 1969.

139. Bernstock, L., and Hirson, C.: Thrombotic thrombocytopenic purpura: Remission on treatment with heparin. Lancet 1:28, 1960.

140. Carmichael, D. S., and Medley, D. R. K.: Heparin in thrombotic microangiopathy. Lancet 1:1421, 1966.

141. Richardson, J. H., and Smith, B. T.: Thrombotic thrombocytopenic purpura: Survival in pregnancy with heparin sodium therapy. J.A.M.A. 203:518, 1968.

142. Kwaan, H. C., Gallo, G., et al.: The nature of the vascular lesion in thrombotic thrombocytopenic purpura. Ann. Intern. Med. 68:1169, 1968.

143. Jobin, F., and Delâge, J. M.: Aspirin and prednisone in microangiopathic haemolytic anaemia. Lancet 2:208, 1970.

144. Zacharski, L. R., Walworth, C., et al.: Antiplatelet therapy for thrombotic thrombocytopenic purpura. New Engl. J. Med. 285:407, 1971.

145. Gasser, C., Gautier, E., et al.: Hämolytisch-uräemische syndrome: Bilaterale Nierenrindennekrosen bei akuten erworkenen hämolytischen Anämien. Schweiz. Med. Wochenschr. 85:905, 1955.

146. Tune, B. M., Leavitt, T. J., et al.: The hemolytic-uremic syndrome in California: A review of 28 nonheparinized cases with long-term follow-up. J. Pediatr. 82:304, 1973.

147. Gianantonio, C. A., Vitacco, M., et al.: The hemolytic-uremic syndrome. J. Pediatr. 64:478, 1964.

148. Piel, C. F., and Phibbs, R. H.: The hemolytic-uremic syndrome. Pediatr. Clin. North Am. 13:295, 1966.

149. Brain, M. C.: The haemolytic-uraemic syndrome. Semin. Hematol. 6:162, 1969.

150. Kaplan, B. S., Katz, J., et al.: An analysis of the results of therapy in 67 cases of the hemolytic-uremic syndrome. J. Pediatr. 78:420, 1971.

151. Lieberman, E., Heuser, E., et al.: Hemolytic-uremic syndrome: Clinical and pathological considerations. New Engl. J. Med. 275:227, 1966.

152. McLean, M. M., Jones, C. H., et al.: Haemolytic-uraemic syndrome. A report of an outbreak. Arch. Dis. Child. 41:76, 1966.

153. Ruthven, I. S., and Fyfe, W. M.: The haemolytic uraemic syndrome — An epidemic disease? Scot. Med. J. 13:162, 1968.

154. Avalos, J. S., Vitacco, M., et al.: Coagulation studies in the hemolytic-uremic syndrome. J. Pediatr. 76:538, 1970.

155. Katz, J., Lurie, A., et al.: Coagulation findings in the hemolytic-uremic syndrome of infancy: Similarity to hyperacute renal allograft rejection. J. Pediatr. 78:426, 1971.

156. Lanzkowsky, P., and McCrory, W.: Disseminated intravascular coagulation as a possible factor in the pathogenesis of thrombotic microangiopathy (hemolytic-uremic syndrome). J. Pediatr. 70:460, 1967.

157. Gilchrist, G. S., Ekert, H., et al.: Heparin therapy

in the haemolytic-uraemic syndrome. Lancet *1*:1123, 1969.

157a. Harker, L. A., and Slichter, M. D.: Platelet and fibrinogen consumption in man. New Engl. J. Med. *287*:999, 1972.

158. Gianantonio, C. A., Vitacco, M., et al.: The hemolytic-uremic syndrome: Renal status of 76 patients at long-term follow-up. J. Pediatr. *72*:757, 1968.

159. Lieberman, E.: Hemolytic-uremic syndrome. J. Pediatr. *80*:1, 1972.

160. Vitacco, M., Avalos, J. S., et al.: Heparin therapy in the hemolytic-uremic syndrome. J. Pediatr. *83*:271, 1973.

161. Beckert, R. S., and Flynn, F. J., Jr.: Toxoplasmosis. Report of two new cases, with a classification and with a demonstration of the organisms in the human placenta. New Engl. J. Med. *249*:345, 1953.

162. Weller, T. H., and Hanshaw, J. B.: Virologic and clinical observations on cytomegalic inclusion disease. New Engl. J. Med. *266*:1233, 1962.

163. Emanuel, I., and Kenny, G. E.: Cytomegalic inclusion disease of infancy. Pediatrics *38*:957, 1966.

164. Colebatch, J. H.: Clinical picture of severe generalized viral infection in the newborn. Med. J. Aust. *1*:377, 1955.

165. Nahmias, A. J., Alford, C. A., et al.: Infection of the newborn with herpes hominis. Adv. Pediatr. *17*:185, 1970.

166. Whitaker, J. A., Sartain, P., et al.: Hematologic aspects of congenital syphilis. J. Pediatr. *66*:629, 1965.

167. Saxoni, F., Lapatsanis, P., et al.: Congenital syphilis: A description of 18 cases and re-examination of an old but ever-present disease. Clin. Pediatr. (Philadelphia) *6*:687, 1967.

168. Silverman, W. A., and Homan, W. E.: Sepsis of obscure origin in the newborn. Pediatrics *3*:157, 1949.

169. Smith, R. T., Platou, E. S., et al.: Septicemia of the newborn. Current status of the problem. Pediatrics *17*:549, 1956.

170. Hamilton, J. R., and Sass-Kortsak, A.: Jaundice associated with severe bacterial infection in young infants. J. Pediatr. *63*:121, 1963.

171. Kalinowski, S. Z., and Walker, J. M.: Thrombocytopenic purpura in tuberculosis. Br. J. Tuberc. *50*:239, 1956.

172. Levy, M., and Cooper, B. A.: Thrombocytopenic purpura associated with tuberculosis lymphadenitis. Can. Med. Assoc. J. *90*:373, 1964.

173. Cohen, P., and Gardner, F. H.: Thrombocytopenia as a laboratory sign and complication of gram-negative bacteremic infection. Arch. Intern. Med. *117*:113, 1966.

174. Perlman, E. C.: Purpura and cerebral manifestations following measles: Report of 2 cases. Arch. Pediatr. *51*:596, 1934.

175. Ackroyd, J. F.: Three cases of thrombocytopenic purpura occurring after rubella. Quart. J. Med. *18*:299, 1949.

176. Reimann, H. A.: Thrombocytopenia in acute infections. J.A.M.A. *206*:649, 1968.

177. Corrigan, J. J., Ray, W. L., et al.: Changes in the blood coagulation system associated with septicemia. New Engl. J. Med. *279*:851, 1968.

178. Eisenstein, E. M.: Congenital amegakaryocytic thrombocytopenic purpura. Clin. Pediatr. (Philadelphia) *5*:143, 1966.

179. Bell, A. D., Mold, J. W., et al.: Study of transfused platelets in a case of congenital hypoplastic thrombocytopenia. Br. Med. J. *2*:692, 1956.

180. Emery, J. L., Gordon, R. R., et al.: Congenital amegakaryocytic thrombocytopenia with congenital deformities and a leukemoid blood picture in the newborn. Blood *12*:567, 1957.

181. Shaw, S., and Oliver, R. A. M.: Congenital hypoplastic thrombocytopenia with skeletal deformities in siblings. Blood *14*:374, 1959.

182. Nilsson, L. R., and Lundholm, G.: Congenital thrombocytopenia associated with aplasia of the radius. Acta Paediatr. *49*:291, 1960.

183. Dignan, P. S. J., Mauer, A. M., et al.: Phocomelia with congenital hypoplastic thrombocytopenia and myeloid leukemoid reactions. J. Pediatr. *70*:561, 1967.

184. Rodriguez, S. U., Leikin, S., et al.: Neonatal thrombocytopenia associated with antepartum administration of thiazide drugs. New Engl. J. Med. *270*:881, 1964.

185. Watson, C. J., Schultz, A. L., et al.: Purpura following estrogen therapy with particular reference to hypersensitivity to (diethyl) stilbestrol and with a note on the possible relationship of purpura to endogenous estrogens. J. Lab. Clin. Med. *32*:606, 1947.

186. Cooper, B. A., and Bigelow, F. S.: Thrombocytopenia associated with the administration of diethylstilbestrol in man. Ann. Intern. Med. *52*:907, 1960.

187. Lindenbalm, J.: Thrombocytopenia in alcoholics. Ann. Intern. Med. *68*:526, 1968.

188. Post, R. M., and Desforges, J. F.: Thrombocytopenia and alcoholism. Ann. Intern. Med. *68*:1230, 1968.

189. Cooper, L. Z., Green, R. H., et al.: Neonatal thrombocytopenic purpura and other manifestations of rubella contracted in utero. Am. J. Dis. Child. *110*:416, 1965.

190. Vossaugh, P., Leikin, S., et al.: Neonatal thrombocytopenia in association with rubella. Acta Haematol. (Basel) *35*:158, 1966.

191. Zinkham, W. H., Medearis, D. N., Jr., et al.: Blood and bone marrow findings in congenital rubella. J. Pediatr. *71*:512, 1967.

192. Oski, F. A., and Naiman, J. L.: Effect of live measles vaccine on the platelet count. New Engl. J. Med. *275*:352, 1966.

193. Paul, M. H., Currimbhoy, Z., et al.: Thrombocytopenia in cyanotic heart disease. Circulation *24*:1013, 1961.

194. Wedemeyer, A., and Lewis, J. H.: Improvement in hemostasis following phlebotomy in cyanotic patients with heart disease. J. Pediatr. *83*:46, 1973.

195. Schulman, I., Pierce, M., et al.: Studies on thrombopoiesis. I. A factor in normal human plasma required for platelet production: Chronic thrombocytopenia due to its deficiency. Blood *16*:943, 1960.

196. Abildgaard, C. F., Simone, J. V., et al.: Chronic thrombocytopenia due to "thrombopoietin" deficiency: A progress report. Blood *30*:546, 1967.

197. Schulman, I.: Unpublished observations.

198. Schulman, I., Smith, C. H., et al.: Vascular hemophilia. Pediatrics 18:347, 1956.

199. Nilsson, I. M., Blombäck, M., et al.: On an inherited autosomal hemorrhagic diathesis with antihemophilic globulin (AHG) deficiency and prolonged bleeding time. Acta Med. Scand. 159:35, 1957.

200. Cornu, P., Larrieu, M. J., et al.: Transfusion studies in von Willebrand's disease: Effect on bleeding time and factor VIII. Br. J. Haematol. 9:189, 1963.

201. Weiss, H. J.: The use of plasma and plasma fractions in the treatment of a patient with von Willebrand's disease. Vox Sang. 7:267, 1962.

202. Spaet, T. H., and Zucker, M. B.: Mechanism of platelet plug formation and role of adenosine diphosphate. Am. J. Physiol. 206:1267, 1964.

203. Weiss, H. J.: Platelet aggregation, adhesion and adenosine diphosphate release in thrombopathia (platelet Factor 3 deficiency)—A comparison with Glanzmann's thrombasthenia and von Willebrand's disease. Am. J. Med. 43:570, 1967.

204. Weiss, H. J.: von Willebrand's disease—Diagnostic criteria. Blood 32:668, 1968.

205. Salzman, E. W.: Measurement of platelet adhesiveness. A simple in vitro technique demonstrating an abnormality in von Willebrand's disease. J. Lab. Clin. Med. 62:724, 1963.

206. Holmberg, L., and Nilsson, I. M.: Two genetic variants of von Willebrand's disease. New Engl. J. Med. 288:595, 1973.

207. Corby, D. G., Zirbel, C. L., et al.: Thrombasthenia. Am. J. Dis. Child. 121:140, 1971.

208. Glanzmann, E.: Hereditare hamorrhagische Thrombasthenie: Ein Beitrag zur Pathologie der Blutplattchen. J. Kinderheilkd. 88:113–120, 1963.

209. Hardisty, R. M., Dormandy, K. M., et al.: Thrombasthenia: Studies on three cases. Br. J. Haematol. 10:371–387, 1964.

210. Cronberg, S., Nilsson, I. M., et al.: Investigation of a family with members with both severe and a mild degree of thrombasthenia. Acta Paediatr. Scand. 56:189–197, 1967.

211. Caen, J., Castaldi, P. A., et al.: Congenital bleeding disorders with long bleeding time and normal platelet count. I. Glanzmann's thrombasthenia (report of 15 patients). Am. J. Med. 41:4, 1966.

212. Weiss, H. J., and Kochwa, S.: Studies of platelet function and proteins in 3 patients with Glanzmann's thrombasthenia. J. Lab. Clin. Med. 71:153, 1968.

213. Nachman, R. L.: Thrombasthenia: Immunologic evidence of a platelet protein abnormality. J. Lab. Clin. Med. 67:411, 1966.

214. Yankee, R. A., Grumet, F. C., et al.: Platelet transfusion therapy: The selection of compatible platelet donors for refractory patients by lymphocyte HL-A typing. New Engl. J. Med. 281:1208–1212, 1969.

215. Holmsen, H., and Weiss, H. J.: Hereditary defect in the platelet release reaction caused by a deficiency in the storage pool of platelet adenine nucleotides. Br. J. Haematol. 19:643, 1970.

216. Holmsen, H., and Weiss, H. J.: Further evidence for a deficient storage pool of adenine nucleo-

tides in platelets from some patients with thrombocytopathia—"Storage pool disease." Blood 39:197, 1972.

217. Weiss, H. J.: Platelet aggregation, adhesion and adenosine diphosphate release in thrombopathia (platelet Factor 3 deficiency): A comparison with Glanzmann's thrombasthenia and von Willebrand's disease. Am. J. Med. 43:570, 1967.

218. Hardisty, R. M., and Hutton, R. A.: Bleeding tendency associated with "new" abnormality of platelet behavior. Lancet 1:983, 1967.

219. Hirsch, J., Castelan, D. J., et al.: Spontaneous bruising associated with defect in interaction of platelets with connective tissue. Lancet 2:18, 1967.

220. O'Brien, J.: Platelets: Portsmouth syndrome? Lancet 2:258, 1967.

221. Sahud, M. A., and Aggeler, P. M.: Platelet dysfunction: Differentiation of a newly recognized primary type from that produced by aspirin. New Engl. J. Med. 280:453, 1969.

222. Ulitin, O. N., and Karaca, M.: A study on the pathogenesis of thrombopathia using the platelet osmotic-resistance test. Br. J. Haematol. 5:302, 1959.

223. Weiss, H. J., and Eichelberger, J. W.: The detection of platelet defects in patients with mild bleeding disorders: Use of a quantitative assay for platelet Factor 3. Am. J. Med. 32:872, 1962.

224. Johnson, S. A., Monto, R. W., et al.: A new approach to the thrombocytopathies: Thrombocytopathy A. Thromb. Diath. Haemorrh. 2:279, 1958.

225. Corby, D. G., and Schulman, I.: The effects of antenatal drug administration on aggregation of platelets of newborn infants. J. Pediatr. 79:307, 1971.

226. Mull, M. M., and Hathaway, W. E.: Altered platelet function in newborns. Pediatr. Res. 4:229, 1970.

227. Hathaway, W. E.: Platelet function. Adv. Pediatr. 19:237, 1972.

228. Weiss, H. J., Aledort, L. M., et al.: The effect of salicylates on the hemostatic properties of platelets in man. J. Clin. Invest. 47:2169, 1968.

229. Weiss, H. J., and Aledort, L. M.: Impaired platelet-connective tissue reaction in man after aspirin ingestion. Lancet 2:495, 1967.

230. Zucker, M. B., and Peterson, J.: Inhibition of adenosine diphosphate–induced secondary aggregation and other platelet functions by acetylsalicylic acid. Proc. Soc. Exp. Biol. Med. 127:547, 1968.

231. O'Brien, J. R.: Effects of salicylates on human platelets. Lancet 1:779, 1968.

232. Stuart, M. J., Murphy, S., et al.: Platelet function in recipients of platelets from donors ingesting aspirin. New Engl. J. Med. 278:1105, 1972.

233. Casteels-Van Daele, M., and Degaetano, G.: Purpura and acetylsalicylic acid therapy. Acta Paediatr. Scand. 60:203, 1971.

234. Singer, R.: Aspirin, a probable cause for secondary post-tonsillectomy hemorrhage. Arch. Otolaryngol. (Chicago) 42:19, 1945.

235. Kaneshire, M. M., Mielke, C. H., Jr., et al.: Bleed-

ing time after aspirin in disorders of intrinsic clotting. New Engl. J. Med. 281:1039, 1969.

236. Quick, A. J.: Salicylates and bleeding: The aspirin tolerance test. Am. J. Med. Sci. 252:265, 1967.

237. Czapek, E. E., Deykin, D., et al.: Platelet dysfunction in glycogen storage disease Type I. Blood 41:235, 1973.

238. Corby, D., Pildes, R., et al.: Platelet defect in glycogen storage disease (GSD). Clin. Res. 19:207, 1971.

239. Stewart, J. H., and Castaldi, P. A.: Uraemic bleeding: A reversible platelet defect corrected by dialysis. Quart. J. Med. 36:409, 1967.

240. Rabiner, S. F., and Hiodek, O.: Platelet Factor 3 in normal subjects and patients with renal failure. J. Clin. Invest. 47:901, 1968.

241. Horowitz, H. I., Cohen, B. D., et al.: Defective ADP-induced platelet Factor 3 activation in uremia. Blood 30:331, 1967.

242. Rabiner, S. F., and Molinas, F.: The role of phenol and phenolic acids on the thrombocytopathy and defective platelet aggregation of patients with renal failure. Am. J. Med. 49:346, 1970.

243. Horowitz, H. I., Stein, I. M., et al.: Further studies on the platelet-inhibitory effect of guanidinosuccinic acid and its role in uremic bleeding. Am. J. Med. 49:336, 1970.

244. Bean, R. H. D.: Thrombocytosis in auto-immune disease. Bibl. Haematol. 23:43, 1965.

245. Marchasin, S., Wallerstein, R. D., et al.: Variation of the platelet count in disease. California Med. 101:95, 1964.

246. Morowitz, D. A., Allen, L. W., et al.: Thrombocytosis in chronic inflammatory bowel disease. Ann. Intern. Med. 68:1013, 1968.

247. Levin, J., and Conley, C. L.: Thrombocytosis associated with malignant disease. Arch. Intern. Med. (Chicago) 114:497, 1964.

248. Gross, S., Keeler, V., et al.: The platelets in iron deficiency anemia. I. The response to oral and parenteral iron. Pediatrics 34:315, 1964.

249. Slater, P. P., and Sherlock, E. C.: Splenectomy, thrombocytosis, and venous thrombosis. Am. Surg. 23:549, 1957.

250. Lipson, R. L., Bayrd, E. D., et al.: The post-splenectomy blood picture. Am. J. Clin. Pathol. 32:526, 1959.

251. Charlesworth, D., and Torrence, H. B.: Splenectomy in idiopathic thrombocytopenic purpura. Br. J. Surg. 55:437, 1968.

252. Hirsch, J., and Dacie, J. V.: Persistent post-splenectomy thrombocytosis and thromboembolism: A consequence of continuing anaemia. Br. J. Haematol. 12:44, 1966.

253. Wollstein, M., and Kreidel, K. V.: Blood picture after splenectomy in children. With special reference to platelets. Am. J. Dis. Child. 51:765, 1936.

254. Sanyal, S. K., Yules, R. B., et al.: Thrombocytosis, central nervous system disease, and myocardial infarction pattern in infancy. Pediatrics 38:629, 1966.

255. Spach, M. S., Howell, D. A., et al.: Myocardial infarction and multiple thromboses in a child with primary thrombocytosis. Pediatrics 31:268, 1963.

256. Spaet, T. H., Bauer, D., et al.: Hemorrhagic thrombocythemia: A blood coagulation disorder. Arch. Intern. Med. (Chicago) 98:377, 1956.

257. Spaet, T. H., Lejnieks, I., et al.: Defective platelets in essential thrombocythemia. Arch. Intern. Med. (Chicago) 124:135, 1969.

258. Bensinger, T. A., Logue, G. L., et al.: Hemorrhagic thrombocythemia. Control of post-splenectomy thrombocytosis with melphalan. Blood 36:61, 1970.

259. Robertson, J. H.: Uracil mustard in the treatment of thrombocythemia. Blood 35:288, 1970.

IV

INVASIVE
AND
STORAGE
DISORDERS

Chapter 22

The Leukemias and Reticuloendothelioses

by Alvin M. Mauer, Beatrice C. Lampkin,
and Nancy B. McWilliams

The leukemias are malignancies of the blood-forming organs. The reticuloendothelioses (Letterer-Siwe disease, Hand-Schüller-Christian disease, eosinophilic granuloma of bone, and related disorders of the reticuloendothelial system) are more difficult to define, but do appear to represent proliferative disorders of that collection of fixed and wandering macrophages which are derived from the blood monocytes. These two forms of proliferative disorders, the leukemias and the reticuloendothelioses, will be discussed in this chapter. The various forms of leukemia will be presented first.

CLASSIFICATION

The blood-forming organs are responsible for the production of several types of cells. In their formation several stages of maturation and degrees of differentiation occur. Therefore, it is to be expected that the defects induced by the malignant transformation in leukemia could result in a variety of clinically and morphologically distinguishable types of leukemia, depending upon the cell line involved and the severity of the maturation defect that had occurred.

A classification of the leukemias of childhood is presented in Table 22–1. One method of classifying these diseases is to divide them into acute and chronic leukemia, based primarily on time of survival in the untreated patient and correlated with the degree of immaturity of the cell type. The advent of prolonged survival in many appropriately treated patients demands more precise definition of these diseases for purposes of treatment and for considerations of etiology, pathophysiology, and clinical characteristics. A more accurate and useful classification would most likely be based on the stem line from which the malignant cells have been derived.

The cell type from which the so-called lymphoid leukemias are derived has not yet been completely established. It is assumed that the cells represent malignant transformation of the lymphocytes of the immune system. The information concerning chronic lymphocytic leukemia is quite consistent with that conclusion. The cells in that disease are sufficiently differentiated to have some of the characteristic features of lymphocytes, most often of the B cell or bone marrow–derived cell line (1, 2). Surface immunoglobulins (1) and receptor sites for complement (2) are present on the cell membranes of lymphocytes from patients with chronic lymphocytic leukemia. Furthermore, abnormalities of immunoglobulin formation can occur in that disease. In acute lymphoblastic leukemia, however, little cell differentiation takes place, and thus the surface receptors characteristic of B or T cells are not regularly developed. For example, complement receptor sites cannot be demonstrated on the cell surface of acute leukemic lymphoblasts (2). In addition, these cells do not respond to mitogens

665

TABLE 22–1. CLASSIFICATION OF THE
LEUKEMIAS OF CHILDHOOD

1. Lymphoid cell line
   a. Acute lymphoblastic leukemia
   b. Chronic lymphocytic leukemia

2. Myeloid cell line
   a. Acute myeloblastic leukemia
   b. Erythroleukemia
   c. Eosinophilic leukemia
   d. Promyelocytic leukemia
   e. Monoblastic leukemia
      (1) Naegeli type
      (2) Schilling type
   f. Chronic myelocytic leukemia
      (1) Juvenile form
      (2) Adult form (Ph^1 chromosome-positive)

3. Undifferentiated
   a. Acute "stem cell" leukemia

such as phytohemagglutinin by cell division, a characteristic of lymphocytes of T cell or thymus-derived type. Functional deficits in either of these two categories of immunologic response have not been described as a feature of acute lymphoblastic leukemia. Recent studies of acute lymphatic leukemia cells, though suggestive that the blasts are of T cell origin in some cases, do not provide sufficient data for a definitive conclusion (2a, 2b, 2c). Therefore, the assignment of the cells of acute lymphoblastic leukemia to the lymphoid system for their derivation is based mostly on morphologic resemblance and the lack of any features which would suggest myeloid cell line origin. Further studies may clarify the question of specific cell line derivation for this form of acute leukemia.

It should be further appreciated that the cells in acute lymphoblastic leukemia are not completely uniform in appearance from patient to patient. On morphologic grounds alone, Amiel (3) has proposed four classifications of acute lymphoblastic leukemia: prolymphoblastic, macrolymphoblastic, microlymphoblastic, and prolymphocytic, in order of their presumed degree of increasing differentiation. He has further correlated these morphologically distinctive types with response to treatment, microlymphoblastic being the most sensitive, and prolymphoblastic the most resistant. We have had no experience with this form of subdivision of acute lymphoblastic leukemia.

In another study Fraumeni and his coworkers (4) reviewed the characteristics of leukemia in 1263 patients classified by their morphologic cell type. They found differences in survival and some epidemiologic features, such as distribution by age among patients classified as having either acute lymphoblastic or acute undifferentiated (stem cell) leukemia. These two forms of leukemia are morphologically so similar that they are usually considered as one group for analysis in most studies. Again, therefore, there is indication that the acute form of leukemia called lymphoblastic may contain subgroups that may be of importance with regard to treatment and etiology.

In children it is the acute form of leukemia of the lymphoid derivation that is seen almost exclusively. Although there are occasional reports of chronic lymphocytic leukemia, or what appears to be a closely allied condition, in children, it is hard to be sure that these conditions truly represent the same disease that is seen in adults, generally in the elderly (5, 5a,b).

The myeloid forms of leukemia presumably all represent malignant transformation of the same stem cell line, the differences in appearance and characteristics of the clinical course being related to the degree and type of differentiation typical of the transformation process. It is intriguing to consider whether the characteristics of the derivative cell line are related in some way to the characteristics of a specific etiologic agent in producing the transformation. Of interest in this respect is the observation that, in Fanconi's anemia in which an increased risk of leukemia occurs, the form of the disease expressed is monoblastic (4). In another condition in which a similar increased risk of leukemia occurs, Down's syndrome, there is no difference in the distribution of types of leukemia seen from that found in children in general when matched for age of onset (6). Much, therefore, remains to be learned about the morphologic expression of leukemia and its possible relationship to etiology.

As in adults, two forms of chronic myelocytic leukemia occur, separable by the presence or absence of the Philadelphia chromosome. The characteristics of these two forms will be discussed in the section on chronic myelocytic leukemia.

In the study by Fraumeni and his co-workers (4), the distribution of the type of acute leukemia in children was 43.9 per cent lymphoblastic, 24.6 per cent undifferentiated, 23.8 per cent myeloblastic, and 7.8 per cent monoblastic. The other forms of acute myeloid leukemia are too infrequent to be compared. Usually, lymphoblastic and undifferentiated (stem cell) leukemias are considered together, although a good case has been made by these authors to regard them as potentially different. The proportion of the various forms of acute leukemia varies from one report to another, primarily because of classification by subjective morphologic assessment. Although criteria have been devised to differentiate the two major forms of acute leukemia, lymphoblastic and myeloblastic (7), there is of necessity variability in the application of these criteria.

ACUTE LEUKEMIA

In this section acute lymphoblastic and myeloblastic leukemia will be discussed. Although there are important distinguishing features of these two forms of acute leukemia, in general the clinical course and the approach to, if not the specifics of, management have enough in common to consider them together. The critical differences in treatment and prognosis will be mentioned. Because these differences are important, every effort should be made to differentiate these two forms at the time of diagnosis. The distinction usually can be made on morphologic grounds using ordinary Wright's stained smears of blood and bone marrow (7), but occasionally some additional help can be gained from special histochemical techniques (8).

Morphologic Considerations in the Differential Diagnosis of the Forms of Acute Leukemia

It is important to discriminate between the acute lymphoblastic, myeloblastic, and undifferentiated forms of leukemia, since selection of therapeutic protocols depends upon such differential diagnosis.

The classification should be based on the findings in the marrow, unless the blast count in peripheral blood is in excess of 20,000 per mm³. This is because in unusual cases the presence of leukemic cells of any type in the marrow may induce a so-called "leukoerythroblastic" response by the remaining normal elements of the marrow. In this response (which occurs as a result of many different kinds of marrow invasion, including fibrosis, granulomatosis, and solid tumor invasion, as well as leukemia), nucleated red cell precursors, myeloblasts, and early granulocyte precursors, megakaryocyte fragments, and "tear drop" red cells are present in the peripheral smear. The presence of myeloblasts in the blood may incorrectly suggest the diagnosis of acute myeloblastic leukemia. Inspection of the marrow will frequently reveal the typical cells of acute lymphoblastic leukemia.

Morphologic characteristics are the mainstays of correct diagnosis. Examples are found in Color Plate I. The important points are that the nuclear chromatin tends to be clumped in lymphoblasts and spongy in myeloblasts; the nuclear : cytoplasmic ratio is higher in lymphoblasts than in myeloblasts; and the nucleoli are more numerous and their borders more distinct or "punched out" in myeloblasts than in lymphoblasts. True Auer rods, which are abnormal lysosomes, are present in myeloblasts but not in lymphoblasts. (Sometimes red-staining mitochondria may line up in the hof of the lymphoblast nucleus like a small chain of beads. These must be distinguished from solid Auer rods which are thicker and uninterrupted.) Finally, the cytoplasm tends to be blue and nongranular in lymphoblasts, when it is visible at all, and blue-grey with occasional granules in myeloblasts.

There are two forms of acute monoblastic leukemia. The first, the so-called Naegeli type, is in fact acute myeloblastic leukemia in which some of the myeloblasts bear a resemblance to monoblasts. The nuclei tend to be folded and ovoid, and the nuclear : cytoplasmic ratio even lower than in the usual myeloblast.

The Schilling type of acute monoblastic leukemia is a distinct entity. The morphology is clearly monoblastic, with ovoid folded nuclei and multiple nucleoli. Clinical expression includes marked gum invasion with gingival hypertrophy and a fulminating course.

Acute stem cell leukemia is usually a diagnosis made in morphologic desperation. The blast cells defy clear-cut classification. They are variably sized primitive cells with foamy nuclei and with distinct and indistinct nucleoli. Occasionally the nucleoli are large and bluish in the Giemsa stain and resemble the nucleoli of primitive reticulum cells.

Special histochemical stains may be useful in the differential diagnosis of the acute leukemias when the morphology after ordinary Giemsa staining is uncertain, but usually the histochemical stains are merely confirmatory (8). The myeloperoxidase stain may be positive in blasts of uncertain lineage, and thereby reveal that they are myeloblasts or monoblasts. The stain may also highlight Auer rods [which contain myeloperoxidase activity (9)] when none are visible by ordinary microscopy. The PAS stain for glycogen is less useful but, when positive, suggests the lymphatic origin of the blast cells. Sudanophilia is more evident in myeloblasts. The reader is referred to the excellent monograph by Hayhoe and coworkers for further use of these techniques (8).

Etiology

Although specific etiologic agents or factors have not been directly linked to the causation of leukemia, over the past few years increasing clarity concerning several relationships has developed. These relationships involve both host factors and environmental agents. It may very well be that an interaction of provocative environmental agents and a susceptible host is responsible for the development of leukemia.

Much of the evidence for relationships of both host and environmental factors in the development of leukemia has come from epidemiologic research observations (10, 11). This kind of research has provided information indicating the likely causal relationship of some agents and host factors by a careful demonstration of statistically significant association. It also has provided equally important evidence against certain hypotheses, such as horizontal transmission of leukemia by infectious agents (12). An important aspect of this research now is to determine the mechanisms by which these factors lead to the development of leukemia. These studies are currently being actively pursued.

ENVIRONMENTAL FACTORS. The best documented environmental factor related to leukemogenesis is *ionizing irradiation*. The evidence has come from studies of individuals who received therapeutic irradiation to the spine for ankylosing spondylitis (13) and of the populations exposed to the atomic bomb explosions at Hiroshima and Nagasaki (14). In both these population groups, there was a dose-related incidence of leukemia, with a linear increase in leukemia occurring with increasing exposure to the ionizing irradiation. In neither study, however, was it possible to assess the risk of leukemia at very low dose rates; thus the possibility of a "threshold effect" was not excluded. In both groups the maximal occurrence of leukemia was about three to five years after the exposure. Also, in both groups the increase in leukemic incidence was caused by increases in both acute and chronic forms of myeloid leukemia.

The mechanisms by which ionizing irradiation can cause malignant transformation are certainly not obvious (15). The necessary somatic mutation leading to malignant transformation could be related to direct alteration of the cell subject to modification by cellular or environmental events. It also could result from activation of a latent oncogenic virus harbored within the cell (15a).

Color Plate I. Photomicrographs of blood, marrow and spinal fluid smears in leukemia, lymphosarcoma and neuroblastoma.
1. Peripheral blood. Acute lymphatic leukemia.
2. Peripheral blood. Acute myeloblastic leukemia. Note Auer rod.
3. Peripheral blood. Leukoerythroblastosis. Acute lymphatic leukemia.
4. Bone marrow. Acute lymphatic leukemia.
5. Bone marrow. Acute myeloblastic leukemia.
6. Bone marrow. Neuroblastoma. Note rosette formation.
7. Blast cell. Acute undifferentiated leukemia.
8. Peripheral blood. Acute lymphatic leukemia, lymphosarcoma type. Note fissured lymphocytes.
9. Spinal fluid. Acute myeloblastic leukemia.

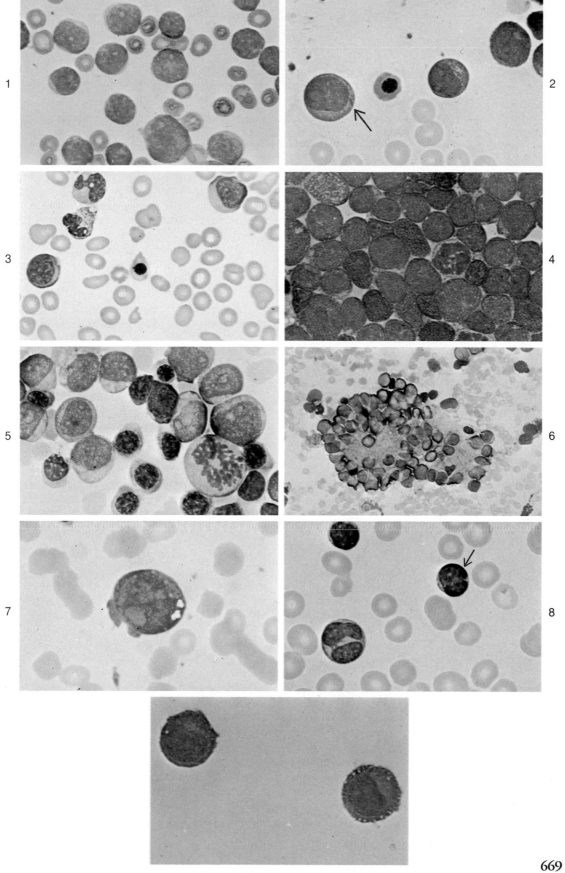

Color Plate I. *See opposite page for legend.*

In either case, a hereditable mutation must result, endowing the cell with the capacity for further cell division, but with phenotypic characteristics which permit escape from the physiologic control mechanisms that govern growth in that tissue. Thus chromosomal alteration should be involved.

During its passage through the cell, a particle of ionizing radiation deposits energy along its path. The energy is absorbed in large part by the production of excited molecules or free radicals (16). Much of this absorbed energy is subsequently dissipated as heat. Some of the free radical formation may institute chemical reactions harmful to the cell by interacting with critical molecules. Of importance in leukemogenesis is the possibility of inactivation of DNA either by causing physical breaks interfering with strand continuity or by destroying bases on both complementary strands (17). The effectiveness of repair mechanisms is an important factor which influences the eventual degree of permanent alteration borne by the radiated cell (18). Although the postirradiation events that lead to the damage require only a microsecond, the subsequent alteration of the cell may persist. Irradiation can induce chromosomal breaks and gaps, as well as the structural abnormalities that occur with rearrangements of the fractured chromosomes, such as inversions or translocations. These abnormalities have been found in survivors of the atomic bomb explosions (19, 20), indicating that such changes are in fact found in a population with a radiation-related increase in the risk of leukemia.

Not all cell lines in acute leukemia have chromosomal abnormalities demonstrable by current techniques, and where aneuploidy does occur, it is not necessarily characteristic of laboratory-induced postirradiation changes. Thus the direct causal relationship between the observed chromosomal changes induced by irradiation and the leukemic transformation of the cell is not established. Of particular interest in radiation leukemogenesis is the observation that, in induced tumors in animals, filterable agents can be found having the characteristics of C-type viral particles which can subsequently induce tumor formation upon transmission to nonirradiated animals (21).

There are apparent host factors operative in radiation leukemogenesis. In the atomic bomb experience, the risk for males was greater than for females. The reason for this sex difference is unknown. It would also seem that patients with a proliferative defect in a cell line, such as presumably exists in polycythemia vera, are particularly susceptible to an additional mutagenic challenge from irradiation (22, 22a).

Other factors may modify the effectiveness of a dose of irradiation in the induction of a leukemic mutation. There is, for example, a cell cycle (23) and total proliferative activity (24) dependency on sensitivity to irradiation-induced cell death. Extrapolating these observations to radiation leukemogenesis, one might expect to find similar variation in responsiveness of the affected tissue, a possibility which needs testing. Some drugs increase radiation sensitivity of cells (25), and others have the potential for decreasing radiation injury (16). Events occurring after irradiation, such as the stress of anemia (26), may potentiate the development of leukemia in rats. The role of all these possible modifying factors has not been evaluated for potential significance in human leukemia.

What is the extent of the role of radiation leukemogenesis in human disease at present? The environmental hazard of the atomic bomb will hopefully not be reproduced again, and irradiation therapy for nonmalignant diseases, such as rheumatoid spondylitis, has been curtailed. The major sources today are background—an irreducible exposure to earth and cosmic irradiation sources—and diagnostic roentgenographic studies. There is no evidence that variation in irradiation from earth (27) or cosmic (28) sources is related to variation in leukemic mortality. The data related to diagnostic irradiation, however, are conflicting. There are three areas of concern: preconceptual, in utero, and postnatal exposure.

The conflicts regarding the effect of preconceptual or in utero irradiation on leukemic incidence have arisen because of the discrepancy between observations based on the atomic bomb studies and those based on surveys of leukemic incidence in children born to parents having preconceptual irradiation or in those who were exposed in utero because of diagnostic irradiation for the mother (11, 29). In the atomic bomb studies, no increase in frequency of leukemia has been observed in these two particular exposure groups, in contrast to the reported increase seen after diagnostic studies. The suggestion has been made that factors related to the *indications* for the diagnostic studies may have a primary or contributory role in leukemogenesis.

A recent study (30) has indicated an association between diagnostic irradiation and leukemia in adult males. The increased incidence was related to acute and chronic forms of myeloid leukemia. The authors concluded, however, that only a small proportion of the irradiated population develops leukemia, and only a small proportion of leukemia cases can be accounted for by diagnostic irradiation.

In summary, irradiation has a relationship to the onset of leukemia, chiefly to the acute and chronic myeloid forms. The mechanism may be an indirect one, such as the activation of a latent oncogenic virus. However, the available evidence indicates that irradiation is a minor factor in the etiology of leukemia at present.

Chemical carcinogens have been implicated as a potential environmental factor because of early observations of leukemia after benzene exposure (11). Chemical carcinogens characteristically are bound to the DNA of the target cell (31, 32) and may achieve this state by an activation process, perhaps involving free radical formation. The attachment of the carcinogen to the DNA may directly modify the DNA, cause alterations which decrease the fidelity of DNA copies, or cause the formation of altered RNA which, by means of the reverse transcription pathway, in turn produces altered DNA for integration into host DNA. Chemical carcinogens may also activate latent oncogenic viruses (33) or perhaps allow for proliferation of neoplastic cells, either by blunting the host immune system or by selective inhibition of normal cell proliferation.

Among the list of agents purported to be causally linked to leukemogenesis, the evidence is best for benzene (11). At present there is no indication that chemicals are responsible for anything but a minor segment of the leukemia incidence. As with irradiation, the risk of chemically induced leukemia may be greater in conjunction with certain host factors. An indication of the potential importance of the association has been the observation of an increased frequency of acute leukemia in patients with multiple myeloma treated with melphalan (34). It may be that, in the future, patient populations can be defined in whom drugs having leukemogenic potential can be avoided.

Most research concerning the etiology of leukemia is now directed toward the role of *oncogenic viruses.* It is interesting that the impetus for studies in radiation and chemical leukemogenesis came primarily from epidemiologic studies in humans. In viral leukemogenesis, however, the epidemiologic studies have been uniformly disappointing. Information concerning viral leukemogenesis has come instead almost entirely from animal studies.

The emergence of knowledge concerning the role of viruses in animal tumors is an oft-told tale and has recently been succinctly summarized by Epstein (35). It does not need repeating here. Of greater interest are the studies which have developed the concepts of how the RNA and DNA tumor viruses induce malignant transformation and human epidemiologic studies which have tested the hypothesis for an infectious, transmissable agent as a causative factor in leukemia.

From animal studies, the most likely candidate for the leukemogenic virus or group of viruses is the RNA virus of the C type (36). An important aspect of the linkage between this class of oncogenic viruses and the actual transformation of a cell to a line having hereditably malignant features is the discovery of the "reverse" transcriptase system (36a,b, 37, 37a). This system may explain how an RNA strand might serve as a template for the formation of a complementary DNA strand by means of the polymerase enzyme, "reverse" transcriptase. The virus carries the RNA template and the necessary enzyme and makes the DNA strand within the infected cell. The DNA strand can then serve as a template for further reproduction of itself and subsequently be incorporated into the genome of the cell itself. In that position it can then serve to produce more tumor virus RNA for continuation of the viral strain. It also can become inactive in the cell genome, only to appear in active form spontaneously upon serial passage of the infected cell line in tissue culture. The appearance of the virus can also be called forth by exposure of the cell line to some physical or chemical agents.

Active production of C-type particles has been seen in some animal tumor cells by means of the electron microscope. None has ever been convincingly demonstrated in human malignant tissue as yet, in spite of extensive search. Recently it has been demonstrated that somatic and germ cells of vertebrates, with primary evidence being obtained in the mouse, rat, and chicken, contain the genetic information for producing C-type RNA tumor virus in an unexpressed form (38). This information has led to the speculation that this information has been part of the genetic construct of vertebrates since early in evolution. The endogenous virogenes (genes for production of the C-type viruses) and oncogenes (the portion of the virogene responsible for transforming a normal cell into a tumor cell) are maintained in an unexpressed form by repressors in normal cells. Various agents, such as irradiation, chemical carcinogens, and perhaps even exogenous viruses, may transform cells by switching on the endogenous oncogenic information. This interesting hypothesis has the attractiveness of unifying the several concepts for environmental factors on leukemogenesis. It also obviously casts the role of the oncogenic virus as something other than that of an infectious transmissable agent.

All these studies have been performed in lower animals. In the past two years proteins with reverse transcriptase activity have been detected in human leukemic cells (37a). In addition, terminal transferase, an enzyme formerly thought to be restricted to thymic tissue, has also been detected in human leukemic cells (38a). It has also been claimed that DNA complementary to animal RNA tumor viruses may be found in leukemic cells and other human tumor tissues (39). That only the leukemic member of pairs of identical twins harbored the DNA complementary to oncorna virus RNA is held as evidence against a virogene or oncogene hypothesis and evidence for the acquisition of a leukemia-inducing exogenous agent (39a). Such an agent might cause leukemia induction directly in marrow cells, or it might induce an alteration in the thymus that would secondarily induce leukemia in cells that pass through the thymus. Needless to say, these developments relating RNA viruses to human malignant disease are being pursued with a sense of real excitement.

The accumulating evidence indicates that the relationship of viruses to leukemia may not be as transmissable or infectious agents. What are the results of epidemiologic studies? The most quoted of the reports which purported to indicate an infectious agent as a cause of leukemia was that based on a study conducted in Niles, Illinois (40). Many subsequent studies, however, have failed to show any significant clustering effect either by time or place (41–43). The apparent clusters that have been reported can be accounted for by random distribution of events (42). There is also no evidence for transmission of leukemia from mother to child (11) in a vertical manner, as has been observed in some animal tumors. There have been recent reports that an excessive incidence of cancer has occurred in children born of mothers having viral infections during pregnancy (44, 45). These studies need confirmation and detailed analysis before a causal relationship can be accepted.

The one DNA virus that has been studied in relationship to leukemogenesis has been the Epstein-Barr virus of infectious mononucleosis (46). This virus does result in proliferation of lymphoid cells in vivo and permits the lymphocyte to be carried as a proliferating cell line in tissue culture (47). It has also been demonstrated that the virus can be recovered from certain lymphoid cell lines after treatment with the drug 5-bromodeoxyuridine (48). Thus the entire viral genome may persist in the nuclei of at least a proportion of lymphoid cells. The relationship of the virus to lymphoid cells suggests the possibility that it induces malignant transformation. Despite the fact that acute leukemia and infectious mononucleosis have been seen concurrently (49), prospective studies have failed to indicate an etiologic role for the Epstein-Barr virus in acute lymphoblastic leukemia (50).

In summary, the relationship of oncogenic viruses to leukemogenesis is still incompletely understood. As the information is currently developing, there is no indication that a transmissable, infectious agent is responsible. The most attractive hypothesis now, that of the oncogene, would suggest that the affected cells carry the information for malignant transformation, requiring activation or switching on by some intracellular event probably related to environmental factors.

HOST FACTORS. There are several observations which indicate the importance of genetic or at least prenatal influences on subsequent development of leukemia in children (51). Children early in the birth order or born to older mothers have a higher risk of leukemia (52, 53). In this context it is interesting to recall that a greater risk for Down's syndrome is also present in children born to older mothers. There is an increased incidence of leukemia in Down's syndrome (22) and furthermore an increased incidence of Down's syndrome among siblings of patients with leukemia (54). In identical twins, a concordance rate of 17 per cent for leukemia exists if the twins are under the age of 6 years when the disease occurs (55). The frequency of leukemia in nontwin siblings has been reported to be four times greater than that in the general population (22), but other studies have not confirmed this increased risk (55). The reported increase could be due to unrecognized, genetically determined diseases predisposing to leukemia in certain families (55). The incidence of acute myeloblastic and lymphoblastic leukemia in white and nonwhite children in the United States is consistent with the hypothesis that the myeloid form has a common etiology in white and nonwhite children, but that nonwhite children either are not exposed to or are protected against agents causing lymphoblastic leukemia (56).

In addition to these general indications of the importance of genetic or prenatal factors, there are specific identifiable congenital conditions predisposing to acute leukemia (22, 57). These conditions are characterized by chromosomal abnormalities, such as the aneuploidy of Down's syndrome or the excessive breaks and chromosomal reconstructions found in Fanconi's anemia and Bloom's syndrome. The exact mechanism by which these abnormalities are related to the malignant transformation of leukemia is not known, but chromosomal changes are also characteristic of irradiation and chemical carcinogenesis. Recently, Swift (58) has studied purported heterozygotes for Fanconi's anemia and found a threefold increase in malignancy. Thus,

hitherto unrecognized genetic predisposition to cancer, including leukemia, may exist in given populations. It is of obvious importance to identify those conditions which may not have easily recognizable features but which may carry a greater risk for leukemia, so that prospective longitudinal studies may be performed.

The syndromes associated with defective immune systems are usually associated with a greater risk of lymphoma, but leukemia may also occur. Two mechanisms which may cause this relationship are inherent abnormalities of the cell line associated with the defective immune state, and the failure of eradication of hypothetical random malignant mutations when the "immune surveillance system" is deficient (57a).

Thus the importance of genetic and prenatal factors in the development of leukemia is amply demonstrated. As preventive measures are developed, it will be increasingly important to develop tools for identification of individuals with an excessive risk for leukemia. Currently, the epidemiologic approach is the strongest tool available.

Incidence

The peak incidence for acute leukemia in children is between the ages of one and five years. Mortality figures for white boys and girls are 6.0 and 5.2 per 100,000 in the United States during that age (59). In the same age group, nonwhite boys and girls in the United States have mortality figures of 3.1 and 2.6 per 100,000. The difference is related to the increased incidence of acute lymphoblastic leukemia in white children, there being no difference in acute myeloblastic leukemia (56). The risk of acute leukemia in white children during the first ten years of life is 1 in 2880 (22). The peak incidence for acute lymphoblastic leukemia in white children is at three to four years of age; no such peak is seen for acute myeloblastic leukemia (4,60). This peak incidence had not been seen for nonwhite children, but in recent years has become apparent (10).

A decrease in mortality from leukemia for children in the United States has been evident since 1960 (61). The distribution of cases by age has not changed, however, and the peak incidence remains at four years of age. Miller (61) has speculated that the decrease may be related to a decreased exposure to a leukemogen in the environment. The one factor for which a decrease in exposure has occurred has been ionizing irradiation because of a growing awareness of the potential dangers of diagnostic and therapeutic irradiation. He also predicts little further decrease if that change has been responsible, because efforts to reduce exposure may have reached their limit.

Pathophysiology

At the time of diagnosis, the patient has a burden of leukemic tissue which occupies the space of normal hemopoiesis, the bone marrow. In most patients the production of normal blood cells has virtually ceased. The pathogenesis of the disease results from the leukemia-related cessation of hemopoiesis, and, with the exception of leukemic cell proliferation in the central nervous system, little else in the way of life-threatening interference with organ function occurs.

The mechanism by which leukemic cells replace normal marrow cells is not completely clear. The best explanation from available information is that a clone of leukemic cells develops, perhaps from a single cell mutation. This clone, although having a longer generation time than normal cells (62–64), does not produce an end stage cell, such as the neutrophil or erythrocyte. Therefore, even though the population is slowly dividing, accumulation of cells can occur.

An alternative concept for the replacement of normal cell elements by leukemic cells is the possible presence of a leukemogenic agent capable of transforming many normal cells to leukemic cells. If the normal cell line affected is the marrow stem cell, then this mechanism could account for the disappearance of normal hematopoiesis as well as the crowding of the marrow with abnormal cells. This alternate hypothesis has not been seriously considered in recent years, but new recognition of its feasibility has come from the observations of Fialkow and his co-workers (65). In a child receiving a marrow transplant for leukemia, evidence was presented for leukemic transformation

of the donor cells after successful implantation.

Furthermore, methods are now becoming available to assess changes in normal marrow cells as infiltrating leukemic cells make their appearance. Evaluation of normal committed and uncommitted stem cells in animals with developing leukemia should permit investigators to determine if marrow function is damaged by mechanisms other than physical replacement. It would be extremely important to determine if leukemic cells have the capacity to impair normal marrow cell proliferative capacity, for this would greatly enhance replacement by the malignant cell line. Studies of this kind are not available in human leukemia as yet.

Another important aspect of the interrelationship between normal and malignant cells for which we have too little information is the mechanism by which normal hemopoiesis returns after chemotherapeutic remission induction. From the absence of normal karyotypes in replaced bone marrow during relapse and their return in remission (66), it would seem that normal hemopoietic cells are absent from the marrow during disease activity and return as remission develops. An alternative might be that quiescent stem cells are present in relapsed marrows which are neither dividing nor differentiating. In that case both functions would return with the decrease in the number of leukemic cells. However, a recent study of myeloid colony-forming units in the bone marrow of patients with acute myeloblastic leukemia has indicated that normal stem cells are absent in relapse and return during remission (67). The most probable mechanism for return of normal hemopoiesis in acute lymphoblastic and myeloblastic leukemia would therefore be reseeding of the marrow by normal stem cells, followed by the formation of differentiated marrow cells. If this explanation is correct, then it would be important to know the source of these stem cells—whether they are residual in the marrow or return to the marrow from other tissue sites by way of the blood.

It has been rather consistently observed that, after several courses of chemotherapeutic agents and several reinduction regimens, the rate and completeness with which return of hemopoiesis occurs are markedly diminished. Many patients die with depleted, hypoplastic marrows during a terminal attempt at reinduction with a new drug.

There are two observations of stem cell function in animals which may serve as possible explanations for failure of marrow recovery after eradication of leukemic cells. If repeated reseeding of the marrow site by stem cells is necessary for hemopoietic recovery during remission induction, a similar exhaustion of stem cell capabilities may occur, as has been observed in the serial transplantation of a stem cell colony through irradiated host mice (68). After the third or fourth transfer, repopulation of the host marrow with normal hemopoietic cells is markedly incomplete. The mechanism for the loss of stem cell function is not known. Finally, stem cells injured by irradiation and alkylating agents have impaired capacity to undergo differentiation to erythroid cells (69). Thus there may be an imposed limitation to chemotherapy by the needs of the host for a normally responding hemopoietic stem cell compartment.

Another aspect which has been little studied is the relationship of the marrow architecture to remission induction. The bone marrow is a complex organ, dependent for normal function on the structure of its supporting tissue and vascular system. The marrow has the capacity to restore its normal architecture, even after severe physical disruption (70). Presumably it can restore itself as well after recovery from leukemic cell infiltration, but further studies are needed to evaluate and understand this aspect of a remission induction. Bone marrow infarcts occur in acute lymphoblastic leukemia (71), and the relationship of the marrow vasculature to the whole process of marrow recovery needs thoughtful study. Eventual loss of normal architecture and the capacity for restoration might be a major limiting factor in the treatment of this disease.

An important question in the pathophysiology of leukemia is what happens to the leukemic cells during a drug-induced disease remission. Some estimation of the total number of leukemic cells present at the time of recognizable disease activity have been made (72), although the methods have all been indirect. There have also been some calculations of the reduction in number necessary to provide for a remission (73). The number of cells present at the time of full disease activity is calculated to be 1×10^{12} leukemic cells, and a reduction of 99.99 per cent is necessary to provide for disease remission. These figures are approximations, but provide some basis for further speculation.

There are several lines of evidence to indicate that some leukemic cells do indeed survive the induction phase of chemotherapy and persist into remission. There has been morphologic evidence presented by Nies and co-workers (74) and Mathé and co-workers (75) that leukemic cells can still be found in patients with complete bone marrow remission. The most common site was the kidney, with other places of residual cell nests being the liver, testes, bowel, lung, central nervous system, and lymph nodes. In some patients, in fact, the first indication of disease activity after a remission may be growth of leukemic cells in one of these areas before any changes in blood or bone marrow are seen. Thus their importance as potential foci for relapse seems assured.

Another line of evidence that leukemic cells persist in remission and are the cause of relapse has been the demonstration that chromosomal abnormalities, when present, are consistent throughout the course of the disease (66). This finding would indicate that a single population line was responsible for the entire disease course. This conclusion is not incontestable, as will be discussed shortly.

These residual cells do not seem to be altogether dormant during remission. One indication for their continued proliferative activity is that, if suppressive drug therapy is not continued through remission, the disease relapse occurs earlier. Thus leukemic cells probably continue to divide and, if not restrained by drug treatment, would more rapidly repopulate the hemopoietic tissue.

The most important site of leukemic cell sequestration from the standpoint of frequency and symptomatology is the central nervous system. There are three important questions which should be raised about this site. The first question already seems reasonably answered: why do leukemic cells proliferate in the central nervous system while they are responding to drug therapy elsewhere? The answer is that with the exception of corticosteroids, the drugs in common use for this disease penetrate the central nervous system poorly, thus allowing for unsuppressed cell growth. Therefore the central nervous system provides a sanctuary area for the leukemic cells.

A more complex second question is less clearly answered; when does the leukemic cell move into the central nervous system? It has been assumed that the event might occur at any time during the course of the disease. Even during remission a wandering cell might penetrate the central nervous system and begin division in that protected environment. This random timing of central nervous system metastases seemed supported by the observation that the frequency of symptomatic disease in the central nervous system increased with prolonged survival of the patient population.

Recently, however, there has been reason to challenge this concept. When irradiation in tumoricidal doses has been given at the time of the initial induction regimen after diagnosis, the incidence of subsequent central nervous system leukemia has been markedly reduced (76). If these findings are confirmed, it would indicate that the leukemic cell penetration of the central nervous system occurs early, perhaps by the time of diagnosis, and that symptomatic central nervous system disease is delayed by factors determining growth rates for these cells in that environment. It is also possible, however, that changes induced by the irradiation make the tissues an inappropriate host for subsequent leukemic cell seeding and proliferation. This point is important for both therapeutic and conceptual standpoints and needs further study and clarification.

The third question deals with the relationship of central nervous system disease and subsequent marrow relapse. Does this sanctuary area provide a site for development of drug resistance and the reseeding of the bone marrow with malignant cells? While the available information is not completely in accord, the results of most studies of the relationship of central nervous system disease to marrow relapse would indicate that these two areas behave independently. On the other hand, the longer initial remissions observed with irradiation of the central nervous system (76) may be evidence of the importance of the central

nervous system as a site for reseeding leading to relapse.

At some time after a successful induction and maintenance of a remission, the disease recurs in most patients. Here again are critical questions. Does the disease always recur from regrowth of dormant cells which have survived from the original population? Is it possible that in some patients a new malignant cell population is responsible for the disease?

The simplest answer, of course, is that residual cells from the original clone return to proliferative activity after becoming drug-resistant. The evidence for the persistence of leukemic cells during remission has been discussed (74, 75). The similarity of chromosome patterns has been noted in newly diagnosed and relapsed leukemic cell populations (66). The basis for this concept is that a single critical mutation occurred as a consequence of some leukemogenic agent producing, as the population grew, a self-replicating clone of cells (77). The observed cell kinetic pattern for leukemic cell populations would support this concept, as will be discussed shortly (78). Certainly this concept is the most hopeful from the standpoint of current methods of therapy, because it would mean that eradication of the leukemic cells would leave behind a normal host, just as surely as would removal of a localized bowel carcinoma.

However, disconcerting contrary evidence is appearing. The most disturbing observation clinically was that of Fialkow and his co-workers (65), already mentioned. The finding of apparent leukemic transformation of the transplanted donor marrow in the leukemic host leads to the conclusion that the environment of the leukemic sibling contained a leukemogenic agent still capable of transforming normal cells to a malignant population.

With regard to the evidence of similarity of chromosome pattern in relapsing leukemia (66), one must consider the observation that identical twins developing leukemia in utero had an identical chromosome pattern (79). The suggestion has been made that such findings might be explained by crossing of a leukemic cell line, arising in one twin, to the other twin through placental vascular communications. Thus this finding could still be explainable by a clonal hypothesis. On the other hand, in studies of radiation-induced mouse leukemia (80) it was found that consistent chromosome changes were elicited by the injection of cell free filtrates of the leukemic tissue. The interpretation of this study was that a leukemogenic agent acting on genetically homogeneous hosts produced identical cell changes. Thus, a continuously present leukemogenic agent acting on a particular host produced identical cell changes. Therefore, a continuously present leukemic agent might produce consistent chromosome changes in genetically similar cells.

We must conclude that it is not presently clear whether recurrence of leukemic cell infiltration always indicates development of drug resistance in the old, dormant cell line, as formerly assumed. In some patients, perhaps, especially those in whom the relapse occurs late in the remission, a new leukemic transformation of normal cells may be the responsible event leading to relapse.

IMMUNE RELATIONSHIPS. There is a growing body of knowledge concerning the importance of host immune responses in tumor growth. Basic to the mechanism involved is the appearance of a "new" antigen on the malignant cell which can be distinguished by the host, with the subsequent development of cellular and humoral immunity to the antigen and an immunologic attack upon the malignant cell membrane. No loss of HL-A antigens has been found from the leukemic leukocytes (81). Some studies have failed to demonstrate new antigens (82), but others have given evidence that antigens are available on the leukemic cell surface which can be related to immunologic reactivity of the patient (83–86). The nature and derivation of these antigens is not known as yet. Of interest in this regard is the observation that host lymphocytes respond in a mixed leukocyte reaction to exposure to autochthonous mononucleosis cells, a response not dependent upon the EB virus antigen (87). Thus the "new" antigens may be cell-derived and related to exposure of material ordinarily covered up on the cell surface. In fact, the so-called leukemia antigens may merely reflect alterations in membrane structure related to cell maturity.

The relationship of the host immune response to the clinical characteristics of the disease is the subject of current study. It has been reported that patients with increased numbers of lymphocytes in their bone marrows during remission survive longer (88). This original report alluded to the possibility that the marrow lymphocytosis might be indicative of a host response to the malignant cell population. Although this conclusion has been supported (89), refutations have appeared (90). If confirmed, this finding could represent an indication of beneficial immunologically mediated host response to leukemic cells.

The possibility has been raised of extending remission duration by means of exogenous stimulation of the host's immune defense against the leukemic cells. This has been based on extension of animal studies indicating enhancement of host resistance through evolution of immunologic, cell-mediated defense mechanisms. This approach is not a simple one, with confounding problems — eliciting blocking antibodies with antigenic stimulation, the relationship of malignant cell population mass, the ability of the malignant tissue to resist immunologic rejection — yet to be fully explained.

Stimulation of the immunologic defense of the host in human leukemia has been attempted with such nonspecific adjuncts as BCG with or without the specific stimuli of pooled irradiated leukemic cells (91). Final evaluation of these attempts is still not possible. Confirmatory trials have failed to substantiate the improved remission times claimed, but have been themselves criticized because of possibly inadequate initial reduction of leukemic cell mass and the use of an antigenically inferior adjunct agent. Such studies must be continued. If any emphasis were needed, recent evaluation of the results of treatment of Burkitt's lymphoma have indicated the probable strong contributing component of host defenses, presumably immunologically mediated (92). Furthermore, preliminary results of a recent British study have shown improved remission duration in patients with acute myelogenous leukemia treated with serial injections of their own killed leukemic cells (92a). Another approach to immunotherapy of leukemia is made possible by the developing technology of bone marrow transplantation. Leukemic mice treated with total body irradiation and isologous marrow have a better survival than similar mice supported with syngeneic marrow (92b). It is believed that the engrafted marrow actually carries out a graft-versus-tumor reaction. Such a conclusion may be supported by Thomas's experience with bone marrow transplantation in patients with leukemia. Marrow transplantation to leukemic patients from identical twins have been largely unsuccessful. Leukemia rapidly recurs. However, when homologous marrow is used, prolonged remission may be observed in a few cases (92c).

CHROMOSOMAL CHANGES. As has been mentioned, there is a relationship between chromosomal aneuploidy (93), excessive chromosome breakage (94), and an increased risk of leukemia. Therefore, it is only natural that the chromosomal patterns of leukemic cells would be determined in an effort to understand the pathogenesis of the malignant transformation. In studies of both acute lymphoblastic and myeloblastic leukemias, approximately 50 per cent of the patients have been found to have aneuploid leukemic cell lines (95, 96). There is no consistent pattern to the aneuploidy. In most cases the aneuploid cell line is stable and persists throughout the disease. In patients with normal karyotypes in their leukemic cell lines, there is usually no progression to abnormal lines. Occasionally, however, rapidly changing chromosome constitution can be seen (97). In patients with an underlying aneuploidy, such as Down's syndrome (94), the leukemic cell line may have only the expected aneuploidy of the somatic cell or have an additional leukemic cell line with specific aneuploidy. In approximately one-half of patients with a "preleukemic" state of disordered myelopoiesis, an aneuploid line may be recovered from the marrow before frank leukemia develops (98). No prognostic significance has been attributed to the karyotype findings in acute lymphoblastic leukemia. In acute myeloblastic leukemia, the presence of normal karyotypes, even admixed with an abnormal line, is indication of a better prognosis than if no normal karyotypes are found (99).

Grossly normal karyotypes can be found in one-half of patients with acute leukemia. No specific pattern is characteristic of the aneuploidy when it does occur. Therefore, chromosomal aneuploidy is not an essential prerequisite of malignant transformation. Although the possibility must be considered that submicroscopic gene involvement may induce gross chromosomal changes leading to the initiation of leukemia, it seems more likely that the chromosomal changes represent secondary phenomena (100). The escape of leukemic cells from normal growth controls is more likely due to gene malfunction, and the karyotypic changes are merely epiphenomena related to intracellular alterations associated with the transformation process.

CELL PROLIFERATION CHARACTERISTICS. Although early concepts of cell proliferation led to the proposal that malignancy in general is due to rapid, uncontrolled cell growth, indications that leukemic cell growth rates were less than that of normal blood cell precursors were presented by Astaldi and Mauri in 1953 (101). With the advent of radioisotopically labeled DNA and RNA precursors shortly thereafter, methods became available for specific studies of leukemic cell proliferative characteristics.

The mitotic cell cycle consists of mitosis (M); the interphase between mitosis and DNA synthesis (G_1); DNA synthesis (S); and the period between S and M (G_2). The total time required from one mitosis to a subsequent mitosis is the generation time. Another measure which is sometimes used is the time required for a dividing population to double in number. If all cells divide in a similar fashion within the population and no loss of cells occurs, the doubling and generation time are the same. In most cell populations, however, not all cells are engaged in proliferative activity (are in G_0), and some loss of cells by death or removal to a nonreproductive end-stage cell does occur. Therefore, in most situations, the population doubling time is slower than the cell generation time.

Three phases of the cell cycle can be demonstrated as an overall assessment of population proliferative activity. The mitotic index can be determined (102), as has been done by Astaldi and Mauri (101). The percentage of cells in DNA synthesis can be determined autoradiographically after exposure of the cells to tritiated thymidine (labeling index with ^{3}HT). The ^{3}HT is specifically incorporated into DNA only during the DNA synthetic phase of the cell cycle and remains with the cell in the nuclear DNA (103). Another assessment of DNA synthetic activity within the cell population can be obtained by measuring the rate of incorporation of ³H- or ¹⁴C-labeled thymidine into DNA by means of liquid scintillation counting techniques. It is possible to determine the content of cellular DNA by microspectrophotometry, coupled with ³HT labeling and autoradiography. This technique can give information about the distribution of cells within the DNA synthetic phase, as labeled cells progress from nearly normal DNA content to cells almost finished with the S phase and having nearly twice the normal DNA content. Cells in G_2 are found to have twice normal DNA content, but are unlabeled on autoradiography because DNA synthesis has been completed.

Several methods have been used to assess the timing of the generation cycle. The most difficult and time consuming has been the measurement of labeling patterns of mitotic figures after a single in vivo injection of ³HT. The label is incorporated rapidly into nuclei of cells in DNA synthesis and is available for only about 20 to 30 minutes (104). Thus "flash" labeling is obtained of that cohort of cells in DNA synthesis at the time of the injection. The labeled cells subsequently complete DNA synthesis and proceed to the following phases of the generation cycle. Their progress can be followed by serial samples of the cell population. A clear marker for observation of the progress is the appearance and disappearance of the labeled phase in the mitotic cycle, where the labeled cells can be distinguished by their altered appearance. A typical result is shown in Figure 22–1. The time for the first appearance of labeled mitotic figures after injection represents the time needed to pass through G_2. The interval between the midpoint of appearance to midpoint of disappearance of labeled mitotic figures represents the time required for DNA synthesis. When the next wave of mitotic figures appears, the generation time for these cells is indicated. Serial determination of grain counts in labeled cells offers another method for the measurement of generation time. The label, once incorporated, becomes diluted in daughter cells by one-half during each mitotic division (105). Therefore, by determination of the half-times for decrease of the mean grain counts in the labeled cells, the generation time should be derived. Unfortunately, this method is not suitable for the study of leukemic cell populations. There is some label reutilization and, furthermore, some entry

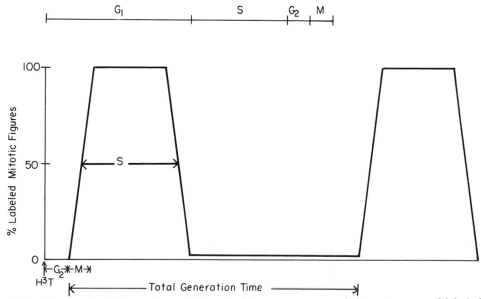

Figure 22–1. Phases of mitotic cycle as determined by appearance and disappearance of labeled mitotic figures.

of cells into a prolonged rest phase (G_0), which affects the rate at which the concentration of label decreases in the cell population.

A more rapid measure of DNA synthesis time can be obtained with a double DNA labeling technique. ^{3}HT is injected in vivo, and at some time thereafter, but within the expected S time, marrow is aspirated and incubated with ^{14}CT in vitro. Cells labeled with ^{3}HT and ^{14}CT can be distinguished by means of special autoradiographic techniques. From the ratio of ^{3}HT-labeled cells to doubly labeled cells and the elapsed time between labeling procedures, the DNA synthesis time can be determined.

Several recent review articles that offer details about cell kinetics in acute leukemia are available (106–109). From studies of the generation cycle with the labeled mitotic index technique (110, 111), the times for leukemic cell division are generally longer than those of normal hemopoietic cells. In some studies of acute myeloblastic leukemia, however, similar generation times have been reported (109). In childhood leukemias the generation time is in the range of 50 to 70 hours, with S about 20 hours, G_2 about 2 hours, M about 2 hours, and G_1 about 30 to 35 hours. Some slight variations from patient to patient have been observed in these studies.

From the earliest studies of the patterns of cell proliferation in acute leukemia, there has been indication that the leukemic cell population is not uniform with respect to proliferative activity. Labeling indices with ^{3}HT indicated that leukemic cells in blood had a lesser degree of proliferative activity than the bone marrow cell population (112). Even in the bone marrow, two functionally different cell populations are discernible (113–115). One population of larger cells with fine nuclear chromatin is the proliferative compartment. The other, comprised of smaller cells with dense nuclear chromatin, is a compartment of cells that exhibits no proliferative activity. The smaller cells appear to arise from the larger cells, as some of these cells drop out of the proliferative cycle to become resting cells.

It was observed by Gavosto and his coworkers (116) that the larger cell compartment was non–self-maintaining in that the loss of cells to the resting compartment was greater than the birth rate of the larger cells.

Therefore, a source of cells coming into proliferative activity had to be found. Subsequently, it was demonstrated that small, resting leukemic cells were capable of reentering the proliferative phase and thus could serve as a stem cell compartment for the larger cells (78). The cell population was in a dynamic equilibrium between the resting and proliferative phases. The resting cells would thus be only temporarily out of phase (in G_0). This population of resting cells, less sensitive to phase-dependent chemotherapeutic agents but capable of return to proliferative activity, has obvious importance for design of therapy regimens. Furthermore, in considering the pathogenesis of acute leukemia, these findings are compatible with a single cell mutation forming a self-maintaining clone of malignant cells.

There are several indications that the leukemic cells respond to growth control mechanisms. One of the earliest indications was the observation that proliferative activity was similar in various marrow sites sampled, either simultaneously (114) or during different times of the day (110). This finding suggests that systemic humoral substances were responsible for proliferation control, not local environmental conditions (64).

It was also observed that considerable variation in proliferative activity occurs from patient to patient and even in the same patient during different phases of his disease (110, 117, 118). In general, the least degree of proliferative activity occurs at the time of diagnosis, when from the duration of symptoms one would expect that the longest growth period for the cell population had been possible. On the other hand, when the patient is studied in a subsequent relapse, proliferative activity of the cells is greater. At this time the duration of symptoms, if any, is short, and it would be expected that the duration of population growth would also be short. The proliferative activity varies inversely with the number of resting leukemic cells.

The most likely explanation for these findings is that, with progressive duration of growth, there is an increasing number of cells entering into a resting phase. The nature of the mechanisms controlling the change in proliferative activity is not known, but, because of the similarity of samples obtained from various marrow sites, the agents would most likely be systemic and humoral rather than local environmental determinants. In many respects, the system resembles the changes in growth rates observed in broth-grown bacteria or in cells grown in tissue culture with increasing population density.

The leukemic cell growth control mechanisms can be perturbed by chemotherapeutic manipulation (119), an exciting potential tool for treatment. With certain agents that have effects on the population control mechanisms, resting cells can be recruited into proliferative activity. Similar recruitment has been reported with extracorporeal irradiation of blood leukemic cells (120), but has not been possible by reduction of the blood leukemic cell concentration by exchange transfusion (119) or leukapheresis (121). Because of the relative resistance of resting cells to cycle-dependent chemotherapeutic agents, the possibility that the therapist might "goad" these cells into a drug-sensitive, proliferative state presents a challenging opportunity.

Recently a new tool for study of growth regulation of cells in acute myeloblastic leukemia has become available. By means of in vitro culture methods, the influence of normal growth factors for myeloid cells can be assessed in malignant cell populations (122, 123, 124). The studies are already making clear that the leukemic myeloblasts are dependent upon factors supporting growth and differentiation of normal myeloid cells. Also, these leukemic cells respond to normal factors in some cases by altering their growth and maturation characteristics. In a rat leukemia, the exposure to normal control factors has reversed the lack of maturation and restored a normal pattern of differentiation (125). Further definition of the relationship of normal myeloid growth factors to the leukemic cell in acute myeloblastic leukemia is awaited with obvious interest. Leukemic patients do have factors in their urine which support normal myeloid growth and differentiation, so the lack of these factors could not be the simple explanation for the observed defect in differentiation in acute myeloblastic leukemia (126, 127). Similar techniques applied to acute lymphoblastic leukemia would be an important advance in our study of that disease.

Clinical Presentation

Children with newly diagnosed acute leukemia present themselves in a fairly uniform manner (128, 129). In two-thirds of the children, symptoms and signs of their disease have been present for less than six weeks. The symptoms in the beginning are usually nonspecific. There may be a history of a viral respiratory infection or exanthem from which the child has never seemed fully to recover. Anorexia, irritability, and lethargy are common manifestations of early disease. Later, pallor, bleeding, and fever develop in most of the children, and one of these signs or a combination of them is the usual immediate cause for presentation to a physician.

On examination pallor is found in most of the patients, and in about one-half there are petechiae or mucous membrane bleeding. Fever is present in about one-fourth of the children at the time of diagnosis. Signs of an upper respiratory tract infection may also be found. In some patients other infectious causes for fever may be evident. Lymphadenopathy is usually not prominent, but may be very impressive. Splenomegaly is to be expected in two-thirds of the cases. When palpable, the spleen is usually less than 6 cm. below the costal margin. Massive splenomegaly is not common and is particularly unusual in acute myelocytic leukemia. Hepatomegaly is less frequent and less striking. Bone tenderness is present in about one-third of the patients, probably due to periosteal invasion and subperiosteal hemorrhage.

There are some less common forms of presentation. Occasionally bone pain or arthralgia may be the major complaint. Signs of increasing intracranial pressure may indicate early meningeal involvement. In acute myeloblastic leukemia, the solid tumor form, a chloroma, may be the initial finding. These problems will be discussed in greater detail under the heading Clinical Complications.

Laboratory Findings

The primary laboratory findings of interest are, of course, those changes in the blood which are usually definitive for diagnosis. The findings reflect the failure of the marrow to produce normal blood cells, as well as the presence in almost all cases of the abnormal leukemic blast cell.

The white blood count at diagnosis is quite variable. In an unselected group (128) and in our own experience, from one-fourth to one-third of the patients have white blood counts less than 5000 per mm³. About one-third to one-half of the patients have total white blood counts in the "normal" range of 5000 to 20,000 per mm³. Distinctly increased counts from 20,000 to 1,000,000 per mm.³ are found in one-third to one-fifth of the patients. Counts greater than 100,000 per mm.³ may be found at diagnosis in one-fifth to one-twentieth of the patients. It is of interest that a greater proportion of our patients had lesser leukocyte concentrations at diagnosis than in the unselected series gathered from a whole Canadian province between 1948 and 1960 (128). Perhaps the lesser leukocyte concentrations reflect earlier diagnosis. This explanation is somewhat supported by the finding that about one-third of the patients in the older series had hemoglobin values below 5 g. per 100 ml., while one-fifth of the patients in our series collected after 1960 were that low. One-half of the patients in the older series had values between 5 and 10 g. per 100 ml., while three-fourths of our series were in that range. Relatively few patients in either series had values greater than 10 g. per 100 ml.

Almost all the patients have thrombocytopenia, whether clinical bleeding manifestations are present or not.

In our experience, all patients who have had blood leukocyte counts greater than 5000 per mm.³ have also had easily detectable leukemic blast cells in blood smears at the time of diagnosis. No doubt an occasional exception might be found, but as a clinical observation, patients suspected of having leukemia from the history and physical examination can usually be confirmed from blood smear alone, if adequate numbers of leukocytes are present. If leukopenia is present, however, some patients will not have easily detectable leukemic blast cells in the blood smear. A buffy coat smear and a bone marrow examination are needed for definitive diagnosis. Further discussion of this problem is found below in the section Diagnosis.

Bone marrow examination may be made by aspirate, with subsequent preparation of smears for staining, or by needle or surgical biopsy. An aspirated specimen is adequate in most cases, but occasionally a biopsy is needed if the marrow is hypocellular and inadequate for diagnosis by simple aspirate. In our experience the needle biopsy technique of Jamshidi and Swaim (130) has been excellent for obtaining marrow specimens in children.

In general, almost complete replacement of normal cell elements by leukemic blast cells is found at the time of diagnosis. Sometimes lesser percentages are found, but greater than 6 per cent blast cells in a marrow specimen should lead to a serious consideration of acute leukemia (131). Rarely, a disparity of samples from different sites can be found, probably indicating an early stage of the disease process (132). Thus, if the clinical findings strongly suggest leukemia but the initial marrow sample is not conclusive, another sample should be obtained.

Inadequate sample by aspiration may be caused by hypocellularity or by reticulin fibrosis or bone infarction (133). These latter two findings are characteristic of acute lymphoblastic leukemia and may be associated with a poor prognosis. Aspiration at a different site or marrow biopsy may be needed for a diagnostic sample. Gaucher's cells have been found in some marrow samples in acute leukemia (134) and are most likely a secondary phenomenon rather than an indication of an underlying genetic defect.

Serum proteins may be altered in acute leukemia (135). An increase in gamma globulins is characteristic of acute myeloblastic but not lymphoblastic leukemia. An increase of α_2-globulin is found in acute lymphoblastic leukemia. In both forms a decrease in serum albumin is found.

Viscosity of blood may be affected by increased concentration of leukemic cells which have little deformability (136). The increased viscosity of blood with marked increase in rigid leukemic blast cells may contribute to clinical manifestations in some instances.

Fetal hemoglobin levels are increased in about one-half of children with acute leukemia of both types (137). The increases are in the range of 2 to 7 per cent. In a few patients with acute myeloblastic or histiomonocytic leukemia, marked increases in the range of 10 to 50 per cent may be found.

Muramidase is a lysosomal enzyme of broad distribution in tissues. In blood and bone marrow it is found in neutrophilic granulocytes, monocytes, and monoblasts. Increased levels of serum and urine muramidase activity have been found in acute monoblastic and myelomonoblastic leukemia. The levels are variable in acute myeloblastic leukemia, and decreased in acute lymphoblastic leukemia (138). The determination can be of some diagnostic help at times.

Another urinary excretion product which bears some relationship to disease activity is the aminoimidazolecarboxamide level (139). There is a positive correlation of the urinary excretion of this purine intermediate with marrow blast content. Methotrexate administration invalidates the observation, because this drug causes increased excretion. Another positive correlation with marrow blast cell content is found in the serum copper level (140).

Diagnosis

The diagnosis is rarely difficult and is generally accomplished from the blood smear. Two problems may present superficial difficulties.

An occasional patient with infectious mononucleosis or a similar illness may bear a resemblance to the patient with acute leukemia, especially if there is the added complication of thrombocytopenic purpura or immunohemolytic anemia. The morphology of the leukocytes is characteristic, however, and the marrow findings distinctly different. Serologic tests for mononucleosis are of great value.

Another problem is the patient with pancytopenia. If leukemic blast cells are not found in the blood and the marrow aspirate is inadequate for diagnosis because of hypocellularity, a biopsy specimen should resolve the problem.

An occasional patient may have a course extending over months, during which a gradual increase in marrow monoblasts occurs, culminating in a fulminant leukemia of the monoblastic (histocytic) form. During the evolution of this malignancy, the clinical course is characterized by pancytopenia, fever, and nonspecific symptoms of lethargy, weakness, irritability, and anorexia. Increased fetal hemoglobin levels and increased serum vitamin B_{12} levels may be helpful clues indicating the nature of the final outcome. It has recently been suggested that enumeration of marrow colony-forming cells or measurement of the capacity of marrow cells to differentiate in culture may discriminate between patients with refractory pancytopenia and preleukemic pancytopenia (67, 140a, b, c).

In the more usual situation of differentiation between the acute course of aplastic anemia and acute leukemia, roentgenographic changes in the skeleton may indicate leukemia. The skeleton is normal in aplastic anemia, whereas typical roentgenographic manifestations may be present in children with acute leukemia (141). A rapid response of blood cell values to corticosteroid therapy in what was assumed to be aplastic anemia should warn one that the probable diagnosis is acute leukemia (142).

The differential diagnosis of the ordinary types of acute leukemia is described above.

Clinical Complications

Clinical complications occur during the course of acute leukemia because of the loss of normal bone marrow function due to replacement by leukemic cells, infiltration of other organs, and side effects of therapy. In this section the problems arising from marrow replacement and organ infiltration will be discussed, as well as treatment of these problems. In the next section, specific measures for treatment of acute leukemia will be presented, along with the complications of therapy.

ANEMIA. Anemia is a regular feature of acute leukemia. There appear to be several mechanisms, each of which may contribute to a greater or lesser extent in each patient. In the treated patient, marrow suppression by chemotherapy may affect red cell production. Blood loss can be a contributory factor.

Studies of patients with measurements of iron turnover for assessment of marrow red cell production and determination of red cell survival with ^{14}C-glycine and ^{51}chromium have been performed (143–145). The results have indicated that both shortened red cell survival and decreased marrow production contribute in variable proportions to the anemia. The mechanisms for the shortened red cell survival are unknown, but may be related to both intrinsic and extrinsic factors (146). Unlike some patients with lymphoma or chronic lymphocytic leukemia, immunohemolytic anemias are not usually seen in acute leukemias as part of the disease pattern.

The normal regulatory mechanisms for red cell production are intact in the patients with appropriate production of erythropoietin in response to the anemia (147). The most likely explanation for the failure of marrow response is the unavailability of erythropoietin-sensitive stem cells because of marrow replacement with leukemic cells. Some patients with acute myeloblastic leukemia have been reported to have inappropriately low urinary erythropoietin excretion in response to their anemia (147).

Treatment for the anemia is by blood transfusion. If blood loss has been recent and significant, whole blood should be used in amounts to be determined by clinical judgment. If a compromised blood volume is not a problem, then the hemoglobin level of the patient should be increased to greater than 10 g. per 100 ml. by giving packed red cells. It has been our practice to maintain the hemoglobin values at levels greater than 10 g. per 100 ml. during the induction period.

BLEEDING. The major cause for bleeding in acute leukemia is thrombocytopenia. There is a correlation between frequency of hemorrhagic episodes and the blood platelet concentration, although no definite threshold value has been demonstrated (148). In general, however, serious bleeding episodes are unusual if the platelet count is greater than 20,000 per mm.³, and rare with counts greater than 50,000 per mm.³ In patients with acute myeloblastic leukemia, defective function of platelets has also been demonstrated (149). The nature of the defects as indicated by platelet aggregation studies is consistent with abnormalities of both membrane reactivity and the release reaction. These functional defects may aggravate a bleeding tendency in some patients with acute myeloblastic leukemia.

Treatment of thrombocytopenic bleeding is by the administration of freshly drawn platelet concentrate. The infusion of 8 to 10 concentrates, each prepared from 500 ml. of whole blood, per 100 pounds body weight will usually increase the platelet count to levels greater than 40,000 per mm.³, which is sufficient to stop bleeding (150). The effectiveness of the platelet transfusion is usually limited to one or two days, so that repeated infusions may be necessary to carry a patient through a period of severe thrombocytopenic bleeding. The availability of platelet transfusion has greatly reduced the frequency with which bleeding is the immediate cause of death in acute leukemia (151). Although repeated transfusion of platelets from unmatched donors in the patient receiving immunosuppressive chemotherapy results in sensitization in only about 10 per cent of cases (152), it may be ncessary to use an HL-A matched donor for selected situations (152a).

At the risk of stating the obvious, aspirin should not be used for fever control in the thrombocytopenic patient. Not only will platelet function be altered by this drug, but also gastrointestinal bleeding will be provoked.

Occasionally unexplained plasma factor deficiencies have been associated with acute leukemia (153). In the patient in whom the bleeding cannot be explained on the basis of thrombocytopenia, further studies of the coagulation mechanism are recommended in order to uncover any other defects. Liver diseases related to drug therapy or infection may be associated with bleeding due to a decrease in the availability of the liver-produced clotting factors. In acute promyelocytic leukemia, there is a unique bleeding problem caused by the elaboration and release of leukocyte procoagulant, resulting in disseminated intravascular coagulation.

The incidence of disseminated intravascular coagulation related to sepsis is surprisingly unusual in patients with acute leukemia. This may be owing to the fact that, during times of increased risk of bacterial infection, the blood granulocyte concentration is usually markedly decreased. Since this cell is an important adjunct in the development of disseminated intravascular coagulation during sepsis, its absence greatly retards the evolution of the process (154). Although an unusual cause of clinical bleeding problems in acute leukemia, the presence of disseminated intravascular coagulation has been demonstrated in some patients (155) and successfully treated with heparin (156).

INFECTION. Infectious disease is currently the major problem in the management of clinical complications of acute leukemia and is the most common cause of death (157, 158, 159). Bacterial infections are the most common problem during disease relapse, with gram-negative bacteria currently the most frequent infecting organisms. There has been an increasing incidence of fungal infection during the past few years, associated with longer survival and more intensive chemotherapeutic regimens. During remission and in association with more intensive maintenance regimens, some nonbacterial infections are more common causes of disease and death (160). *Pneumocystis carinii* infections are more frequently seen under these circumstances (158, 160).

The two major factors involved in the predisposition to infection are the immunoglobulin response and the deficiency of leukocyte number and function. Immunoglobulin levels are decreased in relationship to institution of chemotherapy and the intensity of maintenance chemotherapy (161, 162). Antibody response to antigenic challenge is likewise blunted in the patients receiving chemotherapy (163, 164). The serum complement levels are variable and tend to fluctuate with the course of the disease, but do not seem to be a major factor in the reduction of host resistance (165, 166).

There is a definite relationship between incidence and severity of bacterial infections and the level of circulating blood leukocytes (167). An absolute neutrophil concentration of less than 500 per mm.^{3} generally occurs prior to a serious bacterial or fungal infection (158). It is in this range of blood neutrophil concentrations that infections with *Pseudomonas aeruginosa* are found. The importance of functioning neutrophils can be seen from the observation that most infecting *Pseudomonas* organisms are resistant to serum factors alone (168).

Leukocyte mobilization into inflammatory sites is defective (169). The most obvious cause for the defect is the reduction of circulating blood leukocytes, but in acute myeloblastic leukemia, a qualitative defect

in the available blood cells may also be present (170). Chemotherapy also may inhibit the local inflammatory response (171).

There are some indications that the neutrophils in patients with acute leukemia may have functional deficits with respect to bactericidal activity and the metabolic response to phagocytosis (172, 173). These observed abnormalities are unexplained and need confirmation and extension. In acute myeloblastic leukemia, a defect of neutrophils for the killing of *Candida albicans* has been reported (174), which may be correlated with the observation of myeloperoxidase deficiency in the cells of some patients (175).

In patients with acute leukemia, there is also a diminution of reticuloendothelial phagocytic function (176). Chemotherapy seems to have little effect on this aspect of body defenses. Another aspect of host defense that may be impaired by immunosuppressive chemotherapy is the production of interferon by lymphocytes (177).

Bacterial infections are the most common causes of death during disease activity. The three bacteria most frequently causing death are *Pseudomonas aeruginosa*, *Escherichia coli*, and *Staphylococcus aureus* (158). It is well to remember that, along with those infectious agents usually considered to be pathogens, in patients with acute leukemia such opportunistic pathogens as *Aeromonas hydrophila* (178) and *Listeria monocytogenes* (179) can be the offending organisms. Also, multiple organisms may be recovered in these patients during an episode of sepsis (180).

The most common clinical picture includes sepsis and pneumonia (158). All the usual bacterial infections of childhood may be seen, but special consideration should be given by the clinician to such unusual infections as perirectal abscesses (181), hepatic abscesses (182), and acute appendicitis (183) because of the importance of establishing such diagnoses for treatment and the sometimes difficult clinical problems posed by these entities.

Special attention should be given to *Pseudomonas* infections. The mortality rate is high, and survival is determined not so much by treatment as by the severity of the patient's clinical picture (184). About one-half of hospitalized leukemic patients become carriers of *Pseudomonas aeruginosa*

(185, 186). In addition to a blood granulocyte concentration of less than 500 to 1000 per mm.³ (158, 185), other common antecedent factors are chemotherapy and antibiotic administration (184, 185). In the carriers who subsequently become infected, the same type of organism recovered from stool or throat specimens has been recovered from the site of infection (186).

Viral infections are a common problem during both remission and relapse, but are less frequent causes of death in patients with leukemia (158). Viral infection has become a more important cause of death during remission maintained with the more intensive and immunosuppressive maintenance regimens (160). The usual viral infections caused by such organisms as rhinoviruses, adenovirus, and enteroviruses are not more frequent or severe than in the general population (159). However, infections caused by herpes viruses, vaccinia, and measles can be prolonged and severe in patients with leukemia under treatment.

Cytomegalovirus infections are difficult to document because of the frequency with which virus excretion is found in normal populations. Serial studies of virus excretion and antibody titers for cytomegalovirus have been done (187, 188). Patients excreting virus have a greater frequency of episodes of pneumonitis and fever with rash, but no greater incidence of hepatitis, fever of unknown origin, or upper respiratory tract infections (188). The clinical syndromes thought to be associated with the virus resulted in fourfold antibody titer increases only during hematologic remission. Therefore, this index of infection was not useful during relapses. Antibody titer increase may follow transfusion of fresh blood, indicating that this may be one source of infection with the virus (187). A serious and potentially fatal syndrome resulting from infection with the virus includes high fever, cough, tachypnea, vomiting, and diarrhea. Physical findings include progressive hepatosplenomegaly and sometimes a nonspecific rash. Pancytopenia and bilateral pneumonitis are associated with the syndrome (189). Treatment of cytomegalovirus infection with corticosteroid, fluoxyuridine, and cystosine arabinoside have been attempted, but adequate trials for evaluation are not available. When possible,

chemotherapy should be stopped to allow for adequate host defense response.

Varicella (190), herpes zoster (191), and herpes simplex (192) can produce serious and even fatal infections in children with acute leukemia. Chemotherapy causing immunosuppression is probably the major factor involved in the severity of the clinical course (193), but the nature of the underlying disease is also important (194). In the face of these infections, chemotherapy should be stopped if at all possible. Cytosine arabinoside has been an effective adjunct in the management of herpes zoster infections in some patients.

The association of infectious mononucleosis and acute leukemia has been of interest because of some earlier proposals that acute lymphoblastic leukemia may be a malignant form of EB virus infections. Recent evidence, however, has indicated that concurrent leukemia and infectious mononucleosis may occur (49), and no reason for an etiologic implication exists (50). The clinical course of the disease is as would be expected in a nonleukemic individual.

Australia antigen has been found in about 10 per cent of patients with acute leukemia. This finding is usually related to previous transfusion (195).

Even attenuated viruses, like measles vaccine (196) and vaccinia (197), can produce serious, sometimes fatal diseases. Live virus vaccine should be avoided in immunosuppressed patients.

Fungal infections are an increasing cause of serious infection in patients with acute leukemia (158–160). In a recent review of autopsies of patients dying of acute leukemia, severe fungal infections were found in 28 per cent (198). Oral moniliasis is the most common fungal disease and is to be expected in patients receiving both steroids and antibiotics. Treatment with nystatin may offer some help in containing the infection, but clearing does not occur until antibiotics and steroids are discontinued. Systemic or visceral candidiasis may occur as well, the diagnosis being made by blood cultures or a rise in anti-*Candida* antibodies (199).

Aspergillosis usually produces progressive pneumonitis (200, 201), but cerebral abscesses can also occur (202). Predisposing factors are corticosteroid therapy, cytotoxic therapy, and leukopenia (201). The presence of progressive pulmonary infiltrates responding poorly to antibiotic therapy should be reason to consider aspergillosis as a cause. Positive serum *Aspergillus* precipitation may be found, but may also be negative in the face of invasive fungal disease. Lung biopsy and culture may be necessary to establish the diagnosis. Both pulmonary and cerebral involvement with phycomycosis may also be found (203).

The treatment of systemic or visceral fungal infections is best accomplished with amphotericin B (159). The best prognosis is found in those patients who experience an improvement in their leukemic status.

Toxoplasmosis may be an unusual infection in acute leukemia. The source of the infecting organism may be blood transfusions, especially leukocyte transfusions (204). The clinical course consists of combinations of the following findings: fever, hepatosplenomegaly, abnormal liver function tests, a macular rash, and pancytopenia (204, 205). The diagnosis sometimes may be made from examination of the bone marrow aspirate (205). Treatment with sulfadiazine and pyrimethamine is recommended.

Pneumocystis carinii pneumonia is a problem of increasing frequency, especially in children in remission in whom intensive chemotherapy regimens are being used (160). The clinical picture is of progressing dyspnea and tachypnea, cough, fever, and finally, a reduction in arterial oxygen saturation with developing cyanosis. The roentgenographic features are usually those of a bilateral diffuse, interstitial pneumonitis. Other patterns, such as localized infiltration, may be seen. Diagnosis may require lung biopsy, although the clinical findings can be quite suggestive (206, 207). Sometimes because of the severity of the patient's illness, a clinical trial of sulfadiazine and pyrimethamine is indicated, almost as a diagnostic procedure.

Mycoplasma can be recovered frequently from children with acute leukemia. After immunologic suppression, these organisms may enter the blood stream (208). They do not frequently cause significant disease in patients with acute leukemia.

General management of the patient at risk who has a decreased granulocyte concentration and is receiving immunosuppressive chemotherapy requires good clinical judgment, careful evaluation of febrile episodes, and specific therapy for infections (159). Prophylactic antibiotics are of no value and may be harmful, for they permit overgrowth of antibiotic-resistant organisms. In protected environments, whether of the enclosed variety (209–211) or of a laminar air flow design (212), there has been a significant reduction in the number of infections during granulocytopenic states. Thus far, no improvement in remission rate or overall survival has occurred in these protected patients. In the child with acute lymphoblastic leukemia, response to treatment is usually prompt, and hence such measures are rarely indicated.

Granulocyte transfusions for infected neutropenic patients have been performed with cells from patients with chronic myelocytic leukemia (213) or normal cells prepared from a donor by means of a cell separator apparatus (159). The degree of histocompatibility between donor and recipient influences the percentage recovery of the transfused cells (214). If the cell separator is used, the best results are obtained with multiple transfusions over several days. This method is not feasible except at centers where such facilities are available.

NEUROLOGIC COMPLICATIONS. The neurologic complications of acute leukemia are largely owing to central nervous system infiltration by the leukemic cells. Symptomatic disease from this complication occurs sometime during the course of the disease in approximately one-half the patients. There has been an increasing incidence during the past few years, probably attributable to the increasing duration of survival after diagnosis (215). The median time for the first episode is nine months. The risk of central nervous system disease is about 4 per cent per month for the first two years, then 2 per cent per month thereafter. The first episode may occur as late as four years after diagnosis. Neither age, sex, nor hematologic status of the patient seems to influence the frequency of this complication, and there is no relationship to chemotherapeutic regimen. Obviously inadequate regimens lead to decreased incidence of central nervous system disease, because inadequately treated patients die of systemic relapse before central nervous system relapse can occur.

The origin of the disease process is in the arachnoid (216). The earliest evidence is seen in the walls of superficial arachnoid veins, progressing with extension into the deep arachnoid surrounding blood vessels as they course through the brain. There may be eventual invasion of brain parenchyma, with destruction of the pia-glial membranes. Arachnoid fibrous and brain parenchyma alterations, such as gliosis, necrosis, cerebral hemorrhage, and degenerative encephalopathy, may result. The chromosomal constitutions of leukemic cells in the marrow and cerebral spinal fluid are identical, suggesting the metastatic nature of this complication (217).

The most common presenting manifestations of CNS leukemia are related to increased intracranial pressure (218, 219). Vomiting, headache, papilledema, and lethargy are frequent findings. Convulsions and nuchal rigidity are less common. Prolonged or severe pressure increase may cause sixth cranial nerve involvement, with diplopia and strabismus. Seventh cranial nerve involvement with unilateral facial paralysis is another uncommon associated disorder, which may precede the symptoms and signs of increased intracranial pressure in some patients. A special form of CNS leukemia is the hypothalamic involvement which results in excessive weight gain, behavior disturbance, and hirsutism (218–220). In some children the only manifestation may be rapid weight gain, so that this finding should indicate the need for further studies when it is unexplained.

The spinal fluid findings (218, 219) are abnormal in 95 per cent of the patients with this complication. The most frequent abnormality is an increase in pressure (90 per cent), with 85 per cent of patients having a pleocytosis which results from the presence of leukemic blast cells. These cells can be identified with certainty by centrifuging the spinal fluid, resuspending the cells in a drop of serum, and then making cover slip smears for staining with Wright's stain (see Color Plate I. A cytocentrifuge may also be used for preparation of the cells for staining and identification (221). One-half of the affected patients have decreased spinal fluid glucose concentration, but three-fourths of them have normal spinal fluid protein values (218).

Uncommon and sometimes confusing CNS manifestations may occur, such as central pontine myelinolysis (222), the findings of multifocal leukoencephalopathy (223), or diabetes insipidus (224). Local tumor in the spinal canal in an epidural location may produce paraplegia (225).

Currently, the most widely utilized treatment for CNS leukemia is intrathecal methotrexate. This route of administration provides an effective spinal fluid drug concentration that cannot be achieved by oral or parenteral routes. The dose given ranges from 0.2 to 0.5 mg. per kg. body weight. Intrathecal methotrexate may control CNS leukemia, even when the drug has become ineffective in controlling bone marrow and blood leukemic cell growth. In a regimen of 0.2 mg. per kg. given every other day for four doses, control was achieved in 85 per cent of episodes (226). Symptomatic improvement was found as early as the first lumbar puncture to as late as 18 days after beginning treatment. In general, the spinal fluid abnormalities returned to normal within a week. Rapid symptomatic improvement may be achieved with dexamethasone given in doses of 0.2 mg. per kg. body weight per day, but no change in spinal fluid findings can be expected (227).

CNS leukemia tends to recur within a median time of about three months (226). Recurrence is more frequently found in patients who have greatly increased numbers of cells in the spinal fluid (219). Remission maintenance therapy with intrathecal methotrexate given every six to eight weeks has been advocated (228). In view of the progressively increasing toxicity experienced by those patients, however, it would seem that this treatment is worse than the disease.

Complications of intrathecal methotrexate have been reported (229), including paraplegia and even death (230). The cause of these uncommon drug-related reactions is unknown but may be related to the preservative used in the solutions of the drug (229). Another avoidable complication is severe marrow depression caused by the slow leak of methotrexate into the circulation from the deposit in the spinal fluid. In patients with limited marrow reserve, therefore, we have given prophylactic folinic acid in a dose equal to the intrathecal dose of methotrexate.

Another drug which can be used intrathecally with effect is cytosine arabinoside in a dose of 5 to 70 mg. per square meter body surface area (231, 232). Seventy per cent of patients responded in one study (231), with vomiting being a frequent drug-related complication. Orally administered pyrimethamine has been reported to have been effective in one patient with acute myeloblastic leukemia and CNS leukemia (233). Further studies are needed before this method can be recommended.

Irradiation therapy has also been used, either alone (234) or in conjunction with intrathecal methotrexate therapy (235). Low-dose (160 R.) irradiation does not provide longer remission periods for the intrathecal methotrexate treated patient (235). When used alone, irradiation in doses greater than 500 R. can provide effective control with a low frequency of recurrence. When irradiation is the sole agent for treatment of CNS leukemia, the preferred dose is 1200 R. (234).

Hemorrhage also can cause neurologic signs and symptoms. Multiple hemorrhage in peripheral nerves may cause the clinical picture of mononeuritis multiplex (236). A spinal subdural hemorrhage can result in cord compression (237). Intracranial subdural hematomas may occur (238). In each of these situations, the generalized findings of thrombocytopenic bleeding are to be expected. A massive and usually fatal form of intracerebral hemorrhage is characteristic in patients with a blastic crisis during the course of their leukemia, in whom white blood counts greater than 300,000 per mm.^{3} were found (239, 240). In these patients both thrombocytopenia and the plugging of the vessels with relatively nondeformable leukemic blast cells contribute to the bleeding.

Bacterial meningitis is surprisingly rare in leukemia (218). We have seen only one instance of bacterial meningitis as part of a terminal episode of sepsis with *Pseudomonas aeruginosa*. When bacterial meningitis does occur, it may be confused with CNS leukemia (241). Therefore, each spinal fluid sample from the diagnostic lumbar puncture done in the symptomatic patient should be cultured. Viral meningitis is also an unusual complication (242). In these instances, the differentiation from CNS leukemia can be made by looking at the stained preparations of the spinal fluid cells to distinguish the leukemic blast cell from the small lymphocyte expected in viral infections.

HYPERURICEMIA. This complication is seen almost exclusively in acute lymphoblastic leukemia and can be markedly exacerbated by the institution of chemotherapy. As a consequence of rapid lysis of leukemic cells by drug treatment, degradation of nucleic acids to uric acid can cause a sudden and potentially serious increase in serum and urine uric acid levels. As a result of the uric acid load, nephropathy with renal failure (243), gouty arthritis (244), or a syndrome consisting of anorexia, nausea, persistent vomiting, weakness, and lethargy (245) may occur.

The hyperuricemia may be prevented by prophylactic administration of allopurinol, a xanthine oxidase inhibitor which impairs the conversion of water-soluble hypoxanthine to relatively less soluble uric acid (246, 247). The drug is generally routinely given for the first few days of remission induction in doses of 10 mg. per kg. body weight in three or four divided doses. If 6-mercaptopurine, which is metabolized by the same pathway as is allopurinol, is used in the induction regimen, it is recommended that its dose level be reduced to one-fourth the usual dose to avoid excessive marrow suppression. Few induction regimens currently involve 6-mercaptopurine administration. Therefore this problem rarely arises.

In patients with marked hyperuricemia at the time of diagnosis (serum levels greater than 10 mg. per 100 ml.), a treatment regimen designed to provide a urine pH greater than 7.0 is recommended (248). At a pH in this range, uric acid will not precipitate in the urine, and uric acid nephropathy can be prevented. Intravenous infusion of 5 per cent glucose solution at a rate of 3000 ml. per square meter body surface per day will result in adequate urine flow. Sodium bicarbonate adequate to increase the CO_2 content of serum 10 mEq. per liter over a 24-hour period should be given. A useful formula to increase the serum CO_2 is 0.058 g. sodium bicarbonate for each kilogram body weight for each mEq. increase required. Urinary alkalinization can be further promoted by giving acetazolamide in a dose of 150 mg. per square meter body surface per 24 hours. If nephropathy is already evident, mannitol diuresis with peritoneal dialysis (249) or removal of excess uric acid with the artificial kidney (250) might be attempted.

METABOLIC ABNORMALITIES. There are several metabolic abnormalities which may develop during the course of acute leukemia in an occasional patient. These abnormalities occur during active disease and are not to be expected during remission.

Hypercalcemia associated with nausea, vomiting, generalized severe myalgia, and hypertension (251) may occur, perhaps as a consequence of the production of a parathormone-like substance by leukemic cells (252). Symptomatic response can be obtained by increased fluid administration and phosphate solution given by mouth. Osteoporosis with metastatic calcification in various organs may result.

Hypocalcemia has also been reported (253), but the mechanism is not always clear. The patients are usually in an advanced state of their disease at the time of symptomatic hypocalcemia, and the signs and symptoms in addition to those resulting from the leukemia are mental confusion, stupor, coma, nausea, vomiting, weakness, and the specific signs of hypocalcemia, such as muscle twitching, seizures, carpopedal spasm, and a positive Chvostek's sign. Symptomatic improvement can be obtained by calcium administration. Recently, hypocalcemic tetany has been observed in patients with high white counts undergoing remission induction. The high phosphate load liberated by dying leukemia cells appears to lower serum calcium to significantly depressed levels (253a). Similarly, dangerous hyperkalemia may also occur.

Hypoglycemia is an uncommon complication and has been described in far advanced disease only (254). The expected signs of hypoglycemia are present, such as mental confusion, stupor, and seizures. Symptomatic response can be obtained by glucose administration. The mechanism is unknown. Care must be taken to exclude factitious hypoglycemia, which occurs when blood with a greatly increased leukocyte concentration is obtained (255).

In a few patients, chronic lactic acidosis has been associated with acute leukemia in an active state (256). This complication has been associated with widespread tissue hypoxia or massive, rapidly progressing leukemia. Management includes metabolic correction and control of the leukemic process.

HEART. At autopsy the heart has been found to be involved in about one-half (257) to two-thirds (258) of patients. The pathology may include both leukemic infiltration and hemorrhage. Symptomatic heart disease is uncommon and occurs in less than 5 per cent of patients with acute leukemia (258). One of the more serious complications is pericardial infiltration, which may be a presenting feature (259) and which has occurred during remission (260). Irradiation has been reported to be effective in control of this complication (261).

URINARY TRACT. Renal complications in acute leukemia other than uric acid nephropathy are not common symptomatic problems (262–264). Enlargement may occur as a consequence of leukemic infiltration. Hematuria, hypertension, or renal failure may occur when the kidneys are infiltrated. Local irradiation is the treatment of choice. In about one-half of the patients with renal enlargement, no significant infiltration with leukemic cells is found (263). Proximal tubular hypertrophy of unknown cause has been described as one mechanism for this noninfiltrative renal enlargement (264a).

Hematuria may also result from bladder infiltration (265). Priapism has occurred in boys with both acute lymphoblastic leukemia (266) and acute myeloblastic leukemia (267). Local irradiation has been advocated for relief of discomfort. Response may take several days.

Testicular infiltration is found in about two-thirds of patients at autopsy (268). It may occur at a time when the patient is in apparent blood and bone marrow remission and present as painless enlargement of the testicle (269, 270). Both orchidectomy and tumoricidal irradiation have been recommended for management of testicular involvement in those patients who are otherwise free of systemic disease.

GASTROINTESTINAL TRACT. Complications in this organ system can result from leukemic infiltration, infection, or drug toxicity (271). Infiltration of the esophagus has been associated with dysphagia (272). Extensive leukemic infiltration has been reported in a patient who was in apparent blood and bone marrow remission (273). One of the most serious problems is the necrotizing lesion of the large bowel, which may be confined to the cecum (274) or be more diffuse (275). This lesion may result from shock, chemotherapy (especially methotrexate), hemorrhage, or local trauma. In its most severe form, pneumatosis cystoides can occur (276). In almost all cases, bacteremia results. This requires vigorous supportive measures to control shock, fluid loss, and hemorrhage. Antibiotic treatment for gram-negative organisms must be started after blood cultures are obtained.

Hepatic fibrosis is more commonly an autopsy finding of no clinical significance, but in an occasional patient it may cause hepatic dysfunction during life (277, 278). Among possible causative factors, chemotherapy with methotrexate and 6-mercaptopurine are implicated.

BONES AND JOINTS. Bone pain is a common manifestation of acute leukemia (279). Roentgenographic changes are less common, but may include periosteal reaction, intramedullary osteolytic mottling, and transverse metaphyseal lucent bands. No correlation between initial radiologically evident bone disease and prognosis has been found (280). The bone pain when related to leukemic infiltration of the periosteum responds well to 600 R. irradiation to the local site. Bone necrosis may also produce bone pain and is more frequently associated with acute lymphoblastic leukemia (281). It occurs usually at a time of leukopenia, does not respond to irradiation therapy with relief of pain, and tends to be related to a poor response to chemotherapy. Arthritis with pain and swelling of the joint is less frequent but may be a presenting manifestation at times, causing some initial confusion in diagnosis (282).

LUNGS. The pulmonary complications in acute leukemia are most often of infectious origin, as has been discussed (283, 284). Leukemic infiltration may occur, but is most often found only on microscopic examination in a peribronchial distribution. Pulmonary hemorrhage is found in about one-half of patients at autopsy (284). It occurs as a consequence of thrombocytopenia and may be sufficiently severe to cause or contribute significantly to death. The roentgenographic distinction between hemorrhage, infiltration, and infection can be difficult or impossible, and all considerations should be given to the diagnosis of infection as the most likely disease process.

EYES. The most common ocular findings are those of hemorrhage and papilledema. Leukemic infiltrates are uncommon, but may involve the iris (285) and be associated with the development of glaucoma (286). The use of irradiation has been successful in alleviating the glaucoma. Severe loss of vision has been described in patients in whom a retinal pigment epitheliopathy was found (287).

MISCELLANEOUS. Several miscellaneous complications should briefly be mentioned. In some patients thymic enlargement occurs (288), which may be associated with pleural effusion (289). Involvement of the inner ear may result in vertigo or hearing loss (290). The evolution of a monoclonal gammopathy has been described in acute lymphoblastic leukemia, for which the mechanism and significance are unknown (291, 292). There appear to be no clinical consequences of this paraprotein formation.

Infiltration of the breast has occurred in girls with acute lymphoblastic leukemia (293) and acute myeloblastic leukemia (294). In acute myeloblastic leukemia, local tumor formation (myeloblastoma, chloroma) has been described in breast and ovary during apparent blood and bone marrow remission (295). The term "chloroma" is used to describe the greenish color of this solid mass, which is presumed to result from the verdoperoxidase of the malignant cells. The tumor may be a presenting feature of the disease; a more frequent clinical finding is proptosis (296). Rib involvement, with a clinical picture resembling florid rickets with its characteristic rosary, has been described (297).

Oral findings most frequently are those of bleeding or infection. Thrush is particularly common in the child who is in relapse and receiving corticosteroids and antibiotics. Mucous membrane ulceration may be a manifestation of drug toxicity, especially with methotrexate. Gingival hypertrophy is characteristic of acute myeloblastic and monoblastic leukemia (298, 299).

Therapy

A child with acute leukemia lived only about three months after diagnosis until aminopterin, a folic acid antagonist, was introduced as treatment in 1948 (300, 301). Eight drugs presently are commonly used in the treatment of acute leukemia (Table 22–2). The sites of action of some of them in the cell cycle are shown in Figure 22–2. With these drugs the median survival time has increased about tenfold. This increase is a reflection of better management of complications of the disease, as well as better methods of specific therapy.

AVAILABLE DRUGS. Doses, route, and schedule of administration of the drugs commonly used in the treatment of leukemia and the incidence of remission attained by these drugs are given in Table 22–2. The drugs do not exhibit cross-resistance.

An accepted definition of a complete remission is 5 per cent or less abnormal blasts in the marrow and 40 per cent or less of lymphocytes plus blasts in the marrow. The patient must be free of symptoms and physi-

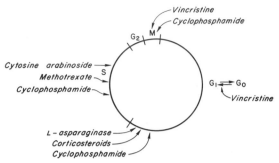

Figure 22–2. Representation of the sites of action of chemotherapeutic agents on the cell cycle.

cal findings attributable to the disease, and the complete blood cell count must be within normal limits (302). Until recently, infiltration of the central nervous system (CNS) with leukemic cells was not considered a relapse if the other indices were normal. Clearly this view is rapidly being revised.

Prednisone is of particular value in the treatment of patients with ALL, not only because an initial remission may occur in 50 per cent or more of the patients, but also because corticosteroids do not depress the marrow. Prednisone must be given daily in order to obtain the greatest number of remissions (302). Increasing the dose to more than 2 mg. per kg. per day does not increase the number of patients who enter remission

TABLE 22–2.   DRUG DOSAGE, ROUTE, INTERVAL OF ADMINISTRATION, AND RESPONSE TO AVAILABLE CHEMOTHERAPEUTIC AGENTS

DRUG	ROUTE	INTERVAL	DOSE (MG./M²)	COMPLETE REMISSION OF 5% ABNORMAL BLASTS IN MARROW — ALL	AML	REFERENCE
Prednisone	Oral	Daily	60	40–60%	14–20%	302, 303, 305
Vincristine	Intravenous	7 days	1.5–2.0	57–85%	36%	306, 307
Methotrexate	Oral	Daily	3.3	22%	11%	312
	Intravenous	14 days	100–200	—	—	
	Intramuscular	4 to 7 days	15	—	—	
6-Mercaptopurine	Oral	Daily	70–90	27%	9%	312
Cyclophosphamide	Oral	Daily	100	31.5%*		321
	Intravenous	7 to 14 days	450	10.2%*		
Cytosine arabinoside	Intravenous or subcutaneous	Variable	Variable	26%	25–100%	323, 324, 325
Daunorubicin	Intravenous	Daily	45–60	43–60%	60%	326, 327, 328
L-Asparaginase	Intravenous	Variable	Variable	43–70%	12%	330

*A small number are children with AML.

(302). The median time required for a remission is 28 days (303). Continuous administration of prednisone beyond the induction period does not appear to be of value (304). A second remission can be obtained with prednisone alone in approximately 46 per cent of patients with ALL (303). The induction of remission in children with AML is uncommon (305).

With the exception of obesity, side effects of prednisone are not commonly seen (Table 22–3).

Vincristine is a natural alkaloid of the periwinkle plant (*Vinca rosea* Linn). It is effective in inducing a remission in approximately 55 to 85 per cent of children with ALL and in a lesser number of children with AML (306, 307). The median time required to obtain a remission is 28 days. Eighty per cent respond by 42 days and 90 per cent by 56 days after starting therapy (307). Most investigators have reported that vincristine in a dose of 1.5 to 2.0 mg. per M^2 per week does not maintain remission (307, 308). However, the results of a study from Australia indicate that this drug may prolong a remission (309).

Neurotoxicity is the major side effect of vincristine, and occasionally the drug has to be discontinued because of severe abdominal pain and distention, which in children is usually secondary to constipation. Use of a stool softener during therapy with vincristine appears to reduce constipation (306). Vincristine has a minimal depressive effect on the bone marrow.

Methotrexate acts primarily through competitive inhibition of dihydrofolic acid reductase, the enzyme required to catalyze the reduction of folic acid to tetrahydrofolic acid (310). The reduced form of this vitamin is necessary for the de novo synthesis of both DNA and RNA. Methotrexate is well absorbed from the gastrointestinal tract (311). Following a single injection, one-half is cleared from the plasma within 2½ hours by a combination of glomerular filtration and active tubular excretion (311). Therefore, methotrexate may accumulate in patients with renal disease.

Methotrexate alone is a poor induction agent in both ALL and AML (312). If a remission is obtained, the median time for maintenance of the remission with oral methotrexate given daily is 5 to 6 months,

TABLE 22–3. SIDE EFFECTS OF CHEMOTHERAPEUTIC AGENTS

PREDNISONE

Cushingoid appearance	Urinary frequency
Hypertension	Hyperuricemia
Monilia	Diabetes mellitus (rarely)

6-MERCAPTOPURINE

Bone marrow depression	Hepatotoxicity (rarely)
Nausea and vomiting (occasional)	

METHOTREXATE

Mouth ulcers	Megaloblastic marrow
Anorexia	Necrotizing enteropathy
Nausea	Hepatotoxicity (rarely)
Vomiting	Pneumonitis
Bone marrow depression	Osteoporosis

CYCLOPHOSPHAMIDE

Alopecia	Bone marrow depression
Anorexia	Hemorrhagic cystitis
Nausea	Bladder fibrosis
Vomiting	

CYTOSINE ARABINOSIDE

Mouth ulcers	Vomiting
Bone marrow depression	Megaloblastic marrow
Anorexia	Alopecia
Nausea	

VINCRISTINE

Major Side Effects Secondary to Neurotoxicity:

Paresthesias	Sensory loss
Slapping gait	Constipation
Hoarseness	Abdominal pain
Muscle weakness	Loss of DTR's

Other Side Effects:

Severe local reaction	
Fever	Minimal bone marrow
Alopecia	depression
Jaw pain	Hyponatremia (rarely)

L-ASPARAGINASE

Hypersensitivity reactions	Nausea
Azotemia	Vomiting
Weight loss	Anorexia
Low cholesterol triglycerides	?Disseminated intravascular coagulation
Nonketotic hyperglycemia	?Depression of synthesis of coagulation factors
Elevated blood ammonia	other than fibrinogen

but it is 9 to 12 months when the drug is given every two weeks intravenously or twice weekly, either intramuscularly or orally (312, 313, 314). These data show that the schedule of administration of this drug is important.

Methotrexate toxicity is observed most commonly in the rapidly replicating tissues of the gastrointestinal mucosa and bone marrow. The drug must be stopped temporarily if mouth ulcers occur or if the marrow is significantly depressed. Other less common side effects which require discontinuation of the drug are acute hepatitis; a pulmonary syndrome consisting of severe dyspnea, nonproductive cough, hypoxemia and bilateral pulmonary infiltrates; and osteoporosis (312–315).

6-Mercaptopurine is a purine analog which inhibits de novo purine synthesis. It is excreted through the kidney and metabolized in the liver (316). A remission can be obtained in approximately 27 per cent of children treated with 6-mercaptopurine alone (312) and can be maintained for about eight months with this drug alone (317).

Bone marrow depression is the major side effect of 6-mercaptopurine. Occasionally hepatitis develops (318), and the drug must then be discontinued.

Cyclophosphamide is a synthetic polyfunctional alkylating agent. It distributes throughout most body fluids and is excreted by the kidneys (319). The compound is inactive until it is converted in vivo to an active metabolite (320).

Cyclophosphamide alone is not a good inducing agent in either ALL or AML (321). The drug appears to be more effective when given daily than when given in weekly injections. It is of questionable value for maintenance treatment. The median duration of remission with cyclophosphamide maintenance is three to four months (321).

Bone marrow depression and hemorrhagic cystitis are the two most serious side effects of this drug (321). Usually the bone marrow depression is not severe, particularly if the drug is given orally and, following interruption of therapy, recovery of the marrow occurs. However, the occurrence of hemorrhagic cystitis may necessitate permanent discontinuation of this drug. All patients on cyclophosphamide should be kept well hydrated and receive the drug early in the day so that the metabolites of cyclophosphamide do not remain in the bladder in a concentrated form for a long period of time.

Cytosine arabinoside is a synthetic antimetabolite, a pyrimidine antagonist. It has a half-life of less than 30 minutes and is rapidly degraded to uracil arabinoside, an inactive metabolite (322). Cytosine arabinoside can induce a remission in approximately 30 per cent of children with ALL and in 25 per cent of children with AML (323–325).

As with methotrexate, the side effects of cytosine arabinoside are primarily related to inhibition of DNA synthesis in replicating tissue (Table 22–3) (323–325).

Daunorubicin is a term adopted as the generic name for daunomycin, an antibiotic isolated from *Streptomyces peucetius* and rubidomycin, an antibiotic isolated from *S. coeruleorubidus* (328). They appear to be identical compounds. Daunorubicin is effective in both ALL and AML. An approximate 50 per cent remission rate can be obtained in patients with either type of leukemia (326, 327, 328).

Daunorubicin causes profound bone marrow depression, particularly of the myeloid series. In addition cardiotoxicity, manifested by hypotension, dyspnea, and death, has been found in patients who have received a total dose of 25 mg. per kg. or more. Electrocardiographic changes may not occur or may occur late. The ECG changes are nonspecific and may be ST depression and T wave inversion (326–328).

L-*Asparaginase* is an enzyme which is usually obtained from *Escherichia coli*. Some leukemic cells require L-asparagine for growth. L-Asparaginase has the ability to eliminate this amino acid and thus kill leukemic cells which are dependent upon L-asparagine (329). L-Asparaginase is a very effective drug in inducing remission in patients with ALL, but not in AML (330).

As seen in Table 22–3, the side effects of L-asparaginase are numerous (329, 330). Significant bone marrow depression does not appear to occur. Some of the side effects, such as decreased synthesis of protein, disturbances of hepatic function, and fatty metamorphosis of the liver, are attributed to changes secondary to depletion of L-asparagine. Other side effects, such as hypersensitivity which may be manifested as anaphylaxis, are attributed to impurities of the enzyme preparation or the enzyme itself. Serious anaphylactoid reactions have been reported in at least 15 per cent of patients treated (330).

The induction of a remission does not appear to depend upon the dose of the drug. However, the toxic manifestations may be decreased if the drug is given weekly over a two-week period. It has been recommended that the therapy should not extend beyond two weeks, because of the promptness of response by patients who are sensitive to the drug and the marked toxicity of the agent (331). The toxicity and efficacy of L-asparaginase may vary, depending upon the source of the enzyme preparation.

DRUG EFFECTS ON THE CELL CYCLE. Most of the chemotherapeutic agents kill leukemic cells by affecting some phase of the mitotic cycle. The phases of the mitotic cycle and a summary of the in vivo effect on the mitotic cycle of most of the chemotherapeutic agents are illustrated in Figure 22-2. Methotrexate and cytosine arabinoside inhibit DNA synthesis (S period) (332-334); corticosteroids and L-asparaginase inhibit the entry of cells into the S period and cause lysis of lymphoblasts (333-336); vincristine arrests blasts in mitosis (M), which were in DNA synthesis at the time the drug was given (333, 334). In addition, vincristine appears to block the entry of resting (G_0) cells into the mitotic cycle (G_1) (333, 334, 337). Although further studies are necessary, cyclophosphamide appears to have several effects on the mitotic cycle — inhibition of DNA synthesis, arrest of cells in mitosis, and inhibition of entry of cells into the S period (334). In a preliminary report, daunorubicin has been reported to be cytocidal for myeloblasts, but cells in the S phase were reported to be particularly sensitive (338). The effect of 6-mercaptopurine on the mitotic cycle has not been studied in vivo.

Leukemic cells can be synchronized in the S phase after a rapid injection of 5 mg. per kg. of cytosine arabinoside intravenously (333, 334). Synchronization may be defined as an increase in the number of cells in a particular phase of the mitotic cycle. Recently it has been possible to take advantage of the synchronizing effect of cytosine arabinoside on the mitotic cycle to induce remission in nine children with AML (325). Further studies are necessary in order to plan rational approaches to therapy based on knowledge of the effect of drugs and the time of the effect on the mitotic cycle of leukemic cells. A recent review concerning cell kinetics and chemotherapy is available for further details (339).

DRUG TREATMENT PLAN. The basic aspects of drug treatment involve remission induction and remission maintenance. Combinations of prednisone with vincristine, 6-mercaptopurine, methotrexate, or cy-clophosphamide induce remissions in 80 to 90 per cent of patients with acute lymphoblastic leukemia. The addition of a third or fourth drug to this form of induction regimen does not increase the percent achieving a remission and does add to morbidity and mortality. The combination of prednisone and vincristine induces remission rapidly, almost always within four to six weeks. The remission must be maintained (340); otherwise it will culminate in a relapse within a median time of six to eight weeks.

Initially maintenance therapy was administered in a sequential fashion. Single agents were used until relapse occurred. Then after another remission induction, another single-agent maintenance regimen was used. With this form of treatment, it may be expected that about 15 per cent of patients with acute lymphoblastic leukemia will achieve seven years of complete remissions, and one-third will survive three years from diagnosis (341). A second form of remission maintenance has been with cyclic drug therapy (342-344). After induction, the remission is maintained by changing drugs at fixed intervals, usually between six weeks and three months. Although it was hoped that the development of drug resistance would be delayed, the median survival times with this therapy regimen proved to be no greater than with the sequential treatment.

Currently most treatment regimens use a form of maintenance which involves multiple drug administration. The two most promising methods have been reported by investigators from St. Jude Hospital (345-347, 347a) and in a preliminary form by Leukemia Cooperative Group B (348). Both groups of investigators have used an induction regimen of prednisone and vincristine.

Various combinations of cyclophosphamide, vincristine, methotrexate, and 6-mercaptopurine were used for maintenance in the first three groups of patients (41 children) treated at St. Jude Hospital. These drugs were given at full dosage whenever the blood count was 2000 or higher. Prophylactic CNS therapy, consisting of 1200 R. in 11 days, was given to the entire CNS in some of these patients. A 17 per cent five-year cure rate was achieved with this therapy. A five-year cure was defined as an initial continuous remission lasting five years. CNS prophylaxis in the dosage given had no significant effect on the appearance of CNS leukemia. In these studies, the majority of children who remained in continuous remission for two years were still in remission five years later. Five patients in a group of 26 who were treated the most intensively were in a complete remission at five years.

On the basis of the results of these early studies, these investigators have continued to use a combination of 6-mercaptopurine, methotrexate, and cyclophosphamide for maintenance, but in addition they have administered a course of prednisone and vincristine every ten weeks. A more intensive course of prophylactic therapy to the CNS was also given. Of 35 patients treated in this manner, 20 of 30 who attained remission and received all initial phases of therapy have been in continuous complete remission for 23 to 30 months. A 50 per cent five-year cure rate has been projected for this group of patients, since the majority of children in the first three groups who remained in complete remission longer than two years were also in remission at five years. With this therapy there was an increased incidence of viral and other nonbacterial infections, such as *Pneumocystis carinii*. Two deaths occurred during remission from viral infections. In addition, growth retardation occurred, but after chemotherapy was stopped, catch-up growth did occur in some patients.

The therapy which has given the best results as reported by Leukemia Cooperative Group B differed from the program at St. Jude Hospital in the following manner: instead of combination therapy with 6-mercaptopurine, methotrexate, and cyclophosphamide, intensive courses of methotrexate were given without the other two drugs. "Staccato" administration of prednisone and vincristine was given. Intensive chemotherapy was continued for eight months, and then all therapy was stopped. Ten cases of a small number of patients treated in this manner have remained in complete remission for 36 months. These ten patients represent 27 per cent of children who completed the eight months of therapy. If induction failures and relapses during methotrexate administration are taken into account, 18 per cent remained in remission for this period of time. The median survival for all patients was over four years.

Recipes for treatment of acute leukemia are dangerous for text books because of the lag between writing and publication. Advances are continuous, and the physician caring for children with acute leukemia should keep up with current literature for the best current form of therapy.

TREATMENT OF ACUTE MYELOBLASTIC LEUKEMIA. Sequential therapy as outlined for patients with ALL may be beneficial in some patients with AML. Until recently, however, the incidence of a complete remission in children with AML generally did not exceed 20 per cent, and the median survival was only one month (301). With the introduction of cytosine arabinoside and daunorubicin in the therapy of leukemia, over 50 per cent of the patients achieved a remission, and median survival time in most studies has increased to six months (325, 327). This remission rate can be expected with either cytosine arabinoside (325) or daunorubicin alone (327), or cytosine arabinoside in combination with daunorubicin (349), thioguanine (350), 6-mercaptopurine (351), or cyclophosphamide (352).

Once a remission occurs, it is not clear whether or not chemotherapy plays an effective role in maintenance. Certainly daunorubicin cannot be used because of its cardiotoxicity, and attempts with cytosine arabinoside alone have not been productive. Remission maintenance regimens thus are a real need for management of patients with AML.

IMMUNOTHERAPY. Mathé in 1969 reported an increase in length of remission in patients who received regular immunization with either BCG, pooled irradiated leukemic cells, or BCG and irradiated leukemic cells (353). The patients were treated with a variety of drugs and were in complete remission before receiving immunotherapy. Seven of the 20 patients treated have remained in remission three years after stopping chemotherapy; four for more than four years, and one for 5½ years (354). A recent report by an English Leukemia Study Group failed to confirm the efficacy of BCG in treatment of ALL (355). This lack of confirmation, however, may not mean that BCG is ineffective, since scarification was not used by the British group, and the strain of BCG was not the same as the one used by Mathé. As mentioned earlier, another English group has gathered encouraging results by immunization with BCG and killed leukemic cells (92a). Further studies are necessary to determine the efficacy of the various forms of immunotherapy (592).

BONE MARROW TRANSPLANTATION. Attempts at treatment of acute leukemia have been made by marrow engraftment with HL-A matched donor cells. Immunosuppressive preparation with whole body irradiation (356) and cyclophosphamide (357) has been used. Results so far have indicated the possibility of engraftment, but median survival after the attempt has been about two months (357). Long-term post-transplant survival has been observed in an occasional patient (356). Complications of the procedure have been failure of engraftment, infection, graft-versus-host reaction (358), and, most disturbing of all, recurrence of the leukemic process in the donor cells (359). Recently an immunosuppressive regimen with antilymphocyte antiglobulin has been reported (360), which may, if confirmed, have fewer associated complications. More experience is needed with this form of therapy before its eventual role in treatment can be assessed.

Emotional Effects of Leukemia

It would be well for anyone caring for children with acute leukemia to read some of the comments available concerning the emotional impact of a fatal disease (361–363) – the aspects of management (364–369) and the effect on the family (370, 371) and on the physician (372, 373). Not all people have taken the same approach to caring for children with fatal illnesses, and it is best to read widely before formulating one's own resolution to this problem.

The first conference with the parents after the diagnosis is confirmed is an important time for the physician. A meeting should be set up with both parents at a time when the physician and parents can have sufficient undisturbed time to explain the diagnosis and its significance adequately. The parents want honesty from the physician and an explanation in a manner that can be understood by them. A description of the disease and a discussion of future plans for management should be given. Prognosis should be discussed, not in absolutes or median sur-

vival times but in the range of possibilities that might occur. The parents should be prepared for the consequences of long survival, as well as the less likely possibility of quick death. The parents' concern about the etiology of this disease involves mostly a consideration of familial predisposition and potential contagiousness of the disease. They should be firmly reassured on both points.

The physician should recognize that an almost universal response on the part of parents is one of guilt. Are they responsible for having passed the leukemia to the child as part of some genetically determined predisposition? If they had taken the child earlier to the doctor, could the disease have been cured? Has any action on their part contributed to the development of the disease in their child? The physician cannot anticipate all possible reasons the parents may have for this guilt feeling, but he should, gently and with understanding, open the way for current and future exploration of this area with the parents.

The problem of what to tell the child is a difficult one, not amenable to dogmatic recommendations for each and every situation. It is wise to discuss the point with the parents, evaluate the child and his reactions and understanding, and then decide in concert with the parents how the disease should be explained to the child. In any case, absolute and consistent truthfulness should be observed in what the child is told. As a generalization, the older child responds best to an open and honest discussion of his disease and its implications. Of critical importance are the attitudes of physicians, nurses, and supporting staff. Though it is obviously important to inform parents of the serious nature of the illness and of the relatively low probability of permanent success, it is equally vital to express a sense of determination to bend every effort to achieve a permanent remission. This honest but firm attitude on the part of the staff is usually successfully projected to parents and can even be transmitted to children who are often astonishingly capable of accepting serious diagnoses if they are convinced that their parents, physicians, nurses, and supporting staff stand squarely behind them. Much has been written about the care of the child dying of cancer and of other serious diseases. In our view, the most essential contribution to emotional support as death approaches is the capacity of the physician and the entire staff to remain at their patient's side. Terror is the consequence of abandonment.

CHRONIC MYELOCYTIC LEUKEMIA

Chronic myelocytic leukemia is a form of leukemia which is characterized by increased numbers of myeloid cells in all stages of maturation in both the blood and bone marrow. This disease is uncommon in children and accounts for less than 5 per cent of all cases of childhood leukemia (374). When chronic myelocytic leukemia occurs in adults, a consistent chromosome abnormality has been found in dividing myeloid, erythroid, and megakaryocytic precursors in over 85 per cent of patients (375). The chromosome abnormality consists of deletion of the long arms of a small group G chromosome. This abnormal chromosome has been called the Philadelphia (Ph[1]) chromosome, and until recently it was thought to be chromosome number 21 (375). However, Prieto and associates have presented evidence to suggest that the abnormal chromosome is actually number 22 (376). A Ph[1] chromosome is not found in other tissues of the body; thus it provides a marker of the leukemic population. Development of chronic myelocytic leukemia from an abnormal stem cell has been suggested because of the presence of the Ph[1] chromosome in most marrow cells at the time of diagnosis.

Further evidence for clonal origin was reported recently by Fitzgerald and co-workers (377). These authors studied a 69-year-old man who was a constitutional XY/XXY sex chromosomal mosaic. The Ph[1] chromosome was found in the 46,XY cell line and not in the 47,XXY cell line. In the event of multicellular origin, the Ph[1] chromosome would be expected in both cell lines.

Assuming that an abnormal clone does develop from a stem cell, it is not known whether the stem cell in question was abnormal from birth and remained dormant for years, or whether a mutation secondary to some stimulus occurred in a normal stem cell (378). Several sets of identical twins have been shown to have a discordant oc-currence of the Ph[1] chromosome, suggesting an acquired defect (379, 380). However, two families have been reported in whom several members had chronic myelocytic leukemia, and the chromosomal abnormality was found in nondiseased siblings (381, 382). These findings would suggest that in some families the defect may be inherited. The Ph[1] chromosome is found during remission in most patients (383). Nevertheless, a few adults have been described who did not have this chromosomal abnormality in their marrow following extensive chemotherapy (384, 385). This finding suggests that in at least some patients a normal stem cell compartment may coexist with abnormal cells, and that perhaps the abnormal stem cell compartment that gives rise to chronic myelocytic leukemia can be eradicated.

In most patients with chronic myelocytic leukemia, the terminal phase of the disease is characterized by an increasing number of abnormal immature myeloid precursors in the blood and bone marrow (blastic transformation). Many of these blasts contain a Ph[1] chromosome along with other chromosomal abnormalities if a Ph[1] chromosome was present prior to the transformation. This finding suggests that mutations resulting in transformation to blasts are more likely to occur in chromosomes in the clone of cells containing the Ph[1] chromosome than in normal stem cells (386).

The total body granulocyte pool is increased in chronic myelocytic leukemia (387), and the disappearance half-time ($t\frac{1}{2}$) of labeled leukocytes in chronic myelocytic leukemia is increased strikingly when compared to normal DF[32]P-labeled autologous cells (388). The release of granulocytes from the marrow to the circulation is defective, as illustrated by impaired leukocytosis after endotoxin stimulation (389). A progressive decrease in the $t\frac{1}{2}$ of labeled autologous cells with DF[32]P occurs as the patient with chronic myelocytic leukemia goes into remission (388). A decrease in tissue migration of granulocytes could explain the increase in $t\frac{1}{2}$ seen in chronic myelocytic leukemia. Data to suggest an impaired ability of leukocytes from patients with chronic myelocytic leukemia to migrate across the vessel wall were recently reported by Banerjee and co-workers (390).

Spontaneous cyclic fluctuations of the leukocyte count in patients with chronic myelocytic leukemia similar to that seen in normal subjects have been reported by several authors (391–394). In addition to the fluctuation in granulocytes, spontaneous fluctuations of platelet counts coincident with the fluctuations in granulocyte counts have been found in two patients with chronic myelocytic leukemia (394). These observations indicate that the proliferation of chronic myelocytic leukemic cells is not autonomous, but some feedback mechanism does exist (394). As the disease progresses, an overshoot in the production of granulocytes and platelets occurs. This increase in oscillations suggests that the feedback control mechanism becomes less effective with time (394). Recently King-Smith and Morley have proposed a model of computer-simulated granulopoiesis, in which two nonlinear feedback loops control granulocyte oscillation under normal situations (395). One loop, representing granulocyte production, is responsible for the underlying oscillating behavior of the system. The other loop, controlling granulocyte release, damps out the oscillations. On the basis of this model, the oscillations seen in chronic myelocytic leukemia could be explained by the loop controlling granulocyte release (394). However, if, as mentioned by Shadduck et al., oscillations were due solely to variation in cell release from the marrow, an increase in marrow granulocyte cells at about the time of the nadir of the blood granulocyte count would be expected (393). In like manner, a relatively normal marrow would be expected at the height of leukocytosis. Such was not the case in the patient reported by Shadduck. Instead granulocytic hyperplasia of the marrow occurred concomitantly with the increase in the blood granulocyte count, and the marrow appeared normal when the white count was 9500. These results suggest that the oscillations in that patient were related to variations in cell production (393).

Recent studies of colony-forming capacity in chronic myelocytic marrows suggest that the marrow stem cell pool may be markedly increased in certain patients (393a). This must contribute to the increased cell production rate.

There are two types of chronic myelocytic leukemia in children—the adult type and the juvenile type (396–399). Most children with chronic myelocytic leukemia have the adult type (399).

Adult Type

This form of chronic myelocytic leukemia is usually found in older children, but well-documented instances in infancy have been recorded (400). The onset of symptoms is insidious. Hepatosplenomegaly may be found on routine physical examination, or pallor may be observed by the parents. Purpura and other bleeding manifestations at the time of diagnosis are uncommon.

The physical examination usually reveals moderate pallor and extreme hepatosplenomegaly. Lymphadenopathy of a moderate degree is common. There may be unexplained fever. Bone-associated myeloid tumors may occur. A curious feature which we have seen in two patients and which has also been described by others (397) is an arthropathy resembling rheumatoid arthritis. Rather striking joint effusions may also occur (397). Retinopathy may be found, and priapism has been reported (401, 402). Rarely skin nodules, deafness, and loss of vestibular function may be found (402).

On laboratory examination a hemoglobin of about 9 g. per 100 ml. is usually found. The anemia is generally normochromic, normocytic, with some poikilocytosis. Thrombocytopenia is not common, and, in fact, there may be thrombocytosis. The white blood cell concentration is increased and may be greater than 100,000 per mm^3. The usual range of leukocyte concentration is from 100,000 to 500,000 per $mm.^3$ (396).

On differential count of blood leukocytes, all forms of myeloid cells from myeloblasts to mature neutrophils are found. There are no characteristic morphologic abnormalities. A constant absolute eosinophilia and basophilia are present. The bone marrow aspirate is hypercellular and consists primarily of myeloid cells. The erythroid precursors are relatively reduced in number. Megakaryocytes are present and may appear to be increased. The serum concentration of vitamin B_{12} is increased strikingly. This increase is related to an increase of capacity of the serum to bind vitamin B_{12} due to increased levels of transcobalamin I. Another protein, transcobalamin II, appears to bind B_{12} proportionately less when added to sera from patients with chronic myelocytic leukemia in relapse. The B_{12} binding abnormalities return toward normal when remission of the disease occurs (403–405).

The alkaline phosphatase activity of the

neutrophils is decreased (399, 406, 407). An increased alkaline phosphatase activity may be seen when a concurrent disease, such as ulcerative colitis, or a complication, such as bronchopneumonia, develops (408). Although not many determinations have been reported, the fetal hemoglobin concentrations are in the normal range with rare exceptions (397, 409). On chromosomal analysis, the Philadelphia chromosome is found (396, 397). The terminal event may be infectious or hemorrhagic in character. Conversion to a clinical and hematologic picture resembling acute myeloblastic leukemia or even promyelocytic leukemia may occur (410). Conversion to the acute blastic form may happen early in the course of the disease (410).

Prognosis is difficult to determine with any degree of confidence because of the limited number of patients. The disease usually runs a course of months, but patients may live for several years after conversion to blastic crisis. A comparison of the adult and juvenile forms of chronic myelocytic leukemia is seen in Table 22–4. Most of the children with the juvenile form are 1 to 2 years of age.

Juvenile Type

Clinical presentation in this group of children frequently involves recurrent infections, an eczematoid rash of the face, and lymphadenopathy which may be suppurative. *Staphylococcus aureus* is usually grown from the exudate.

At times, blood counts during the early symptomatic phases are not helpful. Hepatosplenomegaly is a frequent finding, however, and it is striking how much this clinical picture resembles chronic granulomatous disease of childhood and its manifestations. After several weeks or months of symptoms, purpura and mucosal bleeding may occur. Pallor is found. The enlargement of the liver and spleen is moderate. Respiratory tract infections are a common problem.

The laboratory findings are usually conclusive by the time purpura has appeared. The hemoglobin concentration is reduced, and thrombocytopenia can be demonstrated on blood smear and direct count. The white blood count is increased and is most often in the range of 50,000 cells per mm^3. Leukocyte counts ranging from 15,000 to 190,000 per mm^3 have been reported, but it is unusual for the count to be greater than 100,000 per mm^3 (396–398, 400).

On differential count, all myeloid forms are present—myeloblasts through mature neutrophils. An absolute eosinophilia is frequently found, and an absolute basophilia may be found. There may be monocytosis (396). The cells do not have any striking morphologic abnormalities. The bone

TABLE 22–4. FEATURES OF ADULT AND JUVENILE TYPES OF CHRONIC MYELOCYTIC LEUKEMIA (374, 396–403, 409, 413–415)

FEATURE	ADULT TYPE	JUVENILE TYPE
Age of maximal incidence (year)	10–12	1–2
Philadelphia chromosome	Almost always	Never
Fetal hemoglobin values	2–7%	30–70%
Splenomegaly	Usually marked	Mild to moderate
Lymphadenopathy with suppuration	Occasional	Frequent
Skin rash	None	Frequent eczematous rash of face
White blood cell count at onset	Frequently over 100,000 per mm^3	Rarely over 100,000 per mm^3
Thrombocytopenia at onset	Uncommon	Usually present
Blast forms in blood	Infrequent	Often present
Megakaryocytes in marrow	Often increased	Usually decreased
Complete remission with therapy	Frequent	Rare
Alkaline phosphatase in neutrophils	Decreased	Decreased or lower limit of normal
Serum vitamin B$_{12}$ level	Increased	Increased
Maximum nucleated red cells (10^3 per mm^3.)	0.25–0.5	1–18
Monocytes in blood	Normal to increased	Increased

marrow is cellular, with a predominance of myeloid cells. At the time of diagnosis, no lack of maturation is evident. Erythroid cells are present but relatively reduced in number. Megakaryocytes are scarce.

The alkaline phosphatase activity of neutrophils is frequently decreased, but may be normal (399). Fetal hemoglobin concentration ranges from 30 to 70 per cent (397, 400, 411–415). With progression of the disease, the level of fetal hemoglobin increases (411, 413, 416). Chromosomal analysis usually reveals aneuploidy, but a Philadelphia chromosome is not found (397). The studies may be done with blood if dividing myeloid cells are present; otherwise, marrow aspirates are needed, since only the marrow cell lines carry the defect. This form of chronic myelocytic leukemia has been reported in two sets of infant siblings (417), but in most reports only one child has been reported from a single family.

Children with the juvenile form of chronic myelocytic leukemia have a subnormal level of Hb A$_2$ (412), increased G6PD activity (415), reduced carbonic anhydrase in red cells (412, 413, 415), a decreased titer of the erythrocyte I antigen (397, 412), an oxygen dissociation curve displaced to the left, and a normal amount of 2,3-DPG (418). All these findings are characteristic of fetal red cells. In addition, the ratio of glycine to alanine in γ136 was found to be typical of the neonatal pattern on structural analysis of the γ chain of fetal hemoglobin in one child with chronic myelocytic leukemia (418). On the basis of these findings, Weatherall and others suggested that the fetal-like red cells in juvenile chronic myelocytic leukemia may represent abnormal proliferation of a stem cell line in which normal differentiation processes have not occurred (413, 418). Indeed, Altman and his co-workers have shown that the colony-forming cells in juvenile chronic myelocytic leukemia blood develop into monocytes in culture, whereas adult-type chronic myelocytic leukemia blood gives rise to mature granulocytes in culture. These authors have concluded that the juvenile disease should be classified as a variant of myelomonocytic leukemia (418a).

In 1965 Randall and co-workers reported a leukemia-like disease in nine related children (419). The hematologic and clinical findings were similar to those found in patients with the juvenile form of chronic myelocytic leukemia. The age of onset in these children was between 5 months and 4 years. The clinical findings were increasing lethargy, pallor, and growth retardation. On physical examination, there was massive splenomegaly and moderate hepatomegaly.

Anemia and leukocytosis were present, with early myeloid cell forms being found on blood smear. On bone marrow examination, a hyperplastic specimen was found, with all cell lines being present including megakaryocytes.

In three children the disease ended quickly with an early death. Two children recovered, and in four the condition remained unchanged or slightly improved. Therapy did not alter the course of the disease demonstrably.

No other similar familial disease has been reported, and from the observations of Randall and co-workers, it is even difficult to classify this condition as a leukemia. Further reports and studies may help clarify this puzzling disease complex.

Treatment of Chronic Myelocytic Leukemia

Antileukemic therapy may be withheld from patients who are asymptomatic and have minimal elevation of white blood count, minimal splenomegaly, and normal hemoglobin levels. With the development of anemia, splenomegaly, and related symptomatology, treatment should be instituted.

The drug of choice for children with the adult form of chronic myelocytic leukemia is busulfan, an alkylating agent. The initial dose is 0.06 to 0.1 mg. per kg. per day (397). The drug should be decreased to about one-half the initial dose when the white blood cell count becomes one-half the initial count, or, if the count were very high, when the count reaches 15,000 to 20,000 per mm^3. The drug must be carefully monitored for marrow suppression, and not infrequently the drug must be stopped temporarily. During the early stages of treatment, a complete blood count should be obtained weekly. As a rough guide, the number of leukocytes is halved every three weeks. A fall in the white blood cell count may continue for several weeks after discontinuation of the drug. Occasionally the platelet count decreases before the white blood count, and the drug has to be discontinued because of a decrease in the platelet count.

The longest remissions have occurred in patients who have developed marrow hypoplasia and whose marrow upon recovery has not contained the Ph¹ chromosome (386). Maintenance of the hematologic remission is possible with small daily doses of busulfan.

Patients not responding to busulfan may respond to hydroxyurea (420). This drug has been reported to be as effective as busulfan and may be utilized as primary therapy of chronic myelocytic leukemia.

The drug of choice for treatment of the juvenile form of chronic myelocytic leukemia is not known because of the few patients reported and the lack of response to drugs in most of the reported cases. Busulfan may be tried, as in the children with the adult form of the disease. However, this drug is usually ineffective (396, 397).

The overall remission rate in patients with the blastic phase of chronic myelocytic leukemia is very low (421). The same drugs that are useful in the treatment of acute myeloblastic leukemia should be considered in treatment of a blastic crisis. However, recently a remission was induced with prednisone and vincristine in 30 per cent of a small series of patients in the blastic crisis. Chromosomal analysis was done in 28 patients prior to therapy. Those patients who had a hypodiploid cell line responded better to this therapy (422). Perhaps chromosomal studies should be done on all patients in blastic crisis prior to starting chemotherapy in order to have a better guideline for selection of the chemotherapeutic agent.

THE CHRONIC MYELOPROLIFERATIVE SYNDROMES

As mentioned earlier in this chapter, the combination of anemia, "teardrop" red cells, abnormal platelets, myeloblastosis, and erythroblastosis describes a condition known as leukoerythroblastosis. This morphology usually reflects bone marrow invasion or replacement by fibrosis, cancellous bone, infectious granuloma, solid tumor, or

leukemia. The latter two are by far the most common, but myelofibrosis with myeloid metaplasia, osteosclerosis, fungal or mycobacterial infection, and occasionally rheumatoid arthritis are other less common causes. These are discussed in Chapter 5. Polycythemia vera is very uncommon in childhood and, when present, may be associated with chromosome abnormalities and consumption coagulopathy (422a). The etiology of the consumption process is uncertain and may be related to the high blood viscosity rather than to the thrombocytosis and bizarre platelet morphology observed in the disease. This suggestion is made because mild acceleration of the turnover of clotting factors may also be observed in the high viscosity syndromes observed in congenital heart disease and overtransfusion in the newborn period (Chapter 28).

EOSINOPHILIC LEUKEMIA

Eosinophilic leukemia may be defined as a very rare form of leukemia in which there is a marked increase in eosinophils, eosinophilic precursors, and myeloblasts in the blood, bone marrow, and other tissues. Only about 16 cases of this type of leukemia have been described in the pediatric age group (423). Eosinophilic leukemia may be impossible to diagnose when the patient is first seen, since persistent marked eosinophilia may be seen in various disorders, such as Löffler's endocarditis, polyarteritis nodosa, disseminated collagen disease, and parasitic invasion such as that which occurs in trichinosis and visceral larva migrans, and perhaps as a response to nonspecific antigenic stimulation (423–427).

The diagnosis of eosinophilic leukemia is made by excluding other causes of persistent eosinophilia and by following the course of the disease. The clinical course most commonly is measured in months before death (426). Most of the signs and symptoms of patients with eosinophilic leukemia are similar to those found in other forms of leukemia. However, involvement of the heart, lung, central nervous system, and skin is more common than in other forms. Intractable congestive heart failure is commonly present and may not be related to the anemia. In addition to tachycardia, a gallop rhythm, systolic and diastolic murmurs, and a friction rub may be heard, and there may be peripheral edema and ascites. Heart failure is the most common terminal complication (428). Endocardial fibrosis, eosinophilic infiltrates in the myocardium, and areas of scarring and necrosis, as well as mural and small arterial thrombi have been found at autopsy (423, 424, 426, 428).

Pulmonary manifestations, such as transient, bilateral, reticular densities and persistent infiltrates, have been found frequently in these patients. At autopsy, eosinophilic infiltration is present with or without bacterial or viral pneumonia as a superimposed complication (426).

The central nervous system manifestations have ranged from simple drowsiness to coma, convulsions, delirium, or hemiplegia. The skin manifestations may vary from small subcutaneous tumors to dermatitis herpetiformis and serpiginous and maculopapular eruptions, which are all involved by eosinophilic infiltrates (426).

With rare exception, patients with eosinophilic leukemia present with leukocytosis, over 60 per cent of the granulocytes being eosinophils (426). Ackerman has described morphologic abnormalities of the eosinophils which may be helpful. These changes include asynchronous nuclear cytoplasmic maturation, an increase in cell size, and variation in size, shape, and number of eosinophilic granules (429). However, similar atypical eosinophils may be present in patients with visceral larva migrans. Anemia and thrombocytopenia are found in the majority of patients. However, there has been one case of eosinophilic leukemia which presented with erythrocytosis (430). Leukocyte alkaline phosphatase staining has been normal in the few patients studied (426), and one patient had a large acrocentric chromosome and another a Ph^1 chromosome (431, 432). Most patients who have died with so-called eosinophilic leukemia have not had terminal myeloblastic transformation (426).

The main nonmalignant disorders that may simulate eosinophilic leukemia, along with differential points to help separate each entity, are shown in Table 22–5 (426, 433). Children with parasitic infestation frequently have a history of pica or have a

TABLE 22–5. COMPARISON OF FEATURES OF EOSINOPHILIC LEUKEMIA WITH LÖFFLER'S ENDOCARDITIS, POLYARTERITIS NODOSA, DISSEMINATED EOSINOPHILIC COLLAGEN DISEASE, AND VISCERAL LARVA MIGRANS

FEATURE	EOSINOPHILIC LEUKEMIA	LÖFFLER'S ENDOCARDITIS	POLYARTERITIS NODOSA	DISSEMINATED EOSINOPHILIC COLLAGEN DISEASE	VISCERAL LARVA MIGRANS
Age	Any age	Any age	20–50 years	Any age	1–3 years
Sex, male:female	3:1	3:1	3:1	Only male	1:1
Cardiac failure	++	+++			
Respiratory distress	+	+	+	+	+
CNS manifestations	+	+	+		
Hepatosplenomegaly	+++	++	+	+	+
Eosinophilia	+++	++	+	+	+++
Immature granulocytes	+++			+	
Blast forms	+			+?	
Normoblasts	+				
Anemia	+++		+	+	Iron deficiency
Thrombocytopenia	++			+	
Eosinophilic infiltrates:					
Mature	++	++	+	+	+
Immature	++				
Mural thrombi	++	+++		+	
Arteriolar thrombosis	++	++			
Vasculitis		++	+++		++
Prognosis	Fatal	Often fatal	Occasionally fatal	Often fatal	Recovery if removed from source of parasites

*Modified from Benvenisti, D. S., and Ultmann, J. E.: Ann. Intern. Med. Med. 71:731, 1969.

pet at home, in addition to the findings in the table listed for visceral larva migrans. They also have hyperglobulinemia, increased isohemagglutinin titers, an anti–gamma globulin factor, and a positive serologic test for *Ascaris* and *Toxocara canis* or *catis* (433–435).

As seen in the table, blast forms and normoblasts are characteristically present, and anemia and thrombocytopenia are more common in eosinophilic leukemia than they are in Löffler's endocarditis, polyarteritis nodosa, disseminated eosinophilic collagen disease, or visceral larva migrans. In addition, vasculitis is not found in eosinophilic leukemia.

Occasionally persistent marked eosinophilia is found in an asymptomatic child in whom the known causes of eosinophilia are excluded. An example of such a case was recently reported by Rickles and Miller (423). These authors postulated that profound eosinophilia, even with myeloid immaturity, may represent a leukemoid response to nonspecific antigenic stimulation rather than a true form of leukemia (423).

Unless from the history, physical examination, and serologic tests a diagnosis of visceral larva migrans is evident, the following tests should be done in all children with persistent marked eosinophilia: stool for ova and parasites, bone marrow examination with direct chromosomal analysis of bone marrow cells, determination of quantity of fetal hemoglobin, leukocyte alkaline phosphatase, quantitation of immunoglobulins, antinuclear antibody, latex fixation, and a liver biopsy in order to demonstrate tissue infiltration by immature cells of predominantly eosinophilic type. By doing such studies, it may become possible to definitely conclude whether or not eosinophilic leukemia is a distinct entity.

Therapy for this form of leukemia is unknown. Perhaps cytosine arabinoside or daunorubicin or both should be tried in patients in whom a diagnosis of eosinophilic leukemia is established if myeloblasts are prominent. If myeloblasts are few in number, particularly if a Ph[1] chromosome is present, busulfan should be tried.

BASOPHILIC LEUKEMIA

The existence of basophilic leukemia has been questioned, since basophilia is frequently seen in chronic myelocytic leukemia, and since in at least two patients in whom chromosomal analyses were done a Ph[1] chromosome was found (436). Several patients who initially were thought to have basophilic leukemia died with erythroleukemia (437). In order to separate basophilic leukemia from other forms, an excessive number of basophils and myeloblasts must be present in the blood and bone marrow (438, 439). The leukocyte alkaline phosphatase staining of granules may be low, normal, or high (439).

Basophilic leukemia has been reported in only one child (440). It may be confused with systemic mast cell disease (439). The symptoms of systemic mast cell disease, such as flushing, urticaria, nausea, vomiting, diarrhea, palpitation, and peptic ulceration, have not been described in patients with basophilic leukemia (441). In addition, basophils and mast cells, although similar morphologically, can be distinguished by the light microscope. Mast cells are larger, the granules are smaller, more uniform, and usually do not cover the nucleus. The nucleus is usually small, oval, or round and eccentrically placed, whereas the nucleus of the basophil frequently is lobulated (439).

The clinical course of basophilic leukemia may be rapid, as in acute leukemia, or more protracted, as in chronic leukemia. The drug of choice for treatment of this form of leukemia is unknown. Clinical improvement has been reported after irradiation of the spleen and after use of busulfan (439).

MONOCYTIC LEUKEMIA

Leukemia which is characterized by monocytes and monocytic precursors in the blood and bone marrow may be divided into an acute form and a chronic form. In the acute form monoblasts, promonocytes, and monocytes, are the predominant cells in the blood, bone marrow, or both (442–444). The distinguishing features in addition to the usual findings of acute leukemia are gum hypertrophy, fever, stomatitis, and hemorrhages (443–444). Ulceronecrotic lesions of the perirectal area also are seen more often than in other forms of leukemia (445, 446). Usually the serum muramidase level is increased, and large quantities of this enzyme are excreted in the urine (447, 448). Often hypokalemia is present, and a combined glomerular-tubular dysfunction has been found in some patients (449, 450). Acute monoblastic leukemia (Schilling type, in which monocytic and histiocytic cells predominate, as opposed to the Naegeli type, which is myelomonoblastic in type) is uncommon in children (451). Patients with acute monoblastic leukemia typically have a short unremitting course and are resistant to therapy (451). Cytosine arabinoside or daunomycin or both should be used in an attempt to induce a remission.

Chronic monocytic leukemia is very rare in children but may be suspected in a patient with persistent monocytosis. Known causes of monocytosis, such as tuberculosis, brucellosis, lymphomas, and connective tissue diseases, must be excluded (452, 453). A progressive normocytic, normochromic anemia and/or neutropenia and/or thrombocytopenia are frequently present. Minimal to moderate hepatosplenomegaly and lymphadenopathy may be found (446, 453). There may be aneuploidy of the chromosomes (454). In spite of these clinical and laboratory findings, a diagnosis of chronic monocytic leukemia cannot be made until there is a preponderance of abnormal blasts in the blood or bone marrow or both. Thus the diagnosis of chronic monocytic leukemia is made retrospectively. The abnormal blasts may be monoblasts only, or both monoblasts and myeloblasts. A small number of abnormal blasts may be present for weeks or months before they become the predominant cells. One adult has been described as having had monocytosis for 11 years and another for 9 years before the development of acute leukemia (453, 455).

Treatment of chronic monocytic leukemia should be symptomatic and supportive until the acute form develops. Cytosine arabinoside and daunomycin are the drugs of choice for treatment of the acute stage.

ACUTE PROMYELOCYTIC LEUKEMIA

Acute promyelocytic leukemia is a subclass of acute myeloblastic leukemia, which is characterized by preponderance of promyelocytes filled with azurophilic granules in the blood and bone marrow (456–460).

Except for severe bleeding manifestations that cannot be corrected by giving platelets, other clinical findings are similar to those found in patients with acute myeloblastic leukemia.

Recently Rachmilewitz and co-workers reported high serum vitamin B_{12} levels in five patients with this form of leukemia. In three patients an increased serum vitamin B_{12} binding capacity was observed (461). It has been postulated that the promyelocytes are responsible for the increased serum vitamin B_{12} concentrations, since Simons and Weber (462) and Corcino et al. (463) have shown that vitamin B_{12}–binding proteins appear to be synthesized by granulocytes.

Most commonly the coagulation abnormalities consist of prolonged prothrombin and partial thromboplastin times, thrombocytopenia, fibrinogenopenia, and low levels of Factor V. Decreased levels of plasminogen and Factors VII to X, a shortened euglobulin lysis time, and fibrinogen degradation products in serum have also been reported (456, 458–460, 464, 465). The pathogenesis of the coagulation abnormalities has been attributed to decreased synthesis of fibrinogen and Factor V by the liver, fibrinolysis, or disseminated intravascular coagulation. Decreased production seems very unlikely, since Factor VIII may also be found to be decreased, and liver function tests are usually normal. From reports of results of studies in the literature, it is not clear whether or not the abnormal coagulation studies seen in patients with acute promyelocytic leukemia are secondary to disseminated intravascular coagulation or primary fibrinolysis (459, 464). One reason for the inability to solve this problem is that the treatment with heparin has resulted in variable response. Some authors have found a significant decrease in bleeding manifestations and diminution of the coagulation abnormalities with heparin therapy (459, 460). Other authors have reported only minimal response to heparin (465). In like manner, variable responses have been reported after giving epsilon aminocaproic acid, an inhibitor of fibrinolysis (466, 467). Although this problem is not resolved, there is in vitro evidence that there is a marked increase in thromboplastic activity in promyelocytes over the amount found in normal leukocytes and in myeloblasts from patients with acute myeloblastic leukemia (468). Gralnick and associates have postulated that disseminated intravascular coagulation is initiated by a procoagulant that is released from pro-myelocytes, and that the procoagulant is related to the turnover and destruction of promyelocytes (460). This hypothesis is also suggested by the fact that coagulation ab-normalities disappear after the leukemic mass is decreased and the patient enters remission (464).

Recently, Tan, Wages, and Gralnick have reported a correlation between light and electron microscopic findings of acute pro-myelocytic leukemic cells and response to chemotherapy and heparin therapy (460). By light microscopy they divided the gran-ules seen in acute promyelocytic leukemic cells into three sizes—small, medium, and large. The patients who had the larger gran-ules frequently had granules in the intracel-lular marrow space. These patients re-sponded less well to heparin and to chemotherapy. By electron microscopy spherical, rod, and splinter forms of gran-ules were present. The granules were lyso-somes, and their ultrastructural features were similar to Auer bodies. The promyelo-cytes in the cases responsive to heparin were usually uniform in size, and splinter-shaped lysosomes were not frequently found. In two patients with long-term re-mission (12 and 10 months), it was difficult to distinguish malignant promyelocytes from drug-affected promyelocytes during remission. The promyelocytes present in remission contained fewer azurophilic gran-ules than did the promyelocytes before che-motherapy.

Further studies are necessary to under-stand the abnormal coagulation in patients with acute promyelocytic leukemia before successful therapy can be given to control or stop the bleeding complications. The che-motherapeutic agents of choice are the same as those used in the treatment of acute myeloblastic leukemia.

ERYTHROLEUKEMIA

Erythroleukemia is a variant of acute myeloblastic leukemia in which there is ab-normal proliferation of erythroid precursors as well as myeloid precursors (469). This type of leukemia accounts for only about 2 per cent of all forms of leukemia in children (470).

The natural course of the disease appears to involve three stages: (1) predominantly erythroblastic proliferation in the marrow, (2) mixed erythroblastic-myeloblastic prolif-eration (stage called "erythroleukemia"), and (3) predominantly myeloblastic prolif-eration. Some authors use the term "di Gug-lielmo's disease" or "erythremic myelosis" to describe the first phase (469).

The presenting signs and symptoms of erythroleukemia, which is the most com-mon stage in children, vary little from typi-cal acute leukemia. However, there may be a longer antecedent course of nonspecific symptoms of malaise, weight loss, and unex-plained fever. Usually the presenting symp-toms are related to anemia. However, some patients present with infection, and a smaller number present with easy bruising or petechiae. On physical examination, the prominent features include pallor, spleno-megaly, petechiae, and purpura. The splen-omegaly may be massive. Hepatomegaly is also usually present, but is less striking. Fever may be present with or without obvi-ous cause (471).

The laboratory findings vary with the stage of the disease. Early, the only blood findings may be anemia, leukopenia, and thrombocytopenia. A helpful diagnostic fea-ture, if present, is the finding of a dispropor-tionate number of nucleated red blood cells for the minimal reticulocytosis. The anemia may be macrocytic, and the nucleated red cells are megaloblastic. There is striking anisocytosis and poikilocytosis. Giant eosin-ophilic granules have been reported in one patient, and ring-shaped granulocytes have been reported in another patient (472, 473).

As the disease progresses, blast cells re-sembling myeloblasts, myelomonoblasts, or monoblasts are seen, and the white count may become elevated. Auer rods may be seen in the nonerythroid blasts. Early, the bone marrow may be cellular, with all cell types present. Megakaryocytes are few, even early in the disease, and disappear as progression occurs (469). As in the blood, the characteristic cell is the morphologi-cally abnormal erythroid precursor. The cells are present in all stages of maturation. The nuclear chromatin is open and poorly organized. A resemblance to megaloblastic erythroid cells can be seen. The nuclei may have budding, and two or three nuclei per cell may be seen. Sometimes the nucleus may resemble a cloverleaf. The cytoplasm of the red cell precursors may stain with PAS (474). The alkaline phosphatase stain may be decreased in the circulating neutrophils (474).

With progression of the disease, more and more immature myeloid precursors are present in the marrow. The patient may die while both abnormal red and white precursors are abundant in the marrow, or the disease may progress to a predominance of myeloid precursors in the marrow prior to death. As in other forms of leukemia, death is usually secondary to infection or to bleeding.

Immunologic aberrations may be seen in about one-third of patients with erythroleukemia. The abnormalities reported include hypergammaglobulinemia, an increased tendency to form rheumatoid factor, LE factor, positive serologic tests for syphilis, and erythrocyte autoantibodies and isoantibodies. The significance of the immunologic aberrations is unclear (475).

The quantity of fetal hemoglobin usually is normal but may be increased, and occasionally Hb H has been found (476, 477). A_2 hemoglobin has been reported to be decreased (478). Red cell enzyme studies have been done in a few patients with erythroleukemia. Two red cell populations have been suggested on the basis of the results of the red cell enzyme pattern (479, 480). The levels of G6PD, hexokinase, and 6-phosphogluconate dehydrogenase were increased, but the levels of phosphohexose isomerase, phosphofructokinase, pyruvate kinase, and glutathione reductase were either subnormal or lower than would be expected for the degree of reticulocytosis. In one of these patients studied, 50 per cent of the red blood cells were nonagglutinable by anti-A and anti-A_1 sera. The patient's blood group before the disease was discovered was A_1. Two populations of red cells thus were separated by anti-A serum. The abnormal enzyme pattern was seen in the abnormal red cell population (479).

Patients with erythroleukemia have hyperferremia, an increased number of sideroblasts and ringed sideroblasts (iron in mitochondria of sideroblasts), and unusually rapid iron clearance but slow incorporation of iron into nonnucleated red cells. Thus these patients have ineffective erythropoiesis (483). A defect in heme synthesis and, in some patients, in globin synthesis has been demonstrated in vitro on bone marrow suspensions (484, 485). Also, ^{51}Cr survival time of the red cells may be decreased. The level of plasma erythropoietin is increased (486–488).

Correction of the anemia by transfusion of red cells results in a decrease in red cell precursors in the blood and bone marrow, a decrease in plasma iron turnover, and a decrease in serum erythropoietin (488, 489). Thus, the red cell precursors in this disease are not autonomous, but respond to changes in the concentration of erythropoietin of plasma (486–489). This lack of autonomy has been interpreted by Schwartz and coworkers to suggest that the red cell precursors are not neoplastic (489). However, the abnormal morphology of the red cell precursors, an increase in fetal hemoglobin, the presence of Hb H in some patients, various enzyme changes in the red cells, and chromosomal abnormalities in the red cell precursors as well as in the myeloblasts suggest that the red cell precursors in erythroleukemia are abnormal.

Erythroleukemia has developed in patients with polycythemia vera and in a patient with paroxysmal nocturnal hemoglobinuria (490, 491). Both paroxysmal nocturnal hemoglobinuria and polycythemia vera are acquired abnormalities of red cells, and in both there is an increased incidence of acute myeloblastic leukemia. Therefore, an association with erythroleukemia is a logical link in the progression of the disease to acute myeloblastic leukemia.

Various chromosomal abnormalities have been found in the marrow in about one-half of patients with erythroleukemia. Aberrations have been of three types — aneuploidy, increased polyploidy, and chromosomal breakage. Hypoploidy appears to be the most frequent abnormality found (481). Clonal evolution has been described in one patient with di Guglielmo's syndrome who initially had an extra ?A chromosome (482). Initially in this patient an extra ?A group chromosome was seen in most metaphases. One month prior to death there were three distinct abnormal cell lines, but trisomy of an ?A group was present in all three cell lines. This patient was followed with chromosome analyses throughout all phases of the di Guglielmo syndrome (erythremic myelosis, erythroleukemia, and acute myeloblastic leukemia). During the first stage of the disease, when the patient had a severe anemia but myeloblastic proliferation was not present, an extra ?A group chromosome was seen in most metaphases. One month before the patient's death, there were three distinct abnormal cell lines, but there was persistence of trisomy of ?A chromosome in each cell line. Since the trisomy of ?A group was present in all three lines, a clonal evolution from a common stem cell containing this extra chromosome was postulated.

The morphologic aberration in the red cell precursors is similar to that in patients with megaloblastic anemia secondary to a vitamin B_{12} or folic acid deficiency. However, the serum vitamin B_{12} level is usually either normal or increased, and the clearance of injected folic acid from the serum is normal, thus excluding a folic acid deficiency (492). As expected, the anemia in patients with erythroleukemia does not respond to administration of either vitamin B_{12} or folic acid, or to a combination of these vitamins (492). In addition, white cell changes, such as hypersegmented neutrophils and giant metamyelocytes, are not commonly seen. The morphologic aberration that is seen in patients with B_{12} or folic acid deficiency is secondary to decreased rate of DNA synthesis (493, 494). A disturbance in DNA synthesis has also been reported in two patients with erythremic myelosis (495). Therefore, a defect in DNA synthesis has been suggested to result in the morphologic aberration seen in the red cell precursors in patients with erythroleukemia. The cause of the disturbance in DNA synthesis is unknown.

Presently, therapy of acute erythroleukemia is very disappointing, but better results may be expected with the use of cytosine arabinoside or daunorubicin or both.

CONGENITAL LEUKEMIA

Congenital leukemia is a rare disease which is clinically evident at birth or apparent within the first few weeks of life (496, 497). The usual form of the disease is a poorly differentiated acute myeloblastic leukemia (496, 498), but undifferentiated stem cell (499), erythroleukemia (500), acute lymphoblastic leukemia (501), and

acute histiocytic leukemia (502) also have been reported. Congenital acute myeloblastic leukemia is more common in infants with Down's syndrome than in the general population of infants (93, 503, 504).

The clinical picture of leukemia in the neonate is different from that seen in older children. When the disease is evident at birth, purpura and hepatosplenomegaly are almost invariably present. The infant may be pale, and in about one-half the reported cases nodular skin infiltrates were present. Icterus is uncommon. Usually there is marked leukocytosis, and myeloblasts and promyelocytes are seen on the blood smear. Anemia, if present at birth, is usually not marked but develops during the neonatal period. Platelets usually are reduced in number. The bone marrow is hypercellular with a preponderance of early myeloid forms.

The disease may not be apparent at birth, but signs and symptoms of leukemia develop in the first few days or weeks thereafter. Before definitive indications of leukemia, there may be an antecedent period of failure to gain weight, diarrhea, or low-grade fever. Purpura or infiltrative skin nodules may be the first clinical indications of a blood dyscrasia (506). Hepatomegaly is most often found, but splenomegaly is not a necessary component of the physical findings.

The blood findings are anemia, leukocytosis, and thrombocytopenia. Again the characteristic leukemic cells are the myeloblast and promyelocyte. The bone marrow is hyperplastic and consists primarily of immature myeloid cells.

The etiology of congenital leukemia is just as obscure as that of other types of leukemia. An intrauterine factor seems to inhibit the leukemic process in the fetus, since the symptoms are slight immediately after birth but progress rapidly afterwards (504, 507).

The differential diagnoses include leukemoid reactions secondary to hemolytic disease of the newborn, myeloid metaplasia, congenital syphilis, intrauterine viral disease, other severe infections, and folic acid deficiency (496, 497, 508–510, 512).

Spontaneous and permanent remissions may occur in infants with congenital leukemia and Down's syndrome (504, 505, 507, 511). The course of the disease in infants

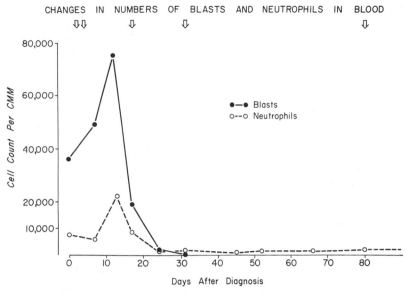

CHANGES IN NUMBERS OF BLASTS AND NEUTROPHILS IN BLOOD

Figure 22–3. Laboratory findings in an infant with mongolism and transient ineffective granulopoiesis mimicking congenital myeloblastic leukemia. Arrows indicate bone marrow examinations, days 6, 8, 21, 35, and 84.

who do not have Down's syndrome is most often short, and is characterized by hemorrhage and infection. Most of these patients die within the first few days or weeks of their illness (496). However, transient spontaneous remissions have been reported in at least two infants who did not have Down's syndrome (497, 513). The incidence of permanent remissions in patients with Down's syndrome is not known, and the child with Down's syndrome may die with unremitting signs of leukemia and at autopsy have the expected infiltration with leukemic blood cells.

Spontaneous and permanent remissions in infants with congenital leukemia and Down's syndrome are not understood. Also, it is not known why Down's syndrome predisposes to leukemia and at the same time the prognosis of congenital leukemia is improved. In most patients in whom spontaneous remissions have been reported, the leukemic cells have disappeared from the blood and marrow by 4 months of age (504). For this reason, a passively transferred stimulatory substance from the mother has been suggested as a cause for congenital leukemia in patients who have spontaneous and permanent remissions (504). Recently, Killman has postulated that leukemia in these infants may have arisen in a clone of stem cells which had a limited proliferative

potential. Thus far, there are no studies to support or confirm either possibility (514). It has also been suggested that these patients do not have leukemia but instead have transient ineffective regulation of granulopoiesis (510, 511). The results of kinetic and electron microscopic studies on serial blood and bone marrow samples from a male infant with congenital leukemia and Down's syndrome seen at Children's Hospital Medical Center suggested this possibility (507). This infant at 4 days of age had 36,500 myeloblasts per mm.^{3} in his blood and less than 15 per cent myeloblasts in his marrow. The clinical and laboratory data over a ten-week period are shown in Figure 22–3. A spontaneous remission was evident by 2 months of age and presently, five and one-half years later, the child is in remission.

Further studies are necessary to define the nature of the abnormal myelopoiesis which may be seen in infants with Down's syndrome.

There appears to be no question that infants with congenital leukemia but not Down's syndrome should be treated with chemotherapy. The chemotherapy used should be the same as in the older child. However, it is questionable whether or not the child with Down's syndrome and a clinical and hematologic picture like congenital leukemia should initially be started on chemotherapy. Certainly if marked hematologic or clinical deterioration occurs, chemotherapy should be started.

RETICULOENDOTHELIOSIS

General Description

The reticuloendothelial system is comprised of a diffuse anatomic network with a wide spectrum of physiologic activity, both phagocytic and metabolic. Fixed and wandering macrophages or histiocytes and their presumed progenitor, the monocyte, are the principal cells involved in this complex system (515, 516). The reticuloendothelial system may be involved in a number of pathologic processes, which Dargeon (517) has divided into the lipid storage diseases, infectious granulomas, and reticuloendotheliosis.

Reticuloendotheliosis is the name given to a group of diseases of unknown etiology whose clinical manifestations are legion, whose outcome is variable, but whose histologic appearance shares the common denominator of histiocytic proliferation or reticuloendothelial hyperplasia (505). It may involve any organ with a reticuloendothelial component. Microscopically the lesions of reticuloendotheliosis are characterized by focal aggregates of large, pale-staining histiocytes or large mononuclear cells in association with eosinophils, lymphocytes, plasma cells, giant cells, and occasionally polymorphonuclear leukocytes. In localized forms of the disease or in relatively new lesions in disease of long standing, the prominent adventitial cell is the eosinophil. In the chronic forms of the disease, there may be accumulation of lipids within the cytoplasm of histiocytes, giving them a foamy appearance (518).

Though primarily a disease of infants and young children, congenital and adult cases have been described (519–525). The disease is more common in males, with a ratio of approximately 3:2 (525, 526), and the majority of cases occur in Caucasians.

Classification

Before presenting the classification of the reticuloendothelioses, it is important to review briefly the history of this fascinating and controversial group of diseases. Although the reticuloendotheliosis marquee is studded with names, those of Smith (527) and Kay (528) who made early observations of the disease are not included in the eponymic litany in use today. Hand (529) in 1921 published a paper dealing with defects of membranous bones, exophthalmos, and polyuria in childhood, in which he made reference to two cases previously described by himself (530), as well as to those of Kay (528), Christian (531), and Schüller (532), all of which dealt with a similar clinical syndrome.

Letterer in 1924 (533) and Siwe in 1933 (534) described patients with widespread disease, including fever, lymphadenopathy, hepatosplenomegaly, and purpura. Letterer's patient had, in addition, purulent otitis media, while Siwe's patient had a destructive lesion of the fibula. Pathologically both revealed reticuloendothelial hyperplasia. Abt and Denenholz in 1936 (535) observed a similar case and proposed the term "Letterer-Siwe disease" to describe the entity. Wallgren in 1940 (536) described two cases with disseminated disease and proposed that Letterer-Siwe and Hand-Schüller-Christian diseases were both manifestations of a similar pathologic entity.

The lesion now known as eosinophilic granuloma of bone was described by Lichtenstein and Jaffe (537) and by Otani and Ehrlich in 1936 (538). In 1942 Green and Farber (539) and subsequently Jaffe and Lichtenstein (540) concluded that this lesion was part of the same basic disease process as Hand-Schüller-Christian and Letterer-Siwe diseases. Lichtenstein (541) in 1953 proposed the term "histiocytosis X" to integrate the three conditions as related manifestations of a single nosologic entity. Although the unitarian theory has been disputed by some authors (542–544), it forms at the present a workable background for this group of diseases.

Eosinophilic granuloma of bone is the most localized and benign form of the disease complex. There is no involvement of skin, viscera, or soft tissues. It is more common in older children and young adults (525, 545).

The lesion is usually unifocal, but multiple lesions may be present. Any bone may be involved, but skull lesions are seen most

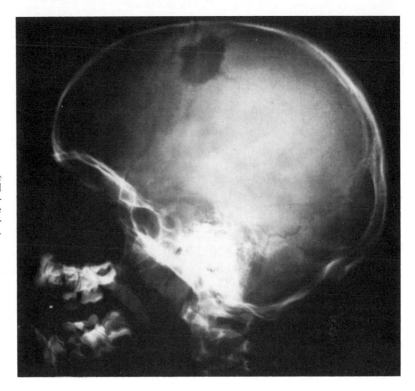

Figure 22–4. Characteristic punched-out lesions in the skull of a patient with reticuloendotheliosis. Both tables of bone are involved, and no marginal sclerosis or periosteal reaction is seen.

commonly (545–547). Of the long bones, the femur is most often affected (546).

The roentgenographic appearance is that of localized rarefaction in the involved bone. Skull lesions have a characteristic punched-out appearance and involve both tables of the bone (Fig. 22–4), without evidence of marginal sclerosis or periosteal reaction. In vertebral body lesions there are loss of height and development of vertebra plana, with the affected vertebra appearing much more dense than its neighbors. Long bone lesions usually affect the diaphysis, beginning in the medullary cavity. The cortex may be eroded, and periosteal new bone formation may be seen simulating malignant tumor of bone (546, 548).

Hand-Schüller-Christian disease has been referred to as the disseminated form of reticuloendotheliosis (517). It occupies an intermediate position in the spectrum of clinical severity and tends to run a chronic course. The age at onset is usually 1 to 3 years, but it may occur in older children and adults (525, 545). Skeletal lesions, again with a predilection for the skull, are found, but in addition visceral or soft tissue lesions are present, especially involving skin, lungs, and ear. The time-honored notion that a triad of exophthalmos, diabetes in-

sipidus, and skeletal lesions characterizes the disorder is erroneous, and the simultaneous occurrence of these findings is rare (525, 545, 547, 549).

Letterer-Siwe disease is predominantly a disease of infancy; it frequently runs a fulminant course, and has been referred to as the malignant form of reticuloendotheliosis (517). At the onset, lesions are confined to skin, soft tissues, and viscera, but skeletal involvement may occur as the disease progresses. Letterer-Siwe disease has been described in both live-born (519, 550) and stillborn infants (521), in siblings (551, 552), and in monozygous twins (553, 554).

In compiling this traditional classification, it must be remembered that it is, at best, tenuous, and that transitional forms may occur in which solitary eosinophilic granuloma of bone may progress to a clinical picture of Hand-Schüller-Christian disease with multiple skeletal lesions and diabetes insipidus.

Etiology

The etiology of reticuloendotheliosis remains obscure. Infectious agents—viral, bacterial and fungal—have been assiduously investigated as possible etiologies, but none has fulfilled Koch's postulates. Case reports (555) of positive cultures from bone or soft tissue lesions may be found in the literature, in addition to a number of reports of the salubrious effect of antibiotics in reticuloendotheliosis (554, 556, 557).

The electron microscopic finding of rod-like structures in the cytoplasm of histiocytes from biopsy material of patients with reticuloendotheliosis has stirred a wave of controversy regarding their significance. Basset et al. have suggested that they are viral in origin (558) and noted their resemblance to cytoplasmic particles seen in association with rabies, Yaba monkey virus, and Shope virus (559). Cancilla et al. (560) and Gianotti et al. (561) reject the viral theory, however, as these same rodlike structures can be found in the Langerhans' cells of normal epidermis. While the presence of these structures in all types of reticuloendotheliosis lends support to the unitarian theory of the disease, their exact function in its pathogenesis remains uncertain.

Other proposed etiologies have included abnormalities of cholesterol metabolism, allergic reaction, neoplasia, and genetic factors. In regard to the latter, Juberg et al. (553) reviewed the literature on Letterer-Siwe disease in twins, sibships, and offspring of consanguineous marriages and concluded that at least some instances of the disease may result from a single autosomal recessive gene with slightly reduced penetrance. Support for this theory has recently come from Freundlich et al. (552), reporting on four infant sibs from two consanguineous families.

Clinical Features

The clinical manifestations of reticuloendotheliosis are myriad. The presenting signs in 68 patients with the Hand-Schüller-Christian variant are listed in Table 22–6.

Skeletal lesions most frequently involve the skull and may be accompanied by soft tissue swelling. Limping, pain, or pathologic fracture may call attention to a lesion in one of the long bones, most commonly the femur. Neurologic deficit or torticollis may point to a lesion of the cervical spine (562). Lesions of the mastoid or petrous portions of the temporal bone with extension into the middle ear are usually associated with a refractory chronic otitis media, and after skeletal lesions, otitis was the most frequently observed manifestation of the disease. Exophthalmos, with or without associated visual disturbances, may be unilateral or bilateral and is almost always associated with destructive orbital lesions. The signs of diabetes insipidus may develop insidiously, may be the presenting complaint, or may develop later in the course of the disease (545). The diabetes insipidus may be complete, or the deficiency in antidiuretic hormone formation may be only partial (563). Other manifestations of hypothalamic dysfunction include growth retardation and delayed puberty (515). Braunstein et al. (563) have recently reported detailed studies of pituitary function in Hand-Schüller-Christian disease. Complete growth hormone deficiency or a blunted growth hormone response to provocative stimuli was found in seven of eight short children with the disease and in three patients with post-

TABLE 22–6.   INITIAL MANIFESTATIONS OF HAND-SCHÜLLER-CHRISTIAN DISEASE

	Avioli et al. (549)	Avery et al. (525)	Oberman (545)	Lucaya (547)	Total
Age	1–12 years	6 months–40 years	2weeks–16 years	0–51 months	
Total patients	10	29	17	12	68
Bone lesions	9	27	17	12	65
Otitis	4	6	11	8	29
Dermatitis	6	3	8	6	23
Hepatomegaly	7	4	4	5	20
Lymphadenopathy	5	2	7	5	19
Anemia	6	1	4	7	18
Diabetes insipidus	5	3	5	2	15
Splenomegaly	4	3	1	4	12
Exophthalmos	3	5	1	2	11
Triad	2	3	1	1	7

pubertal onset. Assessment of gonadotropin function, pituitary-thyroid axis and pituitary-adrenal axis was within normal limits in the patients evaluated in this series. Panhypopituitarism has been reported (564), however, but is considered rare.

Central nervous system manifestations include seizures (547, 565), papilledema with increased intracranial pressure and communicating hydrocephalus (566), mental retardation (547), and cerebellar ataxia (567). The rash characteristically involves the scalp, face, and trunk, but may be generalized. It may be scaly and resemble seborrheic dermatitis. It may also be purpuric or maculopapular with ulceration and hemorrhage. Lymphadenopathy and hepatosplenomegaly are most common in the Letterer-Siwe variant, but may also occur in Hand-Schüller-Christian disease. Jaundice and ascites are rare complications.

Pulmonary involvement in reticuloendotheliosis may vary from isolated eosinophilic granuloma (568, 569) with a benign clinical course to diffuse infiltration with a fulminant course. It occurs in some 20 per cent of patients with generalized disease and may precede the appearance of other lesions by a matter of up to eight years (570). The radiographic appearance may be that of diffuse cystic change, punctate nodular infiltrations, or extensive fibrosis (571). While some patients with pulmonary involvement are asymptomatic, complications are common, with spontaneous pneumothorax developing in 20 to 50 per cent (570). With severe involvement, there may be chronic respiratory failure with pulmonary fibrosis, emphysema, and eventual cor pulmonale.

Involvement of the oral cavity is manifest by gingival ulcerations and loosening or exfoliation of teeth secondary to mandibular lesions. Infiltration of such organs as the gastrointestinal tract (545, 572), kidney (573), and bladder (574) may give rise to specific findings related to their function, but these instances are rare. Anemia may occur as a result of blood loss from thrombocytopenia or secondary to enlargement of the spleen with trapping of red cells. Bone marrow infiltration with immature histiocytes occurs in about 10 per cent of cases (575). Finally, systemic manifestations, such as fever, poor appetite, malaise, and pallor, are commonly seen.

Treatment

Solitary eosinophilic granuloma of bone may be successfully treated by curettage, radiation, or a combination of the two (546). Ochsner (548) found 500 to 1500 R. to be particularly useful in managing mandibular, vertebral, or pelvic lesions.

Local radiation therapy to so-called "hazardous sites" (517) may be used in widespread disease, but chemotherapy is the treatment of choice. Steroids, antimetabolites, and aklylating agents have been used alone or in combination. In a disease with such great variability, results are difficult to assess, but there is no question that treatment is effective and improves overall survival (526). Beier et al. in 1963 (576) were the first to report the successful treatment of Letterer-Siwe disease with vinblastine sulfate. Since then a number of reports on the use of this drug have appeared in the literature (524, 547, 577–580), and results are encouraging. The initial dose is 0.1 mg. per kg., and this should be increased at weekly intervals to a total of 0.4 mg. per kg. Steroids may be added in the severely ill child and may rapidly reduce the systemic toxicity of the disease (575).

A recent cooperative study (581) comparing vincristine, vinblastine, and cyclophosphamide gave similar results for all drugs, but the authors concluded that the small patient number and study design precluded any meaningful conclusions regarding relative efficacy. Studies are in progress using combination chemotherapy, but the rarity of the disease and its unpredictable course will continue to plague investigators trying to extract meaningful data on its optimal therapy.

Prognosis

Prognosis in reticuloendotheliosis is dependent on three principal factors: age at onset, extent of the disease, and localization of the disease (526). The worst prognosis is for infants under the age of 6 months, with a 70 per cent mortality reported by Lahey in his collected series of 69 patients (526), Only 20 per cent of the patients, however, were in this age group. Under the age of 3 years, the mortality rate was approximately

50 per cent in Lahey's series, while a 34 per cent mortality was reported by Lucaya (547) in children between 2 months and 3 years. No deaths in children with onset of disease over the age of 3 were reported by Lahey (526), Lucaya (547), Oberman (545), or Avery (525), but fatalities, though rare, may occur (549, 582) in the older child.

The extent of the disease may be assessed by a scoring system for the number of organ systems involved, as proposed by Lahey (526) and modified by Lucaya (547). One point is assigned for involvement of each of the following: skeleton, skin, lung, liver, spleen, pituitary, hemopoietic system, ears, and lymph nodes. Both Lahey and Lucaya have employed the scoring system in evaluating 91 patients. In these two series, mortality was 0 to 5 per cent with scores of 2 or less, 14 to 34 per cent with a score of 3 to 4, 57 to 75 per cent with a score of 5 to 6, and 100 per cent with a score of 7 or above.

Although this system allows for an intelligent evaluation of prognosis, one must still take into account which systems contribute to the score. Hepatosplenomegaly, especially in the presence of hepatic dysfunction, pulmonary lesions, and involvement of the hemopoietic system are frequently associated with severe disease and suggest a poor prognosis. Skeletal or pituitary lesions, on the other hand, are associated with a favorable outcome, even though the diabetes insipidus is permanent.

LYMPHOHISTIOCYTOSIS

Lymphohistiocytosis (familial hemophagocytic reticulosis, histiocytic medullary reticulosis) is an uncommon, familial, progressively fatal disease of infants and young children of both sexes that is pathologically different from reticuloendotheliosis and histiocytic leukemia.

In 1939 Scott and Robb-Smith (583) described four patients with an illness characterized by fever, anemia, leukopenia, hepatosplenomegaly, and lymphadenopathy. The pathologic features were unique in that, in addition to widespread histiocytic infiltration, may of the histiocytes displayed erythrophagocytosis. The authors introduced the term "histiocytic medullary reticulosis" to describe the disorder.

In 1952 Farquhar and Claireaux (584) described two children in the same family with severe progressive disease, whose pathologic findings were those of reticuloendothelial hyperplasia and severe erythrophagocytosis. They called the disease "familial haemophagocytic reticulosis" and believed it to be the same entity described by Scott and Robb-Smith.

Nelson et al. in 1961 (585) introduced the term "generalized lymphohistiocytic infiltration" to describe three siblings who succumbed to an illness characterized by fever, pancytopenia, hepatosplenomegaly, meningitis, and pneumonia within four days to six months after onset of symptoms. At autopsy, lymphocytes and histiocytes were found to have infiltrated many organs and, again, marked erythrophagocytosis was present. The authors felt that this was a previously undescribed disease, but noted its similarity to what was termed "familial Letterer-Siwe disease" by Falk and Gellei (586).

There seems little doubt at this time that the familial form seen in children and the adult form are similar if not identical diseases.

The etiology is unknown, but genetic factors with an autosomal recessive mode of inheritance are suggested by the occurrence of the disease in siblings and in cousins. Boake et al. (587) have suggested a possible viral etiology because of the simultaneous occurrence of the disease in father and son. Simultaneous occurrences have also been reported by Mozziconacci (588) and by Nelson (585).

The finding of lymphocyte depletion in some organs (589–591) at autopsy suggests that a cellular immune defect might also be operative in the pathogenesis of this disease. Chih-Fei et al. have speculated that the disease is closely related to leukemia because of the invasive proliferation of histiocytes into many organs and even into the blood.

The clinical manifestations of the disease in young adults have been summarized by Chih-Fei et al. (591) in their study of 18 cases. The onset was usually acute, with fever, fatigue, and weight loss. Hepatosplenomegaly occurred in almost all patients, and there was progressive pallor with development of hemorrhagic manifestations late in the course of the illness. Pulmonary manifestations occurred in about half the patients, with cough and rales on auscultation. Diarrhea and abdominal distention were observed in about one-third of patients. Total duration of the disease was less than five months.

Additional clinical manifestations reported in children include generalized lymphadenopathy, meningitis with a lymphocytic response in the cerebrospinal fluid (585, 588–590), polyneuritis and papilledema (588), and periorbital edema (585).

A definitive diagnosis may be made by bone marrow examination and the finding of large numbers of abnormal-appearing histiocytes whose abundant cytoplasm may be loaded with erythrocytes or fragments thereof, platelets, and, less commonly, normoblasts and neutrophilic granulocytes (591).

At the present time, there is no successful treatment of the disease. Vincristine, prednisone, cyclophosphamide, nitrogen mustard, triethylenemelamine, and 6-mercaptopurine have all been used, but the results have been dismal with, at best, temporary remissions. Splenectomy has also failed to alter the inexorably downhill course.

References

1. Aisenberg, A. C. and Bloch, K. J.: Immunoglobulins on the surface of neoplastic lymphocytes. New Engl. J. Med. 287:272, 1972.
2. Shevach, E. M., Herberman, R., et al.: Receptors for complement and immunoglobulin on human leukemic cells and human lympho blastoid cell lines. J. Clin. Invest. 51:1933, 1972.
2a. Chin, A. H., Saiki, J. H., et al.: Peripheral blood T- and B-lymphocytes in patients with lymphoma and acute leukemia. Clin. Immunol. Immunopathol. 1:499, 1973.
2b. Borella, L., and Sen, L.: T cell surface markers on lymphoblasts from acute lymphocytic leukemia. J. Immunol. 3:1257, 1973.
2c. Kersey, J. H., Sabad, A., et al.: Acute lymphoblastic leukemic cells with T (thymus-derived) lymphocyte markers. Science 182:1355, 1973.
3. Amiel, J. L.: The different significance of remissions in acute lymphoblastic leukaemia, without treatment, with chemotherapy and with active immunotherapy, In The Nature of Leukaemia. Vincent, P. C. (ed.), Sydney, Australia, V. C. N. Blight, 1972, pp. 241–256.
4. Fraumeni, J. F., Jr., Manning, M. D., et al: Acute childhood leukemia: Epidemiologic study by cell type of 1,263 cases at the Children's Cancer Research Foundation in Boston, 1947–65. J. Natl. Cancer Inst. 46:461, 1971.
5. Sardermann, H.: Chronic lymphocytic leukemia in an infant. Acta Paediatr. Scand. 61:213, 1972.

5a. Casey, T. P.: Chronic lymphocytic leukemia in a child presenting at the age of two years and eight months. Aust. Ann. Med. 17:70, 1968.
5b. Darte, J. M. N., McClure, P. D., et al.: Congenital lymphoid hyperplasia with persistent hyperlymphocytosis. New Engl. J. Med. 284:431, 1971.
6. Rosner, F., and Lee, S. L.: Down's syndrome and acute leukemia: Myeloblastic or lymphoblastic? Report of forty-three cases and review of the literature. Am. J. Med. 53:203, 1972.
7. Boggs, D. R., Wintrobe, M. M., et al.: The acute leukemias. Analysis of 322 cases and review of the literature. Medicine (Baltimore) 41:163, 1962.
8. Hayhoe, F. G. J., Quaglino, D., et al.: The cytology and cytochemistry of acute leukaemias: A study of 140 cases. London, Her Majesty's Stationery Office, 1964.
9. Freeman, J. A.: Origin of Auer bodies. Blood 27:499, 1966.
10. Fraumeni, J. F., Jr., and Miller, R. W.: Epidemiology of human leukemia: Recent observations. J. Natl. Cancer Inst. 38:593, 1967.
11. Fraumeni, J. F., Jr.: Clinical epidemiology of leukemia. Semin. Hematol. 6:250, 1969.
12. Miller, R. W.: The viral etiology of leukemia: An epidemiologic evaluation, In Proceedings of the International Conference on Leukemia-Lymphoma. Zarafonetis, C. J. D. (ed.), Philadelphia, Lea & Febiger, 1968, pp. 23–29.
13. Court Brown, W. M., and Doll, R.: Leukaemia and aplastic anaemia in patients irradiated for ankylosing spondylitis. Medical Research Council, Special Report Series, No. 295. London, Her Majesty's Stationery Office, 1957.
14. Bizzozero, O. J., Jr., Johnson, K. G., et al.: Radiation-related leukemia in Hiroshima and Nagasaki, 1946–1964. I. Distribution, incidence and appearance time. New Engl. J. Med. 274:1095, 1966.
15. Cole, L. J., and Nowell, P. C.: Radiation carcinogenesis: The sequence of events. Science 150:1782, 1965.
15a. Kaplan, H. S.: On the natural history of the murine leukemias. Cancer Res. 27:1325, 1967.
16. Little, J. B.: Cellular effects of ionizing radiation. New Engl. J. Med. 278:308, 1968.
17. Hutchinson, F.: The molecular basis for radiation effects on cells. Cancer Res. 26:2045, Part I, 1966.
18. Dewey, W. C., Miller, H. H., et al.: Chromosomal aberrations and mortality of x-irradiated mammalian cells: Emphasis on repair. Proc. Natl. Acad. Sci. 68:667, 1971.
19. Bloom, A. D., Neriishi, S., et al.: Cytogenetic investigation of survivors of the atomic bombings of Hiroshima and Nagasaki. Lancet 2:672, 1966.
20. Bloom, A. D., Neriishi, S., et al.: Chromosome aberrations in leucocytes of older survivors of the atomic bombings of Hiroshima and Nagasaki. Lancet 2:802, 1967.
21. Kaplan, H. S.: Induction of murine leukaemia: Interaction of viruses, target cells, host factors, and exogenous agents, In The Nature of Leu-

kaemia. Vincent, P. C. (ed.), Sydney, Australia, V. C. N. Blight, 1972, pp. 13–22.

22. Miller, R. W.: Persons with exceptionally high risk of leukemia. Cancer Res. 27:2420, Part I, 1967.

22a. Modan, B.: *The Polycythemic Disorders.* Springfield, Illinois, Charles C Thomas, Publisher, 1971, p. 70.

23. Chaffey, J. T., and Hellman, S.: Differing responses to radiation of murine bone marrow stem cells in relation to the cell cycle. Cancer Res. 31:1613, 1971.

24. Little, J. B.: Differential response of rapidly and slowly proliferating human cells to X irradiation. Radiology 93:307, 1969.

25. Dewey, W. C., Sedita, B. A., et al.: Radiosensitization of X chromosome of Chinese hamster cells related to incorporation of 5-bromodeoxyuridine. Science 152:519, 1966.

26. Gong, J. K.: Anemic stress as a trigger of myelogenous leukemia in rats rendered leukemia-prone by x-ray. Science 174:833, 1971.

27. Segall, A.: Leukemia and background radiation in northern New England. Blood 23:250, 1964.

28. Craig, L., and Seidman, H.: Leukemia and lymphoma mortality in relation to cosmic radiation. Blood 17:319, 1961.

29. Miller, R. W.: Cancer research by the Atomic Bomb Casualty Commission. J. Natl. Cancer Inst. 47:5 (Aug.), 1971.

30. Gibson, R., Graham, S., et al.: Irradiation in the epidemiology of leukemia among adults. J. Natl. Cancer Inst. 48:301, 1972.

31. Miller, J. A.: Carcinogenesis by chemicals: An overview—G. H. A. Clowes Memorial Lecture. Cancer Res. 30:559, 1970.

32. Miller, J. A., and Miller, E. C.: Chemical carcinogenesis: Mechanisms and approaches to its control. J. Natl. Cancer Inst. 47:5 (Sept.), 1971.

33. Price, P. J., Suk, W. A., et al.: Type C RNA tumor viruses as determinants of chemical carcinogenesis: Effects of sequence of treatment. Science 177:1003, 1972.

34. Kyle, R. A., Pierre, R. V., et al.: Multiple myeloma and acute myelomonocytic leukemia. Report of four cases possibly related to melphalan. New Engl. J. Med. 283:1121, 1970.

35. Epstein, M. A.: The possible role of viruses in human cancer. Lancet 1:1344, 1971.

36. Dalton, A. J.: RNA tumor viruses—Terminology and ultrastructural aspects of virion morphology and replication. J. Natl. Cancer Inst. 49:323, 1972.

36a. Baltimore, D.: RNA-dependent DNA polymerase in virions of RNA tumor viruses. Nature (Lond.) 226:1209, 1970.

36b. Temin, H. M., and Mizutani, S.: RNA-dependent DNA polymerase in virions of Rous sarcoma virus. Nature (Lond.) 226:1211, 1970.

37. Temin, H. M.: The RNA tumor viruses—Background and foreground. Proc. Natl. Acad. Sci. USA 69:1016, 1972.

37a. Gallo, R. C.: RNA-dependent DNA polymerase in viruses and cells: Views on the current state. Blood 39:117, 1972.

38. Todaro, G. J., and Huebner, R. J.: The viral on-cogene hypothesis: New evidence. Proc. Natl. Acad. Sci. USA 69:1009, 1972.

38a. McCaffrey, R., and Baltimore, D.: Detection of reverse transcriptase in cell extracts. Presented at the American Society of Hematology, Hollywood, Florida, December 3–6, 1972. Blood 40:933, 1972.

39. Baxt, W., Hehlmann, R., et al.: Human leukaemic cells contain reverse transcriptase associated with a high molecular weight virus-related RNA. Nature [New Biol.] 240:72, 1972.

39a. Baxt, W., Yates, J. W., et al: Leukemia-specific DNA sequences in leukocytes of the leukemic member of identical twins. Proc. Natl. Acad. Sci. USA 70:2629, 1973.

40. Heath, C. W., Jr., and Hasterlik, R. J.: Leukemia among children in a suburban community. Am. J. Med. 34:796, 1963.

41. Stark, C. R., and Mantel, N.: Temporal-spatial distribution of birth dates for Michigan children with leukemia. Cancer Res. 27:1749 (Part I), 1967.

42. Glass, A. G., Hill, J. A., et al.: Significance of leukemia clusters. J. Pediatr. 73:101, 1968.

43. Glass, A. G., and Mantel, N.: Lack of time-space clustering of childhood leukemia in Los Angeles County, 1960–1964. Cancer Res. 29:1995, 1969.

44. Fedrick, J., and Alberman, E. D.: Reported influenza in pregnancy and subsequent cancer in the child. Br. Med. J. 2:485, 1972.

45. Adelstein, A. M., and Donovan, J. W.: Malignant disease in children whose mothers had chickenpox, mumps, or rubella in pregnancy. Br. Med. J. 4:629, 1972.

46. Levine, P. H., Stevens, D. A., et al.: Infectious mononucleosis prior to acute leukemia: A possible role for the Epstein-Barr virus. Cancer 30:875, 1972.

47. Nilsson, K., Klein, G., et al.: The establishment of lymphoblastoid lines from adult and foetal human lymphoid tissue and its dependence on EBV. Int. J. Cancer 8:443, 1971.

48. Gerber, P.: Activation of Epstein-Barr virus by 5-bromodeoxyuridine in "virus-free" human cells. Proc. Natl. Acad. Sci. USA 69:83, 1972.

49. Stevens, D. A., Levine, P. H., et al.: Concurrent infectious mononucleosis and acute leukemia. Am. J. Med. 50:208, 1971.

50. Miller, G., Shope, T., et al.: Prospective study of Epstein-Barr virus infections in acute lymphoblastic leukemia of childhood. J. Pediatr. 80:932, 1972.

51. MacMahon, B.: Epidemiologic aspects of acute leukemia and Burkitt's tumor. Cancer 21:558, 1968.

52. MacMahon, B., and Newill, V. A.: Birth characteristics of children dying of malignant neoplasms. J. Natl. Cancer Inst. 28:231, 1962.

53. Stark, C. R., and Mantel, N.: Maternal-age and birth-order effects in childhood leukemia: Age of child and type of leukemia. J. Natl. Cancer Inst. 42:857, 1969.

54. Miller, R. W.: Down's syndrome (mongolism), other congenital malformations and cancers among the sibs of leukemic children. New Engl. J. Med. 268:393, 1963.

55. Miller, R. W.: Deaths from childhood leukemia and solid tumors among twins and other sibs in the United States, 1960–67. J. Natl. Cancer Inst. 46:203, 1971.

56. Stark, C. R., and Oleinick, A.: Urban or rural residence and histologic type distribution in 21,000 childhood leukemia deaths in the United States, 1950–59. J. Natl. Cancer Inst. 37:369, 1966.

57. Miller, R. W.: Relation between cancer and congenital defects in man. New Engl. J. Med. 275:87, 1966.

57a. Good, R. A.: Relations between immunity and malignancy. Proc. Natl. Acad. Sci. USA 69:1026, 1972.

58. Swift, M.: Fanconi's anaemia in the genetics of neoplasia. Nature (Lond.) 230:370, 1971.

59. Iversen, T.: Leukaemia in infancy and childhood. A material of 570 Danish cases. Acta Paediatr. Scand. (Suppl. 167) 55:29, 1966.

60. Cutler, S. J., Axtell, L., et al.: Ten thousand cases of leukemia: 1940–62. J. Natl. Cancer Inst. 39:993, 1967.

61. Miller, R. W.: Decline in U. S. childhood leukaemia mortality. Lancet 2:1189, 1969.

62. Saunders, E. F., Lampkin, B. C., et al.: Variation of proliferative activity in leukemic cell populations of patients with acute leukemia. J. Clin. Invest. 46:1356, 1967.

63. Killmann, S. A.: Acute leukemia: The kinetics of leukemic blast cells in man. An analytical review. Ser. Haematol. 1:38, 1968.

64. Mauer, A. M., Lampkin, B. C., et al.: Cell kinetic patterns in human acute leukemia — Evidence for control mechanisms. Unifying concepts of leukemia. Bibl. Haematol. 39:1014, 1973.

65. Fialkow, P. J., Thomas, E. D., et al.: Leukaemic transformation of engrafted human marrow cells in vivo. Lancet 1:251, 1971.

66. Reisman, L. E., Mitani, M., et al.: Chromosome studies in leukemia. I. Evidence for the origin of leukemic stem lines from aneuploid mutants. New Engl. J. Med. 270:591, 1964.

67. Greenberg, P. L., Nichols, W. C., et al.: Granulopoiesis in acute myeloid leukemia and preleukemia. New Engl. J. Med. 284:1225, 1971.

68. Lajtha, L. G., and Schofield, R.: Proliferative capacity of hemopoietic stem cells, In Recent Results of Cancer Research. Normal and Malignant Cell Growth. Fry, R. J. M., Griem, M. J. et al. (eds.), New York, Springer-Verlag, 1969, pp. 10–20.

69. Boggs, D. R., Marsh, J. C., et al.: Factors influencing hematopoietic spleen colony formation in irradiated mice. III. The effect of repetitive irradiation upon proliferative ability of colony-forming cells. J. Exp. Med. 126:871, 1967.

70. Maloney, M. A., and Patt, H. M.: Bone marrow restoration after localized depletion. Cell Tissue Kinet. 2:29, 1969.

71. Kundel, D. W., Brecher, G., et al.: Reticulin fibrosis and bone infarction in acute leukemia. Implications for prognosis. Blood 23:526, 1964.

72. Skipper, H. E., and Perry, S.: Kinetics of normal and leukemic leukocyte populations and relevance to chemotherapy. Cancer Res. 30:1883, 1970.

73. Hart, J. S., Shirakawa, S., et al.: The mechanism of induction of complete remission in acute myeloblastic leukemia in man. Cancer Res. 29:2300, 1969.

74. Nies, B. A., Bodey, G. P., et al.: The persistence of extra-medullary leukemic infiltrates during bone marrow remission of acute leukemia. Blood 26:133, 1965.

75. Mathé, G., Schwarzenberg, L., et al.: Extensive histological and cytological survey of patients with acute leukaemia in "complete remission." Br. Med. J. 1:640, 1966.

76. Aur, R. J. A., Simone, J., et al.: Central nervous system therapy and combination chemotherapy of childhood lymphocytic leukemia. Blood 37:272, 1971.

77. Ohno, S.: Genetic implication of karyological instability of malignant somatic cells. Physiol. Rev. 51:496, 1971.

78. Saunders, E. F., and Mauer, A. M.: Reentry of non-dividing leukemic cells into proliferative phase in acute childhood leukemia. J. Clin. Invest. 48:1299, 1969.

79. Hilton, H. B., Lewis, I. C., et al.: C group trisomy in identical twins with acute leukemia. Blood 35:222, 1970.

80. Wald, N., Upton, A. C., et al.: Radiation-induced mouse leukemia: Consistent occurrence of an extra and a marker chromosome. Science 143:810, 1964.

81. Kourilsky, F. M., Dausset, J., et al.: A qualitative study of normal leukocyte antigens of human leukemic leukoblasts. Cancer Res. 28:372, 1968.

82. Rudolph, R. H., Michelson, E., et al.: Mixed leukocyte reactivity and leukemia: Study of identical siblings. J. Clin. Invest. 49:2271, 1970.

83. Mann, D. L., Rogentine, G. N., et al.: Detection of an antigen associated with acute leukemia. Science 174:1136, 1971.

84. Gutterman, J. U., Mavligit, G., et al.: Antigen solubilized from human leukemia: Lymphocyte stimulation. Science 177:1114, 1972.

85. Leventhal, B. G., Halterman, R. H., et al.: Immune reactivity of leukemia patients to autologous blast cells. Cancer Res. 32:1820, 1972.

86. Rosenberg, E. B., Herberman, R. B., et al.: Lymphocyte cytotoxicity reactions to leukemia-associated antigens in identical twins. Int. J. Cancer 9:648, 1972.

87. Junge, U., Hoekstra, J., et al.: Stimulation of peripheral lymphocytes by allogeneic and autochthonous mononucleosis lymphocyte cell lines. J. Immunol. 106:1306, 1971.

88. Skeel, R. T., Henderson, E. S., et al.: The significance of bone marrow lymphocytosis of acute leukemia patients in remission. Blood 32:767, 1968.

89. Skeel, R. T., Bennett, J. M., et al.: Bone marrow lymphocytosis in acute leukemia: A second look. Blood 35:356, 1970.

90. Breslow, N., and Zandstra, R.: A note on the relationship between bone marrow lymphocytosis and remission duration in acute leukemia. Blood 36:246, 1970.

91. Mathé, G., Amiel, J. L., et al.: New results of active immunotherapy of acute lymphoblastic leukemia, *In* Proceedings of the Fifth International Symposium on Comparative Leukemia Reasarch, Padova-Venice, Italy, 1971, p. 12 (abstract).

92. Ziegler, J. L.: Burkitt's lymphoma: Treatment, cell kinetics and immunology, In Proceedings of the Fifth International Symposium on Comparative Leukemia Research, Padova-Venice, Italy, 1971, p. 7 (abstract).

92a. Crowther, D., Powles, R. L., et al.: Management of adult acute myelogenous leukemia. Br. Med. J. *1*:131, 1973.

92b. Bortin, M. N., Rimm, A. A., et al.: Graft versus leukemia: Quantitation of adoptive immunotherapy in murine leukemia. Science *179*:811, 1973.

92c. Thomas, E. D., Buckner, C. D., et al.: Marrow grafting in patients with acute leukemia. Transplant. Proc. 5:917, 1973.

93. Conen, P. E., and Erkman, B.: Combined mongolism and leukemia. Report of eight cases with chromosome studies. Am. J. Dis. Child. *112*:429, 1966.

94. Schroeder, T. M., and Kurth, R.: Spontaneous chromosomal breakage and high incidence of leukemia in inherited disease. Blood 37:96, 1971.

95. Sandberg, A. A., Takagi, N., et al.: Chromosomes and causation of human cancer and leukemia. V. Karyotypic aspects of acute leukemia. Cancer 22:1268, 1968.

96. Whang-Peng, J., Freireich, E. J., et al.: Cytogenetic studies in 45 patients with acute lymphocytic leukemia. J. Natl. Cancer Inst. *42*:881, 1969.

97. Gunz, F. W., Ravich, R. B. M., et al.: A case of acute leukemia with a rapidly changing chromosome constitution. Ann. Genet. *13*:79, 1970.

98. Nowell, P. C.: Marrow chromosome studies in "preleukemia." Further correlation with clinical course. Cancer 28:513, 1971.

99. Sakurai, M., and Sandberg, A. A.: Prognosis of acute myeloblastic leukemia: Chromosomal correlation. Blood *41*:93, 1973.

100. Sandberg, A. A.: The chromosomes and causation of human cancer and leukemia. Cancer Res. 26:2064(Part I), 1966.

101. Astaldi, G., and Mauri, C.: Recherches sur l'activité proliférative de l'hémocytoblaste de la leucémie aiguë. Rev. Belge Pathol. 23:69, 1953.

102. Japa, P.: A study of the mitotic activity of normal human bone marrow. Br. J. Exp. Pathol. 23:272, 1942.

103. Hughes, W. L.: The metabolic stability of deoxyribonucleic acid, In *The Kinetics of Cellular Proliferation.* Stohlman, F., Jr. (ed.), New York, Grune & Stratton, 1959, pp. 83–96.

104. Rubini, J. R., Cronkite, E. P., et al.: The metabolism and fate of tritiated thymidine in man. J. Clin. Invest. 39:909, 1960.

105. Cronkite, E. P., Greenhouse, S. W., et al.: Implication of chromosome structure and replication on hazard of tritiated thymidine and the interpretation of data on cell proliferation. Nature (Lond.) *189*:153, 1961.

106. Cronkite, E. P.: Kinetics of leukemic cell proliferation. Semin. Hematol. *4*:415, 1967.

107. Killmann, S. A.: Acute leukemia: The kinetics of leukemic blast cells in man. An analytical review. Ser. Haematol. 2:38, 1968.

108. Killmann, S. A.: Kinetics of leukaemic blast cells in man, In *Clinics in Haematology. Acute Leukaemia.* Vol. 1. Roath, S. (ed.), London, W. B. Saunders Company, 1972, pp. 95–113.

109. Greenberg, M. L., Chanana, A. D., et al.: The generation time of human leukemic myeloblasts. Lab. Invest. 26:245, 1972.

110. Saunders, E. F., Lampkin, B. C., et al.: Variation of proliferative activity in leukemic cell populations of patients with acute leukemia. J. Clin. Invest. 46:1356, 1967.

111. Wagner, H. P., Cottier, H., et al.: Variability of proliferative patterns in acute lymphoid leukemia of children. Blood 39:176, 1972.

112. Mauer, A. M., and Fischer, V.: Comparison of the proliferative capacity of acute leukemia cells in bone marrow and blood. Nature (Lond.) *193*:1085, 1962.

113. Gavosto, F., Pileri, A., et al.: Proliferation and maturation defect in acute leukaemia cells. Nature (Lond.) *203*:92, 1964.

114. Mauer, A. M., and Fisher, V.: Characteristics of cell proliferation in four patients with untreated acute leukemia. Blood 28:428, 1966.

115. Killmann, S. A.: Proliferative activity of blast cells in leukemia and myelofibrosis. Morphological differences between proliferating and nonproliferating blast cells. Acta Med. Scand. *178*:263, 1965.

116. Gavosto, F., Pileri, A., et al.: Non-self maintaining kinetics of proliferating blasts in human acute leukemia. Nature (Lond.) *216*:188, 1967.

117. Foadi, M. D., Cooper, E. H., et al.: DNA synthesis and DNA content of leukocytes in acute leukemia. Nature (Lond.) *216*:134, 1967.

118. Pileri, A., Gabutti, V., et al.: Proliferative activity of the cells of acute leukemia in relapse and in steady state. Acta Haematol. (Basel) 38:193, 1967.

119. Lampkin, B. C., Nagao, T., et al. Synchronization and recruitment in acute leukemia. J. Clin. Invest. 50:2204, 1971.

120. Chan, B. W. B., and Hayhoe, F. G. J.: Changes in proliferative activity of marrow leukemic cells during and after extracorporeal irradiation of blood. Blood 37:657, 1971.

121. Reich, L., Ohara, K., et al.: Effect of massive leukapheresis on proliferation in acute myeloblastic leukemia (AML) (abstract). Proc. Am. Assoc. Cancer Res. *12*:25, 1971.

122. Paran, M., Sachs, L., et al.: *In vitro* induction of granulocyte differentiation in hematopoietic cells from leukemic and non-leukemic patients. Proc. Natl. Acad. Sci. USA 67:1542, 1970.

123. Iscove, N. N., Senn, J. S., et al.: Colony formation by normal and leukemic human marrow cells in culture: Effect of conditioned medium from human leukocytes. Blood 37:1, 1971.

124. McCulloch, E. A., and Till, J. E.: Regulatory

mechanisms acting on hemopoietic stem cells: Some clinical implications. Am. J. Pathol. 65:601, 1971.

125. Ichikawa, Y.: Further studies on the differentiation of a cell line of myeloid leukemia. J. Cell. Physiol. 76:175, 1970.

126. Foster, R. S., Jr., Metcalf, D., et al.: Bone marrow colony-stimulating activity in sera of children with acute leukemia. A sequential analysis. Cancer 27:881, 1971.

127. Metcalf, D., Chan, S. H., et al.: Colony-stimulating factor and inhibitor levels in acute granulocytic leukemia. Blood 38:143, 1971.

128. Meighan, S. S.: Leukemia in children. Incidence, clinical manifestations, and survival in an unselected series. Cancer 16:656, 1963.

129. Meighan, S. S.: Leukemia in children. Incidence, clinical manifestations, and survival in an unselected series. J.A.M.A. 190:578, 1964.

130. Jamshidi, K., and Swaim, W. R.: Bone marrow biopsy with unaltered architecture: A new biopsy device. J. Lab. Clin. Med. 77:335, 1971.

131. Ibbott, J. W., Whitelaw, D. M., et al.: The significant percentage of blast cells in the bone marrow in the diagnosis of acute leukaemia. Can. Med. Assoc. J. 82:358, 1960.

132. Raney, R. B., and McMillan, C. W.: Simultaneous disparity of bone marrow specimens in acute leukemias. Am. J. Dis. Child. 117:548, 1969.

133. Kundel, D. W., Brecher, G., et al.: Reticulin fibrosis and bone infarction in acute leukemia. Implications for prognosis. Blood 23:526, 1964.

134. Witzleben, C. L., Drake, W. L., Jr., et al.: Gaucher's cells in acute leukemia of childhood. J. Pediatr. 76:129, 1970.

135. Fahey, J. L., and Boggs, D. R.: Serum protein changes in malignant diseases. I. The acute leukemias. Blood 16:1479, 1960.

136. Lichtman, M. A.: Rheology of leukocytes, leukocyte suspensions, and blood in leukemia. Possible relationship to clinical manifestations. J. Clin. Invest. 52:350, 1973.

137. Miller, D. R.: Raised foetal haemoglobin in childhood leukaemia. Br. J. Haematol. 17:103, 1969.

138. Wiernik, P. H., and Serpick, A. A.: Clinical significance of serum and urinary muramidase activity in leukemia and other hematologic malignancies. Am. J. Med. 46:330, 1969.

139. Lulenski, G., Donaldson, M., et al.: Urinary aminoimidazolecarboxamide levels in children with acute leukemia. Pediatrics 45:983, 1970.

140. Tessmer, C. F., Hrgovcic, M., et al.: Long-term serum copper studies in acute leukemia in children. Cancer 30:358, 1972.

140a. Golde, D. W., and Cline, M. J.: Human preleukemia. Identification of a maturation defect in vitro. New Engl. J. Med. 288:1083, 1973.

140b. Metcalf, D.: Human leukemia. Recent tissue culture studies on the nature of myeloid leukaemia. Br. J. Cancer 27:191, 1973.

140c. Preleukaemia. Lancet 1:1427, 1973.

141. Shackelford, G. D., Bloomberg, G., et al.: The value of roentgenography in differentiating aplastic anemia from leukemia masquerading as aplastic anemia. Am. J. Roentgenol. 116:651, 1972.

142. Melhorn, D. K., Gross, S., et al.: Acute childhood leukemia presenting as aplastic anemia: The response to corticosteroids. J. Pediatr. 77:647, 1970.

143. Wetherley-Mein, G., Epstein, I. S., et al.: Mechanisms of anaemia in leukaemia. Br. J. Haematol. 4:281, 1958.

144. Nathan, D. G., and Berlin, N. I.: Studies of the rate of production and life span of erythrocytes in acute leukemia. Blood 14:935, 1959.

145. Bowie, E. J. W., Kiely, J. M., et al.: The anemia of leukemia. J. Nucl. Med. 3:423, 1962.

146. Troup, S. B., Swisher, S. N., et al.: The anemia of leukemia. Am. J. Med. 28:751, 1960.

147. Zaizov, R., and Matoth, Y.: The pathogenesis of anemia in acute leukemia. Isr. J. Med. Sci. 7:1025, 1971.

148. Gaydos, L. A., Freireich, E. J., et al.: The quantitative relation between platelet count and hemorrhage in patients with acute leukemia. New Engl. J. Med. 266:905, 1962.

149. Cowan, D. H., and Haut, M. J.: Platelet function in acute leukemia. J. Lab. Clin. Med. 79:893, 1972.

150. Alvarado, J., Djerassi, I., et al.: Transfusion of fresh concentrated platelets to children with acute leukemia. J. Pediatr. 67:13, 1965.

151. Han, T., Stutzman, L., et al.: Effect of platelet transfusion on hemorrhage in patients with acute leukemia. An autopsy study. Cancer 19:1937, 1966.

152. Goldfinger, D., and McGinniss, M. H.: Rh-incompatible platelet transfusions—Risks and consequences of sensitizing immunosuppressed patients. New Engl. J. Med. 284:942, 1971.

152a. Yankee, R. A., Grumet, F. C., et al.: Platelet transfusion therapy: The selection of compatible platelet donors for refractory patients by lymphocyte HL-A typing. New Engl. J. Med. 281:1208, 1969.

153. Gralnick, H. R., and Henderson, E.: Acquired coagulation factor deficiencies in leukemia. Cancer 26:1097, 1970.

154. Komp, D. M., and Donaldson, M. H.: Sepsis in leukemia and the Shwartzman reaction. Am. J. Dis. Child. 119:114, 1970.

155. Gralnick, H. R., Marchesi, S., et al.: Intravascular coagulation in acute leukemia: Clinical and subclinical abnormalities. Blood 40:709, 1972.

156. Edson, J. R., Krivit, W., et al.: Intravascular coagulation in acute stem cell leukemia successfully treated with heparin. J. Pediatr. 71:342, 1967.

157. Viola, M. V.: Acute leukemia and infection. J.A.M.A. 201:923, 1967.

158. Hughes, W. T.: Fatal infections in childhood leukemia. Am. J. Dis. Child. 122:283, 1971.

159. Levine, A. S., Graw, R. G., Jr., et al.: Management of infections in patients with leukemia and lymphoma: Current concepts and experimental approaches. Semin. Hematol. 9:141, 1972.

160. Simone, J. V., Holland, E., et al.: Fatalities during remission of childhood leukemia. Blood 39:759, 1972.

161. Kiran, O., and Gross, S.: The G-immunoglobulins in acute leukemia in children. Hematologic

and immunologic relationships. Blood 33:198, 1969.

162. Ragab, A. H., Lindqvist, K. J., et al.: Immunoglobulin pattern in childhood leukemia. Cancer 26:890, 1970.

163. Silver, R. T., Utz, J. P., et al.: Antibody response in patients with acute leukemia. J. Lab. Clin. Med. 56:634, 1960.

164. Ogra, P. L., Sinks, L. F., et al.: Poliovirus antibody response in patients with acute leukemia. J. Pediatr. 79:444, 1971.

165. Miller, J. N., Meyers, R. L., et al.: Serum complement levels in children with acute lymphocytic leukemia. J. Pediatr. 64:134, 1964.

166. Yoshikawa, S., Yamada, K., et al.: Serum complement level in patients with leukemia. Int. J. Cancer 4:845, 1969.

167. Bodey, G. P., Buckley, M., et al.: Quantitative relationships between circulating leukocytes and infection in patients with acute leukemia. Ann. Intern. Med. 64:328, 1966.

168. Young, L. S., and Armstrong, D.: Human immunity to Pseudomonas aeruginosa. I. In-vitro interaction of bacteria, polymorphonuclear leukocytes, and serum factors. J. Infect. Dis. 126:257, 1972.

169. Perillie, P. E., and Finch, S. C.: The local exudative cellular response in leukemia. J. Clin. Invest. 39:1353, 1960.

170. Holland, J. F., Senn, H., et al.: Quantitative studies of localized leukocyte mobilization in acute leukemia. Blood 37:499, 1971.

171. Hersh, E. M., Wong, V. G., et al.: Inhibition of the local inflammatory response in man by antimetabolites. Blood 27:38, 1966.

172. Strauss, R. R., Paul, B. B., et al.: The metabolic and phagocytic activities of leukocytes from children with acute leukemia. Cancer Res. 30:480, 1970.

173. Skeel, R. T., Yankee, R. A., et al.: Hexose monophosphate shunt activity of circulating phagocytes in acute lymphocytic leukemia. J. Lab. Clin. Med. 77:975, 1971.

174. Rosner, F., Valmont, I., et al.: Leukocyte function in patients with leukemia. Cancer 25:835, 1970.

175. Catovsky, D., Galton, D. A. G., et al.: Myeloperoxidase-deficient neutrophils in acute myeloid leukaemia. Scand. J. Haematol. 9:142, 1972.

176. Groch, G. S., Perillie, P. E., et al.: Reticuloendothelial phagocytic function in patients with leukemia, lymphoma and multiple myeloma. Blood 26:489, 1965.

177. Rytel, M. W., and Balay, J.: Impaired production of interferon in lymphocytes from immunosuppressed patients. J. Infect. Dis. 127:445, 1973.

178. Pearson, T. A., Mitchell, C. A., et al.: Aeromonas hydrophila septicemia. Am. J. Dis. Child. 123:579, 1972.

179. Delta, B. G., and Pinkel, D.: Listeriosis complicating acute leukemia. J. Pediatr. 60:191, 1962.

180. Bodey, G. P., Nies, B. A., et al.: Multiple organism septicemia in acute leukemia. Analysis of 54 episodes. Arch. Intern. Med. (Chicago) 116:266, 1965.

181. Sehdev, M. K., Dowling, M. D., Jr., et al.: Perianal and anorectal complications in leukemia. Cancer 31:149, 1973.

182. Dehner, L. P., and Kissane, J. M.: Pyogenic hepatic abscesses in infancy and childhood. J. Pediatr. 74:763, 1969.

183. Johnson, W., and Borella, L.: Acute appendicitis in childhood leukemia. J. Pediatr. 67:595, 1965.

184. Fishman, L. S., and Armstrong, D.: Pseudomonas aeruginosa bacteremia in patients with neoplastic disease. Cancer 30:764, 1972.

185. Schimpff, S. C., Moody, M., et al.: Relationship of colonization with Pseudomonas aeruginosa to development of Pseudomonas bacteremia in cancer patients. Antimicrob. Agents Chemother. 10:240, 1970.

186. Bodey, G. P.: Epidemiological studies of Pseudomonas species in patients with leukemia. Am. J. Med. Sci. 260:82, 1970.

187. Caul, E. O., Dickinson, V. A., et al.: Cytomegalovirus infections in leukaemic children. Int. J. Cancer 10:213, 1972.

188. Henson, D., Siegel, S. E., et al.: Cytomegalovirus infections during acute childhood leukemia. J. Infect. Dis. 126:469, 1972.

189. Cangir, A., Sullivan, M. P., et al.: Cytomegalovirus syndrome in children with acute leukemia. Treatment with floxuridine. J.A.M.A. 201:612, 1967.

190. Pinkel, D.: Chickenpox and leukemia. J. Pediatr. 58:729, 1961.

191. Bacon, G. E., Oliver, W. J., et al.: Factors contributing to severity of herpes zoster in children. J. Pediatr. 67:768, 1965.

192. Nishimura, K., Nagamoto, A., et al.: Extensive skin manifestations of herpesvirus infection in an acute leukemic child. Pediatrics 49:294, 1972.

193. Bodey, G., McKelvey, E., et al.: Chickenpox in leukemic patients — Factors in prognosis. Pediatrics 34:563, 1964.

194. Finkel, K. C.: Mortality from varicella in children receiving adrenocorticosteroids and adrenocorticotropin. Pediatrics 28:436, 1961.

195. Sutnick, A. I., London, W. T., et al.: Australia antigen (a hepatitis-associated antigen) in leukemia. J. Natl. Cancer Inst. 44:1241, 1970.

196. Mitus, A., Holloway, A., et al.: Attenuated measles vaccine in children with acute leukemia. Am. J. Dis. Child. 103:243, 1962.

197. Davidson, E., and Hayhoe, F. G. J.: Prolonged generalized vaccinia complicating acute leukaemia. Br. Med. J. 2:1298, 1962.

198. Mirsky, H. S., and Cuttner, J.: Fungal infection in acute leukemia. Cancer 30:348, 1972.

199. Preisler, H. D., Hasenclever, H. F., et al.: Anti-Candida antibodies in patients with acute leukemia. Am. J. Med. 51:352, 1971.

200. Berkel, I., Say, B., et al.: Pulmonary aspergillosis in a child with leukemia. Report of a case and a brief review of the pediatric literature. New Engl. J. Med. 269:893, 1963.

201. Meyer, R. D., Young, L. S., et al.: Aspergillosis complicating neoplastic disease. Am. J. Med. 54:6, 1973.

202. Amromin, G., and Gildenhorn, V. B.: Massive ce-

rebral Aspergillus abscess in a leukemic child. Case report. J. Neurosurg. 35:491, 1971.

203. Meyer, R. D., Rosen, P., et al.: Phycomycosis complicating leukemia and lymphoma. Ann. Intern. Med. 77:871, 1972.

204. Siegel, S. E., Lunde, M. N., et al.: Transmission of toxoplasmosis by leukocyte transfusion. Blood 37:388, 1971.

205. Abell, C., and Holland, P.: Acute toxoplasmosis complicating leukemia. Diagnosis by bone marrow aspiration. Am. J. Dis. Child. 118:782, 1969.

206. Esterly, J. A., and Warner, N. E.: Pneumocystis carinii pneumonia. Twelve cases in patients with neoplastic lymphoreticular disease. Arch. Pathol. 80:433, 1965.

207. Sedaghatian, M. R., and Singer, D. B.: Pneumocystis carinii in children with malignant disease. Cancer 29:772, 1972.

208. Murphy, W. H., Bullis, C., et al.: Isolation of mycoplasma from leukemic and nonleukemic patients. J. Natl. Cancer Inst. 45:243, 1970.

209. Levitan, A. A., and Perry, S.: The use of an isolator system in cancer chemotherapy. Am. J. Med. 44:234, 1968.

210. Jameson, B., Gamble, D. R., et al.: Five-year analysis of protective isolation. Lancet 1:1034, 1971.

211. Bodey, G. P., Gehan, E. A., et al.: Protected environment-prophylactic antibiotic program in the chemotherapy of acute leukemia. Am. J. Med. Sci. 262:138, 1971.

212. Bodey, G. P., Freireich, E. J., et al.: Studies of patients in a laminar air flow unit. Cancer 24:972, 1969.

213. Eyre, H. J., Goldstein, I. M., et al.: Leukocyte transfusions: Function of transfused granulocytes from donors with chronic myelocytic leukemia. Blood 36:432, 1970.

214. Graw, R. G., Jr., Eyre, H. J., et al.: Histocompatibility testing for leucocyte transfusion. Lancet 2:77, 1970.

215. Evans, A. E., Gilbert, E. S., et al.: The increasing incidence of central nervous system leukemia in children. Cancer 26:404, 1970.

216. Price, R. A., and Johnson, W. W.: The central nervous system in childhood leukemia. I. The arachnoid. Cancer 31:520, 1973.

217. Mastrangelo, R., Zuelzer, W. W., et al.: Chromosomes in the spinal fluid: Evidence for metastatic origin of meningeal leukemia. Blood 35:227, 1970.

218. Hyman, C. B., Bogle, J. M., et al.: Central nervous system involvement by leukemia in children. Blood 25:1, 1965.

219. Hardisty, R. M., and Norman, P. M.: Meningeal leukaemia. Arch. Dis. Child. 42:441, 1967.

220. Barak, Y., and Liban, E.: Hypothalamic hyperphagia, obesity and disturbed behaviour in acute leukemia. Acta Paediatr. Scand. 57:153, 1968.

221. Komp, D. M.: Cytocentrifugation in the management of central nervous system leukemia. J. Pediatr. 81:992, 1972.

222. Rosman, N. P., Kakulas, B. A., et al.: Central pontine myelinolysis in a child with leukemia. Arch. Neurol. 14:273, 1966.

223. Kanner, S. P., Wiernik, P. H., et al.: CNS leuke-

mia mimicking multifocal leukoencephalopathy. Am. J. Dis. Child. 119:264, 1970.

224. Miller, V. I., and Campbell, W. G., Jr.: Diabetes insipidus as a complication of leukemia. A case report with a literature review. Cancer 28:666, 1971.

225. Wilhyde, D. E., Jane, J. A., et al.: Spinal epidural leukemia. Am. J. Med. 34:281, 1963.

226. Hyman, C. B., Bogle, J. M., et al.: Central nervous system involvement by leukemia in children. II. Therapy with intrathecal methotrexate. Blood 25:13, 1965.

227. Mitus, A.: Dexamethasone. Its effectiveness in the treatment of the acute symptoms of meningeal leukemia. Am. J. Dis. Child. 117:307, 1969.

228. Sullivan, M. P., Vietti, T. J., et al.: Remission maintenance therapy for meningeal leukemia: Intrathecal methotrexate vs. intravenous bisnitrosourea. Blood 38:680, 1971.

229. Saiki, J. H., Thompson, S., et al.: Paraplegia following intrathecal chemotherapy. Cancer 29:370, 1972.

230. Back, E. H.: Death after intrathecal methotrexate. Lancet 2:1005, 1969.

231. Wang, J. J., and Pratt, C. B.: Intrathecal arabinosyl cytosine in meningeal leukemia. Cancer 25:531, 1970.

232. Halikowski, B., Cyklis, R., et al.: Cytosine arabinoside administered intrathecally in cerebromeningeal leukemia. Acta Paediatr. Scand. 59:164, 1970.

233. Geils, G. F., Scott, C. W., Jr., et al.: Treatment of meningeal leukemia with pyrimethamine. Blood 38:131, 1971.

234. Kim, T., Nesbit, M. E., et al.: The role of central nervous system irradiation in children with acute lymphoblastic leukemia. Radiology 104:635, 1972.

235. Cook, J. C., and Considine, B., Jr.: Low-dose radiation therapy for leukemic involvement of the central nervous system. Radiology 104:649, 1972.

236. Brun, A., Caviness, V., et al.: Hemorrhages into peripheral nerves in association with leukemia. J. Neuropathol. Exp. Neurol. 23:719, 1964.

237. Wolcott, G. J., Grunnet, M. L., et al.: Spinal subdural hematoma in a leukemic child. J. Pediatr. 77:1060, 1970.

238. Belmusto, L., Regelson, W., et al.: Intracranial extracerebral hemorrhages in acute lymphocytic leukemia. A problem resulting from the chemotherapeutic modifications of acute leukemia. Cancer 17:1079, 1964.

239. Fritz, R. D., Forkner, C. E., Jr., et al.: The association of fatal intracranial hemorrhage and "blastic crisis" in patients with acute leukemia. New Engl. J. Med. 261:59, 1959.

240. Freireich, E. J., Thomas, L. B., et al.: A distinctive type of intracerebral hemorrhage associated with "blastic crisis" in patients with leukemia. Cancer 13:146, 1960.

241. Skeel, R. T., Wright, L. J., et al.: Group D streptococcal meningitis masked by meningeal leukemia. Am. J. Dis. Child. 117:334, 1969.

242. Rupprecht, L. M. T., and Naiman, J. L.: Meningitis due to mumps virus in a child with acute leukemia. Pediatrics 46:942, 1970.

243. Weintraub, L. R., Penner, J. A., et al.: Acute uric acid nephropathy in leukemia. Report of a case treated with peritoneal dialysis. Arch. Intern. Med. (Chicago) *113*:111, 1964.

244. Whitaker, J. A., Shaheedy, M., et al.: Gout in childhood leukemia. J. Pediatr. *63*:961, 1963.

245. Sinks, L. F., Newton, W. A., Jr., et al: A syndrome associated with extreme hyperuricemia in leukemia. J. Pediatr. *68*:578, 1966.

246. DeConti, R. C., and Calabresi, P.: Use of allopurinol for prevention and control of hyperuricemia in patients with neoplastic disease. New Engl. J. Med. *274*:481, 1966.

247. Krakoff, I. H., and Murphy, M. L.: Hyperuricemia in neoplastic disease in children: Prevention with allopurinol, a xanthine oxidase inhibitor. Pediatrics *41*:52, 1968.

248. Holland, P., and Holland, N. H.: Prevention and management of acute hyperuricemia in childhood leukemia. J. Pediatr. *72*:358, 1968.

249. Barry, K. G., Hunter, R. H., et al.: Acute uric acid nephropathy. Treatment with mannitol diuresis and peritoneal dialysis. Arch. Intern. Med. (Chicago) *111*:452, 1963.

250. Firmat, J., Vanamee, P., et al.: The artificial kidney in the treatment of renal failure and hyperuricemia in patients with lymphoma and leukemia. Cancer *13*:276, 1960.

251. Stein, R. C.: Hypercalcemia in leukemia. J. Pediatr. *78*:861, 1971.

252. Neiman, R. S., and Li, H. C.: Hypercalcemia in undifferentiated leukemia. Cancer *30*:942, 1972.

253. Jaffe, N., Kim, B. S., et al.: Hypocalcemia—A complication of childhood leukemia. Cancer *20*:392, 1972.

253a. Zusman, J., Brown, D. M., et al.: Hyperphosphatemia, hyperphosphaturia and hypocalcemia in acute lymphoblastic leukemia. New Engl. J. Med. *289*:1335, 1973.

254. Jaffe, N., and Kim, B. S.: Hypoglycemia and hypothermia in terminal leukemia. Pediatrics *48*:836, 1971.

255. Hanrahan, J. B., Sax, S. M., et al.: Factitious hypoglycemia in patients with leukemia. Amer. J. Clin. Pathol. *40*:43, 1963.

256. Field, M., Block, J. B., et al.: Significance of blood lactate elevations among patients with acute leukemia and other neoplastic proliferative disorders. Am. J. Med. *40*:528, 1966.

257. Sumners, J. E., Johnson, W. W., et al.: Childhood leukemic heart disease. A study of 116 hearts of children dying of leukemia. Circulation *40*:575, 1969.

258. Roberts, W. C., Bodey, G. P., et al.: The heart in acute leukemia. A study of 420 autopsy cases. Am. J. Cardiol. *21*:388, 1968.

259. Jaffe, N., Traggis, D. G., et al: Acute leukemia presenting with pericardial tamponade. Pediatrics *45*:461, 1970.

260. Armata, J., Zajaczkowski, J., et al.: Pericardial involvement during remission in acute leukemia. Haematologia *5*:425, 1971.

261. Haddy, T. B.: Cardiac irradiation in childhood leukemia. Am. J. Dis. Child. *108*:559, 1964.

262. Frei, E., III, Bentzel, C. J., et al.: Renal complications of neoplastic disease. J. Chronic Dis. *16*:757, 1963.

263. Frei, E., III, Fritz, R. D., et al.: Renal and hepatic

264. Persky, L., Newman, A. J., et al.: Urologic manifestations of childhood leukemia. J. Urol. *107*:1073, 1972.

264a. Rubissow, M. J., Holliday, M. A., et al.: Proximal tubular hypertrophy in a case of acute leukemia of childhood: A study of microdissection. Am. J. Clin. Pathol. *53*:843, 1970.

265. Troup, C. W., Thatcher, G., et al: Infiltrative lesion of the bladder presenting as gross hematuria in child with leukemia: Case report. J. Urol. *107*:314, 1972.

266. Vadakan, V. V., and Ortega, J.: Priapism in acute lymphoblastic leukemia. Cancer *30*:373, 1972.

267. Jaffe, N., and Kim, B. S.: Priapism in acute granulocytic leukemia. Am. J. Dis. Child. *118*:619, 1969.

268. Givler, R. L.: Testicular involvement in leukemia and lymphoma. Cancer *23*:1290, 1969.

269. Haggar, R. A., MacMillan, A. B., et al.: Leukemic infiltration of testis. Can. J. Surg. *12*:197, 1969.

270. Finklestein, J. Z., Dyment, P. G., et al.: Leukemic infiltration of the testes during bone marrow remission. Pediatrics *43*:1042, 1969.

271. Prolla, J. C., and Kirsner, J. B.: Gastrointestinal lesions and complications of the leukemias. Ann. Intern. Med. *61*:1084, 1964.

272. Al-Rashid, R. A., and Harned, R. K.: Dysphagia due to leukemic involvement of the esophagus. Am. J. Dis. Child. *121*:75, 1971.

273. Everett, C. R., Haggard, M. E., et al.: Extensive leukemic infiltration of the gastrointestinal tract during apparent remission in acute leukemia. Blood *22*:92, 1963.

274. Wagner, M. L., Rosenberg, H. S., et al.: Typhlitis: A complication of leukemia in childhood. Am. J. Roentgenol. *109*:341, 1970.

275. Gildenhorn, H. L., Springer, E. B., et al.: Necrotizing enteropathy: Roentgenographic features. Am. J. Roentgenol. *88*:942, 1962.

276. Jaffe, N., Carlson, D. H., et al.: Pneumatosis cystoides intestinalis in acute leukemia. Cancer *30*:239, 1972.

277. Wetherley-Mein, G., and Cottom, D. G.: Portal fibrosis in acute leukemia. Br. J. Haematol. *2*:345, 1956.

278. Hutter, R. V. P., Shipkey, F. H., et al.: Hepatic fibrosis in children with acute leukemia. A complication of therapy. Cancer *13*:288, 1960.

279. Thomas, L. B., Forkner, C. E., Jr., et al.: The skeletal lesions of acute leukemia. Cancer *14*:608, 1961.

280. Aur, R. J. A., Westbrook, H. W., et al.: Childhood acute lymphocytic leukemia. Am. J. Dis. Child. *124*:653, 1972.

281. Nies, B. A., Kundel, D. W., et al.: Leukopenia, bone pain, and bone necrosis in patients with acute leukemia. A clinicopathologic complex. Ann. Intern. Med. *62*:698, 1965.

282. Schaller, J.: Arthritis as a presenting manifestation of malignancy in children. J. Pediatr. *81*:793, 1972.

283. Klatte, E. C., Yardley, J., et al.: The pulmonary manifestations and complications of leukemia. Am. J. Roentgenol. *89*:598, 1963.

enlargement in acute leukemia. Cancer *16*:1089, 1963.

284. Bodey, G. P., Powell, R. D., Jr., et al.: Pulmonary complications of acute leukemia. Cancer 19:781, 1966.

285. Deitch, R. D., and Wilson, F. M.: Leukemic reticuloendotheliosis with presenting ocular complaints. Report of a case. Arch. Ophthalmol. 69:560, 1963.

286. Fonken, H. A., and Ellis, P. P.: Leukemic infiltrates in the iris. Successful treatment of secondary glaucoma with x-irradiation. Arch. Ophthalmol. 76:32, 1966.

287. Clayman, H. M., Flynn, J. T., et al.: Retinal pigment epithelial abnormalities in leukemic disease. Am. J. Ophthalmol. 74:416, 1972.

288. Davis, L. A., and McCreadie, S. R.: The enlarged thymus gland in leukemia in childhood. Am. J. Roentgenol. 88:924, 1962.

289. Mainzer, F., and Taybi, H.: Thymic enlargement and pleural effusion: An unusual roentgenographic complex in childhood leukemia. Am. J. Roentgenol. 112:35, 1971.

290. LaVenuta, F., and Moore, J. A.: Involvement of the inner ear in acute stem cell leukemia. Report of two cases. Ann. Otol. (St. Louis) 81:132, 1972.

291. Stoop, J. W., Zegers, B. J. M., et al.: Monoclonal gammopathy in a child with leukemia. Blood 32:774, 1968.

292. Lindqvist, K. J., Ragab, A. H., et al.: Paraproteinemia in a child with leukemia. Blood 35:213, 1970.

293. Kennedy, B. J., Borenstein, R., et al.: Breast involvement in acute lymphatic leukemia. Daunorubicine-induced remission; *Pneumocystis carinii* pneumonia. Cancer 25:693, 1970.

294. Larson, S. M., Graff, K. S., et al.: Positive gallium 67 photoscan in myeloblastoma. J.A.M.A. 222:321, 1972.

295. Gralnick, H. R., and Dittmar, K.: Development of myeloblastoma with massive breast and ovarian involvement during remission in acute leukemia. Cancer 24:746, 1969.

296. Lusher, J. M.: Chloroma as a presenting feature of acute leukemia. A report of two cases in children. Am. J. Dis. Child. 108:62, 1964.

297. Austin, J. H. M.: Chloroma. Report of a patient with unusual rib lesions. Radiology 93:671, 1969.

298. Curtis, A. B.: Childhood leukemias: Initial oral manifestations. J. Am. Dent. Assoc. 83:159, 1971.

299. Lynch, M. A., and Ship, I. I.: Oral manifestations of leukemia: A postdiagnostic study. J. Am. Dent. Assoc. 75:1139, 1967.

300. Farber, S., Diamond, L. K., et al.: Temporary remissions in acute leukemia in children produced by folic acid antagonist 4-aminopteroyl-glutamic acid (Aminopterin). New Engl. J. Med. 238:787, 1948.

301. Pierce, M. I., Borges, W. H., et al.: Epidemiological factors and survival experience in 1770 children with acute leukemia. Cancer 23:1296, 1969.

302. Leikin, S. L., Brubaker, C., et al.: Varying prednisone dosage in remission induction of previously untreated childhood leukemia. Cancer 21:346, 1968.

303. Vietti, T. J., Sullivan, M. P., et al.: The response of acute childhood leukemia to an initial and second course of prednisone. J. Pediatr. 66:18, 1965.

304. Hyman, C. B., Borda, E. C., et al.: Prednisone in childhood leukemia. Comparison of interrupted with continuous therapy. Pediatrics 24:1005, 1959.

305. Wolff, J. A., Brubaker, C. A., et al.: Prednisone therapy of acute childhood leukemia: Prognosis and duration of response in 330 treated patients. J. Pediatr. 70:626, 1967.

306. Evans, A. E., Farber, S., et al.: Vincristine in the treatment of acute leukemia in children. Cancer 16:1302, 1963.

307. Karon, M., Freireich, E. J., et al.: The role of vincristine in the treatment of childhood acute leukemia. Clin. Pharmacol. Ther. 7:332, 1966.

308. Henderson, E. S.: Treatment of acute leukemia. Semin. Hematol. 6:271, 1969.

309. Colebatch, J. H., Baikie, A. G., et al.: Cyclic regimen for childhood leukemia. Lancet 2:869, 1968.

310. Bertino, J. R., Gabrio, B. W., et al.: Dihydrofolic reductase in human leukemic leukocytes. Biochem. Biophys. Res. Commun. 3:461, 1960.

311. Henderson, E. S., Adamson, R. H., et al.: The metabolic fate of tritiated methotrexate. II. Absorption and excretion in man. Cancer Res. 25:1018, 1965.

312. Frei, E., III, Freireich, E. J., et al.: Studies of sequential and combination antimetabolite therapy in acute leukemia, 6-mercaptopurine and methotrexate, from the Acute Leukemia Group B. Blood 18:431, 1961.

313. Nagao, T., Lampkin, B. C., et al.: Maintenance therapy in acute childhood leukemia. J. Pediatr. 76:134, 1970.

314. Acute Leukemia Group B. Acute lymphocytic leukemia in children. Maintenance therapy with methotrexate administered intermittently. J.A.M.A. 207:923, 1969.

315. Ragab, A. H., Frech, R. S., et al.: Osteoporotic fractures secondary to methotrexate therapy of acute leukemia in remission. Cancer 25:580, 1970.

316. Loo, T. L., Luce, J. K., et al.: Clinical pharmacologic observations on 6-mercaptopurine and 6-methylthiopurine ribonucleoside. Clin. Pharmacol. Ther. 9:180, 1968.

317. Freireich, E. J., Gehan, E., et al.: The effect of 6-mercaptopurine on the duration of steroid-induced remission in acute leukemia: A model for evaluation of other potentiating useful therapy. Blood 21:699, 1963.

318. Clark, P. A., Hsia, Y. E., et al.: Toxic complications of treatment with 6-mercaptopurine. Two cases with hepatic necrosis and intestinal ulceration. Br. Med. J. 1:393, 1960.

319. Oliverio, V. T., and Zubrod, C. G.: Clinical pharmacology of the effective antitumor drugs. Ann. Rev. Pharmacol. 5:335, 1965.

320. Foley, G. E., Friedman, O. M., et al.: Studies on the mechanism of action of cytoxan—Evidence of activation in vivo and in vitro. Cancer Res. 21:57, 1961.

321. Pierce, M., Shore, N., et al.: Cyclophosphamide therapy in acute leukemia of childhood. Cancer 19:1551, 1966.

322. Finkelstein, J. Z., Scher, J., et al.: Pharmacologic studies of tritiated cytosine arabinoside (N⁵C–63878) in children. Cancer Chemother. Rep. 54:35, 1970.

323. Ellison, R. R., Holland, J. F., et al.: Arabinosyl cytosine: A useful agent in the treatment of acute leukemia in adults. Blood 32:507, 1968.

324. Howard, J. P., Albo, V., et al.: Cytosine arabinoside. Results of a cooperative study in acute childhood leukemia. Cancer 21:341, 1968.

325. Lampkin, B. C., McWilliams, N. B., et al.: The advantage of cell synchronization in therapy of myeloid leukemias in children. Blood 38:802, 1971.

326. Bernard, J., Paul, R., et al.: *Rubidomycin. Recent Results in Cancer Research*. Vol. 20. New York, Springer-Verlag, 1969.

327. Boiron, M., Weil, M., et al.: Daunorubicin in the treatment of acute myelocytic leukaemia. Lancet 1:330, 1969.

328. Jones, B., Holland, J. F., et al.: Daunorubicin (NSC 82151) in the treatment of advanced childhood lymphoblastic leukemia. Cancer Res. 31:84, 1971.

329. Oettgen, H. F., Stephenson, P. A., et al.: Toxicity of *E. coli* L-asparaginase in man. Cancer 25:253, 1970.

330. Capizzi, R. L., Bertino, J. R., et al.: L-asparaginase: Clinical, biochemical, pharmacological, and immunological studies. Ann. Intern. Med. 74:893, 1971.

331. Pratt, C. B., Simone, J. V., et al.: Comparison of daily versus weekly L-asparaginase for the treatment of childhood acute leukemia. J. Pediatr. 77:474, 1970.

332. Ernst, P., and Killmann, S. A.: Effect of antileukemic drugs on cell cycle of human leukemic blast cells in vivo. Acta. Med. Scand. 186:239, 1969.

333. Lampkin, B. C., Nagao, T., et al.: Drug effect in acute leukemia. J. Clin. Invest. 48:1124, 1969.

334. Lampkin, B. C., Nagao, T., et al.: Synchronization and recruitment in acute leukemia. J. Clin. Invest. 50:2204, 1971.

335. Ernst, P., and Killmann, S. A.: Perturbation of generation cycle of human leukemic blast cells by cytostatic therapy in vivo: Effect of corticosteroids. Blood 36:689, 1970.

336. Saunders, E. F.: The effect of L-asparaginase on the nucleic acid metabolism and cell cycle of human leukemia cells. Blood 39:575, 1972.

337. McWilliams, N. B., Mauer, A. M., et al.: Dose dependent vincristine effects. Clin. Res. 19:494, 1971.

338. Killmann, S. A., and Ernst, P.: An analysis of the relationship of leukemia cell kinetics to chemotherapy. Unifying concepts of leukemia. Bibl. Haematol. 39:1037, 1973.

339. Lampkin, B. C., McWilliams, N. B., et al.: Cell kinetics and chemotherapy of acute leukemia, Semin. Hematol. 9:211, 1972.

340. Pinkel, D., Hernandez, K., et al.: Drug dosage and remission duration in childhood lymphocytic leukemia. Cancer 27:247, 1971.

341. Lampkin, B. C., McWilliams, N. B., et al.: Treatment of acute leukemia. Pediatr. Clin. North Am. 19:1123, 1972.

342. The Australian Cancer Society's Childhood Leukaemia Study Group: Cyclic drug regimen for acute childhood leukaemia. Lancet 1:313, 1968.

343. Krivit, W., Brubaker, C., et al.: Maintenance therapy in acute leukemia of childhood. Comparison of cyclic vs. sequential methods. Cancer 21:352, 1968.

344. Zuelzer, W. W.: Implications of long-term survival in acute stem cell leukemia of childhood treated with composite cyclic therapy. Blood 24:477, 1964.

345. Aur, R. J. A., Simone, J., et al.: Central nervous system therapy and combination chemotherapy of childhood lymphocytic leukemia. Blood 37:272, 1971.

346. George, P., Hernandez, K., et al.: A study of "total therapy" of acute lymphocytic leukemia in children. J. Pediatr. 72:399, 1968.

347. Pinkel, D.: Five-year follow-up of "total therapy" of childhood lymphocytic leukemia. J.A.M.A. 216:648, 1971.

347a. Simone, J.: Acute lymphocytic leukemia in childhood. Semin. Hematol. 11:25, 1974.

348. Glidewell, O. J., and Holland, J. F.: Clinical trials of the Acute Leukemia Group B in acute lymphocytic leukemia of childhood. Unifying concepts of leukemia. Bibl. Haematol. 31:1053, 1973.

349. Crowther, D., Bateman, C. J. F., et al.: Combination chemotherapy using L-asparaginase, daunorubicin and cytosine arabinoside in adults with acute myelogenous leukaemia. Br. Med. J. 4:513, 1970.

350. Gee, T. S., Yu, K. P., et al.: Treatment of adult acute leukemia with arabinosylcytosine and thioguanine. Cancer 23:1019, 1969.

351. Bailey, C. C., Israels, M. C. G., et al.: Cytosine arabinoside in the treatment of acute myeloblastic leukaemia. Lancet 1:1268, 1971.

352. Freedman, M. H., Finklestein, J. Z., et al.: The effect of chemotherapy on acute myelogenous leukemia in children. J. Pediatr. 78:526, 1971.

353. Mathé, G., Amiel, J. L., et al.: Active immunotherapy for acute lymphoblastic leukemia. Lancet 2:697, 1969.

354. Mathé, G.: Experimental basis and first clinical controlled trials of leukemia active immunotherapy, In *Progress in Immunology*, Amos, B., (ed.), New York, Academic Press, 1971, pp. 959–969.

355. Preliminary Report to the Medical Research Council by the Leukaemia Committee and the Working Party on Leukaemia in Childhood: Treatment of acute lymphoblastic leukaemia, comparison of immunotherapy (BCG), intermittent methotrexate, and no therapy after a five month intensive cytotoxic regimen (Concord Trial). Br. Med. J. 4:189, 1971.

356. Thomas, E. D., Buckner, C. D., et al.: Allogeneic marrow grafting for hematologic malignancy using HL-A matched donor-recipient sibling pairs. Blood 38:267, 1971.

357. Graw, R. G., Jr., Yankee, R. A., et al.: Bone marrow transplantation from HL-A matched

donors to patients with acute leukemia. Toxicity and antileukemic effect. Transplantation 14:79, 1972.

358. Krüger, G. R. F., Berard, C. W., et al.: Graft-versus-host disease. Morphologic variation and differential diagnosis in 8 cases of HL-A matched bone marrow transplantation. Am. J. Pathol. 63:179, 1971.

359. Thomas, E. D., Bryant, J. I., et al.: Leukemic transformation of engrafted human marrow. Transplant. Proc. 4:567, 1972.

360. Mathé, G., Schwarzenberg, L., et al.: Bone marrow transplantation after antilymphocyte globulin conditioning—Split lymphocyte chimerism. Transplant. Proc. 4:551, 1972.

361. Howell, D. A.: A child dies. J. Pediatr. Surg. 1:2, 1966.

362. Evans, A. E.: If a child must die . . . . New Engl. J. Med. 278:138, 1968.

363. Kübler-Ross, E., Wessler, S., et al.: On death and dying. J.A.M.A. 221:174, 1972.

364. Toch, R.: Management of the child with a fatal disease. Clin. Pediatr. 3:418, 1964.

365. Vernick, J., and Karon, M.: Who's afraid of death on a leukemia ward? Am. J. Dis. Child. 109:393, 1965.

366. Green, M.: Care of the child with a long-term, life-threatening illness: Some principles of management. Pediatrics 39:441, 1967.

367. Karon, M., and Vernick, J.: An approach to the emotional support of fatally ill children. Clin. Pediatr. 7:274, 1968.

368. Easson, W. M.: Care of the young patient who is dying. J.A.M.A. 205:203, 1968.

369. Burgert, E. O., Jr.: Emotional impact of childhood acute leukemia. Mayo Clin. Proc. 47:273, 1972.

370. Ablin, A. R., Binger, C. M., et al.: A conference with the family of a leukemic child. Am. J. Dis. Child. 122:362, 1971.

371. Lascari, A. D., and Stehbens, J. A.: The reactions of families to childhood leukemia. An evaluation of a program of emotional management. Clin. Pediatr. 12:210, 1973.

372. Schowalter, J. E.: Death and the pediatric house officer. J. Pediatr. 76:706, 1970.

373. Wiener, J. M.: Attitudes of pediatricians toward the care of fatally ill children. J. Pediatr. 76:700, 1970.

374. Cooke, J. V.: Chronic myelogenous leukemia in children. J. Pediatr. 42:537, 1953.

375. Nowell, P. C., and Hungerford, D. A.: Chromosome studies in human leukemia. II. Chronic granulocytic leukemia. J. Natl. Cancer Inst. 27:1013, 1961.

376. Prieto, F., Egozcue, J., et al.: Identification of the Philadelphia (Ph-1) chromosome. Blood 35:23, 1970.

377. Fitzgerald, P. H. Pickering, A. L., et al.: Clonal origin of the Philadelphia chromosome and chronic myeloid leukemia: Evidence from a sex chromosome mosaic. Br. J. Haematol. 21:473, 1971.

378. Killman, S. A.: A biased view on the relapse and remission phase of acute myeloid leukemia, In The Nature of Leukaemia. Vincent, P. C., and Glight, V. C. N. (eds.), Sydney, Australia, Government Printer, 1972, p. 205.

379. Woodliff, H. J., Dougan, L., et al.: Cytogenetic studies in twins, one with chronic granulocytic leukaemia. Nature (Lond.) 211:533, 1966.

380. Goh, K., Swisher, S. N., et al.: Chronic myelocytic leukemia in identical twins: Additional evidence of the Philadelphia chromosome as postzygotic abnormality. Arch. Intern. Med. (Chicago) 120:214, 1967.

381. Tokuhata, G. K., Neely, C. L., et al.: Chronic myelocytic leukemia in identical twins and a sibling. Blood 31:216, 1968.

382. Wiener, L.: A family with high incidence of leukemia and unique Ph¹ chromosome findings. Blood 26:871, 1965.

383. Whang, J., Frei, E., et al.: The distribution of the Philadelphia chromosome in patients with chronic myelogenous leukemia. Blood 22:664, 1963.

384. Tough, I. M., Jacobs, P. A., et al.: Cytogenetic studies on bone marrow in chronic myeloid leukaemia. Lancet 1:844, 1963.

385. Speed, D. E., and Rawler, S. D.: Chronic granulocytic leukaemia. The chromosome and the disease. Lancet 1:403, 1964.

386. Baikie, A. G.: What is a leukaemic remission. The evidence from cytogenetic studies, In The Nature of Leukaemia. Vincent, P. C., and Glight, V. C. N (eds.), Sydney, Australia, Government Printer, 1972, p. 231.

387. Craddock, G. G.: Some aspects of leukokinetics in myeloproliferative disease. Scand. J. Haematol. 1:13, 1965.

388. Cartwright, G. E., Athens, J. W., et al.: Blood granulocyte kinetics in conditions associated with granulocytosis. Ann. N.Y. Acad. Sci. 113:963, 1964.

389. Marsh, J. C., and Perry, S.: The granulocytic response to endotoxin in patients with hematologic disorders. Blood 23:581, 1964.

390. Banerjee, L. K., Senn, H., et al.: Comparative studies on localized leukocyte mobilization in patients with chronic myelocytic leukemia. Cancer 29:637, 1972.

391. Morley, A. A.: A neutrophil cycle in healthy individuals. Lancet 2:1220, 1966.

392. Morley, A. A., Baikie, A. G., et al.: Cyclic leukocytosis as evidence for retention of normal homeostatic control in chronic granulocytic leukaemia. Lancet 2:1320, 1967.

393. Shadduck, R. K., Winkelstein, A., et al.: Cyclic leukemic cell production in chronic myelocytic leukemia. Cancer 29:399,, 1972.

393a. Craddock, C. G., Hays, E. F., et al.: Granulocyte-monocyte colony-forming capacity of human marrow: A clinical study. Blood 42:711, 1973.

394. Vodopick, H., Rupp, E. M., et al.: Spontaneous cyclic leukocytosis and thrombocytosis in chronic granulocytic leukemia. New Engl. J. Med. 286:284, 1972.

395. King-Smith, E. A., and Morley, A.:Computer simulation of granulopoiesis: Normal and impaired granulopoiesis. Blood 36:254, 1970.

396. Reisman, L. E., and Trujillo, J. M.: Chronic granulocytic leukemia of childhood. J. Pediatr. 62:710, 1963.

397. Hardisty, R. M., Speed, D. E., et al.: Granulocytic leukaemia in childhood. Br. J. Haematol. 10:551, 1964.

398. Bernard, J., Seligmann, M., et al.: La leucémie myéloide chronique de l'enfant (étude de

vingt observations). Arch. Fr. Pediatr. *19*:881, 1962.

399. Rosen, R. B., and Mishiyama, H.: Leukocyte alkaline phosphatase in chronic granulocytic leukemia of childhood. Ann. N.Y. Acad. Sci. *155*:992, 1968.

400. Bloom, G. E., Gerald, P. S., et al.: Chronic myelogenous leukemia in an infant. Serial cytogenetic and fetal hemoglobin studies. Pediatrics *38*:295, 1966.

401. Ritz, N. D., and Purfar, M.: Chronic myeloid leukemia with priapism in an eight-year-old child. N.Y. J. Med. *64*:553, 1964.

402. Pochedly, C.: Unusual manifestations of chronic granulocytic leukemia in a child. Cancer *24*:1017, 1969.

403. Beard, M. F., Pitney, W. R., et al.: Serum concentrations of vitamin B$_{12}$ in patients suffering from leukemia. Blood *9*:789, 1954.

404. Mendelsohn, R. S., et al.: Identification of the vitamin B$_{12}$ binding protein in the serum of normals and of patients with chronic myelocytic leukemia. Blood *13*:740, 1958.

405. Hall, C. A., and Finkler, A. E.: Measurement of the amounts of the individual vitamin B$_{12}$ binding proteins in plasma: Abnormalities in leukemia and pernicious anemia. Blood *27*:618, 1966.

406. Mitus, W. J., Bergna, L. J., et al.: Alkaline phosphatase of mature neutrophils in chronic forms of the myeloproliferative syndrome. Am. J. Clin. Pathol. *30*:285, 1958.

407. Kaplow, L. S.: A histochemical procedure for localizing and evaluating leukocyte alkaline phosphatase activity in smears of blood and marrow. Blood *10*:1023, 1955.

408. Rosen, C. B., and Teplitz, R. L.: Chronic granulocytic leukemia complicated by ulcerative colitis: Elevated leukocyte alkaline phosphatase and possible modifier gene deletion. Blood *26*:148, 1965.

409. Miller, D. R.: Raised foetal haemoglobin in childhood leukaemia. Br. J. Haematol. *17*:103, 1969.

410. Ben-Zee, D., Schwartz, S. O., et al.: Promyelocytic leukemia as a terminal manifestation of chronic granulocytic leukemia. Report of a case. Blood *27*:863, 1966.

411. Beaven, G. H., Ellis, M. J., et al.: Studies on human fetal hemoglobin. II. Fetal hemoglobin levels in healthy children and adults and in certain hematologic disorders. Br. J. Haematol. *6*:201, 1960.

412. Weatherall, D. J., and Brown, W. J.: Juvenile chronic myeloid leukemia. Lancet *1*:526, 1970.

413. Weatherall, D. J., Edwards, J. A., et al.: Hemoglobin and red cell enzyme changes in juvenile chronic myeloid leukemia. Br. J. Med. *1*:679, 1968.

414. Fox, A. M.: Case of juvenile chronic myeloid leukemia. Lancet *1*:368, 1970.

415. Cao, A.: Juvenile chronic myeloid leukemia. Lancet *1*:1002, 1970.

416. Stoppoloni, G., and Di Torro, R.: Juvenile chronic myeloid leukemia. Lancet *1*:1176, 1970.

417. Holton, C. P., and Johnson, W. W.: Chronic myelocytic leukemia in infant siblings. J. Pediatr. *72*:377, 1968.

418. Maurer, H. S., Vida, L. N., et al.: Similarities of the erythrocytes in juvenile chronic myelogenous leukemia to fetal erythrocytes. Blood *39*:778, 1972.

418a. Altman, A. J., Palmer, C. G., et al.: Juvenile "chronic granulocytic" leukemia: A panmyelopathy with prominent monocytic involvement and circulating monocyte colony-forming cells. Blood *43*:341, 1974.

419. Randall, D. L., Reiquam, W., et al.: Familial myeloproliferative disease. A new syndrome simulating myelogenous leukemia in childhood. Am. J. Dis. Child. *110*:479, 1965.

420. Kennedy, B. J.: Hydroxyurea in chronic myelocytic leukemia. Cancer *29*:1052, 1972.

421. Galton, D. A. G.: Chemotherapy of chronic myelocytic leukemia. Semin. Hematol. *6*:323, 1969.

422. Canellos, G. P., De Vita, V. T., et al.: Hematologic and cytogenetic remission of blastic transformation in chronic granulocytic leukemia. Blood *38*:671, 1971.

422a. Natelson, E. A., Lynch, E. C., et al.: Polycythemia vera in childhood. Am. J. Dis. Child. *122*:241, 1971.

423. Rickles, F. R., and Miller, D. R.: Eosinophilic leukemoid reaction. J. Pediatr. *80*:418–428, 1972.

424. Bentley, H. P., Reardon, A. E., et al.: Eosinophilic leukemia. Am. J. Med. *30*:310, 1061.

425. Conrad, M. E.: Hematologic manifestations of parasitic infections. Semin. Hematol. *8*:267, 1971.

426. Benvenisti, D. S., and Ultmann, J. E.: Eosinophilic leukemia. Ann. Intern. Med. *71*:731, 1969.

427. Pierce, L. E., Hosseinian, A. H., et al.: Disseminated eosinophilic collagen disease. Blood *29*:540, 1967.

428. Brockington, I. F., Luzzatto, L., et al.: The heart in eosinophilic leukemia. Afr. J. Med. Sci. *1*:343, 1970.

429. Ackerman, G. A.: Eosinophilic leukemia. A morphologic and histochemical study. Blood *24*:372, 1964.

430. Thomas, J. R.: Eosinophilic leukemia presenting with erythrocytosis. Blood *22*:639, 1963.

431. Goh, K. O., Swisher, S. N., et al.: Cytogenetic studies in eosinophilic leukemia: The relationship of eosinophilic leukemia to chronic myelocytic leukemia. Ann. Intern. Med. *62*:80, 1965.

432. Gruenwald, H., Kiossoglou, K. A., et al.: Philadelphia chromosome in eosinophilic leukemia. Am. J. Med. *39*:1003, 1965.

433. Huntley, C. C., Costas, C., et al.: Visceral larva migrans syndrome: Clinical characteristics and immunologic studies in 51 patients. Pediatrics *36*:523, 1965.

434. Huntley, C. C., Costas, M. C., et al.: Anti-gammaglobulin factors in visceral larva migrans. J.A.M.A. *197*:552, 1966.

435. Kazan, I. G.: Serologic diagnosis of visceral larva migrans. Clin. Pediatr. *7*:508, 1968.

436. Shohet, S. B., and Blum, S. F.: Coincident basophilic chronic myelogenous leukemia and pulmonary tuberculosis. Cancer *22*:173, 1968.

437. Mau, R. C., and Hoagland, H. C.: A myeloproliferative disorder manifested by persistent

basophilia, granulocytic leukemia and erythroleukemic phases. Cancer 28:662, 1971.

438. Casey, A. E., Nettles, T. E., et al.: Basophilic leukemia. South. Med. J. 39:325, 1946.

439. Kyle, R. A., and Pease, G. L.: Basophilic leukemia. Arch. Intern. Med. (Chicago) 118:205, 1966.

440. Mitrakul, C., Othaganonda, B. O., et al.: Basophilic leukemia. Report of a case. Clin. Pediatr. (Phila.) 8:178, 1969.

441. Rupe, C. E.: Mast cells in non-neoplastic diseases of man and their relationship to the basophilic leucocyte. Ann. N.Y. Acad. Sci. 103:436, 1963.

442. Dameshek, W.: Acute monocytic leukemia: Review of the literature and case reports. Arch. Intern. Med. (Chicago) 46:718, 1930.

443. Clough, P. W.: Monocytic leukemia. Bull. Johns Hopkins Hosp. 51:148, 1932.

444. Osgood, E. E.: Monocytic leukemia. Arch. Intern. Med. 59:931, 1933.

445. Lynch, M. J.: Monocytic leukemia. Can. Med. J. 70:670, 1954.

446. Sinn, C. M., and Dick, F. W.: Monocytic leukemia. Am. J. Med. 20:588, 1956.

447. Osserman, E. F., and Lawlor, D. P.: Serum and urinary lysozyme (muramidase) in monocytic and monomyelocytic leukemia. J. Exp. Med. 124:921, 1966.

448. Wiernik, P. H., and Serpick, A. A.: Clinical significance of serum and urinary muramidase activity in leukemia and other hematologic malignancies. Am. J. Med. 46:330, 1969.

449. Muggia, F. M., Heinemann, H. O., et al.: Lysozymuria and renal tubular dysfunction in monocytic and myelomonocytic leukemia. Am. J. Med. 47:351, 1969.

450. Pruzanski, W., and Platts, M. E.: Serum and urinary proteins, lysozyme (muramidase) and renal dysfunction in man and myelomonocytic leukemia. J. Clin. Invest. 49:1694, 1970.

451. Dubowitz, V.: Acute monocytic leukemia with response to methotrexate. Arch. Dis. Child. 39:289, 1964.

452. Maldonado, J. E., and Hanlon, D. G.: Monocytosis: A current appraisal. Proc. Mayo Clinic 40:248, 1965.

453. Pretlow, T. G.: Chronic monocytic dyscrasia culminating in acute leukemia. Am. J. Med. 46:130, 1969.

454. Knospe, W. H., and Gregory, S. A.: Smoldering acute leukemia. Arch. Intern. Med. (Chicago) 127:910, 1971.

455. Wechsler, L., and Zahavi, J.: The latent period of acute leukemia. Isr. J. Med. Sci. 2:355, 1966.

456. Ghitis, J.: Acute promyelocytic leukemia. Blood 21:237, 1963.

457. Hillestad, L. L.: Acute promyelocytic leukemia. Acta Med. Scand. 159:189, 1957.

458. Rosenthal, R. L.: Acute promyelocytic leukemia associated with hypofibrinogenemia. Blood 21:495, 1963.

459. Didisheim, P., Trombold, J. S., et al.: Acute promyelocytic leukemia with fibrinogen and Factor V deficiencies. Blood 23:717, 1964.

460. Tan, H. T., Wages, B., et al.: Ultrastructural studies in acute promyelocytic leukemia. Blood 39:628, 1972.

461. Rachmilewitz, D., Rachmilewitz, C. A., et al.: Acute promyelocytic leukemia: A report of five cases with a comment on the diagnostic significance of serum vitamin B_{12} determination. Br. J. Haematol. 22:87, 1972.

462. Simons, K., and Weber, T.: The vitamin B_{12} binding protein in human leukocytes. Biochem. Biophys. Acta 117:201, 1966.

463. Corcino, J., Drauso, I., et al.: Release of vitamin B_{12} binding protein by human leukocytes in vitro. J. Clin. Invest. 49:2250, 1970.

464. Gralnick, H. R., Bagley, J., et al.: Heparin treatment for the hemorrhagic diathesis of acute promyclocytic leukemia. Am. J. Med. 52:168, 1972.

465. Rand, J. J., Moloney, W. C., et al.: Coagulation defects in acute promyelocytic leukemia. Arch. Intern. Med. (Chicago) 123:39, 1969.

466. Nilsson, I. M., Sjoerdsma, A., et al.: Antifibrinolytic activity and metabolism of epsilon aminocaproic acid in man. Lancet 1:1322, 1960.

467. Ben-Zee, D., Schwartz, S. O., et al.: Promyelocytic-myelocytic leukemia as a terminal manifestation of chronic granulocytic leukemia. Blood 27:863, 1966.

468. Gralnick, H. R., Bagley, J., et al.: The hemorrhagic diathesis of acute promyelocytic leukemia: pathogenesis and treatment. Program XIII Internatl. Congress Hematol., 1970, p. 52.

469. Scott, R. B., Ellison, R. R., et al.: A clinical study of 20 cases of erythroleukemia (di Guglielmo's syndrome). Am. J. Med. 37:162, 1964.

470. Pierce, M. I., Borges, W. H., et al.: Epidemiological factors and survival experience in 1770 children with acute leukemia. Cancer 23:1296, 1969.

471. Sheets, R. L., Drevets, C. C., et al.: Erythroleukemia (di Guglielmo's syndrome). A report of clinical observations and experimental studies in 7 patients. Arch. Intern. Med. 111:295, 1963.

472. Finkel, H. E., and Brauer, M. J.: Giant eosinophilic granules in the chronic di Guglielmo syndrome. New Engl. J. Med. 274:209, 1966.

473. Staven, P., Hjort, P. F., et al.: Ring-shaped nuclei of granulocytes in a patient with acute erythroleukemia. Scand. J. Haematol. 6:31, 1969.

474. Hayhoe, F. G. J., Quaglino, D., et al.: The cytology and cytochemistry of acute leukaemias. A study of 140 cases. London, Her Majesty's Stationery Office, 1964.

475. Finkel, H. E., Brauer, M. J., et al.: Immunologic aberrations in the di Guglielmo syndrome. Blood 28:634, 1966.

476. White, J. C., Ellis, M., et al.: An unstable hemoglobin associated with some cases of leukaemia. Br. J. Haematol. 6:171, 1960.

477. Beaven, G. H., Ellis, M. J., et al.: Studies on human foetal haemoglobin. II. Foetal haemoglobin levels in healthy children and adults and in certain haematological disorders. Br. J. Haematol. 6:201, 1960.

478. Aksoy, M., and Erdem, S.: Decrease in the concentration of haemoglobin A_2 during erythroleukaemia. Nature (Lond.) 213:522, 1967.

479. Kahn, A., Vroclans, M., et al.: Differences in the two red-cell populations in erythroleukemia. Lancet 2:933, 1971.

480. Emerson, P. M., and Garrow, D. H.: Differences in the two red-cell populations in erythroleukaemia. Lancet 2:1150, 1971.

481. Heath, C. W., Jr., Bennett, J. M., et al.: Cytogenetic findings in erythroleukemia. Blood 33:453, 1969.

482. Krompotic, E., Silberman, S., et al.: Clonal evaluation in di Guglielmo syndrome. Genet. 11:225, 1968.

483. Baldini, M., Fudenberg, H., et al.: The anemia of the di Guglielmo syndrome. Blood 14:334, 1959.

484. Seiner, M., Baldini, M., et al.: Heme synthesis in "refractory" anemia with ineffective erythropoiesis. Blood 22:810, 1963.

485. Necheles, T. F., and Dameshek, W.: The di Guglielmo syndrome: Studies in hemoglobin synthesis. Blood 29:550, 1967.

486. Adamson, J. W., and Finch, C. A.: Erythropoietin and regulation of erythropoiesis in di Guglielmo's syndrome. Blood 36:590, 1970.

487. Gabuzda, T. G., Shute, H. E., et al.: Regulation of erythropoiesis in erythroleukemia. Arch. Intern. Med. (Chicago) 123:60, 1969.

488. Roloff, J. N., and Lukens, J. N.: Dissociation of erythroblastic and myeloblastic proliferation in erythroleukemia. Am. J. Dis. Child. 123:11, 1972.

489. Schwartz, A. D., Zelson, J. H., et al.: Acute myelogenous leukemia with compensatory but ineffective erythropoiesis: di Guglielmo's syndrome. J. Pediatr. 77:653, 1970.

490. Eastman, P., Wallerstein, R. O., et al.: Conversion of polycythemia vera to chronic di Guglielmo's syndrome. J.A.M.A. 204:1141, 1968.

491. Carmel, R., Cottman, C. A., Jr., et al.: Association of paroxysmal nocturnal hemoglobinuria with erythroleukemia. New Engl. J. Med. 283:1329, 1970.

492. Adams, J. F., and Seaton, D. A.: Pathogenesis of megaloblastic anemia in di Guglielmo's disease. Scottish Med. J. 5:145, 1960.

493. O'Brien, J. S.: The role of the folate coenzymes in cellular division. A review. Cancer Res. 22:267, 1962.

494. Beck, W. S.: The metabolic basis of megaloblastic erythropoiesis. Medicine (Baltimore) 43:715, 1964.

495. Gavosto, F., Maraini, G., et al.: Radioautographic investigations on DNA and protein metabolism in 2 cases of the di Guglielmo's disease. Blood 16:1122, 1960.

496. Pierce, M.: Leukemia in the newborn infant. J. Pediatr. 54:691, 1959.

497. Van Eys, J.: Transient spontaneous remission in a case of untreated congenital leukemia. Am. J. Dis. Child. 118:507, 1969.

498. Bernhard, W. G., Gore, I., et al.: Congenital leukemia. Blood 6:990, 1951.

499. Anatassea-Vlachou, C., Cassimos, J., et al.: A case of stem cell leukemia occurring in an infant 38 days old. Ann. Paediatr. (Basel) 196:310, 1961.

500. Bjure, J., Fichtelius, K. E., et al.: On the problem of congenital hemopathies (congenital myeloid and erythemic blood picture). Acta Paediatr. (Uppsala) 49:358, 1960.

501. Wagner, H. P., Tönz, O., et al.: Congenital lymphoid leukaemia case report with chromosomal studies. Helv. Paediatr. Acta 23:591, 1968.

502. Whorton, C. M.: Congenital histiocytic leukemia. Lab. Invest. 9:199, 1960.

503. Krivit, W., and Good, R. A.: Simultaneous occurrence of mongolism and leukemia: Report of a nationwide survey. A.M.A. J. Dis. Child. 94:289, 1957.

504. Engel, R. R., Hammond, D., et al.: Transient congenital leukemia in 7 infants with mongolism. J. Pediatr. 65:303, 1964.

505. Vogel, J. M., and Vogel, P.: Idiopathic histiocytosis: A discussion of eosinophilic granuloma, the Hand-Schüller-Christian syndrome, and the Letterer-Siwe syndrome. Semin. Hematol. 9:349, 1972.

506. Reimann, D. L., Clemmens, R. L., et al.: Congenital acute leukemia. Skin nodules, a first sign. J. Pediatr. 46:415, 1955.

507. Nagao, T., Lampkin, B. C., et al.: A neonate with Down's syndrome and transient abnormal myelopoiesis: Serial blood and bone marrow studies. Blood 36:443, 1970.

508. Schunk, G. J., and Lehman, W. L.: Mongolism and congenital leukemia. J.A.M.A. 155:250, 1954.

509. Lahey, M. E., Beier, F. R., et al.: Leukemia in Down's syndrome. J. Pediatr. 63:189, 1963.

510. Brough, A. J., Jones, D., et al.: Dermal erythropoiesis in neonatal infants: A manifestation of intrauterine viral disease. Pediatrics 40:627, 1967.

511. Ross, J. D., Moloney, W. C., et al.: Ineffective regulation of granulopoiesis masquerading as congenital leukemia in a mongoloid child. J. Pediatr. 63:1, 1963.

512. Gordon, H. W.: Myeloid metaplasia masquerading as neonatal leukemia. Am. J. Dis. Child. 118:932, 1969.

513. Ambs, E., Biren, P., et al.: Problematik der sogenannten Angeborenen Leukamien (Leukamien, Leukamoide Reaktionen, Reticulosen). Z. Kinderheilkd. 83:171, 1965.

514. Killman, S. A.: A biased view on the relapse and remission phases of acute myeloid leukaemia, In The Nature of Leukaemia. Vincent, P. C. (ed.), Sydney, Australia, V.C.N. Blight, 1972, p. 205.

515. Saba, T. M.: Physiology and physiopathology of the reticuloendothelial system. Arch. Intern. Med. (Chicago) 126:1031, 1970.

516. Volkman, A.: The origin and fate of the monocyte. Ser. Haematol. 3:62, 1970.

517. Dargeon, H. W.: Considerations in the treatment of reticuloendotheliosis — The Janeway lecture, 1964. Am. J. Roentgenol. 93:521, 1965.

518. Kissane, J. M., and Smith, M. G.: Pathology of Infancy and Childhood. St. Louis, Mo., C. V. Mosby Co., 1967.

519. Hertz, C. G., and Hambrick, G. W.: Congenital Letterer-Siwe disease. Am. J. Dis. Child. 116:553, 1968.

520. Bonstein, H.: Un cas de maladie de Letterer-Siwe chez le nouveau-né. Schweiz. Z. Allg. Pathol. 18:1257, 1955.

521. Ahnquist, G., and Holyoke, J. B.: Congenital Letterer-Siwe disease (reticuloendotheliosis) in a term stillborn infant. J. Pediatr. 57:897, 1960.

522. Davidson, C.: Xanthomatosis and the central nervous system (Schüller-Christian syndrome). Arch. Neurol. Psychiat. *30*:75, 1933.

523. Tannhauser, S. J.: *Lipoidosis*. 3rd ed. New York, Grune & Stratton, 1958, pp. 345–424.

524. Siegel, J. S., and Coltman, C. A.: Histiocytosis X: Response to vinblastine sulfate. J.A.M.A. *197*:403, 1966.

525. Avery, M. E., McAfee, J. G., et al.: The course and prognosis of reticuloendotheliosis (eosinophilic granuloma, Schüller-Christian disease and Letterer-Siwe disease). Am. J. Med. *22*:636, 1957.

526. Lahey, M. E.: Prognosis in reticuloendotheliosis in children. J. Pediatr. *60*:664, 1962.

527. Smith, T.: Skull-cap showing congenital deficiencies of bone. Trans. Pathol. Soc. (Lond.) *16*:224, 1864–1865.

528. Kay, T. W.: Acquired hydrocephalus with atrophic bone changes, exophthalmos and polyuria. Pennsylvania Med. J. *9*:520, 1905–1906.

529. Hand, A.: Defects of membranous bones, exophthalmos and polyuria in childhood; is it dyspituitarism? Am. J. Med. Sci. *162*:509, 1921.

530. Hand, A.: General tuberculosis. Trans. Pathol. Soc. Phila. *16*:282, 1893.

531. Christian, H. A.: Defects in membranous bones, exophthalmos and diabetes insipidus; an unusual syndrome of dyspituitarism. Med. Clin. North Am. *3*:849, 1920.

532. Schüller, A.: Uber eigenartige Schädeldefekte im Jugendalter. Fortschr. Röntgenstr. *23*:12, 1915–1916.

533. Letterer, E.: Aleukämische Retikulose. Ein Beitrag zu den proliferativen Erkrankungen des Retikuloendothelialapparates. Frankfurt. Z. Pathol. *30*:377, 1924.

534. Siwe, S. A.: Die Reticuloendotheliose—ein neues Krankheitsbild unter den Hepatosplenomegalien. Z. Kinderheilkd. *55*:212, 1933.

535. Abt, A. F., and Denenholz, E. J.: Letterer-Siwe's disease. Splenohepatomegaly associated with widespread hyperplasia of nonlipoid-storing macrophages: Discussion of the so-called reticuloendotheliosis. Am. J. Dis. Child. *51*:499, 1936.

536. Wallgren, A.: Systemic reticuloendothelial granuloma. Am. J. Dis. Child. *60*:471, 1940.

537. Lichtenstein, L., and Jaffe, H. L.: Eosinophilic granuloma of bone. Am. J. Pathol. *16*:595, 1940.

538. Otani, S., and Ehrlich, J. C.: Solitary granuloma of bone simulating primary neoplasm. Am. J. Pathol. *16*:479, 1940.

539. Green, W. T., and Farber, S.: "Eosinophilic or solitary granuloma" of bone. J. Bone Joint Surg. *24*:499, 1942.

540. Jaffe, H. L., and Lichtenstein, L.: Eosinophilic granuloma of bone. Arch. Pathol. *37*:99, 1944.

541. Lichtenstein, L.: Histiocytosis X. Integration of eosinophilic granuloma of bone, "Letterer-Siwe disease," and "Schüller-Christian disease" as related manifestations of a single nosologic entity. Arch. Pathol. *56*:84, 1953.

542. Siwe, S.: The reticuloendothelioses in children. Adv. Pediatr. *4*:117, 1949.

543. Otani, S.: A discussion on eosinophilic granuloma of bone, Letterer-Siwe disease, and Schüller-

544. Lieberman, P. H., Jones, C. R., et al.: A reappraisal of eosinophilic granuloma of bone, Hand-Schüller-Christian syndrome and Letterer-Siwe syndrome. Medicine (Baltimore) *48*:375, 1969.

545. Oberman, H. A.: Idiopathic histiocytosis. A clinicopathologic study of 40 cases and review of the literature on eosinophilic granuloma of bone, Hand-Schüller-Christian disease and Letterer-Siwe disease. Pediatrics *28*:307, 1961.

546. Fowles, J. V., and Bobechko, W. P.: Solitary eosinophilic granuloma of bone. J. Bone Joint Surg. *52B*:238, 1970.

547. Lucaya, J.: Histiocytosis X. Am. J. Dis. Child. *121*:289, 1971.

548. Ochsner, S. F.: Eosinophilic granuloma of bone. Experience with 20 cases. Am. J. Roentgenol. *97*:719, 1966.

549. Avioli, L. V., Lasersohn, J. T., et al.: Histiocytosis X (Schüller-Christian disease): A clinico-pathological survey, review of ten patients and the results of prednisone therapy. Medicine (Baltimore) *42*:119, 1963.

550. Cohen, D. M., Mitchell, C. B., et al.: Letterer-Siwe disease in a newborn. Arch. Pathol. *81*:347, 1966.

551. Rogers, D. L., and Benson, T. E.: Familial Letterer-Siwe disease. Report of a case. J. Pediatr. *60*:550, 1962.

552. Freundlich, E., Amit, S., et al.: Familial occurrence of Letterer-Siwe disease. Arch. Dis. Child. *47*:122, 1972.

553. Juberg, R. C., Kloepfer, H. W., et al.: Genetic determination of acute disseminated histiocytosis X (Letterer-Siwe syndrome). Pediatrics *45*:753, 1970.

554. Bierman, H. R.: Apparent cure of Letterer-Siwe disease. Seventeen-year survival of identical twins with nonlipoid reticuloendotheliosis. J.A.M.A. *196*:368, 1966.

555. Fisher, R. H.: Multiple lesions of bone in Letterer-Siwe disease: Report of a case with culture of a paracolon Arizona bacilli from bone lesions and blood, followed by response to therapy. J. Bone Joint Surg. *35A*:445, 1953.

556. Lightwood, R., and Tizard, J. P.: Recovery from acute infantile non-lipoid reticuloendotheliosis (?Letterer-Siwe's disease). Acta Paediatr. *43* (Suppl. 100):453, 1954.

557. Aronson, R. P.: Streptomycin in Letterer-Siwe's disease. Lancet *1*:889, 1951.

558. Basset, F., and Turiaf, M. J.: Identification par la microscopie électronique de particules de nature probablement virale dans les liaisons granulomateuses d'une histiocytose X pulmonaire. C.R. Acad. Sci. (Paris) *261*:3701, 1965.

559. Basset, F., and Nezelof, C.: L'histiocytose X. Microscope électronique. Culture "in vitro" et histo-enzymologie. Discussion à propos de 21 cas. Revue Fr. Etud. Clin. Biol. *14*:31, 1969.

560. Cancilla, P. A., Lahey, M. E., et al.: Cutaneous lesions of Letterer-Siwe disease. Cancer *20*:1986, 1967.

561. Gianotti, F., Caputo, R., et al.: Ultrastructural

study of giant cells and "Langerhans cell granules" in cutaneous lesions and lymph-node and liver biopsies from four cases of subacute disseminated histiocytosis of Letterer-Siwe. Arch. Klin. Exp. Dermatol. 233:238, 1968.

562. Davidson, R. I., and Shillito, J.: Eosinophilic granuloma of the cervical spine in children. Pediatrics 45:746, 1970.

563. Braunstein, G. D., and Kohler, P. O.: Pituitary function in Hand-Schüller-Christian disease. Evidence for deficient growth-hormone release in patients with short stature. New Engl. J. Med. 286:1225, 1972.

564. Ezrin, C., Chaikoff, R., et al.: Panhypopituitarism caused by Hand-Schüller-Christian disease. Can. Med. Assoc. J. 89:1290, 1963.

565. Rube, J., De La Pava, S., et al.: Histiocytosis X with involvement of brain. Cancer 20:486, 1967.

566. Feinberg, S. B., and Langer, L. O.: Roentgen findings of increased intracranial pressure and communicating hydrocephalus as insidious manifestations of chronic histiocytosis-X. Am. J. Roentgenol. 95:41, 1965.

567. McWilliams, N. B.: Personal observation.

568. Farinacci, C. J., Jeffrey, C., et al.: Eosinophilic granuloma of the lung: Report of 2 cases. U.S. Armed Forces Med. J. 2:1085, 1951.

569. Mazzitello, W. F.: Eosinophilic granuloma of the lung. New Engl. J. Med. 250:804, 1954.

570. Weber, W. N., Margolin, F. R., et al.: Pulmonary histiocytosis X: A review of 18 patients with reports of 6 cases. Am. J. Roentgenol. 107:280, 1969.

571. Keats, T. E., and Crane, J. F.: Cystic changes of the lungs in histiocytosis. Am. J. Dis. Child. 88:764, 1954.

572. Pops, M. A., and Campbell, T.: Gastrointestinal bleeding from ileal ulcerations in histiocytosis X. Arch. Intern. Med. (Chicago) 122:271, 1968.

573. Adams, P., and Kraus, J. E.: Eosinophilic granuloma, an unusual case with involvement of the skin, lungs and kidneys. Arch. Dermatol. Syph. 61:957, 1950.

574. Brown, E. W.: Eosinophilic granuloma of the bladder. J. Urol. 83:665, 1960.

575. Mauer, A. M.: Textbook on Pediatric Hematology. New York, Blakiston Division, McGraw-Hill Book Co., 1969, p. 398.

576. Beier, F. R., Thatcher, L. G., et al.: Treatment of reticuloendotheliosis with vinblastine sulfate. J. Pediatr. 63:1087, 1963.

577. Winkelmann, R. K., and Burgert, E. O.: Therapy of histiocytosis X. Br. J. Dermatol. 82:169, 1970.

578. Esterly, N. B., and Swick, H. M.: Cutaneous Letterer-Siwe disease. Am. J. Dis. Child. 117:236, 1969.

579. Al-Rashid, R. A.: Successful treatment of an infant with Letterer-Siwe disease with vinblastine sulfate. Clin. Pediatr. 9:494, 1970.

580. Sharp, H., White, J. G., et al.: "Histiocytosis X" treated with vinblastine sulfate. Cancer Chemother. Rep. 39:53, 1964.

581. Starling, K. A., Donaldson, M. H., et al.: Therapy of histiocytosis X with vincristine, vinblastine and cyclophosphamide. Am. J. Dis. Child. 123:105, 1972.

582. Ekert, H., and Campbell, P. E.: Histiocytosis X: A review of experience at the Royal Children's Hospital, Melbourne, 1948–1963. Aust. Paediatr. J. 3:139, 1966.

583. Scott, R. B., and Robb-Smith, A. H. T.: Histiocytic medullary reticulosis. Lancet 2:194, 1939.

584. Farquhar, J. W., and Claireaux, A. E.: Familial haemophagocytic reticulosis. Arch. Dis. Child. 27:519, 1952.

585. Nelson, P., Santamaria, A., et al.: Generalized lymphohistiocytic infiltration. Pediatrics 27:931, 1961.

586. Falk, W., and Gellei, B.: The familial occurrence of Letterer-Siwe disease. Acta Paediatr. 46:471, 1957.

587. Boake, W. C., Card, W. M., et al.: Histiocytic medullary reticulosis: Concurrence in father and son. Arch. Intern. Med. (Chicago) 116:245, 1965.

588. Mozziconacci, P., Nezelof, C., et al.: La lymphohistiocytose familiale. Arch. Fr. Pediatr. 22:385, 1965.

589. Buist, N. R., Jones, R. N., et al.: Familial haemophagocytic reticulosis in first cousins. Arch. Dis. Child. 46:728, 1971.

590. MacMahon, H. E., Bedizel, M., et al.: Familial erythrophagocytic lymphohistiocytosis. Pediatrics 32:868, 1963.

591. Chih-Fei, Y., Chung-Hang, T., et al.: Histiocytic medullary reticulosis. Chinese Med. J. 80:466, 1960.

592. Bast, R. C., Jr., Zbar, B., et al.: BCG and cancer. New Engl. J. Med. 290:1413, 1458, 1974.

Chapter 23

Malignant Lymphoma

by Jeffrey A. Gottlieb

INTRODUCTION

Although the first medical description of malignant lymphoma appeared in 1832 when Thomas Hodgkin published his paper entitled "On Some Morbid Appearances of the Absorbent Glands and Spleen" (1), it was not until 1865, when Wilks added a number of cases to the literature, that the illness was first referred to as Hodgkin's disease (2). It is of interest to note that in 1926 Fox discovered the seven specimens originally described by Hodgkin in the Hunterian Museum and found that three, including one of the two children in the series, had disseminated tuberculosis rather than Hodgkin's disease (3). The term "lymphosarcoma" was used in an ill-defined manner by Virchow in 1863, but it was not until 1893 that Kundrat characterized lymphosarcoma as a disease that was both pathologically and clinically distinguishable from leukemia and Hodgkin's disease (4). The addition of reticulum cell sarcoma as a further division of malignant lymphoma was made by Oberling in 1928 (5), and the most recent of the clinical lymphoma syndromes, that of Burkitt's tumor, was first described by Denis Burkitt in 1958 (6).

Over the past two decades, considerable interest in almost all aspects of the malignant lymphomas has led to a rapid increase in our ability to characterize and understand the clinical courses of these diseases, with a resulting pronounced improvement in treatment. It is the purpose of this chapter to emphasize the developments of the patho-physiologic concepts which have made such progress possible. Because much of the research pertinent to the malignant lymphomas as a whole has begun with studies of Hodgkin's disease, this entity will be dealt with in the greatest detail, although the other non-Hodgkin's lymphomas, including Burkitt's tumor, will also be emphasized.

HODGKIN'S DISEASE*

Definition

The term "malignant lymphoma" is used to describe malignant tumors of reticular tissue, composed of primitive reticular cells and their histiocytic lymphocytic derivatives. For a lymphoma to be characterized as Hodgkin's disease, the neoplastic element must include malignant histiocytes with characteristic features of the Reed-Sternberg cells described below. Since mononuclear inflammatory cells are usually associated with malignant histiocytic proliferation, these inflammatory cells, rather than the neoplastic histiocytes, often form the bulk of the tumor. The characteristics and proportion of these various inflammatory cells are essential to the further pathologic subdivisions of this disease (7).

---

*For complete reviews of the subject, the reader is referred to Kaplan, H. S.: *Hodgkin's Disease.* Cambridge, Harvard University Press, 1972; Smithers, D. (ed.): *Hodgkin's Disease.* London, Churchill Livingstone, 1973; and Rosenberg, S. A. (ed.): Hodgkin's Disease and other lymphomas. Clin. Haematol. 3, No. 1, 1974.

Etiology

While the exact etiology of Hodgkin's disease remains elusive, many recent studies have emphasized the possible causal relationship of several viral and immunologic interactions. The initial clinical descriptions of this disease, which included a history of fever, weight loss, night sweats, as well as an often accompanying leukocytosis, suggested to many early investigators that the illness had an infectious origin. When early pathologic studies failed to uncover an infectious agent, these theories were discarded. However, triggered by the initial observation of Burkitt, in which he noted that the tumor subsequently named after him had a geographic distribution suggesting possible vector transmission (8), an infectious etiology for all lymphomas was reexamined. The discovery of high antibody titers against the Epstein-Barr virus (a new herpes-like virus) in patients with Burkitt's tumor (9) further suggested an infectious etiology. While subsequent studies have been somewhat disappointing because of the finding of this same virus in association with other neoplastic and non-neoplastic conditions (10), the hypothesis that Hodgkin's disease may be due to a virus of low virulence persists. According to these theories, viruses cause antigenic alterations on the surface of lymphocytes. These changes then lead to a chronic immune reaction (not unlike a graft-versus-host reaction), with the resultant appearance of neoplastic cells (11, 12). In keeping with this hypothesis, a new tumor antigen has recently been described in the splenic cells of three patients with Hodgkin's disease (13). In addition, there is well-established evidence that oncogenic viruses may induce lymphoma by an immunologic mechanism in experimental animal models. Thus, if mice are injected with foreign lymphoid cells, they usually develop a severe graft-versus-host reaction which rapidly leads to death. However, if the lymphoid cells injected have only minimal genetic differences, or if the graft-versus-host reaction is attenuated with immunosuppressive drugs, a chronic reaction is established, which is associated with a prolonged survival. In this setting, a number of the mice develop a histiocytic lymphoma which has been shown to be of host cell origin and which contains an associated oncogenic virus. This suggests that the chronic graft-versus-host reaction activates a latent virus, leading to the development of the malignancy (14).

The increased incidence of lymphoreticular neoplasms arising in patients undergoing chronic immunosuppression (15) (described in greater detail in a later section) also lends further support to the hypothesis that in such a setting, an etiologic agent of low virulence could trigger the events described above, leading to the establishment of a malignant clone. While it is tempting to correlate many of the clinical features of Hodgkin's disease with these theories (11, 12, 16), definite laboratory confirmation of these views must occur before an infectious etiology can be accepted as anything but hypothesis. It is of interest, however, that an "epidemic" of Hodgkin's disease has recently been described by Vianna and his colleagues. Thirty-one cases of Hodgkin's disease have been carefully interlinked in a group of students attending a particular high school in Albany County of New York in the period 1950 through 1970. Personal contact among these students has been well documented, and chance alone as an explanatory mechanism has been seemingly excluded (17). Exploration of other clusterings which suggest an infectious origin of this disease are currently in progress (17a, 18).

Epidemiology

The detailed epidemiologic studies of Hodgkin's disease in the United States by MacMahon have shown this disease to have a bimodal incidence peak. The first peak occurs in children and young adults. In this age group, the disease has a fairly good prognosis, with an epidemiology seemingly more characteristic of an infectious disease. The second peak occurs predominantly in patients over the age of 40 and has a much less optimistic prognosis, with epidemiologic characteristics more suggestive of a classical neoplasm. It has also been shown that the incidence of Hodgkin's disease in the young male (under 14 years) is nearly three times that in females, while in older age groups the incidence in both sexes appears quite similar, thus further emphasizing the difference of the disease in the two age peaks (19). Other epidemiologic features have shown a decreasing trend in the incidence of Hodgkin's disease in children as opposed to an increase in the older age groups, and a peculiar geographic pattern of higher childhood incidence rates in several parts of the United States and the world. For example, at least two nations, Peru (20) and Lebanon (21), have a relatively increased incidence of pediatric Hodgkin's disease, as compared with their adult populations, and excessive mortality from this disease in children has been noted in the west-south-central part of the United States, an area which has the lowest rates of Hodgkin's disease mortality in the older age groups (22).

The epidemiologic features summarized above have led Cole et al. to argue that, if Hodgkin's disease of the young is considered as a separate entity, with its etiology, pathophysiology, and prognosis individually investigated, the results of such research may be more fruitful than if all Hodgkin's disease is considered as one entity. They feel that etiologic studies which focus on the young, where an infectious etiology hypothesis seems more promising, will prevent the overall confusion that may develop if all Hodgkin's disease is studied together (23). The rationale of such a theory is appealing and has led to several on going epidemiologic investigations (24).

Incidence

Each year in the United States, there are approximately 3700 deaths from Hodgkin's disease in all age groups (25). For patients under the age of 15 years, the yearly death rate from this illness is approximately 1.2 per million at risk, thus accounting for slightly less than 2 per cent of all deaths from malignancy in childhood (26). The disease has only rarely been described before the age of 2 (27), with the majority of childhood cases occurring in the second decade of life. In virtually all published series, there is a male predominance in Hodgkin's disease in children, especially in the age group from 4 to 15 years. The reason for this sex distribution discrepancy remains unknown. It is much less evident in late adolescence and young adulthood (19). Recent figures have suggested that the in-

cidence of this disease in children has been slowly decreasing over the last 40 years (19).

Histopathology

The histologic picture of Hodgkin's disease is characterized by a complex mixture of lymphoreticular, plasma, and granulocytic cells on a fibrous matrix. There is often a striking paucity of obviously malignant appearing cells. Reed-Sternberg cells, however, are seen in all types of Hodgkin's disease, and indeed their presence is an essential prerequiste for the diagnosis of this tumor. As shown in Figure 23–1, these cells are atypical histiocytes, which vary in size from 15 to 45 microns and have abundant, slightly basophilic cytoplasm. Their nuclei are usually either bilobed or multilobed and contain large prominent nucleoli, resulting in the often used descriptive term "owl's eyes." Although mononuclear histiocytes with similar histologic characteristics are often observed, few pathologists are willing to make the diagnosis of Hodgkin's disease without the presence of at least some cells with bilobed or multilobed nuclei (7).

While the Reed-Sternberg cell is considered the sine qua non of Hodgkin's disease, it is not pathognomonic for this condition since cells of similar appearance have been reported in many other diseases, some of which are benign (28). Perhaps the most important conditions to be considered in the differential diagnosis in children are infectious mononucleosis and adenopathy associated with chronic diphenylhydantoin (Dilantin) administration. This last entity has occasionally been called pseudolymphoma, since it may be associated with fever, eosinophilia, hepatosplenomegaly, and even arthralgia (29). While the majority of patients developing Reed-Sternberg cells in this setting have a benign, self-limited disease which upon discontinuation of the offending drug will disappear, there are now documented reports of patients who have subsequently developed actual lymphoma. Although the number of such cases is small, the question of diphenylhydantoin carcinogenicity must be considered (30, 30a, 30b). Other diseases rarely associated with Reed-Sternberg–like cells include rubeola,

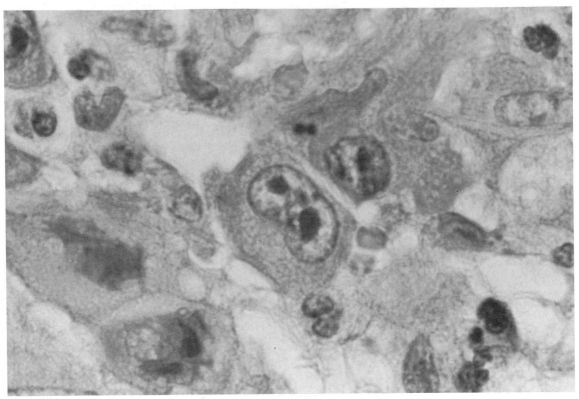

Figure 23–1.   Reed-Sternberg histiocyte. Bilobed cell with prominent nucleoli is readily recognized. Hematoxylin-eosin (× 400).

thymoma, and other non-Hodgkin's lymphomas (28).

The relationship between prognosis and histopathology in Hodgkin's disease was first emphasized by Rosenthal in 1936 (31). Subsequently a number of investigators have put forward schemes of classification in which the peculiarities of the histologic structure were correlated with clinical course. In the 1940's, Jackson and Parker proposed a classification dividing the disease into three forms: paragranuloma, which had a predominant lymphocytic proliferation and was associated with a more prolonged survival; granuloma, in which lymphocytes were less common and which was associated with a varied prognosis; and sarcoma, a rare type associated with the predominant proliferation of neoplastic reticulum cells with a rapidly progressive, downhill course (32). This divisional concept was useful, but the relative infrequency of the paragranuloma and sarcoma subtypes led to assignment of nearly 90 per cent of the patients to the granuloma subtype (33).

Lukes and Butler in the 1960's proposed a new four-part histologic classification which has subsequently proved more useful in its prognostic significance and has therefore become widely accepted (33). The first of the four groups, lymphocyte predominance (Fig. 23–2), contains prominent lymphocyte proliferation and accounts for a larger number of patients than the paragranuloma group of Jackson and Parker. The second division, and perhaps the most important contribution of the Lukes and Butler classification, is the nodular sclerosis group (Fig. 23–3), which had previously been part of the Jackson and Parker granuloma subtype. In this histologic category, there are large, interconnecting, birefringent bands of dense collagen. These interconnecting bands isolate nodules of lymphoid tissue containing occasional Reed-Sternberg cells, with the latter frequently surrounded by a large clear space or lacuna. The extent of the clear space depends on the fixative used in tissue processing. In the third type, mixed cellularity, there is a relatively equal representation of lymphocytes and Reed-Stern-

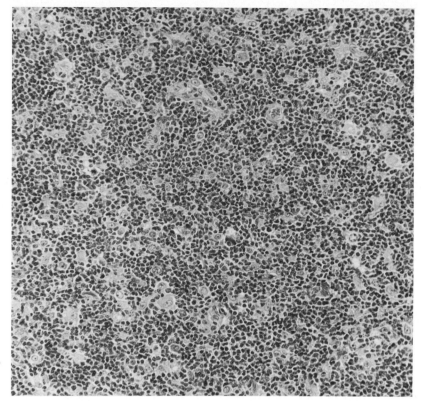

Figure 23–2. Lymphocyte predominance Hodgkin's disease. Many diverse lymphocytes are noted with only occasional Reed-Sternberg cells. Hematoxylin-eosin (× 50).

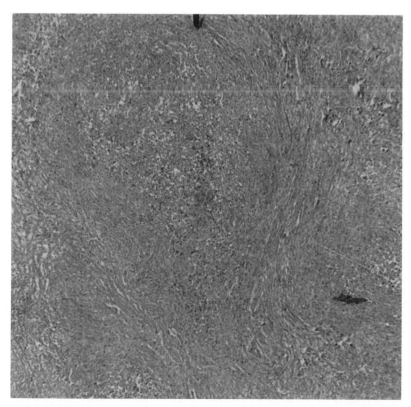

Figure 23–3. Nodular sclerosis Hodgkin's disease. Collagen bands surround small lymphoid nodules. Hematoxylin-eosin (× 9).

berg histiocytes (Fig. 23–4). The final subtype, lymphocyte depletion, has a diffuse reticular fibrosis with few lymphocytes, many Reed-Sternberg cells, and no collagen bands (Fig. 23–5) (33). Many investigators have suggested that the better prognosis associated with the first two of these histologic categories (as emphasized below) may be related to the host reaction to disease, thus "walling off" the tumor with a sheet of lymphocytes in lymphocyte predominance and with collagen bands in nodular sclerosis (11, 16), but laboratory evidence supporting such a theory is lacking.

The relative distribution of these four cell types in childhood, as reported in five recently published large American series, appears in Table 23–1. As shown by this table, the most common cell type is nodular sclerosis, which accounts for approximately half the patients in these series. The lymphocyte predominance and mixed cellularity subtypes have a relatively equal distribution, with lymphocyte depletion a rarity in children. This distribution varies from the pattern observed in elderly patients, in whom the lymphocyte depletion and mixed cellularity subtypes predominate (39).

In several series in which patients have had multiple biopsies over a period of years, there is a suggestion that, as the disease progresses, patients move from lymphocyte predominance and nodular sclerosis categories toward the mixed cellularity and lymphocyte depletion categories (40). However, in all these studies, the effect of therapy must be considered, and whether it is indeed the natural course of the disease to go from lymphocyte predominance to lymphocyte depletion has not yet been well documented. The importance of the new classification of Lukes and Butler becomes apparent when the prognostic significance is examined. Thus Butler has shown that the median survival for children with lymphocyte predominance is 8.4 years; for nodular sclerosis, 4.1 years; for mixed cellularity, 3.3 years; and for lymphocyte depletion, 1.4 years (38). It is important to recognize that other factors, notably extent of disease and

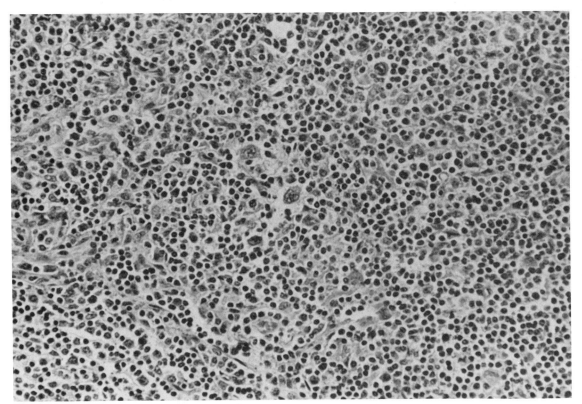

Figure 23–4.   Mixed cellularity Hodgkin's disease. Lymphocytes and histiocytes occur in almost equal numbers. Hematoxylin-eosin (× 100).

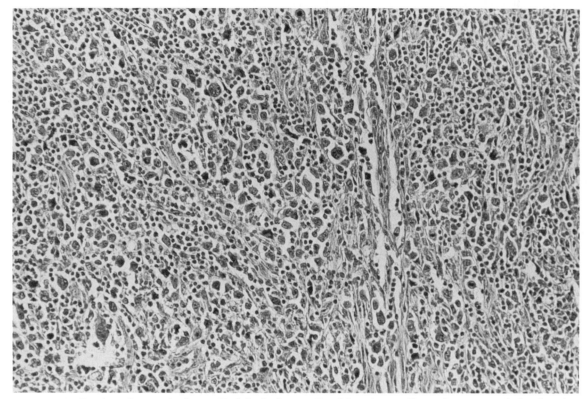

Figure 23–5. Lymphocyte depletion Hodgkin's disease. Reed-Sternberg cells predominate with few lymphocytes. Hematoxylin-eosin (× 100).

age, influence prognosis as well, and these variables are all interlinked, thus making it difficult to isolate one prognostic sign without taking the others into consideration (39).

Recently, Rappaport and Strum noted a small proportion of patients with vascular invasion by the tumor in the lymph node. This was seen more frequently in the lymphocyte depletion subtype and was at least retrospectively associated with an espe-cially unfavorable prognosis (41). These observations could be particularly important with regard to the mode of spread of Hodgkin's disease as discussed below.

Clinical Presentation

Hodgkin's disease usually presents as a painless, enlarged, superficial lymph node,

TABLE 23–1. DISTRIBUTION OF CELL TYPES IN HODGKIN'S DISEASE OF CHILDREN

| | | | HISTOLOGIC DIAGNOSIS | | |
| REFERENCE | | Lymphocyte Predominance | Nodular Sclerosis | Mixed Cellularity | Lymphocyte Depletion |
			(Number of Patients)		
Strum and Rappaport, 1970 (34)	(31 patients)	6	24	1	0
Shah et al., 1972 (35)	(52 patients)	12	19	18	3
Norris et al., 1972 (36)	(116 patients)	22	67	24	3
Santiago et al., 1970 (37)	(31 patients)	9	10	10	2
Butler, 1969 (38)	(56 patients)	6	23	20	7
Totals	(286 patients)	55(19%)	143(50%)	73(26%)	15(5%)

generally in the cervical area. An antecedent history of the node waxing and waning
in size is not uncommon, and frequently
such patients will have received antibiotics
for presumed lymphadenitis. While cervical
adenopathy predominates as the presenting
sign in children (having been found in approximately 90 per cent of childhood cases),
other lymph nodes, including those in the
axillary and inguinal regions, may also be
involved in 10 to 20 per cent of cases. Enlargement of the spleen or liver is relatively
unusual at initial presentation, and pulmonary complaints are also relatively rare in
Hodgkin's disease (as opposed to the non-
Hodgkin's lymphomas). However, asymptomatic mediastinal adenopathy, visible on a
chest x-ray, can be expected in approximately one-quarter of patients with occasional pleural effusions as well. Rarely, the
initial complaint will stem from skeletal or
central nervous system involvement (34, 37,
42, 43).

The extent of the patient's systemic symptoms at diagnosis is extremely important
with regard to the current staging categories
described below. Specifically, the occurrence of fever, night sweats, or weight loss
of 10 per cent or more of the normal body
weight has been shown to effect prognosis
adversely (39). The etiology of fever and
night sweats in Hodgkin's disease is poorly
understood. One theory, proposed by
Young and Hodas, suggests that the fever is
due to an α-globulin present in the urine of
febrile patients, presumably produced by
their tumor cells (44). This globulin disappears with the cessation of fever, usually as
a result of therapy. Studies using cyclohex-
imide, a specific protein synthesis inhibitor
(45), have been shown to decrease the
amount of this globulin, suggesting that it
may be possible to decrease the fever without otherwise affecting the tumor.

The etiology of the weight loss associated
with this malignancy is also unknown. The
psychosomatic effects of having cancer are
hardly applicable as an explanation for the
often pronounced weight loss seen in very
young patients with lymphoma. It has recently been observed that some cachectic
patients have increased levels of catabolic
hydrolyzing enzymes, but the mechanism
for this increase remains obscure (46).

Pruritus, seen in approximately 15 per
cent of adults, particularly in young women
with mediastinal nodular sclerosis, has
been recorded relatively infrequently in
childhood. In the past this symptom has
been associated with a poor prognosis. Recently, the prognostic significance of this
symptom has been questioned, and currently the presence of pruritus no longer
qualifies a patient for a "symptomatic" staging. The itching tends to disappear with effective therapy (47).

Laboratory Findings

Routine laboratory tests are relatively
unrevealing at the initial presentation of
most children with Hodgkin's disease. Mild
degrees of anemia may be observed early
and have been noted to correlate in some
series with visceral involvement. Leukocytosis with an eosinophilia and relative lymphopenia is not uncommon, and the latter
may correlate with impaired cellular immunity (see below). Nonspecific elevation of
several acute phase-reactive proteins is a
common occurrence. The elevation of fibrinogen with the associated elevation of
the erythrocyte sedimentation rate is perhaps the most consistent finding in early
Hodgkin's disease of childhood (48). Similarly, an elevation of the α_2-globulins with
a concomitant increase in haptoglobin and
serum copper is also frequently observed
(49). Low levels of serum iron have been
reported in a number of children with this
disease, but the reason for this finding is not
understood (48). While none of the above
tests can be considered specific for Hodgkin's disease, an overall pattern of the abnormalities described above may raise suspicion of the likelihood of this diagnosis.

In the absence of specific organ involvement, serum enzyme studies are usually
within normal limits. The alkaline phosphatase may be elevated when the liver or
bones are involved. However, the lack of
correlation of serum alkaline phosphatase
activity with such organ involvement is well
established (50). Decreased levels of pyridoxal phosphate, along with abnormalities
of tryptophan metabolism, which revert to
normal with complete remission have also
been observed. As such, they may serve as a
reversible biochemical indicator of the degree of activity of Hodgkin's disease (51).

In the past decade, considerable research

has dealt with the problem of the immune status of the patient with Hodgkin's disease. While anergy to a variety of skin tests as a manifestation of impaired delayed hypersensitivity has been seen in approximately one-quarter of patients at presentation, this characteristic currently seems to have little prognostic significance by itself. Skin test reactivity as well as the absolute peripheral lymphocyte count may correlate, however, with the extent of disease and with each other. Thus, both the mean absolute lymphocyte count and the incidence of skin test reactivity to certain antigen doses tend to fall in more advanced stages, and both are generally increased in earlier stages (52). Similar studies have shown an impairment in the ability of peripheral leukocyte cultures from patients with Hodgkin's disease to undergo phytohemagglutinin-induced lymphocyte transformation (53).

Although the association of anergy in Hodgkin's disease has been known for several decades, the reason for anergy in this disease is still poorly understood. Several hypotheses regarding the etiology of Hodgkin's disease hinge on the implication that the patient with this illness may have impaired immune surveillance and thus be more susceptible to the growth of a malignant clone of cells. Whether anergy increases the susceptibility of a patient to develop Hodgkin's disease or is a manifestation of this illness remains controversial. Nevertheless, the increased frequency of opportunistic infections in these patients has been attributed in part to the inadequate host defense systems documented by these studies.

Mode of Spread

The initial presentation of Hodgkin's disease, as discussed above, most commonly involves cervical lymph nodes. As the disease progresses, an increased frequency of mediastinal and axillary adenopathy is observed, followed by involvement of the para-aortic lymph nodes, spleen, and finally liver. Observations concerning the frequency of involvement of various anatomic sites have led to some important hypotheses regarding the mode of dissemination in this illness. The theory of unifocal origin with contiguous spread, in which one group of lymph nodes becomes involved by spread from other previously involved nodes in close proximity, has strongly influenced the therapeutic philosophy adopted by most clinicians (54). Gilbert initially demonstrated the so-called "prophylactic" effect of extended field radiation in Hodgkin's disease (54a). Peters was one of the first in North America to note that the radiation of the lymph nodes adjacent to those nodes known to be involved with Hodgkin's disease led to an improved duration of the disease-free state and ultimately of survival (55). This concept of treating the extended field as opposed to the involved field (discussed in greater detail below) has been further extended by Kaplan (56) and Johnson (57). They have argued that all lymph node–bearing areas may be considered susceptible to spread of Hodgkin's disease, and therefore all nodes require radiotherapy (which has led to the radiotherapeutic approach of total nodal irradiation). The high correlation between left cervical and left supraclavicular adenopathy with para-aortic abdominal adenopathy has led Kaplan to suggest that Hodgkin's disease spreads in a retrograde fashion from the neck to the abdomen via the thoracic duct (54). While such a hypothesis is in keeping with the observed pattern of involvement, evidence to support such retrograde spread of Hodgkin's disease has not yet been produced (58). More recently, Rappaport and Strum have shown that, in some cases of lymphocyte depletion, there is a tendency for vascular invasion within the lymph node (41). Several recent investigations from the Netherlands have also shown an increased incidence of alleged tumor cells in the blood of patients with advanced Hodgkin's disease (59, 60). Thus hematogenous spread may occur in certain cases.

Clinical Staging

In planning a patient's therapeutic program, it is of utmost importance at the time of diagnosis to determine the extent and location of disease. This procedure is called staging. The current staging classification for Hodgkin's disease is summarized in Table 23–2. These definitions were agreed upon at a recent Ann Arbor Symposium (61) and have been proposed to replace the pre-

TABLE 23–2. STAGING CLASSIFICATION OF HODGKIN'S DISEASE AS RECOMMENDED BY THE ANN ARBOR SYMPOSIUM°

Stage I   Involvement of a single lymph node region (I) or of a single extralymphatic organ or site (I_E)

Stage II   Involvement of two or more lymph node regions on the same side of the diaphragm (II) or localized involvement (by direct extension) of an extralymphatic organ or site and one or more lymph node regions on the same side of the diaphragm (II_E)

Stage III Involvement of lymph node regions on both sides of the diaphragm (III), which may also be accompanied by localized involvement (by direct extension) of an extralymphatic organ or site (III_E) or by the involvement of the spleen or both

Stage IV   Diffuse or disseminated involvement of one or more extralymphatic organs or tissues with or without associated lymph node enlargement

All stages are sublcassified as "A" or "B" to indicate the absence or presence, respectively, of these systemic symptoms: (1) unexplained fever, (2) night sweats, and/or (3) weight loss greater than 10 per cent of normal body weight.

°From Carbone, P. P., Kaplan, H. S., et al.: Cancer Res. *31*:1860, 1971.

vious staging definitions suggested at the Rye Conference in 1966 (62). The concept of Hodgkin's disease being a unifocal illness with contiguous disease spread is implied in the adoption of this staging system. Because of their limited involvement, Stages I and II are considered early stages.

In Stages III and IV the extent of spread and amount of tumor is considerable, thus leading to the connotation of "advanced stage" patients.

The major difference between the Ann Arbor classification and the Rye classification is the concept of extranodal involvement by extension (E). Thus patients with a single focus of lung involvement as a direct extension of hilar lymphadenopathy were shown by Musshoff to have the same prognosis as patients with hilar adenopathy alone (63). On the other hand, if the area of lung involvement was not adjacent to the hilar nodes (and thus presumably representing distant spread as opposed to contiguous extension), the prognosis was grave. The same observation has been made in patients with bone and skin involvement by direct extension, but apparently does not apply to liver involvement; in other words, the direct extension of Hodgkin's disease into the liver from lymph nodes in the porta hepatis remains a grave prognostic sign. Patients with a single extranodal focus as their only evidence of Hodgkin's disease were also shown to have an excellent prognosis, and thus are now considered as having early-stage disease rather than late-stage disease, as had been the case in the Rye classification system.

The other major change in the Ann Arbor criteria is the substitution of a 10 per cent body weight loss for pruritus in the symptomatology category, with patients subclassified as "A" or "B," indicating the absence or presence, respectively, of the systemic symptoms listed (47, 61).

In Table 23–3 it is shown that the majority of children present with early-stage disease,

TABLE 23–3. DISTRIBUTION OF STAGING CLASSIFICATION IN HODGKIN'S DISEASE OF CHILDREN

REFERENCE		STAGE			
		Stage I	Stage II	Stage III	Stage IV
			(Number of Patients)		
Shah et al., 1972 (35)	(57 patients)	20	21	6	10
Norris et al., 1972 (36)	(113 patients)	30	50	24	9
Strum and Rappaport, 1970 (34)	(16 patients)	7	5	4	0
Santiago et al., 1970 (37)	(31 patients)	3	8	13	7
Teillet and Schweisguth, 1968 (64)	(72 patients)	22	22	20	8
Total	(289 patients)	82(28%)	106(37%)	67(23%)	34(12%)

and again the opposite is observed in patients over 40 (39). There is an indirect relationship between stage and survival, i.e., the lower the stage, the longer the survival. Thus Butler has shown that the five-year survival rate for Stage I and II disease is 80 per cent; for Stage III, 33 per cent; and for Stage IV, only 14 per cent—clearly emphasizing the importance of this prognostic factor (38).

In addition to its prognostic value, staging is also a critical prerequisite in the planning of each child's therapeutic program. Table 23–4 summarizes the current procedures most frequently utilized to determine accurately the stage of pediatric patients. Tomograms of the mediastinum and lungs are often extremely helpful in determining the extent of hilar lymphadenopathy or pulmonary involvement. Lymphography has been

TABLE 23–4. PROCEDURES IN STAGING CHILDREN WITH HODGKIN'S DISEASE

History and physical examination
Lymph node biopsy establishing diagnosis
Laboratory studies
  a) Complete blood count, including platelet count
  b) Erythrocyte sedimentation rate; fibrinogen, serum copper
  c) Renal and liver function tests
  d) Serum protein electrophoresis

Radiologic studies
  a) Chest x-ray (lateral and posterior anterior views); ? mediastinal tomography
  b) Lymphography
  c) ? Inferior vena cavagram and intravenous pyelogram
  d) Skeletal survey

Nuclear medicine studies
  a) Liver and spleen scan
  b) Bone scan
  c) ? Total-body [67]gallium scan

Bone marrow biopsy and aspiration

Immunologic studies
  a) Skin tests for evaluating delayed hypersensitivity (*Candida*, mumps, PPD, etc.)
  b) ?DNCB sensitization
  c) ? Immunoelectrophoresis

Exploratory laparotomy
  a) Lymph node biopsies
  b) Wedge liver biopsy
  c) Splenectomy
  d) Disease boundary marking for radiotherapy
  e) In girls, oophoropexy

shown practical, even in very young children (e.g., 15 months of age), but it does require an experienced radiologist. Sedation or anesthesia is to be recommended because of the small lymphatic vessel size, as well as the duration of the study (65). Lymphography is useful not only in delineating the extent of para-aortic lymph node involvement but also as a means of subsequently evaluating the response of these lymph nodes to therapy. In 59 lymphograms done in two series of children, 32 (54 per cent) were interpreted as positive, thus clearly indicating the high yield of this procedure (65, 66). Inferior vena cavography and intravenous pyelography were recommended as standard procedures for demonstrating retroperitoneal lymphadenopathy before lymphography was introduced. However, this last procedure has made visualization of the retroperitoneal lymph nodes much more accurate, thus decreasing the importance of the former contrast studies. The pyelogram may be advisable to establish renal anatomy and location before particular operative or radiotherapeutic approaches are begun. A skeletal survey and bone scan will detect almost all cases of bone involvement with Hodgkin's disease. Radioisotopic scanning of the liver and spleen have also proved helpful in detecting tumor involvement of these organs, although false-positives and false-negatives are not uncommon (67, 68). Whole-body scanning with [67]gallium has recently been introduced as a possible superior isotopic procedure (69). For the detection of bone marrow involvement with lymphoma, several studies have shown that aspiration is an inadequate procedure. Percutaneous biopsy of the marrow has therefore recently been recommended in the work-up of all patients with Hodgkin's disease (70).

As emphasized before, immune response tests, while of little help prognostically, can be used to follow a patient's response to therapy. In addition, anergic patients may be more susceptible to opportunistic infections and thus require more careful observation. The reestablishment of delayed hypersensitivity is an encouraging sign that a patient's therapy is effective. Since many small children have not yet developed enough contact with the common skin antigens to evince delayed hypersensitivity, dinitrochlorobenzene (DNCB) is used as a testing agent (52).

Over the last several years, exploratory laparotomy has become part of the staging procedure in many different institutions (71, 71a). This operation permits direct visualization of the liver and spleen as well as open biopsy of the lymph nodes in the para-aortic region and in other areas where involvement is suspected. Splenectomy, which permits whole organ histologic examination, and wedge biopsy of the liver have been found to be the most accurate procedures for assessing tumor involvement of these organs (72). Lymph nodes thought to be suspicious on lymphography can also be biopsied, as well as lymph nodes in regions not visualized by lymphography (e.g., porta hepatis, stomach, splenic hilum, and mesentery). In the female, the ovaries can be removed from the radiotherapeutic port (oophoropexy), so that adequate irradiation can be given often without inducing sterilization (73).

Recent data have shown that the clinical stage of approximately one-third of patients undergoing laparotomy has been altered by the findings of this operation (71, 71a, 74). If the findings at laparotomy influence the therapeutic plan for a patient, the procedure can be extremely useful. If the results of a laparotomy will not change the treatment (such as in the case of bone marrow involvement, when chemotherapy is recommended regardless of the surgical findings), then it is difficult to recommend this procedure. The role of splenectomy in this disease is still controversial. While removal of the spleen permits the most accurate staging and eliminates the need for radiating this organ (and thus also decreasing the risk of radiation-induced damage to the adjacent lung and kidney), the hazards of splenectomy in the young have been emphasized by a number of recent studies (75, 76), and indeed serious infections in the splenectomized Hodgkin's patient have already been well documented (77). Further data must be accumulated before splenectomy can be routinely recommended.

Therapy

The majority of therapeutic advances in Hodgkin's disease have been made in adult populations. While most of the principles learned from these studies seem applicable to childhood, it must be emphasized that relatively few investigations of modern therapeutic concepts have been carried out in children.

The role of surgery in Hodgkin's disease has been predominantly one of biopsy and laparotomy for establishment of diagnosis. Occasional extranodal foci may require surgical intervention to relieve acute symptoms (e.g., intestinal obstruction), but lymph node dissections are contraindicated since radiotherapeutic and chemotherapeutic procedures have been proved more effective.

Radiotherapy has been shown to be an extremely effective treatment modality in Hodgkin's disease. The advent of megavoltage equipment, such as the cobalt-60 unit and the linear accelerator, has made it possible to deliver high doses of radiotherapy capable of killing neoplastic cells with relative sparing of adjacent normal tissues. The studies of Peters (55) and Kaplan (56) have demonstrated that long-term survival with radiotherapy alone in Stage I and II patients can be regularly achieved. Some patients with more advanced disease may also be similarly benefited. In a series limited to children, Young and his co-workers were able to show a five-year survival rate in excess of 80 per cent for patients with localized disease treated with modern aggressive radiotherapy (78).

The exact treatment technique for patients with early-stage disease is still uncertain. Controlled studies in adult populations are currently comparing the effects of treatment of just the tumor-bearing region (involved field) with treatment of the involved field plus the adjacent contiguous lymph nodes (extended field). The results thus far suggest no difference in the overall survival rate between these two groups (79), but patients who are symptomatic (i.e., Stage B) have been shown to have a poor survival when treated only with involved field as opposed to extended field technique (79a). Because of the late effects of irradiation in children, treatment of the involved field may be a more advisable course in children with Stage I and IIA disease, until the several controlled studies still in progress conclusively indicate that a more radical radiotherapeutic approach will be rewarding (79, 79a, 79b).*

Relatively little controversy remains regarding the dose of irradiation required. Kaplan has shown that the incidence of recurrent tumor in an irradiated field is approximately 50 per cent in patients receiving a tumor dose of 2000 R. or less. In patients receiving 3000 to 4000 R., this incidence drops to 11 per cent, and it drops still further (to less than 5 per cent) in patients receiving approximately 4000 R. or more (80). With modern radiotherapeutic equipment, delivery of 4000 R. to tumor-bearing areas is readily accomplished.

In interpreting survival data in Stage I and II patients, it must be emphasized that, in many of the older series, the lack of adequate staging techniques may have inadvertently and unknowingly led to inclusion of patients with disease outside the irradiated fields, who were therefore inadequately treated. The more modern series which utilize the techniques of lymphography and especially laparotomy will undoubtedly exclude the vast majority of these incorrectly staged patients, and thus give more accurate long-term survival rates for "true" Stage I and II patients.

While it is generally accepted that Stage I and II patients should receive radiotherapy as their primary modality of treatment, the efficacy of chemotherapy in this setting must also be emphasized. In a series of patients from Africa treated with chemotherapy alone (due to the unavailability of radiotherapy), Ziegler and his co-workers were able to show, in an actuarially projected survival, children with Stage I and II Hodgkin's disease who may survive more than five years (81). These observations may be especially important in circumstances in which radiotherapy is unavailable or unacceptable.

In patients with disseminated advanced disease, chemotherapy is the usual primary modality of treatment. Since clinical trials in children and in adults suggest no major differences in the two age groups in the sensitivity of Hodgkin's disease to various chemotherapeutic regimens, the response rate to the major single and multiple drug regimens in series composed of both children and adults is shown in Table 23–5. As the table demonstrates, the combination of several agents, each effective when administered alone, has been associated with a pronounced improvement in the complete remission response rate. The most successful combination regimen currently employed is the MOPP protocol, with the acronym derived from the first letters of the four component drugs, as indicated in the table. This combination takes advantage of the dissimilar toxicities of its component parts to utilize near full dosage of the agents involved. Thus, the major dose-limiting toxicity for vincristine is neurotoxicity; for prednisone, gastroenteric and metabolic disturbances; and for nitrogen mustard and procarbazine, myelosuppression. The principles of utilizing agents which are effective alone and which have nonoverlapping toxicities are the main guidelines leading to successful combination chemotherapy, and the MOPP protocol provides an excellent example of these principles (90). Although the data from childhood are limited, MOPP chemotherapy appears capable of producing median survivals in excess of three years, with the majority of these advanced patients still in complete remission (78, 80a). In fact the median survival is approaching six years in one large multi-institutional study limited predominantly to adults (91).

---

*Editor's Note: The controlled studies referred to here are those in progress at Stanford University. Preliminary results of these studies already show that patients treated with total nodal radiation have a significantly lowered relapse rate when compared with patients treated with involved field techniques. Since relapse has ominous prognostic significance (79a), it is concluded that total nodal irradiation in adults is to be preferred to involved field treatment.

In our opinion children with Stages IA and IIA should be treated (after laparotomy) by radiotherapy to the involved areas and to the functionally contiguous regions. For example, a child with left neck and mediastinal disease would receive treatment to a mantle, periaortic nodes to the bifurcation, and to the splenic pedicle.

Though these recommendations are easy to write, they are less simple to deliver. Such treatment requires a highly skilled and experienced radiotherapy staff using modern equipment. Furthermore, we recognize that such a policy may be associated with a greater risk of late sequelae of radiation. A recent review of the results of aggressive radiotherapy and chemotherapy in childhood Hodgkin's disease supports this view (80a), although follow-up of another group of children treated with a combination of aggressive radiotherapy and chemotherapy has not revealed a high incidence of severe radiation sequelae (80b).

TABLE 23-5.   CHEMOTHERAPY OF HODGKIN'S DISEASE

AGENTS	PER CENT ACHIEVING COMPLETE REMISSION	MEDIAN DURATION OF RESPONSE		References
		Maintained	*Unmaintained*	
Prednisone	<10%	<6 mos.	—	Ezdinli et al., 1969 (82)
Nitrogen mustard	<10%	8 mos.	3 mos.	Jacobs et al., 1968 (83)
				Scott, 1963 (84)
				Spear and Patno, 1962 (85)
Cyclophosphamide	11%	4.5 mos.	3 mos.	Livingston and Carter, 1970 (86)
Vincristine	13%	—	—	Bohannon et al., 1963 (87)
Procarbazine	18%	3 mos.	—	DeConti, 1971 (88)
Combinations				
Cyclophosphamide, vincristine, and prednisone	36%	11 mos.	5 mos.	Luce et al., 1971(89)
MOPP*	81%	—	48 mos.	DeVita et al., 1970 (90)
MOPP	72%	>60 mos.	23 mos.	Frei, 1972 (91)

*Mustargen (nitrogen mustard), Oncovin (vincristine), procarbazine, and prednisone.

In patients refractory to MOPP chemotherapy, a number of other active antitumor agents are currently under investigation and seem promising in the treatment of childhood Hodgkin's disease. Notable examples include vinblastine, a periwinkle alkaloid (92); bleomycin, a polypeptide antibiotic (93); adriamycin, an anthracycline antibiotic (94); and bis-chloroethyl-nitrosourea (BCNU), a synthetic chemical (95). The initial studies with these agents in children have shown antitumor activity similar to that observed in larger adult series, and indicate that approximately half the patients treated with these drugs can be expected to achieve remission.

Controversy exists regarding the therapy of patients with intermediate-stage disease (Stages IIB and III). Proponents of radiotherapy and chemotherapy are each able to cite encouraging series in which either modality has been associated with an encouraging response rate. Moore et al. have recently demonstrated that such patients treated with extensive radiotherapy to all lymph node–bearing regions (total nodal radiotherapy) followed by six monthly courses of MOPP chemotherapy appear to be doing better than similar patients receiving either modality alone (96). While this study must still be considered investigational, it suggests that aggressive therapy in this group of patients with moderately advanced disease can be rewarding,* and that therapeutic approaches designed for cure rather than just palliation should be utilized for most, if not all, of these patients.

Complications

Complications from Hodgkin's disease in its early stages are relatively infrequent. Occasionally tumor masses that infiltrate or compress various structures, such as the trachea or superior vena cava, may produce functional impairment, but these are more likely occurrences in advanced disseminated disease. However, as mentioned before, the anergic state of many patients with Hodgkin's disease, along with the further impairment to host defense mechanisms produced by therapy, increases the likelihood of infectious processes in many children with Hodgkin's disease, regardless of stage. The infections encountered are frequently opportunistic and include viral diseases (notably herpes zoster and cytomega-

*Editor's Note: In fact, it is currently our policy to treat patients with advanced disease with a combination of radiotherapy and chemotherapy. It should be emphasized that relapse following chemotherapy usually occurs in areas of previous bulky tumor involvement (91), whereas true local recurrence is rare following adequate radiotherapy (56).

lic inclusion disease), protozoan diseases (including *Pneumocystis carinii* infection and toxoplasmosis), and especially fungal infections (notably candidiasis and cryptococcosis). Other problems, particularly in advanced disease, include hemolytic anemia and thrombocytopenia. Although the etiology of these last two complications is often obscure, enlargement and tumor involvement of the spleen have often been implicated (97). Modern staging techniques with splenectomy done at the time of diagnosis may decrease the incidence of these hematologic complications. On the other hand, the incidence of herpes zoster infection has appeared to increase since splenectomy has been adopted (97a).

In addition to the problems associated with the disease per se, the long-term complications of intensive radiotherapy or chemotherapy or both must also be considered. Late sequelae of radiotherapy include growth retardation, radiation-induced pericarditis, and pneumonitis. Nephritis and enteritis (57) are rare. The onset of a second malignancy, such as acute leukemia, following irradiation or chemotherapy or both has been reported (98). Chemotherapeutic complications include the serious hemorrhagic and infectious complications associated with severe myelosuppression, as well as the risks of carcinogenicity from some of the agents utilized, such as procarbazine (99). In addition, the combination of repeated courses of radiotherapy and chemotherapy commonly leads to an aplastic and severely immunosuppressed state, and the tolerance of such patients to further therapy if their disease recurs is markedly impaired.

Prognosis

Despite the problems just emphasized, the overall survival pattern for patients with Hodgkin's disease in all age groups has been steadily improving over the last several decades. Properly delivered high-energy radiotherapy has offered the distinct possibility of cure in Stage I and II patients, and successful combination chemotherapy has made significant inroads towards improving the percentage of more advanced patients who achieve long-term survival. Thus Smith, in a review of Hodgkin's disease in children written in 1934, recorded a

median survival of only 1.8 years (42). This was in an era when only minimal therapy was available. Butler, reporting in 1968 on the survival of 54 children treated predominantly with modern radiotherapy, recorded a median survival of 3.9 years (38), while Young et al., reporting in 1972 on the results of 38 children receiving intensive wide-field radiotherapy or combination chemotherapy with MOPP or both, noted a median survival of the entire group in excess of five years, with 63 per cent still alive (78, 80a). The results of many modern protocols derived in an era in which cure rather than palliation is the therapeutic philosophy will not be known for a period of time, but if the trend reported above is indicative of these results, median survivals in excess of ten years and even cure can be anticipated, with long-term survival the rule rather than the exception.

NON-HODGKIN'S LYMPHOMA

Definition

The term "non-Hodgkin's lymphoma" refers to all those malignancies of reticular tissue that are not a part of the Hodgkin's disease classification described above. It includes the terms "lymphosarcoma" and "reticulum cell sarcoma," as well as the more modern histologic subtypes described below. Although exhibiting certain characteristics of Hodgkin's disease, the clinical and pathologic behavior of the non-Hodgkin's lymphomas requires special consideration. The epidemiologic features of non-Hodgkin's lymphoma have been the subject of a recent excellent review (99a).

In recent years, new histologic classifications have clarified to a large degree some of the difficulties encountered with older, more cumbersome pathologic subdivisions. Table 23–6 shows the generally accepted current classification for the non-Hodgkin's group of lymphomas. In this new classification, the subdivisions of lymphosarcoma and reticulum cell sarcoma no longer appear and are replaced by the lymphocytic and histiocytic lymphomas, respectively. The mixed cell classification, which lies between the two classes of subdivisions, occurs with such rarity in childhood that it

TABLE 23–6. HISTOLOGIC
SUBDIVISIONS IN NON-HODGKIN'S
LYMPHOMA*

Well-differentiated lymphocytic lymphoma

Poorly differentiated lymphocytic lymphoma

Histiocytic lymphoma

Mixed histiocytic-lymphocytic lymphoma

Undifferentiated lymphoma

Each subdivision is further delineated by the prefix
"nodular" or "diffuse." In childhood, nodular disease
is very uncommon.

*From Rappaport, H., Winter, W. J., et al.: Cancer
9:792, 1956.

will not be further discussed in this chapter.
Undifferentiated histiocytic lymphoma in
children refers essentially to Burkitt's tumor
and will be discussed in a separate section
devoted to that entity (100).

Etiology

The discussion of the etiology of Hodgkin's disease is also appropriate for the lymphocytic and histiocytic lymphomas. One
observation not seen with Hodgkin's disease, however, is the increased incidence of
non-Hodgkin's lymphoma in patients receiving chronic immunosuppressive therapy in transplant programs. In a recent literature review, Penn and Starzl noted that, of
24 mesenchymal neoplasms which arose de
novo in patients with organ homografts,
there were 11 cases of histiocytic or unclas-
sified lymphomas involving the brain. The
incidence of these lesions is thus approximately 80 times greater than that in the
average population of a comparable age
range (15). Many interesting hypotheses
have arisen from these observations. The
decreased ability of the body undergoing
chronic immunosuppression to carry on the
function of immune surveillance has been
one of the foremost of these hypotheses.
This defect may be especially apparent in
the brain, which has relatively few cells
with functional immunologic capacity. It
has also been suggested that, during chronic
immunosuppression, oncogenic viruses are
more likely to be able to express their on-

cogenic capabilities (15). A laboratory animal model supporting this hypothesis has
been discussed previously.

Incidence

In the United States, approximately
10,000 deaths from non-Hodgkin's lymphoma are recorded yearly (25), with a
yearly mortality rate for children of 3.2 per
million. This entity thus accounts for approximately 6 per cent of all deaths from
cancer in childhood. The lymphocytic
varieties outnumber the histiocytic group in
a ratio of approximately 3:1 (26). As in
Hodgkin's disease and for equally inexpli-
cable reasons, there is a male predominance
with a male to female ratio of approximately
3:1, especially in the age group 11 to 15
years. The age distribution in non-
Hodgkin's lymphoma in childhood shows
that the disease occurs from infancy
throughout adolescence, with two slight increases noted in the 4- to 8-year-old group
and in the second decade; however, the
clear-cut peak that is seen between 2 and 5
years in acute leukemia is not observed in
this disease (101, 102).

Histopathology

When the term "lymphosarcoma" was initially introduced, it was used to describe all
non-Hodgkin's lymphomas. In many of the
articles from the older literature, there is
thus no clear distinction between the lymphocytic and histiocytic varieties. In 1956,
Rappaport et al. attempted to clarify this am-
biguity when they proposed the modern
classification of the non-Hodgkin's lymphomas shown in Table 23–6 (100). Their
studies also emphasized that any of the
cytologic types of non-Hodgkin's lymphoma
may have a nodular (follicular) or diffuse
pattern. In the nodular form of the disease, a
definite nodal architecture can be observed
that is frequently apparent from gross observation (Fig. 23–6). In diffuse histology, as
the term implies, nodal architecture is no
longer apparent, and the tumor is composed
of broad bands of cells (Fig. 23–7). Poorly
differentiated and well-differentiated
lymphocytic lymphomas, which were frequently previously referred to as lym-

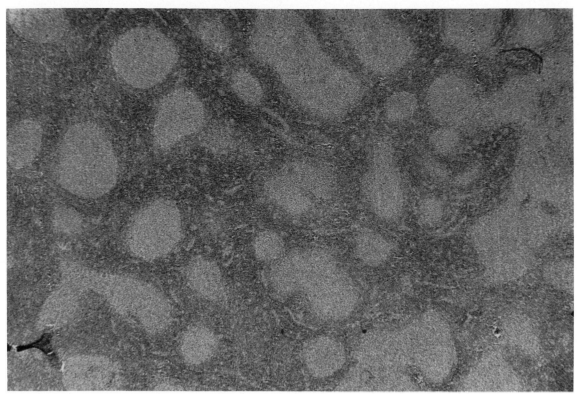

Figure 23-6. Nodular form of non-Hodgkin's lymphoma. The nodules are readily recognizable, even at this low magnification. Hematoxylin-eosin (× 9).

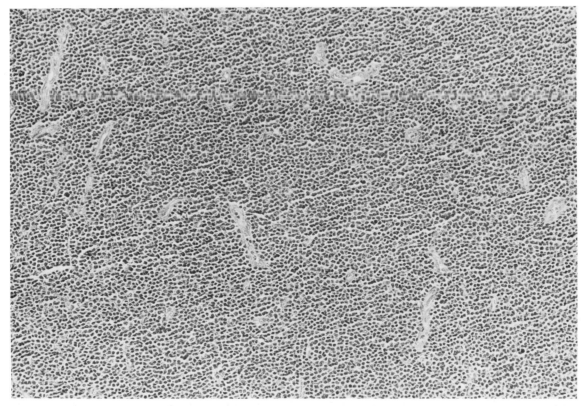

Figure 23-7. Diffuse, well-differentiated lymphocytic lymphoma. Homogeneous proliferation of mature lymphocytes is apparent. Hematoxylin-eosin (× 30).

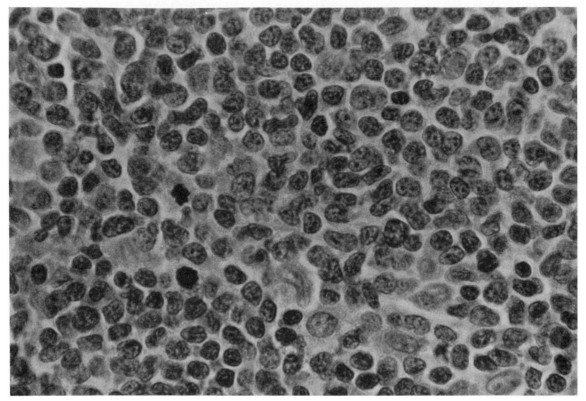

Figure 23–8. Poorly differentiated lymphocytic lymphoma. There is considerable variation in the size and shape of the nuclei. Hematoxylin-eosin (× 240).

phoblastic and lymphocytic lymphomas, respectively, are both tumors composed of lymphocytes with varying degrees of atypical nuclei. These nuclei show immaturity in the poorly differentiated lymphoma (Fig. 23–8), while the well-differentiated tumor is composed of lymphocytes with the morphologic features of more mature cells, usually containing none of the regular cytologic characteristics of malignant cells (Fig. 23–7). There is considerable mitotic activity and variation in nuclear size in the poorly differentiated group, as opposed to the well-differentiated lymphocytic lymphomas, which have nuclear uniformity and few if any mitoses (Fig. 23–7). Nucleoli are more prominent in the former variety. There is considerable disagreement amongst pathologists as to whether the lymphocytic lymphomas can be differentiated microscopically from lymphocytic leukemia involving lymph nodes. This is particularly true in childhood, where the high rate of leukemic transformation (discussed below) may frequently make a distinct separation between lymphomas and leukemia nearly impossible (7).

The histiocytic lymphomas are composed predominantly of neoplastic histiocytes in various stages of maturation and differentiation. Microscopically, these tumors show a wide range of cellular variation, depending upon their degree of differentiation. The nuclei are usually round or slightly oval, often with indented or irregular outlines. While the nucleoli tend to be prominent, the cytoplasm of most cells is pale (Fig. 23–9) (7, 100).

Early observers had noted that nodular lymphocytic lymphomas had a considerably improved prognosis compared with other lymphomas (100). Recent clinical studies, utilizing these new diagnostic categories, have shown that patients with nodular histology, regardless of cell type, do better and have longer survival than their diffuse counterparts (103). As with nodular sclerosing Hodgkin's disease, it is tempting to postulate that the nodular forms are "walled off" by host defense mechanisms, but confirma-

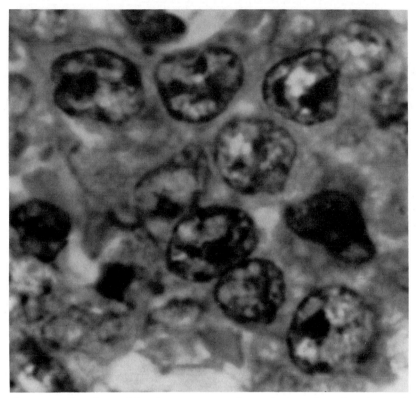

Figure 23–9. Histiocytic lymphoma. The characteristic nuclei are large, indented, and irregular in size. Hematoxylin-eosin (× 400).

tory laboratory data are lacking. Although the histiocytic varieties are generally associated with a graver prognosis than the lymphocytic forms (104), in children the frequency with which the latter transforms to acute leukemia tends to produce a relatively similar overall survival pattern in these two histologic subtypes (101).

In the new classification, the term "giant follicular lymphoma" (frequently referred to under the eponym of Brill-Symmer's disease) is replaced by the nodular form of both well-differentiated and poorly differentiated lymphocytic lymphoma (100). While this disease is more common in older age groups, it is perhaps the one that is most difficult to differentiate from the reactive hyperplasia common in lymph nodes of infected children (102).

Clinical Presentation

As with Hodgkin's disease, many children with non-Hodgkin's lymphoma present with lymph node involvement. However, the proportion presenting with multiple lymph node involvement, as well as with disease in other organs, is much higher in the non-Hodgkin's lymphoma group. As shown in Table 23–7, which is compiled from several childhood series, the presenting tumor is in lymph nodes in only approximately one-third of cases. Another quarter present with intra-abdominal disease, and mediastinal or bone presentations are also quite common. In some sites, such as the stomach or intestines, the frequency of histiocytic and lymphocytic lymphomas appears relatively equal; in other sites, the distribution between the two cell types is unequal, with histiocytic lymphoma accounting for nearly all the patients initially presenting with bone disease, while the opposite is usually the case with pulmonary presentations (108). Symptomatology, apart from organ compression by a particular tumor mass, is also less uniform in the non-Hodgkin's lymphoma group. While fever and weight loss are not uncommon, their

TABLE 23–7.   PRESENTING SITES OF INVOLVEMENT IN
PATIENTS WITH NON-HODGKIN'S LYMPHOMA

		SITE						
REFERENCE		Peripheral Lymph Nodes	Medias- tinum	Intra- abdom- inal	Bone	Head and Neck	Skin and Subcu- taneous	Other
				(Number of Patients)				
Rosenberg et al., 1958 (101)	(69 patients)	30	5	16	10	4	3	1
Pierce, 1960 (102)	(24 patients)	12	4	3	2	0	3	0
Bailey et al., 1961 (105)	(48 patients)	13	10	17	1	5	0	2
Dargeon, 1953 (106)	(62 patients)	18	8	9	10	5	2	10
Maxwell, 1954 (107)	(11 patients)	2	0	4	2	0	0	3
Total	(214 patients)	75(35%)	27(13%)	49(23%)	25(12%)	14(6%)	8(4%)	16(7%)

overall prognostic significance in non-Hodgkin's lymphoma has not been clearly delineated (101).

More than half the patients in many childhood series present with multiple organ involvement, and by history a single site of origin cannot be determined (109). Thus, while the concept of unifocal origin with contiguous spread may be an adequate working hypothesis in Hodgkin's disease, it seems likely that the origin of disease in patients with non-Hodgkin's lymphoma is multicentric, i.e., arises simultaneously in several different areas of the body. Perhaps the most important observation in this regard is the high frequency (up to 50 per cent) of transformation to acute leukemia in patients presenting with lymphocytic lymphomas initially. Nearly all patients with mediastinal disease end with leukemia. By history, such patients may have well-documented nodal or extranodal disease but initially normal bone marrow examinations. After a varying interval, usually less than a year, a frankly leukemic clinical picture develops, with the normal elements of the marrow nearly totally replaced by tumor cells (102, 105–107, 109).

One speculative hypothesis for the etiology of the transformation of the lymphoma to leukemia may be derived from the observations of Folkman and his co-workers. They have recently shown that, in order for a tumor to grow in solid form, an angiogenesis factor must be generated by the tumor, which leads to an ingrowth of blood vessels, without which the tumor cannot enlarge (110). An extrapolation of these data suggests that, if a tumor loses its ability to produce this factor (possibly by de-differentiation), it either stops growing or possibly grows only as single cells suspended in media, such as is seen in leukemic cells suspended in the bone marrow. Thus, transformation to acute leukemia could occur if a lymphoma loses its ability to synthesize tumor angiogenesis factor. Attempts to confirm this hypothesis are in progress.

The staging system devised for Hodgkin's disease is generally used for non-Hodgkin's lymphoma, but many more children will present with Stage III and IV disease instead of the earlier stages, as seen in Hodgkin's disease. The staging procedures are therefore quite similar. Laparotomy has proved beneficial in detecting patients thought to be Stage I and II who had more extensive disease when explored (111). This is particularly true in patients with diffuse histology. Laboratory findings are also similar to those seen in Hodgkin's disease.

Therapy

All three of the major therapeutic modalities — surgery, radiotherapy, and chemotherapy — play a significant role in the treatment of the patient with non-Hodgkin's lymphoma. In patients with unifocal, extranodal presentation, surgical removal followed by radiotherapy has been associated with an excellent prognosis. Thus, patients presenting with lymphoma obstructing the stomach (very rare in children) or intestine (relatively common in children) treated in this manner have long-term survival rates approaching 50 per cent (108). Obviously when the lymphomatous involvement of an organ is only part of a generalized disease pattern, the role of surgery becomes palliative (e.g., relief of obstruction) rather than curative.

Partly because of the more frequent occurrence of widely disseminated disease, the role of radiotherapy in non-Hodgkin's lymphomas has not been as clearly defined as in Hodgkin's disease. Lymphocytic lymphomas of all types and to a lesser extent histiocytic lymphomas are often remarkably radioresponsive, with the rate of tumor regression readily apparent by successive physical examinations 24 hours apart (57). In a recently reported series of adults with Stage I disease receiving 3500 R. or more to the primary tumor site, the four-year survival rate was 85 per cent (112). The need for high total dosage (in excess of 3500 R.) to prevent recurrence was well documented in that study. Despite the use of these high doses, the risk of recurrence remains greater than that seen in Hodgkin's disease, especially in the histiocytic lymphomas (113). Thus, Jones et al. reported a median survival of only 13 months in 26 patients receiving radiotherapy for what appeared to be localized histiocytic lymphoma (114).

Total nodal radiotherapy for adults with Stage III disease has had several limited trials. Johnson and his co-workers at the National Cancer Institute in Bethesda have recently reported on a series of patients treated with this technique, and while their initial reports are encouraging, additional follow-up will be required before this study can be fully evaluated. Because of the widespread pattern of presentation, Johnson has also explored the technique of total body irradiation. In this procedure, the whole body was exposed to cobalt radiotherapy, receiving 5 to 15 R. daily for varying periods of time. Theoretically, all sites of possible lymphomatous involvement were being treated, and again the initial results were encouraging (57). The long-term effects of such a radiotherapeutic program, particularly in children, await further evaluation.

Chemotherapy of non-Hodgkin's lymphoma, like radiotherapy, is also less clearly defined. Single agents, notably vincristine, prednisone, and the alkylating agents, have produced a relatively low percentage of complete remissions.

Combinations of vincristine, prednisone, and cyclophosphamide have produced complete remission rates in the range of 40 to 50 per cent and have improved to some extent the duration of maintained and unmaintained remissions (89). While the improvement with combination chemotherapy has been significant, the saltatory step seen in Hodgkin's disease with the introduction of combination chemotherapy has not yet been clearly achieved in non-Hodgkin's lymphoma. Several new agents, particularly adriamycin (94, 115) and bleomycin (93) (previously mentioned under Hodgkin's disease), have had encouraging trials in pediatric non-Hodgkin's lymphoma. While both of these drugs have serious dose-limiting toxicity (pulmonary fibrosis for bleomycin and cardiomyopathy for adriamycin), the degree of tumor reduction with these agents has been impressive, and in the case of adriamycin, long lasting. The ultimate value of such therapy in pediatric cases is yet to be established.

There does not appear to be any major difference in the response pattern of the various histologic cell types to chemotherapy, although again the nodular forms may do better than their diffuse counterparts. In several series, the patients with histiocytic lymphoma appear to have shorter durations of remission, but these have not proved to be statistically significant. Thus far, no particular regimen or agent has been found with efficacy limited to one histologic cell type (89).

As mentioned above, the tendency for non-Hodgkin's lymphoma in childhood to transform to acute lymphoblastic leukemia is high. Once transformation has taken place, treatment has generally included those agents and regimens effective in the therapy of acute leukemia of childhood. It has been suggested that patients with leukemic transformation are more refractory to chemotherapy than patients with acute leukemia (116). However, when patients with transformed acute leukemia were compared with patients with acute leukemia de novo with a similar total disease duration and extent of prior therapy, the response rate and survival of the two populations were nearly identical (102, 117). This has led investigators to propose that children with diffuse, poorly differentiated, and well-differentiated lymphocytic lymphomas, the types with the highest transformation potential, should be treated with acute leukemia regimens directly after their initial presentation with lymphoma. In one such series still in progress, the patients with lymphoma have fared as well as patients with acute leukemia, and nearly all patients have responded (118). We recommend this approach.

Prognosis

Because of the recent change in histologic classification as well as the recent advent of the currently used aggressive radiotherapeutic and chemotherapeutic approaches, an accurate assessment of prognosis in the non-Hodgkin's lymphomas is difficult. Rosenberg et al. in their 1960 summary of 69 cases of non-Hodgkin's lymphoma in children found a median survival of approximately 10 months, with 17 per cent surviving five years (101). A more recent study suggests the median survival is now approaching 12 to 18 months (118). Results of many on going protocols may be more encouraging, and their results are thus eagerly awaited.

BURKITT'S TUMOR

Definition

Burkitt's tumor is in actuality a subtype of non-Hodgkin's lymphoma, specifically a diffuse undifferentiated lymphoma. The identification of the tumor on the basis of purely morphologic criteria, however, has met with difficulty, especially outside the regions where it is endemic (Africa). Since the diagnosis is usually based on a combination of histologic, cytologic, clinical, and gross anatomic features with no single feature diagnostic by itself (see below) (119), Burkitt's tumor might better be considered as a syndrome.

Etiology

As mentioned earlier in the discussion of etiology of Hodgkin's disease, Burkitt's lymphoma is the lymphoma most commonly linked to a possible viral etiology. The reasons for this linkage are many. In his original description of the tumor, Burkitt noted that it appeared only in central Africa and spared other parts of the continent (6). In particular, it was seen in areas of high temperature and moderate rainfall, which coincided in many ways with the "malaria belt" (8). The idea of an insect vector for viral transmission, therefore, was most appealing. In addition, subsequent studies showed a high correlation between the development of Burkitt's lymphoma and the development of a high titer against the Epstein-Barr virus (9). Extensive studies with Burkitt's tumor cells grown in vitro coupled with investigations of the EB virus itself currently suggest that the EB virus may be an epiphenomenon and not causative (10), and isolation of the causative agent remains an unachieved goal. Thus, while Burkitt's lymphoma has many features suggesting an infectious etiology, the final chapter on proving an infectious origin is yet to be written.

Epidemiology

As mentioned above, this tumor, when first described, was thought to be restricted to the confines of Uganda and the neighboring African nations (8). However, once the syndrome was well defined, other cases in all parts of the world, including a number in the United States (120), were reported. It is of interest to note that a paper written in 1928 by Brown and O'Keefe which described a girl from St. Louis with sarcoma involving both her ovaries and her jaw was probably the first medical description of the disease (121). While the incidence of this disease in the United States is still very low, Burkitt's tumor must often be considered in the differential diagnosis of lymphoma of childhood (120).

In Africa this disease has a peak age incidence in the 4- to 7-year-old group, as opposed to the American patients, in whom the mean age of presentation is usually at the end of the first decade. As expected, Black patients predominate in Africa, but in the United States the diagnosis of Burkitt's tumor has only rarely been made in Blacks. No particular geographic area of the western hemisphere has been noted to have the high incidence recorded in central Africa (6, 120).

Histopathology

As shown in Figure 23–10, Burkitt's tumor has been described as having a "starry sky" pattern. This picture is produced by the numerous macrophages, which contain nuclear and cytoplasmic fragments, as well as intact nuclei, surrounded by the broad sheets of lymphoreticular cells (119). While the starry sky pattern is necessary for the diagnosis, it is not pathognomonic, as it has been seen in all the other types of lymphoma. The tumor cells themselves are primitive undifferentiated cells of relatively uniform size and maturity. They resemble in many cases lymphoblasts, but are frequently more vacuolated than the latter. Special staining, particularly with methyl green pyronin, which stains the chromatin a deep red in Burkitt's tumor,

may be helpful in differentiating this disease from the other lymphomas, which stain much less intensely (120).

Clinical Presentation

Most patients with malignant lymphoma present with lymphadenopathy; however, in the patients originally described by Burkitt in Africa, peripheral lymphadenopathy was conspicuously absent. The majority of his patients presented with involvement to the bones of the jaw or with intra-abdominal disease, notably in the spleen, the para-aortic nodes, and in girls the ovaries (6). In the United States, the presentation pattern in this disease has varied somewhat from that described in Burkitt's original series. For example, there are few jaw tumors in the American patients, and peripheral adenopathy has been a relatively frequent finding. Transformation to acute leukemia and meningeal involvement, both of which were rare in Africa, were seen often in this

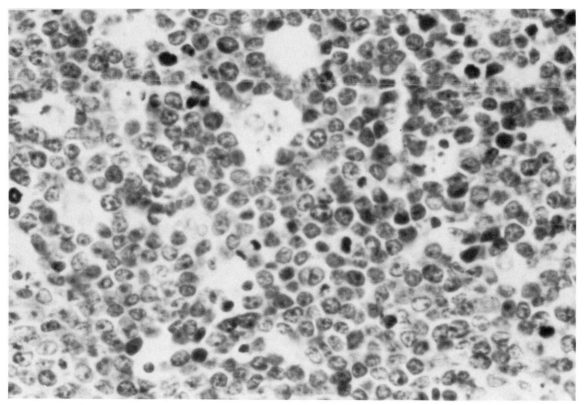

Figure 23–10. Burkitt's tumor. Homogeneous primitive reticular cells surround phagocytic histiocytes, producing the "starry sky" pattern. Hematoxylin-eosin (× 240).

country (120). In both regions, abdominal and retroperitoneal tumors are frequently observed (6, 120).

Fever, anemia, and weight loss are commonly seen, but do not necessarily have the same grave prognostic implications as Hodgkin's disease. While a few patients (15 per cent in one series) (120) may have decreased levels of immunoglobulins, the immunologic studies in the large majority of patients are within normal limits. However, it has recently been demonstrated that patients capable of developing delayed hypersensitivity to an extract made from Burkitt's tumor cells have a better prognosis than patients anergic to such testing. This implies a better host response to the tumor in the group with the favorable prognosis, a finding discussed in greater detail below (122). As mentioned before, one important finding unique among malignant lymphomas is the detection of an elevated antibody titer to the Epstein-Barr virus in patients with Burkitt's tumor. Thus, the mean titer in young American Burkitt's patients was 1:425, compared to a 1:4 titer for normal controls (123).

Because of the unusual pattern of presentation, Ziegler et al. have proposed a staging system somewhat different from that used in Hodgkin's disease (124). As shown by the staging schema in Table 23–8, the two major differences are that involvement of the bones of the face, even when massive, does not warrant a patient with Burkitt's tumor being considered in the advanced stage category, and only central nervous system or bone marrow involvement can qualify a Burkitt's tumor patient for a Stage IV clas-

sification. The prognostic significance of these stages with regard to their response to chemotherapy has been well documented by Ziegler et al., who reported 12 complete remissions in 12 patients with Stage I and II disease, 28 remissions in 38 patients (74 per cent) with Stage III disease, but a response in only 2 of 7 patients (28 per cent) with Stage IV disease (124).

Therapy

Since the majority of patients with Burkitt's tumor had disease presenting regionally, surgery was frequently attempted when the disease was first encountered. However, the massive size of the tumor in a number of patients and the rapid rate of regrowth soon led to exploration of other therapeutic modalities (8). Since radiotherapy was not readily available in Africa, chemotherapeutic programs were extensively evaluated. The first trials, which involved low doses of methotrexate, were unimpressive, but later studies with higher doses of methotrexate did show some response. It was not until the routine use of alkylating agents, however, that chemotherapy for Burkitt's tumor became regularly successful. In one of Burkitt's original studies, single large intravenous doses of cyclophosphamide were associated with long-term survival in approximately 15 per cent of patients (125). Subsequent controlled studies have shown that cyclophosphamide is capable of producing complete disappearance of disease in up to 70 per cent of patients, and if their disease is limited to the early stages, the complete remission rate approaches 100 per cent (124). Currently, intermittent therapy with cyclophosphamide at a dose of 40 mg. per kg. repeated every three weeks has produced the best chemotherapeutic results in the treatment of Burkitt's tumor in this country (120).

While the rate of response to such chemotherapy has been excellent, the duration of response has varied. In a recent review of 130 African Burkitt's tumor patients, Ziegler et al. noted that tumor relapse appeared to have two distinctive patterns. Early relapse was characterized by regrowth at the site of the original tumor and occurred within ten weeks of initial therapy. At relapse, patients with this pattern tended to have generalized

TABLE 23–8.   CLINICAL STAGING OF BURKITT'S TUMOR*

STAGE	EXTENT OF DISEASE
I	Tumor localized to a single extra-abdominal site
II	Tumor involving two or more extra-abdominal sites
III	Intra-abdominal tumor with or without facial involvement
IV	Intra-abdominal tumor (Stage III) with involvement of anatomic sites other than facial

*Revision of staging from Ziegler, J. L., Morrow, R. H., Jr., et al.: Cancer 26:474, 1970.

disease, respond poorly to treatment, and have a poor prognosis. The second pattern of relapse occurred late, beyond the ten-week interval, and generally appeared in uninvolved anatomic sites. Responses to subsequent chemotherapy for these relapses were excellent, and thus the prognosis was good. They further observed that the pattern of relapse did not appear to depend upon the apparent adequacy of the initial chemotherapeutic regimen. The authors speculated that, in the patients with late relapse, reinduction of the tumor may have been responsible for the relapse. In the early relapse group, it was argued that the patients had inadequate therapy from the start which did not eradicate the undetected tumor. Immunologic mechanisms, specifically the adequacy or inadequacy of the host to carry out immune surveillance, were also postulated as a possible explanation of these two patterns. This last hypothesis suggested that the early institution of immunotherapy might be of benefit in Burkitt's tumor patients, especially those with an early relapse pattern (126).

Burkitt's tumor is one of the few diseases that have apparently been cured with drug therapy alone. Although the absolute percentage of long-term survival is difficult to determine because of the inadequacy of follow-up in Africa, it has been estimated that approximately one-fifth of the patients treated with drug therapy in Africa have no further recurrence (125). Why there is complete eradication of all the neoplastic cells with relatively simple drug therapy in this disease and not in other seemingly similar tumors (such as the acute leukemias and other lymphomas) has been the subject of intensive investigation. A number of hypotheses suggest that it is the nature of the host response to tumor, presumably an immunologic response, which accounts for the lengthy survivals in Burkitt's tumor (126, 127). Although these theories are still speculative, they augment the arguments favoring trials with immunotherapy as a means of stimulating the patient's own immune system against tumor. Such trials in the therapy of Burkitt's tumor (128) and, perhaps of even greater importance, in the therapy of acute leukemia (129) are currently under investigation. The concept put forth by Burchenal in 1966 that observations on the response to therapy in Burkitt's tumor may serve as a "stalking horse" for acute leukemia seems even more valid today (127).

CONCLUSIONS

While an improvement in response duration and in survival in all the lymphomas can be anticipated in the decades ahead, it may also be expected that a changing disease pattern may emerge. The long-term effects of intensive chemotherapy or radiotherapy or both, particularly in children, may not be fully realized for another 10 to 20 years. As discussed above, consequences of such aggressive therapy may be grave. Involvement of the central nervous system, which is currently rare in Hodgkin's disease, may become more prevalent, as has been noted in acute leukemia when the duration of survival is prolonged. Transformation to acute leukemia, a process which is limited predominantly to the diffuse lymphocytic lymphoma patients, may become more common in all the lymphomas, either as a direct consequence of long survival or as a consequence of the therapy required to induce these remissions.

As this chapter has emphasized, important studies clarifying the pathophysiology of the malignant lymphomas have been made in the last several years. New observations regarding histologic classifications, staging categories, and patterns of recurrence have led to important therapeutic concepts, many of which are currently under extensive, multidisciplinary testing. During the next decade, a number of these studies will reach their conclusions, hopefully providing information that will increase the likelihood for long-term survival and even cure.

Perhaps the most important research that may come to light in the next several years will concern the etiology of these diseases. The current investigations of an infectious origin, coupled with the more sophisticated immunologic methodologies currently available, may hopefully lead to a fruitful culmination. If the etiology of this disease can be uncovered, it can be anticipated that preventive measures would soon follow, thus making the large body of literature on the treatment of the malignant lymphomas of historic interest only.

References

1. Hodgkin, T.: On some morbid appearances of the absorbent glands and spleen. Trans. Med.-Chir. Soc. Edinb. 17:68, 1832.

2. Wilks, S.: Cases of enlargement of lymphatic glands and spleen (or Hodgkin's disease). Guy's Hosp. Rep. 11:56, 1865.

3. Fox, H.: Presentation of microscopical preparations made from some of the original tissue described by Thomas Hodgkin, 1832. Ann. Med. Hist. 8:370, 1926.

4. Kundrat, H.: Ueber lymphosarkomatosis. Wien Klin. Wochenschr. 6:211, 1893.

5. Oberling, C.: Les reticulo-sarcomes et les reticulo-endothelio-sarcomes de la moelle osseuse (sarcome d'Ewing). Bull. Assoc. Fr. Cancer 17:259, 1928.

6. Burkitt, D.: A sarcoma involving the jaws in African children. Br. J. Surg. 46:218, 1958.

7. Rappaport, H.: Tumors of the hematopoietic system. *Atlas of Tumor Pathology.* Section III, Fascicle 8. Washington D.C., Armed Forces Institute of Pathology, 1966.

8. Burkitt, D. P.: Etiology of Burkitt's lymphoma: Alternative hypothesis to vectored virus. J. Natl. Cancer Inst. 42:19, 1969.

9. Epstein, M. A., and Barr, Y. M.: Cultivation in vitro of human lymphoblasts from Burkitt's malignant lymphoma. Lancet 1:252, 1964.

10. Epstein, M. A.: Aspects of the EB virus. Adv. Cancer Res. 13:383, 1970.

11. Order, S. E., and Hellman, S.: Pathogenesis of Hodgkin's disease. Lancet 1:571, 1972.

12. Schwartz, R. S.: Immunoregulation, oncogenic viruses, and malignant lymphomas. Lancet 1:1266, 1972.

13. Order, S. E., Porter, M., et al.: Hodgkin's disease: Evidence for a tumor associated antigen. New Engl. J. Med. 285:471, 1971.

14. Armstrong, M. Y. K., Gleichman, E., et al.: Chronic allogenic disease. II. Development of lymphomas. J. Exp. Med. 132:417, 1970.

15. Penn, I., and Starzl, F. E.: Malignant tumors arising de novo in immunosuppressed organ transplant recipients. Transplantation 14:407, 1972.

16. Vianna, N. J., and Greenwald, P.: Nature of Hodgkin's disease agent. Lancet 1:733, 1971.

17. Vianna, N. J., Greenwald, P., et al.: Hodgkin's disease: Cases with features of a community outbreak. Ann. Intern. Med. 77:169, 1972.

17a. Klinger, R. J., and Minton, J. P.: Case clustering of Hodgkin's disease in a small rural community with associations among cases. Lancet 1:168, 1973.

18. Clusterings in Hodgkin's disease (editorial). Lancet 2:907, 1972.

19. MacMahon, B.: Epidemiology of Hodgkin's disease. Cancer Res. 26:1189, 1966.

20. Solidoro, A., Guzman, C., et al.: Relative increased incidence of childhood Hodgkin's disease in Peru. Cancer Res. 26:1204, 1966.

21. Azzam, S. A.: High incidence of Hodgkin's disease in children in Lebanon. Cancer Res. 26:1202, 1966.

22. Fraumeni, J. F., and Li, F. P.: Hodgkin's disease in childhood: An epidemiologic study. J. Natl. Cancer Inst. 42:681, 1969.

23. Cole, P., MacMahon, B., et al.: Mortality from Hodgkin's disease in the United States. Evidence for the multiple etiology hypothesis. Lancet 2:1371, 1968.

24. Smithers, D. W.: Hodgkin's disease: One entity or two? Lancet 2:1285, 1972.

25. Silverberg, E., and Grant, R. N.: *Cancer Statistics, 1970.* New York, American Cancer Society, 1970, p. 7.

26. Miller, R. W.: Fifty-two forms of childhood cancer: United States mortality experience, 1960–1966. J. Pediatr. 75:685, 1969.

27. Pitcock, J. A., Bauer, W. C., et al.: Hodgkin's disease in children: A clinicopathological study of 46 cases. Cancer 12:1043, 1959.

28. Strum, S. B., Park, J. K., et al.: Observation of cells resembling Reed-Sternberg cells in conditions other than Hodgkin's disease. Cancer 26:176, 1970.

29. Salzstein, S. L., and Ackerman, L. V.: Lymphadenopathy induced by anticonvulsant drugs and mimicking clinically and pathologically malignant lymphomas. Cancer 12:164, 1959.

30. Is phenytoin carcinogenic? (editorial.) Lancet 2:1071, 1971.

30a. Hyman, G. A., and Sommers, S. C.: The development of Hodgkin's disease and lymphoma during anticonvulsant therapy. Blood 28:416, 1966.

30b. Anthony, J. J.: Malignant lymphoma associated with hydantoin drugs. Arch. Neurol. 22:450, 1970.

31. Rosenthal, S. R.: Significance of tissue lymphocytes in the prognosis of lymphogranulomatosis. Arch. Pathol. 21:628, 1936.

32. Jackson, H., and Parker, F.: Hodgkin's disease. II. Pathology. New Engl. J. Med. 231:35, 1944.

33. Lukes, R. J., and Butler, J. J.: The pathology and nomenclature of Hodgkin's disease. Cancer Res. 26:1063, 1966.

34. Strum, S. B., and Rappaport, H.: Hodgkin's disease in the first decade of life. Pediatrics 46:748, 1970.

35. Shah, N. K., Freeman, A. I., et al.: Hodgkin's disease in children. American Society of Hematology, Abstracts of the December, 1972, meeting. Hollywood, Florida, p. 138.

36. Norris, D. G., Burgert, E. O., et al.: Hodgkin's disease in children. Blood 41:974, 1972.

37. Santiago, P. J., Velez-Garcia, E., et al.: Hodgkin's disease in children: Review of 31 patients. Abstracts of the 13th International Congress of Hematology, Munich, Germany, August, 1970, p. 255.

38. Butler, J.: Hodgkin's disease in children, In *Neoplasia in Childhood.* A Collection of Papers Presented at the Twelfth Annual Clinical Conference, 1967, at The University of Texas M. D. Anderson Hospital and Tumor Institute at Houston, Houston, Texas. Chicago, Year Book Medical Publishers, Inc., 1969.

39. Keller, A. R., Kaplan, H. S., et al.: Correlation of histopathology with other prognostic indicators in Hodgkin's disease. Cancer 22:487, 1968.

40. Butler, J. J.: Histopathology of malignant lymphomas and Hodgkin's disease, In *Leukemia-Lymphoma.* A Collection of Papers Presented

at the Fourteenth Annual Clinical Conference on Cancer, 1969, at The University of Texas M. D. Anderson Hospital and Tumor Institute at Houston, Houston, Texas. Chicago, Year Book Medical Publishers, Inc., 1970.

41. Rappaport, H., and Strum, S. B.: Vascular invasion in Hodgkin's disease: Its incidence and relationship to the spread of the disease. Cancer 25:1304, 1970.

42. Smith, C. A.: Hodgkin's disease in childhood. A clinical study with a résumé of the literature to date. J. Pediatr. 4:12, 1934.

43. Jenkin, R. D. T., Peters, M. V., et al.: Hodgkin's disease in children. Can. Med. Assoc. J. 100:222, 1967.

44. Young, C., and Hodas, C.: Excretion of a cationic protein in the urine of febrile patients with Hodgkin's disease. Proc. Am. Assoc. Cancer Res. 12:37, 1971.

45. Young, C. W., Hodas, S., et al.: Acute effects of anticancer agents on DNA, RNA and protein metabolism in HeLa monolayers. Proc. Am. Assoc. Cancer Res. 5:71, 1964.

46. Schersten, J., and Lundholm, K.: Lysosomal enzyme activity in muscle tissue from patients with malignant tumor. Cancer 30:1246, 1972.

47. Teillet, F., Boiron, M., et al.: A reappraisal of clinical and biological signs of staging in Hodgkin's disease. Cancer Res. 31:1723, 1971.

48. Jaffe, N., and Bishop, Y. M. M.: The serum iron level, hematocrit, sedimentation rate and leukocyte alkaline phosphatase in pediatric patients with Hodgkin's disease. Cancer 26:332, 1970.

49. Hrgovcic, M., Tessmer, C. F., et al.: Serum copper levels in lymphoma and leukemia. Special reference to Hodgkin's disease. Cancer 21:743, 1968.

50. Levine, P. H.: Abnormal blood chemistry values in Hodgkin's disease. Lack of correlation with staging of disease. J.A.M.A. 220:1734, 1972.

51. Chabner, B. A., DeVita, V. T., et al.: Abnormalities of tryptophan metabolism and plasma pyridoxal phosphate in Hodgkin's disease. New Engl. J. Med. 282:838, 1970.

52. Young, R. C., Corder, M. P., et al.: Delayed hypersensitivity in Hodgkin's disease. A study of 103 untreated patients. Am. J. Med. 52:63, 1972.

53. Hersh, E. M., and Oppenheim, J. J.: Impaired in vitro lymphocyte transformation in Hodgkin's disease. New Engl. J. Med. 273:1006, 1965.

54. Rosenberg, S. A., and Kaplan, H. S.: Evidence for an orderly progression in the spread of Hodgkin's disease. Cancer Res. 26:1225, 1966.

54a. Gilbert, R.: Radiotherapy in Hodgkin's disease (malignant granulomatosis): Anatomic and clinical foundations; governing principles; results. Am. J. Roentgenol. 41:198, 1939.

55. Peters, M. V.: A study of survivals in Hodgkin's disease treated radiologically. Am. J. Roentgenol. 63:299, 1950.

56. Kaplan, H. S.: The radical radiotherapy of regionally localized Hodgkin's disease. Radiology 78:553, 1962.

57. Johnson, R. E.: Modern approaches to the radiotherapy of lymphomas. Semin. Hematol. 6:357, 1969.

58. Engeset, E., Hoeg, K., et al.: Thoracic duct cytology in Hodgkin's disease. Int. J. Cancer 4:735, 1969.

59. Halie, M. R., Eibergen, R., et al.: Observations on abnormal cells in the peripheral blood and spleen in Hodgkin's disease. Br. Med. J. 2:609, 1972.

60. Halie, M. R., Seldenrath, J. J., et al.: Curative radiotherapy in Hodgkin's disease: Significance of hematogenous dissemination established by examination of peripheral blood and spleen. Br. Med. J. 2:611, 1972.

61. Carbone, P. P., Kaplan, H. S., et al.: Report of the Committee on Hodgkin's disease staging classification. Cancer Res. 31:1860, 1971.

62. Rosenberg, S. A.: Report of the Committee on the staging of Hodgkin's disease. Cancer Res. 26:1310, 1966.

63. Musshoff, K.: Prognostic and therapeutic implications in staging in extranodal Hodgkin's disease. Cancer Res. 31:1814, 1971.

64. Teillet, F., and Schweisguth, O.: La maladie de Hodgkin chez l'enfant. Etude de 72 observations personelles. Arch. Fr. Pediatr. 25:313, 1968.

65. Musumeci, R., Rossati-Bellani, F., et al.: Usefulness of lymphography in childhood neoplasia. Cancer 29:51, 1972.

66. Grossman, H., Winchester, P. H., et al.: Roentgenographic changes in childhood Hodgkin's disease. Am. J. Roentgenol. 108:354, 1970.

67. Lipton, M. J., DeNardo, G. L., et al.: Evaluation of the liver and spleen in Hodgkin's disease. I. The value of hepatic scintigraphy. Am. J. Med. 52:356, 1972.

68. Silverman, S., DeNardo, G. L., et al.: Evaluation of the liver and spleen in Hodgkin's disease. II. The value of splenic scintigraphy. Am. J. Med. 52:362, 1972.

69. Edwards, C. L., and Hayes, R. L.: Scanning of malignant neoplasms with Gallium 67. J.A.M.A. 212:1182, 1970.

70. Webb, D. I., Ubogy, G., et al.: Importance of bone marrow biopsy in the clinical staging of Hodgkin's disease. Cancer 26:313, 1970.

71. Ultmann, J. E.: Current status: The management of lymphoma. Semin. Hematol. 7:441, 1970.

71a. Hoys, D. M., Karon, M., et al.: Hodgkin's disease technique and results of staging laparotomy in childhood. Arch. Surg. 106:507, 1973.

72. Bagley, C. M., Jr., Roth, J. A., et al.: Liver biopsy in Hodgkin's disease. Clinicopathologic correlations in 127 patients. Ann. Intern. Med. 76:219, 1972.

73. Ray, G. R., Trueblood, H. W., et al.: Oophoropexy: A means of preserving ovarian function following pelvic megavoltage radiotherapy for Hodgkin's disease. Radiology 96:175, 1970.

74. Santiago, P. J., Velez-garcia, E., et al.: Exploratory laparotomy and splenectomy for staging of Hodgkin's disease in children. Abstracts of the Fourteenth International Hematology Congress. São Paulo, Brazil, July, 1972. Abstract No. 584.

75. Horan, M., and Colebatch, J. H.: Relation between splenectomy and subsequent infections. Arch. Dis. Child. 37:398, 1962.

76. Eraklis, A. J., Kevy, S. V., et al.: Hazard of overwhelming infection after splenectomy in childhood. New Engl. J. Med. 276:1225, 1967.

77. Ravry, M., Maldonado, N., et al.: Serious infection after splenectomy for the staging of Hodgkin's disease. Ann. Intern. Med. 77:11, 1972.

78. Young, R. C., DeVita, V. T., et al.: Hodgkin's disease in childhood. American Society of Hematology. Abstracts of December, 1972, meeting. Hollywood, Florida, p. 140.

79. Nickson, J. J., and Hutchison, G. B.: Extensions of disease, complications of therapy and deaths in localized Hodgkin's disease; preliminary reports of a clinical trial. Am. J. Roentgenol. 114:564, 1972.

79a. Rosenberg, S. A., and Kaplan, H. S.: Hodgkin's disease and other malignant lymphomas. Calif. Med. 113:23, 1970.

79b. D'Angio, G. J., and Nisce, L. Z.: Problems with the irradiation of children and pregnant patients. J.A.M.A. 223:171, 1973.

80. Kaplan, H. S.: Evidence for a tumoricidal dose level in the radiotherapy of Hodgkin's disease. Cancer Res. 26:1721, 1966.

80a. Young, R. C., DeVita, V. T., et al.: Hodgkin's disease in childhood. Blood 42:163, 1973.

80b. Smith, K. L., Johnson, D., et al.: Concurrent chemotherapy and radiation therapy in the treatment of childhood and adolescent Hodgkin's disease. Cancer 33:38, 1974.

81. Ziegler, J. L., Bluming, A. Z., et al.: Chemotherapy of childhood Hodgkin's disease in Uganda. Lancet 2:679, 1972.

82. Ezdinli, E. Z., Stutzman, L., et al.: Corticosteroid therapy for lymphomas and chronic lymphocyte leukemia. Cancer 23:900, 1969.

83. Jacobs, E. M., Peters, F. C., et al.: Mechlorethamine HCl and cyclophosphamide in the treatment of Hodgkin's disease and the lymphomas. J.A.M.A. 203:392, 1968.

84. Scott, J. L.: The effect of nitrogen mustard and maintenance chlorambucil in the treatment of advanced Hodgkin's disease. Cancer Chemother. Rep. 27:27, 1963.

85. Spear, P., and Patno, M.: A comparative study of the effectiveness of HN₂ and cyclophosphamide in bronchogenic carcinoma, Hodgkin's disease and lymphosarcoma. Cancer Chemother. Rep. 16:413, 1962.

86. Livingston, R., and Carter, S.: *Single Agents in Cancer Chemotherapy.* New York, IFI/Plenum, 1970.

87. Bohannon, R. A., Miller, D. G., et al.: Vincristine in the treatment of lymphomas and leukemias. Cancer Res. 23:613, 1963.

88. DeConti, R. C.: Procarbazine in the management of late Hodgkin's disease. J.A.M.A. 215:927, 1971.

89. Luce, J. K., Gamble, J. F., et al.: Combined cyclophosphamide, vincristine and prednisone therapy of malignant lymphoma. Cancer 28:306, 1971.

90. DeVita, V. T., Serpick, A. A., et al.: Combination chemotherapy in the treatment of advanced Hodgkin's disease. Ann. Intern. Med. 73:881, 1970.

91. Frei, E., III: Combination cancer therapy: Presidential address. Cancer Res. 32:2593, 1972.

92. Frei, E., III, Franzino, A., et al.: Clinical studies of vinblastine. Cancer Chemother. Rep. 12:125, 1961.

93. Bonadonna, G., DeLena, M., et al.: Clinical trials with bleomycin in lymphomas and in solid tumors. Eur. J. Cancer 8:205, 1972.

94. Wollner, N., Tan, C., et al.: Adriamycin in childhood leukemias and solid tumors. Proc. Am. Assoc. Cancer Res. 12:75, 1971.

95. Young, R. C., DeVita, V. T., et al.: Treatment of advanced Hodgkin's disease with [1,3- bis(2-chloroethyl)-1-nitrosourea] BCNU. New Engl. J. Med. 285:475, 1972.

96. Moore, M. R., Bull, J. M., et al.: Sequential radiotherapy and chemotherapy in the treatment of Hodgkin's disease. Ann. Intern. Med. 77:1, 1972.

97. Lowenbraun, S., Ramsey, H. E., et al.: Splenectomy in Hodgkin's disease for splenomegaly, cytopenias, and intolerance to myelosuppressive chemotherapy. Am. J. Med. 50:49, 1971.

97a. Goffinet, D. R., Glatstein, E. J., et al.: Herpes zoster-varicella infections and lymphoma. Ann. Intern. Med. 76:235, 1972.

98. Ezdinli, E. Z., Sokal, J. E., et al.: Myeloid leukemia in Hodgkin's disease: Chromosomal abnormalities. Ann. Intern. Med. 71:1097, 1969.

99. Kelley, M. G., O'Gara, R. W., et al.: Carcinogenic activity of a new antitumor agent, N-isopropyl-alpha-(2-methyl-hydrazino)-p-toluamide HCl. Cancer Chemother. Rep. 39:77, 1964.

99a. Grundy, G. W., Creagan, E. T., et al.: Non-Hodgkin's lymphoma in childhood: Epidemiologic features. J. Natl. Cancer Inst. 51:676, 1973.

100. Rappaport, H., Winter, W. J., et al.: Follicular lymphoma: A reevaluation of its position in the scheme of malignant lymphomas, based on a survey of 253 cases. Cancer 9:792, 1956.

101. Rosenberg, S. A., Diamond, H. D., et al.: Lymphosarcoma in childhood. New Engl. J. Med. 259:505, 1958.

102. Pierce, M. I.: Lymphosarcoma and Hodgkin's disease in children. Natl. Cancer Conference Proc. 4:559, 1960.

103. Jones, S. E., Rosenberg, S. A., et al.: Non-Hodgkin's lymphoma. II. Single agent chemotherapy. Cancer 30:31, 1972.

104. Newall, J., and Friedman, M.: Reticulum cell sarcoma. Part III: Prognosis. Radiology 97:99, 1970.

105. Bailey, R. J., Burgert, E. O., et al.: Malignant lymphoma in children. Pediatrics 28:985, 1961.

106. Dargeon, H. W.: Lymphosarcoma in childhood. Adv. Pediatr. 6:13, 1953.

107. Maxwell, G. M.: Twelve cases of lymphosarcoma in children. Arch. Dis. Child. 29:155, 1954.

108. Freeman, C., Berg, J. W., et al.: Occurrence and prognosis of extranodal lymphomas. Cancer 29:252, 1972.

109. Jones, B., and Klingberg, W. G.: Lymphosarcoma in children. J. Pediatr. 63:11, 1963.

110. Folkman, J.: Tumor angiogenesis: Therapeutic implications. New Engl. J. Med. 285:1182, 1971.

111. Hanks, G. E., Terry, L. N., Jr., et al.: Contribution of diagnostic laparotomy to staging non-Hodgkin's lymphoma. Cancer 29:41, 1972.

112. Lipton, A., and Lee, B. J.: Prognosis of stage I lymphosarcoma and reticulum cell sarcoma. New Engl. J. Med. 284:230, 1971.

113. Robinson, T., Fischer, J. J., et al.: Reticulum cell sarcoma treated by radiation. Radiology 99:669, 1971.

114. Jones, S. E., Kaplan, H. S., et al.: Non-Hodgkin's lymphomas. III. Preliminary results of radiotherapy and a proposal for new clinical trials. Radiology 103:657, 1972.

115. Gottlieb, J. A., Gutterman, J. U., et al.: Chemotherapy of malignant lymphoma with adriamycin. Cancer Res. 33:3024, 1973.

116. Sullivan, M. P.: Leukemic transformation in lymphosarcoma of childhood. Pediatrics 29:589, 1972.

117. Jones, B., Kung, F., et al.: Chemotherapy of the leukemic transformation of lymphosarcoma. J. Pediatr. 70:442, 1967.

118. Wollner, N., Burchenal, J., et al.: Lymphosarcoma and reticulum cell sarcoma in childhood. Treatment with cyclophosphamide, radiation therapy, and L₂ chemotherapy protocol for acute lymphoblastic leukemia. Abstracts of the Fourteenth International Hematology Congress, São Paulo, Brazil, July, 1972. Abstract No. 529.

119. Rappaport, H., Wright, D. H., et al.: Suggested criteria for the diagnosis of Burkitt's tumor. Cancer Res. 27:2632, 1967.

120. Cohen, M. H., Bennett, J. M., et al.: Burkitt's tumor in the United States. Cancer 23:1259, 1969.

121. Brown, J. B., and O'Keefe, C. D.: Sarcoma of the ovary with unusual oral metastases. Ann. Surg. 87:467, 1928.

122. Bluming, A. Z., Ziegler, J. L., et al.: Delayed cutaneous sensitivity reactions to autologous Burkitt lymphoma protein extracts. Results of a prospective two and a half year study. Clin. Exp. Immunol. 9:713, 1971.

123. Levine, P. H., O'Conor, G. T., et al.: Antibodies to Epstein-Barr virus (EBV) in American patients with Burkitt's lymphoma. Cancer 30:610, 1972.

124. Ziegler, J. L., Morrow, R. H., Jr., et al.: Treatment of Burkitt's tumor with cyclophosphamide. Cancer 26:474, 1970.

125. Burchenal, J. H.: Long-term survivors in acute leukemia and Burkitt's tumor. Cancer 21:595, 1968.

126. Ziegler, J. L., Bluming, A. Z., et al.: Relapse patterns in Burkitt's lymphoma. Cancer Res. 32:1267, 1972.

127. Burchenal, J. H.: Geographic chemotherapy — Burkitt's tumor as a stalking horse for leukemia: Presidential address. Cancer Res. 26:2393, 1966.

128. Ziegler, J. L., Magrath, I. T., et al.: BCG immunotherapy of Burkitt's lymphoma. Proc. Am. Assoc. Cancer Res. 13:38, 1972.

129. Mathé, G., Amiel, J. L., et al.: Active immunotherapy for acute lymphoblastic leukemia. Lancet 1:697, 1969.

Chapter 24

Foam Cells

by Howard R. Sloan and Jan L. Breslow

INTRODUCTION*

The term "foam cell" is frequently used to describe any macrophage containing large amounts of lipid. These cells have been observed in a large variety of disorders characterized by abnormal lipid metabolism; their presence is often considered pathognomonic of the accumulation of abnormal *amounts* of lipid. It is commonly assumed that foam cells or lipid-laden macrophages are a part of the general reticuloendothelial system. The reticuloendothelial system (RES) comprises a large family of cell types that include the phagocytic cells of the serous cavities and the pulmonary alveoli; the sinusoids of the liver, lymph nodes, and spleen; the monocytes of the peripheral blood; the histiocytes of the viscera; the phagocytes of the bone marrow; and the microglia of the central nervous system (1). The cells of the RES are usually divided arbitrarily into fixed and mobile portions; the macrophages in the bone marrow are considered to be an example of the fixed type of reticuloendothelial cell. They represent the most easily obtained cells of this portion of the RES.

The cells of the RES accumulate large amounts of lipid in many diseases; the explanations for this storage process are not fully understood. Several explanations seem reasonable:

1. The reticuloendothelial cells are extremely active metabolically, and they may therefore normally turn over their own lipids at a very rapid rate. A disorder of lipid catabolism may result in the accumulation of endogenous lipid within the reticuloendothelial (RE) cells.

2. The degradation of senescent cells, cellular constituents, and plasma lipoproteins may be a normal function of the RES. The RES may serve as a processing factory for other tissues of the body, including the blood, which may have only a limited ability to degrade their own constituents. If the RE cell is presented with more lipid than it is capable of degrading, then accumulation may result.

3. The RES may also ingest lipids by a specific immunologic mechanism. It is known that glycolipids are potent antigens (2, 3). It is also known that macrophages contain surface sites capable of reacting with antigens. Therefore, antigen-antibody interaction may play a role in the accumulation of lipids in certain disorders.

A comprehensive discussion of the appearance of the entire RES in storage diseases is beyond the scope of this chapter. We will emphasize the techniques used to examine foam cells in the bone marrow and the appearance of these cells in storage diseases. The major features of these diseases will be briefly reviewed.

At this point it would be worth emphasizing that the presence of foam cells, often considered a histologic trademark of Niemann-Pick disease, is not diagnostic of any specific disease. Foam cells must never be termed "Niemann-Pick cells." There is an

---

*For a further discussion, the reader is referred to *Lysosomes and Storage Diseases.* Hers, H. G., and van Hoof, F. (eds.), New York, Academic Press, 1973.

TABLE 24–1. DISEASES WITH FOAM CELLS IN THE BONE MARROW

A. Sphingolipid storage diseases
   1. Niemann-Pick disease
   2. Gaucher's disease
   3. G_{M_1} gangliosidosis
   4. Lactosyl ceramidosis
   5. Fabry's disease

B. Nonpolar lipid storage diseases
   1. Wolman's disease
   2. Cholesteryl ester storage disease
   3. Cerebrotendinous xanthomatosis

C. Hyperlipoproteinemias
   1. Type I
   2. Type II
   3. Type III
   4. Type IV
   5. Type V
   6. Secondary hyperlipoproteinemias

D. Miscellaneous disorders
   1. Tangier disease
   2. Lecithin:cholesterol acyltransferase deficiency
   3. Chronic myelogenous leukemia
   4. Von Gierke's disease

impressively large group of heterogeneous disorders in which foam cells may be observed in the bone marrow; in many cases, these foam cells are indistinguishable from those found in the bone marrow of patients with Niemann-Pick disease. Table 24–1 contains a list of diseases in which foam cells may be observed in the marrow. Foam cells have also been described in the bone marrow of patients with the glycogen storage diseases and the mucopolysaccharidoses.

SAMPLE PREPARATION AND EXAMINATION

Light Microscopy — Minimum Studies

In the evaluation of storage disorders and related diseases, a simple aspiration of the contents of the bone marrow is entirely adequate. In patients of most ages, the marrow obtained from the posterior superior iliac crest is the best sample; in young infants a tibial aspirate may be required.

The most important aspect of the examination of the bone marrow in a patient thought to have a lipid storage disorder is the observation of unstained preparations.

For such studies spicules of the aspirated marrow are transferred to a microscope slide and covered with a coverslip. The sample is spread by the application of gentle pressure on top of the coverslip; a seal is created between the coverslip and the glass slide with vasoline, or preferably, the minimum amount of clear fingernail polish.

The specimen should be examined immediately. It is often most useful to "screen" the entire preparation by examining it under dark-field microscopy. Under these circumstances, the foam cells often appear as large white spheres, measuring approximately 20 to 90 microns in diameter, on a dark background (Color Plate II, *1*). Next the cells are examined by phase contrast microscopy at both 100 and 430 X magnifications. The foam cells appear as large glittering cells (Color Plate II, *2, 7*). The cytoplasm is filled with many droplets, particles, or fibers. There may be a single nucleus or many.

Smears of the aspirated marrow are studied after Wright or Giemsa stains (Color Plate II, *6, 8*). We have examined supravital preparations of many bone marrow aspirates in which large numbers of foam cells were observed; routinely stained smears of the same aspirate revealed only a very small number of these cells.

Light Microscopy — Additional Studies

There are other examinations which may be performed on the supravital preparation. The slide may be viewed under polarization microscopy. With polarizing lenses in place it is possible to scan the entire coverslip for Maltese crosses (Color Plate II, *3*), which indicate the presence of birefringence. The insertion of a $1/4$ wave plate ($1/4$ λ) into the optical system of the microscope permits the determination of the type of asymmetry that is responsible for the birefringence (Color Plate II, *4*). Another approach is Nomarski interference microscopy, which provides an appreciation of the three dimensional appearance of cells (Color Plate II *5, 9*).

Smears of the marrow aspirate may also be fixed in calcium-buffered formalin and stained for iron, collagen, carbohydrates, mucopolysaccharides, and various lipids (4). In the performance of these special staining procedures, smear preparations are preferable to frozen sections of the clot. Embedding the clot in paraffin should be avoided, because this procedure removes most lipids.

It is also possible to examine either supravital preparations or fixed smears by fluorescence microscopy in order to characterize further the chemicals stored within foam cells. When foam cells are irradiated with ultraviolet light, they often emit a greenish-yellow fluorescent color that is thought to be characteristic of ceroids or lipofuscin. This chemical is believed to result from the peroxidation of lipids and is probably not characteristic of any specific lipid class.

Electron Microscopy

Spicules of bone marrow may also be fixed in phosphate-buffered glutaraldehyde for electron miscroscopic examination. In addition, it may be useful to fix a small number of spicules in a digitonin-containing glutaraldehyde solution, which may help to preserve the cholesterol content of the foam cells. Only a few aspirates of bone marrow from patients with storage diseases have been adequately examined by electron microscopy.

MORPHOLOGIC APPEARANCE OF BONE MARROW FOAM CELLS

Foam cells may vary between 20 and 90 μ in diameter, and are usually round or oval in shape. They frequently contain two nuclei and occasionally three or more. The nuclei are usually eccentrically placed, and the nucleolus may be prominent. The most distinguishing characteristic of foam cells is the appearance of the cytoplasm, and it is this feature upon which we will focus our attention.

At this time, examination of supravital preparations is the most useful method for evaluating bone marrow aspirates. Under the phase contrast microscope, the cytoplasm of most foam cells is filled with many small glittering droplets or particles, which usually, but not always, are fairly uniform in size and which give the cell a foamy or "mulberry" appearance (Color Plate II, 2). Many of these droplets are birefringent, and striking Maltese crosses are frequently observed (Color Plate II, 3, 4). These droplets provide the cell with a distinctly rough and granular appearance. Foam cells with this appearance are frequently termed "Niemann-Pick cells"; in fact, however, they are found in the marrow of patients with many different disorders. It seems quite likely that foam cells of this type are present in the bone marrow of patients with all of the disorders listed in Table 24–1, with the exception of Gaucher's disease.

Occasionally foam cells are seen in which the cytoplasmic droplets do not glitter but rather have a homogeneous "ground glass" appearance; these droplets are usually not birefringent. We have observed this type of foam cell in a well-documented case of Niemann-Pick disease (Type C), in G_{M1} gangliosidosis, and in Types I and V hyperlipoproteinemia. It should be noted, however, that the more common, granular type of foam cell has been observed in other patients with each of these disorders. This observation suggests that factors other than the chemical nature of the stored material determine the microscopic appearance of the lipid droplets within foam cells.

In Gaucher's disease the bone marrow contains foam cells that are quite different from those seen in any other disorder. Their appearance under the phase contrast micro-

---

Color Plate II.   Photomicrographs of foam cells.
1. Dark field photomicrograph – Niemann-Pick Disease Type B.
2. Phase contrast photomicrograph – Type I hyperlipoproteinemia.
3. Polarization photomicrograph – Type I hyperlipoproteinemia.
4. Polarization photomicrograph with 1/4 plate – Niemann-Pick Disease Type A.
5. Nomarski photomicrograph – Type I hyperlipoproteinemia.
6. Photomicrograph, Giemsa stained – Niemann-Pick Disease Type B.
7. Phase contrast photomicrograph – Gaucher's Disease Type 1.
8. Photomicrograph, Giemsa stained – Gaucher's Disease Type 1.
9. Nomarski photomicrographs – Gaucher's Disease Type 1.
     (The authors thank Dr. Victor J. Ferrans for photomicrographing several of these cells.)

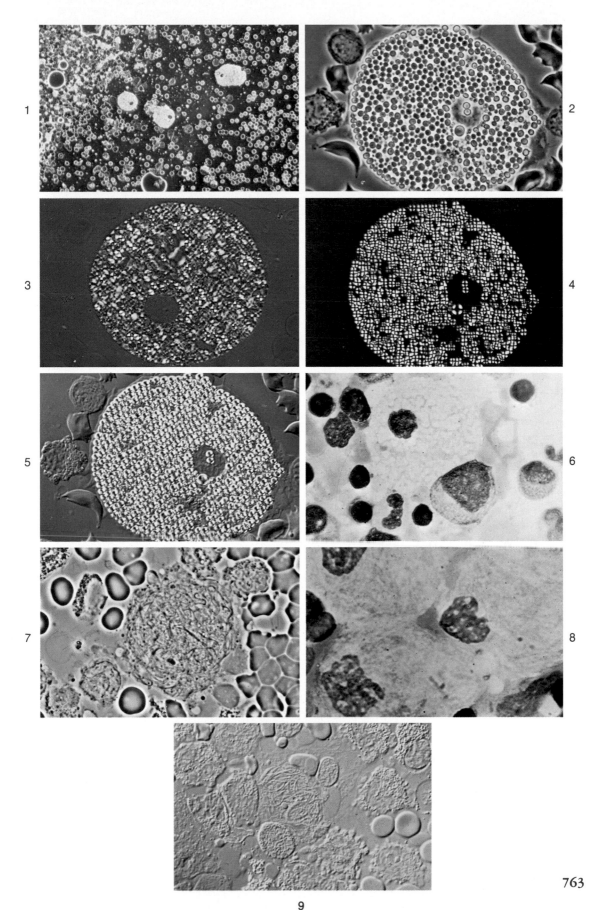

9

Color Plate II. *See Opposite Page for Legend.*

scope is sufficiently unique to permit an almost certain diagnosis. "Gaucher cells" (Color Plate II, 7, 8) are usually between 20 and 100 μ in diameter, with a nucleus that is often eccentric. The cytoplasm appears to be stuffed with many long, undulating fibrils of different lengths. The thickness of these fibrils in a single cell may vary from less than 0.1 μ to more than 1 μ. It has been clearly demonstrated that these fibrils are actually packets of tubules that have been visualized with the electron microscope (2). With the phase microscope, the fibrils appear as clumps of "wrinkled tissue paper" or "crumpled silk." Foam cells in chronic myelogenous leukemia are quite similar in appearance to Gaucher cells; the fibrils, however, tend to have a somewhat coarser appearance.

In routine Giemsa stained preparations of most foam cells, the cytoplasm stains faintly pink and has a foamy, honeycombed or Swiss cheese–like appearance (Color Plate II, 6, 7). No subcellular organization is visible within the cytoplasm. The foam cells observed in Gaucher's disease are an exception to this general rule. The cytoplasm of Gaucher cells contains many wavy fibrils of different lengths (Color Plate II, 8).

The application of lipid staining techniques to the study of foam cells has not proven to be very useful. Unfortunately, there is no histochemical technique that specifically stains only one lipid or one lipid class. Foam cells in many disorders stain positively with the nonspecific fat stain, oil-red-O. Foam cells in Niemann-Pick disease often only stain weakly with Baker's hematoxylin, even though they probably contain large concentrations of phospholipids. Foam cells in G_{M1} gangliosidosis stain weakly with the periodic acid–Schiff (PAS) reaction, although they almost certainly contain significant concentrations of gangliosides. Gaucher cells do stain positively with PAS, and the intracytoplasmic fibrillar material is well visualized following staining with Mallory's trichrome reaction. It is possible that the application of better fixation techniques and the development of more specific lipid histochemical staining reactions may in the future permit a more precise classification of different types of foam cells.

The electron microscopic appearance of the foam cells that occur in most of the diseases listed in Table 24–1 has not been well documented. The foam cells that are found in Gaucher's disease and Niemann-Pick disease have, however, been extensively studied. Under the electron microscope the Gaucher cell is seen to contain characteristic cytoplasmic residual bodies or secondary lysosomes. These have a single limiting membrane surrounding a pale matrix, which is filled with tubular structures that vary between 120 and 750Å in diameter. The tubules may be up to 5 microns in length. Each tubule contains 10 to 12 fibrils twisted around the long axis of the tubule as a right-handed helix (2).

Scattered about the cytoplasm of the foam cells in Niemann-Pick disease are many round or oval residual bodies; they may vary from 0.5 to 5 microns in diameter (5). The residual bodies contain membranous cytoplasmic bodies, which are dense osmiophilic layers alternating with clear osmiophobic layers. Similar membranous cytoplasmic bodies have been observed in foam cells of patients with the hyperlipoproteinemias and in solid tissues of patients with several lipid storage diseases.

At this time only Gaucher's disease can be diagnosed with relative certainty by studying the microscopic appearance of bone marrow foam cells. It seems possible that improved histochemical and electron microscopic techniques may permit the precise differentiation of each lipid storage disorder.

DISORDERS OF LIPID METABOLISM

There are several major classes of disorders characterized by abnormalities of lipid metabolism. We will focus our attention on those disorders of lipid metabolism in which foam cells are observed in the bone marrow. We will also describe other closely related diseases (Table 24–2). It is convenient to classify these diseases as disorders of sphingolipid metabolism, disorders of nonpolar lipid metablism, and disorders of lipoprotein metabolism.

Sphingolipid Storage Diseases
SPHINGOLIPID CHEMISTRY

Sphingolipids contain a family of compounds called sphingosines. The principle naturally occuring member of this family is D (+) *erythro*-1,3-dihydroxy-2-amino-4-*trans*-octadecene; this compound is called

Text continued page 769.

TABLE 24–2. THE TISSUE LIPID STORAGE DISORDERS

	Niemann-Pick Disease Type A	Niemann-Pick Disease Type B	Niemann-Pick Disease Type C
CLINICAL ONSET (YRS.)	1/2	2–4	3–5
LIFE EXPECTANCY (YRS.)	< 4	Unknown	< 15
EARLIEST MANIFESTATIONS	FTT, HSmegaly, PM deterioration	HSmegaly	PM deterioration, HSmegaly
ADDITIONAL ABNORMALITIES			
Cherry Red Spot	+	−	−
Foam Cells	+	+	+
UNIQUE FEATURES	Reticular pulmonary infiltrates, vacuolated lymphocytes	Reticular pulmonary infiltrates	
INHERITANCE	A.R.	A.R.	A.R.
ETHNIC EXTRACTION	Often Jewish		
LIPIDS ACCUMULATED	Sphingomyelin, cholesterol	Sphingomyelin, cholesterol	Sphingomyelin, cholesterol
ENZYME DEFICIENCY	Sphingomyelinase	Sphingomyelinase	?

	Niemann-Pick Disease Type D	Gaucher's Disease Type I	Gaucher's Disease Type II
CLINICAL ONSET (YRS.)	3–5	0–91	1/2
LIFE EXPECTANCY (YRS.)	< 20	Variable	< 2
EARLIEST MANIFESTATIONS	PM deterioration, HSmegaly	HSmegaly, thrombocytopenia & bleeding	PM deterioration, HSmegaly
ADDITIONAL ABNORMALITIES			
Cherry Red Spot	−	−	−
Foam Cells	+	+	+
UNIQUE FEATURES		Bony lesions, reticular pulmonary infiltrates	Head retroflexion, coughing, trismus, laryngospasm, abnormal facies, nystagmus
INHERITANCE	A.R.	A.R.	A.R.
ETHNIC EXTRACTION	Nova Scotian	Often Jewish	
LIPIDS ACCUMULATED	Sphingomyelin, cholesterol	Glucosyl ceramide (GL1a)	Glucosyl ceramide (GL1a)
ENZYME DEFICIENCY	?	GL1a-β-glucosidase	GL1a-β-glucosidase

Abbreviations: FTT, failure to thrive; HSmegaly, hepatosplenomegaly; PM deterioration, psychomotor deterioration; A.R., autosomal recessive; S.L., sex-linked; ACEH, acid cholesteryl ester hydrolase; ATGL, acid triglyceride lipase; AMPS, acid mucopolysaccharides.

Table continued on following page.

TABLE 24–2. THE TISSUE LIPID STORAGE DISORDERS (*Continued*)

	Gaucher's Disease Type III	G_{M1} Gangliosidosis Type I	G_{M1} Gangliosidosis Type II
CLINICAL ONSET (YRS.)	1–3	Birth	1–2
LIFE EXPECTANCY (YRS.)	< 30	< 2	< 10
EARLIEST MANIFESTATIONS	PM deterioration, HSmegaly	PM deterioration, FTT, HSmegaly	PM deterioration
ADDITIONAL ABNORMALITIES			
Cherry Red Spot	–	+	–
Foam Cells	+	+	Variable
UNIQUE FEATURES		Bony lesions, abnormal facies, vacuolated lymphocytes, AMPS in urine	
INHERITANCE	A.R.	A.R.	A.R.
ETHNIC EXTRACTION			
LIPIDS ACCUMULATED	Glucosyl ceramide	Ganglioside G_{M1}	Ganglioside G_{M1}
ENZYME DEFICIENCY	?	G_{M1}-β-galactosidase	G_{M1}-β-galactosidase

	Lactosyl Ceramidosis	Fabry's Disease	Krabbe's Disease
CLINICAL ONSET (YRS.)	1	5–20	1/4–1/2
LIFE EXPECTANCY (YRS.)	< 4	Variable	< 2
EARLIEST MANIFESTATIONS	FTT, PM deterioration, HSmegaly	Fever, joint swelling, peripheral pain and edema, telangiectasias	PM deterioration
ADDITIONAL ABNORMALITIES			
Cherry Red Spot	–	–	–
Foam Cells	+	Variable	–
UNIQUE FEATURES		Renal involvement, cataracts	Optic atrophy
INHERITANCE	Unknown	S.L.	A.R.
ETHNIC EXTRACTION		Often Scandinavian	
LIPIDS ACCUMULATED	Lactosyl ceramide (GL2a)	Trihexosyl ceramide (GL3), dihexosyl ceramide (GL2b)	Galactosyl* ceramide (GL1b)
ENZYME DEFICIENCY	GL2a-β-galactosidase	GL3-α-galactosidase	GL1b-β-galactosidase

*Extensive demyelination with relative increase of GL1b.

TABLE 24–2. THE TISSUE LIPID STORAGE DISORDERS (*Continued*)

	Infantile Metachromatic Leukodystrophy	Juvenile Metachromatic Leukodystrophy	Adult Metachromatic Leukodystrophy
CLINICAL ONSET (YRS.)	1–2	5–10	19–46
LIFE EXPECTANCY (YRS.)	< 10	< 20	Variable
EARLIEST MANIFESTATIONS	PM deterioration	PM deterioration	Dementia
ADDITIONAL ABNORMALITIES *Cherry Red Spot* *Foam Cells*	– –	– –	– –
UNIQUE FEATURES	Nonfunctioning gall-bladder, optic atrophy	Optic atrophy	
INHERITANCE	A.R.	A.R.	A.R.
ETHNIC EXTRACTION			
LIPIDS ACCUMULATED	Sulfatide	Sulfatide	Sulfatide
ENZYME DEFICIENCY	Sulfatidase (aryl-sulfatase A)	Sulfatidase (aryl-sulfatase A)	Sulfatidase (aryl-sulfatase A)

	Metachromatic Leukodystrophy, Multiple Sulfatase Deficiency Form	Tay-Sachs Disease Type I	Tay-Sachs Disease Type II
CLINICAL ONSET (YRS.)	1 2	1/4–1/2	1/4–1/2
LIFE EXPECTANCY (YRS.)	< 12	< 5	< 4
EARLIEST MANIFESTATIONS	PM deterioration	PM deterioration, hypotonia, "hyperacusis"	PM deterioration, hypotonia, hyperacusis
ADDITIONAL ABNORMALITIES *Cherry Red Spot* *Foam Cells*	– –	+ –	+ –
UNIQUE FEATURES	AMPS in urine, bony lesions, granulated lymphocytes	Macrocephaly	Macrocephaly
INHERITANCE	Unknown	A.R.	A.R.
ETHNIC EXTRACTION		Usually Jewish	
LIPIDS ACCUMULATED	Sulfatide	Ganglioside G_{M2}	GL4, ganglioside G_{M2}
ENZYME DEFICIENCY	Arylsulfatase A,B,C	Hexosaminidase A	Hexosaminidase A & B

Table continued on following page.

TABLE 24–2.   THE TISSUE LIPID STORAGE DISORDERS (*Continued*)

	Tay-Sachs Disease Type III	Wolman's Disease	Cholesteryl Ester Storage Disease
CLINICAL ONSET (YRS.)	1–2	Birth	3–19
LIFE EXPECTANCY (YRS.)	< 15	< 1	Variable
EARLIEST MANIFESTATIONS	PM deterioration	FTT, GI symptoms	Hepatomegaly
ADDITIONAL ABNORMALITIES			
Cherry Red Spot	−	−	−
Foam Cells	−	+	+
UNIQUE FEATURES		Adrenal calcification	Hypercholesterolemia
INHERITANCE	Unknown	A.R.	Unknown
ETHNIC EXTRACTION			
LIPIDS ACCUMULATED	Ganglioside G_{M2}	Cholesteryl ester, triglyceride	Cholesteryl ester, triglyceride
ENZYME DEFICIENCY	Hexosaminidase A	ACEH, ATGL	ACEH, ATGL

	Cerebrotendinous Xanthomatosis	Refsum's Syndrome
CLINICAL ONSET (YRS.)	10–51	5–50
LIFE EXPECTANCY (YRS.)	Variable	Variable
EARLIEST MANIFESTATIONS	Cerebellar ataxia, xanthomatosis, dementia	Visual impairment, peripheral neuropathy, ataxia
ADDITIONAL ABNORMALITIES		
Cherry Red Spot	−	−
Foam Cells	+	−
UNIQUE FEATURES		Night blindness, icthyosis, epiphyseal dysplasia, retinitis pigmentosa
INHERITANCE	A.R.	A.R.
ETHNIC EXTRACTION		
LIPIDS ACCUMULATED	Cholesterol, cholestanol	Phytanic acid
ENZYME DEFICIENCY	?	Phytanic acid, α-hydroxylase

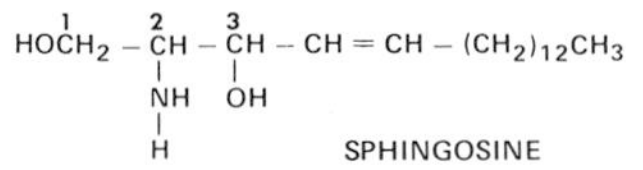

$$HOCH_2 - \overset{2}{C}H - \overset{3}{C}H - CH = CH - (CH_2)_{12}CH_3$$
$$| \quad |$$
$$NH \quad OH$$
$$|$$
$$H \qquad SPHINGOSINE$$

Figure 24–1. Chemical structure of sphingosine.

sphingosine (Fig. 24–1). All sphingosines are aliphatic 2-amino-1,3-diols; variations between members of the sphingosine family occur in the total chain length, degree of unsaturation, and number of additional hydroxyl groups (3).

The fundamental unit of sphingolipids is the N-acyl derivative of sphingosine or its congeners, in which a long-chain fatty acid, R, is attached to the amino group on carbon-2 through an amide linkage. The generic term for this class of compounds is ceramide (Fig. 24–2).

Mammalian sphingolipids contain ceramide as a structural unit, and the distinguishing feature of each is the moiety esterified to the C_1 of ceramide. In the sphingomyelins this group is phosphorylcholine, while in the neutral glycosphingolipids it is a mono- or oligosaccharide (Fig. 24–3). The substituent is galactose-3-sulfate in the sulfatides (Fig. 24–3), and an oligosaccharide containing at least one sialic acid in the gangliosides (Fig. 24–4).

Sphingolipid storage forms the basis for the diagnosis of a sphingolipidosis, and eight major classes have been delineated. Most of these have phenotypically and genotypically distinct subtypes. The storage of sphingolipids may be owing to either excessive production or deficient catabolism. The overwhelming evidence indicates a defect in catabolism in most of the sphingolipidoses. The defect is usually a deficient activity of a lysosomal sphingolipid hydrolase (Fig. 24–5).

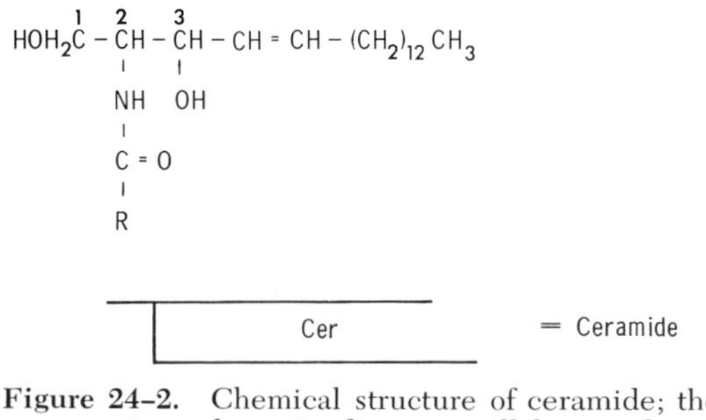

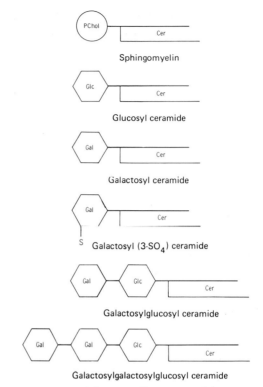

Figure 24–3. Schematic illustration of the structure of sphingolipids. Abbreviations: PChol, phosphorylcholine; Glc, glucose; Gal, galactose; S, sulfate.

Sphingolipid Storage Diseases with Foam Cells

Niemann-Pick Disease

The sphingomyelin lipidoses (Niemann-Pick Disease, NPD) (5) are characterized by the presence of an increased tissue concentration of sphingomyelin. At least four different phenotypes are recognizable:

TYPE A. Type A is characterized by the involvement of both viscera and nervous system in infancy. Before 6 months of age, these patients have hepatosplenomegaly, reticular pulmonary infiltration, mulberry-type foam cells in the bone marrow, cherry-red spots in the retina, and failure to thrive. By age 1 year, evidence of mental retardation is almost invariably present. There ensues a generalized loss of motor and intellectual function, which culminates in death before age 4 years. Tissues from these patients have been shown to be severely deficient in the lysosomal enzyme, sphingo-

$$HOH_2\overset{1}{C} - \overset{2}{C}H - \overset{3}{C}H - CH = CH - (CH_2)_{12} CH_3$$
$$| \quad |$$
$$NH \quad OH$$
$$|$$
$$C = O$$
$$|$$
$$R$$

| Cer | = Ceramide |

Figure 24–2. Chemical structure of ceramide; the accompanying schematic diagram will be employed to designate ceramide throughout this chapter.

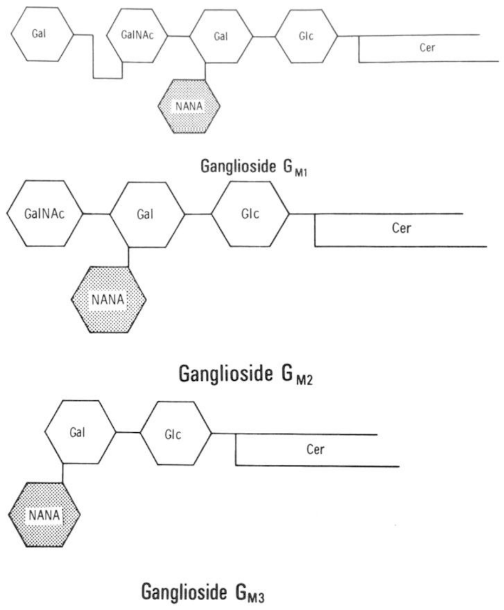

Figure 24–4. Schematic illustration of the structure of three monosialogangliosides. Abbreviations: GalNAc, *N*-acetylgalactosamine; NANA, *N*-acetylneuraminic acid.

myelinase. This enzyme catalyzes the first step in the normal degradation of sphingomyelin.

TYPE B. Type B patients may develop the visceral signs of the disease (hepatosplenomegaly, pulmonary infiltrations, foam cells in the bone marrow) as early as Type A patients. Patients with Type B also have a similar degree of sphingomyelin storage. The nervous system is spared, cherry-red spots do not develop, and vision is normal. Patients may reach adulthood intellectually intact. Sphingomyelinase is also deficient in Type B.

TYPE C. Type C patients have neurovisceral involvement, but follow a more prolonged course than Type A patients. They appear normal for one to two years, then develop neurologic abnormalities and die in childhood or adolescence. Type C patients have less obvious hepatosplenomegaly than Type A or B patients and also a smaller increase in tissue sphingomyelin content. They appear to have normal tissue sphingomyelinase activity. At this time it seems quite possible that Niemann-Pick Disease, Type C, represents a heterogeneous group of diseases.

TYPE D. Type D is similar to type C but found in patients of Nova Scotian ancestry.

It must be reemphasized that microscopic examination of the bone marrow is insufficient evidence upon which to base a diagnosis of Niemann-Pick disease. In many diseases foam cells accumulate in the bone marrow that are morphologically indistinguishable by light microscopy from the cells observed in Niemann-Pick disease. Types A, B, C, and D are autosomal recessive disorders. The Type A gene frequency is unusually high among Jews from Eastern Europe. Heterozygote detection is not reliable. Although there is no specific therapy, intrauterine diagnosis of Type A NPD has been achieved (6).

Gaucher's Disease

Gaucher's disease is characterized by the accumulation within tissues of glucosyl ceramide (2). Three clinical forms have been detected. In all three forms of the disease, distinctive foam cells are observed in the bone marrow. The appearance of the Gaucher cell is sufficiently unique to permit an almost certain diagnosis when unstained preparations of bone marrow are viewed under the phase contrast microscope. The only other condition in which similar foam cells occur is chronic myelogenous leukemia.

TYPE 1. The adult or chronic non-neuronopathic form may manifest itself at any time from birth to old age. Patients with this disease invariably have hepatosplenomegaly; splenomegaly is frequently the most striking feature. Hypersplenism may lead to clinically significant thrombocytopenia; recurrent epistaxis, purpura, or severe bleeding episodes may necessitate splenectomy. Bony lesions are another manifestation of this disease. The marrow cavity is filled with masses of Gaucher cells, and there may be bone pain and pathologic fractures. The commonest radiographic sign is an expansion of the marrow at the lower end of the femur, leaving a radiolucency in the contour of an Erlenmeyer flask.

TYPE 2. The infantile or acute neuronopathic form of Gaucher's disease is usually apparent before 6 months and fatal by 2 years of age. The course of this disease is rapid, with neurologic involvement including strabismus, muscular hypertonicity, persistent retroflexion of the neck, and mental deterioration. Peripheral tissue lipid storage is similar to that in Type 1 Gaucher's disease; hepatosplenomegaly and Gaucher cells in the bone marrow are prominent features.

TYPE 3. A group of individuals have been

THE SPHINGOLIPIDOSES

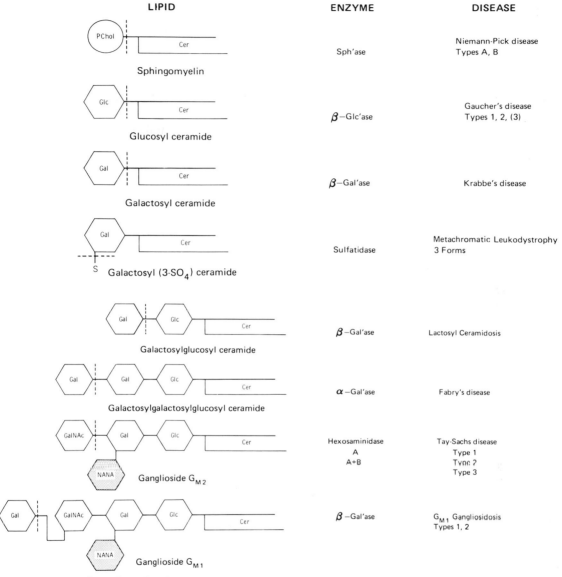

| LIPID | ENZYME | DISEASE |

Sphingomyelin — Sph'ase — Niemann-Pick disease Types A, B

Glucosyl ceramide — β–Glc'ase — Gaucher's disease Types 1, 2, (3)

Galactosyl ceramide — β–Gal'ase — Krabbe's disease

Galactosyl (3-SO$_4$) ceramide — Sulfatidase — Metachromatic Leukodystrophy 3 Forms

Galactosylglucosyl ceramide — β–Gal'ase — Lactosyl Ceramidosis

Galactosylgalactosylglucosyl ceramide — α–Gal'ase — Fabry's disease

Ganglioside G$_{M2}$ — Hexosaminidase A, A+B — Tay-Sachs disease Type 1, Type 2, Type 3

Ganglioside G$_{M1}$ — β–Gal'ase — G$_{M1}$ Gangliosidosis Types 1, 2

Figure 24–5. The sphingolipidoses. A compilation of the lipids accumulated and the apparent enzymatic defects in each of the major classes of the sphingolipidoses.

described who have central nervous system abnormalities and cells in non-neural tissues that have the histologic appearance of Gaucher cells. The clinical course of these patients is, however, subacute, and the onset of cerebral abnormalities may be delayed. Although they usually die in adolescence, some patients have survived into the third decade.

In Type 1 and Type 2 Gaucher's disease, there is deficient activity of tissue glucocerebrosidase, which normally cleaves glucose from glucosyl ceramide. The enzymatic abnormality is less definitively established in Type 3 Gaucher's disease. Types 1, 2, and 3 are autosomal recessive conditions. The gene frequency of Type 1 Gaucher's disease is high among Eastern European Jews. Heterozygote detection may be possible. Although there is no specific therapy, intrauterine diagnosis of Gaucher's disease has been accomplished (7). In Type 1 patients splenectomy may be necessary to prevent bleeding episodes. The underlying disease process is not alleviated by removal of the spleen, and there is no reason to perform a splenectomy before the time when either the hematologic effects of hypersplenism or serious mechanical distress provide a definite indication. Patients may do well for many years with a platelet count below 50,000. There is some evidence that splenectomy may be followed by a more rapid progression of bony involvement (2).

G_{M1} Gangliosidosis

There are two childhood diseases in which ganglioside G_{M1} accumulates (8). TYPE 1 (GENERALIZED GANGLIOSIDOSIS). The symptoms of generalized gangliosidosis are apparent at birth or shortly thereafter. There are psychomotor retardation, weak sucking, poor appetite, and failure to thrive. The infant is dull looking, hypoactive, and hypotonic. The facial abnormalities may include frontal bossing, depressed nasal bridge, and large low-set ears. There is usually a cherry-red spot in the macular region. Hepatosplenomegaly is present by 6 months of age. Musculoskeletal abnormalities include dorsolumbar kyphoscoliosis, short stubby fingers, and flexion contractures of the fingers. The most impressive early radiographic lesion consists of generalized symmetric periosteal new bone formation over the long bones and ribs. By 6 months the most impressive x-ray lesions are beaked lumbar vertebral bodies and long bones widened in the midshaft region with tapering, both proximally and distally. TYPE 2 (JUVENILE G_{M1} GANGLIOSIDOSIS). Patients with this disorder are usually normal for the first year of life. Psychomotor deterioration has its onset between one and two years of age, and death ensues between 3 and 10 years of age. Facies may be normal; there is no cherry-red spot in the macula. Hepatosplenomegaly is absent, and bony abnormalities, if present, are mild.

G_{M1} gangliosidosis Types 1 and 2 appear to be transmitted as autosomal recessive diseases. Ganglioside G_{M1} accumulates in the brain in both disorders; visceral accumulation of ganglioside G_{M1} has been found only in Type 1. Foam cells have been invariably observed in the bone marrow in Types 1 and 2. A mucopolysaccharide similar to keratin sulfate accumulates in the viscera in both disorders. A striking deficiency of ganglioside G_{M1}-β-galactosidase is present in both Types 1 and 2. Although there is no specific therapy, heterozygotes may be detected by β-galactosidase assay, and prenatal diagnosis has been accomplished (9).

Lactosyl Ceramidosis (Galactosylglucosyl Ceramidosis)

A single patient with tissue storage of lactosylceramide has been described (10). The patient showed delayed milestones for the first 2½ years of life and thereafter showed signs of neurologic deterioration. There were hepatosplenomegaly, lymphadenopathy, and foam cells in the bone marrow. A deficiency of galactosylglucosyl ceramide-β-galactosidase was demonstrated.

Fabry's Disease

Patients with Fabry's disease accumulate trihexosyl ceramide (11). The disorder is seen in hemizygous males. The earliest manifestations occur in childhood or early adolescence. Telangiectasias are an early sign and most commonly occur in the area between the umbilicus and the knees. Other clinical signs include bouts of pain and paresthesias of the extremities, edema of the legs, hypohidrosis, albuminuria, and hyposthenuria. Severe renal impairment leads to hypertension and uremia, and death usually results from renal failure or cardiac or cerebrovascular disease. Heterozygous females may express symptoms of the disease as well, although usually in milder form.

The deposition of trihexosyl ceramide occurs in the endothelium and smooth muscle of blood vessels, in ganglion cells, in the heart, kidneys, eyes, and most other tissues. Lipid-laden macrophages are occasionally seen in the bone marrow in this disease. The defect in Fabry's disease is deficient activity of the enzyme trihexosyl ceramide galactosyl-hydrolase, an α-galactosidase. Although there is no specific therapy for Fabry's disease, renal transplantation has aided patients who were dying of chronic renal failure. Fabry's disease has also been diagnosed in utero (12).

Sphingolipid Storage Diseases Without Foam Cells

Krabbe's Disease

Globoid cell leukodystrophy or Krabbe's disease is an autosomal recessive metabolic disorder of the nervous system (13). The onset of the disease is between age 3 and 6 months, with progressive psychomotor deterioration, spastic quadriparesis, and optic atrophy. Death usually occurs by age 2 years. Histopathologic lesions are confined to the nervous system, where there is a paucity of myelin, severe astrocytic gliosis, and massive infiltration of lipid-filled macrophages that have been termed globoid cells. There are no peripheral foam cells in Krabbe's disease. The globoid cells contain galactosyl ceramide. Deficient activities of galactosyl ceramide-β-galactosidase and galactosyl sphingosine-β-galactosidase have been demonstrated. Krabbe's disease has also been diagnosed in utero (14).

Metachromatic Leukodystrophy

Metachromatic leukodystrophy (MLD) represents a group of four inherited autosomal recessive disorders in which myelin degeneration is associated with the accumulation of cerebroside sulfate (15). Infantile MLD usually has its onset between 12 and 18 months of age, and is characterized by progressive paralysis, dementia, and blindness. The disease is usually fatal within two to ten years. Juvenile MLD most commonly has its onset between 5 and 10 years of age. The first symptoms are usually related to poor school performance. The disease is progressive and quite similar to infantile MLD. Patients with the adult form of MLD become symptomatic as early as 19 years of age or as late as 46. Symptoms of dementia may precede motor difficulties by many years. These three forms of MLD are associated with a deficiency in all tissues of the enzyme cerebroside sulfate-sulfatidase. This activity may be conveniently assayed with an artificial substrate; under these circumstances, the enzyme is referred to as arylsulfatase A.

A fourth form of MLD is associated with tissue deficiencies of arylsulfatase A, B, and C, and is called the multiple sulfatase deficiency form of MLD. The clinical onset of psychomotor deterioration is at 1 to 2 years of age; death ensues between 3 and 12 years of age. This disease has certain features in common with the mucopolysaccharidoses, such as thick skin, hepatosplenomegaly, granules in white blood cells, broadening of bones, and increased urinary mucopolysaccharide excretion.

In MLD the main pathologic changes occur in the white matter of the central and peripheral nervous system. Metachromatic material has also been shown in peripheral tissues; the gall bladder is invariably extensively involved. Foam cells have not been observed in the bone marrow in MLD. The infantile form of MLD has been diagnosed in utero (16).

Tay-Sachs Disease

Tay-Sachs disease (TSD), formerly called infantile amaurotic idiocy, is characterized by the tissue accumulation of ganglioside G_{M2} (3). The classic form of the disease (Type 1) has its clinical onset between ages 4 and 6 months. There is progressive psychomotor deterioration, exaggerated extension response to sound (erroneously called hyperacusis), hypotonia, and visual difficulties with a cherry-red spot in the retina. Death occurs by the age of 3 to 4 years. In Type 1 TSD the tissues are deficient in the enzyme ganglioside G_{M2}-hexosaminidase, this enzyme catalyzes the cleavage of the terminal N-acetylgalactosaminyl moiety from ganglioside G_{M2}. This activity, when evaluated with an artificial substrate, is called hexosaminidase A. TSD Type 1 is inherited as an autosomal recessive. The gene frequency is very high in Jews from northeastern Europe, but TSD has been reported in most ethnic groups.

There are two other rare diseases in which ganglioside G_{M2} accumulates. Type 2 is similar clinically to classic TSD, but both hexosaminidase A and B are deficient. Type 3 TSD has a more protracted course than Type 1 TSD.

The major pathologic features of TSD are the accumulation of ganglioside G_{M2} in ganglion cells, ganglion cell destruction, and extensive demyelination associated with reactive gliosis. Although the brain is the site of the most impressive accumulation of G_{M2}, increased concentrations have also been demonstrated in peripheral tissues. A few foam cells may be seen in the spleen or lung. The presence of such cells in a bone marrow aspirate would suggest that TSD was not the proper diagnosis.

Detection of heterozygotes for the TSD gene is possible, and many carriers for this disorder have been identified in high-risk populations (17). Since TSD Type 1 has been diagnosed in utero (18), it should now be possible to reduce significantly the occurrence of this disease.

Nonpolar Lipid Storage Diseases

BIOCHEMISTRY OF THE NONPOLAR LIPIDS

Cholesterol and Cholesteryl Ester Metabolism

Cholesterol is probably synthesized in every tissue (19, 20). Most synthesis occurs in the liver, intestine, and skin. Cholesterol degradation involves alteration of both the side chain and ring structure. The major pathway of catabolism, conversion to bile acids, is limited to the liver. Cholestanol, a compound very similar to cholesterol, is formed in the conversion of cholesterol to bile acids. Tissue cholesteryl esters are derived from three major sources: (1) intestinal absorption: cholesterol from diet, bile, and desquamated intestinal epithelial cells is absorbed by the intestinal mucosal cells; there it is esterified and then secreted into the lymph in chylomicrons; (2) in situ synthesis: all tissues possess enzymes which can esterify cholesterol with a fatty acid; (3) plasma synthesis: cholesterol in plasma may be esterified by the enzyme lecithin:cholesterol acyltransferase (LCAT).

Enzymes that catalyze the cleavage of cholesteryl ester to cholesterol and free fatty acid are found in most tissues. The major portion of this activity is in the lysosomes. Free cholesterol moves across the cell membrane and is transported to the liver, where it is converted to bile acids. Therefore, the inability to hydrolyze cholesteryl esters could seriously disturb the intracellular content of total cholesterol.

Triglycerides

Triglycerides are esters of fatty acids and the trihydroxy alcohol, L-glycerol. Triglycerides are the most abundant fats in nature and are amply present in the diet. Pancreatic lipase converts dietary triglycerides into monoglycerides and fatty acids (21). These enter the intestinal mucosal cell and are immediately reesterified to triglycerides, which are excreted into the lymph as chylomicrons. Tissue triglycerides arise not only from the diet but also from de novo synthe-sis. The liver can convert excess amino acids or carbohydrates into triglycerides and secretes triglycerides into the plasma as a constituent of very low density lipoproteins (VLDL).

The removal of chylomicron and VLDL triglyceride from plasma involves the action of both lipoprotein lipase in muscle and adipose tissue and a "hormone-sensitive" lipase in adipose tissue. Triglycerides are degraded in tissues by lysosomal (acid) enzymes; in addition, liver contains a neutral triglyceride lipase.

Nonpolar Lipid Storage Diseases with Foam Cells

Wolman's Disease

Wolman's disease is an inherited autosomal recessive disorder (20). It expresses itself in the first few weeks of life with diarrhea, hepatosplenomegaly, adrenal calcification, and failure to thrive. Death usually ensues by age 6 months. There is a profound increase in the tissue content of triglycerides and cholesteryl esters. Foam cells are plentiful in the bone marrow. The basic metabolic defect in Wolman's disease seems to be a deficiency of acid hydrolase activity directed toward the catabolism of triglycerides and cholesteryl esters. There is no specific therapy.

Cholesteryl Ester Storage Disease

Cholesteryl ester storage disease is a rare familial disease, probably transmitted as an autosomal recessive (20). The patients are usually asymptomatic, but have hepatomegaly and hypercholesterolemia. Histopathology shows hepatocytes stuffed with lipid; lipid is also seen in the *lamina propria* of the intestine and in foam cells in the bone marrow. Tissue lipid analysis reveals excessive amounts of cholesteryl ester in several tissues. Triglyceride accumulation has also been documented in liver and spleen. The basic defect is a deficiency in many tissues of an acid cholesteryl ester hydrolase and also of an acid trigylceride lipase (22, 23). There is no specific therapy.

Cerebrotendinous Xanthomatosis

The onset of cerebrotendinous xanthomatosis (CTX) is insidious; the first symptoms appear as early as age 10 or as late as age 51 (20). Patients with CTX usually develop progressive cerebellar ataxia, dementia, cataracts, and tendon xanthomas. The most striking pathologic changes usually occur in the cerebellum, tendons, lung, and bone; the cerebrum is histopathologically normal. Lesions appear as granulomas containing needle-shaped, birefringent, crystalline clefts, multinucleated giant cells, and large foam cells. An increased concentration of cholestanol and cholesterol has been observed in apparently normal tissue as well as in organs which are clearly involved in the disease process (24). Plasma cholestanol is also elevated, and the composition of the bile acids is altered. The basic enzyme defect remains to be elucidated; evidence indicates a possible defect in the pathway from cholesterol to bile acids. CTX is transmitted in an autosomal recessive fashion, and there is no specific therapy.

Nonpolar Lipid Storage Diseases Without Foam Cells

Phytanic Acid Storage Disease: Refsum's Syndrome

Refsum's syndrome is a rare disease with autosomal recessive inheritance (25). The onset of clinical symptoms may be in early childhood or as late as the fifth decade. The major features of the disease are peripheral neuropathy, ataxia, retinitis pigmentosa, ichthyosis-like changes in the skin, and epiphyseal dysplasia. Foam cells are not found in the bone marrow. There is a profound tissue accumulation of the 20-carbon branched-chain fatty acid, phytanic acid. There appears to be no endogenous synthesis of this fatty acid, and therefore all of the phytanic acid accumulated originates in the diet. The metabolic defect is a deficiency in the activity of phytanic acid α-hydroxylase, the enzyme that catalyzes the first step in the catabolism of phytanic acid. Significant improvement in clinical manifestations has followed prolonged restriction of phytanic acid precursors in the diet.

The Hyperlipoproteinemias

PLASMA LIPOPROTEIN COMPOSITION AND METABOLISM

Lipoproteins are vehicles which enable water-insoluble lipids to be transported in the blood (26). Lipoproteins are classified on the basis of differences in their size, charge, and rates of flotation in the ultracentrifuge. This latter property is determined by the density of each lipoprotein class. There are four classes of lipoproteins, chylomicrons, very low density lipoprotein (VLDL), low density lipoprotein (LDL), and high density lipoprotein (HDL), each with a characteristic array of proteins and lipids (Table 24–3). Chylomicra are synthesized in the intestinal mucosal cell during fat digestion and serve to transport exogenous (dietary) lipid to the rest of the body. VLDL is synthesized mainly in the liver and transports endogenously synthesized lipid. LDL is thought to arise from the metabolism of VLDL after the removal of much of the glyceride and some of the protein. LDL is the principle carrier of cholesterol in human plasma, and high plasma levels are thought to be atherogenic. HDL is synthesized principally in the liver, and its major function has not been clearly defined. HDL does serve as a cofactor for the cholesterol esterifying enzyme, lecithin:cholesterol acyltransferase, and therefore may play an important role in cholesteryl ester metabolism.

Hyperlipoproteinemia

There are many conditions in which plasma lipoproteins and hence plasma lipids exceed normal values (Table 24–4). It is convenient to think of these conditions either as primary familial disorders or as secondary to other abnormalities (21). There are five major types of familial hyperlipoproteinemia (Table 24–5). Secondary (nonfamilial) hyperlipoproteinemia is most commonly caused by nephrosis, uncontrolled diabetes mellitus, hypothyroidism, biliary obstruction, or multiple myeloma.

TABLE 24–3.   THE PROPERTIES AND COMPOSITION OF THE MAJOR LIPOPROTEIN FAMILIES

	CHYLOMICRONS	VLDL	LDL	HDL
Synonyms		Prebetalipoproteins	β-Lipoproteins	α-Lipoproteins
Range of particle size, Å°	750–10,000	300–500	200–220	75–100
Electrophoretic behavior†	Remain at origin	Pre-beta mobility	Beta mobility	Alpha₁ mobility
Ultracentrifugal behavior‡	D < 0.94; S_f) 400	0.94 < D > 1.006; S_f 20–400	1.006 < D < 1.063; S_f 0–20	1.063 < D < 1.21
Lipoprotein constituents (% of dry weight)				
Protein	1–2	10	25	45–55
Triglyceride	80–95	55–65	10	5–8
Unesterified cholesterol	1–3	10	8	3
Esterified cholesterol	2–4	5	37	15
Phospholipids	3–6	15–20	22	30
Carbohydrate	?	< 1	~ 1	< 1

°As determined by electron microscopy.
†On paper and agarose-gel electrophoresis.
‡Expressed as densities in g. per ml. and in Svedberg flotation units, S_f.

Type I Hyperlipoproteinemia

Familial Type I hyperlipoproteinemia is defined by the presence in the plasma, while the patient is on a normal diet, of massive amounts of chylomicrons; these completely disappear within a few days after fat-free feeding is instituted (21). The chylomicronemia, present from the first few weeks of life, is usually associated with lipemia retinalis, hepatosplenomegaly, bouts of abdominal pain, and pancreatitis. In severe hyperglyceridemia, foam cells are found in reticuloendothelial cells, including bone marrow. The disease is transmitted as an autosomal recessive. The basic defect is a slow clearance of chylomicrons from the circulation owing to a deficiency of lipoprotein lipase activity. The treatment is a low-fat diet (27). This will lower plasma glycerides to a point where xanthomas disappear and pancreatitis will not occur.

TABLE 24–4.   PLASMA LIPID CONCENTRATIONS IN NORMAL SUBJECTS*

AGE	CHOLESTEROL (MG./100 ML.)	TRIGLYCERIDE (MG./100 ML.)
1–9 years	120–230	10–140
10–19 years	120–230	10–140
20–29 years	120–240	10–140
30–39 years	140–270	10–150
40–49 years	150–310	10–160
50–59 years	160–330	10–190

*Based on 90 per cent fiducial limits calculated for small samples.

Type II Hyperlipoproteinemia

Type II hyperlipoproteinemia is defined as an inherited increase in plasma low density lipoprotein concentration (21). The disease is thought to be transmitted as

TABLE 24–5. THE FIVE TYPES OF PRIMARY HYPERLIPOPROTEINEMIA

FEATURES	TYPE I	TYPE II	TYPE III	TYPE IV	TYPE V
Incidence	Very rare	Common	Uncommon	Common	Uncommon
Appearance of plasma°	Cream layer on top; clear below	Clear	Clear, milky or cloudy	Slightly turbid to cloudy	Cream layer on top; turbid below
Cholesterol†	↑	↑	↑	↑ or ↔	↑ or ↔
Triglyceride†	↑↑	↔ or ↑	↑	↑	↑ or ↑↑
Cholesterol/ triglyceride ratio	<0.2	>1.5	Often = 1	Variable	>0.15 and <0.6
Age of detection‡	Infancy	Infancy	>20 years	Variable	>20 years
Signs and symptoms	Eruptive xanthomas, lipemia retinalis, hepatosplenomegaly, abdominal pain	Tendon and tuberous xanthomas, accelerated atherosclerosis	Planar, eruptive, and tuberous xanthomas, accelerated atherosclerosis	Possible accelerated atherosclerosis; abnormal glucose tolerance	Eruptive xanthoma lipemia retinalis, hepatosplenomegaly; abnormal glucose tolerance; abdominal pain
Inheritance	Autosomal recessive	Autosomal dominant	Unclear	Autosomal dominant	Unclear

°After standing at 4°C for 18 hours or more.
†↑, increased; ↑↑, greatly increased; ↔, normal.
‡Based on plasma lipid values.

an autosomal dominant. The heterozygote condition may be found in about 0.5 per cent of the general population. There is variable penetrance, and the disease usually expresses itself in the fourth and fifth decades of life with the development of tendon and tuberous xanthomas and premature coronary, cerebral, and peripheral vascular disease. If both parents are heterozygous for Type II hyperlipoproteinemia, then the children may be homozygous for this trait. Patients with the homozygous conditon are much more severely affected; xanthomas appear in the first decade, and death often occurs from coronary artery disease before adulthood.

Histopathologic examination reveals typical lipid-laden cells in the xanthomas and arteriosclerotic lesions. Foam cells have also been seen in reticuloendothelial tissues, including bone marrow. Treatment consists of a diet low in cholesterol and high in polyunsaturated fats (27). Cholestyramine (16 to 48 g. per day), a resin which binds bile acids, is also quite helpful. The combination of dietary and drug therapy usually results in the normalization of the plasma cholesterol. It has not yet been established that normalizing plasma cholesterol levels in Type II patients will prevent premature coronary artery disease. Preliminary data suggest that therapy is effective.

Type III Hyperlipoproteinemia

Type III hyperlipoproteinemia is a rare familial disorder characterized by the presence of complexes of LDL and glycerides that have the flotation properties of VLDL and the electrophoretic mobility of LDL (21). Clinically these patients exhibit planar xanthomas on the palms, eruptive xanthomas, and premature coronary and peripheral vascular disease. Lipid-laden cells are seen in endothelium, skin, and reticuloendothelial tissues, including bone marrow. The genetic mode has not yet been established. The disorder does not seem to express itself until adulthood, and the basic defect is unknown. Treatment consists of proper diet and drug therapy. Calorie intake is restricted until ideal body weight is achieved. A maintenance diet high in polyunsaturated fats and low in cholesterol is followed (27). A lipid lowering drug such as clofibrate, 2.0 g. per day, may be added to the regimen. Lipid values are usually easily normalized, and within weeks to months there is regression of cutaneous xanthomata and apparent improvement of peripheral blood flow (28).

Type IV Hyperlipoproteinemia

Type IV hyperlipoproteinemia is an inherited disease defined by an isolated increase in plasma VLDL (21). Patients with Type IV patterns often have other medical abnormalities, such as obesity, abnormal glucose tolerance, hyperuricemia, and hypertension. The relationship of Type IV hyperlipoproteinemia to these conditions is unclear. Patients with Type IV seem to have an increased incidence of ischemic heart disease; the relative contribution of elevated blood lipids compared to other associated conditions has not been differentiated. The severity of the hypertriglyceridemia varies with age and body weight. Patients with Type IV patterns may have their triglyceride levels exacerbated by diets high in carbohydrate. Hypertriglyceridemia may lead to lipid storage in RE tissues. Hepatosplenomegaly occurs, and foam cells may be seen upon bone marrow examination. Type IV hyperlipoproteinemia is thought to be an autosomal dominant condition with variable penetrance. The disorder may have its onset in the pediatric age range. The basic defect is unknown. Treatment consists of weight reduction and carbohydrate restriction (27), as well as administration of drugs such as clofibrate and nicotinic acid (29).

Type V Hyperlipoproteinemia

Type V hyperlipoproteinemia is an inherited disease defined as the presence in plasma from fasting individuals of chylomicrons and VLDL (21). The clinical symptoms include abdominal pain, pancreatitis, and hepatomegaly. These patients have a greatly increased incidence of obesity, hyperuricemia, and hyperinsulinemic, nonketotic diabetes mellitus. There is no evidence of accelerated vascular disease. Lipid storage at times of hypertriglyceridemia is seen in the RE system, including Kupffer cells in the liver and macrophages in the bone marrow. Type V rarely occurs in childhood and is aggravated by obesity. About one-third of adult relatives of a Type V proband have Type V; the other two-thirds have normal or Type IV patterns. Treatment consists of caloric restriction until ideal body weight is established. A maintenance diet avoiding excesses of either carbohydrate or fat is then followed (27). Nicotinic acid has been found to be a valuable lipid-lowering agent in this disorder (29).

Hypolipoproteinemia with Foam Cells

Tangier Disease

Tangier disease is a rare autosomal recessive disease which has been detected between 3 and 48 years of age (26). The combination of two features is pathognomonic: a low plasma cholesterol concentration associated with normal or elevated triglyceride levels and enlargement and distinctive orange-yellow coloration of the tonsils. Other clinical features of the disease are hepatosplenomegaly, foam cells in the bone marrow, and peripheral neuropathy. Life expectancy is probably normal. These patients store large amounts of cholesteryl ester in their reticuloendothelial system. The basic defect seems to be an absence of normal HDL in their plasma. In its place there is a small amount of altered HDL. There is no specific therapy.

Hypolipoproteinemia without Foam Cells

Abetalipoproteinemia

Abetalipoproteinemia is an autosomal recessive disease which usually presents in infancy with malabsorption and failure to thrive (26). These patients have low plasma cholesterol and a severe deficiency of triglycerides. In the first decade a typical retinitis pigmentosa and a neurologic picture resembling Friedreich's ataxia develop. Moderate to severe steatorrhea, which begins in infancy, becomes less severe by the fourth or fifth year of life. Fat malabsorption probably accounts for the low plasma levels of both vitamins A and E; folic acid deficiency has also been reported. The presence of acanthocytes in the peripheral blood is a constant feature of abetalipoproteinemia. Disability becomes progressively severe; death has occurred both in early childhood and as late as age 37. The basic defect seems to be the absence of chylomicrons, VLDL, and LDL. There is no specific therapy, but consideration should be given to supplementary administration of vitamins A and E.

Familial Lecithin: Cholesterol Acyltransferase Deficiency (LCAT Deficiency).

LCAT deficiency is an inherited autosomal recessive disorder (30). Corneal opacities, anemia with target cells, proteinuria, and hyperlipemia are constant features of the disease. Associated with the hyperlipemia there is a reduction in the level of plasma cholesteryl esters and an elevation of plasma unesterified cholesterol. Several patients have had progressive renal failure; foam cells have been observed in the bone marrow. The underlying metabolic defect seems to be deficient activity of the enzyme, plasma lecithin:cholesterol acyltransferase. Probands may survive to childbearing age and have offspring. There is no specific therapy.

References

1. Nelson, D. S.: *Macrophages and Immunity.* Vol. 11 In *Frontiers of Biology.* Neuberger, A., and Tatum, E. L. (eds.), New York, John Wiley and Sons, 1969.
2. Fredrickson, D. S., and Sloan, H. R.: Glycosyl ceramide lipidoses: Gaucher's disease, In *The Metabolic Basis of Inherited Disease.* 3rd ed. Stanbury, J. B., Wyngaarden, J. B., et al. (eds.), New York, McGraw-Hill, 1972, p. 730.
3. Sloan, H. R., and Fredrickson, D. S.: G_{M2} gangliosidoses: Tay-Sachs disease, In *The Metabolic Basis of Inherited Disease.* 3rd ed. Stanbury, J. B., Wyngaarden, J. B., et al. (eds.), New York, McGraw-Hill, 1972, p. 615.
4. Pearse, A. G. E.: *Histochemistry—Theoretical and Applied.* Boston, Little, Brown and Co., 1960.
5. Fredrickson, D. S., and Sloan, H. R.: Sphingomyelin lipidoses: Niemann-Pick disease, In *The Metabolic Basis of Inherited Disease.* 3rd ed. Stanbury, J. B., Wyngaarden, J. B., et al. (eds.), New York, McGraw-Hill, 1972, p. 783.
6. Epstein, C. J., Brady, R. O., et al.: *In utero* diagnosis of Niemann-Pick disease. Am. J. Hum. Genet. 24:533–535, 1971.
7. Epstein, C. J., Schneider, E. L., et al.: Prenatal detection of genetic disorders. Am. J. Hum. Genet. 24:214–226, 1972.
8. O'Brien, J. S.: G_{M1} gangliosidoses, In *The Metabolic Basis of Inherited Disease.* 3rd ed. Stanbury, J. B., Wyngaarden, J. B., et al. (eds.), New York, McGraw-Hill, 1972, p. 639.
9. Kaback, M. M., Sloan, H. R., et al.: G_{M1} gangliosidosis, Type 1: *In vitro* detection and fetal manifestations. Pediatr. Res. 6:357, 1972.
10. Dawson, G., Matalon, R., et al.: Lactosyl ceramidosis: Lactosyl ceramide galactosyl hydrolase deficiency and accumulation of lactosyl ceramide in cultured skin fibroblasts. J. Pediatr. 79:423–429, 1971.
11. Sweeley, C. C., Klionsky, B., et al.: Fabry's disease: Glycosphingolipid lipidosis, In *The Metabolic Basis of Inherited Disease.* 3rd ed. Stanbury, J. B., Wyngaarden, J. B., et al. (eds.), New York, McGraw-Hill, 1972, p. 663.
12. Brady, R. D., Uhlendorf, B. W., et al.: Fabry's disease: Antenatal detection. Science 172:174–175, 1971.
13. Suzuki, K., and Suzuki, Y.: Galactosyl ceramide lipidosis: Globoid cell leucodystrophy (Krabbe's disease), In *The Metabolic Basis of Inherited Disease.* 3rd ed. Stanbury, J. B., Wyngaarden, J. B., et al. (eds.), New York, McGraw-Hill, 1972, p. 760.
14. Suzuki, K., Schneider, E. L., et al.: In utero diagnosis of globoid leukodystrophy (Krabbe's disease). Biochem. Biophys. Res. Commun. 45: 1363, 1971.
15. Moser, H. W.: Sulfatide lipidosis: Metachromatic leukodystrophy, In *The Metabolic Basis of Inherited Disease.* 3rd ed. Stanbury, J. B., Wyngaarden, J. B., et al. (eds.), New York, McGraw-Hill, 1972, p. 688.
16. Nadler, H. L., and Gerbi, A. B.: Role of amniocentesis in the intrauterine detection of genetic disorders. New Engl. J. Med. 282:596, 1970.
17. Kaback, M. M., and Zeiger, R. A.: Heterozygote detection for Tay-Sachs disease (TSD) in a sample American-Jewish population. Pediatr. Res. 6:362, 1972.
18. Schneck, L., Valenti, C., et al.: Prenatal diagnosis of Tay-Sachs disease. Lancet 1:582, 1970.
19. Dietschy, J. M., and Wilson, J. D.: Regulation of cholesterol metabolism. New Engl. J. Med. 282:1128, 1179, 1241, 1970.
20. Sloan, H. R., and Fredrickson, D. S.: Rare familial diseases with neutral lipid storage: Wolman's disease, cholesteryl ester storage disease, and cerebrotendinous xanthomatosis, In *The Metabolic Basis of Inherited Disease.* 3rd ed. Stanbury, J. B., Wyngaarden, J. B., et al. (eds.), New York, McGraw-Hill, 1972, p. 808.
21. Fredrickson, D. S., and Levy, R. I.: Familial hyperlipoproteinemia. In *The Metabolic Basis of Inherited Disease.* 3rd ed. Stanbury, J. B., Wyngaarden, J. B., et al. (eds.), New York, McGraw-Hill, 1972, p. 545.
22. Burke, J. A., and Schubert, W. K.: Deficient activ-

ity of hepatic acid lipase in cholesterol ester storage disease. Science 176:309, 1972.

23. Sloan, H. R., and Fredrickson, D. S.: Enzyme deficiency in cholesteryl ester storage disease. J. Clin. Invest. 51:1923–1926, 1972.

24. Salen, G.: Cholestanol deposition in cerebrotendinous xanthomatosis. Ann. Intern. Med. 75: 843, 1971.

25. Steinberg, D.: Phytanic acid storage disease (Refsum's syndrome), In *The Metabolic Basis of Inherited Disease*. 3rd ed. Stanbury, J. B., Wyngaarden, J. B., et al. (eds.), New York, McGraw-Hill, 1972, p. 833.

26. Fredrickson, D. S., Gotto, A. M., Jr., et al.: Familial lipoprotein deficiency (abetalipoproteinemia, hypobetalipoproteinemia, and Tangier disease), in *The Metabolic Basis of Inherited Disease*. 3rd ed. Stanbury, J. B., Wyngaarden,

J. B., et al. (eds.), New York, McGraw-Hill, 1972, p. 493.

27. Levy, R. I., Bonnell, M., et al.: Dietary management of hyperlipoproteinemia. J. Am. Dietetic Assoc. 8:406, 1971.

28. Zelis, R., Mason, D. T., et al.: Effects of hyperlipoproteinemias and their treatment on the peripheral circulation. J. Clin. Invest. 49:1007, 1970.

29. Levy, R. I., Fredrickson, D. S., et al.: Dietary and drug treatment of primary hyperlipoproteinemia. Ann. Intern. Med. 77:267–294, 1972.

30. Norum, K. R., Glomset, J. A., et al.: Familial lecithin:cholesterol acyltransferase deficiency, In *The Metabolic Basis of Inherited Disease*. 3rd ed. Stanbury, J. B., Wyngaarden, J. B., et al. (eds.), New York, McGraw-Hill, 1972, p. 531.

V

GENETICS

Chapter 25

Genetic Aspects of Hematology

by Park S. Gerald

INTRODUCTION

Of all the medical specialties, hematology has perhaps been the most influenced by genetics. In 1944, Neel established the genetic basis for thalassemia and clearly delineated the relationship between thalassemia minor (single defective gene) and thalassemia major (two defective genes) (1). This was soon followed by the discovery that sickle cell trait and sickle cell anemia had a similar genetic relationship (2). By far the greatest impetus to the application of genetics to hematology, however, came with the observation by Pauling, Itano, and co-workers that Hb S was characterized by a genetically determined molecular defect (3). The subsequent use of the abnormal hemoglobins in inferring the fine structure of the hemoglobin gene, and of the nature of mutations in general, is continuing with undiminished enthusiasm to the present day. A comparable rate of development is occurring in the cytogenetic aspects of hematology, especially of leukemia, under the stimulus of the recent discovery of new techniques for identifying chromosomes (4).

The purpose of this chapter is to give the reader a brief introduction to the application of genetics to hematology and a glimpse of the recent explosive growth of human genetics. After a short review of the terminology of mendelian genetics, the reader is presented with an overview covering (1) meiosis, including linkage and recombination, (2) hematologic cytogenetics, and (3) the genetic analysis of mutant protein structures.

ELEMENTARY MENDELIAN GENETICS

To the average person, genetics is exemplified by the phrases dominant and recessive inheritance. The user of these terms is depending upon the concept of paired genetic elements first introduced by Mendel to describe inheritance in plants. Although the principles of mendelian genetics apply to man as well as to any other breeding organism, the inability to plan matings and the limited number of generations available for the observer's scrutiny have effected slight but significant changes in the use of mendelian terminology in human genetics. The areas affected by these changes are reviewed in the following paragraphs.

There are 23 pairs of human chromosomes, including one pair of sex chromosomes and 22 pairs of autosomes. The two members of each pair of autosomes are identical to one another in their microscopic morphology (Fig. 25–1). Each chromosome probably consists of a single DNA double helix that apparently extends without interruption from one end of the chromosome to the other. Each specific region of DNA sequence, located at a specific point on a chromosome and determining a particular function (usually an amino acid sequence of a protein), deserves the label of *gene*. Similar, usually identical, stretches of DNA sequence may be found at a comparable point on each member of a pair of chromosomes. The point on the chromosome where a par-

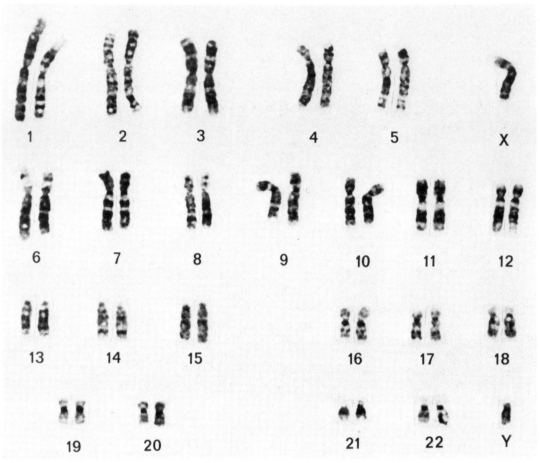

Figure 25–1. Normal male karyotype, stained with Giemsa, after treatment with trypsin. The "banding pattern" is sufficiently distinctive that each chromosome pair can be individually recognized. (This karyotype was supplied by Dr. Kurt Hirschhorn.)

ticular DNA sequence (gene) is found is its *locus*. The two members of a pair of chromosomes are spoken of as *homologous chromosomes*, and the loci found at a comparable point on each are *homologous loci*. In the normal individual, homologous chromosomes have an identical appearance, which reflects the fact that they are composed of a linear series of homologous loci, arranged in an identical linear order.

The pair of genes located at a pair of homologous loci are *alleles* (allelic genes). The behavior of chromosomes during gametogenesis normally guarantees that only one member of each pair of alleles enters a given gamete (segregation). It is this regular segregation of alleles at gametogenesis that provides the clinical basis for determining if two slightly different genes are allelic. It must be emphasized, however, that the

practical difficulty of examining sufficient critical progeny and the confounding effects of nonpaternity and nonmaternity render segregation a relatively inefficient means of determining allelism in human genetics. In consequence, allelism is more and more often being inferred from the amino acid sequence of the gene product. Thus, the genetic defects determining Hb S and Hb C are assumed to be allelic because the proteins differ in a single amino acid residue.

If in a given individual the two genes present at a particular pair of homologous loci are identical, the individual is *homozygous* at that locus. If the two allelic genes are not identical, the individual is *heterozygous*. The combination of two different abnormal (but allelic) genes fits the definition of heterozygosity as accurately as does the combination of one normal and one abnormal gene.

When a given genetically determined feature (usually called the *character* or *phenotype*) in an individual is detectable in the heterozygote, the phenotype is *dominantly inherited*. (It should be noted that the phenotype is determined by the particular tests used, i.e., the individual has the particular phenotype if the particular tests used give positive results. This can be illustrated by sickle cell hemoglobin. If a positive sickling preparation is defined as the phenotype, then the phenotype will be dominantly inherited. On the other hand, if anemia and a hemoglobin electrophoretic pattern with Hb S, moderate levels of Hb F, and no Hb A constitute the phenotype, then recessive inheritance will be observed.) The phenotype will be transmitted, on the average, to half of the progeny of the heterozygote. On the other hand, a phenotype which is expressed only when two mutant genes are simultaneously present is said to exhibit *recessive inheritance.* In human inheritance, the two mutant genes determining a recessively inherited phenotype may not be identical, so that recessively inherited diseases are not necessarily homozygous. Pyruvate kinase deficiency (one of the recessively inherited forms of hemolytic anemia), for example, might result from the presence of two different mutant genes for red cell pyruvate kinase. Each of the two mutant genes would produce a defective form of pyruvate kinase, but the two gene products would not be identical in the nature of their molecular defect.

The preceding remarks apply to autosomal genes; a different situation occurs with sex chromosomal genes. The sex chromosomes X and Y are not known to have any loci in common; that is, none of the loci known to exist on the X chromosome occur on the Y chromosome. (Indeed, no specific gene has been definitely assigned to the Y). The normal female, with two X chromosomes, can be heterozygous or homozygous at loci on the X chromosome. The terms heterozygous and homozygous, however, cannot be applied to the normal male, who has only one X chromosome. Instead, the normal male is said to be *hemizygous* at all loci on the X chromosome. This expression emphasizes that he has only one representative of each X chromosomal locus.

MEIOSIS, RECOMBINATION, AND LINKAGE

Although meiosis is undoubtedly a very complex process with many genetically controlled steps, our present knowledge of it is sufficiently limited that the essentials can be described in simple terms. Meiosis consists of two successive cell divisions (Fig. 25–2). During the first meiotic division, the replicated, homologous chromosomes synapse

Figure 25–2. Schematic representation of normal meiosis (crossing-over is ignored). The individual is heterozygous (genotype A/B) at a hypothetical locus. Prior to first meiotic division, each chromosome has replicated; the two elements (now known as sister chromatids) remain attached at the centromere. Note that meiosis ensures that allelic genes segregate.

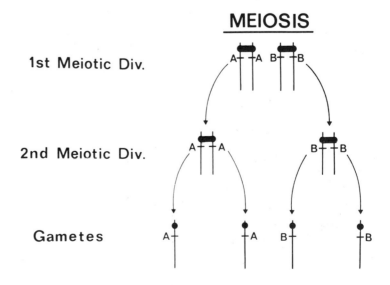

MEIOSIS

1st Meiotic Div.

2nd Meiotic Div.

Gametes

and then separate, one member of each pair
of homologous chromosomes going to each
daughter cell. During the second meiotic
division, each chromosome divides at the
centromere, and sister chromatids separate,
analogous to their behavior in the single
divisional state of mitosis. One further essential must be added to this elementary
description: prior to the first meiotic division, crossing-over occurs between nonsister
chromatids, a phenomenon that will be
taken up during the discussion of recombination.

Normally, meiosis ensures that a *single*
chromatid from each *pair* of homologous
chromosomes enters the gamete. This directly accounts for the segregation of allelic
genes. Occasionally, abnormalities of meiosis occur, and gametes are formed with an
abnormal number of chromosomes. Two different types of meiotic errors are known and
result either from failure of separation of
homologous chromosomes at the first meiotic division or from failure of separation of
sister chromatids at the second meiotic division. These two types of errors are known as
first meiotic division nondisjunction and
second meiotic division nondisjunction.
Either can lead to a gamete with an extra
chromosome or a missing chromosome. (In a
few instances, failure of separation may occur, successively, at both first and second
meiotic division.)

Failure of separation of sister chromatids
also can occur at mitosis; this is designated
mitotic nondisjunction. Alternatively, one
of the chromosomes newly formed by separation of chromatids may fail to be incorporated into the newly created nuclei, a
phenomenon described as anaphase lag
loss. If either of these happens subsequent
to the first mitotic division of the zygote, the
result will be the formation of a mosaic; i.e.,
an individual with a mixture of two cyto-
genetically different cell types. Anaphase
lag loss in a chromosomally abnormal fetus
may well be the principal mechanism leading to formation of mosaicism involving trisomy 21 or XXY.

In Figure 25–2, the chromosomes are depicted as dividing longitudinally at the
centromere but otherwise remaining intact.
This oversimplification was adopted to emphasize the behavior of the centromere. In
reality, exchange of genetic material normally occurs between the chromatids of homol-

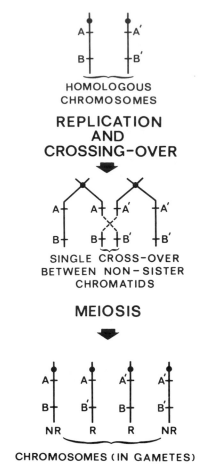

Figure 25–3. Crossing-over between two different
(nonsister) chromatids to produce two recombinant
(R) and two nonrecombinant (NR) gametes.

ogous chromosomes prior to first meiotic
division (Fig. 25–3). These exchanges,
which result from the process known as
crossing-over, are not associated with gain
or loss of chromosomal material, since an
exactly equal exchange occurs.

Crossing-over is most frequently studied
by examination of gene combinations in the
progeny. Assume that two nonhomologous
loci, A and B, are located on the same chromosome and carry the alleles A and A' at
locus A, and B and B' at locus B, so that A
and B are on one chromosome, and A' and
B' are on its homologue (Fig. 25–3). If no
crossing-over occurs, then the gametes will
retain the parental chromosome structure
and will possess either A and B *or* A' and B'.
If a single cross-over occurs between loci A
and B (two nonsister chromatids are involved), then four types of gametes can oc-

cur (Fig. 25–3), two of which have the same combination of genes as the parental chromosomes (and hence are called nonrecombinants) and two of which have new combinations (and hence are called recombinants).

The greater the distance between loci A and B, the more likely crossing-over is to occur between them. If the distance is sufficiently great, however, two cross-overs may occur between A and B, the second of which reverses the effect of the first, so that recombination does not result. For this reason, recombination is a relatively poor measure of the distance between loci when the frequency of recombination between them exceeds about 25 per cent.

Because crossing-over between two nonsister chromatids apparently inhibits crossing-over in the same region between the remaining two chromatids, the maximum value of recombination approaches 50 per cent. It should be noted that, if loci A and B were on different (nonhomologous) chromosomes, their genes would assort independently — that is, the combinations A and B, A and B', A' and B, and A' and B' would all occur equally often. Independent assortment, then, cannot be told from 50 per cent recombination by examining the genotypes of the progeny.

When two loci are located on the same chromosome sufficiently close together that recombinants amount to significantly less than 50 per cent of progeny, their relative juxtaposition can be readily recognized, and the loci are said to be linked. This principle can be used to assess the relative order of three loci. For example, the loci for 6PGD, Rh, and PGM_1 have been examined for the frequency of recombination between each pair of loci (5). The best estimate for the recombination frequency, in the male, between PGM_1 and Rh is 26 per cent, and between Rh and 6PGD is 13 per cent. The recombination frequency between PGM_1 and 6PGD, on the other hand, cannot be distinguished from 50 per cent. It is evident that one arrangement of these three loci — $6PGD:Rh:PGM_1$ — would best comply with the recombination frequencies observed. It should also be noted that the frequency of recombination between any two loci is usually greater in the male than in the female, which probably reflects the difference between meiosis in the male and the female.

Finally, the reader should be introduced to the concept of synteny, as opposed to linkage. If two or more loci are on the same chromosome, then they are syntenic. Loci that are linked together are necessarily syntenic; not all loci that are syntenic, however, will be sufficiently close together to demonstrate the recombination values characteristic of linkage. The creation of the term synteny (and the adjective, syntenic) was necessitated by the development of techniques other than pedigree analysis for assigning genes to chromosomes (such as somatic cell hybridization).

INTRODUCTORY CYTOGENETICS

Human cytogenetics had its effective beginning in 1956 (6), when technical advances made possible a detailed examination of the chromosomes present in individual human cells. Soon thereafter, chromosomal abnormalities were discovered to be associated with specific diseases. The many rapid advances in cytogenetics that have since occurred have largely resulted from additional technical advances. Those of particular importance have been (1) the discovery that a plant substance, phytohemagglutinin, can stimulate peripheral leukocytes to divide (7), (2) the use of tritiated thymidine to analyze the kinetics of human chromosome replication (8), and most recently, (3) the development of staining techniques capable of demonstrating heterogeneity within and between individual chromosomes (9).

Phytohemagglutinin is the term applied to a class of substances which can be extracted from plants, especially their seeds, and which are able to agglutinate red cells. These were first used by Osgood to remove the red cells from uncoagulated whole blood during an attempt to culture leukocytes from human leukemia (10). It was subsequently discovered that the plant extract had the additional property of actively stimulating normal leukocytes to divide and hence contained a phytomitogen (11). Although the name phytomitogen more accurately describes the relevant substance, the expression phytohemagglutinin (PHA) will be employed herein, even though the substance is not employed as an agglutinin, since this is the more generally used term in the current literature. PHA can be obtained from a number of different plants, and its stimulatory properties depend in part upon the source. All forms of PHA appear to stimulate the mitosis only of lymphocytes. The customarily used PHA, which is derived from beans, probably acts primarily upon thymus-derived lymphocytes. By the use of PHA, adequate numbers of metaphases can be obtained from a few drops of blood that have been cultured for three to four days.

The cell cycle of the PHA-stimulated lymphocyte includes a DNA synthesis phase (the S phase) of 6 to 12 hours' duration, which is followed by a delay of three to six hours before mitosis occurs (11). If tritiated thymidine is added to a leukocyte culture, those cells actively synthesizing DNA at that time will incorporate the radioactive label. If colchicine is subsequently added to the culture, cells in the process of division will continue until they reach metaphase, at which point in the cell cycle they will be arrested. By adjusting the time interval between the addition of tritiated thymidine and the addition of colchicine, the incorporation of radioactive thymidine into the chromosomes of colchicine-arrested metaphases can be confined to the last portion of S. Chromosomal regions which are radioactive (as revealed by autoradiography) after this treatment are said to be late-labeling. As will be discussed later, this method reveals an important distinction between the several X chromosomes in cells with more than one X.

While autoradiography of tritiated thymidine-labeled metaphases also permits identification of certain autosomal pairs, it is too laborious a procedure for routine use. Routine identification of individual chromosomes was, until recently dependent upon such morphologic characteristics as the relative length of the chromosome and the position of the centromere. In favorable preparations, certain less constant features, such as secondary constrictions and the presence of satellites, were also of help (Fig. 25–1). Even when conditions are optimal, however, only a few of the chromosome pairs can be confidently recognized when the ordinary Giemsa staining technique is employed.

The first successful identification of all chromosome pairs was achieved by the fluorescence staining technique of Caspersson and co-workers (9). Caspersson utilized quinacrine mustard as the staining agent because it was expected to react preferentially with the DNA base, guanine. Although quinacrine mustard did reveal heterogeneity, the characteristic pattern of fluorescence of the individual chromosomes is now believed to depend upon several other factors in addition to local guanine concentration. The fluorescence pattern has been accepted as the primary standard for identification of each chromosome (12).

Although a number of newer and simpler techniques are now available for chromosome identification, fluorescence staining has several unique features. The distal portion of the long arm of the Y chromosome is the most vividly fluorescent chromosomal region in the male karyotype. [This region of the Y is absent in an occasional normal male (13).] Its fluorescence intensity enables it to be seen even in interphase nuclei, where it is known as the Y body. The presence of the Y body permits recognition of individual Y-containing cells.

The acrocentric chromosomes (nos. 13, 14, 15, 21, and 22) frequently also have distinctive fluorescent features. The centromeric and satellite regions of these chromosomes exhibit a marked variation between individuals in their fluorescence, a variation which is inheritable and which often permits recognition of individual members of a particular chromosome pair. This distinction may be used to follow the inheritance of an individual chromosome within a family.

There are now a number of staining techniques in addition to fluorescence for identifying chromosomes (4). In general they produce a banding pattern which mimics in large part that seen with fluorescence staining but which has the advantage of being visible with conventional light microscopy. Since the banding pattern revealed by each of these techniques depends upon the properties of Giemsa stain, they are collectively referred to as Giemsa banding techniques.

The application of fluorescence staining and Giemsa banding has greatly increased the ability of cytogeneticists to analyze subtle chromosomal changes. It is now apparent that many chromosomal alterations are complex and result from one or more chromosomal breaks. Some of the more common varieties of chromosomal abnormalities are listed in Table 25–1. For a more specific description of the mechanisms involved, the reader should consult one of the many available genetic or cytogenetic texts. The symbolic nomenclature of Table 25–1 conforms to a lengthy set of rules adopted by an informally constituted international group (12). Symbols are also available for specific description of the individual chromosomal bands (12).

Of the several types of chromosomal rearrangements commonly encountered, deletions, reciprocal translocations, and isochromosomes are the varieties presently most important to the hematologist. A deletion results when a portion of one arm of a chromosome is lost as the result of chromosomal breaks. Deletions might be of two kinds, terminal or interstitial. A terminal deletion would result if a single break occurred in a chromosome arm and the portion of the arm distal (relative to the centromere) to the breakpoint were lost. There is some theoretical justification for the belief that terminal deletions may be unstable and not persist as such in subsequent generations of the affected cell. This belief arises from the hypothesis that a definite structure (the telomere) is present on the distal end of each chromosome arm, and its loss, as by terminal deletion, would lead to formation of a chromosome that could not behave normally.

An interstitial deletion, on the other hand, could arise if two different breaks occurred in the same chromosome arm. The segment between the two breaks would be lost, and the more distal and proximal pieces would reunite. While the reunion would reattach the telomere (if such exists) to the chromosome arm and thereby avoid the theoretical objection to terminal deletions, interstitial deletions would be a more complicated event in that two breaks would be required. At present, it can only be stated that interstitial deletions have been observed, while terminal deletions cannot be ruled out. Finally, it should be noted that a deletion might be present in the zygote—and therefore in all cells of the individual—or it might occur in a somatic cell and be present only in a particular organ or tissue.

In modern cytogenetic terminology, dele-

tions are denoted as, for example, 22q–. The lower case letter denotes the chromosome arm (p for short arm and q for long arm), and plus (+) or minus (–) are descriptive of the change in length of the arm in question. This terminology identifies the specific chromosome and chromosome arm from which a segment has been lost. In an individual in whom only one member of a chromosome pair was partially deleted, the more complete description would be 46,XX,22q– or 46,XY,22q–, depending on whether the patient was a female or a male.

Reciprocal translocations, as the name describes, represent an exchange of terminal segments between two different chromosomes. It is presumed that single breaks occurred in each of two different chromosomes in the same cell, with reunion of the broken ends, but not in the original fashion. In the usual circumstance, the mitotic cell is not affected by the exchange, since genes are neither gained nor lost in this process (this point is often emphasized by the descriptive phrase "balanced reciprocal translocation"). During meiosis, however, abnormalities appear, since segregation of genes into haploid sets (half of the total genetic complement) cannot always be achieved, as it is during normal gametogenesis, through segregation of centromeres. Either normal progeny or progeny with several different types of genetic imbalance may be produced.

It is possible that, in a few instances of balanced reciprocal translocation, genes in the region of the breakage and reunion sites may be affected in their function, even though no apparent change in the amount of DNA has occurred. Such alteration in gene function, known as a position effect, has not been specifically demonstrated in man, although it is well known to *Drosophila* cytogeneticists. It might be of extreme importance in understanding chronic myelocytic leukemia, if the most recent cytologic observations recorded in this disease (to be described subsequently) prove to be correct.

The terminology used in describing balanced reciprocal translocations indicates both the chromosome number and the chromosome arms, as t(9q+;22q–). (The "t" designates this as a translocation, and the semicolon specifies that two translocated chromosomes are produced.) In this case the long arm of no. 9 is elongated by

TABLE 25–1. EXAMPLES OF CHROMOSOMAL ABERRATIONS

Type of Chromosomal Aberration and Assumed Mechanism	Verbal Terminology	Examples of Symbolic Terminology
I. Changes in chromosome number		
A. Extra chromosome, resulting from nondisjunction	Trisomy	47,XY,+21 (Male, trisomy 21)
B. Absent chromosome, resulting from nondisjunction or anaphase lag loss	Monosomy	45,XO (Turner's syndrome)
C. Mixture of cells with different karyotypes in the same individual, resulting from mitotic error (anaphase lag loss or mitotic nondisjunction)	Mosaicism	46,XY/47,XY,+21 (Mosaic trisomy 21)
II. Chromosomal rearrangements		
A. Absent chromosomal segment in one chromosome, resulting from break(s) in a single chromosome arm	Deletion (terminal or interstitial)	46,XX,22q− (Partial deletion of long arm of chromosome 22; this specific anomaly is also known as the Ph¹ chromosome when it occurs in patients with chronic myelogenous leukemia)
B. Balanced reciprocal translocation, resulting from breaks occurring simultaneously in two different chromosomes with rejoining of terminal segments to incorrect centromeres	Reciprocal translocation (balanced)	46,XX,t(9q+;22q−) (Reciprocal translocation between long arms of 9 and 22, with elongation of 9 and shortening of 22)
C. Unbalanced translocation, evidenced by one abnormally short or one abnormally long chromosome; about half are inherited from a parent with a balanced reciprocal translocation	Unbalanced translocation	46,XX,17q+ (Translocation of a chromosomal segment to the long arm of 17)
D. Abnormal chromosome whose chromosome arms are identical to one another; hence, one arm is duplicated and the other is missing, possibly resulting from division of the centromere at right angles to its normal divisional plane	Isochromosome	46,XX,i(17q) (Isochromosome of long arm of 17)

the amount of decrease in length of the long arm of no. 22. The expression 46,XX,t(9q+;22q−) would specify the occurrence of a balanced reciprocal translocation in a female. A more specific nomenclature is also available to indicate the probable sites of the original chromosomal breaks.

Isochromosomes represent the third type of rearrangement to be considered. The prefix "iso" emphasizes that in these chromosomes both arms of the rearranged chromosome are genetically identical. This unusual circumstance is believed to arise when a centromere divides at right angles to its normal plane of division. If division in the middle of a centromere could result in formation of two functional centromeres, two different isochromosomes would be produced—one would be an isochromosome composed of two representations of the original short arm [e.g., i(17p)], and the other an isochromosome of the long arm [e.g., i(17q)]. Whatever the reason, usually only one of the two possible isochromosomes is found.

Cytogenetic Aspects of Hematologic Disorders

The first cytogenetic abnormality associated with a hematologic disorder, and still the only specific abnormality exhibiting a high correlation with a specific hematologic disease, is the Philadelphia chromosome (Ph[1]) found in patients with chronic myelocytic leukemia (CML) (14). The Ph[1] chromosome has been presumed to be produced by a deletion of about half the long arm of one of the smallest chromosomes. (As suggested in a preceding section, this might be either a terminal or interstitial deletion.) Since the Ph[1] chromosome was discovered before the current methods for specific identification of chromosomes were available, it was not initially known whether it represented a deletion of no. 21 or no. 22. Nonetheless, most cytogenetic literature appearing prior to 1971 referred to the Ph[1] chromosome as 21q−. The belief that chromosome no. 21 was involved arose from the observation that patients with trisomy 21 (Down's syndrome or mongolism) have an increased incidence of leukemia—although not of the chronic myelocytic type—and,

like patients with CML, have a quantitative alteration in leukocyte alkaline phosphatase activity. Modern staining techniques, however, unequivocally identify the Ph[1] chromosome as 22q−. While the deletion invariably affects chromosome no. 22, it cannot yet be determined whether the chromosomal material missing from 22q consistently comes from the same region of the long arm or whether the loss may occur anywhere within the long arm.

In the patient with CML, the Ph[1] chromosome is found only in the peripheral blood, and not in cells from the skin or other tissues. When chromosome studies are made simultaneously on bone marrow cells (which may be examined directly since many are dividing cells) and on PHA-stimulated peripheral leukocytes, the proportion of metaphases containing the Ph[1] chromosome is usually significantly greater in the bone marrow specimen than in the peripheral leukocyte sample. This is to be expected if the Ph[1] chromosome occurs only in all cells of the bone marrow origin and if the cells which divide after PHA stimulation are lymphocytes. Those metaphases in the peripheral leukocyte preparation which are Ph[1]-positive are presumably the spontaneously dividing myelocytic (leukemic) cells. In support of this, peripheral leukocyte cultures from patients with CML, when cultured without PHA, yield almost solely Ph[1]-positive metaphases.

A few patients with the clinical appearance of CML do not possess the Ph[1] chromosome. It seems likely that these patients represent a different form of the disease, since they apparently have a shorter survival time and a poorer response to chemotherapy, as well as several other differences from the usual Ph[1]-positive patient (15). The apparently specific association between CML and the Ph[1] chromosome raises the question of the nature of the relationship. At present, it is not known whether the chromosomal alteration is a primary or a secondary event. The situation has become even more complicated with the recent report that the Ph[1] chromosome may not be a deletion but may possibly be part of a balanced reciprocal translocation between the long arm of chromosome no. 9 and the long arm of chromosome no. 22, t(9q+;22q−) (16). As was noted in the previous general discussions concerning balanced reciprocal translocations, this would not be expected to produce a change in the amount of DNA. For this presumed balanced reciprocal translocation to have a direct role in the pathogenesis of CML, it might be necessary to consider the possibility of a position effect.

While the Ph¹ chromosome is the only nearly constant cytogenetic feature in CML, a small but significant number of patients with CML may also possess an abnormal chromosome, believed to be an i(17q), in addition to the expected Ph¹ (17). The role such additional chromosomal abnormalities play in the leukemic process is completely unknown at present. The occurrence of this otherwise rare abnormality in a number of different patients with CML is obviously not a chance phenomenon, however.

On the other hand, many patients with acute leukemia of various types have normal chromosomal complements in their bone marrow cells and peripheral leukocytes. Some of these patients may possess cells in their peripheral blood which will divide during leukocyte culture in the absence of phytohemagglutinin. These "spontaneously" dividing cells are very rarely seen in hematologically normal individuals and may be indicative of neoplastic cells in the peripheral blood (17a). Because of this association, a search for spontaneously dividing cells has at times been carried out in patients who have hematologic changes suggestive, but not characteristic, of leukemia. The detection of spontaneously dividing cells under these circumstances is certainly worrisome, but the phenomenon has not yet been sufficiently studied to be considered diagnostic of leukemia in the absence of confirming clinical features.

Those patients with acute leukemia that do exhibit chromosomal changes have no single constant feature. Instead, a wide variation in chromosomal changes (including various aneuploidies and chromosomal rearrangements) may be observed from patient to patient. Within any given patient, the chromosomal complement of the abnormal cells is relatively uniform, especially early in the course of the disease. As the disease progresses, further chromosomal changes occur, so that the abnormal cells may possess simultaneously both the early and the late changes. This has been interpreted to indicate that the neoplastic cells

constitute a clone, within which cells that have acquired additional chromosomal changes increase in proportion until they constitute a subclone. This interpretation implies that the cells of the subclone have a selective advantage over those of the original clone, but it cannot yet be determined whether the advantage is in any way related to the additional chromosomal changes.

The significance of a small percentage of peripheral leukocytes with a consistent chromosomal abnormality in a patient with a hematologic disorder short of frank leukemia is extremely difficult to determine. While some of these patients have later developed overt leukemia, still others have not done so over a reasonable period of observation. If leukemia does not develop during a three-month period of observation, the chance of its occurring later is probably much less (18).

Chronic lymphatic leukemia poses a different problem from the foregoing. In this disease, the peripheral leukocytes apparently do not respond to the mitogenic stimulation of PHA. It is not yet known whether this lack of response is the property of the specific cell type from which the leukemic cell is derived or if it is a consequence of the leukemic process itself. Since chromosome preparations are very difficult to obtain from these cells, little is known about the cytogenetic aspects of this form of leukemia.

In a few of the rarer forms of leukemia and related diseases, possibly specific cytogenetic changes have been reported. A few patients with polycythemia vera, for instance, have been found to have a partial deletion of the long arm of one chromosome no. 20 (19). Since not all patients with polycythemia vera show this cytogenetic abnormality, and since those that do show it frequently have previously received chemotherapy or irradiation, the significance of this observation is somewhat uncertain.

In one group of patients with Burkitt's lymphoma whose tumor cells were studied cytologically with fluorescence staining, the majority had an extra bright band on the end of the long arm of one chromosome no. 14 (20). Again, the relevance of the cytogenetic change to the disease process is unknown.

Fanconi's constitutional aplastic anemia and Bloom's syndrome, both of which are recessively inherited diseases, have still another variety of cytogenetic abnormality. These clinically distinct conditions have in common an increased incidence of chromosomal breaks (22). In association with the breaks is the occurrence of "fusion figures," bizarre arrangements of chromosomes resulting from union of chromatids from two different (nonhomologous) chromosomes. While the cause of the increased breaks is not known, the occurrence of multiple breaks in the same cell would be expected occasionally to result in aberrant reunion with production of fusion figures. Although most of the studies have been done on cultured peripheral leukocytes, the increased chromosomal breakage has also been observed in cultured fibroblasts. The occurrence of increased chromosomal breakage quite naturally suggested the possibility of an underlying error in DNA repair mechanisms, but no abnormality has been found (21).

Other types of chromosomal aberrations have been noted by various observers of these two diseases. The occurrence of achromatic regions in single chromatids has been emphasized by German (21), while endoreduplication (occurrence of a second round of chromosomal division without intervening nuclear division) is stressed by others (22). Finally, as might possibly be expected from the increased incidence of chromosomal breakage, both Fanconi's anemia patients and Bloom's syndrome patients have an increased likelihood of developing malignancy, including leukemia (21).

Cytogenetic variations may be of importance in still other ways in the study of hematologic disorders. The Y chromosome, which forms a distinctive fluorescent body (the Y body) in the interphase nucleus, may be used as a marker to identify male cells after they are transplanted into a female recipient. The Y body is of particular value, since it can be detected in both metaphase and interphase cells. The other fluorescent variants (such as may be found on the short arms and satellite regions of the acrocentric chromosomes) can be readily detected only in metaphase cells but, of course, may be used whatever the sex of the donor and recipient. A significant proportion of individuals with CML and a Ph[1] chromosome will exhibit a morphologic difference (as revealed by fluorescent staining or other techniques) between short arms of the Ph[1]

chromosome and those of the normal no. 22. (The morphologic features of the Ph[1] chromosome are constant from cell to cell in any given patient.) This has been used to determine whether the Ph[1] chromosome is derived from the maternal or paternal no. 22 (23). In those rare instances in which a familial tendency to leukemia is suspected, this technique might be used to determine if the tendency to leukemia could originate from an inherited susceptibility to chromosomal rearrangement in a specific no. 22.

GENE DOSAGE AND THE X CHROMOSOME

Since loci on the X chromosome are not present on the Y chromosome, the XX female has twice as many genes per cell for each X chromosomal locus as the XY male. Once this fact was appreciated, it became obvious that some means must exist to compensate for this difference in gene dosage. The insight into this problem was furnished by the study in mice of X chromosomal genes controlling hair color (Fig. 25–4), and

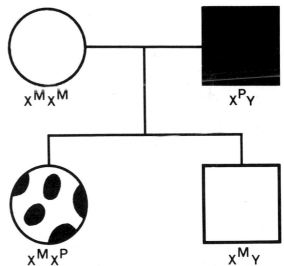

Figure 25–4. Schematic representation of X-linked inheritance of coat color in mice. In male mice with an X-linked coat color gene, the pigment is uniformly distributed over the pelt. In the female progeny of the union between the pigmented male mouse and an unpigmented female, patches of pigment are present. It is reasonable to suggest that the cells of the pigmented patches have the paternal X (X^P) functioning, while the cells of the unpigmented areas have a maternal X (X^M) functioning. This also implies that only one X is functional in any cell.

in man of the X-linked enzyme, glucose-6-phosphate dehydrogenase (G6PD) (24, 25).

From these studies came the generalization regarding X chromosomal behavior, known as the single active X hypothesis (or the Lyon hypothesis) (26). This hypothesis applies with minimal modification to X chromosomal behavior in nearly all placentate mammals. In man, the essential features of X chromosomal behavior in individuals with more than one X include the following:

1. All X chromosomes are active in the embryo during approximately the first 16 days of gestational life.

2. At that time, all except one X chromosome in each cell become inactivated.

3. The choice of which X chromosome remains active (and which become inactive) is independently and randomly determined in each cell.

4. The inactivation is irreversible, so that the same X chromosome remains active in subsequent generations of daughter cells (27).

The concept of the single active X has its physical counterpart in the Barr body. This designation is applied to the densely staining chromatin mass which is found within the nucleus of female cells and which usually is adjacent to the nuclear membrane. This mass is believed to be the inactive, condensed X, since its size usually correlates with the size of any inactive, abnormal X chromosome (e.g., a deleted X or isochromosome X). In cells containing three or more X's, the number of Barr bodies is increased, and the maximal number in a cell is one less than the total number of X's in that cell.

The timing of DNA synthesis, as revealed by autoradiography with tritiated thymidine, brings out a further difference between the X chromosomes of a multiple-X cell. In every nucleated cell, one of the X chromosomes completes DNA synthesis relatively early in S phase; any additional X chromosomes are late-replicating (11). Morphologically abnormal X's are usually late-replicating.

Irreversibility of inactivation of the X chromosome has been clearly demonstrated in tissue culture. Single cells from females heterozygous at X chromosomal loci have been cultured and their cellular descendants shown to express one and the same allele. By this method, five loci on the human X (α-galactosidase deficiency, phosphoglycerate kinase, Hunter's syndrome, glucose-6-phosphate dehydrogenase, and hypoxanthine-guanine phosphoribosyl transferase deficiency) have been tested and irreversible inactivation confirmed (27, 28). The patchy distribution of cellular heterogeneity in intact female animals—such as the pigmentation noted originally in the mouse—is presumably an in vivo demonstration of the same phenomenon and indirectly verifies that other X chromosomal loci, in addition to the aforementioned, undergo irreversible inactivation. Although this is impressive evidence for persistent activity of a single allele at various X chromosomal loci, it still does not prove that the active loci are all on the same X or that all loci on a condensed X are inactivated. [The X-linked blood group locus, Xg, is believed not to be inactivated in XX females (29).] Of more fundamental importance, nothing is known about the molecular basis for inactivation.

Randomness of inactivation is more difficult to study. The proportion of cells exhibiting inactivation of a specific allele in heterozygous human females approximates the 50 per cent expected of random inactivation. Exceptions to random inactivation are regularly observed with certain X chromosomal abnormalities (including inactivation of any isochromosome X, deleted X, or ring X) and inconsistently observed with others (frequently the *normal* X is inactivated in heterozygotes for X-autosome reciprocal translocations). It must be remembered that randomness is usually tested sometime after birth, at a time far removed from the actual inactivation event. Differential survival during the intervening period may significantly distort the ratio of the two cell types (those with an active X of maternal origin and those with an active X of paternal origin), an effect which also could vary from tissue to tissue. Despite these concerns, some insight into cell lineage may be obtained from studies of the ratio of these two cell types.

In the human, inactivation of the X chromosome occurs in the embryo about 16 days after fertilization, when the number of embryonic cells is relatively limited (27). Since inactivation is a random process, it is possible that the proportion of cells with, say, the paternal X active will depart significantly, in a few embryos, from the usual value of approximately 50 per cent. If selective forces do not intervene, then the same proportion will persist into adulthood.

This may affect the expression of certain X-linked diseases in female heterozygotes. Classical hemophilia may be used to illustrate this phenomenon. This X-linked recessive disease results from a deficiency of the antihemophilic factor (AHF) that is produced by the liver. If most of the liver cells in a female heterozygous for this disease had as their functional X the one which carried the hemophilia gene, then very little AHF would be produced. Such a female might appear to have a mild form of hemophilia.

The single active X principle may be used to analyze events occurring in female cells after inactivation of the X. In an XX female heterozygous for an X-linked marker, such as an electrophoretic variant of the enzyme glucose-6-phosphate dehydrogenase (G6PD), malignant transformation originating in a single cell would lead to a line of cells possessing a single type of G6PD, while malignant transformation affecting multiple cells in a random fashion would usually lead to a group of cell lines collectively exhibiting two electrophoretic types of G6PD. Fialkow et al. have found that the leukocytes of patients with CML who could be genetically proved to be heterozygous for G6PD expressed only one of their two G6PD alleles (30). This evidence favors the belief that CML probably arises from a mutation in a single cell. Since these patients expressed in their erythrocytes the same single G6PD allele as was found in their leukocytes, it is probable that CML arises as a mutation in a stem cell that is a precursor to both CML leukocytes and erythrocytes.

Diseases which are X-linked and which exert their effect at the single cell level may be evident even in the heterozygous female. The X-linked disorder chronic granulomatous disease (CGD), for example, is characterized in affected males by lifelong susceptibility to bacterial infection. In these males, the polymorphic leukocytes are able to phagocytose bacteria but lack the normal ability to kill their resident bacteria. This inability appears to be secondary to deficiency of an intracellular enzyme. On the average, half of the polymorphonuclear leukocytes of females heterozygous for this disorder would be expected similarly to lack the ability to kill phagocytosed bacteria. In consequence, those bacterial diseases in which intracellular survival would furnish a persistent focus would predictably be very chronic in heterozygotes for CGD. Consistent with this prediction, persistence of a *Salmonella* infection for at least $3\frac{1}{2}$ years has now been documented in a heterozygote for CGD (31).

GENETICALLY DETERMINED ALTERATIONS IN PROTEIN STRUCTURE

Two important goals of studies of any inherited disease are the determination of both the normal and the mutant DNA sequence, and the pathogenesis of the disease from the abnormal DNA sequence to the final symptoms. Direct determination of the DNA sequence is not practicable at present (although it appears likely that the requisite methods will be available in a surprisingly short time), and indirect methods must be used. In a few instances, the relevant messengers have been isolated, and sequences will soon be available. In general, however, the best approximation to the DNA sequence is the amino acid sequence of its protein product. In this section, the success that has been achieved by this method, particularly as regards the hemoglobin loci, will be once again reviewed from the point of view of the geneticist rather than the hematologist. More details are offered in Chapters 13 and 15.

Hemoglobin Structure

The principal hemoglobin of the fetus is fetal hemoglobin (Hb F, composed of α and γ protein chains combined according to the formula $\alpha_2\gamma_2$). Hemoglobin synthesis begins to shift from fetal hemoglobin to the adult hemoglobins, Hb A ($\alpha_2\beta_2$) and Hb A_2 ($\alpha_2\delta_2$), during late fetal life. This transition is accelerated during the neonatal period, and only a trace amount of Hb F is present thereafter. (The hemoglobins which occur in embryonic life will not be discussed, since so little is known about their structure.)

The mutant forms of hemoglobin (the so-called abnormal hemoglobins) are the principal tools that will be used to analyze hemoglobin genetics. In general, the abnormal hemoglobins differ from the normal hemoglobin in only one of the two kinds of chains present. Hb S, for example, differs from Hb A only in the β chain; Hb S can thus be symbolized as Hb $\alpha_2\beta_2^S$. When the detailed nature of the change is known, then this may be specifically designated. Hb S, for example, would be $\alpha_2\beta_2^{6\ Glu\to Val}$, since this hemoglobin has a valine at the sixth residue of the β chain in place of the normal glutamic acid.

Over 90 per cent of the abnormal hemoglobins examined to date (32) differ from normal hemoglobin at a single amino acid (AA) residue in one protein chain (α, β, γ, or δ). In each instance, it is possible to identify a codon for the normal AA residue which differs by a single RNA base from one of the codons for its AA replacement (33). This rule has proved to be so generally applicable that exceptions are viewed with suspicion. Hb I, for instance, was initially believed to be $\alpha_2^{16\ Lys\to Asp}\ \beta_2$ (34). None of the codons which can be derived from any of the lysine codons by a single base change is a codon for aspartic acid (Table 25-2). This was considered sufficient reason to challenge the analysis of Hb I. Reanalysis justified the concern, for the correct result proved to be glutamic acid rather than aspartic acid (35). As noted in Table 25-2,

replacement of a lysine by a glutamic acid requires only a single base substitution.

Abnormal hemoglobins of the single amino acid substitution type are sufficiently common that individuals possessing two abnormal hemoglobin genes are known. Studies of such individuals provide information concerning the number and relation of the hemoglobin loci. First, there must be at least one pair of homologous loci for each of the common hemoglobin chains (α, β, γ, and δ). This must be so since nearly all individuals are capable of producing all four kinds of hemoglobin chains, and because each chain differs from the rest at many points in its AA sequence. But can there be more than one pair of loci for any one of these chains?

Abnormal hemoglobins characterized by single amino acid substitutions, as we have seen, result from single DNA base changes. It may be assumed that these mutational changes affect only a single gene. Then the individual who has inherited two mutant, allelic hemoglobin genes will not be able to produce any normal hemoglobin chains of that type if there is only one pair of loci for that hemoglobin chain. By this means it has been demonstrated that there is only one pair of loci for β chains and only one pair for δ chains.

The evidence concerning the α chain locus is conflicting at the present time. Some individuals with two mutant α chain genes are known who do not produce any normal α chains (37). A few others have been discovered who produce three kinds of α chains (one normal and two abnormal) (38). It appears likely that some individuals have two pairs of α chain loci and some only one; the relative frequency of these two types is not known. The progeny derived from a mating between these two types ought to have *three* α chain genes, but there is no direct evidence yet concerning this point.

Individuals possessing two mutant γ chain genes are not known, but evidence concerning the γ chain loci is available from another source. Careful analysis of the amino acid composition of the Hb F from neonates reveals that glycine and alanine are not present in integral amounts. Some molecules of the γ chain appear to contain glycine as the 136th residue, while others have alanine (39). (The two γ chains are frequently denoted by $^G\gamma$ and $^A\gamma$.) Since

TABLE 25-2. POSSIBLE AMINO ACID REPLACEMENTS FOR LYSINE DERIVED BY SINGLE BASE SUBSTITUTIONS IN LYSINE CODONS[*]

LYSINE CODONS	POSSIBLE AMINO ACID REPLACEMENTS (WITH CODONS)
AAA	Term.[†](UAA),Gln(CAA),Glu(GAA) Ileu(AUA),Thr(ACA),Arg(AGA) Asn(AAU),Asn(AAC),Lys(AAG)
AAG	Term.(UAG),Gln(CAG),Glu(GAG) Met(AUG),Thr(ACG),Arg(AGG) Asn(AAU),Asn(AAC),Lys(AAA)

[*] From Jukes, T. H., Gatlin, L., et al.: Progr. Nucleic Acid Res. Mol. Biol. *11*:303, 1971.

[†] Term. = termination.

these two amino acids do not differ in their charge, the two types of γ chains do not separate significantly with the usual isolation procedures, and Hb F isolated from normal newborns contains both $^G\gamma$ and $^A\gamma$.

Mutant forms of fetal hemoglobin with abnormal γ chains exist which differ (other than at the 136th residue) from either $^G\gamma$ or $^A\gamma$ by a single amino acid substitution (40). These Hb F variants are generally recognized because they are electrophoretically separable from normal Hb F. Each of these variants has either glycine or alanine at the 136th residue of the γ chain, rather than the mixture found in whole fetal hemoglobin. This is consistent with the mutant γ chain gene being produced by a point mutation in a $^G\gamma$ gene or a $^A\gamma$ gene. Since all newborns have fetal hemoglobin which contains both $^G\gamma$ and $^A\gamma$ chains, the $^G\gamma$ and $^A\gamma$ genes cannot be allelic to one another, and there must be at least one pair of loci for $^G\gamma$ and at least one pair for $^A\gamma$.

The abnormal hemoglobins provide the means of determining if the various hemoglobin loci are linked together. In one large kindred in which both α and β variants were present, no linkage between the mutant genes was evident (41). On the other hand, individuals simultaneously heterozygous for β and δ variants transmit the variants to their progeny in such a way that these loci must be very closely linked (42). From this it is apparent that the α and δ loci also are not linked. Since γ chain variants are primarily studied in newborns, pedigrees providing linkage data regarding the γ chain locus are not available.

Abnormal Hemoglobins Characterized by Absence of One or More Contiguous Amino Acids

Several abnormal hemoglobins are known which have fewer than the expected number of amino acids in either the α chain or the β chain (32). This is the result of the absence of one or more amino acids from the "interior" of the amino acid sequence (i.e., not at the amino or carboxy terminus). These gaps, as they are called, must result from similar gaps in the DNA sequence for the corresponding gene. At the present

time, the genetic aberration which causes the gaps is not known. It is evident, however, that the gaps in the DNA sequence must correspond to the omission of one or more whole codons.

Abnormal Hemoglobins with Elongated Chains

Three abnormal hemoglobins are now known whose amino acid sequence is longer than the normal chains. Two of these (Hb Constant Spring and Hb Wayne) are abnormal in their α chains, and one (Hb Tak) is abnormal in the β chain. The first 141 residues of Hb Constant Spring (Hb CS) are identical to the normal α chain sequence; instead of terminating at the 141st residue, Hb CS extends an additional 31 residues (43). This suggested to the original investigators that the Hb CS might result from a mutation in the termination codon, allowing the post-termination portion of the α chain messenger to be read until a new termination codon was encountered. This speculation was reasonable in that several of the codons for glutamine (CAA, CAG), the 142nd residue in α^{CS}, differ by a single RNA residue from the known termination codons (UAA, UAG, and UGA). The amino acid sequence of α^{CS} may then be used to infer the possible post-termination messenger sequences of the normal α chain messenger (Table 25–3).

This interpretation of the origin of α^{CS} now seems substantiated by the discovery of Hb Wayne (44). This hemoglobin has 146 residues in its α chain, or five more than the normal. In addition, its sequence differs from normal α at amino acid residues 139, 140, and 141. An α messenger sequence can be selected from among those inferred from the α^{CS} amino acid sequence, such that deletion of a single RNA residue would yield a messenger whose product would have the amino acid sequence of α^{Wayne}. Loss of one base from the codon corresponding to the 139th amino acid (lysine) of normal α would result in a frame shift, with the subsequent portion of the α messenger being translated as the terminal portion of α^{Wayne} (Table 25–3) (44).

Table 25–3 provides the probable sequence for a considerable length of the

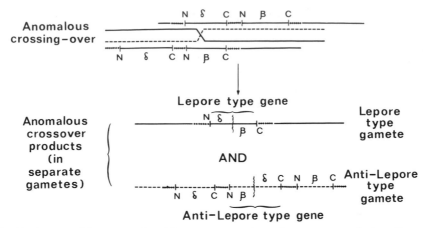

Figure 25–5. Production of Lepore and anti-Lepore type reciprocal crossover products as the result of anomalous crossing-over. (In addition to the two gametes shown, two normal gametes would be derived from the remaining two chromatids not involved in the depicted crossover.) The portion of the DNA sequence depicted as a dotted line is the postulated nontranslated region. The letters "N" and "C" indicate the amino termini or carboxy termini of the delta or the beta chains.

post-termination region of the normal α messenger. The α messenger has been isolated and is now being sequenced, with results consistent with the sequence given in Table 25–3 (45).

With such remarkable success in the analysis of the elongated α chain mutants, it is disappointing to state that no reasonable explanation is available for Hb Tak, the elongated β chain mutant (46). Hopefully, determination of the normal β messenger sequence, which is now in progress, will provide the answer.

Abnormal Hemoglobins Formed by "Fusion" of Two Different Hemoglobin Chains

This group of abnormal hemoglobins has been especially useful in defining the relative position of genes that are known or presumed to be adjacent to one another. Clinical studies of Hb Lepore, the first of these "fused" hemoglobins to be discovered, reveal that heterozygotes for this hemoglobinopathy have two unusual charac-

TABLE 25–3. PROPOSED ALPHA MESSENGER SEQUENCES FOR ABNORMAL HEMOGLOBINS WITH ELONGATED ALPHA CHAINS

AA Residue No.	139	140	141	142	143	144	145	146	147	148
α^A AA sequence	Lys - Tyr - Arg									
α^{CS} AA sequence	Lys - Tyr - Arg - Gln - Ala - Gly - Ala - Ser - Val - Ala - ...									
Possible codons° for α^A messenger inferred from α^{CS} AA sequence	$AA\frac{A}{G}$,$UA\frac{C}{U}$,CGN,$UA\frac{A}{G}$,GCN,GGN,GCN,UCN,GUN,GCN... $\quad AG\frac{A}{G}$,UGA $\qquad\qquad AG\frac{U}{C}$									
Proposed α^A messenger	AAAUACCGUUAAGCUGGAGCCUCGGUAGCN...									
Proposed α^{Wayne} messenger	AAUACCGUUAAGCUGGAGCCUCGGUAG									
α^{Wayne} AA sequence	Asn - Thr - Val - Lys - Leu - Glu - Pro - Arg (Term.)									

°N = unspecified nucleoside (either A,G,C, or U).

teristics — a low proportion of the abnormal hemoglobin (10 to 15 per cent of the total hemoglobin is Hb Lepore) and the red cell morphology typical of a thalassemia heterozygote. Chemical analysis of the Hb Lepore demonstrated that its α chains were normal, and that its non-α chains differed in an unexpected fashion from either β, γ, or δ (47). The N-terminal half or so of the molecule is identical in sequence to the corresponding portion of the normal δ chain, while the remainder is identical to the corresponding portion of the β chain. Since linkage data demonstrates that the δ and β genes are very close together (42), the most reasonable explanation for the structure of the aberrant Lepore chain is that it is the product of a fused δ-β gene. The postulated mechanism producing this mutant gene is known as anomalous crossing-over (47). This mechanism assumes that the δ gene on one chromosome has paired during meiosis with the β gene on the homologous chromosome, with crossing-over occurring within the paired region (Fig. 25–5). Two types of cross-over products are predicted; one chromosome would have a fused gene as well as a normal β and a normal δ gene, and the

other would have only a fused gene. The two fused genes present on the two chromosomes differ in the order of their δ and β segments; that with the δ segment at the N-terminus is designated the Lepore type, and that with the δ segment at the C-terminus is designated the anti-Lepore type. If the relative arrangement of the δ and β genes in the normal chromosome is as given in Figure 25–5, then the cross-over product with the Lepore type gene would lack normal δ and β genes. (If the order of the δ and β genes in the normal chromosome were the reverse of Figure 25–5, then the cross-over chromosome with the Lepore type gene would also contain normal δ and β genes.) The finding that patients inheriting two Lepore-type genes produce neither Hb A nor Hb A_2 (48) indicates that the normal order of the δ and β genes is that depicted in Figure 25–5.

The model of Figure 25–5 also predicts that crossing-over at different points would produce Lepore type genes with different lengths of the δ segment. This prediction has been fulfilled by the discovery both of two additional Lepore type hemoglobins and of two different anti-Lepores (Fig. 25–6) (49).

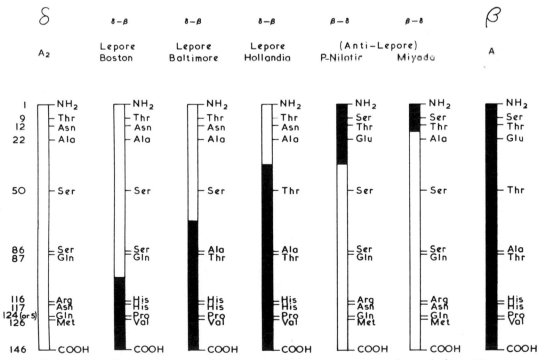

Figure 25–6. Schematic representation of the amino acid sequences in various hemoglobins of the Lepore and anti-Lepore type. (From Badr, F. M. et al.: Nature [New Biol.] 242:107, 1973.)

Hb Kenya has recently been recognized as a probable fused gene product of a new variety (50). As in the Lepore and anti-Lepore hemoglobins, the abnormality in this hemoglobin resides in the non-α chains. The N-terminal half is believed to be identical with the N-terminal portion of both the $^G\gamma$ and $^A\gamma$ chains, while the remainder appears to be indistinguishable from the C-terminal portion of the β chain. The non-α chain is, therefore, the product of a γ-β gene. Since Hb Kenya does not include the C-terminal portion of the γ chain, the feature which distinguishes $^G\gamma$ and $^A\gamma$ from one another (the 136th residue) is absent. The amino acid sequence of Hb Kenya thus does not directly indicate whether the anomalous crossing-over that may have led to its origin occurred in a $^G\gamma$ or a $^A\gamma$ gene. The one individual with Hb Kenya who has been studied so far also possesses Hb S, Hb F, and a less than expected amount of Hb A_2. His maternal ancestor is a Hb S heterozygote. (The paternal ancestor has not been studied.) If the maternal ancestor contributed the Hb S gene (as well as normal δ and γ genes), then it may be presumed that the γ-β gene came from the father.

The investigators of this hemoglobinopathy believe that the low level of Hb A_2 in their patient is evidence that only a single δ gene is present and, hence, that the paternal chromosome with the γ-β gene lacks a δ gene. They have also analyzed the Hb F present in their patient and find it to be of the $^G\gamma$ type, with no $^A\gamma$ present. They speculate that the Hb F is the product of a $^G\gamma$ gene on the paternal chromosome, and that this chromosome lacks any $^A\gamma$ genes (since no Hb F of $^A\gamma$ type is present). Although the information is not sufficient for a final determination, these investigators consider the most probable arrangement of the genes on the normal chromosome to be $^G\gamma$, $^A\gamma$, δ, and β.

References

1. Valentine, W. N., and Neel, J. V.: Hematologic and genetic study of the transmission of thalassemia (Cooley's anemia; Mediterranean anemia). Arch. Intern. Med. 74:185, 1944.
2. Neel, J. V.: The inheritance of sickle cell anemia. Science 110:64, 1949.
3. Pauling, L., Itano, H. A., et al.: Sickle cell anemia, a molecular disease. Science 110:543, 1949.
4. Miller, O. J., Miller, D. A., et al.: Application of new staining techniques to the study of human chromosomes. Progr. Med. Genet. 9:1, 1973.
5. Robson, E. B., Cook, P. J. L., et al.: Linkage data on Rh, PGM₁, PGD, peptidase C and Fy from family studies. Ann. Hum. Genet. 36:393, 1973.
6. Tjio, J. H., and Levan, A.: The chromosome number of man. Hereditas 42:1, 1956.
7. Nowell, P. C.: Phytohemagglutinin: An initiator of mitosis in cultures of normal human leucocytes. Cancer Res. 20:462, 1960.
8. Gilbert, C. W., Muldal, S., et al.: Time-sequence of human chromosome duplication. Nature (Lond.) 195:869, 1962.
9. Caspersson, T., Zech, L., et al.: Analysis of human metaphase chromosome set by aid of DNA-binding fluorescent agents. Exp. Cell Res. 62:490, 1970.
10. Osgood, E. E., and Brooke, J. H.: Continuous tissue culture of leucocytes from human leukemic bloods by application of "gradient" principles. Blood 10:1010, 1955.
11. Miller, O. J.: Autoradiography in human cytogenetics. Adv. Hum. Genet. 1:35, 1970.
12. Hamerton, J. L., Jacobs, P. A., et al.: Paris Conference (1971): Standardization in human cytogenetics. Birth Defects: Orig. Art. Ser. 8:1, 1972.
13. Borgaonkar, D. S., and Hollander, D. H.: Quinacrine fluorescence of the human Y chromosome. Nature (Lond.) 230:52, 1971.
14. Nowell, P. C., and Hungerford, D. A.: Chromosome studies on normal and leukemic leukocytes. J. Natl. Cancer Inst. 25:85, 1960.
15. Whang-Peng, J., Canellos, G. P., et al.: Clinical implications of cytogenetic variants in chronic myelocytic leukemia (CML). Blood 32:755, 1968.
16. Rowley, J. D.: A new consistent chromosomal abnormality in chronic myelogenous leukemia identified by quinacrine fluorescence and Giemsa staining. Nature (Lond.) 243:290, 1973.
17. Lobb, D. S., Reeves, B. R., et al.: Identification of isochromosome 17 in myeloid leukemia. Lancet 1:849, 1972.
17a. Meisner, L. F., Inhorn, S. L., et al.: Cytogenetic analysis as a diagnostic aid in leukemia. Am. J. Clin. Pathol. 60:435, 1973.
18. Nowell, P. C.: Marrow studies in preleukemia. Further correlation with clinical course. Cancer 28:513, 1971.
19. Reeves, R. R., Lobb, D. S., et al.: Identity of the abnormal F-group chromosome associated with polycythemia vera. Humangenetik 14:159, 1972.
20. Manolov, G., and Manolova, Y.: A marker band in one chromosome No. 14 in Burkitt lymphomas. Hereditas 69:300, 1971.
21. German, J.: Genes which increase chromosomal instability in somatic cells and predispose to cancer. Progr. Med. Genet. 8:61, 1972.
22. Bloom, G. E., Warner, S., et al.: Chromosome abnormalities in constitutional aplastic anemia. New Engl. J. Med. 274:8, 1966.
23. Gahrton, G., Lindsten, J., et al.: Tracing of chromosome 22 to parents of patients with chronic

myelocytic leukemia. Exp. Cell Res. 79:246, 1973.

24. Lyon, M. F.: Gene action in the X chromosome of the mouse (*Mus musculus* L.). Nature (Lond.) 190:372, 1961.

25. Beutler, E., Yeh, M., et al.: The normal human female as a mosaic of X-chromosome activity: Studies using the gene for glucose-6-phosphate dehydrogenase deficiency as a marker. Proc. Natl. Acad. Sci. USA 48:9, 1962.

26. Lyon, M. F.: Sex chromatin and gene action in the mammalian X-chromosome. Amer. J. Hum. Genet. 14:135, 1962.

27. Lyon, M. F.: X-chromosome inactivation and developmental patterns in mammals. Biol. Rev. 47:1, 1972.

28. Deys, B. F., Grzeschick, K. H., et al.: Human phosphoglycerate kinase and inactivation of the X chromosome. Science 175:1002, 1972.

29. Race, R. R.: Is the Xg blood group locus subject to inactivation? Proc. 4th Internatl. Congr. Hum. Genet., Sept. 6–11, 1971, pp. 311–314.

30. Fialkow, P. J., Gartler, S. M., et al.: Clonal origin of chronic myelocytic leukemia in man. Proc. Natl. Acad. Sci. USA 58:1468, 1967.

31. Moellering, R. C., and Weinberg, A. N.: Persistent Salmonella infection in a female carrier for chronic granulomatous disease. Ann. Intern. Med. 73:595, 1970.

32. McKusick, V. A.: *Mendelian Inheritance in Man.* 3rd ed. Baltimore, The Johns Hopkins Press, 1971.

33. Vogel, F.: Non-randomness of base replacement in point mutation. J. Mol. Evol. 1:334, 1972.

34. Murayama, M.: Chemical difference between normal human haemoglobin and haemoglobin-I. Nature (Lond.) 196:276, 1962.

35. Beale, D., and Lehmann, H.: Abnormal haemoglobins and the genetic code. Nature (Lond.) 207:259, 1965.

36. Jukes, T. H., Gatlin, L., et al.: Recent studies concerning the coding mechanism. Progr. Nucleic Acid Res. Mol. Biol. 11:303, 1971.

37. Beaven, G. H., Hornabrook, R. W., et al.: Occurrence of heterozygotes and homozygotes for the α-chain haemoglobin variant Hb-J

(Tongariki) in New Guinea. Nature [New Biol.] 235:46, 1972.

38. Hollan, S. R., Szelenyi, J. G., et al.: Multiple α chain loci for human haemoglobins: Hb J-Buda and Hb G-Pest. Nature [New Biol.] 235:47, 1972.

39. Schroeder, W. A., Huisman, T. H. J., et al.: Evidence for multiple structural genes for the γ chain of human fetal hemoglobin. Proc. Natl. Acad. Sci. USA 60:537, 1968.

40. Lorkin, P. A.: Fetal and embryonic haemoglobins. J. Med. Genet. 10:50, 1973.

41. Smith, E. W., and Torbert, J. V.: Study of two abnormal hemoglobins with evidence for a new genetic locus for hemoglobin formation. Bull. Johns Hopkins Hosp. 102:38, 1958.

42. Boyer, S. H., Rucknagel, D. L., et al.: Further evidence for linkage between the β and δ-loci governing human hemoglobin and the population dynamics of linked genes. Am. J. Hum. Genet. 15:438, 1963.

43. Clegg, J. B., Weatherall, D. J., et al.: Haemoglobin Constant Spring—A chain termination mutant? Nature (Lond.) 234:337, 1971.

44. Seid-Akhavan, M., Winter, W. P., et al.: Hemoglobin Wayne: A frame shift variant occurring in two distinct forms (abstract). Am. Soc. Hematol., Dec. 3–6, 1972.

45. Forget, B.: Personal communication.

46. Flatz, G., Kinderlerer, J. L., et al.: Hemoglobin Tak: A variant with additional residues at the end of the β-chains. Lancet 1:732, 1971.

47. Baglioni, C.: The fusion of two peptide chains in hemoglobin Lepore and its interpretation as a genetic deletion. Proc. Natl. Acad. Sci. USA 48:1880, 1962.

48. Weatherall, D. J., and Clegg, J. B.: *The Thalassemia Syndromes.* 2nd ed. Oxford, Blackwell Scientific Publications, 1972.

49. Badr, F. M., Lorkin, P. A., et al.: Haemoglobin P-Nilotic containing a β-δ chain. Nature [New Biol.] 242:107, 1973.

50. Huisman, T. H. J., Wrightstone, R. N., et al.: Hemoglobin Kenya, the product of fusion of γ and β polypeptide chains. Arch. Biochem. Biophys. 153:850, 1972.

Chapter 26

Erythrocyte Blood Groups in Humans

by Fred H. Allen, Jr.

The study of blood groups offers an opportunity to pose important genetic, immunologic, and clinical questions. In this chapter some of these questions and their partial solutions are presented.

Human blood groups can be detected only if some bloods can be distinguished from others. Anti-A typing serum, purchasable from many reputable vendors, will react with (agglutinate) group A_1, A_2, or A_3, or A_1B, A_2B, or A_3B bloods, but will not react with O or B bloods. Because 45 per cent of the population reacts with anti-A, it is a highly efficient test serum for subdividing the population (50 per cent would be maximally efficient for a single reagent). Few other blood typing reagents are as potent, reliable, available, and useful. For the majority of the known blood group specificities, reliable sera for testing are scarce, although the situation has been improving in recent years. The majority of the known antigens are of little help in identifying useful groups in the population—these are the many antigens with frequencies under 1 per cent or over 99 per cent. About 300 specificities have been reported. Most of these belong to one of the 15 to 20 named systems—ABO, MN, P, Rh, and so forth. The vagueness of the words "15 to 20" is owing to the circumstance that not all of the named systems have been fully established as independent of each other. No one has yet been identified, for example, who is both Wr(a+) and Di(a+); the children of such a person would demonstrate whether Wr^a and Di^a segregate independently.

Clinically, antigens A, B, and Rh account for most of the problems because of their relatively great antigenicity and their moderate frequencies. The importance of frequency of blood groups is considerable. Tj^a, of the P system, would probably be tested for routinely in transfusion services if it had a frequency like A or B, but only one person in a million or so is Tj(a−), so it is only a medical curiosity. When someone of this rare type, Tj(a−), needs a transfusion, however, it may be extremely difficult to find a compatible donor. Other rare types pose similar problems. So also do patients with autoimmune hemolytic anemia, whose antibodies, when they are identifiable, usually are directed against antigens of high frequency.

BLOOD GROUP SYSTEMS

A blood group system is a group of antigens that are determined by a single genetic "locus," "locus" being here defined as a DNA sequence short enough that "linkage disequilibrium"* is apparent on statistical analysis of populations in Hardy-Weinberg equilibrium; i.e., not only is all this DNA on one chromosome, but also it is a short enough sequence that cross-overs are so un-

---

*Linkage disequilibrium is illustrated in the Rh system by the very large percentage of D+ in C+ people. C+ people are very much less likely to be D− than are C− people.

TABLE 26–1. INDEPENDENCE OF THE ABO AND Rh SYSTEMS

	A+	A−	Total
Rh+	347	494	841
Rh−	66	93	159
Total	413	587	1000°

°One thousand individuals were studied, and the frequency of Rh and A antigens in this population is shown in the 2 × 2 contingency table.

common that some combinations of antigens are more frequent than would otherwise be expected.

A blood group system may have genetically independent modifiers, dominant or recessive, in addition to the main locus. The genes may also interact with other independent genes to produce hybrid antigens. Sometimes the genes are not expressed because of the absence of a precursor substance, itself determined by still other independent genes. The steps involved in identifying a blood group system are given in detail in the section on the Kell blood groups.

Genetic independence of systems is most easily shown, if relevant data are available, by 2 × 2 contingency tables. The genetic independence of the ABO and Rhesus blood groups is easily demonstrated by the group of observed frequencies in Table 26–1. The observed frequencies are so close to randomness that there is little room for doubt. (Many such observations have removed all possibilities of doubt.) This does not mean that there is no relation between the ABO and Rhesus markers, but only that the principal loci are independent.

SOME TECHNICAL DEFINITIONS

In the *saline agglutination test,* untreated red cells are suspended in a 0.9 per cent sodium chloride solution. Untreated serum is added. Depending on the temperature at which the mixture is held, agglutination would be called "saline," "saline agglutination," agglutination by a "complete antibody," or "cold agglutination." Most, but not all, "saline agglutinins" are IgM molecules, which are large and can span a

considerable distance to bind red cells to each other.

Incomplete antibodies that have blood group specificity are usually IgG molecules of relatively small size. They are, by definition, unable to cause agglutination of saline-suspended red cells, but are bound to red cells of the appropriate phenotype, as can be demonstrated by Coombs' method (the antiglobulin test) and a number of other techniques involving: enzyme treatment of the red cells; addition of albumin, polyvinylpyrrolidone (PVP), or other surface-acting substances; or changes in ionic concentration. These "incomplete" antibodies have also been called "albumin-active" and "monovalent." They have kept the old pros in business for 25 years, and threaten (promise) to keep young pros in business for some time to come. The uncertainties of blood group technology are part of the fascination of this discipline. There is still no perfect laboratory test for blood group compatibility; occasional antibodies are not detectable by any in vitro test.

Isoantibodies in human biology are antibodies produced in response to stimulation by a human (or humanlike) antigen by a person who lacks the corresponding antigens. Anti-Rh is an isoantibody. It is probable, however, that immunization to A and B is often (perhaps usually) initiated by symbiotic microorganisms that carry antigenic determinants identical or nearly identical to human A or B.

The origin of many specific antibodies is obscure. Anti-M^g, for example, is common, although the determinant is apparently very rare. It is, at least, very rare for a human to be M^g-positive, and M^g has not been detected in nonhuman material.

DISTRIBUTION OF ANTIGENS ON CELL MEMBRANES

Recent studies have shown that erythrocytes have a limited number (±1,200,000) of protein islands that presumably harbor the blood group determinants: 810,000 to 1,170,000 A sites on human adult A_1 cells (1), 120,000 A sites on A_2B cells, 70,000 to 85,000 c sites on cc (hr') cells (2), 5800 to

25,600 E (rh″) sites on E+ cells, 10,000 to 202,000 D (Rh₀) sites on Rh+ cells.

For the most part, the cellular distribution of red cell antigens is quite limited, but A, B, and H are found on nearly all cell surfaces, in the plasma, and usually in the saliva and gastric mucoids.

MATURATION OF BLOOD GROUPS

The erythrocytes of newborns are grossly deficient in I and somewhat deficient in A and B antigens, but seem usually to have normal Rh antigens, somewhat hyperreactive MN antigens (3), and notably hyperreactive i antigens. These erythrocytes usually lack Le^a and Le^b, and are poorly endowed with Lutheran antigens. Otherwise, they seem to be quite comparable to the red cells of adults.

Newborns seldom have anti-A or anti-B of their own manufacture, but usually develop both antibodies before they are a year old, if they are group O. If they are group A they will have developed anti-B, and if they are group B they will have anti-A. Human salivary aerosols are a possible source of antigenic stimulation, as are numerous food products. Regardless of the mechanism of their induction, anti-A and anti-B are generally spoken of as "natural" or "nonimmune" isoantibodies. Tj(a−) persons, also called "p," regularly have anti-P (anti-Tj^a) antibodies. As far as is known, no other isoantibody is habitually present in humans who lack the corresponding determinant.

In the following pages, the various blood group systems will be described, not in the order of their discovery or of their clinical importance, *but more or less in the order of their increasing complexity*. Thus I shall start with Diego.

THE DIEGO BLOOD GROUPS

Di^a (Diego) was uncovered by Layrisse, Arends, and Dominguez in 1955 (4) by means of an antibody found in the serum of a mother who had given birth to a child with unexpected erythroblastosis fetalis. The serum of this mother agglutinated (by the Coombs' antiglobulin method) a moderate number of American Indian and Oriental blood samples (up to 35 per cent), but only a rare Caucasian sample.

Twelve years later, anti-Di^b was reported by Thompson, Childers, and Hatcher (5). Many subsequent searches have failed to disclose the phenotype Di(a−b−) (Table 26–2). The Di(a−b−) allele may not exist, or, when homozygous, may give rise to a lethal phenotype, and Di(a+b−) might also be disadvantageous, so we may not know enough about the Diego groups—probably we do not. Study of the other red cell systems indicates, however, that still other phenotypes beyond these three should be looked for. The possibility of various additions is suggested by the complexities of the Lutheran, Kell, and Rh red cell systems.

OTHER "SIMPLE" SYSTEMS

Anti-Do^a (6) and anti-Do^b (7) define the Dombroch system. Anti-Yt^a (8) and anti-Yt^b (9) define the Cartwright system. Anti-Co^a (10) and anti-Co^b (11) define the Colton system. Anti-Sm (12) and anti-Bu^a (13) may define another, though it has not yet been proven independent of Cartwright or Colton. These four systems are like Diego to the extent that only three phenotypes are

TABLE 26–2.   DIEGO PHENOTYPES

| DESIGNATIONS | INCIDENCE | | REACTIONS WITH SERA | |
	Caucasians	Amerindians	Anti-Di^a	Anti-Di^b
Di(a−b+)	1.00	0.90	0	+
Di(a+b+)	0.00	0.10°	+	+
Di(a+b−)	0.00	Rare	+	0
Di(a−b−)	0.00	0.00	0	0

°Approximate value, which varies from 0 in Alaska to 30 per cent in South America.

known, (a—b—) types not having been reported. The antibodies may cause clinical problems, but only rarely. Their real importance is in genetic studies.

Two simple systems, Auberger (14) and Stoltzfus (15), are represented by one antigen each. The phenotype Au(a+) represents the homozygote Au^aAu^a, as well as the heterozygote Au^aAu, while Au(a—) merely represents the absence of Au^a. Sf(a+) and Sf(a—) have a similar relationship in the Stoltzfus system. Again, the antibodies have much more genetic than clinical importance.

Ge1, Ge2, and Ge3 are potentially important antigens in the Gerbich system (16), but in most populations all three are present in nearly everyone. Only in some New Guinea populations have the moderate frequencies been found that make them genetically useful and clinically important.

Cs^a (Cost-Sterling) and Yk^a (York) (17) are part of still another system that has not been much exploited, partly because of lack of publicity. They seem to have little clinical importance, but, because about 8 per cent of Caucasians lack one or both of them, they have value in genetic studies.

Vel 1 and Vel 2 are high-frequency antigens (18), the type Vel:1,—2 being somewhat less rare than Vel:—1—2. Vel antibodies may be hemolytic in vivo and cause severe transfusion reactions.

THE KIDD GROUPS

The antibodies of the Kidd system are notoriously difficult to work with, some more so than others. The original anti-Jk^a produced moderately severe erythroblastosis fetalis in an infant named John Kidd (19). Anti-Jk^b (20) has caused severe transfusion reactions after careful testing had shown the donor to be apparently compatible. In one such case, the anti-Jk^b was detected only

with the help of an AutoAnalyzer hemagglutination apparatus. A few examples of anti-Jk^aJk^b have been found (Table 26–3).

Only anti-Jk^aJk^b is absorbed by leukocytes (21), indicating that the antigen it detects is distinct from Jk^a and Jk^b. The phenotype Jk(a—b—) is probably the result of homozygosity for a silent allele (Jk) at the Kidd locus.

THE ABO GROUPS

After 75 years of intensive study, the ABO groups are still yielding secrets, such as one chromosome producing both A and B (22) and dominant suppressors (23). Although at least three independent loci (H, Y, and ABO) are involved in the expression of the ABO phenotypes, the inheritance of the ABO groups is usually uncomplicated.

A common and informative family has the following features: parents are group A and group B, and children include groups A and B (Fig. 26–1). In such a family it is obvious that the parents are AO and BO, and that O and AB children should occur as often as A's and B's, and that is how it actually occurs. A mating O × AB produces A and B children only. An AB person does (with the rare exception hinted at above) not have an O child or an O parent.

In 1955, however, an apparent type O("Bombay type," actually) mother in Providence, Rhode Island, had a type AB daughter. The mother's red cells were group O, but her serum contained a very strong anti-H and agglutinated all group O bloods in addition to the expected A's, B's, and AB's. Subsequent investigation (24) showed that the mother's ABO genotype was BO (her husband was group A). From these and subsequent data it became obvious that two independent loci were involved in the inheritance of the ABO groups. It was already known that H is the precursor of A

TABLE 26–3. KIDD GROUPS

PHENOTYPE	INCIDENCE	REACTIONS WITH SERA		
		Anti-Jk^a	*Anti-Jk^b*	*Anti-Jk^{a}Jk^b*
Jk(a+b—)	0.27	+	0	+
Jk(a+b+)	0.50	+	+	+
Jk(a—b+)	0.23	0	+	+
Jk(a—b—)	Rare	0	0	0

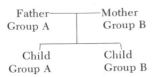

Figure 26–1. A common and informative family.

and B, and that the specificity is determined by oligosaccharides. The *H* gene, now known to be independent of ABO, produces an L-fucosyltransferase which adds L-fucose to the precursor of H. At the ABO locus, the *A* gene produces *N*-acetylgalactosaminyl transferase, and the *B* gene produces D-galactosyl transferase (3). The *O* gene produces no functioning enzyme, as far as is known. The Providence lady had the ABO genotype *BO*, but also had the genotype *hh*, and so produced no H substance. Chemically, B is H with an added terminal D-galactose. In A, the added sugar is *N*-acetyl galactosamine.

Anti-A and anti-B are almost universal in humans lacking the corresponding antigens on their cells. They form after birth from a variety of stimuli, and are of IgM, IgG, and IgA types. Complement fixation is common. Transfusion reactions to ABO-incompatible blood may be so mild as to go unnoticed, but they are often severe enough to lead to renal shutdown in the absence of prompt treatment.

ABO antigens are present on nearly all (some say all) cells of the body. Rarely, however, A or B antigen may be unexpectedly absent from the red cells while present on other cells. The ABO antigens are present also in the saliva of about 75 per cent of humans; this "secretor" state is inherited (25) as a mendelian dominant, independent of the ABO genes. The genes involved are called *Se* (secretor) and *se* (nonsecretor).

Rarely, a change of blood group has been seen in disease, notably malignancy. Presumably this may result from the production of a new transferase or modification of a normal one.

There is a considerable number of variants of the ABO phenotypes. Mostly, these are weak expressions of A or B, and most of them depend on variant genes at the ABO locus. A_2 is a rather common phenotype (nearly 10 per cent), which differs qualitatively as well as quantitatively from A_1. The gene A_2 is recessive to A_1 and dominant to *O*. Persons of group A_2 or A_2B occasionally produce anti-A_1, which agglutinates A_1 cells but not A_2 cells. The other variants are rare and of little clinical importance. Some are caused by independently segregating modifier genes. The most interesting appears to be caused by a dominant suppressor gene at the ABO locus (23).

THE P SYSTEM

Three antigens of the P system have been well studied (3). The phenotypes are best shown in tabular form (Table 26–4). People of p phenotype always have anti-P (anti-Tj^a). Their serum is usually separable into three specific antibodies—anti-P_1, anti-P, and anti-P^k. Anti-Tj^a is a troublemaker. It is a strong complement-binding antibody, responsible for severe clinical problems, which are fortunately rare, as is the p phenotype.

The inheritance of the P system antigens is somewhat obscure. P_1 and P appear to be mendelian dominants dependent primarily on alleles at the P locus. The rare P^k appears, superficially, to be inherited as a recessive, but it seems more likely that P^k is the product of a locus other than the P locus,

TABLE 26–4. PHENOTYPES IN P SYSTEM*

PHENOTYPES		INCIDENCE	REACTIONS WITH SERA			
Current Nomenclature	*Former Nomenclature*		*Anti-P_1 (anti-P)*	*Anti-PP_1P^k (anti-Tj^a)*	*Anti-P*	*Anti-P^k*
P_1	(P+)	0.75	+	+	+	0
P_2	(P−)	0.25	0	+	+	0
p	(Tj(a−))	Very rare	0	0	0	0
P_1^k		Very rare	+	+	0	+
P_2^k		Very rare	0	+	0	+

*Modified from Race, R. R., and Sanger, R.: *Blood Groups in Man.* 5th ed. Philadelphia, F. A. Davis, 1968, p. 153.

and that its expression is dependent on genes at the P locus. The appearance of recessiveness is striking—no parent or child of a P^k+ person has been P^k+; many have been tested.

THE DUFFY SYSTEM

Five antigens have been described. Fy^a was recognized by the first Duffy antibody (26), and Fy^b by the second (27). Anti-Fy3 (28) recognizes something that is shared by Fy(a+) and Fy(b+) people. Anti-Fy4 (29) appears to detect an allele of Fy3. Fy5 (30) is like Fy3 except that it is not produced by persons of the type Rh_{null}. Fourteen phenotypes have been found (Table 26–5). (No other is possible from current evidence.)

The frequencies in the table are for Caucasians. The type Fy(a–b–) results from homozygosity for the gene Fy^4, which may be less than 1 per cent in Caucasians, but is over 80 per cent in Blacks.

An anti-Fy^a titer of 5000 was seen after a transfusion reaction. This antibody is also a rare cause of erythroblastosis fetalis, usually of a mild variety. Anti-Fy^b is usually a weak antibody. Both usually require the Coombs' test for detection.

Fy3 and Fy4 activity on red cells is not destroyed by enzyme treatment, but Fy^a and Fy^b are inactivated, making the cells inagglutinable by the corresponding sera.

Four alleles at the Duffy locus have been defined (Table 26–6). These four alleles are

TABLE 26–6. ALLELES AT THE DUFFY LOCUS

| ALLELES | DETERMINANTS PRODUCED | | | |
	Fy^a	Fy^b	$Fy3$	$Fy4$
Fy^a	+	0	+	0
Fy^b	0	+	+	0
Fy^x	0	Weak	Weak	Unknown
$Fy4$	0	0	0	+

responsible for the first eight phenotypes in the list. The other six are rare Rh phenotypes that react weakly or not at all with anti-Fy5. These six phenotypes indicate some kind of interaction between Duffy and Rh. Fy^a and Fy^b have always been assumed to be allelic. Both the table of alleles and the effect of enzymes suggest that Fy3 and Fy4 are allelic. Fy4 could, however, from present information, be allelic to Fy^a and Fy^b.

THE MN GROUPS

The second blood group system, after ABO, was reported in 1926 (31). Two antibodies, both produced in rabbits by immunization with human blood, were named anti-M and anti-N. Three types were found: M+N+(group MN), M+N–(group M), and M–N+(group N). Tests of families indicated that M and N were inherited as codominant characters. Subsequent studies (32) suggest that N is a precursor of M. N appears to be

TABLE 26–5. DUFFY PHENOTYPES

| DESIGNATIONS | Rh TYPES | INCIDENCE | REACTIONS WITH SERA | | | | |
			Anti-Fy^a	-Fy^b	-$Fy3$	-$Fy4$	-$Fy5$
Fy(a+b–)		0.17	+	0	+	+	+
			+	0	+	0	+
Fy(a+bw)		0.01	+	wk	+	nt	nt
Fy(a+b+)		0.47	+	+	+	0	+
Fy(a–b+)	Ordinary Rh phenotypes	0.35	0	+	+	+	+
			0	+	+	0	+
Fy(a–bw)		Rare	0	wk	wk	nt	nt
Fy(a–b–)		Rare	0	0	0	+	0
Fy(a+b–)	Rh_{null}	Rare	+	0	+	nt	0
Fy(a+b+)	Rh_{null}	Rare	+	+	+	nt	0
Fy(a–b+)	Rh_{null}	Rare	0	+	+	nt	0
Fy(a+b–)	–D–	Rare	+	0	+	nt	wk
Fy(a+b+)	–D–	Rare	+	+	+	nt	wk
Fy(a–b+)	–D–	Rare	0	+	+	nt	wk

Abbreviations: nt = not tested; wk = weakly reactive; 0 = negative. Frequencies for Caucasians.

an essential gene, for, in millions of tests, no M−N− person has been found. M−N+ is a common type. M+Nweak is also common. And M+N+ is almost 50 per cent. Although M−N− has not been found, genes that seem to produce neither M nor N have been observed (33). This suggests that homozygosity for a null allele at the MN locus may be lethal.

S and s (3) are a second allelic pair of antigens in the MN system. S is much more often associated with M than with N ("linkage disequilibrium"), indicating that the genetic loci for MN and Ss are either identical or very closely linked. No "certain" recombinants have been found between MN and Ss. The S−s− group is not uncommon in Africans. Once it was known that S−s− was a possible type, it was soon found in Caucasians, although it is much less frequent than in Africans.

U is another MN antigen (34), almost universally present in humans (over 99 per cent). Most S−s− people are also U−, and no S+ or s+ people have been U−. U is the only MN antigen that is presently detectable (35) on leukocytes, but it is not detectable on the leukocytes of people who have U− erythrocytes.

Many other MN antigens have been described, and they are listed in Table 26-7. Of especial interest is the relatively enormous frequency of "spontaneous" ("natural") antibodies for many of the rare MN antigens in the sera of normal untransfused people. M^g, for example, is a very rare antigen, with an incidence of less than 1 in 10,000. Anti-M^g is found in about 1 per cent of normal sera.

The MN antigens are of minor clinical importance. Anti-U has been responsible for rare cases of severe erythroblastosis fetalis or transfusion reaction. M, S, and s have also been implicated in even rarer clinical problems. Other rare MN antigens may occasionally be troublemakers.

Sialic acid, which is responsible for much of the surface charge of erythrocytes, is also involved in some way with M and N. Treatment of erythrocytes with neuraminidase or other proteolytic enzymes reduces or destroys their reactivity with anti-M and anti-N. Sialic acid appears to be one of the sugars involved in the specificity of M and N, but not of S, s, or U.

From the genetic (and medicolegal and

TABLE 26-7. ANTIGENS OF THE MN SYSTEM

DESIGNATION	FREQUENCY OF ANTIGEN IN CAUCASIANS	DATE OF DISCOVERY
M	0.78	1927
N	0.72	1927
Hu	<0.01	1934
Vw(Gr)	<0.01	1946
S	0.55	1947
s	0.89	1951
He	<0.01	1951
Mi^a	<0.01	1951
U	>0.99	1953
M^c	<0.01	1953
M^g	<0.01	1958
Vr	<0.01	1958
M_1	0.25	1960
Mur	<0.01	1961
M^e	0.78	1961
Ri^a	<0.01	1962
St^a	<0.01	1962
Mt^a	<0.01	1962
Hil	<0.01	1963
Cl^a	<0.01	1963
Ny^a	<0.01	1964
Tm	0.20	1965
U^B	>0.99	1965
Sj	0.02	1966
M^v	0.72	1966
Sul	<0.01	1967

anthropologic viewpoints), the MN system is one of the most important, after only HL-A and Rh. The availability of reliable grouping sera is a major problem in the MN system, as it is in most of the other systems, even in 1974.

THE LUTHERAN SYSTEM

The Lutheran blood groups were simple (36, 37) until Crawford (38) reported the group Lu(a−b−). In her family and a number of others, Lu(a−b−) is inherited as a dominant character owing to an unlinked modifier. This was and still is a phenomenon unique to Lutheran. It has been demonstrated (39) that people of this type are not genetically Lu^{a-b-}, but have common Lutheran genes. Their red cells are not agglutinated by anti-Lu^a or anti-Lu^b, but can specifically absorb anti-Lu^a, anti-Lu^b, or both, depending on the genotype of the individual. More recently (40), families have been found in which the Lu(a−b−) phenotype is inherited by means of a null (amorphic) allele at the Lutheran locus, comparable to the *O* gene of the ABO system. People of this recessive type can produce an antibody that has been called anti-Lu^{a}Lu^b and anti-Lu3. It is nearly impossible to define an antigen corresponding to anti-Lu3. Since people who lack Lu3 also lack all other Lutheran antigens, they can theoretically produce antibody against any one or any combination of these.

The Lutheran system displays also a group of closely related high-frequency antigens that are comparable to a similar group of high-frequency antigens in the Kell system and to the Rh^A, Rh^B, Rh^C, and Rh^D antigens of the Rhesus system. These high-frequency antigens are shown in Table 26–8.

It is evident from the table that Lu5 and Lu10 have an allelic relationship, as do Lu6 and Lu9. Lu9 has been established by family studies (44) to belong to the Lutheran system. There is considerable evidence that the venerable antigen Sw^a (Swann) (48), which has a very low frequency, may also belong to the Lutheran system and have a high-frequency allele (not identified as yet), but unpublished data (49) are against this assumption.

Three additional high-frequency Lutheran antigens (McC., Nob, and Dav.) are under investigation in various laboratories. These could increase the number of named antigens to 16. The testing of rare bloods, such as Lu:−12, with sera recognizing rare antigens will probably add still further to the catalogue of the Lutheran system.

Lutheran antibodies are usually weak. Very few clinical problems have been described, but it would be surprising if rare problems of a serious nature could not arise from incompatibility of at least one of the Lutheran antigens.

Genetic studies indicate that over 99 per cent of humans have Lu2, Lu4, Lu5, Lu6, Lu7, Lu8, Lu11, Lu12, and probably at least three other determinants (Lu13, Lu15, and Lu16).

THE KELL BLOOD GROUPS

Anti-K(K1) was found in the serum of Mrs. Kell, whose child had erythroblastosis fetalis (50). Maternal serum reacted with paternal erythrocytes and with 9 per cent of random samples, and the specificity was obviously different from the few other blood group specificities then known. Subsequent blood grouping tests of many families have shown that Kell is not linked to the previously known ABO, MN, P, Rh, or Lutheran loci. A few years later (51) Mrs. Cellano's serum was found to react with all but 5 of 2500 bloods. Her own red cells and those of the other nonreactors were all K+

TABLE 26–8. HAPLOTYPES (ALLELES) IN THE LUTHERAN SYSTEM*

ALLELES		Lu1	Lu2	Lu4	Lu5	Lu6	Lu7	Lu8	Lu9	Lu10	Lu11	Lu12
Trivial Names:		Lu^a	Lu^b	Bar	Fox	Jan	Gar	Tay	Mul	Sin	Rey	Muc
Frequency:		0.07	0.998	High	High	High	High	High	0.017	Low	High	High
		References		(41)	(42)	(42)	(42)	(43)	(44)	(45)	(46)	(47)
Lu^a	0.03	+	0	+	+	+	+	+	0	0	+	+
Lu^b	±0.95	0	+	+	+	+	+	+	0	0	+	+
Lu^e †	Rare	0	+	0	+	+	+	+	0	0	+	+
Lu^f	Rare	0	+	+	0	+	+	+	0	+	+	+
Lu^m	0.01	0	+	+	+	0	+	+	+	0	+	+
Lu^{am}	0.01	+	0	+	+	0	+	+	+	0	+	+
Lu^g	Rare	0	+	+	+	+	0	+	0	0	+	+
Lu^t	Rare	0	+	+	+	+	+	0	0	0	+	+
Lu^r	Rare	0	+	+	+	+	+	+	0	0	0	+
Lu^k	Rare	0	+	+	+	+	+	+	0	0	+	0
Lu	Rare	0	0	0	0	0	0	0	0	0	0	0

*This table should be compared to Table 26–11 for Kell. Lu3 is in limbo. Numbers are frequencies of antigens and alleles in the Caucasian population.

†Nomenclature beyond *Lu^a*, *Lu^b*, and *Lu* has not been standardized. Other names of alleles are tentative, based on 1973 New York Blood Center information.

(reacted with the serum of Mrs. Kell). Since the probability that six unrelated random persons would all be K+ is only 0.00000053, it was obvious that these six were not random, that being Cellano-negative was somehow related to being Kell-positive. The obvious conclusion that the Kell and Cellano (k, K2) antigens are allelic was subsequently substantiated by many other studies.

Not until 1957 (52) was it known that K—k— persons existed, and data already accumulated showed that this "minus-minus" type was rare. A representative sample of random people in 1957 would have shown, and still would show in 1973, approximately the distribution shown in Table 26–9. Until 1957, Kell was a two-allele (K and k) system. Also in 1957, the studies of Mrs. Penney's serum were reported (53). The antigen detected by her serum, found in 2 per cent of Caucasians, was named Kp^a(K3) (K for "Kell," and p for "Penney"). The superscript (^{a}) was used to designate the first-found of a pair of allelic characters belonging to the Kell system. Kp^b (K4) (Rautenberg) was found almost at the same time, which made things easier (54). The relation of Kp^a to K was shown by a large number of families (55), in which one parent was K+Kp(a+), the other being K—Kp(a—). Without exception, the many children of such matings have been either K+Kp(a—) or K—Kp(a+). The absence of recombinations in such extensive studies shows that K and Kp^a are determined by alleles.

The absence of K+Kp(a+) genes in such extensive studies demonstrates "linkage disequilibrium" and is of considerable genetic interest. The disequilibrium is shown also by population studies illustrated in Table 26–10, which shows a deficit of K+ in a population of Kp(a+) people. The finding of Mr. Rautenberg's serum was almost an-

TABLE 26–10. FREQUENCY OF K+ AMONG 274 Kp(a+) MANITOBANS

	OB-SERVED	EX-PECTED*	χ^2	P
K+	11	23	6.26	0.012
K—	263	251	0.53	
Total	274	274	6.79	0.009

*Frequency of K+ in the same population (55) was 0.0836.

ticlimactic (though not seeming so at the time). The Rautenberg serum, eventually called anti-Kp^b, reacted with almost everyone. However, his own erythrocytes, those of a Kp(b—) brother, and those of two other Kp(b—) people found in random testing were all Kp(a+), indicating the strong probability that Kp^a (Penney) and Kp^b (Rautenberg) are allelic and that, therefore, Kp^b also belongs to the Kell system. In 1958 anti-Js^a was described (56), and in 1963 anti-Js^b (57). Js^a(K6) and Js^b(K7) are allelic by the same criteria as K and k. Recognition of their relation to the Kell system was delayed by the scarcity of double backcross families, with one parent K+Js(a+). But it was shown in 1965 that an anti-Js^b serum did not react with a blood sample of type K—k—Kp(a—b—), indicating the probability that Js^a and Js^b belong to the Kell system (58). Later (59), tests of a number of families in which the rare type K+Js(a+) was found in one parent [the other parent in each case being K—Js(a—)] showed that all of nearly 40 children were either K+Js(a—) or K—Js(a+). None was K+Js(a+), and none was K—Js(a—). This absence of recombinants demonstrated that Js^a (and therefore Js^b also) belongs to the Kell system. Kell was the first system in which three pairs of allelic antigens were demonstrated ("old hat" now) (60).

Further additions to the Kell system have been provided by rare sera that react with nearly all bloods except those that are of the rare type K_o [K—k—K_p(a—b—)Js(a—b—)]. K11, K12, and K14 are in this category; these presumably belong to the Kell system, but no genetic evidence has yet been obtained owing to the rarity of the critical types. K13 has a somewhat stronger position (61), the producer of anti-K13 being a weak (or negative) reactor with all Kell antisera. Ul^a(K10) is a low-frequency antigen belonging to the Kell system by the same criteria as Kp^a and

TABLE 26–9. APPROXIMATE DISTRIBUTIONS OF K(KELL) AND k(CELLANO) ANTIGENS, AS OF 1973

	K+	K—	Total
k+	881	9099	9980
k—	19	1	20
Total	900	9100	10,000*

*Figures are for Caucasian populations. Other populations are much less informative, having much lower frequencies for both K+ and k—.

Js^a (family studies), but no high-frequency allele of Ul^a has yet been identified (62). The allele of Ul^a is being sought, as well as low-frequency alleles of K11, K12, K13, and K14.

Anti-Ku(K5) (63) was present in the serum of Mrs. Peltz, the original K person. It reacts with the red cells of all persons except those of type K$_0$. Attempts to fractionate the serum by absorptions and elutions were unsuccessful, so it was thought to be a monospecific antibody. But it is now evident that, although the Peltz serum did not contain anti-k or anti-Kp^b, it could have contained an antibody directed against any of the six high-frequency Kell antigens subsequently described, or any combination of such antibodies. The work necessary to prove or disprove such a possibility has not yet been done, so the status of Ku is in limbo. In fact, the status of Ku will probably always remain uncertain (same as Lu3).

A weak reagent named anti-K^w (64) was thought to belong to the Kell system because the antibodies were found only in anti-K sera. K^w was also called "K8." Its status is still uncertain. K9, K15, and K16 are revealed by the remarkable McLeod type (65).

McLeod was thought at first to be of the type K$_0$, but his cells had weak expression of k, Kp^b, Js^b, "Ku," K11, K12, K13, and K14. The cells lacked the high-frequency antigens K9, K15, and K16. No other healthy person of this type has been found, but a surprising proportion of patients with chronic granulomatous disease (CGD) have the McLeod type (66), and since in these patients CGD is X-linked, the suspicion cannot be avoided that an X-borne gene could be responsible for the McLeod type.

Anti-K9 was first found in a young boy who, in retrospect, presumably had CGD. He had the McLeod type (67), and his serum reacted with all bloods except his own and McLeod. This serum contained anti-K9 and anti-K15. K9 is absent also in K$_0$ red cells, but K15 is especially strong in K$_0$ cells.

The antigen K15 (68) is the most enigmatic of the Kell antigens. It appears superficially to result from the presence of the K^0 allele at the Kell locus, which produces no other Kell antigens. But nearly all people who do not have K^0 (99 per cent or more) also react very weakly with anti-K15 and have enough K15

on their red cells to absorb all activity from an anti-K15 reagent, and their leukocytes are loaded with K15. (Other Kell antigens are not found on leukocytes.) The only persons who have not had K15 on their leukocytes (out of about 40 tested) are three (of three) boys with X-linked CGD (68). McLeod's leukocytes have normal amounts of K15.

Anti-K16 was considered to be ordinary anti-k until it was absorbed with McLeod's red cells (68). Anti-K16 reacts with all k-positive bloods except McLeod. The interrelations of the Kell antigens are shown in Table 26–11.

The anthropologic and medicolegal value of the Kell system is limited, because of unfavorable frequencies in most populations. K has useful frequencies (±9 per cent K+) in Caucasians, and Js^a has useful frequencies [up to 20 per cent Js(a+)] in Blacks. K+ and Js(a+) are both rare in Orientals and Amerindians. No population has shown a high frequency of Kp^a. All populations tested have high frequencies of K2, K4, K7, K9, K11, K12, K13, and K14.

The antibodies of the Kell system tend to be high-titered and lethal. An anti-k titer of 50,000 has been observed. The most severe forms of transfusion reaction and erythroblastosis fetalis have been caused by antibodies to the antigen K(K1), which is common enough to be of noticeable, though numerically minor, clinical importance. Kell antibodies are next, in clinical importance, after ABO and Rh.

Rh

The Rhesus system was the fourth erythrocyte blood group system to be reported (69, 70). Although Rh does not have the explosive transfusion incompatibility implications of the ABO groups, its paramount importance in erythroblastosis fetalis gives Rh almost equal billing with ABO in overall clinical interest. Anti-D (Rh$_0$) is the only erythrocyte isoantibody apart from anti-I and -i to have demonstrated a titer in excess of 1,000,000. The very powerful anti-Rh$_0$ sera have always contained mostly IgG antibodies, whereas anti-A and anti-B contain mostly IgM. The detection of Rh antibodies has not always been easy. For the first several years of intensive research on the subject, most Rh antibodies were not

TABLE 26–11.   KELL ANTIGENS OF TWELVE HOMOZYGOTES

SHORT NAME	DETECTABLE PHENOTYPES											
k	Weak K15	KL	K16	K5	k	Js^b	Kp^b	—	K11	K12	K13	K14
K	Weak K15	KL	—	K5	K	Js^b	Kp^b	—	K11	K12	K13	K14
k^j	Weak K15	KL	K16	K5	k	Js^a	Kp^b	—	K11	K12	K13	K14
k^p	Weak K15	KL	K16	K5	k	Js^b	Kp^a	—	K11	K12	K13	K14
k^{ul}	Weak K15	KL	K16	K5	k	Js^b	Kp^b	Ul^a	K11	K12	K13	K14
k^{co}	Weak K15	KL	K16	K5	k	Js^b	Kp^b	—	—	K12	K13	K14
k^{bo}	Weak K15	KL	K16	K5	k	Js^b	Kp^b	—	K11	—	K13	K14
k^{sg}	Weak K15	Weak KL	Weak K16	Weak K5	Weak k	Weak Js^b	Weak Kp^b	—	Weak K11	Weak K12	—	Weak K14
k^{sa}	Weak K15	KL	K16	K5	k	Js^b	Kp^b	—	K11	K12	K13	—
k^{pw}	Weak K15	Weak KL	Weak K16	Weak K5	Weak k	Weak Js^b	Weak Kp^a	—	Weak K11	Weak K12	Weak K13	Weak K14
k^{mc}	—	—	—	Weak K5	Weak k	Weak Js^b	Weak Kp^b	—	Weak K11	Weak K12	Weak K13	Weak K14
K^o	K15	—	—	—	—	—	—	—	—	—	—	—

This is not a table of Kell alleles, although it is arranged that way. Rather, it represents the phenotypes of the known homozygotes in the Kell system. The 12 columns bring out allelic relationships (K and k, Kp^a and Kp^b, Js^a and Js^b) and imply the possibility that 12 subloci or closely linked genes could be postulated. On the contrary, each of the 12 columns could represent different antigenic sites on a single long polypeptide chain. The first column gives short names for the various combinations (haplotypes.) K16 (68) is detected by an antibody that was considered to be anti-K2(k) until absorptions with the cells of McLeod showed it to be different. McLeod cells absorb anti-K2, but not anti-K16.

detectable by leading workers in the field. Out of this research there came the "blocking test," the "rapid slide test," the use of albumin and other large-molecular-weight substances, the anti-globulin test of Coombs', and the use of various enzymes—techniques that were to spark the current revolution in immunology. Now, simple tests that can easily be automated make the detection of Rh antibodies very easy and reliable. More than 30 Rh specificities have been reported (Table 26–12), most of which have been proven of occasional clinical importance, but only D is of sufficient importance to require routine laboratory surveillance.

The inheritance of the Rh antigens seems to be quite complicated, involving at least two or three distinct loci, one of which has been postulated by Rosenfield et al. (71) to comprise at least four operator or promotor genes, each with a closely linked structural region. One of these regions can be compared to the principal locus of the Lutheran system. It produces at least four high-frequency D-like antigens (Rh13, Rh14, Rh15, and Rh16), at least two of which have low-frequency alleles (Rh23 and Rh30). With rare exceptions, Rh-positive people have all four of these high-frequency antigens. The null allele, producing the Rh-negative condition, is much more common than Lu_{null}. Otherwise, Rh13, Rh14, and so forth appear to be exactly comparable to Lu^b, Lu4, Lu5, and so on. Rh14, Rh15, and Rh16 also have counterparts within the Rh system itself. Rh21 and Rh2 are usually indistinguishable. So are Rh4 and Rh26. So are Rh5, Rh19, and Rh31. So are Rh3 and Rh24. In each of these series, only rare people lack only one of the antigens—all or none is the rule.

TABLE 26–12. Rh ANTIGENS AND THEIR VARIOUS NAMES

Rh1	Rh_o, D	0.84*		Rh18	Hr	>0.99
Rh2	rh′, C	0.70		Rh19	hr^s	0.97
Rh3	rh″, E	0.30		Rh20	VS, e^s	<0.01
Rh4	hr′, c	0.80		Rh21	C^G	0.70
Rh5	hr″, e	0.97		Rh22	CE	0.01
Rh6	hr, f, ce	0.64		Rh23	D^w	<0.01
Rh7	rh_i, Ce	0.70		Rh24	E^T	0.30
Rh8	rh^{w1}, C^w	0.01		Rh25	LW	>0.99
Rh9	rh^x, C^x	<0.01		Rh26		0.80
Rh10	hr^v, V, ce^s	<0.01		Rh27	cE	0.30
Rh11	rh^{w2}, E^w	<0.01		Rh28	hr^H	<0.01
Rh12	rh^G, G	0.85		Rh29	"total Rh"	>0.99
Rh13	Rh^A	0.84		Rh30	Go^a	<0.01
Rh14	Rh^B	0.84		Rh31	hr^B	0.97
Rh15	Rh^C	0.84		Rh32	Troll	<0.01
Rh16	Rh^D	0.84		Rh33	Rh_o^{Har}	<0.01
Rh17	Hr_o	>0.99		Rh34	Bas.	>0.99

*Frequencies are for Caucasians.

Rh_{null} is a rare phenotype lacking all known Rh antigens, including Rh29. Rh29 is present in all other people and seems to be strongly immunogenic. Rh_{null} can be caused by a recessive homozygote at the Rh locus or a recessive homozygote at an independent locus. In either case, the red cell membrane is apparently defective, for humans with this phenotype have a shortened erythrocyte life span. The anatomic nature of the red cell defect is unknown. The specific molecular anatomy and molecular genetics of Rh likewise are unknown, though theories are abundant.

THE LEWIS SYSTEM

The Lewis blood groups result from gene interactions involving at least three independent loci—*Le* (Lewis), *H* (ABH), and *Se* (Secretor). The Lewis substances, Le^a and Le^b, are plasma antigens and are not on the erythrocytes of newborns. Their presence on red cells is dependent on their presence in plasma, and the Lewis type of erythrocytes can be changed by soaking them in the plasma of a person of different Lewis type. The presence of Lewis substances in saliva is inherited, but the three independent genes shown in Table 26–13 are involved. Le^a is found in the saliva if gene *Le* is present, but Le^b requires the additional presence of both *H* and *Se*. Saliva and erythrocyte types are the same except that the red cell type Le(a−b+) corresponds to the saliva type Le(a+b+). The gene *Le* adds L-fucose to the precursor substance that is common to both ABH and Lewis, but fucose, though a potent inhibitor of anti-H, has little or no effect on anti-Le^a or anti-Le^b.

TABLE 26–13. LEWIS AND SECRETOR GENES AND PHENOTYPES

GENES			PHENOTYPES				
			Erythrocytes			Saliva	
Le	*H*	*Se*	Le^a	Le^b	ABH	Le^a	Le^b
p	p	p	0	+	+	+	+
p	p	a					
p	a	p	+	0	0	+	0
p	a	a					
a	p	p	0	0	+	0	0
a	p	a					
a	a	p	0	0	0	0	0
a	a	a					

Abbreviations: p = gene present; a = gene absent; + = antigen(s) present; 0 = antigens(s) absent.

Lewis antibodies are mostly saline-active agglutinins, somewhat more reactive at cooler temperatures (±15° C). Complement-fixing hemolysin of anti-Le^a specificity has been described as a rare cause of transfusion reaction. No well-documented case of reaction caused by anti-Le^b is known. It has been demonstrated, however, that a unit of plasma from an Le(a−b+) donor neutralizes the circulating anti-Le^b, and that Le(a−b+) red cells (from the same donor) can then be given safely. Adequate in vivo survival studies have not been done in people who have Lewis antibodies.

The Lewis antigens can also be thought of as hybrid antigens. Children with Le(a+) red cells can be born to Le(a−) parents and Le(b+) children can be born to Le(b−) parents. The latter event is less common than expected, so there appears to be an unknown factor in Lewis blood group inheritance. In the plasma and saliva, however, Le^a is inherited as a dominant, and Le^b as a joint product of Le^a and H.

OTHER HYBRID ANTIGENS

Other antigens that can be present in a child while absent in both parents also depend on interactions between the products of genetically independent genes. IA, IB, IH, IP$_1$, Ip, ILe^{bH}, iH, "Luke" (ABO-P interaction), A$_1$Le^b, AD, and Fy5 (Duffy-Rhesus interaction) have been uncovered.

"PUBLICS" AND "PRIVATES"

Well over 100 high-frequency and low-frequency antigens have not been assigned to any of the named systems because enough informative families have not been found. Some of these probably do not belong to any of the named systems, and will eventually achieve system status on their own. The low-frequency ones are of little clinical importance, but the high-frequency ones can pose serious problems when compatible donors are needed for a person having one of the antibodies. Systematic search for these rare negatives has been fruitful, and frozen stocks of some of them are becoming available.

I AND "i"

Apparently all humans have both I (72) and i (73), but fetuses and rare adults have much i and very little I, while nearly all adults have a lot of I on their erythrocytes, and very little i. Anti-I is the common auto-immune cold-reactive agglutinin, which is sometimes seen in very high titer following mycoplasmal pneumonia and which is the most common cause of acquired hemolytic anemia. Anti-i is most commonly found in patients with infectious mononucleosis.

I and i appear to be on the same molecules as H, A, B, Le^a, and Le^b, though the genes are independent. One supposes that, after birth, a sugar molecule begins to be added to these molecules in increasing numbers, thus increasing the I-ness at the expense of the i.

The I-i antibodies, even when they are causing autoimmune hemolytic anemia, are of little significance in transfusion therapy if the patient can be kept warm and if the donor blood is warmed to about 25° C. Compatibility testing should be done at 37°C, with the help of a warm centrifuge.*

ACQUIRED AUTOIMMUNE HEMOLYTIC ANEMIA OF THE "WARM ANTIBODY" TYPE

Many of these patients have autoantibodies of Rh specificity, anti-e being the specificity most frequently identified. Anti-LW has been identified in a few cases, anti-D rarely. Compatibility of the patient's serum with Rh$_{null}$ red cells always suggests Rh specificity of some kind, possibly Rh29, but, in a few cases, the antibody proved instead to be anti-U. Rh$_{null}$, U-negative, and e-negative cells should be in the diagnostic panel when such cases are investigated. If e-negative cells are incompatible, titrations, absorptions, or both with e-negative cells are in order, because e-negatives are fairly common, and an e-negative may be "less incom-

---

*An effective and economic heating device can be obtained from Cote Scientific Products, 52 Clark Street, Medford, Massachusetts 02155.

patible" than an e-positive if the patient has a mixture of antibodies that includes anti-e. Unfortunately, the autoimmune antibody is usually directed against one or more high-frequency antigens. If the specificity of the autoantibody is to be determined, it is essential to make an eluate from washed red cells of the patient. This eluate is usually stronger than the free autoantibody in the plasma, and it is free of any isoantibodies that may be in the plasma. Of course, the identity of any isoantibodies should also be determined.

While this illness is usually cryptogenic, a number of cases have been reported in which the autoimmunity is caused by, or greatly exacerbated by, an incompatible blood transfusion. In such a case, one finds a mixture of isoantibodies and autoantibodies in the patient's serum. In one fulminating case, anti-k (titer 50,000), anti-c (titer 500,000), and anti-Fy^a (titer 5000) were isoantibodies that made finding a "least incompatible" donor very difficult.

DONOR BLOOD PROCESSING

The donor's red cells are typed with anti-A and anti-B. The serum is tested against known A cells and known B cells; if this "back-typing" does not confirm the cell typing, one usually finds a weak form of the antigen in the donor's red cells or an unexpected antibody in the donor serum. The cells are tested with anti-D (Rh$_o$, Rh1) by a technique expected to detect weak variants of D (D^u); therefore D-negatives are usually further tested with a strong anti-D by the Coombs' antiglobulin method. Some automated methods that combine the use of enzymes with a high-molecular-weight additive are sufficiently sensitive that the Coombs' test may be omitted. There is a good deal of evidence that the lowest grade D^u's are not immunogenic (76). Routine testing of donor bloods with anti-C, anti-E, anti-CD, anti-DE, or anti-CDE is useless, wasteful, and a source of confusion. D—C+ or D—E+ blood may be given to any D-negative recipient who has not already been sensitized to C or E. It is easy enough to find C— or E— bloods amongst the D-negatives if they are needed for a particular case.

SOME COMMENTS

The endless fascination of human blood groups stems principally from the intricacies of their inheritance. All the "laws of inheritance" that were considered inviolate as recently as 1950 have since been shown to have exceptions. Two apparently group O parents can have a group A child. A parent who seems to be homozygous for the common R^1 ("Rhesus") gene can have children who appear to be homozygous for R^2 (74). These exceptions have been shown to result from unexpected "null" alleles or from modifying genes that not only are independent of the "blood group" genes themselves but also may be either dominant or recessive in their action. Other unexpected exceptions to the laws result from gene interactions. One common (about 0.79) antigen, ILe^{bH}, for example (75), requires four independent genes to be simultaneously turned on (I, Lewis, secretor, and H). If one parent is a nonsecretor (over 20 per cent frequency) and the other is Lewis-negative (about 5 per cent), both will lack the ILe^{bH} receptor, but they may have a child who has ILe^{bH}, even though it is absent in both parents. The chance that this will happen in such a mating is almost 25 per cent. The medicolegal "value" of blood grouping tests for each of the "markers" is thus somewhat less than was believed before 1950. Since that time, however, the number of markers that can be utilized has increased so greatly that blood group tests can now establish, with reasonable assurance in most cases, that the ostensible parents are in fact the biological parents of a particular child, if, in fact, they are the parents.

"Blood groups" include the various allotypic serum proteins, such as haptoglobin, transferrin, Gm, and so forth; the intracellular proteins, such as hemoglobin, acid phosphatase, phosphoglucomutase, and so forth; and the HL-A antigens. The number of normal genetic markers that are represented by these categories is around 100, about 40 of which are useful (because of favorable frequencies) in a Caucasian population.

If we test different populations with all the available tests, an almost infinite combination of frequencies is observed. One could surely identify a population sample as

Caucasian, African, or Asian. Almost as surely could one distinguish between two unrelated people. Any two neighboring tribes or towns would differ also, though less strikingly. Differences among population groups are thus of great genetic and anthropologic interest. But the similarities of populations are even more striking than the differences. The type k+Kp(b+)Js(b+) in the Kell system, for example, is nearly universal in all human populations so far tested, and so also, with rare exceptions, are all the most common types that have been observed in any single population. The unity of the human species is thus very well illustrated by its blood groups. No population has yet been found to lack antigens of even one of the many known blood group systems, though some populations are quite monomorphic.

In this short presentation I have stressed the aspects of the blood groups that I find exciting. It would not have been possible to make a useful summary of immunohematology in so short a chapter anyway. The authoritative and eminently readable text in this subject is that of Race and Sanger (3), a sixth edition of which is currently being prepared.

References

1. Economidou, J., Hughes-Jones, N. C., et al.: Quantitative measurements concerning A and B antigen sites. Vox Sang. 12:321, 1967.
2. Hughes-Jones, N. C., Gardner, B., et al.: Observations of the number of available c, D, and E antigen sites on red cells. Vox Sang. 21:210, 1971.
3. Race, R. R., and Sanger, R.: Blood Groups in Man. 5th ed. Philadelphia, F. A. Davis, 1968.
4. Layrisse, M., Arends, T., et al.: Nuevo grupo sanguineo encontrado en descendientes de Indios. Acta Med. Venez. 3:132, 1955.
5. Thompson, P. R., Childers, D. M., et al.: Anti-Di^b- first and second examples. Vox Sang. 13:314, 1967.
6. Swanson, J., Polesky, H. F., et al.: A "new" blood group antigen, Do^a. Nature (Lond.) 206:313, 1965.
7. Molthan, L., Crawford, M. N., et al.: Enlargement of the Dombrock blood group system: The finding of anti-Do^b. Vox Sang. 24:382, 1973.
8. Eaton, B. R., Morton, J. A., et al.: A new antibody, anti-Yt^a, characterizing a blood group of high incidence. Br. J. Haematol. 2:333, 1956.
9. Giles, C. M., and Metaxas, M. N.: Identification of the predicted blood group antibody anti-Yt^b. Nature (Lond.) 202:1122, 1964.
10. Heistö, H., van der Hart, M., et al.: Three examples of a new red cell antibody, anti-Co^a. Vox Sang. 12:18, 1967.
11. Giles, C. M., Darnborough, J., et al.: Identification of the first example of anti-Co^b. Br. J. Haematol. 19:267, 1970.
12. Schmidt, R. P., Griffitts, J. J., et al.: A new antibody, anti-Sm, reacting with a high incidence antigen. Transfusion 2:338, 1962.
13. Anderson, C., Hunter J., et al.: An antibody defining a new blood group antigen, Bu^a. Transfusion 3:30, 1963.
14. Salmon, C., Salmon, D., et al.: Un nouvel antigène de groupe sanguin érythrocytaire présent chez 80% des sujets de race blanche. Nouv. Rev. Fr. Hématol. 1:649, 1961.
15. Bias, W. B., Light-Orr, J. K., et al.: The Stoltzfus blood group, a new polymorphism in man. Am. J. Hum. Genet. 21:552, 1969.
16. Rosenfield, R. E., Haber, V., et al.: Ge, a very common red-cell antigen. Br. J. Haematol. 6:344, 1960.
17. Giles, C. M., Huth, M. C., et al.: Three examples of a new antibody, anti-Cs^a, which reacts with 98% of red cell samples. Vox Sang. 10:405, 1965.
18. Sussman, L. N., and Miller, E. B.: Un nouveau facteur sanguin "Vel." Rev. Hématol. 7:368, 1952.
19. Allen, F. H., Diamond, L. K., et al.: A new blood-group antigen. Nature (Lond.) 167:482, 1951.
20. Plaut, G., Ikin, E. W., et al.: A new blood-group antibody, anti-Jk^b. Nature (Lond.) 171:431, 1953.
21. Marsh, W. L., Øyen, R., et al.: Kidd blood-group antigens of leukocytes and platelets. Transfusion (in press).
22. Seyfried, H., Walewska, I., et al.: Unusual inheritance of ABO group in a family with weak B antigens. Vox Sang. 9:268, 1964.
23. Rubinstein, P., Allen, F. H., Jr., et al.: A dominant suppressor of A and B. Vox Sang. 25:377, 1973.
24. Levine, P., Robinson, E., et al.: Gene interaction resulting in suppression of blood group substance B. Blood 10:1100, 1955.
25. Schiff, F., and Sasaki, H.: Der Ausscheidungstypus, ein auf serologischem Wege nachweisbares mendelndes Merkmal. Klin. Wochenschr. 11:1426, 1932. (Translated in Secretion of Blood Group Substances and Lewis System. Vol. II Fort Knox, U.S. Army Medical Research Lab, 1970, p. 336.)
26. Cutbush, M., Mollison, P. L., et al.: A new human blood group. Nature (Lond.) 165:188, 1950.
27. Ikin, E. W., Mourant, A. E., et al.: Discovery of the expected haemagglutinin, anti-Fy^b. Nature (Lond.) 168:1077, 1951.
28. Albrey, J. A., Vincent, E. E. R., et al.: A new antibody, anti-Fy3, in the Duffy blood-group system. Vox Sang. 20:29, 1971.
29. Behzad, O., Lee, C. L., et al.: A new anti-erythrocyte antibody in the Duffy system: anti-Fy4. Vox Sang. 24:337, 1973.
30. Colledge, K. I., Pezzulich, M., et al.: Anti-Fy5, an antibody disclosing a probable association between the Rhesus and Duffy blood group genes. Vox Sang. 24:193, 1973.
31. Landsteiner, K., and Levine, P.: Further observations on individual differences of human blood. Proc. Soc. Exp. Biol. Med. 24:941, 1927.
32. Prokop, O., and Uhlenbruck, G.: Lehrbuch der

menslichen Blud-und Serumgruppen. Leipzig, Thieme, 1963, p. 349.

33. Allen, F. H., Jr.: Some rare types in the MN system and their genetic significance. *Bibliotheca Haematologica,* No. 38, Part I. Basel, S. Karger, 1971, pp. 186–191.

34. Wiener, A. S., Unger, L. J., et al.: Fatal hemolytic transfusion reaction caused by sensitization to a new blood factor, U. J. Am. Med. A. *153*:1444, 1953.

35. Marsh, W. L., Øyen, R., et al.: U antigen in leukocytes. Transfusion (in press).

36. Callender, S. T., and Race, R. R.: A serological and genetical study of multiple antibodies formed in response to blood transfusion by a patient with lupus erythematosus diffusus. Ann. Eugen. (Lond.) *13*:102, 1946.

37. Cutbush, M., and Chanarin, I.: The expected blood-group antibody, anti-Lu^b. Nature (Lond.) *178*: 855, 1956.

38. Crawford, M. N., Greenwalt, T. J., et al.: The phenotype Lu(a−b−) together with unconventional Kidd groups in one family. Transfusion *1*:228, 1961.

39. Stanbury, A., and Francis, B.: The Lu(a−b−) phenotype: An addition example. Vox Sang. *13*:441, 1967.

40. Brown, E., Simpson, S., et al.: The recessive Lu(a−b−) phenotype: A family study. Vox Sang. (in press).

41. Bove, J. R., Allen, F. H., Jr., et al.: Anti-Lu4, a new antibody related to the Lutheran blood group system. Vox Sang. *21*:302, 1971.

42. Marsh, W. L.: Anti-Lu5, anti-Lu6, and anti-Lu7. Three antibodies defining high frequency antigens related to the Lutheran blood group system. Transfusion *12*:27, 1972.

43. MacIlroy, M., McCreary, J., et al.: Anti-Lu8, an antibody recognizing another Lutheran-related antigen. Vox Sang. *23*:455, 1972.

44. Molthan, L., Crawford, M. N., et al.: Lu9, another new antigen of the Lutheran blood-group system. Vox Sang. *24*:468, 1973.

45. Crawford, M. N.: In preparation.

46. Gralnick, M. A., Goldfinger, D., et al.: Anti-Lu11: Another antibody defining a high-frequency antigen related to the Lutheran blood group system. Vox Sang. (in press).

47. Sinclair, M., Buchanan, D. I., et al.: Another antibody related to the Lutheran blood group system (Much.). Vox Sang. *25*:156, 1973.

48. Cleghorn, T. E.: A "new" human blood group antigen, Sw^a. Nature (Lond.) *184*:1324, 1959.

49. Metaxas, M. N.: Personal communication.

50. Coombs, R. R. A., Mourant, A. E., et al.: In-vivo isosensitization of red cells in babies with hemolytic disease. Lancet *1*:264, 1946.

51. Levine, P., Backer, M., et al.: A new human hereditary blood property (Cellano) present in 99.8% of all bloods. Science *109*:464, 1949.

52. Chown, B., Lewis, M., et al.: A "new" Kell blood-group phenotype. Nature (Lond.) *180*:711, 1957.

53. Allen, F. H., and Lewis, S. J.: Kp^a(Penney) a new antigen in the Kell blood group system. Vox Sang. *2*:81, 1957.

54. Allen, F. H., Lewis, S. J., et al.: Studies of anti-Kp^b, a new antibody in the Kell blood group system. Vox Sang. *3*:1, 1958.

55. Dichupa, P. J., Anderson, C., et al.: A further search for hypothetic K^p of the Kell system. Vox Sang. *17*:1, 1969.

56. Giblett, E. R.: Js, a "new" blood group antigen found in Negroes. Nature (Lond.) *181*:1221, 1958.

57. Walker, R. H., Argall, C. I., et al.: Anti-Js^b, the expected antithetical antibody of the Sutter blood group system. Nature (Lond.) *197*:295, 1963.

58. Stroup, M., MacIlroy, M., et al.: Evidence that Sutter belongs to the Kell blood group system. Transfusion *5*:309, 1965.

59. Morton, N. E., Kreiger, H., et al.: Genetic evidence confirming the localization of Sutter in the Kell blood-group system. Vox Sang. *10*:608, 1965.

60. Heistø, H., Guévin, R. M., et al.: Three further antigen-antibody specificities associated with the Kell blood group system. Vox Sang. *24*:179, 1973.

61. Marsh, W. L., Jensen, L., et al.: Anti-K13 and the K:−13 phenotype. A blood-group variant related to the Kell system. Vox Sang. *26*:34, 1974.

62. Furuhjelm, U., Nevanlinna, H. R., et al.: The blood group antigen U1^a (Karhula). Vox Sang. *15*:118, 1968.

63. Corcoran, P., Allen, F. H., Jr., et al.: A new antibody, anti-Ku (anti-Peltz), in the Kell blood group system. Transfusion *1*:181, 1961.

64. Bove, J. R., Johnson, M., et al.: Anti-K^w defining a new antigenic determinant. Unpublished manuscript.

65. Allen, F. H., Krabbe, S. M. R., et al.: A new phenotype (McLeod) in the Kell blood-group system. Vox Sang. *6*:555, 1961.

66. Giblett, E. R., Klebanoff, S. J., et al.: Kell phenotypes in chronic granulomatous disease: A potential transfusion hazard. Lancet *1*:1235, 1971.

67. van der Hart, M., Szaloky, A., et al.: A "new" antibody associated with the Kell blood group system. Vox Sang. *15*:456, 1968.

68. Marsh, W. L.: In preparation.

69. Landsteiner, K., and Wiener, A. S.: An agglutinable factor in human blood recognized by immune sera for the rhesus blood. Proc. Soc. Exp. Biol. Med. *43*:223, 1940.

70. Levine, P., and Stetson, R. E.: An unusual case of intragroup agglutination. J.A.M.A. *113*:126, 1939.

71. Rosenfield, R. E., Allen, F. H., Jr., et al.: Genetic model for the Rh blood-group system. Proc. Natl. Acad. Sci. USA *70*:1303, 1973.

72. Wiener, A. S., Unger, L. J., et al.: Type-specific cold autoantibodies as a cause of acquired hemolytic anemia and hemolytic transfusion reactions: Biologic test with bovine red cells. Ann. Intern. Med. *44*:221, 1956.

73. Marsh, W. L., and Jenkins, W. J.: Anti-i: A new cold antibody. Nature (Lond.) *188*:753, 1960.

74. Ishimori, T., and Hasekura, H.: A Japanese with no detectable Rh blood group antigens due to silent Rh alleles or deleted chromosomes. Transfusion *7*:84, 1967.

75. Tegoli, J., Cortez, M., et al.: A new antibody, anti-ILe^bH, specific for a determinant formed by the combined action of the I, Le, Se and H gene products. Vox Sang. *21*:397, 1971.

76. Schmidt, P. J., Morrison, E. G., et al.: The antigenicity of the D^u blood factor. Blood *20*:196–202, 1962.

Chapter 27

Serum Proteins and Other Genetic Markers of the Blood

by Chester A. Alper and Robertson Parkman

Chapter 26 presents a review of the useful genetic markers on human red cell membranes. This chapter offers a summary of other important genetic markers in human blood, including serum proteins, leukocyte and erythrocyte enzymes, and leukocyte membrane markers (the HL-A system). For all but the HL-A system, the most recent authoritative compilation is that developed by Eloise Giblett.[*]

Study of human allotypes is critically important both clinically and for the purpose of extending our knowledge of the human chromosome. The immediate clinical applications include blood cell transfusion, paternity exclusion, establishment of marrow and organ transplantation, and antenatal diagnosis. The ultimate clinical goal is effective treatment of severe inherited disease by gene replacement or modification either in utero or in early childhood. While the latter goal is certainly distant, immensely valuable biological data are being collected en route as assignment of particular genes to particular chromosomes is in progress.

This chapter is organized into three sections. The first deals with the major serum proteins in some detail. Briefer reviews of blood cell enzymes and the HL-A system then follow.

---

[*]Giblett, E. R.: *Genetic Markers in Human Blood.* Philadelphia, F. A. Davis Co., 1969.

PLASMA PROTEINS

Genetically controlled structural variation among human plasma proteins is the rule and not the exception. For the most part, this variation consists of single amino acid substitutions and is not usually attended by detectable alterations in function. The mutations that gave rise to the variant genes appear to have persisted, in the main, because their bearers have thrived and multiplied, but probably not because of positive evolutionary selective pressure. It is clear that the extent of this genetic heterogeneity of all our proteins is far greater than the meager catalogue we have at present.

Electrophoresis is the most common technique by far for the detection of genetic structural variation in plasma proteins; serologic methods are used in a few instances. Rarely, structurally variant proteins can be detected but not identified by abnormalities in their function or serum concentration. Since electrophoresis is the most widely employed technique for the identification of genetic variants of plasma proteins, it is well to keep in mind that mutations involving a single amino acid substitution produce a change in charge in only a minority of instances.

The extent of variation of individual plasma proteins varies enormously from population to population and from protein to protein. For some proteins and populations, there is remarkable homogeneity and a very low incidence of variants, whereas for others there are two or more "common" types. Variation can be so extensive that no single variant is found in more than half the population. Arbitrary definitions requiring that, in order to qualify as genetic polymorphism, variants of a given protein must be found in more than some arbitrary percentage of some population somewhere have been proposed, but are clearly not useful.

Albumin

Albumin is by far the most plentiful of the plasma proteins. Its concentration is approximately equal to that of the combined concentrations of all the other proteins in plasma (3.5 to 4.5 g. per 100 ml.). It serves to maintain the blood's colloid osmotic pressure, and a great variety of positively and negatively charged and hydrophobic substances bind to it (1). In certain instances, for example for pharmacologic agents, this affords a transport function for albumin. Albumin concentration falls in the presence of acute or chronic inflammatory processes.

Genetic variants of albumin are detected as single electrophoretic bands of a mobility either slower or faster than the usual protein, as is true of the usual variants of hemoglobin A. (Fig. 27–1). All are relatively rare in most populations and occur with a frequency of less than 1 per cent. Rare exceptions have been found in certain American Indian populations in which rather high gene frequencies (up to 0.13) occur. This has been true in the Naskapi and Montagnais tribes of Quebec. There appear to be at least nine electrophoretically detectable albumin variants described in addition to common albumin (2–4). In all instances, the variants are found in concentrations equal to those of common albumin in heterozygotes, except in the case of an unusual albumin variant found in Sweden (5). In the latter instance, the albumin zone was broadened in agarose gel electrophoresis and could be resolved into common albumin and a slower-moving variant of lower concentration. The latter tended to dimerize more readily than common albumin. This variant is of particular clinical interest because of its high incidence in orthopedic patients (5/1550), and the possibility that this variant might be associated with a defect in connective tissue leading to back pain, other bone and joint complaints, and impaired hearing.

Analbuminemia is a rare inherited disorder with virtually complete absence of albumin in serum (6). This characteristic is inherited as an autosomal recessive trait, and the parents of such individuals have normal albumin concentrations. Albumin concentrations in affected persons are not zero, but range from 10 to 40 mg. per 100 ml. Results of studies with isotopically labeled albumin conclusively demonstrate that the defect in this disorder is defective synthesis and not increased catabolism of albumin.

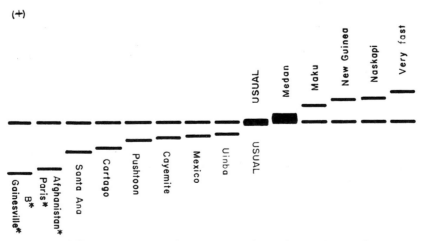

(+)

USUAL Medan Maku New Guinea Naskapi Very fast

Gainesville* B* Paris* Afghanistan* Santa Ana Cartago Pushtoon Cayemite Mexico Uinba USUAL

Figure 27–1. Diagram of albumin variants as they appear in electrophoresis (in starch or agarose gel) at pH 8.6. Variants marked with an asterisk have different mobilities from common albumin at other pH's. [Adapted from (3) and (4).]

Nevertheless, most individuals, particularly males, with hereditary analbuminemia have only mild edema. Thus, hypoproteinemic edema, for example, the anasarca of severely nephrotic patients, is not merely a reflection of the low albumin concentration in their serum. Other processes must be operative as well. In addition, analbuminemic subjects may have developed compensatory mechanisms that minimize edema.

α_1-Antitrypsin

The major inhibitor of trypsin in serum is a protein designated α_1-antitrypsin (7). It also inhibits chymotrypsin, collagenase, elastase, and leukocyte proteases. The mean concentration in the serum of normal individuals is about 250 mg. per 100 ml. Inherited deficiency of α_1-antitrypsin is associated with markedly increased susceptibility to lung and liver disease (8–10).

Although the great majority of individuals in most populations studied have a single major α_1-antitrypsin band on agarose gel electrophoresis at pH 8.6, some serums show variant bands (Fig. 27–2) (11). On crossed immunoelectrophoresis (11) or immunofixation electrophoresis at this pH (12), sera with the common single band also show a minor cathodal component antigenically identical to the major α_1-antitrypsin band. Variant bands also have minor components in positions comparable to that of the minor component of the common protein. Using starch gel or acrylamide gel electrophoresis at an acidic pH, usually around 4.95, the common form and the variants are seen as a series of eight bands migrating ahead of the bulk of the serum proteins (13), as shown in Figure 27–2. The minor components observed at pH 8.6 correspond to the electrophoretically slowest two of these bands. To facilitate specific identification of variants, crossed immunoelectrophoresis into agarose gel containing specific antibody to α_1-antitrypsin is useful (14). The reason for the multiple banding at acid pH of α_1-antitrypsin is unknown, as is the reason for unequal protein distribution among these bands.

The variants are inherited in autosomal codominant fashion. At present, there are at least 19 recognized alleles at the locus for α_1-antitrypsin, a locus called Pi (protease inhibitor) (15). The common form of α_1-antitrypsin is called PiM. The rare variants have been given letter designations that run alphabetically from anode to cathode. Some of the variant gene products are shown in Figures 27–2 and 27–3.

Of particular importance because of the diseases with which they are associated are Pi^Z and $Pi.^S$ The products of these genes are found in lower concentrations than those of the other alleles. The mean concentrations of α_1-antitrypsin of types Pi ZZ, SZ, MZ, and MS are approximately 10 per cent, 30 per cent, 60 per cent, and 70 per cent of Pi MM (8, 15). Other "hypomorphic" alleles exist, such as Pi^P, Pi^{W_1}, and a variant with the electrophoretic mobility of Pi^M at pH 8.6. An allele with no detectable product (Pi^-) has also been identified (16). Individuals homozygous for Pi^Z or Pi^- or heterozygous for Pi^- and Pi^Z, Pi^- and Pi^S, for Pi^Z and Pi^S are prone to develop neonatal hepatitis as infants, cirrhosis as children, and chronic obstructive pulmonary disease as adults. There is some evidence suggesting that heterozygotes for Pi^Z and Pi^S with Pi^M and other non-deficient alleles may be more prone than the general population to de-

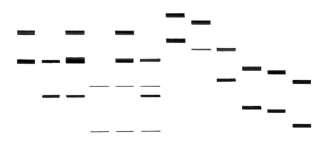

Figure 27–2. Alpha$_1$-antitrypsin (Pi) variants as they appear in starch gel electrophoresis at pH 4.95. Each variant gives rise to a pattern of eight bands, of which only the two major bands are shown in this diagram. Only some of the known variants are shown. [Adapted from (15).]

M   S   MS   Z   MZ   SZ   F   I   P   V   W   X

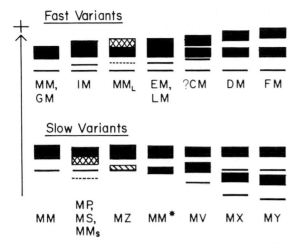

Fast Variants

MM, GM   IM   MM$_L$ EM, LM   ?CM   DM   FM

Slow Variants

MM   MP, MS, MM$_S$ MZ   MM*   MV   MX   MY

Figure 27-3. Diagram of some α_1-antitrypsin (Pi) phenotypes observed in prolonged agarose gel electrophoresis at pH 8.6 and developed by immunofixation with specific antiserum. (Courtesy of Dr. A. Myron Johnson.)

velop chronic obstructive pulmonary disease (17). As can be seen from the Pi gene frequencies given in Table 27-1, such heterozygotes constitute 3 to 5 per cent of many populations, so that if this tendency toward the development of chronic lung disease is true, a very large number of people are at risk.

Although the reason for the low serum concentration of Pi Z and other "deficient" gene products is not fully understood, some clues are available. Alpha$_1$-antitrypsin can be detected in normal or supernormal amounts in hepatocytes in the livers of patients with severe α_1-antitrypsin deficiency. Electron microscopic studies have revealed inclusions in liver cells in such subjects which may represent α_1-antitrypsin. It thus may be that there is defective release of Pi Z (and perhaps other deficient forms of α_1-antitrypsin) from hepatocyte ribosomes. In-

stability of deficient Pi variants in vivo may also occur, but there is little evidence at present for or against this possibility.

The concentration of α_1-antitrypsin may be altered under various physiologic and pathophysiologic circumstances. Alpha$_1$-antitrypsin rises in concentration as part of the acute phase plasma protein response, during estrogen administration, and in pregnancy. There is a selective although variable fall in α_1-antitrypsin (and α_2-macroglobulin) during severe neonatal respiratory distress syndrome (18). In experimental animals it has been shown that α_1-antitrypsin forms an important defense against the administration of proteolytic enzymes, such as trypsin and chymotrypsin. When the capacity of this protein (and that of other protease inhibitors) to complex with and inactivate these enzymes is exceeded, shock and death rapidly ensue (19).

Despite our ignorance of precise mechanisms leading to disease in α_1-antitrypsin deficiency, it seems possible that incompletely inhibited leukocyte proteases and gut proteases may digest lung parenchymal elastin and damage liver. There is no effective therapy for these complications of α_1-antitrypsin deficiency.

α_1-Acid Glycoprotein (Orosomucoid)

This protein binds and appears to inactivate progesterone. Its serum concentration is hormone-sensitive; it rises during pregnancy and in women on oral contraceptive medication and falls if androgens are administered. Alpha$_1$-acid glycoprotein is a marked acute phase reactant, and its level can increase up to five- or six-fold in the presence of acute inflammation.

Alpha$_1$-acid glycoprotein exhibits genetic

TABLE 27-1. SOME *Pi* GENE FREQUENCIES IN VARIOUS POPULATIONS*

POPULATION	Pi^M	Pi^S	Pi^Z	Pi^F	Pi^I	Pi^V	Pi^W
Norwegians	0.946	0.023	0.016	0.013	0.001	0.0004	
Swedes	0.973		0.024	0.003			
Spaniards	0.866	0.112	0.012	0.003	0.001	0.0026	0.0026
Norwegian Lapps	0.992		0.008				
Finnish Lapps	0.9996	0.0003	0.0001				
Finns	0.9955		0.0045				

*Abridged from Fagerhol, M. K., and Laurell, C.-B.: The Pi system—Inherited variants of serum α_1-antitrypsin. Progr. Med. Genet. 7:96–111, 1970, by permission of Grune & Stratton.

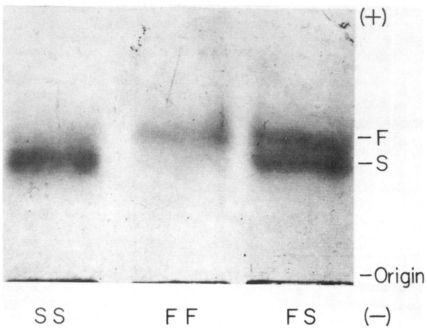

Figure 27–4.   Orosomucoid (Or) patterns obtained with desialidated whole sera after electrophoresis at pH 8.6 and immunofixation with specific antiserum. (From Johnson, A. M., Schmid, K., et al.: J. Clin. Invest. 48:2293, 1969.)

polymorphism of an unusual kind. Alpha$_1$-acid glycoprotein in native serum migrates as multiple bands on electrophoresis (20). If whole serum or purified protein is treated with neuraminidase to remove sialic acid, the electrophoretic behavior of the molecule is greatly simplified. Material from different individuals forms one of three patterns (Fig. 27–4): a major fast band and a minor slow band, a major slow band and a minor fast band, or two bands of approximately equal concentrations (21). The corresponding genotypes are Or^{FF}, Or^{SS}, and Or^{FS}, in which F and S refer to fast and slow. Inheritance is autosomal codominant, but the genes appear to control the relative amounts of Or F and Or S in individuals, all of whom have the same structural genes. Or gene frequencies are given in Table 27–2.

TABLE 27–2.   SOME Or GENE FREQUENCIES IN VARIOUS POPULATIONS*

Ethnic Group	Or^S	Or^F
Bechuana	0.62	0.38
Caucasian American	0.36	0.64
Chinese	0.47	0.53
Congolese	0.47	0.53
Finnish	0.50	0.50
French	0.49	0.51
Indian	0.44	0.56
Amerindian	0.54	0.46
Japanese	0.27	0.73
Nigerian	0.41	0.59
Nyambian˙	0.44	0.56
Swedish	0.67	0.33
Zulu	0.37	0.63

*Abridged from Johnson, A. M., Schmid, K., et al.: J. Clin. Invest. 48:2293, 1969.

Haptoglobin

Haptoglobin is an α_2-glycoprotein occurring in normal serum at a concentration of 30 to 160 mg. per 100 ml. (expressed as hemoglobin-binding capacity) (22, 23). Its concentration rises within one to two days of the onset of acute inflammation or tissue necrosis as part of the acute phase response. Elevated levels are also found in individuals treated with androgens. Only 10 per cent of newborns have detectable serum haptoglobin measured as hemoglobin-binding capacity. However, the haptoglobin rises rapidly after birth and is in the normal adult range by the first month of life.

The most striking property of haptoglobin is its ability to bind with hemoglobin to form a stable complex. Present evidence suggests that the binding site on hemoglobin is on the beta-chain, but that alpha chains are also required for the complex to form. Haptoglobin consists of two kinds of subunits (also designated alpha and beta) (24), and it is the haptoglobin beta chain which bears the globin binding site. Formation of haptoglobin-hemoglobin (Hp-Hb) complexes occurs with half-molecules of hemoglobin ($\alpha\beta$), and saturated complexes consist of one molecule of haptoglobin and two hemoglobin half-molecules.

When the Hp-Hb complex forms in vivo as the result of hemolysis, it is rapidly cleared by the reticuloendothelial system (25, 26). No stimulus to haptoglobin synthesis occurs in response to this removal, and therefore the concentration of serum haptoglobin falls to subnormal levels and may approach zero. In the presence of acute inflammation, because of increased haptoglobin synthesis, the serum level of haptoglobin may be normal or even elevated despite hemolysis in vivo (27). Its concentration will nevertheless be relatively lowered in comparison to those of other positive acute phase reactants such as α_1-antitrypsin, orosomucoid, or α_1-antichymotrypsin. Therefore, in using the measurement of serum haptoglobin as a guide to hemolysis, it is important also to measure one or two other positive acute phase reactants.

Inherited molecular variation in human haptoglobin is one of the best understood of the genetic polymorphisms among the serum proteins, owing largely to the work of Smithies and his colleagues. Initially it was noted that, when hemoglobin was added to sera from various individuals, the mixtures subjected to starch gel electrophoresis, and the resulting gels stained for peroxidase with a benzidine-hydrogen peroxide reagent, three strikingly different common patterns were seen (Fig. 27–5) (28). It soon became evident that the patterns reflected polymorphism in haptoglobin, and that the benzidine reagent detected the known peroxidase activity of the hemoglobin-haptoglobin complex. The patterns were named as in Figure 27–5, and the postulated codominant alleles for haptoglobin were designated Hp^1 and Hp^2. Haptoglobin 1–1 occurs as a single molecular species with a molecular weight of about 85,000; haptoglobin 2–1 consists of some material identi-

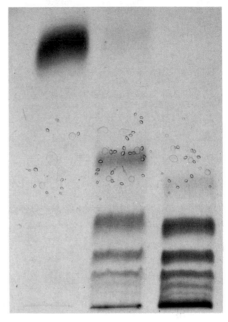

(+)

1-1   2-1   2-2

Figure 27–5. Common haptoglobin types in polyacrylamide gel electrophoresis at pH 8.0. Individual serum samples were saturated with hemoglobin, and patterns were developed by a benzidine–hydrogen peroxide reagent.

cal to Hp 1–1 in electrophoretic mobility and molecular size and heavier protein species, indicating the presence of polymers of the basic 85,000 molecular weight unit. Haptoglobin 2–2 consists only of polymers. Because of the sieving action of starch gel during electrophoresis, the polymers are retarded in proportion to their size, so that dimer, trimer, and so on are seen.

Subsequently, it was shown that all types of haptoglobin are comprised of two types of polypeptide chains designated alpha and beta; each molecule has a pair of each type. When haptoglobin was purified from individual sera, resolved into its constituent polypeptide chains, and examined in starch gel electrophoresis (29), the original polymorphism was found in the alpha-chains, and, furthermore, the 1α chains showed polymorphism (Fig. 27–6). The two kinds of 1α chains were called $1\alpha F$ (fast electrophoretic mobility) and $1\alpha S$ (slow electrophoretic mobility), and the genes were designated $Hp^{1\alpha F}$ and $Hp^{1\alpha S}$. Thus three com-

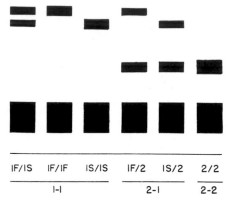

Figure 27–6. A diagram of the electrophoretic patterns of purified haptoglobin of various types in acid urea starch gels in the presence of reducing agent. Subunits are visualized, and the alpha chain is seen to be highly polymorphic.

TABLE 27–3. *Hp* GENE FREQUENCIES IN VARIOUS POPULATIONS*

POPULATION	Hp^{1S}	Hp^{1F}	Hp^2
Nigerian	0.258	0.473	0.27
Caucasian (Italy)	0.252	0.118	0.63
Caucasian (India)	0.104	0.046	0.85
Korean	0.321	0	0.68
Japanese	0.227	0.003	0.77
Chinese	0.341	0	0.66
Thai	0.236	0	0.76
Eskimo (Baffin Island)	0.239	0	0.76
Amerindian (U.S.)	0.374	0	0.63
Amerindian (Chile)†	0.774	0	0.23

*Abridged from Shim, B. S., and Bearn, A. G.: The distribution of haptoglobin subtypes in various populations, including subtype patterns in some non-human primates. Am. J. Hum. Genet. 16:477–480, 1964, by permission of Grune & Stratton.

†Hp^2 frequency includes one Hp^{2FF} individual.

mon alleles at the haptoglobin locus were defined that produced six common phenotypes. Gene frequencies in several populations are given in Table 27–3.

The structural and genetic bases for the haptoglobin polymorphism were further elucidated when the amino acid composition of Hp 1αF was shown to differ from that of Hp 1αS by a single amino acid, lysine, in place of asparagine or glutamine (30) (Fig. 27–7). This accounts for the charge difference between the two gene products. The differences between Hp 1α and Hp 2α proved to be more complex. First of all, molecular weight determinations of these isolated polypeptide chains indicate that Hp 2α is about twice the size of Hp 1αF or Hp 1αS. Analysis of peptides produced by partial digestion of the three types of chains reveals many similarities but sufficient differences between the 2α and 1α chains to exclude simple amino acid substitution as an explanation for the overall differences.

The amino and carboxyl terminal peptides found in both Hp 1αF and Hp 1αS are also found in Hp 2α, while Hp 2α contains both peptides which distinguish Hp 1αF from Hp 1αS. In addition, Hp 2α contains a peptide not found in either Hp 1αF or Hp 1αS. The ingenious and most reasonable explanation of these observations is shown in the postulated structure of the various kinds of Hp α chains shown in Figure 27–7. It thus appears that Hp 2α is composed essentially of the Hp 1αF chain joined via a junctional peptide to the Hp 1αS chain. The most likely genetic mechanism to explain the formation of such a polypeptide chain from two different allelic genes is nonhomologous crossing-over of two chromosomes in a heterozygote (Hp^{1F}/Hp^{1S}), with a resultant almost complete gene duplication and an almost complete gene deletion. The postulated genetic mechanism is illustrated in Figure 27–8.

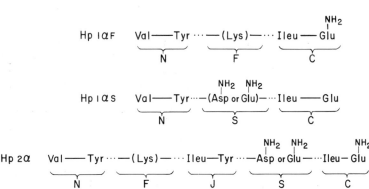

Figure 27–7. Outlines of structures of three common haptoglobin α-polypeptide chains based on studies of chymotryptic peptides. [Adapted from (30).]

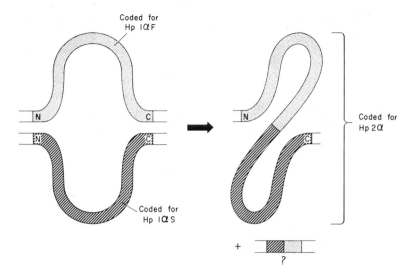

Figure 27–8. Possible mechanism by which $Hp^{2\alpha}$ gene arose by nonhomologous crossing-over in a heterozygote from $Hp^{1\alpha F}$ and $Hp^{1\alpha S}$. [Adapted from (30).]

The genetic event postulated in the origin of the Hp 2 gene must be a rare occurrence. Nevertheless, it was predicted that the same sort of genetic mechanism could, if it occurred in a homozygote (Hp^{1F}/Hp^{1F} or Hp^{1S}/Hp^{1S}), lead to the establishment of two additional types of Hp 2α polypeptide chains. This prediction was confirmed (31) by finding individuals in isolated populations with Hp^{2FF} and Hp^{2SS} instead of the usual Hp^{2FS} (or Hp^{2SF}, since the order of F and S has not yet been established).

In addition to the genetic variants of haptoglobin already described, rare types occur which reflect polymorphism at the beta chain locus, unequal production of 1α and 2α chains in an individual of Type Hp 2–1, and further polymorphism at the alpha chain locus. Since available evidence suggests that the binding of hemoglobin by haptoglobin is via a site on the beta chain of haptoglobin, it is not too surprising that some beta chain variants should be detected by abnormalities in hemoglobin binding. An interesting case is Hp Marburg. This variant was first recognized because of its atypical reactivity with antiserum to haptoglobin. Antiserums to haptoglobin may distinguish the following kinds of antigenic determinants: (1) If the antiserum is made to Hp 2–2 or Hp 2–1, it may contain antibodies specific for the 2α chains, as well as antibodies reacting with all the usual haptoglobin types (32). (2) Most antiserums against haptoglobin of any type react with an antigenic determinant present only on free hapto-

globin, not on haptoglobin bound to hemoglobin (33). The latter site is presumably on the beta chain and appears to be rendered inaccessible when the complex with hemoglobin is formed. Hp Marburg is immunologically similar to free haptoglobin, despite the addition of hemoglobin sufficient to saturate the haptoglobin in the serum in question (34). The most likely interpretation of this phenomenon is that Hp Marburg is a beta chain variant with diminished hemoglobin-binding ability. Such beta chain variants occur independent of the usual (or α) Hp types, and family studies reveal independent segregation, as one would expect from distinct and nonlinked loci.

Relative underproduction of Hp 2α chains in an individual who is Hp 2–1 results in a starch gel or acrylamide electrophoretic pattern termed "Hp 2–1M." In this pattern, there is relatively more material with the mobility of Hp 1–1 and a paucity of slower migrating polymer bands than occur in the usual Hp 2–1. Such patterns are inheritable and occur in highest frequency among Blacks. Genetically determined anhaptoglobinemia appears to be found in such families as a variant of Hp 2–1M. There is a spectrum of patterns between Hp 2–1 and Hp 2–1M which presumably reflects variable degrees of disproportion between 1α chain and 2α chain production.

More rarely, variant haptoglobin patterns are encountered which show duplication of bands and resemble an artificial mixture of

Hp 2–1 and Hp 2–2. These variants may represent a relative underproduction of 1α-chains or, very rarely, true genetic mosaicism in which some liver cells in a single individual presumably produce Hp 2–1, and others produce Hp 2–2.

There is some evidence that one gene for the enzyme catalase may be linked to the Hp α locus, and both appear to be situated on the long arm of chromosome 16 (35).

Ceruloplasmin (Cp)

It is the remarkably rich, deep, and heavenly blue color of this protein that prompted Holmberg and Laurell, who were the first to purify and characterize it, to name it ceruloplasmin (36). Ceruloplasmin is a 7S α$_2$-glycoprotein, with 7 per cent carbohydrate and approximately 160,000 daltons molecular weight. Each molecule of ceruloplasmin contains 8 atoms of copper. It is the presence of the copper which determines the blue color of the protein, since, if one removes the copper to produce apoceruloplasmin, all color disappears. About 90 per cent of the total serum copper is to be found in ceruloplasmin, and the remainder is largely bound to albumin. The copper in ceruloplasmin is not exchangeable in vivo, so that ceruloplasmin does not function as a transport protein for copper (37) (but albumin probably does). Ceruloplasmin is able to catalyze the oxidation of some amines and p-phenylenediamine has been used as a convenient substrate for this enzymatic action (38). The concentration of ceruloplasmin in serum can thus be, and has been, measured by three different methods: as serum copper, as amine oxidase activity, and as the protein part of the molecule by means of specific antibodies.

The concentration of ceruloplasmin in newborn serum is about one third that of normal adult serum and rises to that level within the first year of life. Its concentration is hormone-sensitive, and high serum levels are found in pregnant women and women on oral contraceptives. Elevation of serum ceruloplasmin occurs as part of the acute phase plasma protein response, and if the ceruloplasmin content is sufficiently high, such serum may have a greenish tinge. After the first year of life, low ceruloplasmin concentration is almost always pathognomonic for Wilson's disease (39), providing protein-losing states have been ruled out. Affected persons almost always, and carriers sometimes, have low serum ceruloplasmin concentrations. Although Wilson's disease clearly has a genetic basis, the depression of ceruloplasmin appears to be a secondary phenomenon. A rare primary genetic deficiency of ceruloplasmin without Wilson's disease has been reported (40).

Electrophoretic variants in ceruloplasmin were first detected in starch gel electrophoresis followed by staining for amine oxi-

(+)

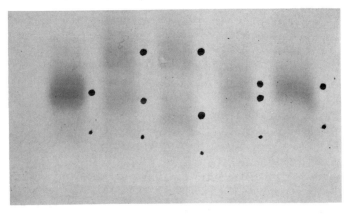

B   AB$_{NH}$ AC   BB$_{NH}$ B

Figure 27–9.   Patterns of ceruloplasmin variants obtained by prolonged agarose gel electrophoresis of serum at pH 8.6 and by immunofixation with specific antiserum. The ink marks indicate the bands.

TABLE 27–4. *Cp* GENE FREQUENCIES
IN A FEW POPULATIONS*

POPULATION	Cp^A	Cp^B	Cp^C	$Cp^{B_{NH}}$
Caucasian (Boston)	0.010	0.983	0.003	0.003
Caucasian (Ann Arbor)	0.006	0.988	–	–
Negro (Boston)	0.052	0.914	0.017	0.017
Negro (Ann Arbor)	0.053	0.943	0.003	–
Oriental (Boston)	–	1.000	–	–

*From (41) and (42).

dase activity (41). Alternatively, they can be tested for by prolonged agarose gel electrophoresis and immunofixation with specific anticeruloplasmin (42). Four known variants, A, B, B_{NH}, and C have been identified, as shown in Figure 27–9. The lettering is from anode to cathode at alkaline pH, and B_{NH} refers to a variant from New Haven. From the gene frequencies of Table 27–4, it is evident that Cp^B is the most common gene in all populations studied, and that it is only Blacks who have high frequencies of other alleles. All of the known variants have amine oxidase activity, by virtue of the original method of detection and the failure to find additional variants by immunochemical means.

Gc-Globulin

The "group-specific component" or Gc-globulin is an α_2-mobility protein in zone electrophoresis occurring in a concentration of about 75 mg. per 100 ml. of normal serum. Its level falls in advanced liver disease (43), and is elevated in pregnancy and during oral contraceptive therapy.

Gc-globulin has a molecular weight of about 51,000 daltons, 4.1S (44). Although the molecule contains 3.3 per cent carbohydrate, there is remarkably no detectable sialic (neuraminic) acid, unlike other serum glycoproteins. At present there is no known function for Gc-globulin.

Extensive genetic polymorphism in Gc-globulin was discovered in 1959 by Hirschfeld (45), who used immunoelectrophoresis for the detection of variants. It was later realized (46) that postalbumin bands which showed considerable variation from serum to serum in starch gel electrophoresis (47)

were, in fact, Gc-globulin. These bands are also seen in polyacrylamide gel electrophoresis. Considerable confusion about the exact number and position of bands in various Gc patterns, both common and rare, has arisen because of the deficiencies of all these techniques. In immunoelectrophoresis, the time needed for diffusion of antigen against antibody militated against sharp delineations of patterns and mobilities. This difficulty was only partially overcome by prolonging the electrophoresis time. The use of polyacrylamide or starch gel electrophoresis, while providing the capability for excellent resolution and fine comparisons of mobility, failed to allow the distinction between Gc-globulin and other proteins of similar electrophoretic mobility. The study of Gc polymorphism has been greatly aided by the application of crossed immunoelectrophoresis (48) and immunofixation electrophoresis (49) to the problem. Figures 27–10 and 27–11 show the common patterns of Gc 1–1, 2–1, and 2–2 in the two latter techniques. It is evident that Gc 1 has two major bands (1A and 1C for anodal and cathodal) and at least one minor band

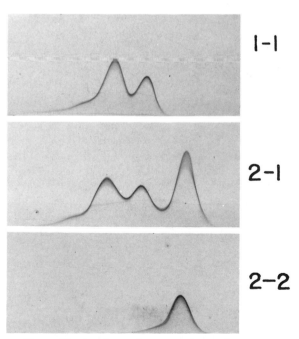

Figure 27–10. Crossed immunoelectrophoresis patterns of the three common Gc phenotypes. The anode for the first separation was at the left, and for the second at the top. Both electrophoreses were carried out at pH 8.6.

(+)

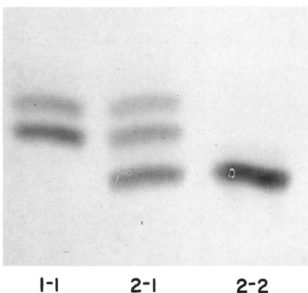

I-I   2-I   2-2

Figure 27–11. The common Gc phenotypes, as developed by prolonged agarose gel electrophoresis at pH 8.6 and immunofixation. Minor components are evident (as they are also in Fig. 27–10) anodal to the major bands.

anodal to 1A. Gc 2, on the other hand, consists of a single major band and a corresponding minor band under a wide variety of electrophoresis conditions. In addition to these major common bands, there appear to be five inherited structurally aberrant bands or sets of bands (Fig. 27–12). In the case of double-banded variants, including Gc 1, there appears to be a spectrum of inherited variation reflected in differences in relative concentration of the two bands (50). The failure to recognize these relationships has led to multiple descriptions (and designations) of some of the variants and to the general impression that there are more structural variants than, in fact, there are. Thus, through the use of immunofixation electrophoresis and crossed immunoelectrophoresis, it is seen that the variants Chip (Chippewa) and N (Norway)

represent extreme concentration variants of Gc 1. Gc Y, Ab (Aborigine), and Eskimo appear to be identical. Gc D (Darmstadt) and J differ only in that both J bands appear to be hypomorphic compared with the common allele product in the same serum.

Some structural work has been done on Gc-globulin. The evidence (51) suggests that the molecule consists of two polypeptide chains of similar size. Gc 1A and 1C appear to differ by at least one amino acid, and one tryptic peptide, at least, is different when Gc 1 and Gc 2 are compared.

Gene frequencies for the common *Gc* alleles are given in Table 27–5. It is apparent that there are fairly marked differences in allele frequencies from ethnic group to ethnic group. Fairly close genetic linkage between the Gc locus and the locus for albumin has been established (52).

(+)

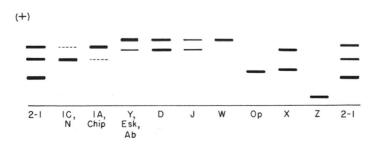

2-I   IC,   IA,   Y,   D   J   W   Op   X   Z   2-I
      N   Chip Esk,
                  Ab

Figure 27–12. Diagrammatic representation of the rare Gc variants as they appear in alkaline gel electrophoresis, with an attempt to relate their electrophoretic positions to the common forms.

TABLE 27–5. *Gc* GENE FREQUENCIES
IN SEVERAL POPULATIONS*

POPULATION	Gc^1	Gc^2
Negro	0.918	0.082
Mongoloid	0.774	0.226
Aborigine	0.879	0.121
Indian	0.700	0.300
Polynesian	0.412	0.588
Lapp	0.802	0.198
Eskimo	0.631	0.369
Caucasian	0.723	0.277

*Adapted from Walter, H., and Steegmüller, H.: Studies on the geographic and racial distribution of the Hp and Gc polymorphisms. Hum. Hered. *19*:209–221 (S. Karger AG, Basel 1969).

Pseudocholinesterase

Plasma contains a 348,000-molecular weight, α_2-mobility, glycoprotein enzyme capable of hydrolyzing acetylcholine (53, 54), among other substrates. This enzyme, acylcholine acylhydrolase, EC 3.1.1.8, or pseudocholinesterase, is of clinical importance because persons deficient in it are subject to apnea if they are given the muscle relaxant, succinylcholine, as an adjunct to anesthesia (55–57). Pseudocholinesterase normally rapidly hydrolyzes this drug, which is essentially a dimer of acetycholine. The small amount of intact drug reaching and depolarizing the motor endplate is responsible for its pharmacologic effect. In the deficient person, much larger concentrations reach the motor endplate, and the resulting paralysis is severe and prolonged.

The physiologic function of pseudocholinesterase is unknown. The serum level is somewhat lower at birth than in later life, but adult levels are attained by 2 months of age (58, 59). The concentration is higher in childhood than in middle and old age (60). Serum levels may be depressed in severe hepatocellular disease, uremia, organic phosphate poisoning (the enzyme is irreversibly inhibited by organic phosphates), carcinoma of the large bowel, and malnutrition (61, 62). Increased serum levels are found in nephrosis (63). The rare individuals with inherited deficiency of pseudocholinesterase activity are healthy and have been recognized for some time (64). Extensive studies of serum from such persons, from their relatives, and from random populations have revealed that several mutant genes may be responsible for deficient enzymic activity (65–68). These studies have involved kinetics of inhibition using various substrates and inhibitors. By this means, usual (U) and atypical (A) pseudocholinesterases could be defined (Table 27–6). The atypical enzyme revealed by these studies is presumably a dysfunctional genetic variant.

A rapid and relatively simple test for the atypical pseudocholinesterase was devised (69) based on its relative resistance to dibucaine. The "dibucaine number" is the ratio of activity in the hydrolysis by serum or plasma of 5×10^{-5} M benzoylcholine in the absence and in the presence of 10^{-5} M dibucaine. When large numbers of random sera were tested in this fashion (60, 68), a trimodal distribution for dibucaine number was found, consistent with homozygous and heterozygous states of a

TABLE 27–6. BEHAVIOR OF USUAL (U) AND ATYPICAL (A) CHOLINESTERASES
WITH TWO DIFFERENT SUBSTRATES AND FIVE CLASSES OF INHIBITORS*

INHIBITORS	SUBSTRATE	
	Benzoylcholine	*α-Naphthyl Acetate*
None	U activity 2–5 times A	U activity 1.3 times A
I. DFP and TEPP	U inhibition = A inhibition	
II. Succinylcholine and decamethonium	Avidity for A greatly reduced; U/A inhibition = 100	
III. Choline, chlorpromazine, physostigmine, dibucaine, neostigmine, RO2–0683	Differential inhibition of U > A increases with potency of inhibitor	Similar to benzoylcholine
IV. Sodium fluoride	U/A inhibition = 5	U/A inhibition < 2
V. Sodium chloride	A/U inhibition = 3	

*From Giblett. E. R.: *Genetic Markers in Human Blood.* Oxford, Blackwell Scientific Publications, 1969, p. 208.

usual gene, E_1^u, and an atypical gene, E_1^a, with a frequency of about 0.02. These findings were confirmed in family studies (68, 70–72). In an analogous test using sodium fluoride as an inhibitor, a fluoride number could be obtained (66, 73). In a study of a large number of random sera, it was found that the dibucaine and fluoride numbers were abnormal in the same sera, but there were exceptions in which the dibucaine number was only slightly decreased, and the fluoride number was markedly reduced. This indicated a third allele at the E_1 locus, E_1^f (74). Family studies confirmed the inheritance of this allele (73, 75).

The possible presence of a silent E_1 allele, without detectable product, was suggested by anomalous findings in some families with E_1^a (68, 70, 71, 76). There were in these families individuals with low dibucaine numbers, suggesting homozygosity for E_1^a, but the family studies indicated that they were, in fact, heterozygotes. Homozygotes for this gene have subsequently been found (76, 77), in which parents and some children have low to low-normal enzyme levels but normal inhibition numbers. This allele has been designated E_1^s (78).

Still another rare variant has been described (79) which, in the homozygous state, results in very low enzyme activity in serum but normal reactivity with an antiserum to pseudocholinesterase activity, indicating another dysfunctional variant at the E_1

locus. This "nearly inactive" gene is thus distinct from E_1^s, which produces little immunoreactive protein (80).

In starch gel electrophoresis at alkaline pH, pseudocholinesterase forms four bands (81, 82), as shown in Figure 27–13. This heterogeneity is primarily in molecular size, rather than charge. The appearance of the usual ($E_1^u E_1^u$), atypical ($E_1^a E_1^a$), intermediate ($E_1^u E_1^a$), silent ($E_1^s E_1^s$), and nearly silent pseudocholinesterase patterns in alkaline starch gel electrophoresis is shown in Figure 27–14.

The E_1^a allele has a frequency of between 0.01 and 0.02 in most Caucasian populations studied (83), but frequencies as high as 0.051 have been observed in non-Ashkenazi Jews (84). The gene has an even lower frequency in most African, Asiatic, native American, and oceanic populations studied. The frequency of E_1^f heterozygotes is around 1 per cent in Europeans and in a mixed Brazilian population. The E_1^s gene frequency is probably even lower than that of E_1^f.

If starch gel electrophoresis of serum is performed at pH 5 to 6, pseudocholinesterase patterns show one (C4) or two (C4 and C5) bands (82). The presence or absence of the C5 band appears to be controlled by a gene at a locus distinct from E_1, designated E_2 (85). This trait is probably inherited as an autosomal dominant, but there appears to be interaction with E_1 expression. Persons who are C5+ (E_2^+) have

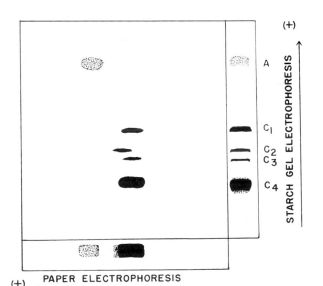

Figure 27–13. Two dimensional paper–starch gel electrophoretic analyses of normal serum for esterase activity. Albumin is indicated by A and pseudocholinesterase by four components, C_{1-4}. It is evident that the C bands have rather similar electrophoretic mobilities in ordinary zone electrophoresis, and that therefore the multiple components seen on starch gel differ primarily in molecular size. [Adapted from (81).]

(+)

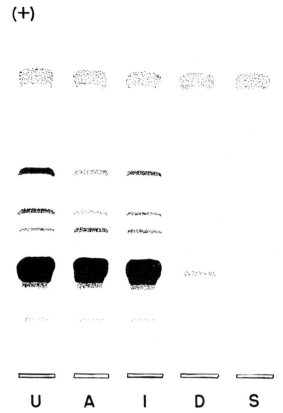

U   A   I   D   S

Figure 27–14. Diagrammatic representation of pseudocholinesterase variant phenotypes in alkaline starch gel electrophoresis stained for esterase activity. The usual (U), atypical (A), intermediate (I), and dysfunctional (D) patterns are shown. (S) = serum albumin.

30 per cent higher enzyme levels than those who are E_2^-. The C5+ phenotype is found in about 10 per cent of Caucasians (86) and in a lower percentage of Blacks.

The E_1 and Tf gene loci are linked and therefore on the same chromosome (87).

Transferrin

Iron is transported in the serum by a 5S β-globulin called transferrin (88). The molecular weight of the molecule is around 75,000, and it contains 5.5 per cent carbohydrate. Each molecule has two binding sites for Fe^{3+}. Iron-free transferrin is colorless, whereas the saturated molecule is salmon pink.

The concentration of transferrin in normal serum has a rather narrow range of 200 to 320 mg. per 100 ml., with a mean of 250.

There is a direct correspondence between the total iron-binding capacity of serum and its transferrin concentration. Both on theoretical and experimental grounds, it has been found that 1 mg. of transferrin binds 1.25 μg. of iron under full saturation (89). The metabolic behavior of transferrin is such that the apoprotein has a $t_{1/2}$ of seven to ten days, but the iron $t_{1/2}$ is of the order of 90 minutes (90), in keeping with the transport function of transferrin for iron.

Transferrin concentration in serum rises in iron deficiency, in the latter portion of pregnancy, and in women on oral contraceptive medication. During any acute or chronic inflammatory state or in the presence of tissue necrosis, transferrin (like albumin) acts as a negative acute phase reactant, and its serum concentration falls.

A very rare and probably inherited deficiency state for transferrin has been described (91, 92). This state is characterized by severe hypochromic, microcytic anemia and death in childhood from excessive iron deposition in tissues, particularly the myocardium, liver, and spleen.

The common form of transferrin has been named Tf C, but some 20 inherited variants have been recognized to date (93). These are distinguished by differences in electrophoretic mobility from Tf C, the more anodal variants being designated B with numerical or geographic subscripts, and the more cathodal variants named D with subscripts. Figure 27–15 shows transferrin patterns containing these variants in association with Tf C or other variants or in the homozygous state. These variants are inherited in mendelian autosomal codominant fashion. In all instances such inheritance patterns suggest that the variants are controlled by mutant alleles at a single locus, Tf. The subunit structure of transferrin is not clearly established, but whether the molecule consists of one polypeptide chain or two, variant gene products migrate as single bands. Thus, if the molecule consists of two subunits, these cannot randomly associate, since the latter process would yield a three-banded pattern in heterozygotes and not the observed pattern of two bands of approximately equal density.

The transferrin variants occur in low frequency in all populations, and individual variants appear to occur in some geographic areas and populations but not others: Tf^{B_2} has a frequency of up to 0.015 in Caucasians;

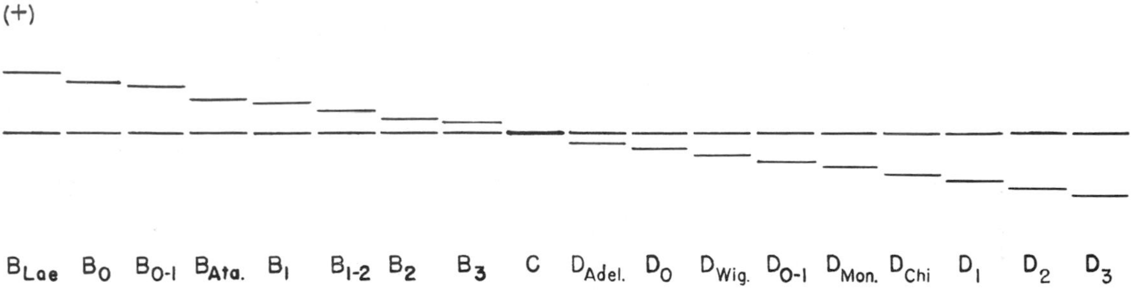

(+)

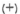

| B_{Lae} | B_O | B_{O-l} | $B_{Ata.}$ | B_l | B_{l-2} | B_2 | B_3 | C | $D_{Adel.}$ | D_O | $D_{Wig.}$ | D_{O-l} | $D_{Mon.}$ | D_{Chi} | D_l | D_2 | D_3 |

Figure 27–15. Diagram of variants of transferrin in relation to transferrin C, as seen in alkaline gel electrophoresis. [Adapted from (93).]

Tf^{D_1}, Tf^{D_2}, and Tf^{D_3} are found in Negroes; and Tf^{B_3} has been found among Japanese, for example. All of the variants studied have had normal function in terms of iron-binding. Structural studies have indicated that the variants are mostly, if not exclusively, the products of single point mutations. For example, there is evidence that Tf B_2 differs from Tf C in that it contains a glutamic acid residue where Tf C has a glycine (94). Tf D_{Chi}, on the other hand, contains an arginine in place of a histidine in Tf C (95). No immunochemical differences between Tf variants have been uncovered.

Lipoproteins

The serum lipoproteins are divisible into two major groups according to their lipid content and apoprotein composition. The high-density lipoproteins (d = 1.093 to 1.149) have Sf values of 2 to 8, molecular weights of 200,000 to 400,000, and electrophoretic mobilities in the α_1-range. The low-density lipoproteins (d = < 1.019 to 1.063) appear to be under separate genetic control and have different apoproteins, more lipid, and molecular weights in excess of 2×10^6. These low-density lipoproteins can be further subdivided into very-low-density (VLDL) with α_2- or pre-β mobility and low-density lipoproteins with β mobility. The whole low-density lipoprotein group of molecules appears to function in the transport of lipids and lipid-soluble material.

The concentrations of the lipoproteins vary under certain pathophysiologic conditions. The α-lipoproteins (high density lipoproteins) may be decreased in patients with chronic renal disease. In thyrotoxicosis there tends to be a decrease in the concentration of low-density lipoproteins, whereas in myxedema their concentration increases. Increases in low-density lipoproteins are also seen in biliary obstruction and diabetic acidosis.

Hereditary deficiency of the β-lipoprotein (96) is a rare disorder inherited as an autosomal recessive characteristic. Affected individuals, in addition to the absence of β-lipoprotein (low-density lipoprotein) from their serum, have neuromuscular disturbances with degenerative changes in the cerebellum and posterolateral columns of the spinal cord, retinitis pigmentosa, malabsorption, and spiculated erythrocytes (acanthocytes) associated with intermittent hemolytic anemia. The striking red cell deformity is at least partially reversible on transfer into normal plasma, or by the intravenous administration of cottonseed oil. Thus the abnormal red cell shape in this disorder is probably a secondary phenomenon. An inherited electrophoretic variant of β-lipoprotein has been documented in one family (97). The variant protein migrated more rapidly than the common type in paper or starch-block electrophoresis, but more slowly in starch gel electrophoresis. On ultracentrifugal analysis, the variant was denser than the common form. The variant was inherited as an autosomal codominant trait.

Polymorphisms in the β-lipoproteins detectable by precipitation (or lack of precipitation) with certain antiserums can be classified into two groups, depending on the source of the antiserum. The Ag determinants (98) are detected by antibodies found in the serum of some patients who have received large numbers of whole blood or plasma transfusions, and particularly in such patients with thalassemia major. The lipoprotein determinants, Lp and Ld, are detected by antiserums prepared in rabbits that have been immunized with whole serum or β-lipoprotein from a single individual (99).

The number of Ag determinants found to date may be as high as six or seven, with two the product of allelic genes. There is some confusion, however, owing to the fact that many of the human reagents have several specificities, and the detection systems are not all ideal. There are Lp specificities, Lp a and Lp x, which are independent of the known Ag determinants but are carried by β-lipoprotein molecules.

There are hereditary influences in the familial hyperlipemias, and the concentration of the low-density lipoproteins may be altered profoundly in affected individuals; however, discussion of this subject is beyond the scope of this chapter.

The high-density or α-lipoprotein is hereditarily absent from the serum of patients with Tangier disease (100). Such patients show deposition of cholesterol esters throughout the reticuloendothelial system. Their serum contains decreased cholesterol, decreased phospholipid, and normal or increased triglyceride. Individuals heterozygous for Tangier disease are asymptomatic, but have decreased concentrations of α-lipoprotein.

C3

The third component of human complement has a critical role in the complement system and is discussed in Chapter 18.

Many of the complement-mediated functions which contribute to the inflammatory response, such as chemotaxis, immune adherence, opsonization of bacteria, and anaphylatoxin generation, are first and in some instances exclusively generated at the C3 step in complement activation. Genetic defects affecting C3, when present in homozygous form, may result in markedly increased susceptibility to infection by pyogenic bacteria.

The serum concentration of C3 may be lowered in patients with systemic lupus erythematosus, membranoproliferative and acute glomerulonephritis, immune complex disease, and advanced chronic liver disease. Deposits of C3 are found in glomeruli in these conditions, usually accompanied by immunoglobulins. C3 concentrations are usually markedly elevated in biliary obstruction. Lesser elevations occur as part of the acute phase response. In newborns, the concentration of C3 is about 60 per cent that of adult serum, and it rises into the normal range within the first few months of life.

C3 exhibits extensive genetic polymorphism (101, 102). Some 20 or more alleles have been identified of which only two are common (103). The most common form is C3 S (for slow), and the second most common type is C3 F (for fast). These and the rare variants are identified by prolonged high voltage electrophoresis of whole serum (Fig. 27–16). Because it is the most abundant of the complement components with a normal range of concentration in serum of 100 to 200 mg. per 100 ml., C3 can be seen directly on protein staining of electrophoretic patterns of serum. To facilitate

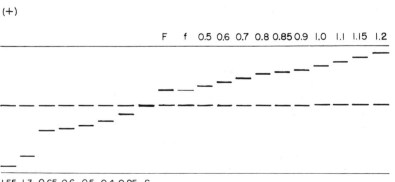

Figure 27–16. Diagram of variants of C3 in relation to C3 S in agarose gel electrophoresis at pH 8.6 with 0.0018 M calcium lactate present. [Adapted from (103).]

TABLE 27-7. C3 GENE FREQUENCIES IN SOME POPULATIONS*

POPULATION	$C3^S$	$C3^F$	$C3^{S0.4}$
Caucasian (USA)	0.77	0.22	0.003
Caucasian (Norway)	0.80	0.19	0.003
Caucasian (Germany)	0.78	0.21	0.003
Negro (USA)	0.92	0.07	–
Negro (Angola)	0.95	0.05	0.001
Oriental (USA)	0.99	–	–
Oriental (Tibet)	1.00	–	–

*The designation for C30.4 is that recently adopted (103). The prior designation was C3 $S_{0.6}$.

this visualization, Ca^{2+} (or Mg^{2+}) is added to the electrophoresis buffer to reduce the migration of C3 and separate it from transferrin and β-lipoprotein (104). Gene frequencies for the more common C3 alleles are given in Table 27-7.

The rare variants have been designated by numbers indicating their relative mobilities with respect to C3 S with Ca^{2+} at 0.0018 M in the gel and electrophoresis buffers (103). One of the more rapid C3 variants was arbitrarily named C3 F1, and the distance from C3 S to C3 F1 is 1.0. Thus, C3 F0.85 migrates 85 per cent of the distance between C3 F1 and C3 S, and C3 S0.65 migrates 65 per cent of this unit distance, but towards the cathode. A number of the C3 variants have been studied functionally, and no abnormality has been found (105). A variant with the electrophoretic mobility of C3 F has been identified (106) which is associated with about half the serum concentration of the other variants. This variant has been named C3 f and has been identified only in heterozygotes with C3 S. The total serum C3 concentration of such persons is normal.

A silent gene, $C3^-$, in heterozygotes results in half normal serum levels (107). Complement-mediated functions are mildly abnormal in such sera, but these individuals are asymptomatic. The homozygous state for $C3^-$ (108), on the other hand, is associated with extreme deficiency of C3; serum complement-mediated functions are severely impaired, and there is a markedly increased susceptibility to infection by pyogenic bacteria. Homozygous C3 deficiency is rare, and only two such patients have been identified.

Low levels of serum C3 are associated with an inherited deficiency of the C3 in-

activator (109). The latter protein is an enzyme which inhibits the hemolytic and other activities of activated C3 and functions as an inhibitor of the properdin or alternate pathway of complement activation by inactivating GBGase. As a result, in homozygous C3 inactivator deficiency (110, 111, 112), there is consumption and relative serum deficiency of properdin Factor B or GBG (see below), C3, and other proteins of this pathway. The single known patient with this disorder has markedly increased susceptibility to infection by pyogenic bacteria, much as the patients homozygous for C3 deficiency and agammaglobulinemic boys.

Glycine-Rich β-Glycoprotein (GBG)

GBG (113) is a 6S protein of serum which functions as properdin Factor B (114). Other names for this protein are C3 proactivator (C3PA) (115), heat-labile factor (HLF), and unknown factor (UF). It occurs in normal serum at a concentration of 12 to 56 mg. per 100 ml. On activation of the properdin or alternate complement pathway, it is cleaved into two fragments, one of α electrophoretic mobility (GAG), and one of γ mobility (GGG) (116). The latter fragment is also known as β_2-glycoprotein II (117).

On electrophoresis of whole fresh serum or plasma and immunofixation with specific antiserum, GBG forms multiple bands (Fig. 27-17). The specific patterns have been shown to be genetically determined by four known alleles, two common and two rare, at a genetic locus designated Gb (118). In homozygotes for the common alleles, Gb^F or Gb^S (F and S stand for fast and slow), there are five roughly equidistant GBG bands. From cathode to anode the ratios of protein in these bands is approximately 6:16:15:6:1. The electrophoretic difference between Gb S and Gb F consists of a shift of an equal distance for each band. The less common variants, Gb F_1 and Gb S_1, are shifted three positions anodally and two positions cathodally with respect to Gb S. On fragmentation of the GBG molecule during complement activation, Gb F and Gb S differences are preserved in the

(+)

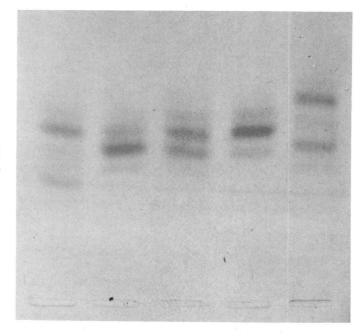

FS₁   SS   FS   FF   F₁S

Figure 27–17. Prolonged agarose gel electrophoretic patterns of GBG variants developed by immunofixation with specific antiserum.

GAG fragments, whereas Gb F₁ and Gb S₁ are found in GGG.

The foregoing observations suggest that the GBG molecule is a random tetramer of two kinds of similar subunits, which we might arbitrarily name A and B. In analogy to the lactate dehydrogenase isozymes, the five GBG bands in the homozygous patterns would consist of A_4, A_3B, A_2B_2, AB_3 and B_4. The band ratios would then be explainable by an unequal input of A and B subunits in an approximate ratio of 1.6. Genetic differences would then be ascribable to a third moiety associated with the tetramer, perhaps a third kind of polypeptide chain. The postulated model for GBG is shown in Figure 27–18.

Gene frequencies for various populations are given in Table 27–8. Since these data were collected, Gb^F_1 has been found rarely in Caucasians, and Gb^S_1 has been found in a few Negroes.

There are only incomplete data available concerning acquired variations in GBG concentration. Strikingly low levels may be seen (along with depressed C3 concentration) in patients with advanced chronic liver disease. There is only modest and inconstant lowering of GBG serum concentration in patients with systemic lupus erythematosus and other diseases in which classic complement activation is thought to occur in vivo. This is surprising since generation of C3b from C3 by any mechanism (including activated C4 and C2) is known to activate the alternate pathway and cleave GBG in vitro (119). Since the level of any plasma protein reflects both

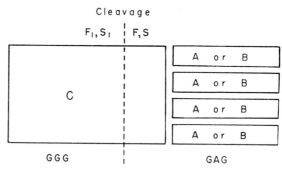

Figure 27–18. A possible model of the GBG molecule deduced from the genetic polymorphism. [Adapted from (118).]

TABLE 27–8. *Gb* GENE FREQUENCIES AMONG RANDOM UNRELATED INDIVIDUALS

	No. Tested	Gb^S	Gb^F	Gb^{F_1}	Gb^{S_1}
Negro	127	0.437	0.512	0.051	—
Caucasian	158	0.709	0.278	—	0.013
Oriental	86	0.890	0.110	—	—

synthetic and catabolic rates, it may be that GBG synthesis is increased in patients with complement activation.

Immunoglobulins

Humoral antibody activity resides in a group of molecules of unique structural heterogeneity, the immunoglobulins (see Chapter 18). The basic structural units of these proteins consist of two kinds of chains, designated heavy and light, held together by disulfide bridges as well as noncovalent forces (120). The structure of IgG1, the most plentiful of the immunoglobulins, serves as a model for this structure and is shown in Figure 27–19. It should be noted that the molecule is symmetrical, and that the light chains and heavy chains about the axis of symmetry are identical in structure. The kind of heavy chain determines the immunoglobulin class: γ, α, μ, δ, and ϵ

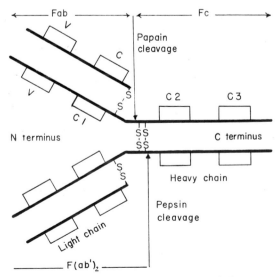

Figure 27–19. A simplified model of the IgG1 molecule.

chains are found in IgG, IgA, IgM, IgD, and IgE, respectively. Subclasses have been identified in IgG (IgG1, 2, 3, and 4) and IgA (IgA1 and IgA2), and there are probably subclasses of the other immunoglobulins as well (121). The light chains in any immunoglobulin molecule are of two types, designated κ and λ. The amino acid sequences of two molecules of the same immunoglobulin subclass are found to be very similar in the C-terminal half of the light chain and the C-terminal three-quarters of the heavy chain. These areas of the molecule have been called constant (C) regions, and the structural bases for the human genetic markers to be discussed are found here. The remaining N-terminal variable (V) regions of both heavy and light chains show marked differences in amino acid sequences from molecule to molecule, even within a single immunoglobulin subclass. This remarkable diversity is undoubtedly related to the specific antibody function of the immunoglobulins.

A useful tool in the study of the structure of immunoglobulins has been limited enzymic cleavage by papain and pepsin (122, 123). Sites of cleavage by these enzymes are shown in Figure 27–19. For a fuller description of the immunoglobulins, their structure and function, see Chapter 18.

The two major unlinked genetic systems are Gm, controlling IgG C-region heavy chain synthesis, and Inv, controlling the C-region of κ chains. The methods for detecting these markers are primarily serologic and require some detailed description.

The Gm system was discovered by Grubb and Laurell (124), who were working with the agglutination of red cells coated with gamma globulin (incomplete Rh antibodies) by serum from patients with rheumatoid arthritis. If the gamma globulin coats were from single individuals, certain of these rheumatoid agglutinins (Ragg's) agglutinated some coated red cells and not others, and agglutination could be inhibited by the serum from certain normal individuals but not others. It later became clear that similar and usually more specific agglutinins were found in some serum from normal subjects (SNagg's) (125). A third source of specific agglutinins is suitably absorbed animal antiserum to purified M-components (struc-

TABLE 27-9. NOMENCLATURE FOR IMMUNOGLOBULIN GENETIC MARKERS (ALLOTYPES)

WHO	Original	WHO	Original
Gm(1)	a	Gm(17)	z
Gm(2)	x	Gm(18)	Rouen 2
Gm(3) = Gm(4)	b^W, b²	Gm(19)	Rouen 3
Gm(4) = Gm(3)	f	Gm(20)	z(S.F.)
Gm(5)	b, b¹	Gm(21)	g
Gm(6)	c, like	Gm(22)	y(? non-a)
Gm(7)	r	Gm(23)	n
Gm(8)	e	Gm(24)	c⁵
Gm(9)	p	–	m
Gm(10)	b^α		
Gm(11)	b^β, b⁰	Inv(1)	l
Gm(12)	b^γ	Inv(2)	a
Gm(13)	b³	Inv(3)	b
Gm(14)	b⁴		
Gm(15)	s	Am(1)	l or +
Gm(16)	t		

turally homogeneous immunoglobulins from patients with multiple myeloma and related disorders) (126). The ability of some human serums to inhibit this kind of agglutination is inherited in mendelian fashion and resides in the immunoglobulins. A heavy chain genetic marker (Am) has more recently been found on IgA2 subclass molecules (127).

In practice, two sources of IgG are used to coat human type O red cells for the detection of Gm and Inv factors. Incomplete anti-Rh (D) (see Chapters 9 and 26) is usually of the IgG1 or IgG3 subclass and renders Rh (D)-positive cells a useful indicator particle. Alternatively, purified M-components can be linked chemically to type O red cells to provide an indicator.

The various known Gm, Inv, and Am factors are listed in Table 27-9. Two major nomenclatures are in use, and some factors originally considered as separate are, in fact, very similar or identical. In our dis-

cussion, we will use the letter nomenclature and deal only with some major markers.

The markers on IgG1 include Gm a, z, x, and f; those on IgG3 are Gm g and the b group as well as c, s, and t, whereas a single marker, Gm n, is known for IgG2 (128). These markers are inherited as gene complexes in a manner analogous to the Rh antigens (Chapter 26). These gene complexes differ in different ethnic groups (129). Table 27-10 lists the Gm and Am gene complexes for the major races of man. It is thus clear that the cistrons coding for IgG subclass and IgA2 heavy chains are very closely linked and perhaps contiguous. From this fact and the many areas of structural homology shared by the C-regions of the heavy chains of the IgG subclass molecules, it seems highly likely that the subclasses arose by gene duplication (130). Largely through the work of Kunkel and his associates (131), who studied rare families with unusual gene complexes arising presumably from unequal homologous chromosomal crossover (similar to the origins of Lepore hemoglobin and Hp 2α), evidence for the following order of cistrons has been obtained: IgA2, IgG4, IgG2, IgG3, IgG1.

Intensive investigation of myeloma proteins has established the structural bases for many of the serologically detected genetic markers. Some of these findings are shown in Table 27-11. It will be noted that in some instances, for example Gm(f) and Gm(z), the markers are determined by the presence of one or another amino acid at the same position in the sequence. In other cases, an alternative sequence at a given position for a marker residue is not recognized as a marker by any specific serologic testing system. Furthermore, this alternative sequence is often shared by other IgG subclasses. The antigen in such cases is termed a "nonmarker." In all the

TABLE 27-10. MAJOR GENE COMPLEXES OF DIFFERENT POPULATIONS*

Population	IgA2,Am	IgG2,Gm	IgG3,Gm	IgG1,Gm
Caucasian	+	n+	b	f non-a
Caucasian	+	n–	b	f non-a
Caucasian and Mongoloid	+	n–	g	z a
Caucasian	+	n–	g	z ax
Negro	–	n–	b	z a
Mongoloid	+	n+	b	f a
Mongoloid	–	n–	b	z a

*Adapted from Natvig, J. B., and Kunkel, H. G.: Adv. Immunol. 16:1, 1973.

TABLE 27–11.   AMINO ACID DIFFERENCES RELATED TO GENETIC MARKERS*

Antigen	Chain	Papain Fragment	Sequence No.	Amino Acids
Gm(a)	$\gamma 1$	Fc	356–358	Asp Glu Leu
Non-a	$\gamma 1, 2, 3$	Fc	356–358	Glu Glu Met
Gm(f)	$\gamma 1$	Fd	214	Arg
Gm(z)	$\gamma 1$	Fd	214	Lys
Gm(g)	$\gamma 3$	Fc	296	Tyr
Non-g	$\gamma 2, 3$	Fc	296	Phe
Gm(b⁰)	$\gamma 3$	Fc	436	Phe
Non-b⁰	$\gamma 1, 2, 3$	Fc	436†	Tyr
Inv(1)	κ	(Fab)	191	Leu
Inv(2)	κ	(Fab)	191	Val

*Adapted from Natvig, J. B., and Kunkel, H. G.: Adv. Immunol. *16*:1, 1973.
†This position may be related to another Gm(b) marker.

examples given, the differences in sequence between markers or between markers and nonmarkers can be explained by point mutations consistent with the genetic code.

Of some interest is the relationship between genetic type and protein concentration. It has been shown that individuals homozygous for Gm(b) have higher IgG3 serum levels than those who are Gm(g) homozygotes (132). Gm(bg) heterozygotes have intermediate levels. Similar though less pronounced relationships hold for other Gm markers.

Since there is specific transport of maternal IgG of all subclasses across the placenta into the fetal circulation, and some fetal blood leaks into the maternal circulation, particularly during the final trimester of pregnancy, it is not surprising that SNagg's arise in both the infant and the pregnant woman (133) to different genetic markers on each other's immunoglobulins. These antibodies are for the most part transient and probably harmless. Most are IgM and, if they are maternal, do not cross the placenta. There is some suggestion, however, that the rare IgG SNagg produced by the mother during pregnancy may be responsible for the syndrome of transient hypogammaglobulinemia. Although it may be that all infants who themselves lack maternal immunoglobulin genetic markers produce antibodies to these antigens during the latter part of the first year of life, these tend to disappear gradually over the next two or three years (134). Nevertheless, SNagg's can be found in 1 or 2 per cent of the healthy, untransfused normal population.

Recent evidence has been obtained for linkage between the *Pi* locus and the *Gm-Am* gene complex (135).

Other Serum Protein Genetic Markers and Deficiency States

Some enzymes, primarily of tissue origin, are found in serum or plasma. Because their electrophoretic patterns vary depending upon the tissue of origin and because the relative contributions of different tissues vary in health and disease, reliable genetic typing is made difficult. Such enzymes include lactate dehydrogenase and alkaline phosphatase.

Some genetic deficiency states of plasma proteins have already been discussed in this chapter. They include albumin, transferrin, α_1-antitrypsin, C3, C3 inactivator, β-lipoprotein, α-lipoprotein, haptoglobin, ceruloplasmin, and pseudocholinesterase. All are rare. Inherited deficiencies of clotting factors are discussed elsewhere (Chapter 19).

Additional deficiency states are known. Most are rare but one, that for β_2-glycoprotein, is sufficiently common in the populations studied that it constitutes a useful genetic marker (136). Persons homozygous for inherited deficiency of β_2-glycoprotein are of the genetic constitution Bg^D/Bg^D. They are entirely healthy. Heterozygotes (Bg^N/Bg^D) have half normal levels. In a study of 260 random sera it was shown that the Bg^D gene frequency was about 0.03.

Hereditary angioneurotic edema (Chapter 18) is associated in 80 per cent of affected kindred with levels of C$\overline{1}$ inhibitor that range from about 5 to 30 per cent of the normal level (137). This trait is inherited as an autosomal dominant, and thus affected persons are heterozygotes. In the remaining 20 per cent of families with hereditary angioneurotic edema, the C$\overline{1}$ inhibitor is dysfunctional and is present in normal or supernormal concentrations. There are at least four electrophoretically distinguishable, inherited, dysfunctional C$\overline{1}$ inhibitors. This trait, too, is inherited as an autosomal dominant.

Deficiency states have been reported for the complement components, C2 (138), C6 (139), and C7 (140) in man. Most affected persons who are homozygotes appear to be entirely healthy, although some authors have suggested an association between C2 deficiency and a lupuslike illness (141). Heterozygotes for these deficiency states have approximately half normal levels of protein.

There is evidence for a common genetic polymorphism in the sixth component of human complement (142). Preliminary findings suggest polymorphism in many of the other complement proteins. Structural polymorphism for human C4 occurs (143), although its genetic basis remains obscure.

BLOOD CELL ENZYMES

Chapters 10, 11, 16, and 18 describe the presently known clinical disorders associated with deficiencies in quality or quantity of blood cell enzymes. Several recent reviews and textbooks contain summaries of the blood cell enzymes that exhibit polymorphism (144–146) and the application of linkage analysis and somatic cell hybrids to determination of synteny (see Chapter 25) and chromosome mapping (147–149). Therefore, in this section of the chapter only selected examples of blood cell enzyme heterogeneity will be presented. For a complete review the reader should consult the references cited above.

Red Cell Acid Phosphatase

During his extensive studies of blood cell enzymes in human diseases, Valentine and his co-workers (150) discovered that red cell acid phosphatase activity is higher in young cells (reticulocytes) than in an older cell population. Oski et al. (151) and Choremis and co-workers (152) reported that red cell acid phosphatase activity is decreased in Caucasians with G6PD deficiency, and it has been proposed that glutathione levels influence the activity of this enzyme in human cells. However, the relationship between G6PD and acid phosphatase activity has not been confirmed in subsequent studies (153).

Starch gel electrophoresis patterns of acid phosphatase activity (144) (zymograms) usually reveal six different phenotypes of varying frequency, one of which (CC) is extremely rare. The phenotypes are the result of heterozygosity for three alleles labeled A, B, and C. These alleles are responsible for differences in activity as well as structure. For example, type BB individuals tend to have approximately 50 per cent more activity than type AA individuals, and type AB individuals have intermediate activity (145).

Rare acid phosphatase types have also been discovered (144).

Phosphoglucomutase (PGM) (145)

The conversion of glucose-1-phosphate to glucose-6-phosphate, an important step in glycogen metabolism, is catalyzed by phosphoglucomutase. Glucose-1,6-diphosphate is an intermediate in the reaction. The enzyme is present in red cells, although glycogen is virtually absent in these cells. Two different PGM loci control the production of the common red cell PGM electrophoretogram (Fig. 27–20). The phenotypes are designated PGM$_1$1, 2–1, and 2, and are created by the products of two common alleles at the PGM$_1$ locus, termed PGM_1^1 and PGM_1^2, as well as the products of the second PGM locus (PGM$_2$), which has very little variation. Thus the PGM$_1$1 phenotype represents homozygosity for the PGM_1^1 allele, PGM$_1$2 represents

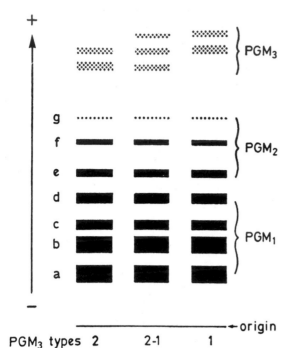

Figure 27–20. Diagram of three types of PGM_3 isozymes, PGM_3 1, PGM_3 2–1, and PGM_3 2, as seen in placental extracts. In each case the PGM_1 isozymes are PGM_1 2–1, and the PGM_2 isozymes are PGM_2 1. [From Harris, H.: *Frontiers of Biology: The Principles of Human Biochemical Genetics.* Vol. 19, Neuberger, A., and Tatum, E. L. (eds.), Amsterdam, North-Holland Publishing Company, 1970, p. 50.]

homozygosity for the PGM_1^2 allele, and PGM 2–1 represents heterozygosity (PGM_1^1/ PGM_1^2). Why each allele is represented by two enzyme bands (such as bands A and C of PGM_1^1) is not clear, but is certainly related to post-translational alteration of enzyme mobility. Some believe that the bands represent the phospho- and dephospho- enzymes.

Even more complexity has been introduced into PGM genetics by the finding of other uncommon alleles at the PGM_1 and PGM_2 loci and by the discovery of a third locus, PGM_3. The potential complexity of a PGM zymogram is bewildering, and careful family studies are often necessary to decipher them. The PGM_3 locus (which contributes a very small fraction of total red cell PGM activity) was detected by examination of PGM zymograms from cells other than red cells that contain much more PGM activity. Placenta is an excellent source of PGM_3, and leukocytes are as well. In fact, it is through linkage studies of

leukocyte PGM_3 that the HL-A system has been tentatively traced to chromosome no. 6, where these histocompatibility loci are probably in close proximity to PGM_3 (see below). Somatic cell hybrid studies have shown that PGM_1 resides on chromosome no. 1. The location of PGM_2 is not known.

Red Cell Adenylate Kinase (AK) (144)

Adenylate kinase catalyzes 2 ADP $\rightleftarrows$ ATP + AMP and thereby contributes to the regulation of ATP metabolism. In muscle the enzyme is known as myokinase.

As occurs in the case of PGM, zymograms of AK activity from red cells are rendered somewhat confusing by post-translational increments in the number of enzyme bands produced by a single allele. Despite this source of difficulty, it has been possible to define four major AK phenotypes, three of which conform to a relatively simple model, such as that which explains acid phosphatase zymograms. There is one AK locus with two common alleles expressed in the red cell. The AK 1 phenotype represents homozygosity for the AK^1 allele. AK 2 phenotype represents homozygosity for the AK^2 allele. The AK 2–1 phenotype is due to heterozygosity AK^1/AK^2. A fourth phenotype, AK 4–1, is rare.

Catalase

Catalase is a heme enzyme that accelerates the breakdown of H_2O_2 to H_2O and O_2. As such this activity should play an important role in the removal of unwanted H_2O_2 from the red cell. Yet homozygous catalase deficiency (acatalasemia) is not associated with oxidative hemolysis, probably because H_2O_2 is mainly disposed of in red cells via the glutathione reductase hexose monophosphate shunt system (154). In some individuals with absent catalase, ulcerating lesions of the oral and nasal mucosa occur (155, 156).

There is no firm evidence for molecular heterozygosity in the catalase system (144). Multiple bands are observed in zymograms, but these represent post-translational artifacts. Aebi and Cantz (157) have shown that the enzyme is age-dependent, being much more active in reticulocytes. The deficiency state is similar to G6PD deficiency in that some catalase activity is observed in young cells, while none is present in old cells. Thus the deficiency appears to be the result of the synthesis of an unstable enzyme protein (158).

Galactose-1-Phosphate Uridyl Transferase

This enzyme catalyzes the reaction Gal-1-P+UDPG → G-1-P+UDPGal. Deficiency of this enzyme and accumulation of Gal-1-P in tissues are responsible for hereditary galactosemia, a syndrome which, when severe, is characterized by anorexia, distension, diarrhea, vomiting, hypoglycemic attacks, jaundice, and chronic liver disease. Cataracts are common, as is mental deficiency in severe cases. The kidneys are also affected (159).

Deficiency of the enzyme appears to be owing to a hypomorphic allele that is associated with decreased production of the normal protein, as is the case in beta thalassemia or pyruvate kinase deficiency. A convenient spot test for the enzyme in red cells makes it possible to screen newborns for the defect with relative ease (160).

One electrophoretic variant (the Duarte variant) has been described and appears to occur in about 10 per cent of the population (161).

Adenosine Deaminase

Red blood cell adenosine deaminase has a molecular weight of approximately 35,000 (162). Genetic polymorphism has been demonstrated by starch gel electrophoresis. The most common form (ADA 1) is found in 95 per cent of persons of European extraction and migrates more anodally than the rarer phenotype (ADA 2) (163). Individuals who are heterozygotes (ADA 2–1) have equal quantities of both phenotypes. Secondary modification of the primary gene product gives rise to two electrophoretically definable proteins that retain their enzymatic activity; therefore, red blood cell hemolysates from homozygous individuals give rise to a three-band pattern

(164). The absence of ADA has been reported in 13 individuals, 12 of whom suffered from the autosomal recessive form of severe combined immune deficiency (SCID) — approximately one-half the reported cases (165). None of the patients had any definable hematologic abnormality. It has been suggested that the absence of ADA is causally related to SCID; the demonstration that ADA is present in the fibroblasts from individuals with SCID and absent red cell ADA makes a causal relationship unlikely (166). The gene loci for red cell ADA are most probably linked to the loci for SCID; therefore, the absence of red cell ADA may provide a method for the in utero diagnosis of SCID (167). Cell fusion studies have assigned adenosine deaminase to chromosome no. 20 (148).

Chromosomal Localization of the Genes for Blood Cell Enzymes by Somatic Cell Hybridization

Though extensive family and population studies of enzyme phenotypes and karyotypes can lead to specific assignment of genes to chromosomes, this technique of linkage analysis is very slow and time consuming. The technique of hybrid cell cultivation has provided a new approach to gene localization. The recent reviews by Ruddle (148, 149, 186) and Grzeschik (146) offer an analysis of progress in this area.

Human and mouse somatic cells grown in culture may be fused together and give rise to a binucleate heterokaryon. Following the first mitosis in the heterokaryon, mononucleated or hybrid daughter cells are formed. These contain chromosomes of parental cell lines. During continued culture of such hybrids, there is progressive loss of the human chromosomes, often to a point at which the human chromosome representation stabilizes. Then the line with a partial complement of human chromosomes may replicate indefinitely. It is this capacity to isolate a few human chromosomes in a living cell and the newer methods of chromosome identification outlined in Chapter 25 which form the fundamental basis of linkage analysis by means of somatic cell hybrids. This approach permits the investigator to determine whether a given enzyme or other protein is invariably associated with a given segment of a particular chromosome.

Usefulness of the hybridization technique was markedly increased by enrichment methods that increase the number of hybrids produced by fusion of parental cells. Drug-resistant mutant cell lines can be utilized to achieve increased hybridization by a process of enzyme complementation. A parental cell line was taken from a patient with Lesch-Nyhan syndrome. The cells were therefore deficient in hypoxanthine-guanine-phosphoribosyltransferase (HGPRT). When exposed to aminopterin to block de novo purine and pyrimidine synthesis, these cells, which cannot incorporate hypoxanthine or guanine, depend upon thymidine kinase (TK) for DNA synthesis. Mouse cell lines can be rendered TK-deficient by exposure to the antimetabolites BUdR and thioguanine. In the presence of aminopterin, they depend upon HGPRT for DNA synthesis. When mixed in culture in the presence of HAT medium (hypoxanthine, thymidine, and aminopterin), only the hybrid cells with complementary enzymes capable of utilization of both hypoxanthine and thymidine will survive. Other conditioning methods, including temperature-dependent mutants, have since been developed.

Even more convenient is the use of enzyme-deficient rodent cells hybridized with normal human cells. One of the retained human chromosomes must contain the gene for the enzyme if the medium is such that the enzyme deficiency would not permit cell survival. The actual linkage or synteny is assigned from the concordant segregation of the chromosome and the enzyme phenotype in cloned hybrids. Table 27–12 provides a list of such assignments, as of 1973. PGM_3 is now thought to be localized to chromosome no. 6.

Chromosome mapping may be performed by the use of spontaneous or random human chromosome rearrangements in human-mouse hybrid lines. The continuation of concordant segregation of a phenotype with a fragment of a given chromosome permits such autosomal localization. A tentative map of human chromosome no. 1 is presented in Table 27–13.

TABLE 27–12. ASSIGNMENTS OF GENES TO CHROMOSOMES*

Chromosome 1	PGM_1, 17190; PGD, 17220; Pep C, 17000
Chromosome 2	IDH, 14770; MOR, 15425
Chromosome 3	—
Chromosome 4–5	Adenine B^+, 10265
Chromosome 6	MOD, 15420; IPO-B, 14745; PGM3, HL-A, Gb, MLC
Chromosome 7	MPI, 15455; PK_3, 17905
Chromosome 8–9	—
Chromosome 10	GOT, 13825
Chromosome 11	LDH-A, 15000; Es-A_4, 13340; KA, 14875
Chromosome 12	LDH-B, 15010; Pep B, 16990; $GlyA^+$ (serinehydroxymethylase?), 13845
Chromosome 13	—
Chromosome 14	NP, 16405
Chromosome 15	
Chromosome 16	APRT, 10260, $Hp\alpha$
Chromosome 17	TK, 18830
Chromosome 18	Pep A, 16980
Chromosome 19	GPI, 23575
Chromosome 20	ADA, 10270
Chromosome 21	IPO-A, 14744; AVP, 10745
Chromosome 22	—
Chromosome X	HGPRT, 30800; PGK, 31180; GPD, 30590; α-Gal, 30150
Chromosome Y	—

*These genes were assigned or confirmed by cell hybrid analysis. Each trait is identified by McKusick's human gene catalogue number. IPO-A and B used here agree with the original designation of Brewer. (From Ruddle, F. H.: Nature (Lond.) 242:167, 1973.)

THE HL-A SYSTEM*

In most species, histocompatibility antigens are determined by a series of multiallelic systems; however, one system defines the major histocompatibility region (MHR), i.e., the H-2 system in mice, the Ag-B locus in rats, and the B locus in chickens. In man the MHR is composed of both serologically defined (SD) and lymphocyte-defined (LD) antigens (168). The SD or HL-A antigens are defined in a complement-dependent, antibody-mediated lymphocytotoxicity assay in which the monospecific antisera are obtained from multiparous females, multitransfused individuals, or specifically immunized donors (169). The LD antigens are defined in mixed lymphocyte culture (MLC), in which the blastogenesis of a mixture of lympho-

*For an excellent recent review, see Seminars in Hematology, Vol. 11, No. 3, 1974.

TABLE 27-13. CHROMOSOME NO. 1°

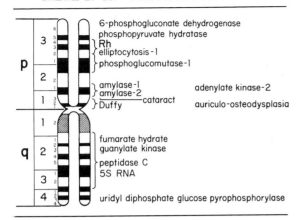

6-phosphogluconate dehydrogenase
phosphopyruvate hydratase
Rh
elliptocytosis-1
phosphoglucomutase-1
amylase-1
amylase-2
cataract
Duffy
adenylate kinase-2
auriculo-osteodysplasia
fumarate hydrate
guanylate kinase
peptidase C
5S RNA
uridyl diphosphate glucose pyrophosphorylase

°Courtesy of Dr. V. A. McKusick.

cytes from two individuals is compared to their separate spontaneous rates of division; the test may be done with both lymphocyte populations capable of responding (two-way MLC) or with one population having been treated with x-ray or mitomycin C, so that one cell population is stimulated by the other (one-way MLC). A ratio of greater than 2 (stimulated/control) in either test is considered to demonstrate a lack of MLC identity between the two lymphocyte donors (170).

The HL-A locus is further divided into two subloci, the first and second; the possible antigenic specificities are presented in Table 27-14. Antigens designated with the prefix HL-A are specificities that have been accepted as unique by WHO, while anti-

TABLE 27-14. HL-A SPECIFICITIES

First Sublocus	Second Sublocus
HL-A1	HL-A5
HL-A2	HL-A7
HL-A2, A28	HL-A8
HL-A3	HL-A12
HL-A9	HL-A13
HL-A10	HL-A14
HL-A11	HL-A17
HL-A28	HL-A27
W-19	W-5
W-19.6	W-10
W-23	W-15
W-24	W-16
W-25	W-18
W-26	W-21
W-29	W-22
W-30	
W-31	
W-32	

gens with a W prefix are provisional specificities. Within any given family, these two subloci are inherited jointly, although occasional crossing-over between them has been demonstrated (171). In large population studies, some degree of linkage disequilibrium has been established, i.e., HL-A 1,8 (172).

Chemical isolation and analysis of the HL-A antigens has progressed slowly. In acrylamide electrophoresis, purified HL-A antigens contain a glycoprotein with a molecular weight of 34,000 and a protein molecular weight of 11,000, identical with beta$_2$-microglobulin. The specificity of the antigen resides in the glycoprotein component (173). HL-A antigens are found on lymphocytes, granulocytes, platelets, fibroblasts, and reticulocytes, but not mature red blood cells (174). Sensitization to HL-A antigens can be produced by transfusion even with washed red blood cells.

Within families, siblings who are HL-A–identical are usually nonstimulating in MLC; thus, the HL-A and the MLC are on the same chromosome and are closely linked. However, there is evidence that recombination between the MLC and HL-A occurs at a higher frequency than that between the two HL-A subloci. Recent evidence seems to demonstrate that there are MLC loci associated with each of the HL-A subloci, and that the MLC locus associated with the second sublocus is the major determinant of MLC responsiveness (175). The degree of polymorphism at the MLC loci would appear to be as great as that for the HL-A locus, since random HL-A–identical pairs are rarely MLC-nonreactive. Additionally, rare HL-A–nonidentical pairs have been shown to be nonreactive in MLC (176).

Lymphocytes that have been activated in one-way MLC are capable of the specific destruction of suitable PHA-stimulated lymphocytes, i.e., cell-mediated lysis (CML). The presence of MLC differences is necessary for the production of "killer" lymphocytes. However, in experiments using donor pairs in which recombinations between HL-A and MLC have occurred, the cytotoxicity appears to be directed towards the HL-A antigens, especially those of the second subloci (175).

MLC and CML appear to be the in vitro correlates of in vivo lymphocyte sensitization and graft rejection or graft-versus-host disease. Thus, in determining donor status for bone marrow transplantation, MLC and CML nonreactivity are obligatory, while HL-A identity is not necessary. One patient with combined immunodeficiency has been successfully reconstituted with bone marrow from an MLC-nonreactive uncle that differed at all four HL-A alleles (177).

Recent evidence from human bone marrow transplantation patients with aplastic anemia has demonstrated that in vivo cytotoxic lymphocytes can be generated between HL-A–identical and MLC-nonreactive sibling pairs (178). These cytotoxic lymphocytes are capable of graft rejection and probably fatal graft-versus-host disease; the antigens involved may not be linked to the MHR. Pedigree studies have shown that HL-A and PGM_3 are linked (179), and somatic cell hybridization has assigned PGM_3 to chromosome no. 6 (179a). Thus the genes for HL-A and the MHR are probably on chromosome no. 6.

In mice the control of the immunologic response to certain synthetic polypeptide antigens and susceptibility to certain leukemic viruses are linked to certain alleles of the MHR. Since in man the basis of some diseases may be either an increased susceptibility to a particular infectious agent or an increased reactivity to a particular antigenic stimulus, much effort has been directed toward determining associations between certain diseases and the patients' MHR. Patients with psoriasis have an increased frequency of W-17 and HL-A13 and decreased frequency of HL-A12 (180); those with ankylosing spondylitis, increased W-27 (181); those with adult celiac disease, increased HL-A1,8 (182); those with autoimmune chronic hepatitis, increased HL-A1,8 (183); and those with childhood acute lymphoblastic leukemia, increased HL-A2 and decreased HL-A9 (184). An increased frequency of the MLC allele associated with HL-A7 has been shown in patients with multiple sclerosis (185).

References

1. Schultze, H. E., and Heremans, J. F.: *Molecular Biology of Human Proteins.* Vol. I. New York, Elsevier, 1966, p. 183.
2. Scheurlen, P. G.: Über Serumeiweissenveränderungen beim Diabetes mellitus. Klin. Wochenschr., 33:198, 1955.
3. Weitkamp, L. R., Shreffler, D. C., et al.: An electrophoretic comparison of serum albumin variants from nineteen unrelated families. Acta Genet. 17:399, 1967.
4. Weitkamp, L. R., and Buck, A. A.: Phenotype frequencies for four serum proteins in Afghanistan: Two "new" albumin variants. Humangenetik 15:335, 1972.
5. Laurell, C.-B., and Niléhn, J. E.: A new type of inherited serum albumin anomaly. J. Clin. Invest. 45:1935, 1966.
6. Bennhold, H., Peters, H., et al.: Über einen Fall von kompletter Analbuminämie ohne wesentliche klinische Krankheitzeichen. Verh. Dtsch. Ges. Inn. Med. 60:630, 1954.
7. Schultze, H. E., Heide, K., et al.: α_1-Antitrypsin aus Humanserum. Klin. Wochenschr. 40:427, 1962.
8. Eriksson, S., and Laurell, C.-B.: A new abnormal serum globulin α_1-antitrypsin. Acta Chem. Scand. 17:5150, 1963.
9. Eriksson, S.: Pulmonary emphysema and alpha$_1$-antitrypsin deficiency. Acta Med. Scand. 175: 197, 1964.
10. Sharp, H. L., Bridges, R. A., et al.: Cirrhosis associated with alpha$_1$-antitrypsin deficiency: A previously unrecognized inherited disorder. J. Lab. Clin. Med. 73:934, 1969.
11. Axelsson, U., and Laurell, C.-B.: Hereditary variants of serum α_1-antitrypsin. Am. J. Hum. Genet. 17:466, 1965.
12. Laurell, C.-B., and Ericksson, S.: The electrophoretic α_1-globulin pattern of serum in α_1-antitrypsin deficiency. Scand. J. Clin. Lab. Invest. 15:132, 1963.
13. Fagerhol, M. K., and Braend, M.: Serum prealbumins: Polymorphism in man. Science 149: 986, 1965.
14. Fagerhol, M. K., and Laurell, C.-B.: The polymorphism of "prealbumins" and α_1-antitrypsin in human sera. Clin. Chim. Acta 16: 199, 1967.
15. Fagerhol, M. K., and Laurell, C.-B.: The Pi system — Inherited variants of serum α_1-antitrypsin. Progr. Med. Genet. 7:96, 1970.
16. Talamo, R. C., Reed, C. E., et al.: α_1-Antitrypsin deficiency: A variant with no detectable α_1-antitrypsin. Science 181:70, 1973.
17. Lieberman, J.: Heterozygous and homozygous α_1-antitrypsin deficiency in patients with pulmonary disease. New Engl. J. Med. 281: 279, 1969.
18. El-Bardeesy, M. W., and Johnson, A. M.: Serum proteinase inhibitors in infants with hyaline membrane disease. J. Pediatr. 81:579, 1972.
19. Ohlsson, K.: Interactions in vitro and in vivo between dog trypsin and dog plasma protease inhibitors. Scand. J. Clin. Lab. Invest. 28:219, 1971.
20. Schmid, K., Binette, J. P., et al.: The polymorphic forms of α_1-acid glycoprotein of normal Caucasian individuals. J. Clin. Invest. 43:2347, 1964.
21. Johnson, A. M., Schmid, K., et al.: Inheritance of human α_1-acid glycoprotein (orosomucoid) variants. J. Clin. Invest. 48:2293, 1969.
22. Polonovski, M., and Jayle, M.-F.: Sur la préparation d'une nouvelle fraction des protéines

plasmatiques, l'haptoglobine. C. R. Acad. Sci. (Paris) 211:517, 1940.

23. Nyman, M.: Serum haptoglobin. Scand. J. Clin. Lab. Invest. 11(Suppl. 39):87, 1959.

24. Smithies, O., Connell, G. E., et al.: Gene action in the human haptoglobins. I. Dissociation into constituent polypeptide chains. J. Mol. Biol. 21:213, 1966.

25. Laurell, C.-B., and Nyman, M.: Studies on the serum haptoglobin level in hemoglobinemia and its influence on renal excretion of hemoglobin. Blood 12:493, 1957.

26. Allison, A. C., and ap Rees, W.: The binding of haemoglobin by plasma proteins (haptoglobins): Its bearing on the "renal threshold" for haemoglobin and the aetiology of haemoglobinuria. Br. Med. J. 2:1137, 1957.

27. Whitten, C. F.: Studies on serum haptoglobin: A functional inquiry. New Engl. J. Med. 266:529, 1962.

28. Smithies, O.: Zone electrophoresis in starch gels: Group variations in the serum proteins of normal human adults. Biochem. J. 61:629, 1955.

29. Connell, G. E., Dixon, G. H., et al.: Subdivision of the three common haptoglobin types based on 'hidden' differences. Nature (Lond.) 193:505, 1962.

30. Smithies, O., Connell, G. E., et al.: Chromosomal rearrangements and evolution of haptoglobin genes. Nature (Lond.) 196:232, 1962.

31. Nance, W. E., and Smithies, O.: New haptoglobin alleles: A prediction confirmed. Nature (Lond.) 198:869, 1963.

32. Korngold, L.: Antigenic differences among human haptoglobins. Int. Arch. Allergy. 23:268, 1963.

33. Korngold, L.: The effect of hemoglobin on the haptoglobin–anti-haptoglobin reaction. Immunochemistry 2:103, 1965.

34. Cleve, H., and Deicher, H.: Haptoglobin "Marburg"; Untersuchungen über eine seltene erbliche Haptoglobin-Variante mit zwei verschiedenen Phänotypen innerhalb einer Familie. Humangenetik 1:537, 1965.

35. Robson, E. B., Polani, P. E., et al.: Probable assignment of the alpha locus of haptoglobin to chromosome 16 in man. Nature (Lond.) 223:1163, 1969.

36. Holmberg, C. G., and Laurell, C.-B.: Investigations in serum copper. II. Isolation of the copper containing protein, and a description of some of its properties. Acta Chem. Scand. 2:550, 1948.

37. Gitlin, D., and Janeway, C. A.: Turnover of the copper and protein moieties of ceruloplasmin. Nature (Lond.) 185:693, 1960.

38. Holmberg, C. G., and Laurell, C.-B.: Oxidase reactions in human plasma caused by ceruloplasmin. Scand. J. Clin. Lab. Invest. 31:103, 1951.

39. Scheinberg, I. H., and Gitlin, D.: Deficiency of ceruloplasmin in patients with hepatolenticular degeneration (Wilson's disease). Science 116:484, 1952.

40. Cox, D. W.: Factors influencing serum ceruloplasmin levels in normal individuals. J. Lab. Clin. Med. 68:893, 1966.

41. Shreffler, D. C., Brewer, G. J., et al.: Electrophoretic variation in human serum ceruloplasmin: A new genetic polymorphism. Biochem. Genet. 1:101, 1967.

42. Alper, C. A., and Johnson, A. M.: Immunofixation electrophoresis: A technique for the study of protein polymorphism. Vox Sang. 17:445, 1969.

43. Kitchin, F. D., and Bearn, A. G.: Quantitative determination of the group specific protein in normal human serum. Proc. Soc. Exp. Biol. Med. 118:304, 1965.

44. Cleve, H., Prunier, J. H., et al.: Isolation and partial characterization of the two principal inherited group-specific components of human serum. J. Exp. Med. 118:711, 1963.

45. Hirschfeld, J.: Immunoelectrophoretic demonstration of qualitative differences in normal human sera and their relation to the haptoglobins. Acta Path. Microbiol. Scand. 47:160, 1959.

46. Schultze, H. E., Biel, H., et al.: Über die Gc-Komponenten von Hirschfeld. I. Lage im Stärkegel-Elektrophoresebild. Naturwissenschaften 49:16, 1962.

47. Smithies, O.: An improved procedure for starch-gel electrophoresis: Further variations in the serum proteins of normal individuals. Biochem. J. 71:585, 1959.

48. Cleve, H., Kitchin, F. D., et al.: A faster migrating Gc-variant: Gc Darmstadt. Humangenetik 9:26, 1970.

49. Johnson, A. M., Alper, C. A., et al.: Unpublished observations.

50. Johnson, A. M., and Alper, C. A.: Unpublished observations.

51. Bowman, B. H., and Bearn, A. G.: The presence of subunits in the inherited group-specific protein of human serum. Proc. Natl. Acad. Sci. USA 53:722, 1965.

52. Weitkamp, L. R., Rucknagel, D. L., et al.: Genetic linkage between structural loci for albumin and group specific component. Am. J. Hum. Genet. 18:559, 1966.

53. Surgenor, D. M., and Ellis, D.: Preparation and properties of serum and plasma proteins. Plasma cholinesterase. J. Am. Chem. Soc. 76:6049, 1954.

54. Haupt, H., Heide, K., et al.: Isolierung und physikalisch-chemische Charakterisierung der Cholinesterase aus Humanserum. Blut 14:65, 1966.

55. Bourne, J. G., Collier, H. O. J., et al.: Succinylcholine (succinoylcholine). Muscle relaxant of short action. Lancet 1:1225, 1952.

56. Evans, F. T., Gray, P. W. S., et al.: Sensitivity to succinylcholine in relation to serum cholinesterase. Lancet 1:1229, 1952.

57. Kalow, W.: Heritable factors recognized in man by the use of drugs, In Pharmacogenetics. Philadelphia, W. B. Saunders Co., 1962, p. 69.

58. McCance, R. A., Hutchinson, A. O., et al.: The cholinesterase activity of the serum of newborn animals and of colostrum. Biochem. J. 45:493, 1949.

59. Lehmann, H., Cook, J., et al.: Pseudocholinesterase in early infancy. Proc. R. Soc. Med. 50:147, 1957.

60. Kalow, W., and Gunn, D. R.: Some statistical data on atypical cholinesterase of human serum. Ann. Hum. Genet. 23:239, 1959.

61. Waterlow, J.: Liver choline-esterase in malnourished infants. Lancet 1:908, 1950.

62. Wetstone, H. J., LaMotta, R. V., et al.: Studies of cholinesterase activity. V. Serum cholinesterase in patients with carcinoma. Ann. Intern. Med., 52:102, 1960.

63. Kunkel, H. G., and Ward, S. M.: Plasma esterase activity in patients with liver disease and nephrotic syndrome. J. Exp. Med. 86:325, 1947.

64. Forbat, A., Lehmann, H., et al.: Prolonged apnoea following injection of succinyldicholine. Lancet 2:1067, 1953.

65. Davies, R. O., Marton, A. V., et al.: The action of normal and atypical cholinesterase of human serum upon a series of esters of choline. Can. J. Biochem. Physiol. 38:545, 1960.

66. Harris, H., and Whittaker, M.: Differential inhibition of human serum cholinesterase with fluoride. Recognition of two new phenotypes. Nature (Lond.) 191:496, 1961.

67. Bamford, K. F., and Harris, H.: Studies on "usual" and "atypical" serum cholinesterase using α-naphthyl acetate as substrate. Ann. Hum. Genet. 27:417, 1964.

68. Kalow, W., and Staron, N.: On distribution and inheritance of atypical forms of human serum cholinesterase, as indicated by dibucaine numbers. Can. J. Biochem. Physiol. 35:1305, 1957.

69. Kalow, W., and Genest, K.: A method for the detection of atypical forms of human serum cholinesterase. Determination of dibucaine numbers. Can. J. Biochem. Physiol. 35:339, 1957.

70. Harris, H., Whittaker, M., et al.: The pseudocholinesterase variants. Esterase levels and dibucaine numbers in families selected through suxamethonium sensitive individuals. Acta Genet. 10:1, 1960.

71. Bush, G. H.: Prolonged apnoea due to suxamethonium. Br. J. Anaesth. 33:454, 1961.

72. Telfer, A. B. M., MacDonald, D. J. F., et al.: Familial sensitivity to suxamethonium due to atypical pseudocholinesterase. Br. Med. J. 1:153, 1964.

73. Harris, H., and Whittaker, M.: The serum cholinesterase variants. A study of twenty-two families selected via the "intermediate" phenotype. Ann. Hum. Genet. 26:59, 1962.

74. Motulsky, A. G.: Pharmacogenetics. Progr. Med. Genet. 3:49, 1964.

75. Lehmann, H., Liddell, J., et al.: Two further pseudocholinesterase phenotypes as causes of suxamethonium apnoea. Br. Med. J. 1:1116, 1963.

76. Liddell, J., Lehmann, H., et al.: A "silent" pseudocholinesterase gene. Nature (Lond.) 193:561, 1962.

77. Hart, S. M., and Mitchell, J. V.: Suxamethonium in the absence of pseudocholinesterase. A case report. Br. J. Anaesth. 34:207, 1962.

78. Simpson, N. E., and Kalow, W.: The "silent" gene for serum cholinesterase. Am. J. Hum. Genet. 16:180, 1964.

79. Goedde, H. W., Gehring, D., et al.: On the problem of the "silent gene" in pseudocholinesterase polymorphism. Biochim. Biophys. Acta 107:391, 1965.

80. Hodgkin, W. E., Giblett, E. R., et al.: Complete pseudocholinesterase deficiency: Genetic and immunologic considerations. J. Clin. Invest. 44:486, 1965.

81. Harris, H., Hopkinson, D. A., et al.: Two dimensional electrophoresis of pseudocholinesterase components in human serum. Nature (Lond.) 196:1296, 1962.

82. Harris, H., Hopkinson, D. A., et al.: Genetical studies on a new variant of serum pseudocholinesterase detected by electrophoresis. Ann. Hum. Genet. 26:359, 1963.

83. Giblett, E. R.: Genetic Markers in Human Blood. Oxford, Blackwell Scientific Publications, 1969, p. 208.

84. Szeinberg, A., Pipano, S., et al.: Frequency of atypical pseudocholinesterase in different populations in Israel. Proc. 2nd Congr. Eur. Anaesth., Copenhagen. Acta Anaesth. (Suppl. 24):199, 1966.

85. Harris, H., Robson, E. B., et al.: Evidence for non-allelism between genes affecting human serum cholinesterase. Nature (Lond.) 200:1185, 1963.

86. Robson, E. B., and Harris, H.: Further data on the incidence and genetics of the serum cholinesterase phenotype C5+. Ann. Hum. Genet. 29:403, 1966.

87. Robson, E. B., Sutherland, I., et al.: Evidence for linkage between the transferrin locus (Tf) and the serum cholinesterase locus (E₁) in man. Ann. Hum. Genet. 29:325, 1966.

88. Holmberg, C. G., and Laurell, C.-B.: Studies on the capacity of serum to bind iron. A contribution to our knowledge of the regulation mechanism of serum iron. Acta Physiol. Scand. 10:307, 1945.

89. Schade, A., Reinhart, R., et al.: Carbon dioxide and oxygen in complex formation with iron and siderophilin, the iron-binding component of human plasma. Arch. Biochem. Biophys. 20:170, 1949.

90. Katz, J. H.: Iron and protein kinetics studied by means of doubly labeled human crystalline transferrin. J. Clin. Invest. 40:2143, 1961.

91. Heilmeyer, L., Keller, W., et al.: Kongenitale Atransferrinämie bei einem sieben Jahre alten Kind. Dtsch. Med. Wochenschr. 86:1745, 1961.

92. Goya, N., Miyazaki, S., et al.: A family of congenital atransferrinemia. Blood 40:239, 1972.

93. Giblett, E. R.: Genetic Markers in Human Blood. Oxford, Blackwell Scientific Publications, 1969, p. 126.

94. Wang, A. C., Sutton, H. E., et al.: A chemical difference between transferrins B₂ and C. Am. J. Hum. Genet. 18:454, 1966.

95. Wang, A. C., Sutton, H. E., et al.: Human transferrins C and D_Chi: An amino acid difference. Biochem. Genet. 1:55, 1967.

96. Salt, H. B., Wolff, O. H., et al.: On having no beta-lipoprotein: A syndrome comprising a-beta-lipoproteinaemia, acanthocytosis, and steatorrhoea. Lancet 2:325, 1960.

97. Seegars, W., Hirschhorn, K., et al.: Double beta-

lipoprotein: A new genetic variant in man. Science 149:303, 1965.

98. Allison, A. C., and Blumberg, B. S.: An isoprecipitation reaction distinguishing human serum protein types. Lancet 1:634, 1961.

99. Berg, K.: A new serum type system in man—The Lp system. Acta Path. Microbiol. Scand. 59:369, 1963.

100. Fredrickson, D. S., Altrocchi, P. H., et al.: Tangier disease: Combined clinical staff conference at the National Institutes of Health. Ann. Intern. Med. 55:1016, 1961.

101. Alper, C. A., and Propp, R. P.: Genetic polymorphism of the third component of human complement (C′3). J. Clin. Invest. 47:2181, 1968.

102. Azen, E. A., and Smithies, O.: Genetic polymorphism of C′3 (β_{1C}-globulin) in human serum. Science 162:905, 1968.

103. Alper, C. A., Azen, E. A., et al.: Statement on the polymorphism of the third component of complement in man (C3). Vox Sang. 25:18, 1973.

104. Laurell, C.-B., Laurell, S., et al.: Buffer composition in paper electrophoresis. Considerations on its influence, with special reference to the interaction between small ions and proteins. Clin. Chem. 2:99, 1956.

105. Colten, H. R., and Alper, C. A.: Hemolytic efficiencies of genetic variants of human C3. J. Immunol. 108:1184, 1972.

106. Alper, C. A., and Rosen, F. S.: Studies of a hypomorphic variant of human C3. J. Clin. Invest. 50:324, 1971.

107. Alper, C. A., Propp, R. P., et al.: Inherited deficiency of the third component of human complement (C′3). J. Clin. Invest. 48:553, 1969.

108. Alper, C. A., Colten, H. R., et al.: Homozygous deficiency of C3 in a patient with repeated infections. Lancet 2:1179, 1972.

109. Alper, C. A., Rosen, F. S., et al.: Inactivator of the third component of complement as an inhibitor in the properdin pathway. Proc. Natl. Acad. Sci. USA 69:2910, 1972.

110. Alper, C. A., Abramson, N., et al.: Increased susceptibility to infection associated with abnormalities of complement-mediated functions and of the third component of complement (C3). New Engl. J. Med. 282:349, 1970.

111. Alper, C. A., Abramson, N., et al.: Studies in vivo and in vitro on an abnormality in the metabolism of C3 in a patient with increased suceptibility to infection. J. Clin. Invest. 49:1975, 1970.

112. Abramson, N., Alper, C. A., et al.: Deficiency of the C3 inactivator in man. J. Immunol. 107:19, 1971.

113. Boenisch, T., and Alper, C. A.: Isolation and properties of a glycine-rich β-glycoprotein of human serum. Biochim. Biophys. Acta 221:529, 1970.

114. Alper, C. A., Goodkofsky, I., et al.: The relationship of glycine-rich β-glycoprotein to Factor B in the properdin system and to the cobra factor-binding protein of human serum. J. Exp. Med. 137:424, 1973.

115. Götze, O., and Müller-Eberhard, H. J.: The C3-activator system: An alternate pathway of complement activation. J. Exp. Med. 134:90s, 1971.

116. Boenisch, T., and Alper, C. A.: Isolation and properties of a glycine-rich γ-glycoprotein of human serum. Biochim. Biophys. Acta 214:135, 1970.

117. Haupt, H., and Heide, K.: Isolierung und Eigenschaften eines β_2-glykoproteins aus Humanserum. Clin. Chim. Acta 12:419, 1965.

118. Alper, C. A., Boenisch, T., et al.: Genetic polymorphism in human glycine-rich beta-glycoprotein. J. Exp. Med. 135:68, 1972.

119. Müller-Eberhard, H. J., and Götze, O.: C3 proactivator convertase and its mode of action. J. Exp. Med. 135:1003, 1972.

120. Edelman, G. M., Cunningham, B. A., et al.: The covalent structure of an entire γG immunoglobulin molecule. Proc. Natl. Acad. Sci. USA 63:78, 1969.

121. Natvig, J. B., and Kunkel, H. G.: Human immunoglobulins: Classes, subclasses, genetic variants, and idiotypes. Adv. Immunol. 16:1, 1973.

122. Porter, R. R.: Hydrolysis of rabbit γ-globulins and antibodies with crystalline papain. Biochem. J. 73:119, 1959.

123. Franklin, E. C.: Structural units of human 7S gamma globulin. J. Clin. Invest. 39:1933, 1960.

124. Grubb, R., and Laurell, A. B.: Hereditary serological human serum groups. Acta Pathol. Microbiol. Scand. 39:390, 1956.

125. Ropartz, C., Lenoir, J., et al.: Possible origins of the anti-Gm sera. Nature (Lond.) 188:1120, 1960.

126. Litwin, S. D., and Kunkel, H. G.: Genetic factors of human gamma globulin detected by rabbit antisera. Transfusion 6:140, 1966.

127. Kunkel, H. G., Smith, W. K., et al.: Genetic marker of the γA2 subgroup of γA immunoglobulins. Nature (Lond.) 223:1247, 1969.

128. Kunkel, H. G., Yount, W. J., et al.: Genetically determined antigen of the Ne subgroup of gamma globulin: Detection by precipitin analysis. Science 154:1041, 1966.

129. Natvig, J. B., and Kunkel, H. G.: Genetic markers of human immunoglobulins. The Gm and Inv systems. Ser. Haematol. 1:66, 1968.

130. Giblett, E. R.: Genetic Markers in Human Blood. Oxford, Blackwell Scientific Publications, 1969, p. 3.

131. Natvig, J. B., Kunkel, H. G., et al.: Genetic studies on the heavy chain subgroups of gamma G globulin, In Gamma Globulins. Killander, J. (ed.), Nobel Symp. 3. New York, Interscience Publishers, 1967, p. 313.

132. Yount, W. J., Kunkel, H. G., et al.: Studies of the Vi (γ2c) subgroup of γ-globulin. A relationship between concentration and genetic type among normal individuals. J. Exp. Med. 125:177, 1967.

133. Fudenberg, H. H., and Fudenberg, B. R.: Antibody to hereditary human γ-globulin (Gm) factor resulting from maternal-fetal incompatibility. Science 145:170, 1964.

134. Fudenberg, H. H., Pink, J. R. L., et al.: Basic Immunogenetics. New York, Oxford University Press, 1972, p. 48.

135. Gedde-Dahl, T., Jr., Fagerhol, M. K., et al.: Au-

tosomal linkage between the *Gm* and *Pi* loci in man. Ann. Hum. Genet. 35:393, 1972.

136. Cleve, H.: Genetic studies on the deficiency of β_2-glycoprotein I of human serum. Humangenetik 5:295, 1968.

137. Rosen, F. S., Alper, C. A., et al.: Genetically determined heterogeneity of the C1 esterase inhibitor in patients with hereditary angioneurotic edema. J. Clin. Invest. 50:2143, 1971.

138. Klemperer, M. R., Woodworth, H. C., et al.: Hereditary deficiency of the second component of complement (C'2) in man. J. Clin. Invest. 45:880, 1966.

139. Leddy, J. P., Frank, M. M., et al.: Hereditary deficiency of the sixth component of complement (C6) in man. J. Clin. Invest. 52:50a, 1973.

140. Boyer, T.: Personal communication.

141. Agnello, V., DeBracco, M. M., et al.: Hereditary C2 deficiency with some manifestations of systemic lupus erythematosus. J. Immunol. 108:837, 1972.

142. Alper, C. A., Hobart, M. J., et al.: Polymorphism of the 6th component of complement, In *Electrofocusing*. Arbuthnott, J. (ed.), Edinburgh, Blackwell, 1974 (in press).

143. Rosenfeld, S. I., Ruddy, S., et al.: Structural polymorphism of the fourth component of human complement. J. Clin. Invest. 48:2283, 1969.

144. Giblett, E. R.: *Genetic Markers in Human Blood.* Oxford, Blackwell Scientific Publications, 1969.

145. Harris, H.: The principles of human biochemical genetics. New York, American Elsevier, 1970.

146. Grzeschik, K. H.: Utilization of somatic cell hybrids for genetics studies in man. Humangenetik 19:1, 1973.

147. Harris, H., and Hopkinson, D. A.: Average heterozygosity per locus in man: An estimate based on the incidence of enzyme polymorphisms. Ann. Hum. Genet. 36:9, 1972.

148. Ruddle, F. H.: Linkage analysis in man by somatic cell genetics. Nature (Lond.) 242:165, 1973.

149. Ruddle, F. H.: Linkage analysis using somatic cell hybrids, In *Advances in Human Genetics.* Vol. 3. Harris, H., and Hirschhorn, K. (eds.), New York, Plenum Press, 1972.

150. Valentine, W. N., Tanaka, K. R., et al.: Erythrocyte acid phosphatase in health and disease. Am. J. Clin. Pathol. 36:328, 1961.

151. Oski, F. A., Shahidi, N. T., et al.: Erythrocyte acid phosphomonoesterase and glucose-6-phosphatase dehydrogenase deficiency in Caucasians. Science 139:409, 1963.

152. Choremis, C., Kattamis, C., et al.: Erythrocyte acid phosphomonoesterase in glucose-6-phosphate dehydrogenase deficient Greeks. Lancet 1:108, 1964.

153. Scheltini, F., Meloni, T., et al.: Red cell acid phosphatase in normal and G6PD-deficient Sardinian subjects. Acta Haematol. (Basel) 33:230, 1965.

154. Jacob, H. S., Ingbar, S. H., et al.: Oxidative hemolysis and erythrocyte metabolism in hereditary acatalasia. J. Clin. Invest. 44:1187, 1965.

155. Bütter, R., Frei, J., et al.: Observations in two Swiss families with acatalasia. Enzymol. Biol. Clin. (Basel) 2:1, 1963.

156. Takahara, S.: Progressive oral gangrene probably due to lack of catalase in the blood (acatalasemia), report of nine cases. Lancet 2:1101, 1952.

157. Aebi, H., and Cantz, M.: Über die celluläre Verteilung der Katalase im Blut homozygoter und heterozygoter Defektträger (Akatalasie). Humangenetik 3:50, 1966.

158. Matsubara, S., Suter, H., et al.: Fractionation of erythrocyte catalase from normal, hypocatalatic and acatalatic humans. Humangenetik 4:29, 1967.

159. Bondy, P. K.: Disorders of carbohydrate metabolism. In *Duncan's Diseases of Metabolism.* 7th ed. Bondy, P. K., and Rosenberg, M. D. (eds.), Philadelphia, W. B. Saunders Co., 1974, p. 221.

160. Beutler, E., and Baluda, M. C.: A simple spot screening test for galactosemia. J. Lab. Clin. Med. 68:137, 1966.

161. Beutler, E., Baluda, M., et al.: The genetics of galactose-1-phosphate uridyl transferase deficiency. J. Lab. Clin. Med. 68:646, 1966.

162. Edwards, Y. H., Hopkinson, D. A., et al.: Adenosine deaminase isozymes in human tissues. Ann. Hum. Genet. 35:207, 1971.

163. Spencer, N., Hopkinson, D. A., et al.: Adenosine deaminase polymorphism in man. Ann. Hum. Genet. 32:9, 1968.

164. Hopkinson, D. A., and Harris, H.: The investigation of reactive sulfhydryls in enzymes and their variants by starch gel electrophoresis. Studies on red cell adenosine deaminase. Ann. Hum. Genet. 33:81, 1969.

165. Giblett, E. R., Anderson, J. E., et al.: Adenosine-deaminase deficiency in two patients with severely impaired cellular immunity. Lancet 2:1067, 1972.

166. Hirschhorn, R., Parkman, R., et al.: Unpublished observations.

167. Green, H., and Chan, T. S.: Pyrimidine starvation induced by adenosine in fibroblasts and lymphoid cells: Role of adenosine deaminase. Science 182:836, 1973.

168. Kissmeyer-Nielsen, F., and Thorsby, E.: *Human Transplantation Antigens.* Copenhagen, Munksgaard, 1970.

169. Terasaki, P., and McClelland, S. D.: Microdroplet assay of human serum cytotoxins. Nature (Lond.) 204:998, 1964.

170. Bach, F. H., and Kirschhorn, K.: Lymphocyte interaction: A potential *in vitro* histocompatibility test. Science 143:813, 1964.

171. Eijsvoogel, V. P., van Rood, J. J., et al.: Position of a locus determining mixed lymphocyte reaction distinct from the known HL-A loci. Eur. J. Immunol. 2:413, 1972.

172. Svejgaard, A., Thorsby, E., et al.: Genetics of the HL-A system. A population and family study. Vox Sang. 18:97, 1970.

173. Grey, H. M., Kubo, R. T., et al.: The small subunit of HL-A antigens is B_2-microglobulin. J. Exp. Med. 138:1608, 1973.

174. Harris, R., and Zervas, J. D.: Reticulocyte HL-A antigens. Nature (Lond.) 221:1062, 1969.

175. Eijsvoogel, V. P., du Bois, M. J. G. J., et al.: Position of a locus determining mixed lymphocyte reaction (MLR), distinct from known HL-A loci, and its relation to cell-mediated lympholysis (CMC), In *Histocompatibility Testing*. Dausset, J., and Colombani, J. (eds.), Copenhagen, Munksgaard, 1973, pp. 501–508.

176. Mempel, W., Grosse-Wilde, H., et al.: Identity for the strong MLC-locus in HL-A different unrelated pairs. Blut 27:336, 1973.

177. Koch, C., Henriksen, K., et al.: Bone marrow transplantation from an HL-A non-identical but mixed lymphocyte-culture identical donor. Lancet 1:1146, 1973.

178. Parkman, R., and Rosen, F. S.: Unpublished observations.

179. Lammus, L. U., Svejgaard, A., et al.: PGM$_3$:HL-A is another linkage in man. Nature [New Biol.] 231:109, 1971.

179a. Jongsma, A., van Someran, H., et al.: Localization of genes in human chromosomes by studies of human–chinese hamster somatic cell hybrids. Humangenetik 20:195, 1973.

180. White, S. H., Newcome, V. D., et al.: Distribution of HL-A antigen frequency in psoriasis. New Engl. J. Med. 287 :740, 1972.

181. Schlosstein, L., Terasaki, P. I., et al.: High association of an HL-A antigen, W27, with ankylosing spondylitis. New Engl. J. Med. 288: 704, 1973.

182. Stokes, P. L., Asquith, P., et al.: Histocompatibility antigens associated with adult coeliac disease. Lancet 2:162, 1972.

183. Mackay, I. R., and Morris, P. J.: Association of autoimmune active chronic hepatitis with HL-A1,8. Lancet 2:793, 1972.

184. White, S. H., Newcome, V. D., et al.: Disturbance of HL-A antigen frequency in psoriasis. New Engl. J. Med. 287:740, 1972.

185. Jersild, G., Hansen, G. S., et al.: Histocompatibility determinants in multiple sclerosis, with special reference to clinical course. Lancet 2:1221, 1973.

186. Ruddle, F. H., and Kucherlapati, R. S.: Hybrid cells and human genes. Sci. Amer. 231:36, 1974.

VI

BLOOD TRANSFUSION THERAPY

Chapter 28

Red Cell Transfusion and Phlebotomy

by Frank A. Oski

When one ponders the uses and abuses of transfusion therapy, the words of Woody Hayes, the successful head football coach of Ohio State University, are worthy of recall for the purpose of paraphrasing. When Hayes was asked to explain his seeming overreliance on a rushing attack as the foundation of his football offense, he remarked, "When you throw a pass three things can happen, and only one of them is good." Similarly, when a patient is transfused, many things can happen, and only one of them is good. The transfusion of blood and blood products is like all other forms of medical therapy, and thus the clinician, in making a decision, should be thoroughly aware of the indications, contraindications, and undesirable side effects of his chosen course of action.

INDICATIONS FOR TRANSFUSION

There are three primary types of clinical situations in which transfusion therapy is indicated. They are:

1. The maintenance or restoration of an adequate circulating blood volume to prevent or combat shock.

2. The replacement of a specific blood component, such as a plasma protein or a formed blood element (erythrocytes, leukocytes, or platelets), because its deficiency has produced or is likely to produce adverse clinical manifestations.

3. The removal of harmful substances by exchange transfusion.

In this discussion, attention will be focused on the use of whole blood or red cell preparations and their storage and survival characteristics. For a lucid and more detailed presentation of this material, the reader should consult Mollison's text, *Blood Transfusion in Clinical Medicine* (1).

Acute Hemorrhage

The acute loss of 10 per cent of the circulating blood volume is not generally associated with any significant alterations in the circulation. A hemorrhage resulting in a 20 per cent decrease in the blood volume will not produce a decrease in blood pressure in the supine patient (2). When the blood volume has been reduced by 30 to 40 per cent, clinical evidence of shock will be observable in most patients (3). This will be reflected by a fall in right auricular pressure (central venous pressure), decreased cardiac output, a fall in arterial pressure, an increase in heart rate, and constriction of the veins and venules primarily in the skin, muscles, kidney, and gastrointestinal tract. Symptoms and signs include pallor, sweating, thirst, light-headedness, restlessness, and air hunger. One of the more reliable signs of peripheral vasoconstriction is the temperature of the nose; if a patient lying in a reasonably warm room has a cold nose, then circulatory failure should be strongly suspected.

A useful guide to the volume of blood loss in acute hemorrhage is the systolic blood pressure. In an adult, if this is below 100 mm. Hg, the blood volume is probably less than 70 per cent of normal (4). Other standards must be applied in infants and children. A guide for suspecting a hemorrhage of 30 per cent or more of the blood volume for children under 4 years of age is a systolic blood pressure of less than 65 mm. Hg; for children 5 to 8 years of age, 75 mm. Hg; for children 9 to 12 years of age, 85 mm. Hg; and for children 13 to 16 years of age, a systolic pressure of less than 90 mm. Hg.

The blood volume of premature infants is approximately 105 ml. per kg. (5), while in the term infant the blood volume is close to 85 ml. per kg. (6). By 3 months of age, the blood volume is similar to that of the normal adult, 70 to 75 ml. per kg.

The pulse rate is a less reliable guide than the blood pressure as an indicator of the magnitude of a hemorrhage. In general, a persistent pulse rate of over 100 per minute in an adult is associated with a 20 per cent reduction in blood volume. Standards for infants and children are close to the following: newborn, greater than 170 per minute; 1 to 11 months, greater than 160 per minute; 1 to 2 years, greater than 130 per minute; 2 to 6 years, greater than 120 per minute; 6 to 10 years of age, greater than 110 per minute.

Estimation of the hemoglobin level is not a reliable indication of the extent of hemorrhage. A period of 24 to 36 hours may elapse before the plasma volume is restored to normal and sufficient hemodilution has occurred to reflect the extent of blood loss. Even after the loss of 10 per cent of the blood volume, only one-half the decrease has been replaced at the end of 24 hours (7). A reduced hemoglobin or hematocrit within three to six hours of hemorrhage suggests a blood loss of greater than 20 to 25 per cent of the blood volume, while a normal hemoglobin level six hours after a hemorrhage suggests that the blood loss has not been substantial. In patients in shock or preshock, hemoglobin determinations must be performed on central venous blood. Capillary samples from vasoconstricted extremities will result in falsely elevated hemoglobin or hematocrit determinations as a consequence of stasis and hemoconcentration.

Treatment of Acute Blood Loss

When the history and physical examination indicate that the patient has sustained a significant acute loss of blood, then replacement therapy with whole blood, colloid, or saline is indicated. When the loss of blood is less than 20 per cent of the blood volume, but may reoccur, then transfusion is also justified. In such circumstances, blood of any storage age is suitable. When the amount of blood to be transfused in a period of 24 hours is equal to or greater than the patient's blood volume, then the age of the transfused blood becomes important in terms of the alterations in coagulation factors, platelets, and oxygen transport mechanisms it may produce. Blood stored for periods in excess of 48 hours lacks adequate numbers of functional platelets and has insufficient quantities of Factor VIII (8). The use of specific component therapy rather than reliance on fresh whole blood is an effective means of managing coagulation disturbances produced by massive transfusions of whole blood. The problems produced by 2,3-diphosphoglycerate-depleted blood will be discussed in a later section of the chapter.

When whole blood is not immediately available, then plasma, "plasma protein solutions" (9), or saline may be used to restore the blood volume. The infusion of a volume of saline equal to the volume of blood lost will not restore the blood volume, but infusions of much greater quantities can effectively restore the circulation to normal. Pruitt and co-workers (7) bled five subjects 20 per cent of their blood volume and replaced it with buffered saline. The amount infused was equal to: (the volume of red cells removed × 4) + (the volume of plasma removed × 1.3). No significant reduction in the subject's blood volume was observed immediately after the infusion or at 24 hours after the bleed.

Transfusions following hemorrhage should be administered until the central venous pressure has been restored to normal or, if such information is not available, until the blood pressure and pulse have returned to a satisfactory level and the signs of peripheral vascular insufficiency have disappeared. The infusions initially may be administered rapidly. In adults in shock, the acute infusion of 500 ml. in a period of three to four minutes produces no difficulty.

Treatment of Anemia

Packed red cells should be used in all situations in which only a red cell mass deficit exists. This is the usual situation in most patients with chronic anemia. Whole blood should be reserved for those clinical situations characterized by hypovolemia that is accompanied by signs of circulatory insufficiency. Table 28–1 describes what the patient will receive when either whole blood or packed cells are administered from blood stored in acid-citrate-dextrose for a period of 21 days. The adverse effects of whole blood include the unnecessary increase in the intravascular volume, the presence of potentially antigenic plasma proteins, and the administration of large quantities of potassium, sodium, ammonia, and citrate. It has been estimated that 80 to 90 per cent of all transfusions administered in the United States should be in the form of packed red blood cells (10).

The rapid correction of red cell mass deficits, i.e., anemia, is rarely necessary at hemoglobin levels above 6 g. per 100 ml. Increases in cardiac output (11) or elevations in the blood lactate to pyruvate ratio (12) rarely are observed in adults at rest until the hemoglobin concentration falls below 6 g. per 100 ml. In the absence of physical stress or associated pulmonary or cardiac disease, most patients can tolerate hemoglobin values of 3 to 6 g. per 100 ml. without developing signs of congestive heart failure.

The decision to transfuse an anemic pa-

TABLE 28–1. COMPARISON OF WHAT IS ADMINISTERED WHEN WHOLE BLOOD OR PACKED CELLS ARE ADMINISTERED (21-DAY STORAGE)

	WHOLE BLOOD	PACKED RED BLOOD CELLS
Volume	517.5 ml.	300 ml.
Red blood cell mass	200.0 ml.	200 ml.
Citrate	67.5 ml.	22 ml.
Plasma	250.0 ml.	78 ml.
Albumin	12.50 g.	4 g.
Globulin	6.25 g.	2 g.
Total protein	48.75 g.	36 g.
Hemoglobin	30.00 g.	30 g.
Hematocrit	39%	70%
Plasma sodium	45 mEq.	15 mEq.
Plasma potassium	15 mEq.	4 mEq.
Plasma acid (citric-lactic) pH 6.6	80 nanoEq.	25 nanoEq.
Plasma ammonia	2159 μg.	680 μg.
Protein antigens	Maximal	Minimal
Protein antibodies	Maximal	Minimal

tient should not be made on the basis of the hemoglobin concentration alone, but should include an assessment of the patient's cardiac and pulmonary status, his level of physical activity, and the prospects of correcting the anemia with hematinic agents, such as iron, folic acid, or vitamin B_{12}. Patients with iron deficiency, the most common form of severe anemia in childhood, rarely will require a transfusion.

When, in the judgment of the physician, a transfusion is required, the amount of packed red cells to be administered can be determined by formula No. 1 (see below). This formula can be further simplified by assuming that the patient's blood volume is approximately 75 ml. per kg., and that the concentration of hemoglobin within the packed cells is 22 to 24 g. per 100 ml. The formula will be formula No. 2. Another popular formula, based on the same principles, employs the hematocrit and is formula No. 3.

$$\text{(1)} \quad \text{volume of cells} = \frac{\text{patient's weight (kg.)} \times \text{blood volume (ml./kg.)} \times (\text{Hb desired} - \text{Hb observed})}{\text{hemoglobin concentration of packed cells (g./100 ml.)}}$$

$$\text{(2)} \quad \text{volume of cells} = \frac{\text{patient's weight (kg.)} \times 75 \times (\text{Hb desired} - \text{Hb observed})}{24}$$

$$\text{(3)} \quad \text{volume of cells} = \text{patient's weight (kg.)} \times \text{increment in Hct desired}$$

When packed red cells are administered to an anemic patient in incipient heart failure, their rate of administration should not exceed 2 ml. per kg. per hour (13). The administration of ethacrynic acid or furosemide, rapidly acting diuretic agents, prior to the transfusion is a valuable means of decreasing the chances of producing circulatory overload. Ethacrynic acid should never be added to the red cell suspension, since it is a potentially hemolytic agent (14).

In severely anemic patients in frank congestive heart failure, exchange transfusion with packed red cell suspensions has been demonstrated to be an effective means of both correcting anemia and improving the cardiac status (15). The use of ethacrynic acid followed by packed red cell transfusion has been shown to be equally effective (16). The choice of exchange transfusion or diuretic plus simple transfusion is generally determined by the urgency of the situation. In patients requiring emergency surgery, the use of exchange transfusion will decrease the waiting time to operation.

Removal of Harmful Substances

In the newborn, exchange transfusions are employed for the removal of bilirubin and sensitized cells in infants with hemolytic disease, in the treatment of isoimmune neonatal thrombocytopenia, in the treatment of neonates with disseminated intravascular coagulation (17), and in an attempt to improve oxygen unloading in the infant of very low birth weight (18).

With the exception of its proven value in the treatment of hyperbilirubinemia, the other uses of exchange transfusion during this period of life must still be considered experimental. The techniques, hazards, and choice of blood for exchange transfusion in infants with red cell isoimmunization are described in Chapter 9.

In older infants and children, exchange transfusion has been utilized in the management of poisonings with nondialyzable substances, for the removal of inhibitors in patients with hemophilia, for the treatment of the painful crisis of sickle cell anemia, for the management of cerebral occlusions in patients with sickle cell anemia (19), and as an adjunct to the treatment of patients with acute hepatic failure from a variety of causes, including Reye's syndrome.

In such circumstances, a two-blood-volume exchange transfusion should be employed to effectively cleanse 90 per cent of the circulation. The blood used should be as fresh as possible and not over five days of age.

PARTIAL EXCHANGE TRANSFUSION IN POLYCYTHEMIC STATES

Partial exchange transfusion is a useful technique for the management of patients with an increased red cell mass that has produced hyperviscosity of the blood and associated symptoms. In pediatric patients, such polycythemia is rarely encountered except in the newborn period and in children with various forms of cyanotic heart disease.

Blood viscosity varies very little with hematocrit over the range of 0 to 40 per cent (20). The relative increase in viscosity at a hematocrit of 50 per cent, as compared to that of 25 per cent, is insignificant in the circulation. In regions in the circulation where cell-cell interaction is important, shear rates are high, and cells do not aggregate, while in regions of low shear rate, cell-cell interaction is minimal. Once the hematocrit rises above 50 per cent, the viscosity begins to rise rapidly, and at a hematocrit of 60 per cent, it is four times greater than at a hematocrit of 40 per cent.

During the first week of life, a venous hemoglobin value of 22.0 g. per 100 ml. or greater, or a venous hematocrit of more than 65 per cent, should be regarded as polycythemia. Other conditions that may cause or be associated with polycythemia are listed in Table 28–2. The symptoms observed in such infants appear to be primarily a consequence of the associated increase in blood viscosity produced by the high hematocrit, although some of these infants have rigid red cells which will produce a greater than expected viscosity at any given hematocrit reading (21).

Respiratory distress, cyanosis, congestive heart failure, convulsions, priapism, jaundice, thrombocytopenia, renal vein throm-

TABLE 28–2. NEONATAL POLYCYTHEMIA

May be caused by placental hypertransfusion:
  Twin to twin transfusion
  Maternal-fetal transfusion
  Delayed cord clamping
    Intentional
    Unassisted home delivery

May be associated with:
  Placental insufficiency
    Infants small for gestational age
    Postmaturity
    Toxemia of pregnancy
    Placenta praevia
  Endocrine and metabolic disorders
    Congenital adrenal hyperplasia
    Neonatal thyrotoxicosis
    Maternal diabetes
  Miscellaneous
    Down's syndrome
    Hyperplastic visceromegaly (Beckwith's syndrome)

bosis, hypoglycemia, and hypocalcemia all appear to be more common among infants with polycythemia, although many infants with polycythemia are asymptomatic.

It still remains unclear if efforts should be made to reduce the hematocrit in infants who are asymptomatic. Treatment of infants with symptoms should be designed to reduce the venous hematocrit to less than 60 per cent. This can be readily accomplished by the performance of a partial exchange transfusion, using fresh frozen plasma. The formula shown below may be employed to approximate the volume of exchange required to reduce the hematocrit to the desired level.

Unless the infant can be demonstrated to be hypervolemic, simple phlebotomy should not be performed to reduce the hematocrit. Most of these infants have a reduced cardiac output as a consequence of their hyperviscosity, and further reduction in blood volume may, in fact, aggravate the symptoms (22).

In patients with cyanotic heart disease, polycythemia, if severe, may be a liability and produce undesired physiologic effects. Clinical manifestations may include headaches, irritability, anorexia, and excessive dyspnea. Although thrombotic lesions are found in patients with cyanotic heart disease, particularly in the vessels of the central nervous system, they appear to be more common among children with iron deficiency and high hematocrits rather than a consequence of polycythemia alone (23, 24). Iron deficiency should always be treated in such patients. Alterations in red cell indices, particularly in the mean corpuscular volume (MCV), serve as an excellent clue to the presence of iron deficiency complicating polycythemia.

In the patient with cyanotic heart disease and symptomatic polycythemia, cautious attempts at partial exchange transfusion should be employed using the formula described above. Reduction of high hematocrits in such patients can be expected to produce a decrease in peripheral vascular resistance and increases in stroke volume, systemic blood flow, and oxygen transport (25). Acute phlebotomy without fluid replacement can result in reduced stroke volume and systemic blood flow, and may lead to vascular collapse, seizures, and cerebral vascular occlusions. Reduction of hematocrit in polycythemic patients with cyanotic heart disease may also improve associated coagulation abnormalities (26), since consumption of clotting factors is sometimes associated with the high viscosity state.

HAZARDS OF TRANSFUSION THERAPY

The use of blood or blood products carries a significant risk to the recipient. It has been estimated that approximately 5 per cent of all transfusions administered to adults are associated with some form of adverse reaction. Studies conducted at the Boston Children's Hospital Medical Center have demonstrated an incidence of 1.7 per cent. The use of erythrocytes or other specific components rather than whole blood

$$\text{volume of exchange (ml.)} = \frac{\text{blood volume} \times (\text{observed Hct} - \text{desired Hct})}{\text{observed Hct}}$$

(assume a blood volume of 100 ml. per kg.)

will reduce the number of undesirable side effects.

The adverse effects may be immediate and include hemolytic transfusion reactions, febrile reactions, allergic reactions, infections from bacterial contamination, air embolism, and circulatory overload. The adverse effects that are delayed in their appearance include the delayed hemolytic reaction, isoimmunization to both cellular and plasma antigens, hemosiderosis, and the transmission of diseases such as hepatitis, cytomegalovirus disease, and malaria. No statistics are currently available as to the true incidence of delayed undesirable side effects, but it may be as high as 10 per cent in situations in which blood is obtained from commercial donors.

Hemolytic Reaction

A hemolytic transfusion reaction can be defined as the occurrence of clinical and laboratory signs of red cell destruction following transfusion. Antibodies which are hemolytic in vitro characteristically bring about intravascular destruction, with consequent rupture of red cells within the blood stream and liberation of hemoglobin. Those antibodies which are nonhemolytic in vitro bring about destruction which is predominantly extravascular, but the process is characteristically accompanied by some degree of hemoglobinemia.

The administration of group-incompatible blood or contaminated blood is usually associated with the onset of symptoms before much blood has been introduced, and, if the transfusion is stopped, no serious harm may result. The symptoms observed include restlessness, anxiety, flushing of the face, precordial oppression and pain, an increase in pulse and respiratory rate, generalized tingling sensations, and pain in the back and thighs. Nausea and vomiting may follow and cyanosis; shock with cold, clammy skin; coma; and a failing pulse may develop. A chill, followed by a rise of temperature to 105°F or higher, and possibly delirium may ensue.

A hemorrhagic tendency due to intravascular coagulation may develop within minutes after the transfusion of incompatible blood. As noted previously, hemoglobi-

nemia can be detected by examining the plasma, followed by jaundice, hemoglobinuria, oliguria, or even anuria.

The management of such reactions is governed by the patient's condition. Since shock may be an important factor in the development of renal shutdown, hypovolemia must be prevented. The rapid infusion of mannitol (1.5 to 2.0 g. per kg.) has been recommended as a means of maintaining renal blood flow and glomerular filtration. If intravascular coagulation is present, the judicious use of heparin therapy is warranted.

Alkalinization of the urine has always been recommended, based upon animal studies which have demonstrated that precipitation of heme pigments in the kidney is favored by an acid reaction. This procedure is of little value once the kidneys have been injured, since renal ischemia rather than pigment precipitation is the etiologic factor in renal failure. The management of renal insufficiency in this situation is the same as that for renal failure of other etiologies.

Allergic Reactions

These are relatively frequent but seldom serious. They are characterized by urticaria, pruritus, diffuse rash, and occasionally facial and periorbital edema. After they develop, parenteral antihistamine should be administered. Parenteral steroids or epinephrine or both is the treatment of choice if laryngospasm is present. In known reactors, antihistamines may be given orally or parenterally prior to transfusion, but under no circumstances should they be injected into the unit of blood.

Plasma Reactions

Plasma protein reactions have been identified in patients with antibodies to the immunoglobulin IgA. These reactions are severe and striking. They resemble anaphylaxis, with flushing, abdominal pain, diarrhea, chills, and fever. These patients can be transfused with blood that is washed by a continuous flow process or that has been previously frozen.

Febrile (Nonhemolytic) Reactions

This type of reaction has an incidence of 0.08 per cent in children who have not been previously transfused, and 3.8 per cent in the multitransfused recipient. The signs and symptoms may vary from mild chilliness and slight temperature elevation to severe chills and higher fever. There may also be muscle aches and pains, flushing, nausea, and vomiting. This reaction often cannot be distinguished from a hemolytic reaction, except that there is no hemoglobinemia or hemoglobinuria. It has been attributed to bacterial pyrogens, plasma sensitivity, citrate sensitivity, circulatory overload, and white cell antibodies. The latter etiology is the only one that has been confirmed by clinical and laboratory findings. As noted in a previous section, the patient should be evaluated for leukoagglutinins and treated with leukocyte-poor blood.

References

1. Mollison, P. L.: *Blood Transfusion in Clinical Medicine.* 5th ed. Oxford, Blackwell Scientific Publications, 1972.
2. Wallace, J., and Sharpey-Schafer, E. P.: Blood changes following controlled hemorrhage in man. Lancet 2:393, 1941.
3. Howorth, S., and Sharpey-Schafer, E. P.: Low blood pressure phases following haemorrhage. Lancet 1:19, 1947.
4. Grant, R. T., and Reeve, E. B.: Observations on the general effects of injury in man, with special reference to wound shock. Spec. Rep. Ser. Med. Res. Coun. (Lond.), No. 277, 1951.
5. Sisson, T. R. C., Lund, C. J., et al.: The blood volume of infants. J. Pediatr. 55:163, 1959.
6. Usher, R., Shepard, M., et al.: The blood volume of the newborn infant and placental transfusion. Acta Paediatr. 52:497, 1963.
7. Pruitt, B. A., Moncrief, J. A., et al.: Effect of buffered saline solution upon the blood volume of man after acute measured hemorrhage. Annual Res. Progr. Report, U.S. Army Surgical Research Unit, Texas, 1965.
8. Preston, A. E.: The Factor VIII activity in fresh and stored plasma. Br. J. Haematol. 13:42, 1967.
9. Ricketts, C. R.: Molecular composition of transfusion dextran. Br. Med. J. 2:1423, 1966.
10. Greenwalt, T. J.: Can current transfusion practices be improved? Med. Counterpoint 1:6, 1969.
11. Whitaker, W.: Some effects of severe chronic anemia on the circulatory system. Quart. J. Med. 25:175, 1956.
12. Siebert, D. J., and Ebaugh, F. G., Jr.: Assessment of tissue anoxemia in chronic anemia by the arterial lactate/pyruvate ratio and excess lactate formation. J. Lab. Clin. Med. 69:177, 1967.
13. Duke, M., Herbert, V. D., et al.: Hemodynamic effects of blood transfusion in chronic anemia. New Engl. J. Med. 271:975, 1964.
14. Lieberman, J., and Kaneshiro, W.: Ethacrynic acid with packed red cells. Lancet 1:911, 1971.
15. Fullerton, W. J., and Turner, A. G.: Exchange transfusion in treatment of severe anaemia in pregnancy. Lancet 1:75, 1962.
16. Harrison, K. A., Ajabor, L. N., et al.: Ethacrynic acid and packed-blood-cell transfusion in the treatment of severe anaemia in pregnancy. Lancet 1:11, 1971.
17. Delivoria-Papadopoulos, M., Miller, L. D., et al.: Effect of exchange transfusion on altering mortality in: (1) infants weighing less than 1250 grams at birth and (2) infants with severe respiratory distress (RDS). Pediatr. Res. 7:63, 1973.
18. De Lemos, R. A., McLaughlin, G. W., et al.: Abnormal partial thromboplastin time and survival in respiratory distress syndrome: Effect of exchange transfusion. Pediatr. Res. 7:168, 1973.
19. Stockman, J. A., Nigro, M. A., et al.: Occlusion of large cerebral vessels in patients with sickle cell anemia. New Engl. J. Med. 287:846, 1972.
20. Merrill, E. W.: Rheology of the blood. Physiol. Rev. 49:863, 1969.
21. Gross, G. P., Hathaway, W. E., et al.: Hyperviscosity in the neonate. J. Pediatr. 82:1004, 1974.
22. Gersony, W. M.: Persistence of the fetal circulation: A commentary. J. Pediatr. 82:1103, 1973.
23. Martelle, R. R., and Linde, L. M.: Cerebrovascular accidents with tetralogy of Fallot. Am. J. Dis. Child. 101:206, 1961.
24. Rudolph, A. M., Nadas, A. S., et al.: Hematologic adjustments to cyanotic congenital heart disease. Pediatrics 11:454, 1953.
25. Rosenthal, A., Nathan, D. G., et al.: Acute hemodynamic effects of red cell volume reduction in polycythemia of cyanotic congenital heart disease. Circulation 42:297, 1970.
26. Ikenacho, H. N. C., Fletcher, D. J., et al.: Consumption coagulopathy in congenital heart disease. Lancet 1:231, 1973.

Chapter 29

The Storage of Erythrocytes

by Sherwin V. Kevy

ANTICOAGULANT SOLUTIONS

Blood must be stored at a temperature in the range of 1° to 6°C. At this temperature, the rate of glycolysis is 40 times slower than it is at 37°C. Despite this reduction in the rate of glycolysis, sufficient lactic acid is produced to cause a progressive fall in pH which interferes with enzyme function halting glycolysis. There is also a progressive loss of red cell viability throughout this period, with an associated decline in the concentrations of red cell adenosine triphosphate (ATP) and 2,3-diphosphoglycerate (2,3-DPG).

Acid Citrate Dextrose (ACD) and Citrate Phosphate Dextrose (CPD)

The first advancement in preservative solutions occurred in 1943 when Loutit and Mollison published their work demonstrating the superiority of ACD solutions over sodium citrate for the preservation of whole blood (1). This became the universal anticoagulant until the late 1960's. In recent years, CPD has replaced ACD as the most commonly used anticoagulant for the preservation of whole blood in the liquid state, although the latter is still more widely used in plasmapheresis systems. The components of the two solutions are described in Table 29–1. Citrate phosphate dextrose solution has a higher pH, 20 per cent less citrate, and is virtually isotonic as compared with ACD. The relative hypotonicity of ACD is responsible for damage to the red cells during the first 100 ml. of collection during an ordinary donation. This has been termed the "lesion of collection" by Gibson et al. (2).

As shown in Table 29–2, whole blood collected in CPD has a higher pH on the 21st day of storage than ACD on the 7th day, and a slightly lower potassium on the 14th day as compared with ACD on the 7th day of storage.

The first clinical criterion of a well-preserved unit of blood is autologous in vivo

TABLE 29–1.   A COMPARISON OF ACD AND CPD SOLUTIONS

ACD Solution	CPD Solution
67.5 ml. of solution for the collection of 450 ml. of blood	63.0 ml. of solution for the collection of 450 ml. of blood
Each 67.5 ml. contains 540 mg. citric acid (hydrous)	Each 63.0 ml. contains 206 mg. citric acid (hydrous)
1.49 g. sodium citrate (hydrous)	1.66 g. sodium citrate (hydrous)
1.65 g. dextrose (hydrous)	140 mg. sodium biphosphate
	1.61 g. dextrose (hydrous)

TABLE 29–2. A COMPARISON OF BIOCHEMICAL PARAMETERS OF ACD AND CPD BLOOD STORED AT 1–6°C*

Days Stored	0	7	14	21	28
			pH		
ACD	7.00	6.79	6.73	6.71	6.71
CPD	7.20	7.00	6.89	6.84	6.78
		Potassium (mEq./l.)			
ACD	10	22	33	47	72
CPD	4	10	21	30	40
		Inorganic Phosphate (mM/L.)			
ACD	0.6	1.5	2.2	3.0	3.4
CPD	3.6	3.6	4.2	4.9	5.5
		2,3-DPG (μM/g. Hgb.)			
ACD	12.8	9.1	4.12	1.7	1.0
CPD	13.2	14.1	9.8	3.2	1.2
		ATP (μM/g. Hgb.)			
ACD	3.9	3.8	3.5	2.5	1.2
CPD	4.1	3.9	3.7	3.1	2.9

*Findings represent average values obtained by analysis of 20 units.

survival of the red cell. Standards have been set forth by the National Research Council and adopted by the Food and Drug Administration Bureau of Biologics for blood collected in plastic blood packs. This requires that in three of four infusions, at least 70 per cent of the infused cells must be present in the circulation 24 hours post transfusion and display normal survival characteristics. If this criterion is not met, six additional survivals must be done, and the average of ten survivals must be 70 per cent or greater, with any values more than two standard deviations from the mean disregarded. Several comparisons have been published of the post-transfusion survival of the red cells stored in CPD and ACD. After 21 days of storage as whole blood, Orlina and Josephson found an average survival of 79.4 per cent for red cells stored in CPD, as compared with 74.8 per cent for red cells preserved in ACD (3). Button has shown an average survival of 82.0 ± 8.1 per cent at 21 days for CPD, and 81.0 ± 7.9 per cent at 21 days for 123 units collected in ACD. The average survival of 130 units of CPD on the 28th day of storage is 75.4 ± 8.9 per cent. Although the latter survival is slightly lower than those originally recorded by Gibson, it suggests that the viability might be slightly better maintained in CPD than ACD (4). The survival of red cells separated by either centrifugation or sedimentation within the first 24 hours of collection and stored as packed red cells (hematocrit 70 per cent) for 21 days is 81.7 per cent in CPD and 82.4 per cent in ACD.

Any dating period, be it 21 days or 28 days, is practical provided that the red cell antigenicity is maintained throughout this period. Utilizing the plastic blood pack system, segments can be made from the donor tubing which provide multiple 0.5-ml. samples of donor blood for use in crossmatching. The anticoagulant present in the segments permits a better preservation of red cells and their antigenicity than is possible with the clotted pilot tube. A comparative study is summarized in Table 29–3.

Comparable titers were obtained in the CPD segments and in the plastic bags; however, the clotted samples were hemolyzed

TABLE 29–3. PRESERVATION OF RED CELL ANTIGENICITY OF CPD BLOOD IN THE PLASTIC PACK AND PLASTIC SEGMENT COMPARED WITH THE CLOTTED PILOT TUBE AFTER VARYING PERIODS OF STORAGE*

Red Cell Antigen	Rh$_o$ (D)					rh' (C)					hr' (c)				
Days Stored	0	7	14	21	28	0	7	14	21	28	0	7	14	21	28
CPD plastic segment	42	42	33	32	26	37	37	32	34	30	39	34	31	25	16
CPD plastic bag	44	37	34	32	27	36	33	36	30	32	38	38	34	27	22
Clotted pilot tube	38	37	27	22	13	36	33	19	17	14	27	22	19	7	0

Red Cell Antigen	Kell					M					P				
Days Stored	0	7	14	21	28	0	7	14	21	28	0	7	14	21	28
CPD plastic segment	30	24	20	16	15	50	45	45	41	38	15	10	8	7	5
CPD plastic bag	24	22	20	19	17	51	49	45	43	41	15	12	10	6	8
Clotted pilot tube	25	18	14	6	0	47	42	34	29	24	12	8	2	0	0

*A numerical scoring system was used rather than the titer of the antiserum with the cells: 4+ = 10; 3+ = 8; 2+ = 5; 1+ = 3; + microscopic = 2. The numbers in the table represent the sum of the degree of agglutination at several dilutions.

and demonstrated marked loss of antigenicity for Kell (K), hr' (c), and P after 14 days. By the 28th day, negative reactions were obtained for these antigens. In contrast, red cells preserved in the segments and in the plastic bag retained a 3+ reaction for Kell, M, rh_0 (D), rh' (C), and hr' (c) with undiluted antiserum. Only in the case of the P antigen did the reactivity with undiluted antiserum diminish to a 2+ reaction in the CPD segments on the 28th day of storage.

In 1965, Kevy et al. (5) compared the serum pH in children massively transfused with blood preserved in CPD and ACD solutions. The duration of storage of these CPD bloods was on the average three days greater than that of the ACD blood. A definite correlation existed between the volume of blood administered in relation to the recipient's blood volume and the depression of serum pH. This trend was more marked in the ACD group, although the size of the sampling did not allow a statistical comparison.

The importance of using a medium for the preservation of whole blood which will maintain a more physiologic pH was not confirmed until several years later, when Chanutin and Curnish (6) and Benesch and Benesch (7) almost simultaneously made the observation that hemoglobin–organic phosphate complexes in red cells play a role in the release of oxygen from HbO_2. In the human, red cell 2,3-DPG and Hb are virtually equimolar. 2,3-DPG lowers the affinity of hemoglobin for oxygen and does so at concentrations commonly found in red cells (see Chapter 13). Akerblom (8) concluded in 1968 that the shift to the left in the oxygen dissociation curve in stored ACD blood, as described by Valtis and Kennedy (9), was owing to the depletion of 2,3-DPG. Red cell 2,3-DPG is much better maintained in CPD than in ACD. This is true not only of whole blood but also of packed cells separated within two hours of collection at a hematocrit of 70 per cent and stored for 21 days. After one week's storage in CPD, the 2,3-DPG content is normal or slightly above normal, whereas in ACD the level has fallen by almost 60 per cent. Dawson (10) not only has confirmed the correlation of 2,3-DPG and P_{50} but also has demonstrated that the favorable effect of CPD is mainly owing to its higher pH.

The direct effect of 2,3-DPG-depleted erythrocytes on metabolism and tissues has not been demonstrated. Present knowledge of tissue oxidation on a molecular basis suggests that oxidation in the mitochondria is not affected, whereas oxidation in the microsomes is probably oxygen-dependent within the relevant tension range. If the diminished oxygen transporting capacity of 2,3-DPG-depleted cells cannot be compensated for by an increase in blood flow, there should be an effect on tissue oxygenation. This effect will persist until in vivo regeneration of 2,3-DPG occurs. Normally, 24 to 36 hours are required for this process to become complete (11, 12).

Heparin

Blood packs are available for the collection of heparinized blood which contain 2250 units of heparin in 30 ml. of buffered isotonic saline. These cells deteriorate rapidly during refrigerator storage owing to the rapid consumption of glucose. The post-transfusion survival is not more than 60 per cent three to five days after collection. Heparinized blood may be salvaged if it is collected into a double pack system which contains ACD or CPD in the secondary unit. The transfer must be made within 24 hours of collection. Post-transfusion survival studies of these converted units have shown that the percentage of viable red cells falls to 70 per cent within 12 days (13). Plasma pH, hemoglobin, and potassium levels were within the same range as those of ACD blood stored for a similar period. The use of heparinized blood in surgery requiring extracorporeal circulation or for exchange transfusions or neonatal transfusions should no longer create an economic or logistic problem to the hospital blood bank. Our present experience indicates that whole blood collected in CPD and stored for as long as five days can be converted to heparinized blood by the addition of 2250 units of heparin followed by 5 ml. of a 10 per cent solution of calcium gluconate. Care must be taken to see that the blood is well mixed by inversion prior to the addition of the calcium. An analysis of over 100 units so converted reveals that the calcium level varies between 10 and 14 mg. per 100 ml.

ACD-Adenine, CPD-Adenine

The addition of adenosine or adenine to the ACD solution is useful in prolonging the storage period of erythrocytes. Fischer and co-workers reported that the addition of small amounts of adenine and guanosine to the inosine substrate was more effective and could prolong the useful storage period of red cells to 42 days (14). Other workers have demonstrated that an inosine-adenine combination was as effective as the inosine-adenine-guanosine formula in regenerating the ATP content of stored erythrocytes (15, 16). Simon (17) has demonstrated that small amounts of adenine (0.5 to 0.75 μM per ml. ACD blood) were more effective than large supplements of inosine in maintaining erythrocyte viability and ATP content. These effects have been confirmed by Swedish investigators who have reported on the effect of transfusion of blood collected in ACD with adenine to over 7000 recipients (18).

The effect of adenine on maintenance of ATP content was further confirmed by Bishop (19) and by Beutler and Duron (20). The survival values obtained by Shields would suggest that adenine could increase the preservative effect of ACD or CPD solution or both for storage periods as long as six weeks (21).

Studies conducted by four investigators indicate that the yield and survival of platelets prepared from purine fortified blood are equal to those of ACD or CPD solution. In vitro studies have demonstrated that this material is as effective as either anticoagulant alone for the preparation of cryoprecipitates. Studies utilizing the segment technique described in the preceding paragraphs have demonstrated that red cell antigenicity has been adequately maintained throughout the periods of storage. At present, this anticoagulant combination is not licensed for use in the United States because of the toxicity studies carried out in laboratory animals. Crystalline deposition in animals massively infused with this material has been identified as 2,8-dioxyadenine, although the amount of such material administered to these animals is far in excess of the amount they would receive from as much as 30 units of whole blood administered within a 24-hour period.

Rejuvenation of Red Cells

The erythrocyte obtains its energy from glucose and therefore must have the capacity to phosphorylate sugar, first in the hexokinase reaction and later in the phosphofructokinase reaction. These steps are extremely sensitive to changes in pH and, as the pH falls during storage, the utilization of glucose diminishes. This is the principal reason that the red cell is unable to maintain its 2,3-DPG and ATP content. This loss of ATP during storage can be used as a guide to the viability of transfused cells. An ATP content of less than 15 per cent of normal is invariably associated with less than the accepted survival of at least 70 per cent of the transfused red cells (22).

Solutions have been devised by several investigators to rejuvenate red cells during their final days of normal storage, as well as outdated whole blood (23). The principal components of these solutions include (1) adenine, which has been demonstrated to greatly improve both the ATP content and red cell viability; (2) inosine, which enhances the erythrocyte's capacity to maintain 2,3-DPG content; (3) ascorbic acid, which permits maintenance of 2,3-DPG concentration as well as viability (24); and (4) pyruvate, which in the presence of an alkaline medium enhances 2,3-DPG content and prevents loss of ATP.

Valeri and Zaroulis (25) have applied the technique of rejuvenation to their frozen blood program. Red cells were incubated at 37°C for 60 minutes with various rejuvenating solutions and then stored in high concentrations of glycerol at −70°C. These cells had normal oxygen transport function and 24-hour post-transfusion survivals of up to 80 per cent after thawing and washing. The thawing and washing procedure removes not only the added glycerol but also all materials used for rejuvenation, and thus conforms to federal regulations concerning administration of potentially toxic substances.

RED CELL PREPARATIONS

Washed Red Cells

There are many who believe that washed cells are indicated for the transfusion of patients undergoing hemodialysis, those awaiting organ transplant, and those who have recurrent, febrile, nonhemolytic reactions.

An extensive comparison of batch washing (BW) and a continuous-flow (CF) technique has been done by Button et al. (26). Blood and sedimented red cells stored for up to 21 days prior to being washed by either technique were found to have an average post-transfusion survival of greater than 70 per cent. An average plasma protein dilution of 1:25,000 was obtained with the CF technique, as compared with 1:600 with the conventional batch wash. Both hepatitis-associated antigen (HBAg) and cytomegalovirus (CMV) were undetected in any of the washed cell preparations. Cytomegalovirus and HBAg were present in all of the first-wash supernatants from the BW cells, and once in the supernatant from the second wash. Neither HBAg nor CMV could be detected in the CF wash after one third of the wash solution had passed through the cells. The absence of detectable HBAg, even by radioimmunoassay in CF-washed red cells, cannot be accepted as evidence of safety. However, as with frozen red cells, the decrease in hepatitis is probably owing to the dilutional effect of washing.

Most distressing has been the failure of washing techniques to remove significant numbers of white cells. This has been documented by counting the white blood cells pre and post wash, by noting the occurrence of severe febrile reactions in granulocyte-sensitive patients, and by lymphocyte culture.

Leukocyte-Poor Red Cells

Recognition that white cell antibodies were responsible for a significant number of febrile nonhemolytic transfusion reactions led to the development of a number of techniques for the preparation of leukocyte-poor blood. The methods in use in most transfusion services result in a sacrifice of a proportion of red cells and leave a significant contamination of white cells (usually lymphocytes), but the resulting component has generally been adequate for the intended purpose. Statistics from the Boston Children's Hospital Medical Center reveal that 29 per cent of all chronically transfused children develop leukoagglutinins. This is by far more common in patients with thalassemia than in patients with either sickle cell anemia, aplastic anemia, or leukemia. Our approach has been to give these children granulocyte-free blood, using the leukocyte filter (Leuko-Pak). This is prepared from freshly collected, noncooled (30° to 37°C), heparinized whole blood. If the unit of blood has cooled below 30°C, the blood bag should be placed in a centrifuge bag and immersed for 45 to 60 minutes in a 37°C water bath before filtration. Units so prepared show a reduction of 70 per cent of the leukocytes and anywhere from 85 to 96 per cent of the granulocytes. In 20 multitransfused patients who have had both demonstrable leukoagglutinins and febrile transfusion reactions, blood prepared in this manner has resulted in an 82 per cent decrease in febrile transfusion reactions.

Recently, more attention has been given to the fact that transfusion of blood products containing white cells and platelets may sensitize recipients to HL-A antigens, thus compromising leukocyte and platelet survival and possibly affecting allograft survival as well. Unfortunately, the dose of antigenic material necessary to produce an antibody response in the human has not been established. Thus, efforts to reduce exposure are hampered because the end point is unknown.

As alluded to in the preceding paragraphs, the initial efforts to prepare leukocyte-poor blood were directed at minimizing febrile, nonhemolytic transfusion reactions. Methodology for the preparation of HL-A–poor red cells has primarily been based upon the use of either frozen red cells or washed red cells. The latter method has been demonstrated to be entirely unsatisfactory for the production of white cell–free blood. More recently, a report of the combined studies revealed that white cell–poor red cells can be satisfactorily prepared without resorting to frozen red cells (27, 28). The methodology employed and the resulting yield of both red cells and decrease in white cells are shown in Table 29–4. As noted, nylon filtration combined with differential centrifugation, as well as double centrifugation (upright and then inverted), provides excellent removal of leukocytes and platelets. This latter procedure allows for the recovery of other components.

TABLE 29–4. PER CENT REDUCTION OF CELLS IN VARIOUS LEUKOCYTE-POOR BLOODS*

METHOD	ANTICOAGULANT	WHITE BLOOD CELLS	PLATELETS	RBC MASS
Nylon filtration	Heparin	65%	87%	12%
Upright centrifugation (light spin for platelets) plus inverted centrifugation (5200 × g for 9 minutes)	ACD or CPD	87%	97%	30%
Nylon filtration plus inverted centrifugation	Heparin	97%	97%	32%
Frozen red cells—Huggins Original technique	ACD	87%	96%	28%
New technique	or	80%	89%	19%
Continuous flow	CPD	91%	97%	25%

* Summarizes the results obtained when preparing leukocyte-poor blood by the most commonly used techniques.

Frozen Red Cells

Many notable achievements have been made during the past decade in the techniques of red cell freezing and processing. It is now possible to store red cells in the frozen state for ten years with excellent post-thaw yield and survival. Two basic techniques with minor variations are being used: low-glycerol fast freezing (liquid nitrogen, −150°C), and high-glycerol slow freezing (−85°C) (29–32).

The manipulations that the red cell must undergo in collection, storage in the liquid state, storage in the frozen state, and freeze, thaw, and post-thaw red cell washing procedure result in what is called a "preservation injury." This manifests itself in the form of irreversibly damaged red cells that are removed from the recipient's circulation within 24 hours of transfusion, as quantitated by in vivo measurements of red cell survival.

All the techniques of red cell freezing currently in clinical use have an in vivo survival of at least 90 per cent for red cells stored six months or less. Red cells frozen and thawed by the Huggins' dilution agglomeration procedure demonstrate a marked fall in therapeutic effectiveness after 18 months of storage, whereas other techniques show no change after storage for as long as seven years (33). In all instances, the preserved cells have levels of ATP and 2,3-DPG and oxyhemoglobin dissociation characteristics after thawing equal to or slightly better than immediately prior to freezing.

Despite these accomplishments, there is considerable controversy as to how frozen storage of red cells should be applied. There are those who believe that it is applicable to less than 2 per cent of donor blood, whereas others favor its use for more than 80 per cent of all donor blood.

References

1. Loutit, J. F., and Mollison, P. L.: Advantages of a disodium citrate glucose mixture as a blood preservative. Br. Med. J. 2:744, 1943.
2. Gibson, J. G., II, Murphy, W. P., et al.: The influence of extracellular factors in the collection of blood in ACD on maintenance of red cell viability during refrigerated storage. Am. J. Clin. Pathol. 26:855, 1956.
3. Orlina, A., and Josephson, A.: Comparative viability of blood stored in ACD and CPD. Transfusion 9:62, 1969.
4. Gibson, J. G., II: Personal communication.
5. Kevy, S. V., Gibson, J. G., II, et al.: A clinical evaluation of the use of citrate phosphate dextrose solution in children. Transfusion 5:427, 1965.
6. Chanutin, A., and Curnish, R. R.: Effect of organic and inorganic phosphates on the oxygen equilibrium of human erythrocytes. Arch. Biochem. Biophys. 121:96, 1967.
7. Benesch, R. E., and Benesch, R.: The influence of organic phosphates in the oxygenation of hemoglobin. Fed. Proc. 26:673, 1967.
8. Akerblom, O., de Verdier, C. H., et al.: Restoration of defective oxygen-transport function of stored red cells by addition of inosine. Scand. J. Clin. Lab. Invest. 21:245, 1968.

9. Valtis, D. J., and Kennedy, A. C.: Defective gas transport function of stored red cells. Lancet *1*:119, 1954.

10. Dawson, R. B., Kocholaty, W. F., et al.: Hemoglobin function and 2,3-DPG levels of blood stored at 4°C. in ACD and CPD. pH effect. Transfusion *10*:299, 1970.

11. Beutler, E., Meul, A., et al.: Depletion and regeneration of 2,3-diphosphoglyceric acid in stored red blood cells. Transfusion *9*:109, 1969.

12. Valeri, C. R., and Hirsch, N. M.: Restoration in vivo of erythrocyte adenosine triphosphate, 2,3-diphosphoglycerate, potassium ion, and sodium ion concentrations following the transfusion of acid-citrate-dextrose–stored human red blood cells. J. Lab. Clin. Med. *73*:722, 1969.

13. Button, L. N., Gibson, J. G., II, et al.: The salvage of heparinized blood with acid citrate dextrose. Transfusion *3*:37, 1963.

14. Fischer, H., Feber, E., et al.: Preservation of blood in the liquid state; practical importance of some new media. Presented at the 10th Congress of the International Society of Blood Transfusion, Stockholm, Sweden, 1964.

15. Gabrio, B. W., Donohue, D. M., et al.: Erythrocyte preservation. V. Relationship between chemical changes and viability of stored blood treated with adenosine. J. Clin. Invest. *34*:1509, 1955.

16. Donohue, D. M., Finch, C. A., et al.: Erythrocyte preservation. VI. The storage of blood with purine nucleosides. J. Clin. Invest. *35*:562, 1956.

17. Simon, E. R.: Red cell preservation: Further studies with adenine. Blood *20*:485, 1962.

18. de Verdier, C. H., Garby, L., et al.: Adenine in blood preservation: Post transfusion viability and biochemical changes. Transfusion *4*:331, 1964.

19. Bishop, C.: Some in vitro effects of adenine added to stored blood. Transfusion *4*:265, 1964.

20. Beutler, E., and Duron, O.: The preservation of red cell ATP in adenine containing citrate dextrose preservative mixtures. Presented at the 10th Congress of the International Society of Blood Transfusion, Stockholm, Sweden, 1964.

21. Shields, C. E.: Comparison studies of whole blood stored in ACD and CPD and with adenine. Transfusion *8*:1, 1968.

22. Valeri, C. R.: *Preservation of Red Cells.* National Academy of Sciences, 1974, p. 265.

23. Beutler, E.: Rejuvenation of liquid-stored red cells, In *Preservation of Red Cells.* National Academy of Sciences, 1973, p. 195.

24. Wood, L., and Beutler, E.: The effect of ascorbic acid on the 2,3-DPG level of stored blood. Clin. Res. *20*:186, 1972.

25. Valeri, C. R., and Zaroulis, C. G.: Rejuvenation and freezing of outdated stored human red cells. New Engl. J. Med. *287*:1307, 1972.

26. Button, L. N., Kevy, S. V., et al.: The effects of continuous-flow washing on stored red blood cells. Transfusion *12*:84, 1972.

27. Tenczar, F. J.: Comparison of inverted centrifugation, saline washing, and dextran sedimentation in the preparation of leukocyte-poor red cells. Transfusion *13*:183, 1973.

28. Miller, W. V., Wilson, M. J., et al.: Simple methods for the production of HL-A antigen–poor red cells. Transfusion *13*:189, 1973.

29. Tullis, J. L.: Red cell storage in the frozen state, In *The Red Blood Cell.* Bishop, C., and Surgenor, D. M. (eds.), New York, Academic Press, 1964.

30. Meryman, H. T. (ed.): *Review of Biological Freezing. Cryobiology.* New York, Academic Press, 1966.

31. Hogman, C. F., and Akerblom, O.: Practical aspects on the use of frozen blood, In *International Symposium on Modern Problems of Blood Preservation.* Stuttgart, Gustav Fischer Verlag, 1969.

32. Valeri, C. R., and Brodine, C. E.: Current methods for processing frozen red cells. Cryobiology *5*:129, 1968.

33. Valeri, C. R., and Runck, A. H.: Long-term frozen storage of human red blood cells. Transfusion *9*:5, 1969.

Chapter 30

Platelet Transfusion

by Robert I. Handin

The observation that platelet transfusion can temporarily raise the platelet count and stop hemorrhage in thrombocytopenic patients is not new. Duke first demonstrated this in 1910 when he infused fresh whole blood into three patients with life-threatening hemorrhage due to thrombocytopenia and noted both a rise in platelet count and a decrease in the time necessary to stop blood flow from an ear lobe puncture (1). However, increased use of platelet transfusions awaited the development of reliable methods of anticoagulating blood and separating it into its major components. Progress has been slow, since preparing platelets for transfusion presents problems not encountered with red cell transfusion.

Several units of blood must be processed to obtain sufficient platelets for a single transfusion. Platelets have a short life span, which necessitates frequent transfusion to maintain a given platelet count, and they require special handling to prevent damage during preparation and storage. Methods to assess the need for a platelet transfusion or to measure its effectiveness have not been clearly defined. Since methods for preparing and administering platelets change periodically, the emphasis here will be on general principles, recent developments, and future areas for improvement rather than on technical details.

PROCUREMENT

Platelets are usually prepared from single units of blood by differential centrifugation.

Ideally, blood that is destined to be used to prepare platelet concentrates should be kept at room temperature (22° to 25°C) prior to and during separation of platelets, as it increases the subsequent yield (2). When blood is chilled, platelets sphere and develop surface projections which may change their buoyant density (3). In addition, there is a tendency for platelets kept at 4°C to clump, especially if they are rewarmed during centrifugation (4). Unfortunately, it is standard blood bank practice to chill blood upon collection, although there is no firm evidence that a short period at room temperature will adversely affect red cells or plasma proteins.

Platelet-rich plasma is first prepared by low-speed centrifugation for varying periods of time. Most blood banks then concentrate the platelets by high speed centrifugation and resuspend the platelets in 10 to 50 ml. of plasma. One convenient centrifugation scheme is shown in Table 30–1, although there are a number of alternatives (5). The high gravitational force necessary to sediment the platelets results in the release of ADP into the plasma, causing the platelets to aggregate when the platelet button is dispersed. Formerly, EDTA was used as an anticoagulant, since it prevents platelet clumping. However, EDTA has adverse effects on the platelet membrane and is not satisfactory for red cell preservation (3, 6).

There are now several methods available to prevent platelet clumping when other anticoagulants are employed. Aster and Jandl reported that, when ACD was used as

TABLE 30–1. PREPARATION OF PLATELET CONCENTRATES

1. Collect whole blood in triple pack in either ACD or CPD anticoagulant.
2. Centrifuge whole blood at $4500 \times g^*$ for 3 minutes† and express platelet-rich plasma into transfer pack.
3. Centrifuge platelet-rich plasma at $4500 \times g^*$ for 5 minutes. Remove all but last 5 ml. of plasma into second transfer pack.
4. Let platelet button sit undisturbed for 45 to 60 minutes.
5. Gently resuspend platelets and add desired amount of plasma, usually 25 to 30 ml.

*Based on Sorvall RC-3 with HG-4 rotor.
†Times given will vary slightly with each centrifuge, as they include acceleration, time at top speed, and deceleration. Alternatives for other centrifuges are given in (5).

an anticoagulant, platelet clumping could be prevented by adding excess citric acid to lower the pH to 6.5 prior to high-speed centrifugation (2). This approach was successful since platelets do not respond well to aggregating agents at this low pH. Various modifications of the acidification technique have been introduced, and there are platelet packs available which contain a transfer pack with extra ACD.

This acidification step complicates platelet preparation and requires special bags or manipulations to provide the extra ACD. There has also been concern regarding the subsequent yield of cryoprecipitate from acidified plasma (7). Fortunately, the same goal can be achieved by allowing the centrifuged platelets to sit in a small volume of unacidified plasma for 30 minutes prior to being resuspended (8). It was initially postulated that a plasma enzyme inactivated and released ADP, and, subsequently, this plasma ADPase has been purified (9).

With the advent of CPD anticoagulant, which provides blood with a higher pH and more ionized calcium, platelet clumping again became a problem (10). However, several investigators have now shown that platelet concentrates can also be prepared from blood collected in CPD by letting the platelets sit 45 to 60 minutes before resuspension (11). When they are properly collected and resuspended, there is no significant difference in the recovery and subsequent life span of platelets collected in normal amounts of ACD, extra ACD, or CPD. The most important variables seem to

be maintenance of a constant temperature during preparation, preferably room temperature, and patiently waiting 45 to 60 minutes before resuspending the platelet button.

Institutions that prepare large numbers of platelet concentrates often rely on two-unit plasmapheresis of selected donors rather than single-unit blood donations. There are a number of advantages to plasmapheresis, including more efficient screening of donors for hepatitis-associated antigen, the ability to schedule collections in advance, and a decrease in the number of donors needed for a single transfusion. In addition, it is possible to optimize the separation procedures for platelets and return the plasma and red cells to the donor. Tullis et al. have described a continuous-flow system for platelet procurement using a modification of the Cohn fractionator (12). It is now available commercially using disposable equipment and can be used to obtain rapidly the equivalent of six to eight platelet units from a single donor (13). Szymanski and colleagues have recently reported extensive experience with the technique in a large blood center and have platelet yields that are equivalent to those obtained by conventional centrifugation (14). Another continuous-flow system, the Aminco Celltrifuge, can be used to prepare platelets, although it is usually set up to isolate granulocytes.

Platelet-rich plasma prepared by differential centrifugation of whole blood contains 70 per cent of the original platelets in 200 to 250 ml. of plasma. Subsequently, an additional 5 to 10 per cent of the platelets are lost preparing the platelet concentrate (Table 30–2). The newer continuous-flow systems also have an overall yield of 65 per cent but collect the platelets in a small volume without the need for recentrifugation.

It is obvious that separation procedures that lose one-third of the platelets could be

TABLE 30–2.

	VOLUME (ML.)	NUMBER OF PLATELETS $\times 10^{11}$	% YIELD
Whole blood	500	1.25	100
Platelet-rich plasma	250	0.85	70
Platelet concentrate	30	0.80	65

improved. Recently, workers in several laboratories have reported that the addition of 5 to 10 ng. per ml. of PGE_1, a potent inhibitor of platelet aggregation, increased the yield of platelets from whole blood by 15 to 20 per cent (15, 16). In addition, the presence of PGE_1 during centrifugation makes the platelets refractory to the effects of released ADP, and they can be resuspended immediately. The PGE_1 does not affect the subsequent survival of red cells or the platelets. While the use of PGE_1 is obviously a research tool, it could be of future benefit when the potential hazards have been completely defined.

Platelets are usually administered through a conventional nylon blood transfusion filter. Although special filters have been designed for platelet transfusion, they appear to have no particular advantage. Morrison has shown that an average of 3 per cent of the platelets are trapped in the filter and that repeated passage through the filter does not affect subsequent recovery and life span (17). There is increasing concern over the debris that accumulates in stored blood and the possible effects of these aggregates on the microcirculation (18). As new filters with smaller pore size are developed for red cell transfusion, the effect of filters on platelets may have to be reevaluated.

Since it is well known that some clotting proteins and platelets are activated by contact with glass, early platelet transfusions were carried out with siliconized glass equipment. The development of "inert" plastic bags for blood transfusion which are more convenient for transfusion has produced several unexpected problems. Murphy and Gardner pointed out that platelet viability during storage could be affected by the type of polyvinyl chloride (PVC) used to construct the platelet bags (19). In addition, Rubin and Jaeger have reported a high concentration of diethylhexyl phthalate in transfused blood (20). Phthalate is a "plasticizer" added to the PVC to keep the material pliable. Platelets effectively take up the phthalate ester and contain the highest concentrations of any of the blood cells (21). There is, to date, no firm data that phthalates are toxic, but they are present in transfused blood products and are deposited in body tissues following transfusion. It is also possible that the phthalates themselves adversely affect platelet function and viability during storage. However, they are present in all types of PVC, including those that are least harmful to stored platelets.

TRANSFUSION

Platelet transfusions are usually indicated if a patient is bleeding from mucous membranes or into the gastrointestinal or genitourinary tract. Skin bleeding, such as petechiae or ecchymoses, is so common in patients with severe thrombocytopenia that their presence alone should not be an indication for transfusion. The most feared complication is central nervous system bleeding, which was a frequent terminal event in thrombocytopenic patients before the advent of platelet transfusions.

As shown by Gaydos et al., the risk of bleeding correlates roughly with the patient's platelet count (22). Patients with platelet counts above 50,000 per mm.^{3} do not generally bleed; between 20,000 and 50,000 per mm.^{3}, there is a moderate risk; and below 20,000 per mm.^{3}, the patient is at serious risk. Bleeding is unpredictable, and some patients with platelet counts below 10,000 per mm.^{3} for long periods may not bleed. Ingestion of antiplatelet drugs, such as aspirin, or the presence of a disease that produces functionally abnormal platelets will, of course, increase the risk of bleeding at a given platelet count.

Factors other than the platelet count also contribute to the risk of hemorrhage. For example, patients with idiopathic thrombocytopenic purpura who have a young platelet population that functions more efficiently will bleed less often than patients with aplastic anemia who have the same platelet count. Patients with acute leukemia have the greatest difficulty with bleeding, and factors such as leukostasis or direct invasion of blood vessels by abnormal white cells may provoke bleeding. In most cases, the decision to transfuse can be made by examining both the patient and the platelet count. However, because the potential for bleeding is great in patients with platelet counts less than 10,000 per mm.^{3}, some centers routinely support these patients with prophylactic transfusions (23).

The best indication that a transfusion has been successful is a sustained rise in the recipient's platelet count. There are no experimental data to show that transfusions which do not raise the platelet count are effective in stopping hemorrhage. This point was elegantly demonstrated in a series of experiments on irradiated thrombocytopenic dogs who developed spontaneous bleeding into the lymphatics (24). The rate of hemorrhage could be readily quantitated by measuring the output of red cells into the thoracic duct lymph. The lymphatic red cell count could be reduced only by the infusion of viable platelets that raised the peripheral blood platelet count (25).

This approach to evaluating hemostasis is impractical clinically but does stress the importance of the platelet's role in maintaining endothelial integrity. It is the loss of this function that leads to the spontaneous hemorrhage and capillary fragility seen in severely thrombocytopenic patients (26). Roy and Djerassi, using the identical dog model, have reported that only a small rise in platelet count is necessary to stop the flow of red cells into the lymphatics (27). A much larger increment in platelet count is needed to improve the bleeding time, which is a measure of the ability of the animal to form hemostatic plugs in injured vessels. The only reliable clinical measurement of a hemostatic effect in man is shortening of the bleeding time, since there is no direct way to assay the important platelet-endothelial interaction.

Following transfusion, a large portion of the infused platelets immediately leaves the circulation and is sequestered in a normal splenic pool. Thus, the average recovery of ^{51}Cr-labeled platelets infused into normal volunteers is only 65 per cent and may be much lower in patients with splenomegaly. In clinical practice, the recovery of transfused platelets is much lower and averages 25 to 39 per cent (23). Precise calculation of platelet recoveries in thrombocytopenic recipients is difficult, since estimates of blood volume may be inaccurate in these chronically bleeding patients. Platelet counts are accurate to within 10 per cent under ideal circumstances, and larger errors are not uncommon.

In the absence of alloimmunization or splenomegaly, the recipient's platelet count should rise 10,000 to 15,000 per unit transfused per M.^{2} To raise the platelet count from 5000 to 50,000 per mm.^{3} in a 1 M.^{2} child would require three to four units of fresh platelet concentrate.

The subsequent life span of platelets transfused to normal individuals is eight to ten days. Host factors such as sepsis, endotoxemia, or disseminated intravascular coagulation can shorten the survival of transfused platelets. For unexplained reasons, patients with acute leukemia have shortened platelet survival in the absence of overt infection or intravascular coagulation (28, 29). It is also possible that hemorrhage per se might shorten platelet life span. However, the number of platelets that are "consumed" to nurture the endothelium of a thrombocytopenic individual is quite small and should not affect the overall survival.

While it is desirable to keep the platelet count above 20,000 per mm.^{3}, one must always consider the real risks of alloimmunization, as well as the fact that bleeding is often episodic and unpredictable. The nature of the underlying disease is also important when planning transfusion therapy. Patients with acute leukemia will require intensive treatment for short periods of time during relapse. When in remission, they may not need any support. In contrast, patients with congenital thrombocytopenia or severe aplasia may require continuous platelet support for many months or years.

PRESERVATION

Platelet transfusion therapy would be simplified if a satisfactory method for preservation of viable and functional platelets were available. Since this goal has not been achieved, most patients continue to receive platelets within four to eight hours of collection. Currently platelets are being stored for up to 72 hours at either 4° or 22°C in various hospitals, although there is no consensus on the optimal temperature or length of storage. It is becoming apparent that a number of technical details, such as the type of container, the volume and pH of the plasma, and the frequency of agitation, may be important for successful platelet storage (30).

An extensive experience has been gained with platelets stored at 4°C, and several studies have shown that the post-transfusion recovery and subsequent life span are diminished (31). However, storage at 4°C appears to preserve some hemostatic function, as measured by aggregation and adhesiveness (32). One would expect that any hemostatic effect following storage at 4°C would require large numbers of platelets and would be of short duration, as the platelets rapidly leave the circulation. There are several clinical studies that demonstrate a transient hemostatic effect following infusion of platelets stored at 4°C (33, 34).

The reports by Murphy and Gardner that the viability of platelets could be improved by storage at 22°C are of great interest (19, 35). Unfortunately, storage at this higher temperature introduces a number of new problems. Platelets have a higher rate of glycolysis, produce more lactic acid, and become depleted of glycogen. The amounts of lactate produced may exceed the buffering capacity of the plasma, and there are large falls in pH which can be deleterious to the platelets (19). The platelets also lose their ability to aggregate in response to the usual stimuli (36, 37). While some of these changes are reversible, it may take up to 24 hours for transfused platelets to function optimally (36, 37). One group has reported bacteriologic growth and some episodes of sepsis that could be traced to platelets stored at toom temperature (38). However, this has not been noted in any other large centers or blood banks.

There is only one clinical study that directly compares the hemostatic effect of platelets stored at the two temperatures by infusion into thrombocytopenic recipients (39). Becker et al. noted a better immediate hemostatic effect, as measured by a shortening of the bleeding time, after infusion of platelets stored at 4°C. This might have been predicted from the in vitro work on platelet function. Surprisingly, the authors found no significant difference in the immediate recovery or subsequent rate of disappearance of platelets stored at the two temperatures. Vallejos and Freireich have compared the rise in platelet count after transfusion of fresh and room temperature–stored platelets in patients with acute leukemia and found much lower post-transfusion recovery after storage at 22°C for 24 hours (40). These studies suggest that the data obtained from ^{51}Cr survivals in normal volunteers may not be directly applicable to thrombocytopenic patients.

At present, it is difficult to make rational recommendations regarding short-term platelet storage. The best immediate hemostatic effects seem to occur after transfusion with platelets stored at 4°C, while the best survival occurs after storage at 22°C. Since platelet life span is often shortened in the acutely ill thrombocytopenic patient, preservation of normal life span may not be as important as an immediate hemostatic effect. Perhaps, when more is understood about the loss of function during storage at 22°C, this will provide a superior storage method. In practice, platelets stored at either temperature for up to 24 hours are probably of some benefit, although most transfusions will still be given with fresh platelets.

Several attempts have been made to preserve platelets by freezing (41, 42). Although patients can be supported with frozen platelets, the large losses due to freeze-thaw injury, the unpleasant side effects of infused dimethylsulfoxide used as a cryoprotective agent, and the added expense have limited their usefulness. There is one recent report of a method that removes DMSO prior to infusion and provides more viable platelets, but the technique has yet to be tested clinically (43).

IMMUNOLOGY

Following repeated platelet transfusions, there is a decrease in post-transfusion recovery of platelets (44). This refractoriness to platelet transfusions is the result of alloimmunization. Antibodies have been detected in up to 50 per cent of refractory patients using complement fixation techniques (45). The number of patients with detectable antibody may increase as newer, more sensitive tests for antiplatelet antibody are developed (46, 47). Although refractoriness has been described after a single transfusion episode, a decrease in the response to platelets is usually not encountered until six to eight weeks of therapy (48).

Yankee et al. have reported that refractoriness can be overcome by transfusing platelets from HL-A–matched donors. This is most readily accomplished by choosing donors from the immediate family, although unrelated donors have been used successfully (49, 50). The genetics of the HL-A system are such that a panel of at least 5000 donors would be necessary for a reasonable chance to find a successful match. Despite these logistic problems, patients with severe aplastic anemia have been supported with HL-A–matched platelets for several years and continue to respond to platelet transfusions.

Since routine matching for HL-A antigens is impractical, there is no method to prevent alloimmunization from platelet transfusions. It is important to note that sensitization occurs despite the "immunosuppressed" state of many patients with acute leukemia or other hematologic malignancies. Refractoriness can be delayed by limiting the number of donors used for each transfusion and by avoiding unnecessary transfusions. This will decrease the number of antigens to which each patient is exposed.

Splenectomy has been advocated as a method to overcome refractoriness in patients with alloantibody. While splenectomy will improve the post-transfusion recovery of compatible platelets by eliminating normal splenic pooling, neither splenectomy nor corticosteroids improve the response to infusion of platelets in patients with alloantibody (49).

There are a number of other antigenic systems which may be important in platelet transfusion. The clinical significance of the Pl^{A1} antigen has been discussed earlier (see Chapter 21). Since only a small percentage of the population lacks the Pl^{A1} antigen, anti-Pl^{A1} antibody is not a common cause of refractoriness. However, Pl^{A1}–positive infants born to Pl^{A1}–negative mothers may develop neonatal thrombocytopenia due to transplacental passage of anti-Pl^{A1}. They can be readily transfused with maternal platelets that have been washed free of the antibody-containing plasma. Platelet transfusion can be readily repeated if necessary, and exchange transfusion can often be avoided. Most infants recover in 14 to 21 days, and may only need a single transfusion (51).

Transfusion therapy of the rare patient with post-transfusion purpura is more difficult. These patients are usually young women who are Pl^{A1}–negative and develop anti–Pl^{A1} antibody following a transfusion of blood. For unexplained reasons, they will destroy both Pl^{A1}–positive and Pl^{A1}–negative platelets. They have been treated with exchange transfusion and intensive plasmapheresis to try to decrease the titer of antibody (52).

The platelet also has A and B antigens on its surface (53, 54). The clinical significance of this observation is not completely clear, since some workers have found no difference in the recovery of ABO-incompatible platelets (44). However, Aster reported a significant decrease in recovery when infusing A platelets into type B or O recipients (55). Although matching for ABO groups could be readily accomplished, in most blood banks "incompatible" platelets are often administered. The number of red cells that are infused is so low that hemolytic red cell reactions have not been described.

Although Rh antigens are not present on the platelet, their presence on contaminating red cells in the platelet concentrates is a potential problem. Rh-negative recipients could theoretically be sensitized and develop Rh antibody. However, in one recent series, the incidence of sensitization was only 8 per cent (56). In addition, the limited life expectancy of most patients who require platelet support makes this problem less significant.

ADVERSE REACTIONS

The risks associated with platelet transfusion are minimal. With any blood product, there is always a chance of transmitting hepatitis, although the development of tests for hepatitis-associated antigen and the increased use of plasmapheresis donors may help decrease the incidence of this problem. The possible risk of bacterial contamination in platelets stored at room temperature has not yet been fully defined. It should be emphasized that scrupulous care should be taken with units of platelets to be stored at this temperature, and the bag should not be entered until just prior to infusion. The platelets should never be pooled prior to storage.

Since refractoriness is such a common occurrence in the multitransfused patient, the effects of transfusing incompatible platelets must be considered. While incompatible platelets are rapidly removed from the circulation and may not benefit the recipient, there is little systemic reaction associated with their destruction. Patients usually have no symptoms or may have a brief chill or slight elevation in temperature. Yankee has observed that the the infusion of incompatible platelets may also lower the absolute granulocyte count in patients with limited marrow reserve and make them more susceptible to infection (50).

References

1. Duke, W. W.: The relation of blood platelets to hemorrhagic diseases relieved by transfusion. J.A.M.A. 55:1185, 1910.
2. Aster, R. H., and Jandl, J.: Platelet sequestration in man. I. Methods. J. Clin. Invest. 43:843, 1964.
3. Zucker, M. B., and Borrelli, J.: Reversible alterations in platelet morphology produced by anticoagulants and by cold. Blood 9:602, 1954.
4. Kattlove, H. E., and Alexander, B.: The effect of cold on platelets. I. Cold-induced platelet aggregation. Blood 38:39, 1971.
5. Technical Methods and Procedures of the American Association of Blood Banks. 5th ed. 30 N. Michigan Avenue, Chicago, Illinois, 1970.
6. Aster, R. H.: The anticoagulants of choice for platelet transfusions. Transfusion 6:32, 1966.
7. Gilchrist, G. S., and Ekert, H.: Reduction of factor VIII activity in cryoprecipitate obtained from acidified plasma. Transfusion 8:294, 1968.
8. Mourad, N.: A simple method for obtaining platelet concentrates free of aggregates. Transfusion 8:48, 1968.
9. Holmsen, I., and Holmsen, H.: Partial purification and characterization of an ADP phosphohydrolase from human plasma. Thromb. Diath. Haemorrh. 26:177, 1971.
10. Pert, J. H., Zucker, M. B., et al.: Recent advances in preparation of platelet concentrates from ACD and CPD blood. Vox Sang. 13:119, 1967.
11. Tranum, B. L., and Haut, A.: In vivo survival of platelets prepared in CPD anticoagulant. Transfusion 12:108, 1972.
12. Tullis, J. L., Eberle, W. G., II, et al.: Plateletpheresis, Description of a new technic. Transfusion 8:154, 1968.
13. Tullis, J. G., Tinch, R. J., et al.: Plateletpheresis in a disposable system. Transfusion 11:368, 1971.
14. Szymanski, I. O., Patti, K., et al.: Efficacy of the Latham Blood Processor to perform plateletpheresis. Transfusion 12:405, 1973.
15. Becker, G. H., Chalos, M. K., et al.: Prostaglandin E₁ in preparation and storage of platelet concentrates. Science 175:537, 1972.
16. Valeri, C. R., Zaroulis, C. G., et al.: Prostaglandins in the preparation of blood components. Science 175:539, 1972.
17. Morrison, F. S.: The effect of filters on the efficiency of platelet transfusion. Transfusion 6:493, 1966.
18. Solis, R. T., and Gibbs, M. B.: Filtration of microaggregates in stored blood. Transfusion 12:245, 1972.
19. Murphy, S., Sayar, S. N., et al.: Storage of platelet concentrates at 22°C. Blood 35:549, 1970.
20. Jaeger, R. J., and Rubin, R. J.: Migration of a phthalate ester plasticizer from polyvinyl chloride blood bags into stored human blood and its localization in human tissues. New Engl. J. Med. 287:1114, 1972.
21. Jaeger, R. J., and Rubin, R. J.: Di-2-ethylhexyl phthalate, a plasticizer contaminant of platelet concentrates. Transfusion 13:107, 1973.
22. Gaydos, L. A., Freireich, E. J., et al.: Quantitative relation between platelet count and hemorrhage in patients with acute leukemia. New Engl. J. Med. 266:906, 1962.
23. Perry, S., and Yankee, R. A.: Transfusion and preservation, In *The Circulating Platelet*. Johnson, S. A. (ed.), New York, Academic Press, 1971, pp. 541–563.
24. Brecher, G., and Cronkite, E. P.: The effects of platelet transfusions in dogs made pancytopenic by X-radiation. New York J. Med. 53:544, 1953.
25. Jackson, D. P., Sorenson, D. K., et al.: Effectiveness of transfusions of fresh and lyophilized platelets in controlling bleeding due to thrombocytopenia. J. Clin. Invest. 38:1689, 1959.
26. Wojcik, J. D., Van Horn, D. L., et al.: Mechanism whereby platelets support the endothelium. Transfusion 9:324, 1969.
27. Roy, A. J., and Djerassi, I.: Effect of platelet transfusions: Plug formation and maintenance of vascular integrity. Proc. Soc. Exp. Biol. Med. 139:137, 1972.
28. Djerassi, I., Farber, S., et al.: Transfusions of fresh platelet concentrates to patients with secondary thrombocytopenia. New Engl. J. Med. 268:221, 1963.
29. Zucker, M. B., Pert, J. H., et al.: Preservation and clinical use of platelets. Vox Sang. 16:373, 1969.
30. Levin, R. H., and Freireich, E. J.: Effect of storage up to 48 hours on response to transfusions of platelet rich plasma. Transfusion 4:251, 1964.
31. Roy, A. J., Cavins, J., et al.: Circulation of concentrated one day old platelets in vivo. Transfusion 10:52, 1970.
32. Shively, J. A., Gott, C. L., et al.: The effect of storage on adhesion and aggregation of platelets. Vox Sang. 18:204, 1970.
33. Raccuglia, G., and Bethell, F. H.: Platelet transfusions and administration of platelet derivatives in man. II. Evaluation of systemic and hemostatic properties of various preparations. Am. J. Clin. Pathol. 34:505, 1960.
34. Tober, J. R., Jr., and Friedman, I. A.: Platelet transfusion with use of blood in plastic bags from routine storage. J.A.M.A. 172:50, 1960.
35. Murphy, S., and Gardner, F. H.: Platelet preservation: Effect of storage temperature on maintenance of platelet viability—Deleterious effect of refrigerated storage. New Engl. J. Med. 280:1094, 1969.
36. Murphy, S., and Gardner, F. H.: Platelet storage at

22°C: Metabolic, morphologic and functional studies. J. Clin. Invest. 50:370, 1971.

37. Handin, R. I., and Valeri, C. R.: Hemostatic effectiveness of platelets stored at 22°C. New Engl. J. Med. 285:538, 1971.

38. Buchholz, D. H., Young, V. M., et al.: Bacterial proliferation in platelet products stored at room temperature. New Engl. J. Med. 285:429, 1971.

39. Becker, G. A., Tuccelli, T., et al.: Studies of platelet concentrates stored at 22°C and 4°C. Transfusion 13:61, 1973.

40. Vallejos, C. S., Freireich, E. J., et al.: Effect of platelets stored at 22°C for 24 hours in patients with acute leukemia. Blood 42:565, 1973.

41. Cohen, P., and Gardner, F. H.: Platelet preservation. IV. Preservation of human platelet concentrates by controlled slow freezing in a glycerol medium. New Engl. J. Med. 274:1400, 1966.

42. Djerassi, I., Farber, S., et al.: Preparation and in vitro circulation of human platelets preserved with combined dimethylsulfoxide and dextrose. Transfusion 6:572, 1966.

43. Handin, R. I., and Valeri, C. R.: Improved viability of frozen platelets. Blood 40:509, 1972.

44. Freireich, E. J., Kliman, A., et al.: Response to repeated platelet transfusions from the same donor. Ann. Intern. Med. 59:277, 1963.

45. Aster, R. H., Levin, R. H., et al.: Complement fixing isoantibodies in serum of transfused persons. Correlation of antibodies with platelet survival in thrombocytopenic patients. Transfusion 4:428, 1964.

46. Handin, R. I., Piessens, W. F., et al.: Stimulation of non-immunized lymphocytes by platelet-antibody complexes in idiopathic thrombocytopenic purpura. New Engl. J. Med. 289:714, 1973.

47. Hirschman, R. J., and Shulman, N. R.: Utilization of the platelet release reaction to measure ITP factor and platelet antibodies. Trans. Assoc. Am. Physicians 85:325, 1972.

48. Grumet, F. C., and Yankee, R. A.: Long-term platelet support of patients with aplastic anemia. Effect of splenectomy and steroid therapy. Ann. Intern. Med. 73:1, 1970.

49. Yankee, R. A., Grumet, F. C., et al.: Platelet transfusion therapy: The selection of compatible platelet donors for refractory patients by lymphocyte HL-A matching. New Engl. J. Med. 281:1208, 1969.

50. Yankee, R. A., Graff, K. S., et al.: Selection of unrelated compatible platelet donors by lymphocyte HL-A matching. New Engl. J. Med. 288:760, 1973.

51. Adner, M. M., Fisch, G. R., et al.: Use of "compatible" platelet transfusions in treatment of congenital isoimmune thrombocytopenic purpura. New Engl. J. Med. 280:244, 1969.

52. Morrison, F. S., and Mollison, P. F.: Post-transfusion purpura. New Engl. J. Med. 275:243, 1966.

53. Gurevitch, J., and Nelken, D.: ABO groups in blood platelets. J. Lab. Clin. Med. 44:562, 1954.

54. Coombs, R. R. A., and Bedford, D.: The A and B antigens on human platelets demonstrated by means of mixed erythrocyte platelet agglutinations. Vox Sang. 5:11, 1955.

55. Aster, R. H.: Effect of anticoagulant and ABO incompatibility on recovery of transfused human platelets. Blood 26:732, 1965.

56. Goldfinger, D., and McGinniss, M. H.: Rh-incompatible platelet transfusions—Risks and consequences of sensitizing immunosuppressed patients. New Engl. J. Med. 284:942, 1971.

Chapter 31

Granulocyte Transfusion

by Joel M. Rappeport

INTRODUCTION*

Granulocytes and lymphocytes are the newest additions to the field of component blood transfusions and are used as supportive therapy, especially in patients with hematologic malignancies, aplastic anemia, and immunologic deficiency states. Most prior experience has been gained through granulocyte transfusions for bacterial infections, but in certain clinical circumstances lymphocytes are collected from appropriate donors for transfusion therapy in overwhelming viral infections, cancer immunotherapy, or transfer factor therapy for rare immunodeficiency states. The risk of graft-versus-host disease is sufficiently high in patients with altered immunologic function that lymphocyte transfusions and, in fact, transfusion of any blood products in this setting should only be approached by a skilled immunologist. The use of lymphocyte therapy is not discussed further here. Study of the potential use of monocyte transfusions is in a preliminary investigational stage; at present they have no practical application. Comprehensive reviews of prior work in the field of granulocyte transfusions, including indications and methodology, may be found in three recent publications (1–3); hence the references in this chapter will be highly selective.

Indications for granulocyte transfusions should be carefully considered in any pa-

tient in view of the expense of the laborious procurement methods available at present. This expense includes both equipment and extensive donor time. Also, the risk of alloimmunization of the recipient must be considered. In a study conducted at the National Cancer Institute between 1965 and 1971, almost 80 per cent of the patients with hematologic malignancies died of infections (4). More than 50 per cent of the organisms identified were bacterial. Similarly, in aplastic anemia the most common cause of death is infection alone or infection in combination with hemorrhage (5). The same is true for drug-induced agranulocytosis. Bodey demonstrated a quantitative relationship between the absolute circulating granulocyte count and the incidence of infection in leukemic patients (6) in remission and relapse. Both the incidence of infection and the patient days with infection increased markedly when circulating granulocyte counts were less than 500 per mm³. The incidence of infection decreased with increasing granulocyte counts, up to a granulocyte count of 1500 per mm³. This relationship is not seen in the idiopathic benign neutropenias, perhaps because the granulocyte reserve is greater in the latter condition.

With advances in the therapy of both malignancies and aplastic anemia, supportive treatment of these patients becomes more imperative. Attempts to decrease the potential exposure to infection have included protected environments and intestinal sterilization (7). These procedures have decreased the incidence of severe infections by as much as 50 per cent, and patients may be maintained for prolonged periods with-

---

*For a comprehensive recent review, see Boggs, D. R. Transfusion of neutrophils to prevent or treat infection in neutropenic patients. New Engl. J. Med. 290:1055, 1974.

out severe sepsis. However, appropriate cultures should be obtained in any patient with fever and a circulating granulocyte count of less than 1000 per mm.[3] Then the patient should start on appropriate antibiotics and be considered for early institution of daily granulocyte transfusions. Less commonly, patients with granulocyte dysfunction syndromes may be considered for granulocyte transfusions, despite the fact that their absolute PMN count may be normal.

Attempts to evaluate the efficacy of granulocyte transfusions have been hampered by the availability of adequate numbers of cells, complex critically ill recipients, and proper controls. Brecher et al. demonstrated that it is possible to increase the number of circulating granulocytes in lethally irradiated dogs with granulocyte transfusions (8). In these experiments the number of granulocytes did not increase to normal levels, and only a small percentage of cells were recovered from the circulation, but there was migration of cells to peripheral tissues. In human studies involving chronic myelogenous leukemia donors, circulating donor cells identifiable by sex markers, Philadelphia chromosomes, and histochemical staining could be recovered from recipient blood (9, 10). Infused CML cells have been demonstrated morphologically to have ingested the bacterial organism implicated in the recipient's sepsis (9). We have demonstrated that granulocytes obtained from both normal donors and CML donors by continuous-flow centrifugation develop a defect in ingestion in the transfusion bag, but this acquired defect is totally reversible after circulation in the recipient (11). Despite small increments in circulating granulocytes, these cells maintain the ability to migrate to Rebuck skin windows.

Various reports have demonstrated a decrease in the temperature and associated symptoms of infection in febrile, leukopenic patients treated with a single transfusion of CML cells (10, 12). Epstein and co-workers developed a dog model in which lethally irradiated dogs were given a bacterial challenge with intravenous *E. coli* (13). Subsequent leukocyte transfusions produced both prolonged sterility of the blood stream and prolonged life when compared with appropriate controls, and in fact provided the most encouraging evidence that granulocyte transfusions are of value in altering a potentially lethal clinical situation. Some of the effects of multiple normal-donor granulocyte transfusions on human recipients have been examined by Graw and co-workers, who studied two groups of leukopenic patients with documented gram-negative bacterial sepsis (14). One group of 37 patients received appropriate antibiotics alone without granulocyte transfusions. Only 10 patients of this group survived. Thirty-nine patients received both antibiotics and granulocyte transfusions and exhibited a progressive increase in survival, depending on the number of daily transfusions received. In fact, all 12 patients who received four or more daily transfusions survived their episodes of bacterial sepsis. We may conclude, therefore, that if sufficient numbers of functionally intact granulocytes can be obtained for periods of time, recovery may occur in bacterially infected neutropenic patients who would otherwise die.

As in all blood component therapy, certain potential hazards and complications must be considered. The routine problems of ABO compatibility and hepatitis transmission must be dealt with. Malarial parasites have been transmitted in leukocyte transfusions (15), and the risk of transmission of cytomegalovirus is potentially enhanced. Despite partial immunosuppression in many recipients, alloimmunization will commonly occur, making future platelet and granulocyte therapy extremely difficult. Prior development of leukocyte antibodies is probably a contraindication to random granulocyte transfusions, since severe febrile reactions associated with dyspnea and hypotension may occur (16). These reactions may further compromise an already thrombocytopenic patient by further decreasing the platelet count. The reactions may be reduced by prior treatment of the recipient with antihistamines or corticosteroids or both, but these agents may be hazardous since antihistamines interfere with platelet function (17) and corticosteroids may inhibit granulocyte function (18). The selection of an HL-A–matched donor may decrease or eliminate reactions, and in fact an enhanced number of circulating granulocytes can be recovered from such transfusions. However, certain clinical situations, such as marrow transplant preparation, dictate that HL-A–matched donors not be used.

This is discussed in Chapter 5. The chances of finding an HL-A, ABO-compatible CML donor are negligible, and since prolonged therapy may be required, the use of a normal ABO-compatible, HL-A–matched donor may make excessive demands upon the donor involved.

In rare circumstances, when severe immune suppression exists as a result of chemotherapy, engraftment with temporary chimerism and graft-versus-host disease may occur (19). If the immunosuppressed state is either permanent or prolonged, the engraftment could be fatal to the recipient. Graft-versus-host disease may be prevented by administering 5000 R. radiation to the transfusion bag. This dose does not interfere with either platelet or granulocyte function (20, 21).

METHODOLOGY

At present, three methods are available for obtaining human granulocytes for transfusion, each having certain advantages and disadvantages. The technique to be used in any given hospital will depend upon the need for granulocyte transfusions over a prolonged period, as well as the ability of the blood bank to undertake specialized procedures.

Double Plasmapheresis

Prior to the development of the IBM-NCI separator, granulocyte transfusions could only be produced from buffy coat preparations derived by plasmapheresis of ABO-compatible chronic myelogenous leukemia patients with an elevated leukocyte count (22). The technique involves the sequential removal of two units of blood into ACD or CPD double packs. The buffy coat is separated from the red cells by sedimentation at 37°C for one hour. This prevents granulocyte clumping. The yield of granulocytes in the donor pack is high owing to the increased rate of sedimentation of red cells in CML patients. The leukocyte-rich plasma is expressed into the second bag of the double pack, and the white cells are concentrated by centrifugation at 500 rpm. for 20 minutes. The red cells and excess plasma are returned to the donor, while the white cells are administered to the recipient through a standard nylon filter blood administration set. The average number of granulocytes transfused by this method is 7×10^{10}, and this usually results in a detectable increase in the number of circulating granulocytes.

The advantages of this technique are the lack of expensive equipment, the ability to carry out the procedure in any blood bank, and the lack of risk for a nonanemic donor. The technique cannot be relied upon because the availability of an ABO-compatible CML donor with an elevated WBC is very uncertain. Some centers treat their CML patients intermittently with hydroxyurea. The drug is discontinued a few days prior to needed white cell procurement, resulting in a prompt rise of white count. After plasmapheresis, the hydroxyurea is reinstituted until the donor is again needed. Some CML donors may be managed by leukapheresis alone (22). Frequent granulocyte donations decrease the circulating white count, decrease spleen size, and appear to decrease the hypermetabolic symptoms. Since myelosuppressive therapy has little to contribute to the life span of patients with CML (23), and since some patients enjoy their role as essential donors to others more critically ill, an ethical problem rarely if ever exists.

Continuous-Flow Centrifugation

In an attempt to process large volumes of blood for granulocytes from single normal donors, a combined team from the NCI and the IBM Corporation developed the continuous-flow centrifuge, which is based on the principle that granulocytes are less dense than red cells (24). Another corporation also manufactures the instrument (Aminco Centrifuge). By differential centrifugation in a bowel through which a continuous flow of anticoagulated venous blood is peristaltically pumped, leukocytes are concentrated into a buffy coat layer at the plasma red cell interface. This leukoconcentrated material is continuously collected through a port into a transfusion bag, while the leukocyte-poor plasma and red cells are returned to the donor. During a 4-hour period, approximately two blood volumes of the donor may be processed. Since this is a concentration method, significant numbers of red cells, plasma, and platelets contami-

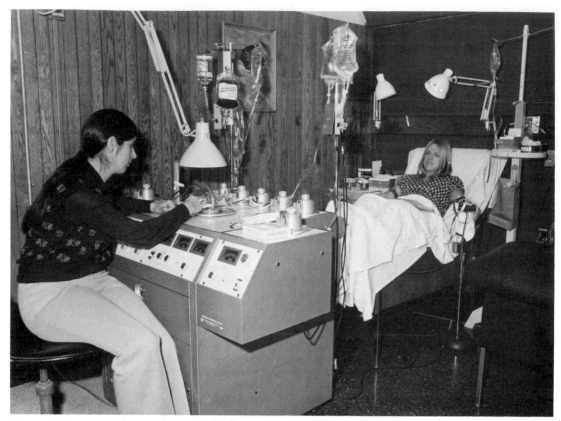

Figure 31–1. A granulocyte donor attached to an Aminco Continuous-Flow Centrifuge, operated by a nurse-technician. The complexity of the equipment and the relative comfort of the donor may be noted.

nate the collected buffy coat. At least an ABO, Rh-compatible donor should be used and, if possible, an HL-A–compatible donor. CML donors can also be therapeutically leukapheresed in this manner.

If the peripheral blood of the normal donor is enriched with granulocytes by oral treatment 12 hours prior to donation with 0.06 mg. dexamethasone per kg. body weight or by 0.1 mg. etiocholanolone per kg. I.M., and if during the procedure hydroxyethyl starch is added to the venous blood as it enters the cell separator at the rate of one ml. of a 6 per cent solution per 12 ml. of blood, with a maximum of 500 ml. used during the procedure (25), as many as 2.2×10^{10} PMN's may be recovered in four hours with a total volume of 450 ml. and an average hematocrit of 20 per cent. The principles and function of the machine have been more extensively reviewed by its designer (2). A view of the instrument with a donor attached to it is shown in Figure 31–1.

The advantages of this method are two-fold. First, both normal donors and CML patients may be leukapheresed, and the centrifuge is also adaptable to other uses, such as plasma exchange, red cell exchange, and lymphocyte and blast cell collections. While granulocyte collections are being made, simultaneous plateletpheresis may be carried out, thereby exposing the recipient to fewer donors, a distinct advantage in the chronically transfused patient. Second, and most important, the functional integrity of the granulocytes obtained in this fashion has been demonstrated.

The disadvantages are not insignificant. Without dexamethasone and hydroxyethyl starch, the latter functioning as a rouleaux-forming agent, the yields from the cell separator are not sufficient. The procedure is relatively inefficient, with only approximately 25 per cent of the available cells being harvested. The yield of cells in any given run is quite variable. The risk of this procedure to the donor are potentially greater than those associated with plasmapheresis alone. The dexamethasone is probably safe given once, but if the donor is used more frequently, subtle symptoms of hyper-adrenocorticism might appear. We have not yet seen complications from the relatively nonallergenic hydroxyethyl starch, which is metabolized by amylase or excreted in the urine over several days (26), but an unusual response to this agent will probably be observed sooner or later. The necessary anti-coagulation might lead to unsuspected gas-trointestinal bleeding. Multiple frequent donations or breakage in tubing with acute blood loss might necessitate red cell trans-fusion, which carries the risk of hepatitis. Inadequate sterilization of reusable equip-ment or breaks in the continuity of the sys-tem might also lead to hepatitis or other infections. Most of these risks are only po-tential problems and occur rarely. Even mild problems of venipuncture difficulty, fatigue, stiff arms, chills, and donor anxiety are infrequent, and they occur less fre-quently in large centers in which the proce-dure is frequently performed. A thorough history, physical examination, and explana-tion to the donor can eliminate many poten-tial problems. The risks to the recipients are as described earlier. The major problem in this procedure is obtaining adequate num-bers of donors who can spend the time nec-essary to provide granulocytes on a daily basis when the patient needs them. Our cur-rent view of granulocyte transfusions with the cell centrifuge technique is a mixed one. If an episode of sepsis occurs in a neutropenic patient, daily granulocyte transfusions may be life-saving. However, the cost of the procedure, the requirement of a team of ex-pert physicians and technicians to operate the instrument and care for the donors, and the initial expense of the machine along with operating costs probably restrict this procedure to highly sophisticated hematol-ogy centers that deal with large numbers of potential recipients.

Continuous-Flow Filtration Leukapheresis

When chronically transfused patients ex-hibit frequent febrile reactions to packed red cells despite ABO compatibility, it is usually found that their sera contain leuko-cyte antibodies, and the reaction between these antibodies and the white cells in the transfused blood produces the febrile reac-tion. An effective way to eliminate such reactions is to collect the donor blood through nylon filters (Leuko-Pak, Fenwal Laboratories, Inc., Morton Grove, Illinois). Granulocytes adhere to these filters and are markedly reduced in numbers in the packed cells. Granulocyte adherence occurs only in the presence of calcium and magnesium ions. Advantage of this principle was taken by Djerassi et al. (27), who noted that granu-locytes from heparinized blood adhere to the nylon filters. When the filters are washed with acidified ACD plasma, calcium and magnesium ions are decreased by che-lation, and the adherent granulocytes are removed. A continuous flow apparatus has been designed in which heparinized donor blood passes through two to four filters in parallel during the collection period. After a two-blood volume leukapheresis, the filters are disconnected from the donor and washed with acidified plasma into transfusion bags, where the liberated granulocytes are con-centrated.

The advantages of this system as com-pared with the cell centrifuge are that su-perior numbers of PMN's are collected from normal donors in a shorter period of time. Also, the donor does not need to receive corticosteroids, etiocholanolone, or hy-droxyethyl starch to enhance the peripheral granulocyte count. Actually, the filtration donor experiences a rise in his peripheral granulocyte count during the procedure owing to the release of a poorly character-ized substance from the PMN's during the process of adhesion (28). This substance is then recirculated to the donor, where it stimulates granulocytosis and assists in the granulocyte collection, since the donor PMN count is increased. However, the sub-stance may also cause a febrile response in the donor. As with the cell separator, these donors also face the risks of anticoagulation, acute blood loss, and infection, although the routine loss of hemoglobin is less than that with the cell separator.

The effects on the recipient are less fa-vorable than those observed when cell centrifuge–derived PMN's are used. Recov-ery in the recipient is decreased, and PMN life span in the circulation is shorter (28). Furthermore, the functional integrity of these cells has not been as carefully docu-mented as has the cell separator–derived cells. Since the purpose of the procedure is to provide an adequate number of *func-tionally intact* cells to the septic neutropenic patient, more investigation is needed in this area. Careful comparative studies of centrifuge and filtration cells are required. Although the product of the centrifuge appears to be of higher quality, the filtration method provides more cells, is less cumbersome, and is less expensive. Our experience would suggest that CML donors should not be placed on the filtration leukapheresis. All such donors whom we have treated in this manner have become temporarily febrile and hypotensive.

In addition to the problems of proper donor selection and obtaining adequate numbers of functional granulocytes, a major problem of preservation must be faced. When large numbers of cells are obtained from CML donors or normal adult donors for recipients who are small children or infants, the contents of one leukapheresis may be divided into two transfusions. One is given immediately and the second may be stored at 4°C for up to 24 hours. Phagocytic function is well protected after such brief storage (29). However, long-term storage and, in particular, cryopreservation remain unsolved problems. Solution of these problems could make granulocyte transfusion a more widely used and probably more successful therapy in critical situations.

References

1. Mathé, G., Amiel, J., et al.: *Bone Marrow Transplantation and Leucocyte Transfusions.* Springfield, Ill., Charles C Thomas, Publisher, 1971.
2. Mathé, G. (ed.): *Les Transfusions de Globules Blancs.* Paris, Centre National de la Recherche Scientific, 1970.
3. Graw, R. G., and Yankee, R. A.: Principles of hematologic supportive care. Med. Clin. North Am. 57:441, 1973.
4. Levine, A. S., Graw, R. G., et al.: Management of infections in patients with leukemia and lymphoma: Current concepts and experimental approaches. Semin. Hematol. 9:141, 1972.
5. Williams, D. M., Lynch, R. E., et al.: Drug-induced aplastic anemia. Semin. Hematol. 10:195, 1973.
6. Bodey, G. P., Buckley, M., et al.: Quantitative relationships between circulating leukocytes and infection in patients with acute leukemia. Ann. Intern. Med. 64:328, 1966.
7. Levine, A. S., Siegel, S. E., et al.: Protected environments and prophylactic antibiotics. New Engl. J. Med. 288:477, 1973.
8. Brecher, G., Wilbur, K. M., et al.: Transfusion of separated leukocytes into irradiated dogs with aplastic marrows. Proc. Soc. Exp. Biol. Med. 84:54, 1953.
9. Shohet, S. B.: Morphologic evidence for the *in vivo* activity of transfused chronic myelogenous leukemia cells in a case of massive staphylococcal septicemia. Blood 32:111, 1968.
10. Eyre, H. J., Goldstein, I. M., et al.: Leukocyte transfusions: Function of transfused granulocytes from donors with chronic myelocytic leukemia. Blood 36:432, 1970.
11. Rappeport, J. M., Kevy, S. V., et al.: A reversible phagocytic defect in leukocyte transfusions (in preparation).
12. Morse, E., Freireich, E. J., et al.: The transfusion of leukocytes from donors with chronic myelocytic leukemia to patients with neutropenia. Transfusion 6:183, 1966.
13. Epstein, R. B., Clift, R. A., et al.: The effect of leukocyte transfusions in experimental bacteremia in the dog. Blood 34:782, 1969.
14. Graw, R. G., Herzig, G. P., et al.: Granulocyte transfusions: Treatment of gram-negative septicemia. New Engl. J. Med. 287:367, 1972.
15. Dover, A. S., and Guinee, V. F.: Malarial transmission by leukocyte component therapy. J.A.M.A. 217:1701, 1971.
16. Goldstein, I. M., Eyre, H. J., et al.: Leukocyte transfusions: Role of leukocyte alloantibodies in determining transfusion response. Transfusion 11:19, 1971.
17. Mills, D. C. B., and Roberts, G. C. K.: Membrane active drugs and the aggregation of human blood platelets. Nature (Lond.) 213:35, 1967.
18. Boggs, D. R., Athens, J. W., et al.: The effect of adrenal glucocorticosteroids upon the cellular composition of inflammatory exudates. Am. J. Pathol. 44:763, 1964.
19. Levin, R. H., Whang, J., et al.: Persistent mitosis of transfused homologous leukocytes in children receiving anti-leukemic therapy. Science 142:1305, 1963.
20. Zuck, T. F., Brown, G. L., et al.: Effects of *in vitro* irradiation on platelet function and lymphocyte viability. Transfusion 13:344, 1973.
21. Rappeport, J. M., and Parkman, R.: Personal communication.
22. Morse, E. E., Carbone, P. P., et al.: Repeated leukapheresis of patients with chronic myelocytic leukemia. Transfusion 6:175, 1966.
23. Galton, D. A.: Chemotherapy of chronic myelocytic leukemia. Semin. Hematol. 6:323, 1969.
24. Freireich, E. J., Judson, G., et al.: Separation and collection of leukocytes. Cancer Res. 25:1516, 1965.
25. McCredie, K., and Freireich, E.: Increased granulocytic collection from normal donors with increased granulocyte recovery following transfusion. Proc. Am. Assoc. Cancer Res. 12:58, 1971.
26. Thompson, W. L., Fukushima, T., et al.: Intravascular persistence, tissue storage, and excretion of hydroxyethyl starch. Surg. Gynecol. Obstet. 130:965, 1970.
27. Djerassi, I., Kim, J. S., et al.: Continuous flow filtration leukapheresis. Transfusion 12:75, 1972.
28. Herzig, G. P., Root, R. K., et al.: Granulocyte collection by continuous flow filtration leukaphersis. Blood 39:554, 1972.
29. McCullugh, J., Weiblen, B., et al.: *In vitro* function and *in vivo* survival of fresh and stored granulocytes collected using the continuous flow centrifuge. Transfusion 13:354, 1973.

Glossary of Abbreviations
and Symbols

A (1) blood group A; (2) adenine; (3) factor in the alternate pathway of activation of complement, properdin factor; (4) antibody; (5) absence of systemic symptoms in Hodgkin's disease

Å angstrom

AA amino acid

A,Ac acetic acid

ACD acid citrate dextrose

ACEH acid cholesteryl ester hydrolase

ACTH adrenocorticotropic hormone, corticotropin

ADA adenosine deaminase

ADH antidiuretic hormone

ADP adenosine diphosphate

Ag a genetic type on β-lipoprotein

AHF antihemophilic factor, factor VIII

AIP acute intermittent porphyria

AK adenylate kinase

ALA δ-aminolevulinic acid

ALL acute lymphocytic leukemia

Alpha (α) heavy chain of IgA

Am a genetic type of IgA

AML acute myelogenous leukemia

AMP adenosine monophosphate

AMPS acid mucopolysaccharides

APRT adenosinephosphoribosyl transferase

AR (1) ascorbate reductase; (2) autosomal recessive

AS heterozygous sickle cell anemia; sickle cell trait

ATGL acid triglyceride lipase

ATP adenosine triphosphate

ATPase adenosine triphosphatase

B (1) blood group B; (2) factor in the alternate pathway of activation of complement, properdin factor; (3) lymphocytes derived from the bone marrow, or from the bursa of Fabricius in avian species; (4) presence of systemic symptoms in Hodgkin's disease

BAL British anti-lewisite, 2,3-dimercaptopropanol

BCB bromcresyl blue

BCG Bacillus Calmette-Guérin

BCNU 1,3–Bis(2–chloroethyl)–1–nitrosourea

BMGR bone marrow granulocyte reserve

BSP Bromsulphalein

BUdR bromodeoxyuridine

BW batch washing

C (1) complement; (2) constant segment gene for immunoglobulin; (3) cytosine

Cb_5R cytochrome b_5 reductase

cAMP cyclic adenosine monophosphate

CF continuous flow

CFU colony-forming unit

CGD chronic granulomatous disease

CGP circulating granulocyte pool

CHBA congenital Heinz body hemolytic anemia

CID cytomegalic inclusion disease

CLL chronic lymphocytic leukemia

CML (1) cell-mediated lysis; (2) chronic myelogenous leukemia

CNS central nervous system

CNSHA congenital nonspherocytic hemolytic anemia

CO carbon monoxide

CoA coenzyme A

COPRO   coproporphyrin

C3PA   C3 proactivator

CPD   citrate phosphate dextrose

^{51}Cr   51-chromium

CRM   cross-reacting material

^{14}CT   carbon-14–labeled thymidine

CTX   cerebrotendinous xanthomatosis

d   density

D   dehydrogenase

DCIP   dichlorophenolindophenol

Delta (δ)   heavy chain of IgD

DFP   di-isopropyl fluorophosphate

DG   dense granules

DHAP   dihydroxyacetone phosphate

DIC   disseminated intravascular coagulation

DMSO   dimethylsulfoxide

DNA   deoxyribonucleic acid

DNCB   dinitrochlorobenzene

DPG   diphosphoglycerate

1,3-DPG   1,3-diphosphoglycerate

2,3-DPG   2,3-diphosphoglycerate

DPGM   diphosphoglycerate mutase

DPGP   diphosphoglycerate phosphatase

DPN, NAD   diphosphopyridine nucleotide, nicotinamide adenine dinucleotide

DPNH, NADH   reduced diphosphopyridine nucleotide, reduced nicotinamide adenine dinucleotide

DTPA   diethylenetriamine pentacetate

DTR   deep tendon reflex

e   electron

E   (1) extralymphatic involvement in Hodgkin's disease; (2) pseudocholinesterase; (3) sheep erythrocytes

EACA   epsilon aminocaproic acid

EB   Epstein-Barr

EC   enzyme commission

ECG   electrocardiogram

EDTA   ethylenediaminetetraacetate, versene

Epsilon (ϵ)   heavy chain of IgE

Es   a functionally silent variant of pseudocholinesterase

ESF   erythropoiesis stimulating factor; erythropoietin

ESR   electron spin resonance

F   fast; electrophoretically fast variant of C3

F(ab)   portion of gamma globulin molecule

Factor I   fibrinogen

Factor II   prothrombin

Factor III   thromboplastin

Factor V   proaccelerin

Factor VII   proSPCA, pro–serum prothrombin converting activity

Factor VIII   antihemophilic factor

Factor IX   Christmas factor, plasma thromboplastin component

Factor X   Stuart factor

Factor Xa   activated Stuart factor

Factor XI   plasma thromboplastin antecedent

Factor XII   Hageman factor

Factor XIII   fibrin stabilizing factor

FAD   flavin adenine dinucleotide

Fb   filamentous bands

Fc   portion of gamma globulin molecule

FDP   fructose diphosphate

Fe   iron

Fe^{+2}   ferro

Fe^{+3}   ferri (met)

FFA   free fatty acid

FIGLU   formiminoglutamic acid

F1,6P   fructose-1,6-diphosphate

F6P   fructose-6-phosphate

FR   fibrin-related antigen

FSF   fibrin stabilizing factor, factor XIII

FSFa   activated fibrin stabilizing factor

FTT   failure to thrive

G   (1) glycogen; (2) guanidine

G$_1$ interphase between mitosis and DNA synthesis

G$_2$ period between DNA synthesis and mitosis

GAG   glycine-rich α-glycoprotein

Gal   galactose

Gal NAc   N-acetylgalactosamine

Gamma (γ)   heavy chain of IgG

Gb   genetic type on properdin factor B (glycine-rich β-glycoprotein, C3 proactivator)

GBG   glycine-rich β-glycoprotein

Gc   group-specific component

GGG   basic fragment of glycine-rich β-glycoprotein (glycine-rich γ-glycoprotein)

GI   gastrointestinal

GL1a   glucosyl ceramide

GL1b   galactosyl ceramide

GL2a   lactosyl ceramide

GL2b   dihexosyl ceramide

GL3   trihexosyl ceramide

GL4   glycosphingolipid

Glc   glucose

Gm   genetic type of gamma globulin

G0   cells not in proliferative activity

GOT   glutamic-oxaloacetic transaminase

G3P   glyceraldehyde-3-phosphate

G6P   glucose-6-phosphate

GPD   glyceraldehyde phosphate dehydrogenase

G3PD   glyceraldehyde-3-phosphate dehydrogenase

G6PD   glucose-6-phosphate dehydrogenase

GPI   glyceraldehyde phosphate isomerase

GR   glutathione reductase

GSH   glutathione, reduced

GSSG   glutathione, oxidized

GTR   granulocyte turnover rate

GVH   graft-versus-host

H   heavy chain of immunoglobulin

HABA   hydroxyaminobenzoic acid

Hb   hemoglobin

HBAg   hepatitis B antigen

HDL   high density lipoproteins

HEMPAS   hereditary erythroblastic multi-nuclearity with a positive acidified serum test

Hg   mercury

Hgb   hemoglobin

HGPRT   hypoxanthine-guanine phosphoribosyltransferase

HK   hexokinase

HL-A   human leukocyte antigens

HLF   heat-labile factor (properdin factor B)

HMP   hexose monophosphate

HPFH   hereditary persistence of fetal hemoglobin

Hp-Hb   haptoglobin-hemoglobin

HS   hereditary spherocytosis

HSmegaly   hepatosplenomegaly

HT   hypertransfusion

3HT   tritiated thymidine

HUS   hemolytic uremic syndrome

i   fetal red cell antigen

I   adult red cell antigen

Ig   immunoglobulin

IM   intramuscular

Inv   genetic type on kappa chain of immunoglobulins

ISC   irreversibly sickled cell

ITP   idiopathic thrombocytopenic purpura

J   subunit of polymeric forms of IgA and IgM

K   light chains of immunoglobulin

KAF   conglutinogen activating factor

Ki   inhibitor concentration at half maximal inhibition

Km   Michaelis constant; substrate concentration at half maximal velocity of reaction

L   light chain of immunoglobulin

Lambda (λ)   light chains of immunoglobulin

LCAT   lecithin:cholesterol acyl transferase

Ld   genetic type on β-lipoprotein

LD   lymphocyte-defined antigen

LDH   lactate dehydrogenase

LDL   low density lipoproteins

LMB   leukomethylene blue, reduced methylene blue, MBH

Lp   genetic type on β-lipoprotein

LPC   lysophosphatidyl choline

LW   a blood group antigen

M   (1) methyl; (2) mitochondria; (3) mitosis

M²   meter squared

MB   methylene blue, oxidized

MCH   mean corpuscular hemoglobin

MCHC   mean corpuscular hemoglobin concentration

MCV   mean corpuscular volume

MGP   marginating granulocyte pool

MHR   methemoglobin reductase

MIF   macrophage inhibitory factors

MLC   mixed lymphocyte culture

MLD   metachromatic leukodystrophy

MOPP   *M*ustargen (nitrogen mustard), *O*ncovin (vincristine), *P*rocarbazine, *P*rednisone

MPS   mucopolysaccharide syndromes

mRNA   messenger RNA

MT   circumferential bundle of microtubules

MTT   a tetrazolium salt

Mu (μ)   heavy chain of IgM

M.W.   molecular weight

n   an index of heme-heme interaction; Hill constant

N   a blood group antigen

NAc   *N*-acetyl

NAD   nicotinamide adenine dinucleotide

NADH   reduced nicotinamide adenine dinucleotide

NADP   nicotinamide adenine dinucleotide phosphate

NADPH   reduced nicotinamide adenine dinucleotide phosphate

NANA   *N*-acetylneuraminic acid

NBT   nitroblue tetrazolium

NIH   National Institutes of Health

NMR   nuclear magnetic resonance

NPD   Niemann-Pick disease

O   blood group O

O.D.   optical density

P   (1) propionic; (2) a red cell antigen; (3) short arm of chromosome

P$_{50}$ partial pressure of oxygen at 50 per cent saturation

PA   phosphatidic acid

PAS   periodic acid Schiff

PBG   porphobilinogen

PC   phosphatidyl choline

PChol   phosphorylcholine

pCO$_2$ partial pressure of carbon dioxide

PCMB   parachloromercuribenzoate

PCV   packed cell volume

PE   phosphatidyl ethanolamine

PEP   phosphoenolpyruvate

Pep C   peptidase C

PF3   platelet factor 3

PFK   phosphofructokinase

PG   prostaglandin ·

2-PG   2-phosphoglycerate

3-PG   3-phosphoglyceric acid

6-PG   6-phosphogluconic acid

PGA   pteroylglutamic acid

6-PGA   6-phosphogluconic acid

6-PGAD   6-phosphogluconic acid dehydrogenase

6-PGD   6-phosphogluconic acid dehydrogenase

PGI   phosphoglucose isomerase

PGK   phosphoglycerate kinase

PGM$_1$ phosphoglucomutase type 1

Ph^1   Philadelphia chromosome

PHA   phytohemagglutinin

Pi   (1) protease inhibitor, genetic types of alpha-1-antitrypsin; (2) inorganic phosphate

PI   phosphatidyl inositol

PIVKA   protein induced by vitamin K antagonists

PK   pyruvate kinase

Pl^{A1}   platelet antigen A1

PM   psychomotor

PMN   polymorphonuclear leukocyte

PMSF   phenylmethanesulfonyl fluoride

PNH   paroxysmal nocturnal hemoglobinuria

pO$_2$ partial pressure of oxygen

PPD   purified protein derivative (tuberculin test)

PPi   high energy inorganic phosphate (pyrophosphate)

Pr   propionic acid

PROTO   protoporphyrin

PRP   platelet-rich plasma

PRPP   phosphoribosyl pyrophosphate

PS   phosphatidyl serine

PSP   phenolsulfon phthalein

PTA   plasma thromboplastin antecedent

PTC   plasma thromboplastin component, factor IX, Christmas factor

PTT   partial thromboplastin time

PVC   polyvinyl chloride

PVP   polyvinylpyrrolidone

Pyr   pyruvate

q   long arm of chromosome

Q   blood flow (ml. per min.)

R   relaxed

R.   rads, a unit of radiation

Ragg's   rheumatoid agglutinins for gamma globulin in rheumatoid sera

RBC   red blood cell

RCV   total red cell volume

RDS   respiratory distress syndrome

RES   reticuloendothelial system

Rh   Rhesus antigen

RNA   ribonucleic acid

R1P   ribose-1-phosphate

R5P   ribose-5-phosphate or ribulose-5-phosphate

RPK   ribosephosphate pyrophosphokinase

RVV   Russell's viper venom

S   (1) slow; (2) electrophoretically slow variant of C3; (3) sulfate; (4) Svedberg unit; (5) DNA synthesis

Sat$_A$ per cent saturation of arterial blood

Sat$_V$ per cent saturation of venous blood

SCID   severe combined immunodeficiency

SCS   surface-connecting system

SD   (1) standard deviation; (2) serum-defined antigen

SDS   sodium dodecylsulfate

SDS-PAGE   sodium dodecyl sulfate–polyacrylamide gel electrophoresis

SEM   standard error of the mean

Sf   Svedberg flotation unit

S.L.   sex-linked

SLE   systemic lupus erythematosus

SM   sphingomyelin

SNagg's   agglutinins for gamma globulin found in normal serum

SOD   superoxide dismutase

SPCA   serum prothrombin converting activity

SS   homozygous sickle cell anemia

t   translocation

T   (1) taut; (2) thymidine; (3) thymus-dependent lymphocytes

T$_3$ 3,5,3-triiodothyronine

T$_4$ thyroxine

TBGP   total blood granulocyte pool

TEM   triethylenemelamine

TEPP   tetraethylpyrophosphate, an inhibitor of cholinesterase

Tf   transferrin

TK   thymidine kinase

TPI   triosephosphate isomerase

tRNA   transfer RNA, 4S RNA

TSD   Tay-Sachs disease

TTP   thrombotic thrombocytopenic purpura

U   uridine

UDP   uridine diphosphate

UDPG   uridine diphosphoglucose

UF   unknown factor, properdin factor B

URO   uroporphyrin

V   (1) vinyl; (2) variable segment gene for immunoglobulin

Vmax   maximal enzyme velocity

VLDL   very low density lipoproteins

W   an HL-A locus

WBC   white blood count

Y   (1) hepatic Y protein, which binds and transfers bilirubin; (2) the fractional saturation of hemoglobin with oxygen (Hill equation)

Z   hepatic Z protein, which binds and transfers bilirubin

INDEX

Note: Page numbers in *italics* refer to illustrations. Page numbers followed by the letter "t" refer to tables.

Abetalipoproteinemia, 223, 227t, 778, 779
  red cell morphology in, *20*
ABO blood group system, 803t, 805, 806, *806*
  and platelet transfusion, 606t, 872
ABO hemolytic disease, 308–310
Abruptio placentae, and disseminated intravascular coagulation, 606, 606t
Acanthocytes
  energy metabolism in, *38*
  in abetalipoproteinemia, 223
  in asplenia, 245
  in liver disease, 223
  in PK deficiency, *329*
Acanthocytosis, 223
Acatalasemia, 840
Acatalasia, 105
ACD (acid citrate dextrose), 860, 860t, 861, 861t, 862
ACD-adenine, 863
Acetyl CoA pathway, in platelets, 628
Acetylcholinesterase, 191t
Acetylsalicylic acid. See *Aspirin.*
Acid citrate dextrose (ACD), 860, 860t, 861, 861t, 862
α_1-Acid glycoprotein, 821, 822, *822*, 822t
Acid phosphatase, red cell, 839
Acid serum lysis test, 270
  in HEMPAS, 276
  in paroxysmal nocturnal hemoglobinuria, 217, 270, 276
Aciduria, orotic, 134
ACTH, 82
Addison's disease, anemia in, 181
Adenine, in preservation of stored blood, 863
Adenine nucleotide metabolism, and platelet constituent release reaction, 629, *629*, 630, 631
Adenine nucleotide precursor, and red cell metabolism, 42, *43*
Adenosine deaminase (ADA), 841
Adenosine triphosphate. See *ATP.*
Adenylate kinase (AK), red cell, 840
Adrenal corticoids. See *Corticosteroids.*
Aeromonas hydrophila infection, in acute leukemia, 685
Afibrinogenemia, congenital, 583, 584
Agammaglobulinemia
  acquired, 538
  congenital, 535–537

Agrammaglobulinemia (*Continued*)
  in intestinal lymphangectasia, 538
  lymphopenia, in, 538
  Swiss type, 539–543
  transient, in infancy, 535
  X-linked, 535–537
Agglutinins, 267
  blood group, 802–817
  cold, characteristics of, 274t
  rheumatoid (Ragg's), 836
  SNagg's, 836, 838
Agranulocytosis, infantile, chronic, 498. See also *Neutropenia.*
ALA. See δ-*Aminolevulinic acid.*
Albumin, 28, 33, 819, *819*, 820
  binding of bilirubin to, 294, *294*
Alder anomaly, 502
Aleutian mink, 511
Alkaline phosphatase, leukocyte, in chronic myelogenous leukemia, 700
  in infection, 502
Alkylating agents
  in Hodgkin's disease, 744, 745t
  in idiopathic thrombocytopenic purpura, 642
  in immunohemolytic anemia, 272
  in leukemia, 693–695
  in lymphohistiocytosis, 716
  in non-Hodgkin's lymphoma, 751
  in reticuloendotheliosis, 716
Alleles, 784
Allergic purpura, 592, 593
Allergic reactions, to red cell transfusion, 858
Allografts. See *Bone marrow transplantation.*
Allopurinol, 689
Alpha (α) chains, 390, 450–484
  elongated, and abnormal hemoglobins, 797, 798, 798t
Alpha thalassemia. See *Thalassemia, alpha.*
Alphamethyldopa, 273
Alymphocytosis, 539–543
Alymphoplasia, thymic, 539–543
Am gene complexes, 837t
Amaurotic idiocy, infantile, 773
Amino acid substitutions, and abnormal hemoglobins, 796, 796t
ϵ-Amino caproic acid
  in disseminated intravascular coagulation, 608

D. E. Craig M.D.